PERIOPERATIVE MEDICINE

ANESTHESIOLOGY: A PROBLEM-BASED LEARNING APPROACH

Series Editor: Magdalena Anitescu, MD

Published and Forthcoming Titles

Pain Management edited by Magdalena Anitescu

Anesthesiology edited by Tracey Straker and Shobana Rajan

Pediatric Anesthesia edited by Kirk Lalwani, Ira Todd Cohen, Ellen Y. Choi, and Vidya T. Raman

Neuroanesthesia edited by David E. Traul and Irene P. Osborn

Cardiac Anesthesia edited by Mohammed M. Minhaj

Critical Care edited by Taylor Johnston, Steven Miller, and Joseph Rumley

Regional Anesthesiology and Acute Pain Medicine edited by Nabil Elkassabany and Eman Nada

Obstetric Anesthesia edited by Rebecca Minehart, Jaime Daly, and Heather Nixon

Professional, Ethical, Legal, and Educational Lessons in Medicine
edited by Kirk Lalwani, Ira Cohen, Ellen Choi, and Berklee Robins

PERIOPERATIVE MEDICINE

A PROBLEM-BASED LEARNING APPROACH

EDITED BY

Deborah C. Richman
STONY BROOK MEDICINE, STONY BROOK, NEW YORK

Debra D. Pulley
WASHINGTON UNIVERSITY SCHOOL OF MEDICINE, ST. LOUIS, MISSOURI

Adriana D. Oprea
YALE SCHOOL OF MEDICINE, NEW HAVEN, CONNECTICUT

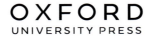

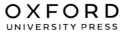

Oxford University Press is a department of the University of Oxford. It furthers
the University's objective of excellence in research, scholarship, and education
by publishing worldwide. Oxford is a registered trade mark of Oxford University
Press in the UK and certain other countries.

Published in the United States of America by Oxford University Press
198 Madison Avenue, New York, NY 10016, United States of America.

© Oxford University Press 2024

All rights reserved. No part of this publication may be reproduced, stored in
a retrieval system, or transmitted, in any form or by any means, without the
prior permission in writing of Oxford University Press, or as expressly permitted
by law, by license, or under terms agreed with the appropriate reproduction
rights organization. Inquiries concerning reproduction outside the scope of the
above should be sent to the Rights Department, Oxford University Press, at the
address above.

You must not circulate this work in any other form
and you must impose this same condition on any acquirer.

CIP data is on file at the Library of Congress

This material is not intended to be, and should not be considered, a substitute for medical or other
professional advice. Treatment for the conditions described in this material is highly dependent on
the individual circumstances. And, while this material is designed to offer accurate information
with respect to the subject matter covered and to be current as of the time it was written, research
and knowledge about medical and health issues is constantly evolving and dose schedules for
medications are being revised continually, with new side effects recognized and accounted for
regularly. Readers must therefore always check the product information and clinical procedures
with the most up-to-date published product information and data sheets provided by the
manufacturers and the most recent codes of conduct and safety regulation. The publisher and the
authors make no representations or warranties to readers, express or implied, as to the accuracy or
completeness of this material. Without limiting the foregoing, the publisher and the authors make
no representations or warranties as to the accuracy or efficacy of the drug dosages mentioned in the
material. The authors and the publisher do not accept, and expressly disclaim, any responsibility
for any liability, loss or risk that may be claimed or incurred as a consequence of the use and/ or
application of any of the contents of this material.

ISBN 978–0–19–090200–1

DOI: 10.1093/med/9780190902001.001.0001

Printed by Integrated Books International, United States of America

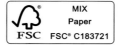

CONTENTS

Preface vii
  Deborah C. Richman, Debra D. Pulley,
  and Adriana D. Oprea
List of Contributors ix

PART I PREOPERATIVE ASSESSMENT

1. Preoperative Process: Phone Triage, Preoperative Clinic, or Virtual Patient Visits   3
   Maureen Keshock and Kenneth Cummings
2. Perioperative Surgical Home Care Model: Utopia or Bureaucracy?   15
   Eileen Campbell and Janine Limoncelli
3. Choosing Wisely: How to Advise the Patient on Preoperative Testing   26
   Jay S. Kersh and BobbieJean Sweitzer
4. My 79-Year-Old Patient for Right Inguinal Hernia Repair Has No Labs on File   46
   Wiebke Ackermann and Barbara Rogers
5. Medication Management: Drug-Eluting Stent 2 Months Ago   53
   Julio Montejano and Angela Selzer
6. Perioperative Management of Medications for Substance Use Disorders   67
   Thomas R. Hickey and Shafik Boyaji
7. Indications for Preoperative C-Spine Imaging for Elective Procedures   78
   Deborah C. Richman
8. Prehabilitation Before Total Hip Replacement   84
   Olivia Belloni, Rashwan Gogue, Luigi Beretta, and Enrico Maria Minnella
9. Cardiopulmonary Exercise Testing   93
   Paris Dove, Emily Traer, Hilmy Ismail, and Bernhard Riedel

PART II AGE

10. Ex-Premie for Interval Hernia Repair at 11 Weeks   117
    Joseph P. Resti and Bettina Smallman
11. Geriatric Assessment: "The Get Up and Go, Got Up and Left"   125
    Kaitlin Willham and Heather E. Nye

PART III ORGAN SYSTEMS

CARDIAC

12. AHA Guidelines Application   139
    Samuel Papke, Michael Benson, and Joshua Zimmerman
13. Perioperative Atrial Fibrillation and Anticoagulation Management   148
    Jing Tao and Adriana D. Oprea
14. Severe Aortic Stenosis: Candidate for a Surgicenter?   162
    Elvera L. Baron and Menachem M. Weiner
15. Does Your Cataract Surgeon Know You Were Admitted for Heart Failure Last Week?   168
    Michael Curtis, Nathaen Weitzel, and Miklos D. Kertai
16. Echo Shows Elevated Pulmonary Artery Pressure   187
    Debra D. Pulley and Anand Lakshminarasimhachar
17. Shoulder Replacement in Patient Who Had a Heart and Lung Transplant   195
    Caroline R. Gross and Zdravka Zafirova

PULMONARY

18. COPD: Still Smoking, Still Wheezing   207
    Wesley Rajaleelan and Jean Wong
19. Severe OSA in the Ambulatory Setting   218
    Sean Love, Chelsey Santino, and Tina Tran
20. COVID-19   227
    Robert Fong

GASTROINTESTINAL

21. Cirrhosis and Truly Elective Major Surgery   249
    Sofia S. Jakab and Adriana D. Oprea

NEUROLOGICAL

22. Patient Has Seizures and Needs "Clearance"   261
    Ramanjot S. Kang, Ashley Mathew, and Shirley Avraham
23. Clinical Application of Perioperative Brain Health   271
    Samuel N. Blacker
24. Restrictive Lung Disease from Parkinson's Disease Rigidity: Is It Real?   282
    Shilpa Rao

25. A 56-Year-Old with a Recent CVA for Elective Surgery: How Soon Is Too Soon? 291
Debra D. Pulley

RENAL

26. Avoiding Exacerbation of Chronic Kidney Disease 297
Emily Y. Xue, David Moore, and Alexander F. Arriaga

HEMATOLOGY

27. Preoperative Anemia Management: Evaluation and Treatment 307
Kenneth Cummings

28. Prolonged PTT in a Healthy Patient 312
Nicole Verdecchia and Khoa Nguyen

ENDOCRINE

29. Elevated Glucose on Admission Fingerstick: How High Can We Go? 323
Lindsay E. Carafone, Colin E. Bauer, Joshua D. Miller, and Steven D. Wittlin

30. Pheochromocytoma and MEN Syndromes 333
Zyad J. Carr, Andrea Farela, and Adriana D. Oprea

PART IV WOMEN'S HEALTH

31. Pregnant Patient for Non-Obstetric Surgery 345
Nayema K. Salimi and Kristen L. Fardelmann

32. Older Primigravida with Twin Pregnancy for Elective Cesarean Delivery 358
Evan Jin, Sangeeta Kumaraswami, and Garret Weber

PART V SURGICAL CONSIDERATIONS

33. Minimally Invasive Surgery and Other Elements of Enhanced Recovery Protocols 373
Lesley Bennici, Morgane Factor, Sunitha M. Singh, and Ana Costa

34. Blood Conservation 381
Seth Perelman and Christian Mabry

PART VI ETHICS AND SHARED DECISION-MAKING

35. When DNR Stands in the OR: Who Benefits? Who Decides? 395
Joseph F. Kras

36. Informed Consent: Do We Really Do This Correctly? 403
Stephen Harden and Nicholas Sadovnikoff

37. Can I Refuse to Anesthetize This Patient? 414
Jeanna D. Blitz

38. Difficult Conversations 423
Laura J. Ostapenko and Katherine A. Hill

PART VII MISCELLANEOUS

39. This Patient Has 17 Allergies: Including "General Anesthesia" 433
Debra D. Pulley

40. Nonverbal Autistic 30-Year-Old for Full Mouth Dental Rehabilitation with Malignant Hyperthermia 439
Jonathan Bacon and Ralph Epstein

41. Patient with AAA with Implanted Spinal Cord (Neuro) Stimulator 452
Meredith Whitacre and Loreta Grecu

42. Patient with Pacemaker-Dependent ICD for Renal Cryoablation 464
Paula Trigo Blanco and Adriana D. Oprea

43. My Friend's Son Requests Surgery for Gynecomastia Caused by the Drugs He Uses for Bodybuilding 476
Adam Adler and Arvind Chandrakantan

44. Perioperative Care of the Cancer Patient 481
Cory W. Helder and Alessia Pedoto

PART VIII PACU

45. Discharge Criteria in Developmentally Disabled Patient with OSA 495
Jonathan L. Wong and Mana Saraghi

46. My Patient Is Twitching Like a Fish Out of Water: Avoiding the Risks of Residual Paralysis 507
Ramon E. Abola

47. My Patient in the PACU Is Not Making Any Sense 514
Joy Steadman

48. The HR Monitor Is Alarming in the PACU: Postoperative Arrhythmias 522
Avi Dobrusin and Muthuraj Kanakaraj

Index 531

PREFACE

We are excited to publish this book on perioperative medicine using a problem-based learning format. The concept started a while ago, due to insufficient literature available to guide busy clinicians in preoperative clinics (like us) who are trying to make potentially life-altering decisions concerning the optimization and suitability of patients who are scheduled to have surgery. As chapters were being written, we faced a few obstacles and had to postpone publication.

- *COVID-19*: As many recall, in December 2019, we heard about a viral outbreak elsewhere in the world but did not know how that was going impact us. As the pandemic continued to spread in the United States, hospitals and ICUs were reaching capacity and elective surgeries were being postponed. Personnel were deployed to ICUs or were furloughed.[1,2]

- *Backlog of surgeries*: After the hospital bed census improved, operating rooms became increasingly busy with increasingly sicker patients due to lack of primary and preventive care during the pandemic.[3]

- *Physician/nurse burnout leading to inadequate staffing*: Although not new, there continues to be an increase in burnout leading to inadequate staffing throughout the healthcare system.[4,5]

We truly thank our authors who have taken time out of their busy lives to research the current literature and transfer their clinical expertise into written words on diverse topics within the perioperative arena. These chapters are organized into sections ranging from general topics (e.g., how to choose a preoperative process, what medications need to be given or withheld), to more focused topics (e.g., evaluation and perioperative care for patients with disorders affecting various organ systems such as the heart and lungs).[*] There is a section on how to handle important conversations including DNR, informed consent, and shared decision-making. We also have a few chapters discussing management of complications that can occur in the PACU.

Throughout these trying times, our focus has been and will continue to be on providing optimal patient care. We therefore dedicate this book to our patients (past, present, and future).

REFERENCES

1. Shaparin N, Mann GE, Streiff A, et al. Adaptation and restructuring of an academic anesthesiology department during the COVID-19 pandemic in New York City: Challenges and lessons learned. *Best Pract Res Clin Anaesthesiol*. 2021;35(3):425–435.
2. Mazzaferro DM, Patel V, Asport N, et al. The financial impact of COVID-19 on a surgical department: The effects of surgical shutdowns and the impact on a health system. *Surgery*. 2022;172(6):1642–1650.
3. Meredith JW, High KP, Freischlag JA. Preserving elective surgeries in the COVID-19 pandemic and the future. *JAMA*. 2020;324(17):1725–1726.
4. Stephenson J. US Surgeon General sounds alarm on health worker burnout. *JAMA Health Forum*. 2022;3(6):e222299.
5. Murthy V. Addressing health worker burnout: The U.S. Surgeon General's advisory on building a thriving health workforce. Office of the U.S. Surgeon General. 2022. https://www.hhs.gov/surgeongeneral/priorities/health-worker-burnout/index.html

---

[*] The cases in this book are fictional and were created to facilitate education.

CONTRIBUTORS

Ramon E. Abola, MD
Stony Brook Medicine

Wiebke Ackermann, MD
Ohio State University Wexner Medical Center

Adam C. Adler, MD, MS, FAAP, FASE
Baylor College of Medicine/Texas Children's Hospital

Alexander F. Arriaga, MD, MPH, ScD
Harvard Medical School, Brigham and Women's Hospital

Shirley Avraham, MD
North American Partners in Anesthesia (NAPA), Somnia Anesthesia

Jonathan Bacon, DDS
Howard University College of Dentistry

Elvera L. Baron, MD, PhD
Case Western Reserve University

Colin E. Bauer, MD
Anesthesia and Analgesia Medical Group, Inc.

Olivia Belloni, MD
IRCCS San Raffaele Scientific Institute

Lesley Bennici, MD
Stony Brook Medicine

Michael Benson, MD
Oregon Health and Science University

Luigi Beretta, MD
IRCCS San Raffaele Scientific Institute

Samuel N. Blacker, MD
University of North Carolina at Chapel Hill

Jeanna D. Blitz, MD, FASA, DFPM
Wake Forest University, Noridian Healthcare Solutions

Shafik Boyaji, MD
Valley Pain Consultants

Eileen Campbell, EdD, APRN, ACNS-BC, CNS-CP
Western Connecticut State University

Lindsay E. Carafone, MD
University of Rochester School of Medicine and Dentistry

Zyad J. Carr, MD
Yale School of Medicine

Arvind Chandrakantan, MD, MBA, FAAP, FASA, FAASM
Baylor College of Medicine/Texas Children's Hospital

Ana Costa, MD
Stony Brook Medicine

Kenneth Cummings, MD, MS, FASA
Cleveland Clinic

Michael Curtis, MD
Stanford Health Care

Avi Dobrusin, MD
Washington University in St. Louis

Paris Dove, MBBS, FANZCA
Fiona Stanley Fremantle Hospitals Group, Perth, Australia

Ralph Epstein, DDS
Stony Brook Medicine

Morgane Factor, MD
Stony Brook Medicine

Kristen L. Fardelmann, MD
Yale School of Medicine

Andrea Farela, MD
Yale School of Medicine

Robert Fong, MD, PhD
University of Chicago

Rashwan Gogue, MD
IRCCS San Raffaele Scientific Institute

Loreta Grecu, MD
Duke University School of Medicine

Caroline R. Gross, MD
Mount Sinai Hospital System

Stephen Harden, MD
Anesthesia Associates of Charleston

Cory W. Helder, MD
New York University Grossman School of Medicine

Thomas R. Hickey, MD
VA Connecticut Healthcare System, Yale School of Medicine

Katherine A. Hill, MD, MS
West Virginia University

Hilmy Ismail, MD, FRCA, FFARCS(I), FANZCA
Peter MacCallum Cancer Centre, University of Melbourne

Sofia S. Jakab, MD
Yale School of Medicine

Evan Jin, MD
Westchester Medical Center

Muthuraj Kanakaraj, MD, MBBS
Washington University in St. Louis

Ramanjot S. Kang, MD
North Texas Orthopedics & Spine Center

Jay S. Kersh, MD
Feinberg School of Medicine, Northwestern University

Miklos D. Kertai, MD, MMHC, PhD
Vanderbilt University Medical Center

Maureen Keshock, MD, MHSA, FASA
Cleveland Clinic Foundation

Joseph F. Kras, MD, DDS, MA, FASA, HEC-C
Washington University in St. Louis

Sangeeta Kumaraswami, MD
Westchester Medical Center, New York Medical College

Anand Lakshminarasimhachar, MD, FRCA
Washington University in St. Louis

Janine Limoncelli, MD
Weill Cornell Medicine/NYP

Sean Love, MD
Johns Hopkins University School of Medicine

Christian Mabry, MD
Prisma Health

Enrico Maria Minnella, MD, PhD
IRCCS San Raffaele Scientific Institute
Dompe farmaceutici S.p.A.

Ashley Mathew, MD
Stony Brook Medicine

Joshua D. Miller, MD, MPH
Stony Brook Medicine

Julio Montejano, MD
University of Colorado School of Medicine

David Moore, MD
Physician Specialists in Anesthesia
Emory St. Joseph's Hospital

Khoa Nguyen, MD
University of Pittsburgh

Heather E. Nye, MD, PhD
San Francisco VA Medical Center

Adriana D. Oprea, MD
Yale School of Medicine

Laura J. Ostapenko, MD, MPP
West Virginia University

Samuel Papke, MD
Oregon Health and Science University

Alessia Pedoto, MD, FASA
Memorial Sloan Kettering Cancer Center

Seth Perelman, MD, FASA
NYU Grossman School of Medicine

Debra D. Pulley, MD
Washington University in St. Louis

Wesley Rajaleelan MBBS, MD
The Ottawa Hospital, University of Ottawa

Shilpa Rao, MD
Yale School of Medicine

Joseph P. Resti, MD
SUNY Upstate Medical University

Deborah C. Richman, MBChB, FFA(SA)
Stony Brook Medicine

Bernhard Riedel, MD, MBA, PhD
Peter MacCallum Cancer Centre, University of Melbourne

Barbara Rogers, MD
Ohio State University Wexner Medical Center

Nicholas Sadovnikoff, MD, FCCM, HEC-C
St. Elizabeth's Medical Center

Nayema K. Salimi, MD
Princeton Medical Center

Chelsey Santino, MD, MS
Johns Hopkins University School of Medicine

Mana Saraghi, DMD
Jacobi Medical Center

Angela Selzer, MD
University of Colorado School of Medicine

Sunitha M. Singh, MD, CPHQ
Stony Brook Medicine

Bettina Smallman, MD, FRCPC
SUNY Upstate Medical University

Joy Steadman, MD
Ascension Providence Hospital

BobbieJean Sweitzer, MD, FACP, SAMBA-F, FASA
University of Virginia, Inova Health

Jing Tao, MD
Memorial Sloan Kettering Cancer Center

Emily Traer, MBChB, MRCS, FRCA, FANZCA
Peter MacCallum Cancer Centre, University of Melbourne

Tina Tran, MD
Johns Hopkins University School of Medicine

Paula Trigo Blanco, MD
Health Alliance Clinton Hospital

Nicole Verdecchia, MD
University of Pittsburgh

Garret Weber, MD
Westchester Medical Center, New York Medical College

Menachem M. Weiner, MD
Icahn School of Medicine at Mount Sinai

Nathaen Weitzel, MD
University of Colorado School of Medicine

Meredith Whitacre, MD
Duke University School of Medicine

Kaitlin Willham, MD
University of California—San Francisco

Steven D. Wittlin, MD
University of Rochester School of Medicine and Dentistry

Jean Wong, MD, FRCPC
Toronto Western Hospital, University Health Network

Jonathan L. Wong, DMD
Coastal Pediatric Dental & Anesthesia

Emily Y. Xue, MD
Brigham and Women's Hospital

Zdravka Zafirova, MD
Mount Sinai Hospital System

Joshua Zimmerman, MD, FASE
University of Utah

PART I

PREOPERATIVE ASSESSMENT

1.

PREOPERATIVE PROCESS

PHONE TRIAGE, PREOPERATIVE CLINIC, OR VIRTUAL PATIENT VISITS

Maureen Keshock and Kenneth Cummings

In the past 30 years, there have been significant changes in the design and setup of preoperative evaluation clinics as more and more patients have planned elective surgery. More than 50 million surgical procedures were performed annually before 2020, when our nation experienced a global pandemic limiting elective surgery.[1] Preoperative clinics are as variable as the patients they serve. However, their value is without question to improve rates of surgical delays, complications, hospital length of stay, cost, and day-of-surgery cancellations.[2,3] The preoperative clinic is associated with the institution's surgical site (hospital or ambulatory surgical center [ASC]) and depends on the culture, goals, and existing resources. In all cases, the preoperative process ensures chart compilation, risk stratification, and compliance with regulatory bodies such as The Joint Commission, American Healthcare Organization (AHCA), and others. However, in some cases, not all patients undergo the same process. It was recognized decades ago that in elective noncardiac patients undergoing surgery, many are free from disease and can bypass the pre-anesthesia evaluation clinic.[4]

The preop process can vary based on surgical case risk and patient risk. Patients may be triaged via a chart review or algorithm to either a preop phone call, in-person clinic, or virtual visit at a single institution with a single delivery model of the pre-anesthesia clinic. Sites with a lower case-mix index may serve the population well with a preop phone call supplemented by an anesthesiology assessment on the day of surgery. The optimal model is yet to be defined but does depend on facility characteristics such as resources, private versus academic setting, procedure mix, patient expectations, and case-mix index.[5]

STEM CASE AND KEY QUESTIONS

The patient is a 61-year-old woman with scapholunate advanced collapse syndrome (SLAC) stage 2 and median nerve compression. She is scheduled for a proximal carpal row carpectomy and open decompression of the median nerve at the wrist. She only takes vitamin D and has no known drug allergies. Her BMI is 41 kg/m². The patient is an information technology (IT) specialist for your institution and would like to have surgery as soon as possible. Her orthopedic surgeon is newly graduated from his upper-extremity fellowship and asks about your preoperative clinic.

The surgeon asks whether his patient can simply have a phone screen prior to her surgery at the ASC.

Ideally, the patient can interact with the preoperative process via an interactive online modality. However, phone screening can incur staffing costs because connecting on the phone with the patient can be cumbersome. You state that your hospital has a process to direct his patient to the best type of visit, either a virtual visit, in-person clinic visit, or no visit necessary. The algorithm will direct the surgeon to schedule the correct patient visit type.

The orthopedic surgeon asks what model preoperative clinic our hospital has.

You answer that we have a hybrid model that sees a large number of patients per year. We identify high-risk patients and prioritize obtaining an accurate history and physical while reducing unnecessary testing. We have a centralized Main Campus, but any sites are accessible to the patient for their visit.

He asks if he should just go ahead and order preoperative labs and ECG.

You answer that our Clinic would honor any test he feels is valid (e.g., COVID-19), but our preoperative clinic has no age-based criteria. Instead, we will triage the patient and use evidence-based guidelines to determine if she needs any lab work or special studies after her pre-op visit to optimize her medical condition best.

Will a virtual visit serve as a complete history and physical (H&P)?

Virtual visits can serve as a complete history and physical if she travels to a site that has a facilitated telemedicine platform. An appointment is required, and a nurse will facilitate using Bluetooth technology to complete the physical. A virtual visit with a mobile-only platform also exists. It is institution-specific whether this suffices for a complete H&P. The virtual visit may be supplemented with a formal heart and lung exam on the day of surgery, as recommended by the American Society of Anesthesiologists.

The surgeon agrees to have his office staff fill out the algorithm. His wife is a busy ophthalmologist who was just made Chief of Staff. The ophthalmologist performs 100 cataract surgeries a week and would like them all to come to the Preanesthesia Clinic.

You answer that medical optimization may not be the service best suited for these patients, but rather an advanced practice provider (APP) who can perform accurate, up-to-date H&Ps might best serve his wife's patient population.

What is the evidence that virtual visits can allow reliable preoperative assessment?

We've seen the rapid rise of telemedicine in many specialties with the onset of COVID-19, and, at this point, there appears to be no compromise to patient health or quality of care.[6] In anesthesia, a recent study involving more than 400 patients with a mobile platform showed no increase in case cancellation rate after a virtual preanesthesia assessment.[6,7]

How does one identify patients who do not need to be seen preoperatively?

It's a combination of patient comorbidities and level of surgical risk. Many healthy patients undergo low-risk surgical procedures and can be assessed by anesthesia on the day of surgery. The prescreening or triage process can be accomplished in various ways, either by telephone, questionnaire, or chart review.

What conditions can be identified by a virtual visit?

Virtual visits that are facilitated and performed with electronic stethoscopes meet the same standards as an in-person visit with a focused physical exam, including heart and lungs. An airway exam is also possible. Lab capability depends on the facility.

A stand-alone virtual visit with a mobile platform can also identify abnormalities but is patient-dependent. For example, some patients have medical devices at home and can incorporate reliable vital signs, including pulse oximetry, blood pressure, pulse, and temperature. Visual observation includes a respiratory rate. General patient appearance and well-being can be established.[8] Close inspection of the pulmonary system includes breathing pattern, skin color, accessory muscle use, symmetric chest rise, auditory wheezing, cough, and change in voice.

Patients can be directed to self-examine and perform radial pulse palpation or expiratory maneuvers to determine the severity of dyspnea.[9] Again, difficult airways can be diagnosed, and dentistry and oral-maxillofacial surgery lead the way.[10,11]

In addition, similar to an in-person visit, a virtual visit can match the appropriate facility to the proposed procedure. During chart review and patient evaluation, suitability for the level of care possible at different facilities can be evaluated and matched.

DISCUSSION

Preoperative clinic models exist on a continuum separated by size and scope. Likewise, there are various ways to triage patients into the chosen delivery model, either by telephone, questionnaire, or preadmission testing visit in the case of a perioperative surgical home model. This chapter focuses on these various mechanisms and delineates the factors that make the preop process *most efficient* through phone triage, in-person, or virtual patient visits.

Preoperative clinic models include but are not limited to the models listed below. In a large health system, local practice models evolve, leading to heterogeneity in staffing as well as variable quality and cost of preoperative evaluation. Therefore, an important role of the perioperative leadership team is to standardize this process as much as possible. Such standardization should be grounded in the latest evidence-based guidelines (where available) and local best practices when evidence or guidelines are lacking.

Among the many goals of a preoperative clinic, ensuring patients are medically optimized for surgery is arguably the most important. This is a rational use of resources because attendance at a preoperative clinic is associated with lower costs from unnecessary testing, reduced cancellations, and even improved in-hospital survival.[3,12–14]

Over time, two separate preoperative processes evolved at our institution (Cleveland Clinic). Our Main Campus location, a large referral center, developed a two-clinic system that involved hospital medicine and anesthesiology input.[15] Although this system was effective and had demonstrable benefits, it was not generalizable across our health system. As a result, a separate network of preoperative clinics was established with central scheduling and credentialing, online clinical guidelines, and designated physician oversight. The Main Campus location was transitioned to this centralized hybrid model to increase standardization, allow patient movement anywhere in the health system, and reduce resource duplication.

NURSE-RUN CLINIC

In this model, the surgery date is set, and, subsequently, the patient is seen in the hospital-run clinic. The nurse-led clinics are effective, but the data quality is low due to the paucity of randomized controlled trials studying this model. The most recent studies of nurse-led clinics show a low day-of-surgery cancellation rate (1%) due to incomplete medical assessment and an accurate assessment of patient readiness for surgery.[16,17] The nurse is an important member of the team who can address multiple educational components of the surgical process. Still, many management decisions need to be made by a licensed, independent practitioner or physician.[18]

ANESTHESIOLOGY-RUN CLINIC

In this model, the surgery date is prioritized, and the clinic is hospital-run.[19] This model comprises the majority of delivery systems nationwide, and they are usually smaller, but not necessarily. Many smaller clinics do not charge capture for a separate evaluation and management code because they provide no separate consultative service or H&P. Instead, anesthesia departments with well-documented evidence-based guidelines will often manage the preop testing. An example of this system would be Stony Brook University Medical Center in New York. The Clinic is responsible for choosing needed labs yet defers to specific service lines that still use historical recommendations (neurosurgery, urology). The patients, in this clinic, represent referrals from combination of private physicians, academic physicians, lab-only visits, or full-service consultations.

SEPARATE ANESTHESIA AND MEDICINE CLINICS

In this model, the surgery date is prioritized, and patients are subsequently triaged to either day-of-surgery evaluation, anesthesia only, medicine only, or both departments. Patients easily get medical optimization at the time of their preanesthesia visit, if necessary. This is convenient for out-of-town patients, but waste is sometimes built into the system because both departments are usually seen. The medical clinic can bill for consultation, and revenue is generated. This works well in a large system with a long history of collaboration, but it may be a legacy system and requires two sets of physicians and clinic support. In fact, a major health system that previously used this model (the Cleveland Clinic) has transitioned away from this to a more hybrid model.

COMBINED ANESTHESIA AND MEDICINE CLINIC

A combined anesthesia and internal medicine clinic is a relatively new hybrid model suited for a large academic center. This model was chosen for a center recently built at the University of Miami.[19] The surgery date is prioritized, and a preop questionnaire is completed. In addition, patients may get a triage phone call from a nurse. We created a Pre-Anesthesia Consultation Clinic (PACC) at the Cleveland Clinic. The triage phone call has been replaced by an algorithm embedded in the electronic medical record (EMR). Patients may or may not need to be seen prior to the day of surgery, but of those who do come to the clinic, all are seen by a resident and attending anesthesiologist or an APP. Consultation by internal medicine specialists is available as needed. In this hybrid model, efficiency is increased by requiring less infrastructure and fewer support staff.

PREOPERATIVE ANESTHESIA AND SURGICAL SCREENING (PASS) CLINIC

This sophisticated preoperative model established at Duke University describes a collaborative clinic that prioritizes managing modifiable risk factors preoperatively. It is a protocol-driven screening center where, if a modifiable risk condition is found, a dialogue occurs between surgeons and anesthesiologists about the window available before the surgery must take place.[1] Thus, the surgery date is flexible yet time-sensitive. Significant resources were used to develop a question algorithm that used existing data points from the EMR to determine phone screen eligibility. The IT team also created a unified scheduling system to complete multiple preoperative initiatives before the proposed surgical date.

COMPREHENSIVE PREOPERATIVE ASSESSMENT AND GLOBAL OPTIMIZATION

Shah and Vetter describe a comprehensive perioperative surgical home model that coordinates the preoperative, intraoperative, postoperative, and post-discharge phases of care.[20] The Perioperative Assessment and Global Optimization (PASS-GO) program aims to influence population health, surgical outcomes, and patient and provider experience. All patients are seen for a preoperative visit, followed by a telephone interview with a nurse in the Command Center.[21] For those cases with the most straightforward status, patients are then stratified by an APP based on comorbidities and surgical risk, and patients get an additional brief phone interview and day-of-surgery evaluation by an anesthesiologist. Patients with American Society of Anesthesiologists (ASA) status of 2 or 3 are seen for an in-person office visit by an APP working with an anesthesiologist or hospitalist where evaluation and management occur. Subsequently, the surgery date and post-acute care discharge planning are confirmed.[20] ASA status 3 and 4 patients are seen for evaluation and management in the same context, where shared-decision planning occurs regarding treatment options followed by definitive surgery date scheduling and post-acute care discharge planning.[22]

OPERATIONS

The following sections further describe the operations of the preoperative process. The ASA 2012 Practice Advisory for Pre-Anesthesia Evaluation states that an anesthesiologist is responsible for medically assessing and optimizing a surgical patient.[23] However, the temporal nature of the proposed procedure is important in considering the extent to which the patient is optimized. Patients scheduled for emergency surgery cannot be seen in a preoperative clinic. The most significant opportunity to add value is for time-sensitive or elective procedures. The "urgent procedures" that need to occur between 6 and 24 hours leave little time for optimization and often bring a burden to the patient and clinic to schedule an appointment.[24]

All stakeholders (hospitals, surgeons, anesthesiologists, and others) must accept the operations and scheduling policies of a preoperative clinic. Seeing patients scheduled for elective cases in a short time frame often precludes the ability to offer substantial medical optimization. It uses resources that could be allocated to complex patients with a longer time interval before surgery. The clinic must serve the hospital's needs by progressing patients through the process efficiently while minimizing delays. Therefore, add-on cases to be done within 48 hours are not seen in our preoperative clinic, and the responsibility for the preoperative evaluation remains with the surgeon.

Once it is determined that a procedure meets the criteria for a preoperative assessment, there are several methods of triage through prescreening that identify which patients are best referred for clinic visits, virtual visits, or anesthesia assessment on the day of surgery.[25] The prescreening methods include but are not limited to phone triage, chart review, or questionnaire—either online or in person. The challenge remains to create a preop process that is flexible enough to both respect patient perspectives and fulfill the goal of medical optimization.

TELEPHONE TRIAGE

Telephone prescreening is ideal for the ASA 1 or 2 patient who is easily assessable by phone and has clear expectations for the upcoming procedure. However, screening involves using unique patient identifiers once contact is made and informing patients that a telephone prescreen will be occurring.[26] A recent systematic review found that telephone prescreening is best accomplished when a structured protocol is used to conduct the telephone prescreening combined with appropriate patient criteria such as specific age range, BMI, risk of surgery, and general health status.[27] The results of the telephone prescreen are then entered into either a paper-based form, electronic questionnaire, or H&P template to be completed on the day of surgery.

The main advantage of a telephone prescreening process is that it permits the preoperative clinic to "assess greater numbers of patients with more complex medical and social issues."[25,26] Badner and colleagues surmised from their study that, in a university setting, most same-day admit or outpatient surgery patients were healthy enough to forego a comprehensive clinic visit.[4] Other advantages of a telephone prescreen include triage to specific clinicians and/or subspecialty consultations if a medical concern is identified. Anesthetic or social issues may also be identified prior to the procedure, thereby increasing efficiency on the proposed procedure date.[26]

Telephone prescreening may also increase clinic efficiency in complex patients when used as a preliminary method to augment a future comprehensive assessment.[28] Ludbrook points to an improvement in the quality of telephone prescreening when a checklist is used for data collection.[29] In multiple studies, telephone prescreening improved efficiencies, including decreasing the clinic no-show rate, and met with high patient satisfaction.[25,28–31]

Limitations do exist with telephone prescreening, including the inability to perform a physical exam and response bias depending on who performs the interview. For example, asymptomatic aortic stenosis is reported at 15% in patients older than 65 years.[29] Although the significance is unclear, improved future technologies could include an anesthesiologist performing a bedside transthoracic echocardiogram on the day of surgery. From an operational standpoint, it is essential to consider the correct staff member of the clinic to conduct a telephone prescreen. A telephone screen could be considered inefficient if it requires a second appointment set up by scheduling. Failure to contact patients with a cold-call attempt was 31.1% in a 2012 study and 6.5% in a scheduled call time.[17] Ideally, the earlier in the system, the better to triage the patient in the most efficient process. However, surgical schedulers are often overwhelmed with fielding large numbers of phone calls, and telephone technology is not patient-driven.

QUESTIONNAIRE

Patient-driven self-assessments that occur early in the perioperative process are most efficient in triage, data sharing, and minimizing costs. One of the earliest investigations was by Badner and colleagues.[4] Patients manually completed a health screening questionnaire in the surgeon's office, which then shared the information with the preadmission clinic. A registered nurse and then a staff anesthesiologist reviewed the information and used it to stratify patients to different types of appointments or same-day surgery evaluations. Edwards points to other researchers who integrated manual screening questionnaires into their preassessment clinic model. The report describes a nurse-based triage tool that "had an accuracy of 81%, specificity of 86%, and a negative predictive value of 93%" compared with a subsequent anesthesiologist evaluation.[25] The patients were routinely seen 2 weeks prior to the surgery date, and the model was better at identifying patients who would suffice with a same-day anesthesia assessment versus a preoperative clinic visit.[31]

Technological improvements allow for outpatient preoperative assessment computer programs. *HealthQuest* (HQ) was a patient-facing questionnaire administered in the surgeon's office with many branch points depending on health status.[32] A sicker patient could be completing more than 30 questions to document their medical condition before their preoperative evaluation. Although not the first computer-assisted preanesthesia tool described, it was original in that it combined medical data with a surgical classification scheme. Information obtained was used to supplement the preoperative visit and stratify patients to a clinic visit or not. Parker and colleagues identified 35.6% of patients at a tertiary referral center who did not need to be seen by an anesthesiologist until the day of surgery. A recent evaluation of an electronic screening tool drew a similar conclusion. This large, prospective study concluded that a web-based tool reliably identified outpatients who could bypass the preoperative clinic and be assessed on the day of surgery.[33]

Digital data sharing integrates institutional electronic health records in a manner that has multiple benefits. For example, an Austrian research team implemented an electronic preoperative care pathway (e-Form) "that allowed all hospitals to access comprehensive patient medical history through a clinic-portal on the health-board intranet."[34] Improvements realized included a reduction in unnecessary testing, cost-effectiveness of their preoperative process, and improved clinical documentation.

Technology will drive applications that permit patients to answer medical health screening questions. Osman's group used a digital tablet to have patients self-administer a preanesthesia health assessment with moderate to good validity and high patient acceptance. Their study occurred in a tertiary women's preoperative clinic. It concluded that their

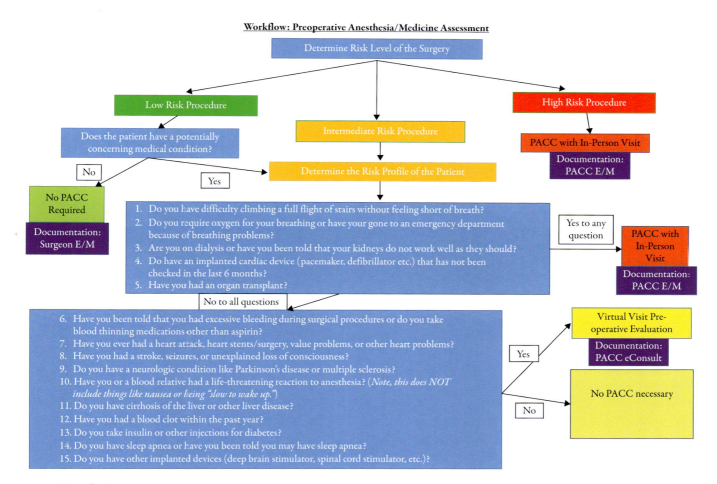

Figure 1.1 Overall triage process.
PACC, Pre-Anesthesia Consultation Clinic; E/M, evaluation/management.

questionnaire was reliable in obtaining a medical history in English-speaking patients.[35] Rubin's group used a patient-facing smartphone application to assess the Duke Activity Status Index (DASI).[36] Patient portals or surgeon's offices are early opportunities to complete a simple, system-based series of yes/no questions that ultimately direct patients to the best perioperative visit type for that patient and procedure.

Electronic decision support algorithms can also direct patients to the appropriate visit type available in each specific health system. For example, the Cleveland Clinic uses a PACC triage questionnaire to automatically assign patients to either in-person, virtual, or no PACC visit. A multispecialty team from internal medicine, anesthesiology, surgery, and IT developed an algorithm for triaging the necessary preoperative evaluation of patients. This triage tool uses simple language so that ancillary staff will feel comfortable completing it. The workflow is shown in Figure 1.1. This workflow is designed to be overly cautious in triaging patients, thus defaulting to an in-person visit if there is any concern about patient safety. The patients were stratified to PACC in-person visits or PACC virtual visits based on (1) patient risk profile (first five questions) and (2) risk level of surgery. The surgical team determines the risk level of surgery at the time of scheduling. Examples of high-risk cases requiring an in-person visit included cardiothoracic, multilevel spinal fusions, total joint revisions, vascular, major urologic, and most open major abdominal cases.

Those patients who do not have a high-risk patient profile (answered "no" to the first five questions) and are not undergoing a high-risk procedure continue along the flowchart to determine if they should be seen in a PACC virtual visit or if no PACC visit is needed. Ten additional questions are used to triage between PACC virtual visits or no PACC visit. If patients respond "no" to the follow-up questions, they are considered low-risk and are triaged to no PACC visit. Conversely, any "yes" answer will generate a recommendation for a virtual visit. Overall, candidates for PACC virtual visits include complex patients undergoing low-risk procedures and relatively healthy patients undergoing intermediate-risk procedures. The underlying algorithm for triaging patients was embedded in the EMR's logic behind each question, allowing the completed questionnaire to generate the recommended visit type automatically. The screenshots shown in Figure 1.2 show the questionnaire and the answer selections that will lead to a recommended PACC visit type (recommendation shown at the bottom of the questionnaire).

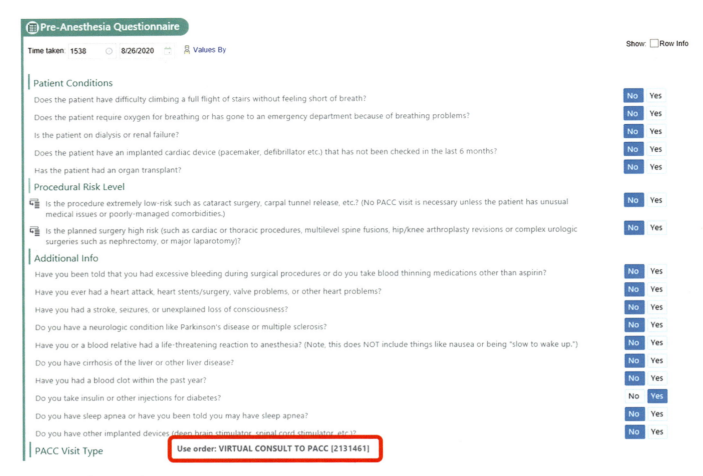

Figure 1.2 Virtual visit consult.

Figure 1.3 shows the algorithm directing the patient to an in-person visit. Again, significant patient conditions were identified in the initial stages of the decision tree.

VIRTUAL VISITS

There is little information regarding the presurgical optimization process and telemedicine visits in a large-scale healthcare system. A virtual visit involves telemedicine—using electronic, digital, web-based, or smartphone-based communication for direct patient care.[37] Telemedicine visits allow two-way audio-video–mediated patient interactions over electronic devices and increase access to the healthcare system when there are concerns for social distancing for patients and caregivers alike.

The technology evolution has led to the distinction of a *telemedicine visit*, where the patient still has to travel to a healthcare site to use high-quality video technology and electronic stethoscopes versus using their own personal tablet, laptop, or cellphone.[38] Patient travel to a healthcare facility is a *facilitated telemedicine visit*, which can even include basic testing done at the site. A *facilitated virtual visit* does require staff to schedule and enable the use of integrated physical exam tools. A *stand-alone telemedicine visit* is virtual but does not have a formal video tower with a digital stethoscope and hand-held video camera. Table 1.1 details the differences and is modified from Bridges' work.[38]

A large variety of equipment is available, and the size and resources of the preoperative clinic may dictate the products and platform chosen. Capital costs for a hospital could range from $1,700 to $7,000, depending on the scale of equipment selected.[39] The most complete towers include point-of-care diagnostics, including 12-lead ECG testing, digital spirometers, and ultrasound probes for cardiac, vascular, or nerve imaging.[38] The towers increase the price significantly but may be offset if the equipment is shared with another service line (e.g., ENT).[40]

The healthcare facility may choose to employ an electronic stethoscope and not the complete video tower. Assisted by a nurse at a site remote from the clinic, the electronic stethoscope is used to conduct heart and lung exams. The video portion of the exam is conducted with tablet technology over a secure connection.

The most common direct-to-consumer device available for a stand-alone telemedicine visit is a smartphone; more than 77% of Americans owned one in 2020.[37] The technical quality of images is reliable and of sufficient quality to enable accurate exams.[41–43] Multiple stand-alone video platforms are available for an institution to choose from, and some institutions have transitioned easily from one platform to another. For example,

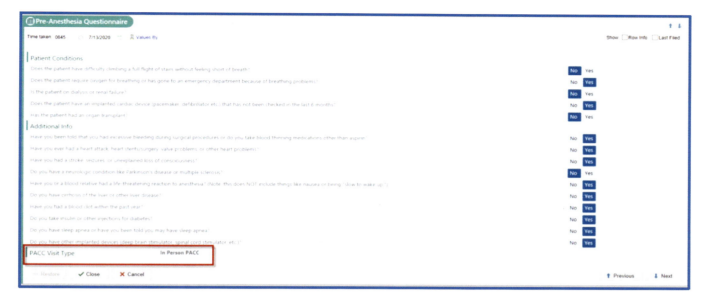

Figure 1.3 In-person PACC visit.
PACC, Pre-Anesthesia Consultation Clinic.

Table 1.1 TELEMEDICINE AND VIRTUAL VISITS

VISIT TYPE	PHONE SETTING	STAND-ALONE TELEMEDICINE VISIT	FACILITATED TELEMEDICINE VISIT
Obtain PMHX, anesthesia history	Yes	Yes	Yes
Medication reconciliation	Yes	Yes	Yes
Airway exam	No	Yes	Yes
Auscultate heart and lungs	No	No	Yes
Face-to-face interaction	No	Yes	Yes
Remote location and staff needed for visit	No	No	Yes
Administrative scheduling support needed	Depends	Yes	Yes
Able to obtain basic testing (ECG, spirometry)	No	No	Yes
Patient visit from home	Yes	Yes	No
Required capital investment	No	No	Yes

PMHX, Past medical history.

Kamdar and associates at the University of California, Los Angeles (UCLA) used a Health Insurance Portability and Accountability Act (HIPAA)-compliant platform, Zoom (Zoom Video Communications Inc., San Jose, CA), in 2017.[44] They were dissatisfied with the inability to photo capture the airway exam and the requirement for email scheduling of the virtual visit so they switched to Vidyo (Vidyo Inc., Hackensack, NJ), which integrated easily within their EMR, EPIC.

HIPAA compliance regarding direct-to-consumer devices requires a business associate agreement (BAA) in place with the healthcare provider.[38] Video conferencing software companies that are motivated to adapt their software to HIPAA-compliant platforms include but are not limited to, Skype for Business, Zoom, and GoToMeeting. But the most critical factor in considering HIPAA compliance is the prevailing governmental regulation at the time, as the COVID-19 pandemic has relaxed HIPAA requirements.[45]

Virtual visits start with staff obtaining informed consent for the visit. Providers use a specific preoperative note template, which includes required virtual visit elements such as total visit time (including the mode and location of patient and provider) and physical exam modifications appropriate for virtual evaluation. Virtual physical exams differ from traditional in-person exams but still include what is appropriate and medically necessary. For example, the respiratory system exam references observation of lip color, respiratory pattern, use of accessory muscles, audible wheezing, or pursed lip breathing. Cardiovascular assessment includes directing patients to self-palpate radial pulse and count their pulse out loud. Patients are asked to comment on the rhythm. New-onset atrial fibrillation has previously been identified in this manner.[46] The airway exam is completed with attention to the 11-point airway exam detailed by the ASA.[47]

The current literature consists of several telemedicine reports from rural and urban settings.[44,48,49] The largest and most recent study highlights patient satisfaction, cost savings, and no adverse effect on day-of-procedure cancellation rates with facilitated visits.[47] Also, stand-alone telemedicine visits are well accepted, incur a negligible capital investment for the institution, and patients feel a telemedicine visit saves them time and money.[50] This contrasts with a recent prospective study where patients were divided in their acceptance of virtual visits. This study from Stanford included comments from patients worried about privacy and not wanting to be videotaped.[51] As technology and security for virtual visits continue to improve and the process becomes more routine, some of these reservations may be mitigated. Hesitance by some to use technology (or not owning a suitable device) is an additional barrier likely to diminish over time as smartphone use is increasingly common.

Multiple authors have also depicted why telehealth has reached a "tipping point" in adopting virtual visits in the setting of preanesthesia assessment.[44,48] A tertiary healthcare system serves patients from various geographic locations, and patient experience is enhanced with patient-centered assessment. Smartphones are ubiquitous and incorporate high-quality cameras into everyday life. Patients are more used to interfacing with their healthcare system via "digital telecommunications including e-mail, mobile phone, and electronic patient portals."[52] Rapid adoption of telehealth visits are supported by recent provisions made by the US Centers for Medicare and Medicaid Services (CMS) governing telehealth and telemedicine.[48]

The Public Health Emergency billing mandates, stipulated by CMS, have prevented any deduction in reimbursement or work-relative value units (wRVUs) for telemedicine visits. This has greatly facilitated the adoption of these visits for both patients and healthcare systems. Like traditional evaluation and management (E&M) coding, the patient visit is categorized as new or established. New patients are those who have not received any services from the healthcare system in the past 3 years. The CMS requirements for documentation of video visits are available on a Medicare fee-for-service supplement published during the pandemic.[53,54] In general, visits are coded based on elements in the note unless the total time spent allows for a higher billing code.[54]

Post-pandemic, federal funding remains for telemedicine. The 2023 Omnibus appropriations bill extends telehealth flexibilities through the end of 2024. Medicare telehealth coverage has shifted from non–HIPAA-compliant platforms to HIPPA-compliant platforms only. Extended flexibilities after the crisis now state that telemedicine visits are billable at the same rate as video as long as they are used as a backup and/or if patients don't have means for video.[55]

Data on the quality of telemedicine visits remain scarce. However, one recent study collected information on outcome and process measures. They included balance measures (unintended consequences) and, consistent with QI methodology, defined patient selection criteria, referral, evaluation, and escalation to an in-person consultation.[56] Experts in the preoperative process must evaluate modern technology to continually improve and define quality.

SUMMARY

The preoperative process has expanded beyond traditional prescreening and can serve as a model for a higher integration standard throughout the healthcare system. This entry point to superior patient care comes from a preoperative clinic model that functions as a collaborative network of providers. Successful acceptance of modern technology depends on all stakeholders seeing value in the proposition. Thus, it is essential to have an evolving workflow to risk-stratify and optimize patients preoperatively.

Experience illustrates that telemedicine incorporating an embedded screening algorithm can successfully evaluate patients in the perioperative setting. This has the advantages of reducing congestion in the preoperative clinic and allowing social distancing in pandemic conditions. Additionally, using an online screening tool reduces the need for clinicians to intervene and manually assign patients to in-person or virtual visits.

CONCLUSION

- Multidisciplinary effort is important to obtain optimal innovation outcomes.
- Virtual visits offer patients convenience while maintaining safety and patient and provider satisfaction.
- There is no one ideal preoperative assessment clinic model.
- The most efficient prescreening process occurs early in the system and is patient-centric.

REVIEW QUESTIONS

Choose the best answer.

1. Preoperative clinics
    a. Are known to decrease patient safety.
    b. Increase preoperative testing and consultations.
    c. Can increase day of surgery delays and cancellations.
    d. Can help increase an institution's rate of advance directive completion.

The correct answer is d.

Although providing information about advance directives (AD) in a preoperative clinic may conjure images of bad outcomes, it is an ideal setting because patients are not in crisis and can calmly consider the issue. The preoperative clinic helps to ensure compliance with regulatory bodies, and there is an increased emphasis on advance care planning before surgeries and procedures, including the completion of AD documents such as the healthcare power of attorney and living wills.[19] The initial legislation that introduced the requirement to provide written information about ADs to adult patients on enrollment to a healthcare facility passed in 1990.[57]

2. New technologies for telehealth

   a. May increase costs.
   b. May decrease costs.
   c. Can be subject to state regulations regarding consent for telehealth visits.
   d. a, b, and c.

The correct answer is d.

Telehealth virtual visits can be a facilitated visit with a large variety of equipment and price points available or use equipment that the patient already owns. Opportunity costs and direct costs not incurred by the patient or institution can be realized with a stand-alone virtual visit. Thus costs can increase or decrease.

Institutions should explore their state's regulations regarding informed consent because telehealth is no different from any other aspect of medicine in that regard. The Center for Connected Health Policy and Health Resources and Services Administration (HRSA) offers a comprehensive source for telehealth information.[58]

3. The Preoperative Anesthesia and Surgical Screening (PASS) clinic at Duke

   a. Would see the patient immediately after the surgery date was scheduled.
   b. Would wait until financial clearance to schedule the PASS clinic date.
   c. Would see the patient for PASS clinic before the surgery date scheduled.
   d. Is a collaborative anesthesia and surgery clinic.
   e. c and d.

The correct answer is e.

This group has created a multidisciplinary clinic that sets a priority on optimizing a patient prior to their elective procedure. After consultation with a surgeon, there are accepted thresholds for wait times to optimize certain medical conditions.[1] It is not absolute, but, for many surgeries, the surgery date is scheduled *after* the completion of an optimization clinic based on standardized protocols. This clinic is in the initial phase, and health outcomes are yet to be defined.

4. A triage algorithm embedded in an electronic medical record

   a. Can fail if it is a unilateral decision.
   b. Must consider the end user.
   c. Can facilitate scheduling appropriate types of preoperative clinic visits.
   d. a, b, and c.

The correct answer is d.

A triage algorithm is a prescreening process that facilitates scheduling a correct visit type for a large preoperative clinic. Prior to the screening algorithm being developed, preoperative clinic providers would spend time manually assigning patients to virtual or in-person PACC visits. Although the benefit of saving time seems obvious, it is crucial to have surgeon input into the process of developing the algorithm so that the value is recognized and utilized in the surgeon's office.

5. A facilitated telemedicine visit is able to support

   a. Accurate airway exam.
   b. Heart and lung auscultation.
   c. ECG and spirometry.
   d. Patient participation from home.
   e. a, b, and c.

The correct answer is e.

A facilitated telemedicine visit is one in which the patient doesn't have to travel to the main preoperative clinic site but still needs to travel to a site with the correct equipment, office staff, and technical support. The secondary site is a better geographic choice than the main clinic. The patient needs to schedule a visit and engage with a healthcare provider who can use modern electronic equipment to send audiovisual data and use a digital stethoscope at the least. The range of point-of-care add-on devices to the main audiovisual tower is increasing and even includes spirometry and ECG.[59]

6. Telemedicine

   a. Can highlight health inequities.
   b. Cannot be HIPAA-compliant.
   c. Must include significant capital investment.
   d. Cannot be incorporated directly into an EMR.

The correct answer is a.

Telemedicine *can* highlight health inequities because not everyone owns a smartphone. Virtual visits can be HIPAA-compliant, but it is most important to be aware of current regulations because, at the time of this writing, all government regulations regarding HIPAA and virtual visits are relaxed due to the public health emergency, but this may revert. Airway exams can be directly incorporated into the EMR. We are emerging from a public health emergency, and, given the absence of government or state standards regarding telemedicine, a preanesthesia clinic must maintain a commitment to meet the need for patient service safely. Preoperative clinics must balance their mission and goals with current state regulatory guidelines.

7. The patient is a 61-year-old man making a virtual visit for lipoma excision in the right axilla, under general anesthesia. He has a BMI of 39 kg/m^2. The patient is borderline hypertensive, on no meds, and has never been told he has sleep apnea. Other comorbidities include depression, reflux, and exercise-induced asthma. His exercise-induced asthma is very mild, and he denies using inhalers. During the virtual visit, the physical exam shows a BP of 135/80, the pulse is regular (per the patient), an airway exam is significant for MP2, and a thick

neck. The color of the skin is normal, and no abnormality is observed in his respiratory system.

The proposed surgery is scheduled at an ASC. The chart image includes an ultrasound showing a benign axilla lipoma measuring 8 × 10 cm and having no suspicious vascularity.

The virtual visit goes well. The provider calls you afterward to ensure that this is an appropriate ASC case. They ask if this case should be moved to a hospital, given the nature of giant lipoma.

You agree to discuss it with the surgeon. Eventually, the case proceeds at a hospital, where it is complicated by a torn axillary artery and excess bleeding with subsequent vascular surgeries to repair the axillary artery.

This case illustrates:

a. A virtual visit is identical to an in-person visit, except the physical exam and critical thinking must still take place.
b. Appropriate imaging should occur preoperatively, which may include MRI in case of large lipomas.
c. It is important to correctly match facility and procedure.
d. All of the above.

The correct answer is d.

Preoperative evaluation is an intersection of patient safety and throughput. Considerations of surgical risk and patient-specific risk factors apply whether an evaluation is virtual or in-person. A structured risk assessment may lead to additional preoperative testing and a safer alignment of patient, procedure, and facility. Despite a general acceptance of virtual preoperative visits, it is crucial to identify those who need additional evaluation and testing.[60]

REFERENCES

1. Aronson S, Murray S, Martin G, Blitz J, Crittenden T, Lipkin ME, Mantyh CR, Lagoo-Deenadayalan SA, Flanagan EM, Attarian DE, Mathew JP, Kirk AD; Perioperative Enhancement Team (POET). Roadmap for transforming preoperative assessment to preoperative optimization. *Anesth Analg.* 2020;130(4):811–819.
2. O'Glasser AY, Taylor CC, Hunter AJ. Beyond the algorithm: Implementation of a hospitalist-led pre-operative clinic assessment before cardiac surgery. *Periop Care Op Room Manage.* 2017;8:1–4.
3. Ferschl MB, Tung A, Sweitzer B, Huo D, Glick DB. Preoperative clinic visits reduce operating room cancellations and delays. *Anesthesiology.* 2005 Oct;103(4):855–859. doi: 10.1097/00000542-200510000-00025. PMID: 16192779.
4. Badner NH, Craen RA, Paul TL, Doyle JA. Anaesthesia preadmission assessment: a new approach through use of a screening questionnaire. *Can J Anaesth.* 1998 Jan;45(1):87–92. doi: 10.1007/BF03012002. PMID: 9466037.
5. Yen C, Tsai M, Macario A. Preoperative evaluation clinics. *Curr Opin Anaesthesiol.* 2010 Apr;23(2):167–172. doi: 10.1097/ACO.0b013e328336f4b9. PMID: 20124896.
6. Bashshur. Telemedicine and the COVID-19 pandemic: Lessons for the future. *Telemed eHealth.* 2020;26(5):571–573.
7. Applegate RL 2nd, Gildea B, Patchin R, Rook JL, Wolford B, Nyirady J, Dawes TA, Faltys J, Ramsingh DS, Stier G. Telemedicine pre-anesthesia evaluation: a randomized pilot trial. *Telemed J E Health.* 2013 Mar;19(3):211–216. doi: 10.1089/tmj.2012.0132. Epub 2013 Feb 5. PMID: 23384334.
8. Mihalj M, Carrel T, Gregoric ID, et al. Telemedicine for preoperative assessment during a COVID-19 pandemic: Recommendations for clinical care. *Best Pract Res Clin Anaesthesiol.* 2020;34(2):345–351.
9. Accorsi TAD, Amicis K, Brígido ARD, Belfort DSP, Habrum FC, Scarpanti FG, Magalhães IR, Silva Filho JRO, Sampaio LPC, Lira MTSS, Morbeck RA, Pedrotti CHS, Cordioli E. Assessment of patients with acute respiratory symptoms during the COVID-19 pandemic by Telemedicine: clinical features and impact on referral. *Einstein (Sao Paulo).* 2020 Dec 7;1–8:eAO6106. doi: 10.31744/einstein_journal/2020AO6106. PMID: 33295428; PMCID: PMC7690926.
10. Dilisio RP, Dilisio AJ, Weiner MM. Preoperative virtual screening examination of the airway. *J Clin Anesth.* 2014;26(4):315–317.
11. Wood EW, Strauss RA, Janus C, Carrico CK. Telemedicine consultations in oral and maxillofacial surgery: A follow-up study. *J Oral Maxillofac Surg.* 2016;74(2):262–268.
12. Blitz JD, Kendale SM, Jain SK, Cuff GE, Kim JT, Rosenberg AD. Preoperative Evaluation Clinic Visit Is Associated with Decreased Risk of In-hospital Postoperative Mortality. *Anesthesiology.* 2016 Aug;125(2):280–294. doi: 10.1097/ALN.0000000000001193. PMID: 27433746.
13. Correll DJ, Bader AM, Hull MW, Hsu C, Tsen LC, Hepner DL. Value of preoperative clinic visits in identifying issues with potential impact on operating room efficiency. *Anesthesiology.* 2006 Dec;105(6):1254–1259; discussion 6A. doi: 10.1097/00000542-200612000-00026. PMID: 17122589.
14. Emanuel A, MacPherson R. The anaesthetic pre-admission clinic is effective in minimising surgical cancellation rates. *Anaesth Intens Care.* 2013;41(1):90–94.
15. Parker BM, Tetzlaff JE, Litaker DL, Maurer WG. Redefining the preoperative evaluation process and the role of the anesthesiologist. *J Clin Anesth.* 2000;12(5):350–356.
16. van Klei WA, Hennis PJ, Moen J, Kalkman CJ, Moons KG. The accuracy of trained nurses in pre-operative health assessment: results of the OPEN study. *Anaesthesia.* 2004 Oct;59(10):971–978. doi: 10.1111/j.1365-2044.2004.03858.x. PMID: 15488055.
17. Grant C, Ludbrook GL, O'Loughlin EJ, Corcoran TB. An analysis of computer-assisted pre-screening prior to elective surgery. *Anaesth Intensive Care.* 2012 Mar;40(2):297–304. doi: 10.1177/0310057X1204000213. PMID: 22417025.
18. Tariq H, Ahmed R, Kulkarni S, Hanif S, Toolsie O, Abbas H, Chilimuri S. Development, Functioning, and Effectiveness of a Preoperative Risk Assessment Clinic. *Health Serv Insights.* 2016 Oct 30;9(Suppl 1):1–7. doi: 10.4137/HSI.S40540. PMID: 27812286; PMCID: PMC5090289.
19. Chandra S Fleisher D, Jaffer A. Developing, implementing, and operating a preoperative clinic in perioperative medicine. 2012.
20. Shah NN, Vetter T. Comprehensive preoperative assessment and global optimization. *Anesthesiol Clin.* 2018;36:259–280.
21. Vetter TR, Uhler LM, Bozic KJ. Value-based Healthcare: Preoperative Assessment and Global Optimization (PASS-GO): Improving Value in Total Joint Replacement Care. *Clin Orthop Relat Res.* 2017 Aug;475(8):1958–1962. doi: 10.1007/s11999-017-5400-z. Epub 2017 Jun 9. PMID: 28600689; PMCID: PMC5498398.
22. Vetter TR, Jones KA. Perioperative surgical home: Perspective II. *Anesthesiol Clin.* 2015;33:771–784.
23. Committee on Standards and Practice Parameters; Apfelbaum JL, Connis RT, Nickinovich DG; American Society of Anesthesiologists Task Force on Preanesthesia Evaluation; Pasternak LR, Arens JF, Caplan RA, Connis RT, Fleisher LA, Flowerdew R, Gold BS, Mayhew JF, Nickinovich DG, Rice LJ, Roizen MF, Twersky RS. Practice advisory for preanesthesia evaluation: an updated report by the American Society of Anesthesiologists Task Force on Preanesthesia Evaluation. *Anesthesiology.* 2012 Mar;116(3):522–538. doi: 10.1097/ALN.0b013e31823c1067. PMID: 22273990.
24. Fleisher LA, Fleischmann KE, Auerbach AD, Barnason SA, Beckman JA, Bozkurt B, Davila-Roman VG, Gerhard-Herman MD, Holly TA, Kane GC, Marine JE, Nelson MT, Spencer CC, Thompson A, Ting

HH, Uretsky BF, Wijeysundera DN. 2014 ACC/AHA guideline on perioperative cardiovascular evaluation and management of patients undergoing noncardiac surgery: executive summary: a report of the American College of Cardiology/American Heart Association Task Force on Practice Guidelines. *Circulation*. 2014 Dec 9;130(24):2215–2245. doi: 10.1161/CIR.0000000000000105. Epub 2014 Aug 1. PMID: 25085962.

25. Edwards AF, Slawski B. Preoperative clinics. *Anesthesiology Clin*. 2016;34:1–15. http://dx.doi.org/10.1016/j.anclin.2015.10.002

26. Digner M. At your convenience: Preoperative assessment by telephone. *J Perioperative Practice*. 2007;17:294–301.

27. Ireland S, Kent B. Telephone pre-operative assessment for adults: A comprehensive systematic review. *JBI Libr Syst Rev*. 2012;10(25):1452–1503. doi: 10.11124/01938924-201210250-00001. PMID: 27819953.

28. Lozada MJ, Nguyen JT, Abouleish A, Prough D, Przkora R. Patient preference for the pre-anesthesia evaluation: Telephone versus in-office assessment. *J Clin Anesth*. 2016 Jun;31:145–148. doi: 10.1016/j.jclinane.2015.12.040. Epub 2016 Apr 15. PMID: 27185698.

29. Ludbrook G, Seglenieks R, Osborn S, Grant C. A call centre and extended checklist for pre-screening elective surgical patients – a pilot study. *BMC Anesthesiol*. 2015 May 19;15:77. doi: 10.1186/s12871-015-0057-1. PMID: 25985775; PMCID: PMC4438626.

30. Hepner DL, Bader AM, Hurwitz S, Gustafson M, Tsen LC. Patient satisfaction with preoperative assessment in a preoperative assessment testing clinic. *Anesth Analg*. 2004 Apr;98(4):1099–1105. doi: 10.1213/01.ANE.0000103265.48380.89. PMID: 15041606.

31. Vaghadia H, Fowler C. Can nurses screen all outpatients? Performance of a nurse based model. *Can J Anaesth*. 1999;46(12):1117–1121.

32. Parker BM, Tetzlaff JE, Litaker DL, Maurer WG. Redefining the preoperative evaluation process and the role of the anesthesiologist. *J Clin Anesth*. 2000 Aug;12(5):350–356. doi: 10.1016/s0952-8180(00)00169-0. PMID: 11025233.

33. van den Blink A, Janssen LMJ, Hermanides J, Loer SA, Straat FK, Jessurun EN, Schwarte LA, Schober P. Evaluation of electronic screening in the preoperative process. *J Clin Anesth*. 2022 Nov;82:110941. doi: 10.1016/j.jclinane.2022.110941. Epub 2022 Aug 5. PMID: 35939972.

34. Flamm M, Fritsch G, Hysek M, Klausner S, Entacher K, Panisch S, Soennichsen AC. Quality improvement in preoperative assessment by implementation of an electronic decision support tool. *J Am Med Inform Assoc*. 2013 Jun;20(e1):e91–6. doi: 10.1136/amiajnl-2012-001178. Epub 2013 Apr 18. PMID: 23599223; PMCID: PMC3715339.

35. Osman T, Lew E, Lum EP, van Galen L, Dabas R, Sng BL, Car J. PreAnesThesia computerized health (PATCH) assessment: development and validation. *BMC Anesthesiol*. 2020 Nov 14;20(1):286. doi: 10.1186/s12871-020-01202-8. PMID: 33189131; PMCID: PMC7666442.

36. Rubin DS, Dalton A, Tank A, Berkowitz M, Arnolds DE, Liao C, Gerlach RM. Development and Pilot Study of an iOS Smartphone Application for Perioperative Functional Capacity Assessment. *Anesth Analg*. 2020 Sep;131(3):830–839. doi: 10.1213/ANE.0000000000004440. PMID: 31567326.

37. Blue R, Yang AI, Zhou C, De Ravin E, Teng CW, Arguelles GR, Huang V, Wathen C, Miranda SP, Marcotte P, Malhotra NR, Welch WC, Lee JYK. Telemedicine in the Era of Coronavirus Disease 2019 (COVID-19): A Neurosurgical Perspective. *World Neurosurg*. 2020 Jul;139:549–557. doi: 10.1016/j.wneu.2020.05.066. Epub 2020 May 16. PMID: 32426065; PMCID: PMC7229725.

38. Bridges KH, McSwain JR, Wilson PR. To Infinity and Beyond: The Past, Present, and Future of Tele-Anesthesia. *Anesth Analg*. 2020 Feb;130(2):276–284. doi: 10.1213/ANE.0000000000004346. PMID: 31397698.

39. Wood EW, Strauss RA, Janus C, Carrico CK. Telemedicine Consultations in Oral and Maxillofacial Surgery: A Follow-Up Study. *J Oral Maxillofac Surg*. 2016 Feb;74(2):262–268. doi: 10.1016/j.joms.2015.09.026. Epub 2015 Oct 3. PMID: 26501427.

40. Shih J, Portnoy J. Tips for Seeing Patients via Telemedicine. *Curr Allergy Asthma Rep*. 2018 Aug 15;18(10):50. doi: 10.1007/s11882-018-0807-5. PMID: 30112587.

41. Park HY, Jeon SS, Lee JY, Cho AR, Park JH. Korean Version of the Mini-Mental State Examination Using Smartphone: A Validation Study. *Telemed J E Health*. 2017 Oct;23(10):815–821. doi: 10.1089/tmj.2016.0281. Epub 2017 Apr 19. PMID: 28422578.

42. Sahin D, Hacisalihoglu UP, Kirimlioglu SH. Telecytology: Is it possible with smartphone images? *Diagn Cytopathol*. 2018 Jan;46(1):40–46. doi: 10.1002/dc.23851. Epub 2017 Nov 8. PMID: 29115040.

43. McBeth P, Crawford I, Tiruta C, Xiao Z, Zhu GQ, Shuster M, Sewell L, Panebianco N, Lautner D, Nicolaou S, Ball CG, Blaivas M, Dente CJ, Wyrzykowski AD, Kirkpatrick AW. Help is in your pocket: the potential accuracy of smartphone- and laptop-based remotely guided resuscitative telesonography. *Telemed J E Health*. 2013 Dec;19(12):924–930. doi: 10.1089/tmj.2013.0034. Epub 2013 Oct 19. PMID: 24138615.

44. Kamdar NV, Huverserian A, Jalilian L, Thi W, Duval V, Beck L, Brooker L, Grogan T, Lin A, Cannesson M. Development, Implementation, and Evaluation of a Telemedicine Preoperative Evaluation Initiative at a Major Academic Medical Center. *Anesth Analg*. 2020 Dec;131(6):1647–1656. doi: 10.1213/ANE.0000000000005208. PMID: 32841990; PMCID: PMC7489226.

45. HIPAA Journal. HIPAA guidelines on telemedicine. https://www.hipaajournal.com/hipaa-guidelines-on-telemedicine/

46. Jaakkola J, Vasankari T, Virtanen R, Juhani Airaksinen KE. Reliability of pulse palpation in the detection of atrial fibrillation in an elderly population. *Scand J Prim Health Care*. 2017 Sep;35(3):293–298. doi: 10.1080/02813432.2017.1358858. Epub 2017 Aug 7. PMID: 28784027; PMCID: PMC5592357.

47. Applegate RL 2nd, Gildea B, Patchin R, Rook JL, Wolford B, Nyiracy J, Dawes TA, Faltys A, Ramsingh DS, Stier G. Telemedicine pre-anesthesia evaluation: A randomized pilot trial. *Telemed J E Health*. 2013 Mar;19(3):211–216. doi: 10.1089/tmj.2012.0132. Epub 2013 Feb 5. PMID: 23384334.

48. Lu AC, Cannesson M, Kamdar N. The Tipping Point of Medical Technology: Implications for the Postpandemic Era. *Anesth Analg*. 2020 Aug;131(2):335–339. doi: 10.1213/ANE.0000000000005040. PMID: 32511105; PMCID: PMC7302096.

49. Mullen-Fortino M, Rising KL, Duckworth J, Gwynn V, Sites FD, Hollander JE. Presurgical Assessment Using Telemedicine Technology: Impact on Efficiency, Effectiveness, and Patient Experience of Care. *Telemed J E Health*. 2019 Feb;25(2):137–142. doi: 10.1089/tmj.2017.0133. Epub 2018 Jul 26. PMID: 30048210.

50. Zetterman CV, Sweitzer BJ, Webb B, Barak-Bernhagen MA, Boedeker BH. Validation of a virtual preoperative evaluation clinic: A pilot study. *Stud Health Technol Inform*. 2011;163:737–739. PMID: 21335890.

51. Fishman M, Mirante B, Dai F, Kurup V. Patient preferences on telemedicine for preanesthesia evaluation. *Can J Anaesth*. 2015 Apr;62(4):433–434. doi: 10.1007/s12630-014-0280-0. Epub 2014 Nov 26. PMID: 25424380.

52. Kamdar N, Jalilian L. Telemedicine: A Digital Interface for Perioperative Anesthetic Care. *Anesth Analg*. 2020 Feb;130(2):272–275. doi: 10.1213/ANE.0000000000004513. PMID: 31934901.

53. Portnoy J, Waller M, Elliott T. Telemedicine in the Era of COVID-19. *J Allergy Clin Immunol Pract*. 2020 May;8(5):1489–1491. doi: 10.1016/j.jaip.2020.03.008. Epub 2020 Mar 24. PMID: 32220575; PMCID: PMC7104202.

54. American Medical Association. CMS payment policies regulatory flexibilities during COVID-19 emergency. https://www.ama-assn.org/practice-management/medicare/cms-payment-policies-regulatory-flexibilitiesduring-covid-19

55. Center for Connected Health Policy. https://www.cchpca.org/2023/03/MEDICARE-TELEHEALTH-POLICIES-POST-PHE-AT-A-GLANCE-FINAL-MAR-2023.pdf

56. Popivanov P, Bampoe S, Tan T, Rafferty P. Development, implementation and evaluation of high-quality virtual preoperative anaesthetic

assessment during COVID-19 and beyond: A quality improvement report. *BMJ Open Qual*. 2022 Oct;11(4):e001959. doi:10.1136/bmjoq-2022-001959. PMID: 36216375; PMCID: PMC9556744

57. Galambos CM. Preserving end-of-life autonomy: The Patient Self-Determination Act and the Uniform Health Care Decisions Act. *Health Soc Work*. 1998;23(4):275–281. PMID 9834880

58. Center for Connected Health Policy. https://www.cchpca.org/

59. Baker J, Stanley A. Telemedicine Technology: a Review of Services, Equipment, and Other Aspects. *Curr Allergy Asthma Rep*. 2018 Sep 26;18(11):60. doi: 10.1007/s11882-018-0814-6. PMID: 30259201.

60. Filipovic MG, Schwenter A, Luedi MM, Urman RD. Modern preoperative evaluation in ambulatory surgery: Who, where and how? *Curr Opin Anaesthesiol*. 2022 Dec 1;35(6):661–666. doi:10.1097/ACO.0000000000001192. Epub 2022 Oct 4. PMID: 36194141.

2.

PERIOPERATIVE SURGICAL HOME CARE MODEL

UTOPIA OR BUREAUCRACY?

Eileen Campbell and Janine Limoncelli

STEM CASE AND KEY QUESTIONS

A 72-year-old male patient presents to the perioperative surgical home (PSH) clinic for preoperative assessment and optimization after being recently diagnosed with hepatocellular liver cancer (HCC). MRI studies reveal that he has a 3.2 cm lesion in the posterior right liver lobe. The patient has a history of pulmonary fibrosis and is oxygen dependent. In addition, the patient's history is significant for pacemaker/automatic internal cardiac defibrillator (ICD) placement, burr hole for brain abscess with need for prolonged ventilation via tracheostomy, atrial fibrillation with anticoagulation, and alcohol-related liver cirrhosis. The surgical plan is to perform a right-sided laparoscopic liver resection. The surgeon has referred the patient to the PSH for further evaluation and management because a general anesthetic will be required for a laparoscopic liver resection. Here we will review this patient's case with a PSH in place and determine what the patient's perspective is of that PSH. Is the PSH perceived by the patient as a utopian place or just another medical entity where there is more red tape and bureaucracy? For the PSH, with the anesthesiologist as leader, to function as control central it is important for the anesthesiologist to understand all the different elements and aspects of not only the patient's comorbidities but also of the proposed procedure as well.

What are the goals of the PSH for this patient?

Typically, the goal of the PSH is described as achieving the "triple aim."[1] The triple aim is improving patient outcomes, increasing patient satisfaction, and decreasing hospital costs.[1] In reality, the expected metrics that a PSH should aim to achieve are more far-reaching, defined, and greater in number.[2]

    Expected metrics from a PSH include[1,2]

    Improved operational efficiencies
    Decreased resource utilization
    Reduced length of stay
    Reduced readmission
    Decreased complication rate
    Decreased mortality
    Improved patient experience

How are these metrics/goals achieved?

The metrics and goals are achieved by increasing patient satisfaction, improving patient outcome and decreasing hospital costs. This triple aim is achieved by employing evidence-based clinical pathways; providing a coordinated, comprehensive, accessible care plan to the patient and their caregiver, and embracing and utilizing new technologies.

What is the entry point for the patient to the PSH?

To begin, once the patient has decided to have surgery, the first appointment should be at the PSH at their institution 2–4 weeks prior to the planned surgery. At the initial visit the patient, ideally with their caregiver, is seen by a member of the perioperative team. Information is collected from the patient and an in-depth education is provided to the patient with respect to their active participation in their surgical process and successful recovery (i.e. incentive spirometry, prehabilitation, preoperative carbohydrate loading drinks, etc.). The processes that begin at the preoperative visit at the PSH are founded on evidence-based clinical pathways that address and achieve the expected quality metrics.[2] This includes preoperative optimization and individualized risk stratification. It is critical to counsel the patient to report any changes in their health status between the time of the PSH evaluation and the date of surgery. Certain conditions may cause surgery to be postponed (e.g., infection with COVID-19, chronic obstructive pulmonary disease [COPD], or congestive heart failure [CHF] exacerbation).

What factors determine the preoperative optimization and risk stratification for this patient?

The patient's current physical status, comorbidities, and the risk of the surgery are reviewed and analyzed to determine if the patient's medical conditions are stable and optimized. Determining optimization status and estimating the risk to the patient is an important role of the PSH.

What is the rationale for an anesthesia plan that includes both general anesthesia and neuraxial techniques for this particular case?

General anesthesia (GA) will allow for complete anesthesia and analgesia. Neuraxial or regional techniques, such as transversus abdominis plane (TAP) block, will provide extended postoperative pain control and may provide an opioid-sparing effect for the patient in the postoperative phase. This is especially important for this patient who may not be able to metabolize opiates because of his dual hepatic disease. Furthermore, in the current social context of an opioid crisis, we are attempting to prevent harm and reduce risk by minimizing the use of opioids. In addition, decreasing postoperative pain will promote adequate chest wall excursion, thereby improving this patient's already compromised pulmonary status. This will hopefully result in a decreased risk for postoperative pulmonary infection and/or reintubation.

What are the risks, benefits, and alternatives that the anesthesiologist must explain to the patient regarding the anesthetic plan?

The patient is evaluated using American Society for Anesthesiology (ASA) risk stratification.[3] ASA risk stratification attempts to predict the relative risk for a patient.[3] A healthy patient with no comorbidities is classified as ASA I.[3] A patient with well-managed medical problems of at least two body systems is classified as ASA II.[3] ASA III[3] patients have major diseases of two or more body systems that are stable and well-controlled. The patient in this discussion is classified as ASA IV[3] based on his multiple comorbidities. ASA IV patients have multiple medical problems that are neither stable nor controlled and/or are patients at the end stage of their disease process. ASA IV indicates an elevated risk of perioperative complications, including death.[3] In addition to risk stratification according to ASA guidelines, the procedure itself is also assigned a risk status. Surgical procedures are classified by the American College of Surgeons as low risk, medium risk, or high risk. The use of both tools provides an estimate of the overall risk that the patient will be exposed to. In this particular case, this is a medium-risk surgery for a high-risk patient.

How does the anesthesiologist explain the potential risks and complications related to the patient's underlying pulmonary fibrosis?

The patient is at high risk of a perioperative complication that may require prolonged intubation and ventilation because of the underlying pulmonary fibrosis and oxygen dependence.[4] The anesthesiologist explains to the patient that people with pulmonary fibrosis are at increased risk of prolonged intubation after surgery, and, even if the patient is extubated after surgery, reintubation may be required. There is a real risk that the patient's pulmonary system will be so compromised by the surgical procedure and the anesthetic agents used that extubation may not be possible and the patient may require lifelong mechanical artificial ventilation. In addition, the anesthesiologist also explains that the patient is at high risk of an intraoperative pulmonary event that could result in permanent mechanical artificial ventilation or even death.[4]

What are the initial consults and evaluations that the PSH team will obtain to assess and/or improve this patient's medical optimization? How will the evaluations be coordinated between the individual providers and then communicated to the patient?

To determine if the patient's medical conditions are optimized for the planned procedure, all of the patient's medical conditions will be evaluated. *Optimization* refers to the concept of a patient being as healthy as possible for surgery despite preexisting disease and illness. The initial preoperative specialty evaluations will be from cardiology and pulmonology. The patient has been treated for atrial fibrillation and an underlying heart block by a cardiologist for many years and has been placed on apixaban for thromboembolic prophylaxis. After being examined by his cardiologist, the cardiologist provided an evaluation that indicated the patient is at an elevated risk for cardiac complications and recommended discontinuation of apixaban 48 hours prior to the procedure. The cardiac evaluation was sent to the surgeon and PSH. The cardiologist also recommends that a cardiac electrophysiologist be involved in the care of the patient because of the presence of the pacemaker device/ICD.

What are the potential problems with a pacemaker and intraoperative electrocautery use?

It is recommended that if monopolar electrocautery is used, it should be used in short bursts of several seconds because the ICD usually requires several seconds of cardiac rhythm detection before pacing or defibrillation occurs. Pauses in the monopolar electrocautery allow for fewer erroneous ICD interventions. The electrocautery dispersion pad should be placed on the patient so that the path of the electromagnetic interference (EMI) does not cross over the ICD generator. It is generally accepted that the electrocautery grounding pad be placed opposite the pacemaker site.

How will the patient's cardiac pacemaker be managed? What is the intraoperative management of an ICD? Why is it important that members of the PSH determine specific information about individual patient devices?

A cardiac electrophysiologist will need to be contacted because the patient's pacemaker will need to be interrogated within 30 days after the procedure. This is done to detect any damage to the device's generator secondary to the use of electrocautery. An ICD is a device that has a pacemaker function for bradyarrhythmia treatment and implantable cardioverter cardiac defibrillator for tachyarrhythmia management. ICDs are becoming more common in our patient population with 1 million patients worldwide receiving an ICD each year. The Heart Rhythm Society (HRS)/American Society of Anesthesiologist (ASA) issued a consensus statement noting that most patients with an ICD do not need a new preoperative evaluation of the ICD due to the fact that most ICDs undergo a telephone interrogation every few months as well as yearly evaluations by a physician.[5]

It is important to determine if a patient who has a pacemaker for bradyarrhythmia is in fact pacemaker dependent (absence of perfusing rhythm without pacing). If the patient is pacemaker dependent, it is necessary to establish a secondary method for pacing the patient should the current pacemaker fail. This can be done by transesophageal, transcutaneous, or transvenous pacing. It is extremely important to anticipate the need for alternative temporary pacing and have all emergency equipment available before the surgical procedure is initiated.

What are the functions of ICDs? What are some of the perioperative considerations regarding the functions of ICDs?

Implanted defibrillators have four functions.[5] They sense atrial or ventricular electrical activity. The device classifies these signals to various programmed rate zones and then delivers tiered therapies to terminate ventricular tachycardia or fibrillation, and it will provide a pacing therapy for bradycardia. The most important aspect of ICD management for the defibrillator function is to deactivate the tachyarrhythmia response of the device to avoid inappropriate pacing or shocks due to EMI from the electrocautery being perceived as a malignant arrhythmia. Once the defibrillator's functions are disabled, it is imperative to have another source available to actively defibrillate the patient if need be. EMI can cause malfunction of both the pacemaker and the defibrillator. The most common cause for malfunction for patients with ICDs is monopolar electrocautery. The EMI from the monopolar cautery can inhibit pacing because the device interprets the electrocautery energy as intrinsic cardiac activity, and EMI can damage the device's generator. In addition, the EMI can be perceived by the ICD as a tachyarrhythmia thus producing an inappropriate tachyarrhythmia therapy (i.e., an electrical shock). Bipolar electrocautery is much safer to use when an ICD is in place because the current is small and the energy travels between the two poles of the instrument's stylus itself, thus electricity does not need to be dispersed outward. This will prevent the ICD from reading the current generated by the electrocautery as a tachyarrhythmia. However, bipolar electrocautery may not be able to achieve the necessary level of hemostasis as monopolar electrocautery, therefore additional measures, such as the use of a laser argon beam, may be needed in the event of severe or prolonged bleeding.

What is the role of magnets for pacemakers and internal defibrillators?

The effect of a magnet on a pacemaker is variable, depending on the device and the manufacturer. Some pacemakers have no response when a magnet is placed, while other pacemakers will be reprogrammed to pace asynchronously. The rate at which the pacemaker paces asynchronously depends on the manufacturer and the battery life of the generator. Patients with pacemakers that are programmed to pace at a slower rate may need this adjusted prior to a surgery in which there will be large hemodynamic swings in order for the heart rate to appropriately increase in the setting of a lower intrinsic sinus ventricular rate. When a ICD is present the magnet inactivates the shock function, while having no effect on the pacemaker. (there is only one magnetic switch per device).

The patient is referred by PSH to a pulmonologist for further evaluation and optimization. The patient has a known history of severe pulmonary fibrosis and is oxygen dependent. The patient's current pulmonary medications are albuterol, tiotropium bromide, and prednisone. What information is needed from a pulmonary evaluation? How will pulmonary optimization be determined?

This patient is being considered for laparoscopic surgery that will require an intraoperative pneumoperitoneum and the steep reverse Trendelenburg position. Based on the results of the patient's pulmonary function tests and response to bronchodilators it is determined that the patient is stable for activities of daily living (ADLs). The pulmonary evaluation determines that the patient is a high-risk candidate for a procedure that involves both GA and laparoscopy, and there is a strong possibility that prolonged intubation and/or reintubation will be necessary during the postoperative course (see Figure 2.1).

In addition, the pulmonology evaluation indicates that the patient has a STOP-BANG score of 5, which represents a high possibility of obstructive sleep apnea (OSA), and therefore the pulmonologist recommends a sleep study to rule out OSA.[6] The STOP-BANG screening tool is a series of questions that determine if a patient is at risk for OSA. In summary, the pulmonologist determines that this patient is a high-risk candidate for the planned procedures and strongly recommends exploration of alternative therapies, such as an interventional radiology procedure.

What are the possible options that an interventional radiologist could offer to this patient? How does the pathophysiology of the patient's disease impact the selection of the interventional approach?

Two possible interventional treatments could be offered to this patient, thermal ablation versus chemoembolization.[7] HCC is a tumor that usually develops in the setting of chronic liver disease and liver cirrhosis. Liver cirrhosis is often the most predominant pathological lesion behind the development and progression of HCC. HCC worldwide is the third most common cause of death related to cancer.[7] HCC is a hypervascular tumor, thus it can rapidly progress and invade surrounding structures.

Many studies support the use of local ablative therapies as an advantageous solution for patients who are not candidates for surgery.[7] Thermal ablative techniques include radiofrequency ablation (RFA) and microwave ablation (MWA). These techniques are generally safe and can be as effective as surgical resection. RFA works by passing electrical currents in the range of radiofrequency waves between the needle electrode and the grounding pads placed on the patient's skin. These currents create heat around the electrode, which, when directed into the tumor, destroys the cancer cells. Patients are often up, ambulating, and back to work 24–72 hours after the procedure. The time needed to achieve pain relief can be variable. Typically pain relief is experienced within 10 days; however, relief may be immediate for some patients or relief may not be experienced until 3 weeks post-procedure. Transarterial chemoembolization (TACE) therapies allow for selective delivery of a chemotherapeutic agent to hepatic tumors, and it protects against ischemic necrosis of normal liver tissue. Many studies show a benefit in combining TACE with one of the thermal ablative techniques. TACE blocks arterial blood flow to a tumor. Iodized oil and gelatin sponge particles are used in TACE to achieve coagulation necrosis. These particles go through multiple arterioportal channels, block the blood flow, and thereby reduce the risk of tumor recurrence.

What are the considerations regarding positioning and effect on treatment related to the procedures that could be performed in the interventional radiology (IR) suite? What diagnostic tests will be needed for a procedure performed by IR?

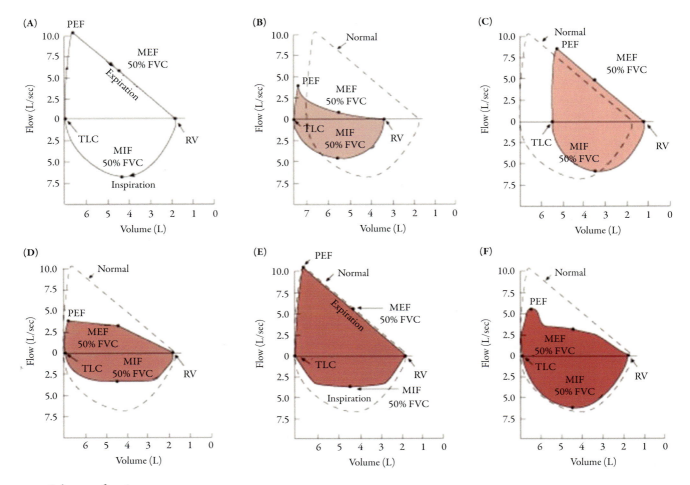

Figure 2.1 Pulmonary function test.

Flow-volume loops.

(A) **Normal**. Inspiratory limb of loop is symmetric and convex. Expiratory limb is linear. Airflow at the midpoint of inspiratory capacity and airflow at the midpoint of expiratory capacity are often measured and compared. Maximal inspiratory airflow at 50% of forced vital capacity (MIF 50% FVC) is greater than maximal expiratory airflow at 50% FVC (MEF 50% FVC) because dynamic compression of the airways occurs during exhalation.

(B) **Obstructive disorder** (e.g., emphysema, asthma). Although all airflow is diminished, expiratory prolongation predominates, and MEF < MIF. Peak expiratory flow is sometimes used to estimate degree of airway obstruction but depends on patient effort.

(C) **Restrictive disorder** (e.g., interstitial lung disease, kyphoscoliosis). The loop is narrowed because of diminished lung volumes. Airflow is greater than normal at comparable lung volumes because the increased elastic recoil of lungs holds the airways open.

(D) **Fixed obstruction of the upper airway** (e.g., tracheal stenosis, goiter). The top and bottom of the loops are flattened so that the configuration approaches that of a rectangle. Fixed obstruction limits flow equally during inspiration and expiration, and MEF = MIF.

(E) **Variable extrathoracic obstruction** (e.g., unilateral vocal cord paralysis, vocal cord dysfunction). When a single vocal cord is paralyzed, it moves passively with pressure gradients across the glottis. During forced inspiration, it is drawn inward, resulting in a plateau of decreased inspiratory flow. During forced expiration, it is passively blown aside, and expiratory flow is unimpaired. Therefore, MIF 50% FVC < MEF 50% FVC.

(F) **Variable intrathoracic obstruction** (e.g., tracheomalacia). During a forced inspiration, negative pleural pressure holds the floppy trachea open. With forced expiration, loss of structural support results in tracheal narrowing and a plateau of diminished flow. Airflow is maintained briefly before airway compression occurs.

TLC, total lung capacity; RV, residual volume; PEF, peak expiratory flow; MIF, maximal inspiratory flow; FVC, forced vital capacity; MEF, maximal expiratory flow.

The patient may be placed prone or in a lateral position. These positioning techniques may place considerable stress on the patient's pulmonary system, and interventions to protect the airway may have to be implemented. These interventions may result in the need for sedation and protection of the airway resulting in risk levels similar to a surgical approach and GA. Prone positioning can place the hepatic flexure of the colon in close proximity to the targeted tumor site thereby making ablation difficult or even unsafe. There is no reliable way to predict this potential complication, and this is explained to the patient.

How does the patient's coexisting chronic alcohol use and liver cirrhosis affect the planned procedure? Should this patient be required to engage in an AA program before they are considered for transplant?

The patient is at risk for acute alcohol withdrawal syndrome (AWS). AWS may result in delirium and seizures.[8] Alcohol withdrawal is a serious medical complication, and efforts to prevent or minimize symptoms should be implemented. This patient is at high risk for AWS. One of the cornerstones of treatment of AWS is the administration of a benzodiazepine.[8] This may further compromise the patient's respiratory status. AWS affects people with a history of heavy alcohol use; as defined by the Center for Disease Control and Prevention, heavy drinking is 15 drinks per week for men and 8 drinks per week for females. Excessive drinking excites and irritates the central nervous system thus causing the body to be dependent on alcohol over a period of time. The neurotransmitters dopamine (DA/5HT) and gamma aminobutyric acid (GABA) and glutamine pathways are affected and suppressed by alcohol. When these neurotransmitters are no longer suppressed, they go into a state of overexcitement, thus causing the symptoms of AWS.[9,10] Some of the symptoms of AWS are agitation, anxiety, chest pain, confusion, delirium, excessive sweating, fever, hallucinations, and seizures. AWS can occur as early as 2 hours after the last drink, but frequently occurs 6–24 hours post drinking. Withdrawal seizures typically occur 24–48 hours after the last drink. This patient is at increased risk of AWS, and participation in a program that supports abstinence may be required if the patient wishes to proceed with the planned procedure.[5.]

As we all know, the demand for liver transplants far outweighs the supply of available organs, both living and cadaver donation. Many people believe that patients with alcoholic cirrhosis have caused their own illness, and this has led to controversy over whether patients with alcohol-related cirrhosis should be candidates for liver transplant.[9] To address this issue many hospitals have incorporated a 6-month alcohol abstinence criterion ("6-month rule") in an effort to select optimal candidates for recipients of a transplant. This 6-month rule serves two primary purposes: (1) it provides time for the liver to recover in absence of alcohol (perhaps even then avoiding the need for transplant), and (2) it allows time to observe the patient to verify that they remain alcohol free, thus reducing the risk of relapse. Everhart et al. determined that 85% of US liver transplant programs and 43% of third-party payers require a defined period of abstinence as part of the waiting list process.

The waters are still murky with respect to the abstinence criteria and selection of liver transplant recipients with a history of alcohol abuse.[9] Some studies have shown that roughly 20% of patients with a history of alcohol use disorder who have received a transplant engage in the use of alcohol after their surgery, with one-third of these patients engaging in repetitive or heavy drinking. A longer duration of abstinence is correlated inversely with the likelihood of relapse, but it does not predict relapse or recovery with 100% accuracy. Chronic stressors and everyday life stressors can cause the patient to be prone to relapse at any future time. Each case of an alcoholic liver cirrhotic patient being a candidate for liver transplant needs to be evaluated individually.

Are there any other options, other than adding or changing medications, that could help optimize this patient for surgery?

Several preoperative strategies could improve this patient's optimization status. Studies have shown that assessing a patient for frailty preoperatively and then prehabilitating that patient are associated with decreased postoperative complications and improved patient outcome.[10] Prehabilitation involves improving the patient's health status prior to the surgical procedure.

Frailty can be difficult to define. It may encompass physical conditions, psychological conditions, or both.[10] Frailty can be "a condition or syndrome which results from a multi-system reduction in reserve capacity to the extent that a number of physiological systems are close to, or past, the threshold of symptomatic clinical failure."[10] One major approach to classify a patient's frailty status is by using the Frailty Index.[10] The Frailty Index consists of 10 questions with a scoring system that can indicate no frailty, risk of frailty, or frank frailty (see Table 2.1). Frailty has been associated with adverse surgical outcomes including, but not limited to, an increase in postoperative complications, increase hospital length of stay, increased number of patients discharged to a skilled nursing

Table 2.1 **FRAILTY SCREENING TOOL**

ITEM	CIRCLE RESPONSE
1. Do you need help getting in or out of bed?	Yes No
2. Do you need help with washing or bathing?	Yes No
3. Without wanting to, have you lost or gained 10 pounds in the last six months?	Yes No
4. Do you have tooth or mouth problems that make it hard to eat?	Yes No
5. Do you have a poor appetite and quickly feel full when you eat?	Yes No
6. Did your physical health or emotional problems interfere with your social activities?	Yes No
7. Would you say your health is fair or poor?	Yes No
8. Do you get tired easily?	Yes No
9. Were you hospitalized in the last 3 months?	Yes No
10. Did you visit an emergency room for a health problem in the past 3 months?	Yes No

Scoring:

A score of 0 indicates no frailty

A score of 1–3 indicates frailty risk

A score of 4 or greater indicates frailty

From Tocchi C, Dixon J, Naylor M, Sangchoon J, McCorkle R. (2014). Development of a frailty index measure for older adults: The Frailty Index for Elders. *J Nurs Measure*. 2014;22(2):223–240, table 7.

facility, and increased mortality rates. Studies have shown that 42–50% of older patients undergoing elective cardiac and noncardiac surgery are frail. The risk of anesthesia-related complications and death is markedly elevated in patients older than 55–64 years, with the highest incidence in patients older than 85 years.[10]

The frailty status of a patient can be improved by influencing modifiable conditions. Nutrition has been shown to play a strong role in frailty modification. Treatment of anemia, resolution of vitamin D deficiency, and protein supplementation to improve sarcopenia have all been shown to affect the frailty index. Preoperative home interventions such as respiratory and muscle strengthening, in addition to relaxation techniques, have been shown to decrease frailty. Instruction in the use of incentive spirometry preoperatively not only decreases the incidence of postoperative pulmonary complications, but it also improves muscle strength, thus further decreasing frailty status as well. The ideal exercise program to decrease frailty index scores has not yet been defined but programs that incorporate exercise 3 times per week using 30- to 45-minute sessions have reported improved postoperative outcomes.

Adopting frailty screening as part of the preoperative evaluation done by the PSH and then implementing a program to decrease a patient's frailty index will most likely be a set of successful, cost effective maneuvers that will be in the best interest of the patient and thus fit precisely into the "triple aim."[11]

What is the role of the PSH for intraoperative and postoperative periods?

The footprint of the PSH continues into the intraoperative and postoperative periods. This is seen in the already mentioned prevention of delay or cancellation of the operative case on the day of surgery. In addition, because elements of the evidence-based clinical pathways are executed, this enables the PSH to measure outcomes and compare those outcomes to national benchmarking data. For example, assigning dedicated personnel to specific cases, standardization of instruments and supplies to decrease variability, and adhering to evidence-based postoperative care plans all lead to the successful endpoint of improving patient care and decreasing hospital costs.[10]

Results from a number of published studies illustrate the positive outcomes related to the implementation of a PSH program. For example, Kaiser Permanente at Baldwin Park Medical Center compared outcomes between 518 patients treated over an 8-month period using a PSH care model and 546 patients cared for using the hospital's traditional model for total knee arthroplasty.[12] The data indicated that the PSH group had shorter hospital length of stay, fewer skilled nursing facility (SNF) admissions, and lower costs of care. All these metrics were achieved without any compromise in the quality of care or reports of decreased patient satisfaction. In addition, Ochsner Hospital in Maryland instituted a PSH program for patients having primary total hip arthroplasty (THA).[13] Their results showed more than a full day decrease in the hospital length of stay of patients in the PSH program. Furthermore, Ochsner Hospital showed that, before the implementation of the PSH, 27% of their THA patients transitioned to a SNF and only 5% were able to be discharged to home care. With the PSH program in place only 17% of patients were discharged to a SNF, while 14% were able to manage home self-care.

What are the fiscal concerns about the implementation of the PSH versus the traditional model; in particular what is the current reimbursements system for PSH healthcare visits?

Fiscal concerns regarding the implementation of a PSH relate to the challenges of demonstrating financial savings or benefits in providing preoperative care in a nontraditional setting.[2] Current reimbursement systems are complex, and billing for the PSH visit has not been universally incorporated. While some services may be rolled into the actual surgical bundle, specific complex activities may be billed separately. Counseling and referral to smoking cessation programs, screening for OSA and other conditions may also be billed. The cost saving of an effective PSH is difficult to determine until retrospective data are examined to evaluate the savings related to lower number of case cancellations on the day of surgery, reduced length of stay for patients who are optimized prior to surgery,[14] and cost savings from standardization of surgical and operative supplies.

What are some of the key steps and who are the stakeholders in starting a PSH in your facility? Are any nonmedical personnel important to have on board?

The triple aim includes improving patient outcomes, increasing patient satisfaction, and decreasing hospital costs.[1] Setting up a PSH requires an investment in physical and human resources. One of the methods that has worked well in implementing successful PSHs is the use of co-management agreements between physicians and the hospital.[14] Co-management agreements are contractual arrangements by which hospitals engage independent or employed physician groups to manage one or more service lines and their quality aspects. The co-management agreements can be used to enable anesthesiologist and surgeons to participate together in service line-specific as well as OR-wide PSH initiatives. Standardizing intraoperative care and the development of evidence-based clinical pathways produces a tremendous amount of savings to the hospital with respect to decreasing expenses for multiple variations of a supply that can be uniformly used. In addition, purchasing large quantities of one specific item provides greater negotiating power for the hospital with vendors. Moreover, a patient who is evaluated in the PSH well before the date of the procedure can benefit from prehabilitation and medical optimization, thus resulting in more and greater savings to the hospital. There are significant savings to the hospital with respect to reductions in case cancellations, delays on the day of surgery, decreased length of stay, decreased complication rates, decreased readmissions, lower numbers of patients discharged to SNF, and, of course, decreased supply costs due to process standardization. Additionally, decreased turnover time between cases and increased first case on-time starts (due to all information needed for the patient being available and not having to wait for an office to open at 8:00 AM to retrieve the results of an evaluation) add up to tremendous savings.

Anesthesiologists as physicians with specific expertise in the perioperative environment must remain relevant to and valued by the patient, surgeons, and healthcare facility. The PSH model allows the anesthesiologist to demonstrate our value throughout the entire continuum of the perioperative process. Increased anesthesiologist involvement evolves into increased surgery efficiencies, increased team participation, better outcomes, and increased patient and family satisfaction.

It is essential when establishing a successful PSH to engage the healthcare executives outside of the perioperative environment. The PSH cannot be successful without endorsement and support from the hospital's executives or the chiefs of various service lines and surgical specialties, often referred to as the "C-suite." When proposing the concept of a PSH, it is beneficial to present a business plan that reflects a return on investment (metrics such as decreased length of hospital stay and decreased complication rates) as well as softer gains such as patient satisfaction. Patient satisfaction is an important metric to follow because it has an impact on reimbursement and referral patterns. The healthcare system has turned from a volume-based payment plan to a value-based payment plan, and this needs to be presented to the healthcare executives to achieve not only their endorsement but financial support as well. Presenting the differences between a traditional preoperative process and a PSH model will help key stakeholders to conceptualize the advantages of a streamlined PSH process (see Figure 2.2).

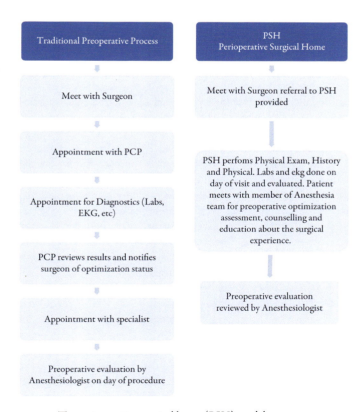

Figure 2.2 The perioperative surgical home (PSH) model.

DISCUSSION

The preoperative team of the PSH is the center of the wheel with respect to evaluating the patient for surgery and ensuring medical optimization of the patient prior to the proposed procedure, as well as providing counseling and education to the patient and caregiver with respect to the surgical procedure. Having a preoperative control center enables the team to request data, such as laboratory work, diagnostic testing, or medical specialty consults and then gather and analyze that data. This ensures that the patient is optimized for the day of surgery and also avoids redundancy of laboratory and diagnostic studies performed by different providers who are not connected through the PSH. In addition, the preparation of the patient by the preoperative team at the PSH enables all data to be present for and easily accessible by the team taking care of the patient on the operative day, thus preventing costly delays of case start time on the day of surgery or the even more costly cancellation of case on day of surgery. Furthermore, elements of evidence-based clinical pathways, such as preoperative carbohydrate loading, correction of iron deficiency anemia, use of incentive spirometer by patient prior to day of surgery, and prehabilitation are initiated by the preoperative PSH team.[15] The process of the PSH from the patient's perspective may be perceived as utopia or bureaucracy. Identifying those elements of the PSH model that, from the patient's perspective, reflect utopia rather than bureaucracy is essential to understanding the differences between the traditional model, a well-managed PSH, and a poorly organized PSH model (see Figure 2.2). Let us look how these different scenarios can play out.

ANTICOAGULATION

Patient's Cardiac Evaluation

Patient's PSH Perspective: Bureaucracy. The patient schedules appointments with the cardiologist, pulmonologist, and their primary care provider. The patient is seen by the individual providers. However, the information is sent individually by each provider to the surgeon and PSH. The cardiologist is concerned about decreasing the risk for a cerebrovascular event related to the discontinuation of novel oral anticoagulant (NOAC) medication. The cardiologist is also concerned about the perioperative management of the patient's implanted cardiac device. The patient is given conflicting directions regarding discontinuing his NOAC by the surgeon, the PSH anesthesiologist, and the cardiologist. The cardiologist recommends discontinuation of the NOAC 48 hours prior to the date of surgery because these are the manufacturer's recommendations and the cardiologist believes that a shorter discontinuation period of apixaban minimizes the risk to the patient. The surgeon recommends discontinuing NOAC 5 days prior to the procedure because of the high risk for bleeding. The PSH anesthesiologist recommends discontinuing the NOAC 72 hours prior to the procedure due to the potential vascular puncture during placement for neuraxial anesthetic and the serious potential complication of an epidural hematoma. The patient is completely confused and quite frankly second-guessing the capability and coordinating efforts of this "team."

Patient's PSH Perspective: Utopia. During the PSH visit, the anesthesiologist directs the PSH staff to schedule appointments for the patient with providers from cardiology, pulmonology, and primary care. The PSH anesthesiologist communicates with all the providers that the patient is scheduled to have a high-risk procedure and the PSH physician will be coordinating the perioperative optimization.

The PSH anesthesiologist receives all the consultations and, after an extensive review, determines that the patient has received conflicting directions and recommendations from each provider. The PSH anesthesiologist arranges a conference call with the providers to resolve the conflicts. The team discusses the case during the conference call, and the recommendations are discussed and aligned into one consistent plan. The plan will be for the patient to discontinue apixaban 72 hours prior to procedure and to resume anticoagulation with low-molecular-weight heparin (LMWH) after the procedure. This plan is communicated directly to the patient by the PSH team. Verbal and written instructions are provided to the patient and his caregiver.

Patient's Pulmonary Evaluation

Patient's PSH Perspective: Bureaucracy: The patient schedules an appointment with the pulmonologist and is evaluated. An additional appointment is scheduled to perform specific pulmonary diagnostic tests to evaluate the patient's pulmonary optimization status. Pulmonary function tests (PFTs) and a sleep study are performed.

The patient is informed by the treating pulmonologist that there is a high risk of pulmonary complications if the patient proceeds with the planned procedure under GA. The patient is informed that there is a risk of pulmonary collapse or decompensation during the procedure which may result in prolonged or permanent mechanical ventilation and/or death. The pulmonologist encourages the patient to return to the surgeon and discuss this elevated risk for the upcoming procedure. The pulmonologist sends reports to the surgeon and the PSH anesthesiologist.

As a result of all these consults and differing results and opinions obtained at the request of PSH, the patient is left confused, frightened, and hopeless. The patient verbalizes that he feels that although there are many providers involved in his case, the care is fragmented and there is no single provider coordinating his care for the planned procedure.

Patient's PSH Perspective: Utopia. The pulmonary evaluation and the results of the pulmonary diagnostics (PFTs and sleep study) are sent to the PSH anesthesiologist and the surgeon. Discussion occurs between the PSH team and the surgeon. Due to the potential high risk of pulmonary failure postoperatively for this patient, the PSH team suggests involving an interventional radiologist in the planning of care for this patient. The surgeon concurs, and an intradisciplinary team meeting takes place. The PSH team includes an RN case coordinator in addition to the anesthesiologist and other team members. After careful review the team decides that the best and safest approach would be a percutaneous thermal tumor ablation performed with local anesthetic and minimal sedation in the IR suite. The PSH team arranges for the RN case coordinator to go to the patient's home to set up a video conference with the patient, his caregiver, and the respective physician team members. Telemedicine is emerging as an essential part of patient care and management in our present age of technology and is frequently implemented by this PSH team. The PSH coordinates a time that works for all stakeholders in the process. During the video conference the patient and the team members discuss the risks related to the strong possibility of postoperative mechanical ventilation, postoperative pneumonia, increased risk of tracheostomy, and other negative outcomes if a laparoscopic hepatectomy is performed. Ultimately the patient elects to proceed with an evaluation by IR to address less invasive tumor therapy.

Patient's Interventional Radiology Evaluation

Patient's PSH Perspective: Bureaucracy. The patient is instructed by the PSH to schedule an appointment with IR. The patient does not have a clear understanding of what the radiology options are, thereby creating confusion at the time of his phone call to schedule an appointment. The clerk scheduling appointments for radiology does not know what area of the radiology department the patient requires for further evaluation (i.e., CT imaging, MRI, IR, flat plate). The patient's experience while attempting to schedule the appointment with the radiology department is frustrating. During the initial call the patient is placed on hold for an extended period and then told that a staff member will return his call with the appointment information. A number of days go by before the patient is scheduled for an appointment with the interventional radiologist. Ultimately, the patient is contacted by the IR department and is scheduled for an evaluation with an attending interventional radiologist. The patient is seen and evaluated by the interventional radiologist who informs the patient that a thermal ablation is an option, but the positioning required for the procedure could lead to respiratory complications. The interventional radiologist recommends that an anesthesiologist be on standby in case the procedure cannot be performed with moderate sedation. The patient is again informed of the increased risks related to the procedure. The recommendations of the interventional radiologist are sent to the PSH department who again contact the surgeon to discuss the case. However, the patient is now reluctant to proceed with any intervention and is exhausted by the preoperative process and the additional testing.

Patient's PSH Perspective: Utopia. Following the video conference between the patient and the PSH team, the PSH administrative assistant schedules the patient for an evaluation with the attending interventional radiologist. All relevant records are provided to the attending interventional radiologist. The patient and his caregiver arrive for the appointment and are surprised to find that the interventional radiologist is already extremely familiar and knowledgeable about the patient's case and is fully aware of the evaluations and studies that have taken place prior to this appointment.

The interventional radiologist discusses possible therapeutic modalities for the patient, including percutaneous thermal tumor ablation under CT guidance. If this approach is deemed reasonable by the team and the patient, then only one course of therapy will be needed. However, the patient's tumor is exophytic and thus a small amount of adjacent kidney would also need to be ablated to ensure clear tumor margins. In addition, placing the patient in the prone position can cause the hepatic flexure of the colon to move adjacent to the targeted tumor site, thus making the ablation difficult or unsafe. An option that would then be available would be chemoembolization of the tumor with a subsequent limited ablation as needed. However, before any of these procedures are further explored, updated imaging would need to be done as well as a discussion of the case at the institution's interdisciplinary tumor conference. The PSH arranges for a follow-up video conference with the patient and the team to discuss decision-making.

Patient's Primary Care Evaluation

Patient's PSH Perspective: Bureaucracy. While at the primary care office a healthcare professional has noticed that the patient has weak hand grip, struggles to get out of their chair, and has temporal wasting. The healthcare provider gives the patient an incentive spirometer (IS) and instructs the patient to read the pamphlet inside on how to use the device; she tells the patient to incorporate the device into his everyday life preoperatively. In addition, the patient is told to exercise and eat a healthier diet. The patient and his caregiver return home and have great difficulty understanding the instructions about the use of the IS and argue about what type of "exercise" the patient should engage in, how long to exercise, and how frequently. Finally, there is great disagreement as to what "eating healthier" means, and both the patient and their caregiver are frustrated, exhausted, and confused yet again.

Patient's PSH Perspective: Utopia. During the PSH visit, the team notices the weak hand grip of the patient, the difficulty the patient has in both achieving a sitting position in the chair as well as difficulty in getting up from chair. The team also inquires if the patient has experienced any recent weight loss. Furthermore, the patient is asked what he typically eats on a given day. After collecting and analyzing the data the PSH team performs a frailty screening. It is clear from the screening that the patient is in frail condition. The patient is given an IS to take home. The staff explains the benefits of using the IS both preoperatively and postoperatively to the patient. The patient is shown how to use the IS and is asked to demonstrate to the PSH staff that he can correctly use the device. The patient is shown a series of gentle home exercises to perform and is given an illustrated and easy to follow brochure with the stated exercises. The patient is taught how often the exercises should be performed throughout the week and well as a targeted time span to perform the exercises. After assessing the patient's daily diet, the importance of nutrition preoperatively to optimize the patient's condition is discussed with the patient. The patient is discharged with protein shakes to be added to his diet as well as a diet brochure indicating foods that are rich in iron, fiber, and protein. The patient and his caregiver are eager to engage in a healthier lifestyle which will be extremely beneficial to the patient as he continues through the perioperative process.

CONCLUSION

- The PHS is a system for coordinating and organizing medical care that is patient-centered, physician-led, and team-based. The care from the PSH team extends throughout the perioperative period and is focused on what is known as the "triple aim" of increased patient satisfaction, improved patient outcome, and decreased hospital costs.

- The communication, commitment, and consistency of PSH team members with respect to the management of the perioperative period strongly impacts how the PSH is perceived by the patient and their caregivers.

- Using evidence-based clinical pathways and standardizing surgical supplies has a strong impact on the cost savings to the hospital with respect to decreasing length of stay, complication rates, and the number of patient admissions to SNFs. These factors are important to relay to the hospital executives who are not caregivers in the perioperative period, but whose support is essential to creating a successful PSH.

- The PSH model is an emerging and growing paradigm in a healthcare system that is struggling to achieve optimal outcomes while controlling costs.

- Anesthesiologists as leaders in this new paradigm will continue to provide expert care through their specialized medical management abilities and broad knowledge of physiology, pharmacology, and medicine relative to other caregivers. The PSH with an anesthesiologist leader will be relevant and involved in the entire perioperative event from the decision to have surgery to the postoperative management of the patient. Finally, not only is it important for anesthesiologists to maintain a broad depth of current medical knowledge but they also must proactively connect to new technologies and utilize new and different options to communicate and treat patients in a complex and evolving healthcare system. The PSH model is an ideal environment for the use of innovative practices such as telemedicine and virtual visits.

REVIEW QUESTIONS

1. The benefit of pulmonary function tests is directed to which of the triple aims?

    a. Decreasing cost.
    b. Decreasing length of stay.
    c. Improving patient outcomes.
    d. All of the above.

The correct answer is d.

Airflow and lung volume measurements are used to help differentiate between obstructive versus restrictive pulmonary disorders, characterize severity, and measure responses to therapy.[16] Most common respiratory disorders can be categorized as obstructive versus restrictive based on airflow and lung volumes. Please see Figure 2.1 for examples and detailed descriptions of flow volume loops and pulmonary disorders. In general, obstructive disorders are characterized by a reduction in airflow, particularly the forced expiratory volume in one second (FEV_1), and the FEV_1 expressed as a percentage of the forced vital capacity (FVC). The degree of reduction in FEV_1 compared with predicted values determines the degree of the obstructive disease.

2. What are the medical conditions where an obstructive pulmonary pattern is observed? Select all that apply.

a. Emphysema.
b. Asthma.
c. Pulmonary fibrosis.
d. Reactive airway disease.

The correct answers are a and c.

Increased resistance to airflow due to abnormalities within the airway lumen can be related to tumors, secretions, or mucosal thickening. An obstructive pulmonary pattern may also be seen when there are changes in the walls of the airway related to the contraction of smooth muscle and edema. In addition, an obstructive pulmonary pattern may be observed in patients who have decreased pulmonary elastic recoil such as emphysema. When there is decreased airflow, we see a longer than usual expiratory time and the air may become trapped due to incomplete emptying, leading to an increase in lung volumes.

3. What pulmonary test results are abnormal in restrictive pulmonary disease?

a. Pulse oximetry.
b. Chest radiography.
c. Flow volume loop.
d. Lung volumes and capacities.

The correct answer is d.

Restrictive diseases are characterized by a reduction in lung volume, in particular a total lung capacity (TLC) of less than 80% of the predicted value. The decrease in the TLC determines the severity of the restriction. The decrease in volumes causes a decrease in airflow. Because the airflow relative to lung volume is increased, the FEV_1/FVC ratio can be normal or even increased.

4. A patient with multiple comorbidities in two body systems that are well managed and stable is classified according to the ASA classification as

a. ASA I.
b. ASA II.
c. ASA III.
d. ASA IV.

The correct answer is b.

The patient is evaluated using the ASA risk stratification.[3] ASA risk stratification attempts to predict the relative risk for a patient. A healthy patient with no comorbidities is classified as an ASA 1. A patient with well-managed medical problems of at least two body systems is classified as an ASA II. ASA III patients have major diseases of two or more body systems that are stable and well-controlled. The patient in our example is classified as an ASA IV based on his multiple comorbidities. ASA IV patients have multiple medical problems that are either not stable or controlled or at end stage. ASA IV indicates an elevated risk of perioperative complications, including death.[3]

5. What is the triple aim?

a. Accountability, fiscal responsibility, and safety.
b. Safety, satisfaction, and accountability.
c. Safety, cost-savings, and physician engagement.
d. Patient outcome, patient satisfaction, and decreasing hospital costs.

The correct answer is d.

The triple aim is improving patient outcome, increasing patient satisfaction, and decreasing hospital costs.[11]

6. Who are key stakeholders in the development and implementation of a PSH?

a. Patient and physicians.
b. Nurses and support personnel.
c. Administrators.
d. All of the above.

The correct answer is d.

It is essential for the successful implementation of a PSH to engage administration leadership, physicians, nursing, and support personnel as well as patients.[14]

7. What are priority considerations for decreasing costs associated with the perioperative environment?

a. Standardization.
b. Surgeon preference.
c. Cost.
d. Increased variability.

The correct answer is a.

Standardization of materials and processes is essential for cost savings.

8. The decision to place a patient on the liver transplant list is influenced by what factors?

a. Patient request.
b. Patient health status.
c. Estimated life expectancy.
d. Availability of a compatible liver.

The correct answer is b.

The decision to place a patient on the liver transplant list is multifactorial, but the patient's overall health status is the most significant factor to consider.

9. Which index is a sensitive predictor of postoperative outcomes?

   a. ASA classification.
   b. Surgical risk classification.
   c. Frailty Index.
   d. Wellness Index.

The correct answer is c.

Frailty has been associated with an adverse surgical outcome, including but not limited to increased postoperative complications, increased hospital length of stay, increased discharge to skilled nursing facility, and increased mortality.

10. When will the patient will need to have his ICD interrogated or evaluated?

    a. Immediately before surgery.
    b. During surgery.
    c. Immediately after surgery.
    d. Within 30 days after surgery.

The correct answer is d.

The Heart Rhythm Society (HRS)/American Society of Anesthesiologist (ASA) issued a consensus statement stating that most patients with an ICD do not need a new preoperative evaluation of the ICD due to the fact that most ICDs undergo a telephone interrogation every few months and well as yearly evaluations by a physician.[5] However, it is recommended that the device be interrogated within 30 days postoperatively if electrocautery was used during the case.

REFERENCES

1. Vetter TR, Goeddel LA, Boudreaux AM, Hunt TR, Jones KA, Pittet J. The perioperative surgical home: How can it make the case so everyone wins? *BMC Anesthesiol.* 2013;13:6–6. doi:10.1186/1471-2253-13-6
2. Raphael DR, Cannesson M, Rinehart J, Kain ZN. Health care costs and the perioperative surgical home: A survey study. *Anesth Analg.* 2015;121(5):1344–1349. doi:10.1213/ANE.0000000000000876
3. ASA physical status classification system. https://www.asahq.org/standards-and-guidelines/statement-on-asa-physical-status-classification-system
4. Mercer M. Anaesthesia for the patient with respiratory disease. *Update Anaesthesia.* 2000;12:51–58. https://resources.wfsahq.org/wp-content/uploads/uia-12-ANAESTHESIA-FOR-THE-PATIENT-WITH-RESPIRATORY-DISEASE.pdf
5. Neelankavil JP, Thompson A, Mahajan A. Managing cardiovascular implantable electronic devices (CIEDs) during perioperative care. *Anesth Patient Safety Foundation.* 2013;28(2):29,32–35. https://www.apsf.org/article/managing-cardiovascular-implantable-electronic-devices-cieds-during-perioperative-care/
6. Mathangi K, Mathews J, Mathangi CD. Assessment of perioperative difficult airway among undiagnosed obstructive sleep apnoea patients undergoing elective surgery: A prospective cohort study. *Indian J Anaesth.* 2018;62(7):538–544. doi:10.4103/ija.IJA_158_18
7. Abdelaziz AO, Abdelmaksoud AH, Nabeel MM, et al. Transarterial chemoembolization combined with either radiofrequency or microwave ablation in management of hepatocellular carcinoma. *Asian Pac J Cancer Prev.* 2017;18(1):189–194. doi:10.22034/APJCP.2017.18.1.189
8. Healthline. Alcohol withdrawal delirium: Causes, symptoms, and treatment. https://www.healthline.com/health/alcoholism/delirium-tremens. Updated 2016.
9. Bramstedt KA, Jabbour N. When alcohol abstinence criteria create ethical dilemmas for the liver transplant team. *J Med Ethics.* 2006;32(5):263–265. doi:10.1136/jme.2005.012856
10. Robinson TN, Wu DS, Pointer L, Dunn CL, Cleveland JCJ, Moss M. Simple frailty score predicts postoperative complications across surgical specialties. *Am J Surg.* 2013;206(4):544–550. doi:10.1016/j.amjsurg.2013.03.012
11. Kwon MA. Perioperative surgical home: A new scope for future anesthesiology. *Korean J Anesthesiol.* 2018;71(3):175–181. doi:10.4097/kja.d.18.27182
12. Qiu C, Cannesson M, Morkos A, et al. Practice and outcomes of the perioperative surgical home in a California integrated delivery system. *Anesth Analg.* 2016;123(3):597–606. doi:10.1213/ANE.0000000000001370
13. Vetter TR, Barman J, Hunter JMJ, Jones KA, Pittet J. The effect of implementation of preoperative and postoperative care elements of a perioperative surgical home model on outcomes in patients undergoing hip arthroplasty or knee arthroplasty. *Anesth Analg.* 2017;124(5):1450–1458. doi:10.1213/ANE.0000000000001743
14. Szokol JW, Chamberlin KJ. Value proposition and anesthesiology. *Anesthesiol Clin.* 2018;36(2):227–239. doi:10.1016/j.anclin.2018.02.001
15. Cannesson M, Mahajan A. Vertical and horizontal pathways: Intersection and integration of enhanced recovery after surgery and the perioperative surgical home. *Anesth Analg.* 2018;127(5):1275–1277. doi:10.1213/ANE.0000000000003506
16. Merck. Overview of tests of pulmonary function: Pulmonary disorders. Merck Manuals Professional Edition Web site. https://www.merckmanuals.com/professional/pulmonary-disorders/tests-of-pulmonary-function-pft/overview-of-tests-of-pulmonary-function

3.

CHOOSING WISELY

HOW TO ADVISE THE PATIENT ON PREOPERATIVE TESTING

Jay S. Kersh and BobbieJean Sweitzer

STEM CASE AND KEY QUESTIONS

A 71-year-old woman presents to the preoperative clinic. Six days earlier, she had a transvaginal ultrasound for dysfunctional uterine bleeding (DUB) which revealed an enlarged uterus with a thickened endometrial stripe. A hysteroscopy with endometrial biopsy was performed the next day, and it was negative for endometrial adenocarcinoma. The patient is scheduled for a total abdominal hysterectomy with possible lymph node dissection in 7 days. The only medical history the patient reports is a 70 pack-year smoking history and hypertension, for which she takes amlodipine.

The patient states that a friend took her to an urgent care clinic 5 weeks ago after 3 days of a "bad" cough, shortness of breath, and fatigue. She remembers that some tests were done, and blood was drawn during the visit, but she does not remember the results. She recalls being told that she had bronchitis and was given antibiotics along with an inhaler. She was sent home with instructions to return if there was no improvement or to go to an emergency department if her condition were to worsen.

What organ systems are of particular importance in this patient anticipating surgery?

Given her recent lower respiratory infection, advanced age, long-standing hypertension, and tobacco use, the patient deserves careful consideration of her cardiovascular, pulmonary, renal, and musculoskeletal systems during the history-taking and physical examination. Auscultation of heart and lungs and measurement of vital signs, as well as an examination of her airway and extremities and a calculation of BMI are all indicated.

What additional questions for the patient are important?

The patient is an elderly, hypertensive tobacco user scheduled for an elevated-risk surgery. One needs to explore details about her history of shortness of breath including duration, relation to activity or deep breathing, history of lung disease, associated chest pressure or tightness, leg swelling, lightheadedness, occupational and environmental exposures, general fatigue, or anxiety. Careful questioning should also reveal the patient's current functional capacity and changes over the past year.

Upon questioning the patient, it is learned that she has become increasingly breathless with progressive limitation of activities for the past several months. She has a cough that is productive of thick, white sputum for several months prior to the urgent care visit. Currently she denies fever or chills. The patient does not report chest pressure or tightness, peripheral edema, or lightheadedness.

What should the examination focus on for this patient?

On examination, the patient appears tired. She is breathing rapidly and using accessory muscles. Vitals signs are: temperature 36.7°C, heart rate 96 beats/minute, BP 158/91 mm Hg, respiratory rate 21 breaths/min, oxygen saturation (SpO$_2$) 92%. She is 5'11" and weighs 58 kg, corresponding to a BMI of 18.4 kg/m^2. Distant breath sounds with mild expiratory wheezing are auscultated bilaterally. Heart sounds are irregularly irregular, and a mid-systolic murmur is auscultated over the right upper sternal border. There is no radiation of the murmur, and no peripheral edema, clubbing, or cyanosis of the extremities.

How should the patient's shortness of breath be evaluated?

An evaluation for dyspnea includes consideration of pulmonary, cardiac, infectious, and metabolic origins (Figure 3.1). The patient has a long history of tobacco use, a chronic productive cough, and a recent lower tract respiratory infection. Given her abnormal oxygen saturation and labored breathing, the patient needs additional testing. She states that she was recently treated for bronchitis as an outpatient. There is no information available from that encounter, so a new evaluation must be initiated.

The patient already had a chest radiograph at the urgent care clinic. Should it be repeated since the results are not available?

This patient warrants follow-up chest radiography. In patients with a lower respiratory infection, such as acute bronchitis or pneumonia, 6-week follow-up chest radiography is indicated if (1) symptoms persist despite appropriate treatment or (2) the patient is older than 50 years with a significant smoking history.[2] A repeat chest radiograph may identify a lung malignancy. Repeat chest radiography shows bilateral hyperinflated lung fields and flattened hemi-diaphragms, without signs of an infiltrate or mass.

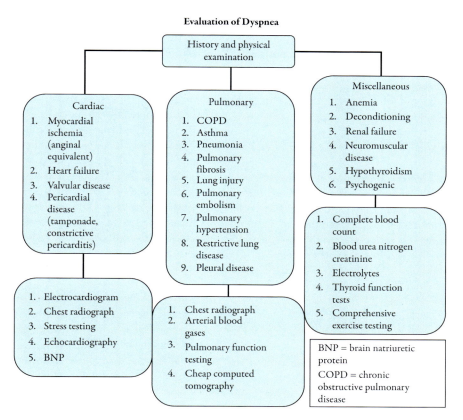

Figure 3.1 Dyspnea workup.
From Sweitzer, BJ. *Preoperative Assessment and Management*. 3rd ed. Wolters-Kluwer; 2018.

What additional evaluation can be done in the preoperative clinic to assess the patient's dyspnea, hypoxia, and risk of pending surgery?

Another useful, noninvasive assessment is determination of the 6-minute walk test (6MWT). It is performed by having the patient walk as far as possible on level ground in 6 minutes. This test is not to be performed on patients who have had unstable angina or a myocardial infarction within the past month. It also should not be performed if the patient's heart rate is greater than 120 beats/minute, systolic BP is greater than 180 mm Hg, or diastolic BP is greater than 100 mm Hg. The test is to be immediately discontinued for chest pain, intolerable dyspnea, leg cramps, staggering, diaphoresis, or pale or ashen appearance. This test can provoke or worsen hypoxemia with exertion. The test is not diagnostic for any heart or lung disease process. Oxygen saturation (SpO_2) should be measured both before and after the walk.

For healthy 55- to 75-year-olds, 659 meters is considered the attainable average distance, with 484–820 meters (m) as the reference range.[3] For all age groups, 6MWT minima are calculated using the following sex-specific equations[4]:

$$Men: 6MWT = (7.57 \times height\ in\ cm) - (5.02 \times age) - (1.76 \times weight\ in\ kg) - 309m$$

*The lower limit of normal is determined by subtracting 153 m.

$$Women: 6MWT = (2.11 \times height\ in\ cm) - (2.29 \times weight\ in\ kg) - (5.78 \times age) + 667\ m$$

*The lower limit of normal is determined by subtracting 139 m.

There is evidence that 325 m of walking distance serves as the threshold for predicting postoperative pulmonary complications (PPC) with 77% sensitivity and 100% specificity, similar to the positive predictive value of a forced expiratory volume in 1 second (FEV_1).[5]

This patient was able to walk 317 m, which is below her calculated prediction of 601 m. Her SpO_2, which began at 94%, dropped to 83% when measured at the completion of her 6MWT. After resting for 2 minutes, the patient's SpO_2 rose to 93%. Improving cardiopulmonary function can potentially lower the risk of PPC, but there is little time to do so for this patient, given the time-sensitive nature of the planned surgery.

Should the patient be referred for pulmonary function testing (PFT) before surgery?

A presumptive diagnosis of obstructive lung disease can be made based on this patient's age, history of tobacco use, and dyspnea at rest. Findings on physical examination of wheezing and hyperresonant lung sounds, along with the chest radiographic findings of overinflation and flattened diaphragms increase the pretest probability of obstructive lung disease, which includes asthma, chronic bronchitis, and chronic obstructive pulmonary disease (COPD). However, a definitive diagnosis of COPD can only be obtained after undergoing spirometric PFT, which has not been shown to reliably predict PPC. Since PFT has not been shown to predict PPC for non-lung resection surgery, PFT is not indicated for this patient before her scheduled surgery.

What additional testing should be performed to evaluate this patient?

Additional testing should be considered based on the patient's symptomatology, physical examination findings, the likelihood of disease, and the anticipated procedure. The data gathered from the history and physical examination suggest that the patient's shortness of breath is caused by a pulmonary process. COPD is highly likely. However, other diagnoses to consider include heart failure (HF), ischemic heart disease, anemia, hypothyroidism, valvular heart disease, and chronic kidney disease (CKD).

What additional testing should be performed to evaluate this patient's irregularly irregular HR?

The American College of Cardiology/American Heart Association (ACC/AHA) guidelines for cardiac evaluation for noncardiac surgery recommend ECG if an arrhythmia is suspected.[7] The patient's ECG showed atrial fibrillation (AF) without other abnormalities. Additional testing for AF includes thyroid function tests, complete blood count (CBC), serum electrolytes, and echocardiography. These tests can be arranged for by the preoperative clinic. The patient will be referred to a cardiologist for management of her AF, which includes rate control in the short term. Longer-term management includes possible rhythm control and anticoagulation.

The patient's electrolyte and thyroid-stimulating hormone concentrations were normal The CBC revealed a white blood cell count of 9,600/μL, a hemoglobin (Hb) of 10.5 g/dL, a hematocrit (Hct) of 31.5%, and a platelet count of 643,000/μL. Serum electrolytes were normal, and serum bicarbonate was 28 mEq/L. Blood urea nitrogen and creatinine were normal.

Does this patient's anemia need further evaluation?

The most likely etiology of her anemia is her DUB, and the most likely type of anemia is iron deficiency anemia (IDA). Iron studies are indicated. Preoperative iron deficiency is associated with increased morbidity and mortality, especially in older patients. The patient's serum iron is 58 mcg/dL, transferrin saturation (T_{SAT}) is 7%, and ferritin is 203 ng/dL. Her erythrocytes are noted to be hypochromic and small. A ferritin of less than 30 ng/dL and a T_{SAT} of less than 20% is diagnostic for IDA. However, in the setting of chronic disease, especially an inflammatory condition such as this patient's chronic bronchitis and possible malignancy, her ferritin can be falsely elevated, even with IDA. Therefore, the T_{SAT} of 7% is consistent with IDA. This patient will benefit from IV iron therapy before surgery.

Should blood typing and an antibody screen (T&S) be performed?

Appropriate preparation for availability of blood products is an important part of the preoperative process. The patient's preoperative Hb concentration, along with the procedure's anticipated blood loss, predicts the need for intra- or postoperative transfusions. The recommendations for preoperative ordering of blood typing, screening for antibodies, and cross-matching of blood are typically tabulated in an institution-specific maximum surgical blood ordering schedule (MSBOS)[6] (Figure 3.2). The MSBOS helps to optimize pretransfusion testing and reduce unnecessary or inadequate blood testing. This patient has DUB and IDA. The planned surgery has the potential for significant blood loss. If the patient continues to have uterine bleeding, even appropriate preoperative IV iron repletion may not correct her anemia. There is a role for tranexamic acid to reduce bleeding, and this needs to be discussed with the gynecologist. A T&S is indicated for this patient.

How should the patient's murmur be evaluated?

This patient has a previously undefined murmur in the setting of dyspnea. The cause(s) of her dyspnea has not yet been established. The character of this murmur, low-pitched and mid-systolic, in an older patient increases the likelihood that the aortic valve is the source of her murmur. Echocardiography is recommended to evaluate this murmur in the setting of dyspnea. Secondarily, given her history of AF, a cardiac thrombus must be ruled out. An assessment of systolic and diastolic function and evaluation for structural abnormalities are indicated to further evaluate her dyspnea, murmur and AF.[7]

Transthoracic echocardiography reveals a left ventricular ejection fraction of 61%. Her aortic valve has three moderately calcified leaflets, but velocities across the valve and the valve orifice are normal. The left atrium is moderately dilated, and there is evidence of mild pulmonary hypertension. All other valves are structurally and functionally normal, and the right ventricular systolic function is normal. There is no thrombus. The patient should be counseled to avoid calcium supplements, which can lead to an acceleration of aortic stenosis (AS) in the setting of a calcified valve.

What is the best way to assess the patient's perioperative risk for major adverse cardiovascular events (MACE)?

The risk stratification process for perioperative MACE can be facilitated by using a risk assessment tool such as the Revised Cardiac Risk Index (RCRI), or a calculator such as the Gupta Perioperative Cardiac Risk Calculator for Myocardial Infarction or Cardiac Arrest (MICA) or the National Surgical Quality Improvement Project (NSQIP) risk assessment tool.

Using the RCRI, or an online calculator, such as MICA or NSQIP, one can determine a patient's risk of MACE. Table 3.1 provides the components of the RCRI, which can be translated to a percentage risk of MACE. The patient has one RCRI risk factor, a high-risk surgery, which translates to a MACE risk of 0.9%. By comparison, the patient's MACE risk according to MICA is 0.7% and is 0.5% according to NSQIP. There is discordance 29% of the time among RCRI, MICA, and NSQIP calculators when determining MACE.[8] MICA and NSQIP appear to be more accurate than the RCRI. For

SURGICAL BLOOD ORDER SCHEDULE

Cardiac Surgery

Case Category	Rec
Heart or lung transplant	T/C 4U
Minimally invasive valve	T/C 4U
Revision sternotomy	T/C 4U
CABG/valve	T/C 4U
Open heart surgery	T/C 4U
Assist device	T/C 4U
Cardiac/major vascular	T/C 4U
Open ventricle	T/C 4U
CABG	T/C 2U
Cardiac wound surgery	T/C 2U
Percutaneous cardiac	T/C 2U
Pericardium	T/C 2U
Lead extraction	T/C 2U
AICD/pacemaker placement	T/S

General Surgery

Case Category	Rec
AP resection	T/C 2U
Intra-abdominal GI	T/C 2U
Whipple or pancreatic	T/C 2U
Liver resection	T/C 2U
Retroperitoneal	T/C 2U
Substernal	T/C 2U
Bone marrow harvest	T/S
Hernia – Ventral/Incisional	T/S
Hernia – Inguinal/Umbilical	No Sample
Appendectomy	No Sample
Abdomen/chest/soft tissue	No Sample
Lap. or open chalecystectomy	No Sample
Thyroid/parathyroid	No Sample
Central venous access	No Sample
Any Breast – except w/flaps	No Sample

Gynecological Surgery

Case Category	Rec
Uterus open	T/C 2U
Open pelvic	T/C 2U
Uterus/ovary	T/S
Total vaginal hysterectomy	T/S
Cystectomy robotic assisted	T/S
Cystoscopy	No Sample
External genitalia	No Sample
GYN cervix	No Sample
Hysteroscopy	No Sample
Superficial wound	No Sample

Neurosurgery

Case Category	Rec
Thoracic/Lumbar/Sacral fusion	T/C 4U
Spine tumor	T/C 2U
Posterior cervical spine fusion	T/C 2U
Spine Incision and Drainage	T/C 2U
Intracranial tumor/aneurysm	T/C 2U
Laminectomy/discectomy	T/S
Spine hardware removal/biopsy	T/S
ACDF	T/S
Extracranial	No Sample
Nerve procedure	No Sample
CSF/shunt procedure	No Sample

Orthopedic Surgery

Case Category	Rec
Thoracic/Lumbar/Sacral fusion	T/C 4U
Pelvic orthopedic	T/C 4U
Open hip	T/C 2U
Femur open	T/C 2U
Above/below knee amputation	T/C 2U
Humerus open	T/S
Fasciotomy	T/S
Shoulder Incision & Drainage	T/S
Tibial/fibular	T/S
Total knee replacement	T/S
Shoulder open	T/S
Knee open	T/S
Thigh soft tissue	No Sample
Ortho external fixation	No Sample
Peripheral nerve/tendon	No Sample
Lower extremity I&D	No Sample
Hand orthopedic	No Sample
Upper extremity arthroscopy	No Sample
Upper extremity open	No Sample
Podiatry/Foot	No Sample
Hip closed/percutaneous	No Sample
Lower extremity arthroscopic	No Sample
Shoulder closed	No Sample
Tibial/fibular closed	No Sample

Otolaryngology Surgery

Case Category	Rec
Laryngectomy	T/C 2U
Facial reconstruction	T/C 2U
Cranial surgery	T/C 2U
Radical neck dissection	T/C 2U
Carotid body tumor	T/C 2U
Mandibular surgery	T/S
Neck dissection	T/S
Mastoidectomy	No Sample
Parotidectomy	No Sample
Facial plastic	No Sample
Oral surgery	No Sample
Sinus surgery	No Sample
Thyroid/parathyroidectomy	No Sample
Suspension laryngoscopy	No Sample
Bronchoscopy	No Sample
Cochlear implant	No Sample
EGD	No Sample
External ear	No Sample
Inner ear	No Sample
Tonsillectomy/adenoidectomy	No Sample
Tympanomastoid	No Sample

Thoracic Surgery

Case Category	Rec
Esophageal open	T/C 2U
Sternal procedure	T/C 2U
Chest wall	T/C 2U
Thoracotomy	T/C 2U
Pectus repair	T/C 2U
VATS	T/S
Mediastinoscopy	T/S
EGD/FOB	No Sample
Central venous access	No Sample

Urology

Case Category	Rec
Cystoprostatectomy	T/C 2U
Urology open	T/C 2U
Nephrectomy	T/C 2U
Lap/Robotic kidney/adrenal	T/S
RRP	T/S
Percutaneous nephrolithotomy	T/S
Robotic RRP	No Sample
External genitalia/Penile	No Sample
TURP	No Sample
Cysto/ureter/urethra	No Sample
TURBT	No Sample

Vascular/Transplant Surgery

Case Category	Rec
Liver transplant	T/C 15U
Thoracoabdominal aortic	T/C 15U
Major liver resection	T/C 4U
Major vascular	T/C 4U
Exploratory lap. vascular	T/C 4U
Kidney pancreas transplant	T/C 2U
Major endovascular	T/C 2U
Above/below knee amputation	T/C 2U
Nephrectomy/kidney transplant	T/C 2U
Organ procurement	T/C 2U
Peripheral vascular	T/C 2U
Vascular wound I and D	T/C 2U
Carotid vascular	T/S
AV fistula	T/S
Peripheral endovascular	T/S
Angio/Arteriogram	No Sample
Peripheral wound I&D	No Sample
1st rib resection/thoracic outlet	No Sample
Superficial or skin	No Sample
Foot/toe amputation/debride	No Sample
Central venous access	No Sample

If the procedure you are looking for is not on this list, then choose the procedure that most closely resembles that procedure.

"Emergency Release blood is available for ALL cases, and carries a risk of minor transfusion reaction of 1 in 1,000 cases.

Figure 3.2 Maximum blood ordering schedule (MSBOS).
From Frank SM, Rothschild JA, Masear CG, Rivers RJ, Merritt WT, Savage WJ, Ness PM. Optimizing preoperative blood ordering with data acquired from an anesthesia information management system. *Anesthesiology.* 2013 Jun;118(6):1286–1297.

demonstration purposes the MACE scores generated by all three calculators are provided.

This patient has risk factors for coronary artery disease (CAD) (age, hypertension, smoking) and dyspnea on exertion (which may be an angina equivalent, especially in a female).

The ACC/AHA guidelines are designed to be followed in a stepwise fashion.[7] Step 1 deals with emergency surgery, Step 2 with an evaluation for an acute coronary syndrome (ACS), and Step 3 with calculation of MACE. ACS includes symptoms at rest and new-onset or worsening symptoms. This

Table 3.1 REVISED CARDIAC RISK INDEX (RCRI)

High-risk surgery	1
History of ischemic heart disease	1
History of congestive heart failure	1
History of cerebrovascular disease	1
Preoperative insulin treatment	1
Preoperative serum creatinine ≥2.0 mg/dL	1
TOTAL	___ out of 6 points

Risk category		MACE Risk
Minimal (Class I)	0	0.4%
Low (Class II)	1	0.9%
Intermediate (Class III)	2	6.6%
High (Class IV)	3-6	11.0%

https://www.mdcalc.com/revised-cardiac-risk-index-pre-operative-risk#evidence

Table 3.2 DUKE ACTIVITY STATUS INDEX (DASI)

Activity	Yes	No
Walking around indoors	1.75	0
Light housework	2.70	0
Perform activities of daily living	2.75	0
Walking 1 block without an incline	2.75	0
Moderate housework (vacuuming, sweeping, carry groceries)	3.50	0
Yard work	4.50	0
Sexual intercourse	5.25	0
Climb a flight upstairs or hill	5.50	0
Moderate sports (golf, bowling, doubles tennis, playing catch)	6.00	0
Strenuous sports (swimming, singles tennis, basketball, skiing)	7.50	0
Heavy work (moving furniture, scrubbing floors)	8.00	0
Short distance run	8.00	0
TOTAL		

VO_2 peak = [0.43 × "yes" total] + 9.6 in mL/kg/min

METS = VO_2 peak/3.5

Fleisher LA, Fleischmann KE, Auerbach AD, Barnason SA, Beckman JA, et al. 2014 ACC/AHA guideline on perioperative cardiovascular evaluation and management of patients undergoing noncardiac surgery: A report of the American College of Cardiology/American Heart Association Task Force on practice guidelines. *J Am Coll Cardiol*. 2014;64(22): e77–137.

---

patient needs further testing to assess her dyspnea on exertion. It is important for this patient not to skip to Step 3 to calculate MACE, which is designed to be used only for asymptomatic patients or those with stable, chronic symptoms.

Are there any tests that can be used before proceeding with stress testing?

Brain natriuretic peptide (BNP) or the N-terminal fragment of BNP (NT-BNP) are useful laboratory tests in patients with dyspnea, known heart disease, or risk factors for heart disease. BNP is released by cardiac myocytes in response to atrial or ventricular distension in patients with HF, AF, and ischemic or valvular disease. This patient has a BNP concentration of 328 pg/mL, which corresponds with her moderately enlarged left atrium and AF. Many patients with HF have chronically elevated concentrations, although normal concentrations are attainable in a patient with well-managed HF. Patients with elevated preoperative BNP (>189 pg/mL) have a 32.8% risk of 30-day postoperative MACE following noncardiac surgery versus 4.0% in those with normal BNP preoperatively.[9]

The patient reports limited activity but thinks she could walk up a flight of stairs "if she had to." What is the best way to determine this patient's functional capacity?

Patients often have difficulty quantifying their maximal activity level. The Duke Activity Status Index (DASI) is a patient-reported survey of activity level (Table 3.2). The DASI data reported by the patient can be used to approximate the patient's metabolic equivalents (METs). Exercise capacity is incorporated into the ACC/AHA guidelines in Step 4, after determination of the patient's risk of MACE (Figure 3.3), to determine if preoperative myocardial ischemia testing is warranted. The rationale is that if patients can achieve a MET level of greater than 4, *without symptoms*, then no further cardiac assessment for *ischemic disease* is indicated. This patient has dyspnea at rest. Other testing, such as echocardiography, as noted above, for evaluation of a murmur, HF, or AF is indicated, independent of the ACC/AHA algorithm, which is primarily designed to determine if stress testing is indicated. An objective measure such as the 6MWT, discussed above, is recommended for objective measurement of functional capacity.

Because this patient may have dyspnea from cardiac ischemia, and it is unclear if she can achieve 4 or greater METS, dobutamine stress testing will assist with determining if she has ischemic heart disease.

Dobutamine stress echocardiography revealed posterolateral apical hypokinesis which occurred at the patient's target HR, and AF was present throughout. The patient's dyspnea did not worsen during the study, and the patient reported no chest pain or lightheadedness. Fifteen minutes after completion of the study, the patient's HR returned to her pretest rate, and the wall motion abnormalities (WMA) normalized.

Should this patient be referred for cardiac catheterization?

The patient's dobutamine stress test was abnormal. The ACC/AHA guidelines recommend *consideration* of coronary

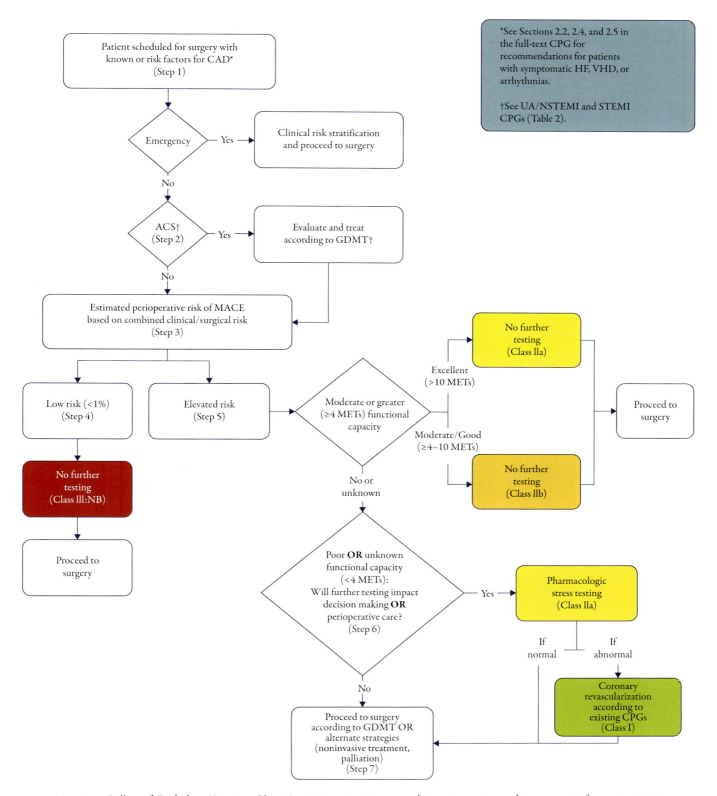

Figure 3.3 American College of Cardiology/American Heart Association stepwise approach to perioperative cardiac assessment for coronary artery disease.
From Fleisher LA, Fleischmann KE, Auerbach AD, Barnason SA, Beckman JA, et al. 2014 ACC/AHA guideline on perioperative cardiovascular evaluation and management of patients undergoing noncardiac surgery: A report of the American College of Cardiology/American Heart Association Task Force on practice guidelines. *J Am Coll Cardiol.* 2014;64(22):e77–137.

angiography after an abnormal stress test.[7] This patient's stress test was only mildly positive, with segmental WMA occurring at 102% of her target HR that resolved with return to her pretest HR. The distribution in the posterolateral apex is suggestive of distal single-vessel CAD with a small area of myocardium at risk. This is not consistent with left main disease. However, the positive findings of ischemia increase her MACE score to 6.6% as determined by RCRI, 1.8% by MICA, and 1% by NSQIP. However, given her active DUB and the likelihood that she may have cancer, delaying surgery for coronary angiography and possible revascularization is not ideal. And, as mentioned, the stress test suggests single-vessel CAD which is not an indication for coronary artery bypass graft (CABG) unless the left main coronary artery is the culprit. Angioplasty requires a 21-day delay in noncardiac surgery to allow 14 days of dual antiplatelet therapy (DAPT) and then typically 7 days off clopidogrel. Placement of a bare metal stent requires 30 days of DAPT, and a drug eluting stent requires 6 months (ideally 1 year) of DAPT. In addition to the time-sensitive nature of surgery, the patient will be at increased risk of worsening DUB upon the initiation of DAPT[10] (Table 3.3). The preferred approach is for the patient to receive goal-directed medical therapy (GDMT) aimed at reducing her risk of MACE. The addition of beta blockers for more than 7 days before surgery with careful titration is reasonable for this patient.[7] Beta blocker therapy will also treat the patient's AF. Additional benefits are provided by a statin, including the potential for spontaneous cardioversion of AF to normal sinus rhythm[11] and the reduction of progression of aortic sclerosis.[7] The patient should also be started on aspirin 81 mg to complete GDMT and further reduce her MACE risk, and this should be continued throughout surgery.[7]

Table 3.3 ISCHEMIC RISK VERSUS BLEEDING RISK WITH DUAL ANTIPLATELET THERAPY

INCREASED ISCHEMIC RISK	INCREASED BLEEDING RISK
Advanced age	History of prior bleeding
Acute coronary syndrome presentation	Oral anticoagulant therapy
Multiple prior myocardial infarctions	Female sex
Extensive coronary artery disease	Advanced age
Diabetes mellitus	Low body weight
Chronic kidney disease	Chronic kidney disease
	Diabetes mellitus
	Anemia
	Chronic steroid or NSAID therapy

Levine GN, Bates ER, Bittl JA, Brindis RG, Fihn SD, et al. 2016 ACC/AHA guideline focused update on duration of dual antiplatelet therapy in patients with coronary artery disease: A report of the American College of Cardiology/American Heart Association Task Force on Clinical Practice Guidelines. *J Thorac Cardiovasc Surg.* 2016 Nov;152(5):1243-1275.

NSAID, nonsteroidal anti-inflammatory drug

Table 3.4 STOP-BANG

Loud Snoring	1
Tired, sleepy, or fatigued during the day	1
Observed apnea while sleeping	1
Active treatment for elevated blood Pressure	1
BMI >35 kg/m²	1
Age >50	1
Neck circumference >40 cm	1
Gender male	1
TOTAL	
Low risk	0–2 points
Intermediate risk	3–4 points
High risk	≥5 points

Chung F, Abdullah HR, Liao P. STOP-Bang questionnaire: A practical approach to screen for obstructive sleep apnea. *Chest.* 2016 Mar;149(3):631–638.

Upon further questioning, the patient reports loud snoring. Does this patient need a polysomnogram?

The STOP-Bang questionnaire (Table 3.4) is a reliable method of assessing the risk of sleep apnea. Using STOP-Bang this patient scores 3 (loud snoring, hypertension, and age >50 years), which indicates an intermediate risk. If the patient has an elevated serum bicarbonate concentration, the likelihood of sleep apnea increases,[12] and this particular patient may have an elevated serum bicarbonate due to chronic carbon dioxide (CO_2) retention from COPD or chronic bronchitis. However, her CO_2 is normal, so polysomnography is not indicated.

This patient has a BMI of 18.4 kg/m². Is she malnourished?

Poor nutritional status is an independent predictor of increased morbidity and mortality.[13] The patient needs to be evaluated for malnutrition. She should be asked about unintentional weight loss of greater than 10% over the past 6 months and if she has consumed less than 50% of all meals over the past week. Additional testing includes an assessment of electrolytes, liver enzyme concentrations, total protein, albumin, prealbumin, transferrin, retinal binding protein, and vitamin D. Deficiencies confirm a diagnosis of severe malnutrition.

According to the European Society of Clinical Nutrition and Metabolism (ESPEN), the patient is considered malnourished based on her BMI of less than 18.5 kg/m².[14] This patient will benefit from preoperative protein supplementation and a dietary consultation to improve her nutritional status.

Is this patient frail?

Anemia, COPD, and malnutrition adversely affect this patient's functional status and negatively impact her daily life. They all contribute to frailty. A useful scale to evaluate for frailty is the Preoperative Frailty Assessment (PFA).[15] It evaluates five criteria: hand grip strength, a timed 15-minute walk, ability to complete activities of daily living, unintentional weight loss, and subjective frequency of exhaustion. The PFA scores frailty on a scale of 1 through 5. Each criterion with a deficiency earns the patient 1 point. A patient is considered pre-frail with scores of 1–2.[15] Frail status is assigned to patients who are scored 3–5 points. This particular patient scores 2 due to frequency of exhaustion and unintentional weight loss of more than 10 pounds over the past year. She is at twice the risk of becoming frail within the next 3 years as compared to a patient who is not pre-frail.[16] The Clinical Frailty Scale (CFS) is a global assessment tool based on clinical assessment of comorbidities (Table 3.5).[17] This patient is scored as Level 5, which is considered mild frailty, on the CFS.

Should surgery be postponed?

Postponement of surgery to allow full assessment of her dyspnea is not necessary. The patient has completed 30 days of treatment for her lower respiratory tract infection. Her dyspnea persists, and new diagnoses have been established. Her persistent cough and dyspnea may benefit from a trial of anticholinergic therapy and a short course of steroids for

Table 3.5 FRAILTY SCORING

Very fit	People who are robust, very active, and motivated. These people commonly exercise regularly. They are among the fittest of their age.
Well	People who have no active disease symptoms but are less fit than category 1. Often they exercise or are very active occasionally.
Managing well	People whose medical problems are well controlled, but they are rarely active beyond walking.
Vulnerable	While not dependent on others for daily help, often symptoms limit activities. A common complaint is being "slowed up" and/or being tired during the day.
Mildly frail	These people often have more evident slowing and need help in high-order instrumental activities of daily living (IADLs). Typically, this impairs shopping and walking outside alone, meal preparation, and housework.
Moderately frail	People need help with all outside activities and with keeping house. Inside, they often have problems with stairs and need help with bathing, and they might need minimal help with dressing.
Severely frail	Completely dependent for all personal care from whatever cause (physical or cognitive). Even so, they seem stable and not at high risk of dying (within ≈6 mo).
Terminally ill	Approaching the end of life. This category applies to people with a life expectancy <6 mo, who are not evidently frail.

Table 3.6 CHA$_2$D$_2$-VASc VERSUS HAS-BLED

Ischemic vs bleeding risk

CHA$_2$DS$_2$-VASc	Point	HAS-BLED	Point
Congestive heart failure (or EF <40%)	1	Hypertension	1
Hypertension	1	Abnormal renal or liver function	1 each
Age >75 years (or 65–74)	2 (or 1)	Stroke	1
Diabetes	1	Bleeding predisposition	1
Stroke/TIA/VTE	2	Labile INR (if on warfarin)	1
Vascular (arterial) disease	1	Elderly (age >65 years)	1
Sex: Female	1	Drug or alcohol abuse	1 each
	9 total		9 total

EF, ejection fraction; TIA, transient ischemic attack; VTE, venous thromboembolism; INR, international normalized ratio

Lip GY, Nieuwlaat R, Pisters R, Lane DA, Crijns HJ. Refining clinical risk stratification for predicting stroke and thromboembolism in atrial fibrillation using a novel risk factor-based approach: The euro heart survey on atrial fibrillation. *Chest*. 2010 Feb;137(2):263–272.

Lane DA, Lip GY. Use of the CHA(2)DS(2)-VASc and HAS-BLED scores to aid decision making for thromboprophylaxis in nonvalvular atrial fibrillation. *Circulation*. 2012 Aug 14;126(7):860–865.

treatment of a possible COPD exacerbation. Surgery may proceed if treatment results in symptomatic improvement of wheezing and cough.

The patient's newly diagnosed AF increases her risk of perioperative hemodynamic instability, MACE, and stroke.[18] She has a CHA$_2$DS$_2$-VASc score (Table 3.6) of 3, which puts her at about a 3.8% annual risk of stroke.[19] The 2014 AHA/ACC/ARS Guidelines for the Management of Patients with Atrial Fibrillation recommend cardioversion, followed by 4 weeks of anticoagulation in patients with AF of unknown duration.[18,20] This patient is currently hemodynamically stable. Cardioversion and anticoagulation should be deferred until after the DUB is surgically treated. The patient should proceed to surgery without delay of further AF management at this time. She will benefit from anticoagulation and rhythm control expeditiously postoperatively.

What options can this patient be offered for anesthesia?

The patient is scheduled for an open abdominal hysterectomy with possible lymph node dissection. If a low transverse incision is an option, then avoiding general anesthesia (GA) may be possible. Avoiding GA can lower the risk of PPC.[21,22] However, a midline incision may require GA. If GA is required, an epidural, or paravertebral, transverse abdominus or erector spinae plane blocks for postoperative analgesia may lower the risk of PPC.[23] These options should be discussed with the patient. She should be informed of the possibility of postoperative intubation with prolonged ventilation given her likely COPD. Extubating to noninvasive positive pressure ventilation should be considered. Complete reversal of neuromuscular blockade using train-of-four monitoring can lower the risk of PPC.[24]

A vaginal hysterectomy can easily be done with a neuraxial technique, but a lymph node dissection cannot be performed via a vaginal approach. A transvaginal approach would also decrease the risk of PPC. Raising this question with the surgeon is important, though vaginal hysterectomy may not be feasible as it is reserved for benign disease. A laparoscopic approach lowers the risk of PPC.[25] The surgeon should be informed of the patient's increased risk of PPC.

How can this patient be optimized?

Several steps can be taken to optimize this patient for surgery. Her dyspnea should be treated with an inhaled corticosteroid, an oral corticosteroid pulse, and an inhaled anticholinergic. An inhaled β_2 agonist may be beneficial, but there is a small risk of tachycardia while her recently started beta blocker dose is being established. Follow-up at 3 days to assess dyspnea symptoms is reasonable.

The patient will also benefit from IV iron therapy. Treating her iron deficiency begins with determining her total iron deficit (TID), as determined by the formula[19]:

$$TID[mg] = ideal\ body\ weight[kg] \\ \times (target\ Hb - actual\ Hb)[g/dL] \\ \times 2.4 + depot\ iron[mg]$$

Depot iron is typically 500–1,000 mg. The TID may be repleted with any one of several IV iron formulations (Table 3.7). Using the patient's body weight of 59.8 kg, current Hb of 10.5 g/dL along with a target Hb of 12.0 g/dL and depot provision of 500 mg, the patient's TID is calculated as 715 mg of IV iron. This can be achieved by giving a one-time preoperative dose of ferric carboxymaltose (Table 3.7).

The newly started beta blocker will provide rate control for her AF and CAD. The newly introduced statin and aspirin will serve as GDMT aimed at reducing her MACE. All of these medications should be continued perioperatively.[7]

Table 3.7 INTRAVENOUS IRON PREPARATIONS.

	IRON DEXTRAN	IRON SUCROSE	FERRIC GLUCONATE	FERUMOXYTOL	FERRIC CARBOXYMALTOSE
FDA approved indication	Iron deficiency in patients whom oral administration is unsatisfactory or impossible.	Iron deficiency anemia in adult and pediatric patients with CKD.	Iron deficiency anemia in adult and pediatric patients with CKD receiving hemodialysis who are receiving supplemental ESA therapy	Iron deficiency anemia in adult patients with chronic kidney disease (CKD).	Iron deficiency anemia in adult patients who have intolerance to oral iron, have had unsatisfactory response to oral iron, or who have non–dialysis-dependent CKD.
Maximum FDA approved single dose	100 mg	400 mg	125 mg	1,020 mg	750 mg
Dosing	Doses less than or equal to 300 mg, slow IVP no faster than 50 mg/minute; or diluted in 100–250 ml NS. A 1000 mg dose is diluted in 250 to 1000 mL of NS. After a test infusion, the solution may be infused over 1 or more hours.	100 mg IVP over 2–5 minutes; 100 mg/100 mL NS over 15 minutes; 200 mg/250 mL NS over 2–4 hours for a TDI of 1,000 mg over a 14-day period 300 mg/250 mL NS infusion over 1.5 hours 400 mg/250 mL NS infusion over 2.5 hours	Administer 125 mg diluted in 100 mL NS over 60 minutes daily for 5 doses maximum per week. May need to continue to a cumulative dose of 1 g.	Up to 510 mg IVP in 60–90 seconds. An infusion of 1,020 mg in 100 mL NS over 15 minutes. Observe patients for signs and symptoms of hypersensitivity during and after administration for at least 30 minutes and until clinically stable.	Up to 750 mg can be delivered in a single dose. Give 2 doses separated by at least 7 days for a total cumulative dose of up to 1,500 mg per course1 Slow IVP at 100 mg (2 mL) per minute over at least 7.5 minutes. For patients weighing less than 50 kg (110 lb), dose at 15 mg/kg body weight. When administered via infusion, dilute up to 750 mg of iron in no more than 250 mL of NS, and administer over at least 15 minutes.

CKD, chronic kidney disease; ESA, erythrocyte stimulating agent; FDA, Federal Drug Administration; IVP, intravenous push; NS, normal saline; TSAT, transferrin saturation.

From http://www.sabm.org/wp-content/uploads/2018/08/IV-IronTable-May-2014.compressed.pdf

Optimizing her nutrition with a daily enteral protein total of 1.2–2.0 g/kg for 7–14 days before surgery can lower morbidity and mortality.[13] The protein should be consumed as 2–3 divided doses, with a minimum of 18 g/meal.[13] For this ~60 kg patient, her total suggested daily protein dose is 72–120 g/day. Per meal, the patient should consume 24–40 g enterally.

All of these interventions can be undertaken before the patient's scheduled surgery. Considering the fact that this surgery is time sensitive and given the active DUB and possible malignancy, taking the above steps should have a significant effect on morbidity and mortality reduction.

DISCUSSION

DYSPNEA

Five weeks ago, this patient visited an urgent care clinic for shortness of breath and cough. She was evaluated and treated for an acute medical problem, but none of that information is accessible at the time of her preoperative visit. The focus of her preoperative clinic visit has been on evaluating her irregular heart rate, her murmur, calculating her risk of MACE, determining the cause of her dyspnea, and optimizing her for surgery.

The preoperative clinic evaluation included a chest radiograph to evaluate resolution of her possible pneumonia. At 6 weeks post-treatment, 60.2% of patients older than 70 years of age demonstrate radiographic resolution of a lower respiratory infectious process. At 12 weeks, the resolution rate increases to 84.2%.[2] A follow-up chest radiograph is not recommended for asymptomatic nonsmokers, regardless of age.[2] Smokers older than 50 years or those of any age without complete resolution of symptoms should have a follow-up chest radiograph.

This patient has risk factors for COPD and a clinical picture consistent with inadequately treated COPD. Findings suggestive of COPD can be present on a chest radiograph, but a definitive diagnosis requires spirometry testing.

The Global Initiative for Obstructive Lung Disease (GOLD) recommends spirometry to diagnose COPD. FEV_1 and forced vital capacity (FVC) are measured. Diagnostic criteria include FEV_1/FVC of less than 0.7 after bronchodilator therapy.[26] Asthma is distinguished from COPD by an increase in FEV_1/FVC after bronchodilator therapy. FEV_1 is used to classify severity. An FEV_1 80% or greater of predicted is consistent with mild COPD. Moderate COPD is present with an FEV_1 50–79%, severe disease has an FEV_1 30–49%, and very severe COPD is determined with an FEV_1 of less than 30% of predicted.[27]

ANEMIA

Burton et al. reported an increased risk of morbidity and mortality due to untreated preoperative anemia with various types of surgeries.[28] Outcomes included increased risk of venous thromboembolism, transfusion requirements, amputation in vascular patients, and reintubation of cervical spine surgery patients within 30 days of surgery. In cancer patients with anemia, a decrease in recurrence-free days was observed.[28] However, they do not endorse universal preoperative screening of patients for anemia. Instead, a selective approach is recommended based on comorbidities, a history of anemia or bleeding, historical procedure-specific blood loss data (>500 cc), historical rate of transfusion of greater than 10%, type of surgery (e.g., aorta, spine), and in any patient who requires cross-matching of blood.[28]

If a procedure carries a significant risk of blood loss, or if the patient reports symptoms of anemia (shortness of breath, easy fatigability, angina), has CKD or liver disease, a chronic inflammatory condition, cancer, or a history of anemia then a preoperative Hb concentration should be obtained. A 2013 study found anemia (Hct <39%) in 47% of patients older than 65 years who had an open vascular or endovascular procedure.[29] Anemia was associated with a 30-day perioperative mortality rate of 2.4% and cardiac event rate of 2.3%.[29] Patients with normal Hct (>39%) had half the mortality and cardiac event rates of those with an Hct of less than 39%.[29] Additionally, for each 1-point drop in Hct below 39%, 30-day mortality risk increased by 4.2%.[29]

IRON DEFICIENCY ANEMIA

Iron deficiency is a common problem in preoperative patients. It is estimated that half of all anemias are due to iron deficiency.[30] Iron studies are indicated if a patient is anemic. If the serum ferritin is less than 30 ng/mL or transferrin saturation (T_{SAT}) is 20% or less, then the patient is iron deficient. Ferritin is an acute phase reactant and can be normal or high in the presence of iron deficiency. This is true for patients with kidney disease or other chronic conditions, including cancer, infections, and chronic inflammation. Some patients with a T_{SAT} of 20–50% and a ferritin of less than 800 ng/mL may respond to IV iron. In this setting a reticulocyte Hb content of less than 28 pg confirms the diagnosis of IDA.[31]

A 2013 systematic review and meta-analysis of randomized controlled trials evaluated red cell transfusion and mean Hb increases in patients who received IV iron therapy. Several different preparations of iron were used, including iron sucrose, iron gluconate, ferric carboxymaltose, and iron dextran. The analysis concluded that Hb concentration increased by a mean of 0.65 g/dL, and there was a significant reduction in the red cell transfusion rates.[32] Additionally, IV iron was generally safe, other than a slight, but significant increase in the risk of infection as compared to oral or no iron supplementation. Every effort should be made to provide IV iron therapy prior to surgery, even if it means postponing surgery.

PERIOPERATIVE BLOOD PRODUCT MANAGEMENT

Patients with a history of previous erythrocyte transfusion or pregnancy may screen positive for antibodies against red cell surface antigens (alloimmunization). The positive result can arise from the presence of a single antibody.[33] Exposure of an alloimmunized patient to incompatible donor blood risks significant hemolytic transfusion reactions. Blood samples that test positive for clinically significant antibodies need extra time for cross-matching and obtaining compatible units. In some cases, it can take hours to days to ensure available blood products for transfusion. If significant blood loss or transfusion is anticipated, then type and screen testing should be done before the day of surgery. Pretransfusion testing can be completed several days to weeks in advance based on individual institutional policies provided the patient has not been pregnant or transfused in the preceding 3 months. If a patient has been pregnant or transfused in the preceding 3 months, a type and screen is only valid for 72 hours.[33]

A proprietary electronic cross-matching has demonstrated a reduction in preoperative blood orders from 40.4% to 25% in one institution and has reduced the ratio of units cross-matched to units given from 2.11:1 to 1.54:1.[34] The process of electronic cross-matching is significantly faster than traditional cross-matching of a blood sample.

VALVULAR HEART DISEASE

The most common cause of murmurs in elderly patients is AS. AS is a disease of aging, and the same risk factors which contribute to CAD contribute to AS. AS is classified as mild if V_{max} is 2.0–2.9 meters/second or there is a mean pressure gradient across the valve of less than 20 mmHg. Moderate AS is present if V_{max} is 3.0–3.9 m/s or if the pressure gradient is 20–39 mm Hg. Severe AS corresponds with a V_{max} of 4 m/s or greater or a pressure gradient of greater than 40 mm Hg.[35] In patients with known valvular disease, a careful history and physical examination searches for syncope, chest pain, dyspnea, lower extremity edema, wheezing, rales, or diminished breath sounds. If any of these are present, an echocardiogram should be performed to assess the degree of valve stenosis and to evaluate ventricular function.[36] In established valvular disease, an echocardiogram is recommended annually to evaluate severe disease even in the absence of symptoms.[36] However, even if AS is severe, the patient may proceed with noncardiac surgery with advanced care, invasive monitoring, and postoperative intensive care management. The combined 30-day mortality and myocardial infarction (MI) risk is 4.4% with moderate AS versus 1.7% without disease, and 5.7% with severe AS versus 2.7% for those without AS.[37]

ATRIAL FIBRILLATION

Patients with AF experience a mortality risk almost double that of those with CAD,[38] and they are at increased risk for thromboembolic stroke. Patients who have preoperative AF experience greater mortality with urgent surgery as compared to elective surgery.[39]

Patients who require anticoagulant therapy need careful consideration of preoperative adjustments to their anticoagulant medication to balance their bleeding and thromboembolic risks. The CHA_2DS_2-VASc (Table 3.6) scoring system is most often used to recommend long-term anticoagulation, but it can also be helpful in guiding anticoagulant bridging therapy. Patients with AF who have a CHA_2DS_2-VASc (Table 3.6) score 2 or greater require anticoagulation due to an increased annual thromboembolic stroke risk.[17] However, their risk of stroke must be balanced against their risk of bleeding while taking an anticoagulant, as determined by the HAS-BLED scale (Table 3.6). Any patient with a HAS-BLED score of 2 or higher is at increased risk for major bleeding on anticoagulation therapy[40] and should seek an alternative to anticoagulation therapy if the CHA_2DS_2-VASc score is less than 2. Bridging should only be considered for patients with CHA_2DS_2-VASc 6 or greater. Direct-acting oral anticoagulants (DOAC) should not be bridged.

ANTICOAGULATION MANAGEMENT

Typically, AF patients have an INR target of 2–3 which requires stopping warfarin 5 days preoperatively to reach an INR of less than 1.5, which is considered acceptable for surgery. Several circumstances increase the risk of excessive warfarin anticoagulation. In addition to the criteria included in HAS-BLED, recent antibacterial or antifungal therapy, malignancy, chemotherapy, and a hospitalization within the past 30 days increase the risk of warfarin over-anticoagulation and increase bleeding risk.[41] The supratherapeutic INR that results usually requires a longer period than the typical 5 days of medication discontinuation. The INR is usually checked at the preoperative encounter and rechecked immediately before surgery.

DOACs such as apixaban, rivaroxaban (factor Xa antagonists), and dabigatran (a factor IIa antagonist) are used frequently due to their ease of administration and reliable anticoagulation effect. DOACs' anticoagulant effects can be monitored with factor Xa assay testing. However, testing is not routinely done preoperatively. Factor testing can be considered for the patient who has not held his DOAC for sufficient time preoperatively when surgery cannot be delayed. Otherwise, universal coagulation testing as a screening test causes unnecessary delays and is a poor predictor of abnormal perioperative bleeding.[42]

MAJOR ADVERSE CARDIOVASCULAR EVENTS

Preoperative MACE risk calculators (RCRI, https://www.mdcalc.com/revised-cardiac-risk-index-pre-operative-risk; *MICA*, https://www.mdcalc.com/gupta-perioperative-risk-myocardial-infarction-cardiac-arrest-mica; *NSQIP*, https://riskcalculator.facs.org/RiskCalculator/PatientInfo.jsp) consider several factors to predict the likelihood of a perioperative cardiac event. Prediction of MACE guides decisions regarding further testing, whether the risk of surgery may outweigh the benefits, or if a less invasive treatment is a better option. Patients with active acute unstable coronary symptoms (e.g., chest pressure or pain, dyspnea, diaphoresis, syncope or presyncope) should not proceed with noncardiac surgery. These patients require appropriate evaluation and treatment to reduce MACE.

There is some overlap among the components of the different MACE risk calculators, but there are also important differences. The RCRI score is generated from six risk factors (Table

3.1), with the type of surgical procedure classified in a binary manner of low-risk or elevated risk. MICA includes 11 different surgical risk categories, and the NSQIP calculator considers several comorbidities and accounts for the risk of specific surgeries by providing an expansive list of procedures.[43]

A patient who presents for emergency surgery and patients with low risk (<1%) for MACE should proceed to surgery. If a patient is at increased risk for MACE (>1%), functional status determines if further stress testing may be of benefit. Patients having cataract surgery are considered to have such a low risk of MACE related to surgery that the ACC/AHA guidelines recommend no further testing, regardless of the calculated risk of MACE or functional capacity.[44]

The Duke Activity Status Index (DASI) is a tool that determines a patient's self-reported activity level, which can then be translated into metabolic equivalents (METs) (Table 3.2). The DASI is easier to perform than cardiopulmonary exercise testing (CPET). However, DASI only predicts peak oxygen uptake per minute (VO_2), whereas CPET directly measures maximum VO_2. In one study of patients undergoing CPET before major cancer surgeries, there was a large difference of agreement and bias between DASI and CPET, suggesting DASI's unreliability in screening that patient population.[45] Any patient who can achieve 4 METs or greater without symptoms should proceed to surgery without further cardiac testing no matter their calculated MACE risk, though goal directed medical management should be optimized (Figure 3.3). If a patient cannot achieve 4 METs or greater, further cardiac testing should *only* be pursued if it will change further management (Figure 3.3).

OBSTRUCTIVE SLEEP APNEA

Patients with sleep apnea experience increased postoperative pulmonary and cardiac complications.[46] Screening for obstructive sleep apnea (OSA) with the STOP-Bang questionnaire is an important step in identifying patients with a high clinical suspicion for OSA. The sensitivity of STOP-Bang in predicting moderate-severe and severe OSA is 93% and 100% respectively.[47] The eight individual components of STOP-Bang contribute 1 point to the score. A score of 0–2 suggests a low likelihood of moderate to severe OSA, supporting no further testing. A score of 3–4 is considered intermediate risk. A score in this range has a greater specificity when it is composed of two STOP items plus either male sex or BMI of greater than 35 kg/m² rather than when a neck circumference of greater than 40 cm or age older than 50 years are added.[48] While the patient is likely to have "some" degree of sleep apnea, there is a relatively lesser chance of moderate to severe sleep apnea as compared to a score 5 or higher. A score of 5 or higher corresponds with a high likelihood of severe OSA, therefore warranting polysomnography testing for diagnosis.

Chung et al. suggest that a serum bicarbonate concentration of greater than 28 mmol/L increases the sensitivity of a STOP-Bang score of 3–4 for predicting the presence of any OSA from 37% to 85.2%, moderate to severe OSA from 30.4% to 81.7%, and severe OSA from 27.7% to 79.7%.[12]

METABOLIC PANEL

Metabolic testing is indicated for patients with malnutrition, diabetes, HF, kidney or liver disease, those taking diuretics, or patients with risk factors for CKD. Electrolyte, blood urea nitrogen, and serum creatinine testing in healthy patients undergoing low- or intermediate-risk surgery is not recommended due to a low abnormal rate and lack of evidence in predicting adverse events.[49]

NUTRITION SCREENING

Nutrition plays a vital role in health maintenance and wellness. In some cases, inadequate nutrition results in malnutrition. The prevalence of malnutrition in developed countries is 15% in the elderly population outside of the hospital, 23–65% in hospitalized patients, and up to 85% in nursing home residents. Individuals with less than 80% expected total body protein concentrations have increased morbidity. A 10% or greater unintentional weight loss is associated with adverse outcomes and prolonged hospitalizations. In lean healthy subjects, greater than 35% weight loss, greater than 30% protein loss, and greater than 70% fat loss from baseline is associated with death.[50]

It can be very difficult to accurately and comprehensively assess the adequacy of nutritional status for various reasons. Therefore, all preoperative assessments must include calculation of BMI using measured height and weight. Any BMI of less than 20 kg/m² should be investigated with a detailed history and physical examination focused on nutritional status. Wischney et al. recommend asking pointed questions about nutritional status based on the Preoperative Nutrition Scale (PONS).[13]

PONS consists of the following questions:

1. Is BMI less than 18.5 kg/m² or less than 20 kg/m² (if older than 65 years of age)?

2. Has there been unintentional weight loss of more than 8 lbs. over the past 3 months or more than 10 lbs. in the past 6 months?

3. Is there less than 50% of normal meal consumption over the past week?

A "Yes" answer to any of the three questions listed above should prompt nutritional intervention.[13] Nutrition intervention helps to reverse the catabolic state of surgery by tipping the metabolic balance in favor of protein synthesis. If a patient screens positive for malnutrition, they should be referred to a nutrition specialist to help the patient meet daily nutrition requirements. The goal is to take in 1.2–2.0 g/kg of protein per day for at least 7–14 days before surgery.[13] Additionally, only 8 hours of solid food fasting time should be adhered to, not a blanket "nothing to eat after midnight" policy.[13] The daily protein goal is to be maintained postoperatively as well. If the patient cannot tolerate oral feedings, then enteral nutrition in the form of immunonutrition or high-protein oral nutrition supplementation should be provided via a feeding tube. If the goal cannot be achieved with enteral feedings, then parenteral nutrition should be provided.[13]

In addition to BMI and weight loss, the fat-free mass index (FFMI) is a useful assessment of lean body mass. FFMI may be better than BMI at predicting poor outcomes. A population-based epidemiological study found 26.1% of COPD patients had normal BMI with corresponding FFMI lower than the lowest 10th percentile of the general population.[51] These patients were at increased risk for overall and COPD-related mortality.[51] Among hospitalized COPD patients, malnutrition was determined by (1) greater than 10% unintentional weight loss over any time period or greater than 5% over the previous 3 months; combined with either (2) a BMI of less than 20 kg/m² if younger than 70 years, a BMI of less than 22 kg/m² if 70 or older; or (3) an FFMI of less than 17 kg/m² in men and less than 15 kg/m² in women. These criteria were compared with a single criterion of a BMI less than 18.5 kg/m² as the determinant of malnutrition. Using FFMI as part of the malnutrition assessment, 21% of patients were considered malnourished.[52] Patients with low FFMI compared with BMI alone were found to be at greater risk for a greater than 7-day hospital stay, and they faced a greater 6- and 9-month mortality risk.[53] The severity of COPD was positively correlated with low FFMI and was negatively associated with unintentional weight loss.[52]

The drawback with FFMI calculation is that it requires measurement of the percentage of body fat. There are many modalities available to measure body fat, and each has its own benefits and drawbacks. The optimal method is the multicompartment model, but its widespread use is limited because it is very labor-intensive and expensive. Dual-energy X-ray absorptiometry (DXA) and computed tomography (CT) use radiation. Air displacement plethysmography and 3-D body scanning are relatively expensive. Hydrostatic weighing in a pool of water requires complete submersion, which may not be possible for some patients. A more practical and cost-effective method of body fat analysis is the portable bioelectrical impedance analyzer. The downside is that accuracy is sacrificed if lower-cost equipment is used. Perhaps the most practical and cost-effective methods of body fat analysis include body circumference measurement and caliper skin fold testing. Both methods of manual body fat measurement incur operator and patient errors with regards to accuracy and precision. Patient shape and fat distribution can affect body circumference measurement, and caliper skin fold testing is not accurate in patients who are extremely thin or extremely obese.

The unit of measure for FFMI is the same (kg/m²) as for BMI, but the values considered normal are lower. Normal FFMI values are 16.7 to 19.8 kg/m² for men and 14.6 to 16.8 kg/m² for women within the normal BMI ranges of 18.5 kg/m² to 24.9 kg/m².[53] The formulas for FFMI calculation are as follows[54]:

$$Fat-Free\ Mass\ Index(FFMI) = FFM[kg]/(height[m])^2$$

$$Normalized\ FFMI = [kg/m^2] = FFM[kg]/(height[m])^2 + 6.1$$

$$Fat-Free\ Mass\ (FFM) = weight[kg]$$

FRAILTY

Makary et al. describes frailty as diminished organ-system reserve and decreased resistance to stressors that predispose to adverse outcomes.[15] As a result of the naturally decreasing organ system reserve that occurs with aging, an elderly patient is at increased risk of being frail. The domains involved in frailty include resistance, shrinkage, weakness, low physical activity, and slowness. All domains can be easily tested in a preoperative clinic setting. Frailty increases postoperative complications, length of stay, falls, functional status, and likelihood of discharge to a place other than home.[55] The *Preoperative Frailty Assessment* has been validated by several studies and has shown a correlation between frailty and increased length of stay, 30-day readmission rate, and 30-day mortality.[56]

Identification of frailty should prompt a geriatrician consult for a comprehensive assessment to determine severity.[57] This process allows for fully informed surgical and anesthetic decisions. It also influences discussions with the patient and caregivers or power of attorney, if applicable. Discussions should include the likelihood of complications resulting from the proposed procedures and the likelihood of discharge to a place other than home. Targeted preoperative interventions to improve frailty or pre-frailty should be specific to the individual patient and may include a preoperative exercise program, and nutritional and psychological interventions[57] (Figure 3.4).

CONCLUSION

- Preoperative testing is customized to the patient's planned procedure and medical problems.

- History and physical examination are invaluable in determining the need for preoperative testing.

- The 6MWT is a practical, cost-effective screening assessment that can uncover numerous undiagnosed cardiopulmonary or neuromuscular disease processes. If a patient cannot walk 325 m, the risk of postoperative pulmonary complications is increased.

- PFT has *not* been shown to be of value in predicting PPC outside of lung resection surgery. PFTs may have a role, in rare circumstances, in establishing diagnoses in patients with symptoms and findings suggestive of progressive severe pulmonary disease such as COPD or interstitial pulmonary fibrosis when clinical diagnosis is not certain.

- Anemia is very common, especially in females, older patients, and those on anticoagulation therapy. Iron deficiency anemia is the most common cause and is associated with a significantly increased risk of mortality. CBC

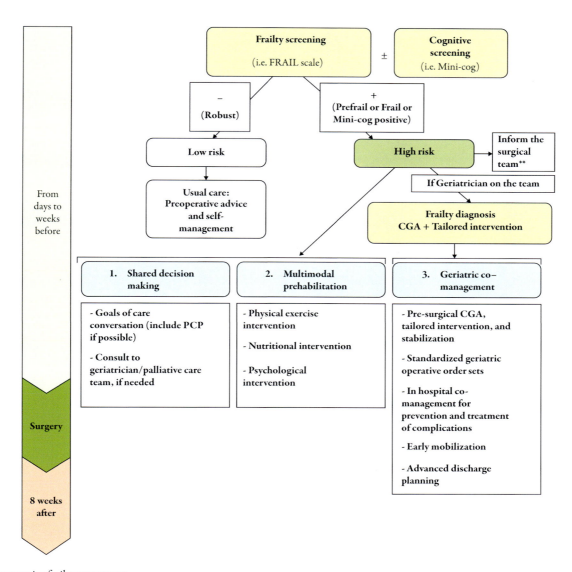

Figure 3.4 Preoperative frailty assessment.
CGA, comprehensive geriatric assessment; PCP, primary care physician.
From Alvarez-Nebreda ML, Bentov N, Urman RD, Setia S, Huang JC, Pfeifer K, Bennett K, Ong TD, Richman D, Gollapudi D, Alec Rooke G, Javedan H. Recommendations for Preoperative Management of Frailty from the Society for Perioperative Assessment and Quality Improvement (SPAQI). *J Clin Anesth*. 2018 Jun;47:33–42.

testing is recommended in those with signs and symptoms of anemia or risk factors for anemia.

- Correcting anemia can reduce blood product utilization and reduce morbidity and mortality.
- CBC testing and blood typing with antibody screening are recommended for procedures associated with expected blood loss more than 500 mL
- Since the prevalence of anemia is higher in the elderly, routine hemoglobin testing is suggested for those older than 65 years, except for cataract surgery.
- Valvular heart disease and murmurs, if symptomatic, progressive, new, or undiagnosed, should be evaluated with a preoperative echocardiogram.
- Effective cardiac risk stratification informs decision-making, including the decision to proceed with surgery, the need for further testing or medication management, and determination of intraoperative management and postoperative care.
- BNP may be used to risk-stratify patients with valvular heart disease, atrial fibrillation, heart failure, ischemic heart disease or dyspnea before noncardiac surgery. A normal BNP is associated with a very low risk of MACE. Establishing a baseline BNP can assist with following patients with heart failure perioperatively.
- In the absence of a personal or family history of bleeding or clotting disorders, qualitative or quantitative platelet deficiency, or a reported history of spontaneous or excessive

bleeding, routine coagulation studies and platelet count are not recommended.

- Atrial fibrillation requires careful consideration of perioperative bleeding risk versus thromboembolic stroke risk. The perioperative anticoagulation therapy plan must take these risks into account when deciding on management.
- Coagulation studies are not required for patients taking direct-acting oral anticoagulants or low-molecular-weight heparin. An INR is recommended for those taking warfarin.
- Undiagnosed and untreated OSA increases morbidity, mortality, and perioperative resource utilization. Screening patients for OSA using a tool such as STOP-Bang is recommended in *all* patients.
- Nutrition screening helps to identify malnutrition. Once malnutrition is identified, preoperative oral nutritional supplementation should be provided for a minimum of 7–14 days before surgery.
- The FFMI is a useful adjunct to BMI. As an indicator of nutritional status, a low FFMI increases postoperative morbidity and mortality risk. Though it is cumbersome to calculate the FFMI, there appears to be utility in doing so because FFMI may be low in the setting of a normal BMI.
- Pre-frail and frail patients are at greater risk of morbidity and mortality. Once frailty is identified, interventions are indicated.

ACKNOWLEDGMENTS

The authors thank the American Board of Internal Medicine Foundation on their success in decreasing unnecessary testing through a successful Choosing Wisely campaign.

REVIEW QUESTIONS

Choose the best answer.

1. An obese (BMI 36 kg/m²) 42-year-old man presents to clinic after referral for an inguinal hernia. He is otherwise healthy. His wife reports snoring at night that she can hear from her office, adjacent to the bedroom. The patient also has a neck circumference of 43 cm. What preoperative testing is needed before a laparoscopic inguinal hernia repair?

   a. Serum bicarbonate.
   b. Pulmonary function testing (PFTs).
   c. Polysomnogram (PSG).
   d. Both a and c.
   e. None of the above.

   The correct answer is d.

   The patient has a STOP-Bang score of 4: male sex, obesity (BMI >35), neck circumference greater than 40 cm, and loud snoring. This puts him in the "intermediate risk" category, and he has a high likelihood of having sleep apnea but possibly not "moderate to severe" or worse. According to Chung et al., elevated serum bicarbonate concentrations are suggestive of a higher probability of "moderate to severe" or "severe" sleep apnea. PFTs require patient participation and are not indicated as his symptoms are not suggestive of lung disease.

2. Which of the following has the potential to increase bleeding while on anticoagulation?

   a. Renal failure.
   b. Hypertension.
   c. Stroke.
   d. Age >65 years.
   e. All of the above.

   The correct answer is e.

   According to the HAS-BLED score, all factors listed above increase the likelihood of bleeding while on anticoagulation therapy. If a patient has two or more risk factors and needs anticoagulation therapy, alternatives to anticoagulation therapy should be considered.

3. All of the following are reasons to discontinue a 6-minute walk test (6MWT), *except*

   a. Hypoxia.
   b. Angina.
   c. Worsening dyspnea.
   d. Staggering.

   The correct answer is a.

   The 6MWT is a nonspecific test that provides information on a patient's cardiopulmonary reserve. If new, activity-induced angina or worsening dyspnea occur during testing, an acute coronary syndrome should be suspected in those with risk factors, and the patient should be taken to an emergency department. If staggering occurs, it can result in injury from a fall. Additionally, staggering reduces the 6MWT's ability to assess cardiopulmonary function as it may be due to neurological or musculoskeletal system dysfunction. If the patient becomes hypoxemic during the 6MWT, the test may continue if there are no associated symptoms, such as angina, dyspnea, or new staggering. The degree of hypoxemia should be noted along with the patient's resting oxygen saturation.

4. Which of the following factors is/are associated with a supratherapeutic warfarin concentration?

   a. Renal failure.
   b. Consumption of leafy green vegetables.
   c. Hospital discharge 6 weeks prior.
   d. Antibiotic.
   e. None of the above.

   The correct answer is d.

According to Jaakkola et al.,[34] recent antibacterial or antifungal therapy, a malignancy, chemotherapy, and a hospitalization within the past 30 days are positive predictors of warfarin over-anticoagulation.

5. The patient you are seeing before a total shoulder arthroplasty is a 68-year-old male tobacco user with poorly controlled hypertension, type 2 diabetes treated with insulin, with stage III chronic kidney disease (baseline serum creatinine 1.5 mg/dL), and a BMI of 30 kg/m². He has a bare metal stent (placed for an MI 15 years prior). He can easily walk up a flight of stairs. What is the appropriate preoperative testing for this patient?

   a. Stress testing.
   b. Hemoglobin A1c.
   c. ECG.
   d. None of the above.

The correct answer is b.

Hemoglobin A1c will determine the degree of blood glucose control. His cardiac risk, as calculated by MICA, NSQIP, and RCRI, is 0.6%, 0.6%, and 6.6%, respectively. Noteworthy is the MACE risk of greater than 1% calculated by the RCRI. The key factor is the greater relative weight of the diabetes mellitus managed with insulin criterion. The NSQIP places less weight on diabetes treated with insulin as it is 1 of 19 criteria. Insulin use is not a factor in the calculation of MACE by MICA.

According to the ACC/AHA Stepwise Approach to Perioperative Cardiac Assessment for CAD, although RCRI assesses MACE risk at 6.6%, the patient requires no further cardiac testing due to his ability to achieve 4 or more METs.

6. Iron studies can diagnose iron deficiency by which of the following?

   a. Transferrin saturation <20%.
   b. Serum ferritin <30 ng/dL.
   c. Serum iron 105 µg/dL.
   d. Either a or b.

The correct answer is d.

The combination of transferrin saturation of less than 20% and serum ferritin less than 30 ng/dL confirm iron deficiency. If either, but not both, is present, iron deficiency may still be likely, but the diagnosis cannot be confirmed. Serum iron can be normal or low in iron deficiency anemia. Ferritin, serum iron, and transferrin saturation can also be high if iron therapy was recently administered because hemoglobin synthesis lags behind iron replacement.

7. Frailty assessment consists of all of the following criteria, *except*

   a. Slowness.
   b. Shrinkage.
   c. Weakness.
   d. Low physical activity.
   e. Malnutrition.

The correct answer is e.

Makary et al. developed the Preoperative Frailty Assessment as a screening tool to identify patients at risk for postoperative complications, morbidity, and mortality due to frailty. Resistance, shrinkage, weakness, low physical activity, and slowness are criteria used to diagnose frailty. Malnutrition can contribute to frailty by resulting in shrinkage, but it can be present independent of frailty.

8. A 58-year-old man presents for inguinal hernia repair. He is not very active, but he reports no chest pain, shortness of breath, or leg swelling with light housework. On preoperative physical examination, you appreciate a loud holosystolic murmur at the right upper sternal border. Upon further questioning, the patient denies having been told about a murmur. What preoperative testing is indicated?

   a. Echocardiogram.
   b. BNP.
   c. ECG.
   d. None.

The correct answer is a.

The patient has a new, loud murmur that should be evaluated with an echocardiogram. Although the patient is asymptomatic, his age and the location of the murmur increase the probability that it is a pathological murmur. Although the patient denies symptoms and endorses a moderate functional capacity, careful questioning may reveal a subtle, progressive decline in functional status. ECG and BNP are useful adjunct tests, but, given the symptomatology, the echocardiogram is the preferred test to diagnose the likely cause of the murmur.[36]

9. A healthy 54-year-old male nonsmoker is recovering from influenza complicated by bacterial pneumonia. He has completed 7 days of antibiotic therapy. When should he have his follow-up chest radiograph?

   a. 2 weeks.
   b. 4 weeks.
   c. 6 weeks.
   d. He does not need a follow-up.

The correct answer is d.

A healthy nonsmoker of any age does not require a chest radiograph after a radiographically diagnosed lower respiratory tract infection.[2] With appropriate therapy and symptom resolution, no imaging is needed. If, however, the patient is a smoker over the age of 50 years, or of any age with persistent symptoms, then a 6-week follow-up chest radiograph is recommended to screen for malignancy or unresolved infection.[2]

10. Which statement regarding pulmonary function testing (PFT) is *most* accurate?

   a. PFT are not predictive of postoperative pulmonary complications (PPC).
   b. PFT should be completed preoperatively if COPD is suspected.
   c. PFT are unnecessary if radiographic evidence of COPD is present.
   d. PFT reduce perioperative morbidity and mortality.

The correct answer is a.

The only definitive diagnosis of COPD is provided by spirometric PFT. GOLD criteria state that a FEV_1/FVC ratio less than 0.7 after bronchodilator therapy establishes a diagnosis of COPD. The FEV_1 is used to determine severity. This allows for appropriate long-term management of COPD, but it does not mandate PFT before time-sensitive surgery. Chest radiography may provide evidence of COPD, but it does not allow for definitive diagnosis. PFT has not been shown to reduce PPC or perioperative morbidity and mortality.

11. Brain natriuretic peptide (BNP) testing is most useful for which of the following?

    a. Heart failure.
    b. Atrial fibrillation.
    c. Valvular heart disease.
    d. Ischemic heart disease.
    e. All of the above.

The correct answer is e.

BNP is released from distended cardiac myocytes. The serum BNP concentration correlates with the degree of tissue stretch and worsens with the severity of cellular trauma. In the presence of renal failure, serum BNP concentrations can be dramatically increased due to decreased clearance. BNP can be falsely low in severe obesity.

12. Which of the following is *not* a cause of dyspnea?

    a. Valvular heart disease.
    b. Hyperparathyroidism.
    c. Renal failure.
    d. Anemia.
    e. Hypothyroidism.

The correct answer is b.

All answers, except for b, can be responsible for dyspnea. Pulmonary congestion due to fluid overload from renal failure or valvular heart disease are known causes of dyspnea. Severe anemia can cause peripheral hypoperfusion due to inadequate oxygen carrying capacity. The resulting systemic acidosis causes dyspnea. Hypothyroidism can be complicated by myxedema coma. Hyperparathyroidism results in hypercalcemia, which is not a direct cause of dyspnea.

13. A 65-year-old woman presents urgently for an open sigmoidectomy for diverticulitis. Her medical history includes an MI 2 years ago, complicated by cardiogenic shock. At the time, she had a drug-eluting stent placed. Her most recent transthoracic echocardiogram reveals an ejection fraction of 32%, and she is medically managed with carvedilol, lisinopril, aspirin, atorvastatin, and furosemide. Her physical examination reveals bilateral lower extremity edema but clear lung fields on chest radiography. She can walk two flights of stairs without symptoms. The most accurate categorization of her MACE risk is:

    a. Minimal risk.
    b. Low risk.
    c. Intermediate risk.
    d. High risk.

The correct answer is d.

This patient is planning intraperitoneal surgery and has ischemic heart disease with heart failure. According to the Revised Cardiac Risk Index (RCRI) she is assigned 1 point for each of these conditions for a total of 3 points. This calculates a MACE risk of 11%, which is considered high-risk. Despite her high MACE risk, the ACC/AHA cardiac evaluation for noncardiac surgery guidelines state that she may proceed to surgery without further cardiac testing because she can achieve a 4 METs level of activity. Aspirin and a statin should be started to reduce her MACE risk.

14. Malnutrition in a 46-year-old healthy man is determined by:

    a. BMI < 18.5 kg/m^2.
    b. <50% meal consumption over the past 5 days.
    c. >8-pound weight loss in the previous 6 months.
    d. All of the above.
    e. None of the above.

The correct answer is a.

According to the Preoperative Nutrition Scale, a BMI of less than 18.5 kg/m^2 in an adult younger than 65 years (<20 kg/m^2 if >65 years of age) identifies malnutrition. Other independent diagnostic criteria include less than 50% meal consumption over the past 7 days or a greater than 8 pound weight loss over the past 3 months. A malnourished patient has an increased risk of morbidity and mortality. They should be referred for a nutrition consultation and provided with 7–14 days of 1.2–2.0 g/kg/day of protein supplementation preoperatively to counterbalance the catabolic state of surgery. The increased protein intake goal should continue into the postoperative period as well.

15. A 66-year-old woman is undergoing repair of an incisional hernia that was a complication of an open cholecystectomy 1 year ago. She has hypertension treated with amlodipine. She denies any chest pain or shortness of breath, but she states that she cannot do anything strenuous due to sciatica pain. She frequently weeds her garden and has sexual relations. She was able to play doubles tennis as recently as 2 years ago. Her physical examination is negative with a BMI of 25 kg/m^2. What preoperative testing is needed?

    a. Stress testing.
    b. 6-minute walk test (6MWT).
    c. Frailty screen.
    d. ECG.
    e. None of the above.

The correct answer is e.

According to the RCRI, this patient has only 1 point for the planned intraperitoneal surgery. Therefore, she is considered low (0.9%) MACE risk. This patient is unlikely to be frail considering her ability to do gardening. Considering the five domains of slowness, resistance, shrinkage, weakness, and low physical activity, her ability to garden and participate in sexual relations suggests that she can attain more than 4 METs. According to the ACC/AHA cardiac evaluation for noncardiac surgery, this patient may proceed to surgery without any further cardiac testing which includes no ECG. The 6MWT is useful to evaluate heart failure, dyspnea, or COPD.

16. Which of the following are useful to screen for sleep apnea?

   a. Neck circumference >40 cm.
   b. Age >50 years.
   c. BMI >35 kg/m^2.
   d. Male sex.
   e. All of the above.

The correct answer is e.

According to Chung et al., the STOP-Bang criteria are loud snoring, daytime tiredness, observed apnea, treatment for hypertension, BMI over 35 kg/m^2, age older than 50 years, neck circumference greater than 40 cm, and male gender. This pushes the score into the intermediate range of 3–4. Patients planning surgeries requiring significant opioids or a surgery that may impair effective ventilation and oxygenation should undergo polysomnography if they score 5 or higher on STOP-bang.

17. The following statement(s) is/are true regarding BNP:

   a. A high BNP is always associated with a high MACE risk.
   b. Perioperative BNP can be used to evaluate patients with heart failure.
   c. BNP is released by the brain in response to myocardial distension.
   d. All of the above.
   e. None of the above.

The correct answer is b.

Preoperative BNP can be used to evaluate systolic or diastolic dysfunction and heart failure. BNP is released from stretched or injured cardiac myocytes, not the brain. An elevated BNP is associated with increased MACE.[9] BNP can be used to follow the course of HF treatment.

18. A 64-year-old man with chronic hypertension and newly diagnosed atrial fibrillation is presenting for surgery to correct a radial fracture malunion. What is his CHA$_2$DS$_2$-VASc score?

   a. 0.
   b. 1.
   c. 2.
   d. 3.
   e. 4.

The correct answer is b.

The patient earns only 1 point for his hypertension. Neither his age nor his sex is worth a point. As a result, he has a low annual risk for thromboembolic events. He does not need anticoagulation with warfarin for his atrial fibrillation. However, once he turns 65 years of age, he will earn another CHA$_2$DS$_2$-VASc point for being 65–74 years of age. At that age, his stroke risk increases from low to high, thus warranting anticoagulation with warfarin.[17]

19. Which of the following statements is *false* regarding iron deficiency anemia (IDA)?

   a. Ferritin can be normal in the presence of iron deficiency.
   b. IDA is associated with an increased perioperative mortality.
   c. IDA is responsible for 50% of all anemias.
   d. All of the above.

The correct answer is d.

All of the above statements are true. IDA is responsible for at least half of all anemias.[24] It increases perioperative morbidity and mortality, and it is very treatable with preoperative IV iron infusions preparations. A serum ferritin of less than 30 ng/dL or transferrin saturation of 20% or lower is diagnostic of iron deficiency. Ferritin is an acute phase reactant so a transferrin saturation of 20% or lower is diagnostic of iron deficiency if the ferritin is less than 800 ng/dL.

20. Which of the following statements regarding functional capacity assessment is/are true?

   a. A patient with low MACE risk must be able to achieve 4 metabolic equivalents (METs) before surgery.
   b. The Duke Activity Status Index (DASI) is not a reliable measure of functional capacity.
   c. Climbing two flights of stairs is a MET level of 4.
   d. All of the above are true.

The correct answer is c.

According to the ACC/AHA cardiac evaluation for noncardiac surgery, a patient without angina with a less than 1% risk of MACE needs no further testing before surgery. The DASI is self-reported and allows for calculation of a $\dot{V}O_2$ max, which can be translated into METs. Walking two flights of stairs is the equivalent of 4 or more METs. These patients do not benefit from further cardiac testing. However, high-risk patients should be medically optimized with aspirin and statin therapy.[7]

REFERENCES

1. Pearse RM, Beattie S, Clavien PA, et al. Global patient outcomes after elective surgery: Prospective cohort study in 27 low-, middle- and high-income countries. *Br J Anaesth*. 2016 Oct 31;117(5):601–609.
2. El Solh AA, Aquilina AT, Gunen H, Ramadan F. Radiographic resolution of community-acquired bacterial pneumonia in the elderly. *J Am Geriatr Soc*. 2004;52(2):224–229.
3. Camarri B, Eastwood PR, Cecins NM, Thompson PJ, Jenkins S Six minute walk distance in healthy subjects aged 55–75 years. *Respir Med*. 2006 Apr;100(4):658–665.
4. Enright PL, Sherrill DL. Reference equations for the six-minute walk in healthy adults. *Am J Respir Crit Care Med*. 1998 Nov;158(5 Pt 1):1384–1387.
5. Keeratichananont W, Thanadetsuntorn C, Keeratichananont S. Value of preoperative 6-minute walk test for predicting postoperative pulmonary complications. *Ther Adv Respir Dis*. 2016 Feb;10(1):18–25.

6. Frank SM, Rothschild JA, Masear CG, Rivers RJ, Merritt WT, Savage WJ, Ness PM. Optimizing preoperative blood ordering with data acquired from an anesthesia information management system. *Anesthesiology*. 2013 Jun;118(6):1286–1297.
7. Fleisher LA, Fleischmann KE, Auerbach AD, et al. 2014 ACC/AHA guideline on perioperative cardiovascular evaluation and management of patients undergoing noncardiac surgery: A report of the American College of Cardiology/American Heart Association Task Force on practice guidelines. *J Am Coll Cardiol*. 2014;64(22):e77–137.
8. Glance LG, Faden E, Dutton RP, Lustik SJ, Li Y, Eaton MP, Dick AW. Impact of the choice of risk model for identifying low-risk patients using the 2014 American College of Cardiology/American Heart Association Perioperative Guidelines. *Anesthesiology*. 2018;129(5):889–900.
9. Malhotra AK, Ramakrishna H. N-terminal pro B type natriuretic peptide in high cardiovascular-risk patients for noncardiac surgery: What is the current prognostic evidence? *Ann Card Anaesth*. 2016 Apr-Jun;19(2):314–320.
10. Levine GN, Bates ER, Bittl JA, et al. 2016 ACC/AHA guideline focused update on duration of dual antiplatelet therapy in patients with coronary artery disease: A report of the American College of Cardiology/American Heart Association Task Force on Clinical Practice Guidelines. *J Thorac Cardiovasc Surg*. 2016 Nov;152(5):1243–1275.
11. Hodgkinson JA, Taylor CJ, Hobbs FD. Predictors of incident atrial fibrillation and influence of medications: A retrospective case-control study. *Br J Gen Pract*. 2011 Jun;61(587):e353–e361.
12. Chung F, Chau E, Yang Y, Liao P, Hall R, Mokhlesi B. Serum bicarbonate level improves specificity of STOP-Bang screening for obstructive sleep apnea. *Chest*. 2013 May;143(5):1284–1293.
13. Wischney PE, Carli F, Evans DC, Guilbert S, Kozar R, et al. Perioperative Quality Initiative (POQI) 2 Workgroup. American Society for Enhanced Recovery and Perioperative Quality Initiative Joint Consensus Statement on nutrition screening and therapy within a surgical enhanced recovery pathway. *Anesth Analg*. 2018 Jun;126(6):1883–1895.
14. Cederholm T, Bosaeus I, Barazzoni R, et al. Diagnostic criteria for malnutrition: An ESPEN Consensus Statement. *Clin Nutr*. 2015 Jun;34(3):335–340.
15. Makary MA, Segev DL, Pronovost PJ, et al. Frailty as a predictor of outcomes in older patients. *J Am Coll Surg*. 2010;210:901.
16. Chow WB, Rosenthal RA, Merkow RP, Ko CY, Esnaola NF; American College of Surgeons National Surgical Quality Improvement Program; American Geriatrics Society. Optimal preoperative assessment of the geriatric surgical patient: A best practices guideline from the American College of Surgeons National Surgical Quality Improvement Program and the American Geriatrics Society. *J Am Coll Surg*. 2012 Oct;215(4):453–466.
17. Rockwood K, Song X, MacKnight C, Bergman H, et al. A global clinical measure of fitness and frailty in elderly people. *CMAJ*. 2005 Aug 30;173(5):489–495.
18. Prasada S, Desai MY, Saad M, et al. Preoperative atrial fibrillation and cardiovascular outcomes after noncardiac surgery. *J Am Coll Cardiol*. 2022 Jun 28;79(25):2471–2485.
19. Lip GY, Nieuwlaat R, Pisters R, Lane DA, Crijns HJ. Refining clinical risk stratification for predicting stroke and thromboembolism in atrial fibrillation using a novel risk factor-based approach: The euro heart survey on atrial fibrillation. *Chest*. 2010 Feb;137(2):263–272.
20. January CT, Wann LS, Alpert JS, et al. American College of Cardiology/American Heart Association Task Force on Practice Guidelines. 2014 AHA/ACC/HRS guideline for the management of patients with atrial fibrillation: A report of the American College of Cardiology/American Heart Association Task Force on Practice Guidelines and the Heart Rhythm Society. *J Am Coll Cardiol*. 2014 Dec 2;64(21):e1–76.
21. Hausman MS, Jewell ES, Engoren M. Regional versus general anesthesia in surgical patients with chronic obstructive pulmonary disease: Does avoiding general anesthesia reduce the risk of postoperative complications? *Anesth Analg*. 2015 Jun;120(6):1405–1412.
22. Rogers JG, Pagani FD, Tatooles AJ, et al. Intrapericardial left ventricular assist device for advanced heart failure. *N Engl J Med*. 2017 Feb 2;376(5):451–460.
23. Hausman MS Jr, Jewell ES, Engoren M. Regional versus general anesthesia in surgical patients with chronic obstructive pulmonary disease: Does avoiding general anesthesia reduce the risk of postoperative complications? *Anesth Analg*. 2015 Jun;120(6):1405–1412.
24. Cammu G. Residual neuromuscular blockade and postoperative pulmonary complications: What does the recent evidence demonstrate? *Curr Anesthesiol Rep*. 2020;10(2):131–136.
25. Chern YJ, You JF, Cheng CC, et al. Decreasing postoperative pulmonary complication following laparoscopic surgery in elderly individuals with colorectal cancer: A competing risk analysis in a propensity score-weighted cohort study. *Cancers (Basel)*. 2021 Dec 28;14(1):131.
26. Global RPH. https://globalrph.com/medcalcs/calculation-of-the-total-iron-deficit-equation-appears-in-cosmofer-pi/
27. Han MK, Muellerova H, Curran-Everett D, et al. GOLD 2011 disease severity classification in COPD Gene: A prospective cohort study. *Lancet Respir Med*. 2013;1(1):43–50.
28. Burton BN, A'Court AM, Brovman EY, Scott MJ, Urman RD, Gabriel RA. Optimizing preoperative anemia to improve patient outcomes. *Anesthesiol Clin*. 2018 Dec;36(4):701–713.
29. Gupta PK, Sundaram A, Mactaggart JN, et al. Preoperative anemia is an independent predictor of postoperative mortality and adverse cardiac events in elderly patients undergoing elective vascular operations. *Ann Surg*. 2013 Dec;258(6):1096–1102.
30. Beattie WS, Karkouti K, Wijeysundera DN, Tait G. Risk associated with preoperative anemia in noncardiac surgery: A single-center cohort study. *Anesthesiology*. 2009 Mar;110(3):574–581.
31. Nalado AM, Mahlangu JN, Duarte R, et al. Utility of reticulocyte haemoglobin content and percentage hypochromic red cells as markers of iron deficiency anaemia among black CKD patients in South Africa. *PLoS One*. 2018;13(10):e0204899.
32. Litton E, Xiao J, Ho KM. Safety and efficacy of intravenous iron therapy in reducing requirement for allogeneic blood transfusion: Systematic review and meta-analysis of randomised clinical trials. *BMJ*. 2013 Aug 15;347:f4822.
33. McWilliams B, Yazer MH, Cramer J, Triulzi DJ, Waters JH. Incomplete pretransfusion testing leads to surgical delays. *Transfusion*. 2012;52:2139–2144.
34. Frank SM, Oleyar MJ, Ness PM, Tobian AA. Reducing unnecessary preoperative blood orders and costs by implementing an updated institution-specific maximum surgical blood order schedule and a remote electronic blood release system. *Anesthesiology*. 2014 Sep;121(3):501–509.
35. Nishimura RA, Otto CM, Bonow RO, et al. 2014 AHA/ACC Guideline for the Management of Patients With Valvular Heart Disease: executive summary: a report of the American College of Cardiology/American Heart Association Task Force on Practice Guidelines [published correction appears in Circulation. 2014 Jun 10;129(23):e650]. *Circulation*. 2014;129(23):2440–2492.
36. Douglas PS, Garcia MJ, Haines DE, et al. ACCF/ASE/AHA/ASNC/HFSA/HRS/SCAI/SCCM/SCCT/SCMR 2011 appropriate use criteria for echocardiography: A report of the American College of Cardiology Foundation Appropriate Use Criteria Task Force, American Society of Echocardiography, American Heart Association, American Society of Nuclear Cardiology, Heart Failure Society of America, Heart Rhythm Society, Society for Cardiovascular Angiography and Interventions, Society of Critical Care Medicine, Society of Cardiovascular Computed Tomography, and Society for Cardiovascular Magnetic Resonance endorsed by the American College of Chest Physicians. *J Am Coll Cardiol*. 2011;57(9):1126–1166.
37. Agarwal S, Rajamanickam A, Bajaj NS, et al. Impact of aortic stenosis on postoperative outcomes after noncardiac surgeries. *Circ Cardiovasc Qual Outcomes*. 2013 Mar 1;6(2):193–200.

38. van Diepen S, Bakal JA, McAlister FA, Ezekowitz JA. Mortality and readmission of patients with heart failure, atrial fibrillation, or coronary artery disease undergoing noncardiac surgery: An analysis of 38 047 patients. *Circulation*. 2011 Jul 19;124(3):289–296.
39. Ge Y, Ha ACT, Atzema CL, et al. Association of atrial fibrillation and oral anticoagulant use with perioperative outcomes after major noncardiac surgery. *J Am Heart Assoc*. 2017 Dec 12;6(12):e006022.
40. Lane DA, Lip GY. Use of the CHA_2DS_2-VASc and HAS-BLED scores to aid decision making for thromboprophylaxis in nonvalvular atrial fibrillation. *Circulation*. 2012 Aug 14;126(7):860–865.
41. Jaakkola S, Nuotio I, Kiviniemi TO, Virtanen R, Issakoff M, Airaksinen KEJ. Incidence and predictors of excessive warfarin anticoagulation in patients with atrial fibrillation: The EWA study. *PLoS One*. 2017;12(4):e0175975.
42. Chee YL, Crawford JC, Watson HG, Greaves M. Guidelines on the assessment of bleeding risk prior to surgery or invasive procedures. British Committee for Standards in Haematology. *Br J Haematol*. 2008 Mar;140(5):496–504.
43. Liu JB, Liu Y, Cohen ME, Ko CY, Sweitzer BJ. Defining the intrinsic cardiac risks of operations to improve preoperative cardiac risk assessments. *Anesthesiology*. 2018 Feb;128(2):283–292.
44. Keay L, Lindsley K, Tielsch J, Katz J, Schein O. Routine preoperative medical testing for cataract surgery. *Cochrane Database Syst Rev*. 2012;(3):CD007293.
45. Li MH, Bolshinsky V, Ismail H, et al. Comparison of Duke Activity Status Index with cardiopulmonary exercise testing in cancer patients. *J Anesth*. 2018 Aug;32(4):576–584.
46. Memtsoudis SG, Stundner O, Rasul R, et al. The impact of sleep apnea on postoperative utilization of resources and adverse outcomes. *Anesth Analg*. 2014 Feb;118(2):407–418.
47. Chung F, Abdullah HR, Liao P. STOP-BANG questionnaire: A practical approach to screen for obstructive sleep apnea. *Chest*. 2016 Mar;149(3):631–638.
48. Chung F, Yang Y, Brown R, Liao, P. Alternative scoring models of STOP-Bang questionnaire improve specificity to detect undiagnosed obstructive sleep apnea. *J Clin Sleep Med*. 2014 Sep 15;10(9):951–958.
49. Czoski-Murray C, Lloyd Jones M, McCabe C, et al. What is the value of routinely testing full blood count, electrolytes and urea, and pulmonary function tests before elective surgery in patients with no apparent clinical indication and in subgroups of patients with common comorbidities: A systematic review of the clinical and cost-effective literature. *Health Technol Assess*. 2012 Dec;16(50):i–xvi, 1–159.
50. Feldman M, Friedman L, Brandt L. *Sleisenger and Fordtran's Gastrointestinal and Liver Disease: Pathophysiology, Diagnosis, Management*, 9. Elsevier; 2009.
51. Vestbo J, Prescott E, Almdal T, Dahl M, Nordestgaard BG, et al. Body mass, fat-free body mass, and prognosis in patients with chronic obstructive pulmonary disease from a random population sample: Findings from the Copenhagen City Heart Study. *Am J Respir Crit Care Med*. 2006 Jan 1;173(1):79–83.
52. Ingadottir AR, Beck AM, Baldwin C, et al. Two components of the new ESPEN diagnostic criteria for malnutrition are independent predictors of lung function in hospitalized patients with chronic obstructive pulmonary disease (COPD). *Clin Nutr*. 2018 Aug;37(4):1323–1331.
53. Kyle UG, Schutz Y, Dupertuis YM, Pichard C. Body composition interpretation: Contributions of the fat-free mass index and the body fat mass index. *Nutrition*. 2003 Jul-Aug;19(7–8):597–604.
54. Good Calculators. https://goodcalculators.com/ffmi-fat-free-mass-index-calculator/
55. Lin HS, McBride RL, Hubbard RE. Frailty and anesthesia: Risks during and post-surgery. *Local Reg Anesth*. 2018;11:61–73.
56. Chao CT, Wang J, Chien KL; COhort of GEriatric Nephrology in NTUH (COGENT) study group. Both pre-frailty and frailty increase healthcare utilization and adverse health outcomes in patients with type 2 diabetes mellitus. *Cardiovasc Diabetol*. 2018 Sep 27;17(1):130.
57. Alvarez-Nebreda ML, Bentov N, Urman RD, et al. Recommendations for preoperative management of frailty from the Society for Perioperative Assessment and Quality Improvement (SPAQI). *J Clin Anesth*. 2018 Jun;47:33–42.

4.

MY 79-YEAR-OLD PATIENT FOR RIGHT INGUINAL HERNIA REPAIR HAS NO LABS ON FILE

Wiebke Ackermann and Barbara Rogers

STEM CASE AND KEY QUESTIONS

Your next patient has arrived for his surgery today at your free-standing ambulatory surgery center. He is a 79-year-old man for a right inguinal hernia repair and has no laboratory tests (labs) available for review. He has hypertension and takes metoprolol and furosemide daily; he has no other diagnoses listed. He lives independently with his wife.

The patient complains that the hernia has been causing him intermittent discomfort and is impacting his daily life. He decided it should be surgically repaired.

What is an inguinal hernia? What are the common presenting symptoms?

Your patient noticed a lump in his right groin area. The lump becomes larger with straining, coughing, and lifting objects. He has been able to push the bulge back in and has purchased a hernia belt from the local drug store.

Are there complications related to an inguinal hernia? When is repair necessary?

An inguinal hernia that is asymptomatic may be treated conservatively. Once the hernia causes symptoms, many people desire surgical repair. The hernia will not resolve spontaneously without surgery and over time it will become larger. If the hernia were to become trapped, or *incarcerated*, emergency surgery would be necessary. Our patient does not want to risk being subjected to an emergency surgical procedure and has planned for today's elective repair.

The patient asks what the surgical repair options are? Are there any complications?

Inguinal hernias can be surgically repaired in an open fashion or laparoscopically. The surgeon may use mesh in the repair. There can be complications related to the actual surgical repair, from the anesthesia, or from patient-derived factors. These complications include bleeding, infection, postoperative urinary retention (POUR), ileus, postoperative nausea and vomiting (PONV), cardiopulmonary complications, chronic postsurgical pain (CPSP), and hernia recurrence.

The patient and surgeon have decided on a laparoscopic repair of his inguinal hernia.

The patient and family are concerned about anesthesia. They wish to avoid general anesthesia (GA). What are his alternatives?

Anesthesia options depend on the type of hernia repair that is planned. The patient is having a laparoscopic repair and will have GA.

Are there any required laboratory tests for this surgery?

Your patient had labs drawn for an annual physical less than a year ago.

Does he need repeat labs for surgery? Does patient age affect the need for labs?

No required laboratory tests are specific to inguinal hernia repair surgery or anesthesia. There is no age-specific required testing. All testing should be based on the patient's history and physical examination. He has hypertension and has been taking a beta blocker and furosemide for more than 5 years. He does not take potassium supplementation. He denies muscle weakness, fatigue, or palpitations.

The examining physician reviews a complete blood count and a chemistry panel in the electronic medical record from 6 months ago. Findings are within normal limits.

Your patient tells you he works full time as a school bus driver, takes care of his two-story house, and push mows his 2-acre yard.

He is wondering if you will be ordering an ECG. What are the indications for a preoperative ECG preoperatively?

An ECG in the electronic medical record from 18 months ago shows normal sinus rhythm with first-degree AV block (PR = 126 ms), normal axis, no ST/T wave abnormalities.

Your patient thinks he has a "urinary problem" and wants to know if you are going to get a urine sample. What are the indications for preoperative urinalysis?

All testing should be based on the patient's history and physical. No urinalysis is routinely needed for surgery.

What is the patient's American Society of Anesthesiologists (ASA) classification? ASA physical status classification system has been used as a risk assessment tool since the 1940s—*see discussion below.*

Is he a candidate for your outpatient surgery center, which is close to his house?

See discussion below.

The patient and family have heard reports of anesthesia causing irreversible cognitive dysfunction. The family knows of elderly friends that "were never the same" after anesthesia.

Although the patient has had surgery before and has had no issues with mentation after surgery, they are very, very concerned.

What can be done to prevent this happening to him?

This is a common concern for elderly surgical patients and their families. As the population in general lives longer, more elderly patients will need surgery. Some of these patients may have mild cognitive impairment that is not yet diagnosed.

Postoperative neurocognitive dysfunction is a condition that happens after surgery and is defined as a new cognitive dysfunction. It can cause memory impairment and difficulty with executive tasks. It differs from delirium in that there is no fluctuation in consciousness. It is more common in patients 60 years old and older. To diagnose cognitive dysfunction, psychometric testing must be done preoperatively. The preoperative results are compared to postoperative results. As yet, there is no convincing evidence that one anesthesia type has lower incidence of postoperative cognitive dysfunction compared to another. Some studies show it may happen more with longer, complex surgeries.

DISCUSSION

HERNIA SURGERY

Inguinal hernias are the *most common type of hernia*, accounting for around 75% of all anterior abdominal wall hernias, with a prevalence of 4% in those over the age of 45. More than 20 million surgeries of inguinal hernia repair are performed worldwide.[1] The inguinal hernia is an abnormal anatomic condition that is more common in men than women. Two-thirds of patients with hernias will have symptoms. Some factors contribute to increase prevalence of abdominal wall hernias in the elderly population, and they include loss of strength of the abdominal wall and the existence of concurrent medical conditions that increase intra-abdominal pressure such as chronic pulmonary disease, prostatic hypertrophy, etc.[2]

An inguinal hernia occurs when abdominal contents (fat or small intestines) extrude through the abdominal wall. There are two types of inguinal hernias, indirect and direct. An indirect inguinal hernia (80%) is a congenital anomaly. They arise from an incomplete closure of the processus vaginalis. Direct hernias are acquired, more common in men, and usually age related (>40). The main risk factors for developing an inguinal hernia are male sex, increasing age, increased intra-abdominal pressure, and abdominal wall laxity. The patient may complain of pain and a groin bulge that worsens with coughing and straining. Over time, the bulge may enlarge. A hernia is considered "reducible" when gentle pressure over the bulge will essentially push it back into the abdomen when the patient lies in a supine position.[2] Rarely, a hernia can be irreducible and can complicate with symptoms of small bowel obstruction—this constitutes a medical emergency.

An inguinal hernia will not resolve without surgery. Therefore, the presence of an inguinal hernia is considered a sufficient cause for a surgical intervention; the probability of an asymptomatic hernia becoming a symptomatic hernia may be as high as 75% in 10 years.[1]

Symptomatic patients should undergo repair. The main goals of elective hernia surgery are symptomatic improvement and prevention of acute surgical emergencies such as incarceration (abdominal contents extrude through the inguinal canal and cannot be reduced) or strangulation (incarcerated hernia not treated in timely fashion). With interruption of the blood supply to the intestine in an incarcerated hernia, this will present as an irreducible and tender tense lump, with the pain often being out of proportion to clinical signs. This presentation frequently accompanied with clinical features of intestinal obstruction. Emergency repair is known to carry significantly higher rates of morbidity and mortality, especially among the elderly.[3] Watchful waiting in the elderly patient with inguinal hernia had been advocated in the past, primary due to concerns in inguinodynia and costs[4,5]; however, most recent evidence shows that elective hernia repair can be safely performed in the elderly patient. The patient and the surgeon should decide when elective repair is the best option. Once the hernia strangulates, surgery is no longer optional: this is a surgical emergency.

Many techniques for hernia repair have been described (>100), such as open with or without mesh and laparo-endoscopic mesh repair techniques.[6] Proponents of laparoscopic inguinal hernia repair cite shorter recovery times. A study by Zanella et al concluded that laparoscopic inguinal hernia repair is cost effective and there is no contraindication to repair in the elderly.[7] Ciftci, in a prospective study in 108 patients older than 75 years, showed that laparoscopic hernia repair was a safe procedure in this population without an increase morbidity or mortality.[8] Similar results were reported by He et al. in a retrospective study of 3,203 cases of laparoscopic hernia repair performed in patients older than 60 years.[9] The Guidelines of the Hernia-Surge Group recommend that the surgical treatment should be tailored based on surgeon expertise, local resources, patient- and hernia-related factors, unilateral versus bilateral hernia, gender, recurrence, scrotal hernia, previous lower abdominal or pelvic surgery, severe cardiopulmonary comorbidities, and incarceration.[2] These guidelines strongly recommend a mesh-based repair technique for patients with inguinal or femoral hernias.[2,10] Surgical treatment is successful in most cases, with an average rate of postsurgical recurrence of 11%. Recurrence rates are as high as 15%, but accurate data are lacking because follow-up periods vary. Highly specialized hernia centers have recurrence rates as low as 1%.[2,11]

The most common postoperative complications of hernia repair include acute pain, bruising, hematoma, and POUR. Urinary retention is more common (12–15%) in males due to preexisting benign prostatic hypertrophy (BPH). Increased

BMI, bilateral repair, and increased length of operative time are other risk factors.[12] Less common are damage to the vas deferens or testicular vessel, leading to ischemic orchitis. Delayed postoperative complications are recurrence (1% within 5 years) and chronic pain (persisting more than 3 months after surgery), with an incidence of 30%; pain may become disabling in 2% of patients. Hernia registries in several countries, as well as the National Surgical Quality Improvement Program (NSQIP), have shown an increased risk of perioperative complications in patients older than 65 years undergoing open and laparoscopic procedures when compared with younger patients.[13–15] Mayer et al. analyzed the data of 24,571 patients undergoing hernia repair and concluded that patients older than 65 years have a higher rate of perioperative complications associated with laparoscopic inguinal hernia surgery, particularly in those over the age of 80.[16] Chlebny et al., in a recent prospective study done in 132 patients undergoing hernia repair in elective and emergency settings, showed that 18 patients developed complications (13.6%), 8 (50%) of those in the emergency surgery group but only 10 (8,6%) in those having elective surgery. They also demonstrated that, in the emergency group, severe medical complications were frequent, whereas in the elective group, severity of surgical and medical complications were classified as mild.[17]

Chronic postoperative pain after inguinal hernia repair is a common complication. Its incidence is lower after laparoscopic procedures (6%) than in open repair (18%).[18] Postsurgical chronic pain interferes significantly with daily activities (10–12%).[19,20] Preventive measures to minimize postsurgical chronic pain include knowledge of risk factors, use of multimodal analgesic techniques, optimization of prosthetic materials (mesh), and meticulous attention to the surgical anatomy and technique.[18]

PERIOPERATIVE MANAGEMENT

Current evidence shows that, although elective hernia repair in the elderly patient carries a mortality rate similar to the general population, the emergent procedure is associated with a higher mortality rate.[21,22] Therefore, every effort should be made to operate early and on an elective basis. The developments in regional anesthesia and perioperative monitoring guarantee much better outcomes in hernia repair regardless of the surgical technique.[17] Main concerns about postoperative adverse events in elderly surgical patients are related to decompensation of cardiac and pulmonary function, as well as deterioration of cognitive function.[23]

Anesthesia options include local infiltration by the surgeon if the hernia is small. Larger hernias are repaired in an open fashion or laparoscopically. For open repair, either regional or general anesthesia can be used. Laparoscopic repair, done in Trendelenburg position with peritoneal insufflation usually requires GA. In the elderly patient with comorbidities, the choice of anesthesia is an important decision. Metanalyses and other studies have not definitively elucidated whether regional anesthesia is more advantageous than GA. Nevertheless, the incidence of hemodynamic and respiratory complications, as well as the use of opioids, has been reported lower with the use of regional anesthesia.[24–26] Regional anesthesia can be used for emergent hernia repair, but it is more common for the patient to have GA.[17]

Cognitive dysfunction after anesthesia and surgery is not a new trend. It was first referenced by Savage in 1887.[27] Patients are increasingly concerned about their brain function. Papers in the 1900s seemed to indicate that people older than 65 have a risk of confusion after surgery. Though this research acknowledges the issue, there is no understanding of why. Some postulate that it is somehow related to hypoxia that may happen during anesthesia and surgery. The term postoperative cognitive dysfunction (POCD) became popular in the 1980s, when patients were tested before and after major surgery and the results were compared. Unfortunately, some of the results only showed data for groups of people and not individuals, so defining predictors of cognitive decline was not possible. There have been studies that look at individual patients, but each study has different definitions for what constitutes POCD. This makes comparing the studies very difficult. Additionally, the term POCD does not have any official description in the International Classification of Disease or the *Diagnostic and Statistical Manual of Mental Disorders* (DSM). Prospective studies that look at patient's cognitive state more than 12 months after surgery are ongoing. In 2018, Evered and colleagues proposed the nomenclature change to *perioperative neurocognitive disorders* (PND) to address the needs of standardization of diagnosis and for the purposes of research.[28] There is yet to be a standardized care plan for avoiding PND, partly because the pathogenesis is not fully understood. There is some evidence that it could be related to an inflammatory reaction that might let macrophages impair the function of the hippocampus.[29] It is not consistent that patients with cognitive dysfunction preoperatively will get worse after surgery. No research has proved one anesthesia technique better than another.[30]

Delirium and PND are different conditions that occur after surgery, and both are common in the elderly. They are defined as a new cognitive dysfunction. Delirium is a short-lived disorder of attention and cognition and therefore easier to detect clinically. It does predispose to the development of PND. PND may persist for weeks or months, there is no fluctuation in consciousness, and it may not be obvious to the physician. Patients and family members will recognize subtle changes. Diagnosis is by standard neuropsychological testing[26] and most accurate if there is a preoperative test available for comparison.[31] Factors that increase the risk of PND are older age; preexisting cognitive decline; preexisting cerebral, cardiac, and vascular disease; alcohol abuse; low educational level; and intra- and postoperative complications. Major risk factors of postoperative delirium include severe illness, baseline dementia, dehydration, and sensory impairment.[26,31] Data from studies comparing the incidence of POCD with general versus regional anesthesia have been rather conflicting, however a recent systematic review published by Davis et al. showed no difference between regional and general anesthesia on postoperative cognitive function.[32]

POCD can significantly impact a patient's surgical recovery. These patients may have a higher rate of mortality and disability, not returning to home, and not returning to the workforce, with associated increased use of financial resources.

Our patient can be reassured that elective surgery is associated with fewer complications and so it is reasonable to proceed to avoid acute complications and allow him to return to his active and social lifestyle.

PREOPERATIVE ASSESSMENT AND TESTING

The ASA physical status classification system has been used as a risk assessment tool since the 1940s. It has been revised and updated over time.[33] Patients can be classified as ASA I through ASA VI, with an E added for emergency. Although there are limitations to the ASA classification system for patients undergoing anesthesia, it is widely used.[34] ASA II classification is used for a patient with mild systemic disease without substantial functional limitations. Accurate ASA classification not only informs risk, but also can reassure clinicians against unnecessary testing.[35,36]

The ASA practice advisory for Preoperative Evaluation,[37] from 2012, recommends that patients receive a preoperative history and physical and that other relevant records are reviewed. The advisory states that "indicated testing" is testing based on a specific clinical reason or purpose. It is not done for the purpose of "screening." The preoperative examination can take place on the day of surgery or days earlier. The advisory says that patients having more invasive procedures may benefit from this evaluation earlier than the day of surgery. Multiple studies have supported earlier literature that there are no absolute requirements for any specific test to be performed before surgery.[38-42] This is supported by regulatory bodies: ASA, The Joint Commission, and various departments of health have no required preoperative testing and the Centers for Medicare & Medicaid Services (CMS) does not have a billing code for preoperative laboratory tests. Testing should be based on patient comorbidities and surgery-specific risks.[38,43] Studies have shown that routine preoperative testing not based on the patients specific comorbidities does not decrease adverse events, and there are no studies that show elderly patients, in particular, benefit from any laboratory test, chest X-ray, or ECG in the absence of a clinical or procedural indication.[44-47] The biggest predictor of an abnormal finding on routine ECG is advanced age. Abnormal finding on a routine preoperative ECG are not associated with worse outcomes in asymptomatic individuals.[48] The 2014 AHA/ACC guidelines give a class III (no benefit) recommendation against performing these for low cardiac risk procedures.[44] An ambulatory hernia procedure carries low cardiac risk.

Despite the long-standing evidence against routine testing, it is pervasive, even for lowest-risk procedures. In a 2015 study of 440,857 patients undergoing cataract surgery, it was discovered that unnecessary preoperative laboratory tests are still frequently ordered. This appears to be more related to the surgeon's preference rather than to actual patient characteristics or needs.[38] It behooves us to move on into 21st-century medicine and assess what really matters. Geriatric syndromes are often found in those older than 65 years.[49] As the population ages, more people over the age of 65 will need a surgical procedure. Although no specific laboratory testing is needed in the elderly, there should be consideration given to frailty, POCD, and the utility of prehabilitation.

Surgery type may affect laboratory tests drawn preoperatively; for example, the need for a type and screen to administer blood products should be drawn when significant blood loss is expected. Preoperative urinalysis for patients who are asymptomatic is generally not needed. This practice leads to unnecessary antibiotics and to antibiotic resistance.[50] In endoscopic urological procedures, the treatment of asymptomatic bacteriuria is recommended and hence this would be one of the few indications for a routine preoperative urine test.[51]

SURGICAL VENUE

Settings for surgical procedures that require anesthesia range from office-based settings and freestanding outpatient surgical centers on one end of the spectrum and large university-based hospitals on the other. Outpatient surgery centers have limited recourse, especially when freestanding. They do not usually have access to resources such as ICU care, overnight observation, radiology support, laboratory support, blood bank access, advanced anesthesia equipment, invasive monitoring, respiratory therapy support, cardiac device technicians, and additional staff for help. Licensing and safety features limit the type of patients that can be treated and the type of surgeries that can be performed in these locations. The decision to perform a surgical procedure in an outpatient surgical center versus a hospital should be based on the type of procedure and the resources available at the two centers. The popularity of outpatient surgery centers has grown significantly in the United States. Providers should know details of their center's eligibility and exclusion criteria, and who to contract with if a hospital transfer is needed.[52]

Advanced age alone does not preclude a patient from care in an outpatient surgical center. However, certain comorbidities, such as severe cardiopulmonary disease, might make an surgery center inappropriate. Certain surgeries themselves, such as those requiring transfusions, may not be appropriate for a surgery center.

Our patient appears to be an ASA 2, with METS of more than 4 and no significant comorbidities. He could appropriately have his surgery in an accredited surgery center. He can be reassured that minor ambulatory surgery has low risk of PND, and a familiar home environment and regular undisturbed sleep cycles are to his advantage.

He had uneventful surgery but was not able to void before discharge. A bladder ultrasound was performed showing that he had less than 150 cc of urine in his bladder, so he was discharged home with instructions "to return to the emergency room ER if you cannot void within 6 hours." He presented to the ER with abdominal pain and was found to have 750 cc of urine in his bladder. An indwelling catheter was placed, and he was referred for urological follow-up. This minor complication was predictable by his history, but no lab testing would have added information or prevented that complication. There are validated screens for predicting POUR, with the International Prostate Symptom Score (IPSS) being one of them.[53] Preoperative tamsulosin initiation to decrease BPH symptoms and POUR has met with mixed results, but no harm.[54,55]

CONCLUSION

- The population is aging, and many of the elderly are presenting for surgeries to improve quality of life.
- Elective hernia repair is safe, even in the elderly, and should be performed to prevent higher-risk emergency incarcerated or strangulated hernia surgeries.
- The basis of preoperative assessment is a thorough history and physical examination.
- There is no requirement for routine laboratory testing for surgery.
- Testing should be done to reduce risk and improve outcomes.
- If laboratory tests are indicated, results from the past 6 months are acceptable if no change in clinical status.[37]

REVIEW QUESTIONS

A 72-year-old man presents to the preoperative clinic prior to an elective shoulder arthroscopy. He has a history of well-controlled diabetes without complications, hypertension (HTN), obesity, and atrial fibrillation. His medications are apixaban, metformin, lisinopril, metoprolol, baby aspirin, and a multivitamin. He uses the treadmill regularly without symptoms. Exam is noncontributory other than an irregularly irregular pulse (70 bpm) and BMI is 39.

1. This patient needs a preoperative ECG.
    a. True.
    b. False.

The correct answer is b.

AHA/ACC guidelines give a class III recommendation—no benefit—for this low cardiac risk procedure. It will only confirm what you already know and not change management in any way.

2. He needs a preoperative Hb A1C.
    a. True.
    b. False.

The correct answer is a.

Elevated A1C is associated with a myriad of peri- and postoperative complications. If it is above the institutional cutoff (usually 8–9) range, surgery will be delayed for better glycemic control and hopefully improved outcomes.

3. He needs a preoperative prothrombin time (PT)/partial thromboplastin time (PTT).
    a. True.
    b. False.

The correct answer is b.

It is commonly believed that anticoagulant therapy is an indication for the PT/PTT test. There may be an abnormality of one or both, but this is not a dose-dependent effect. If the indication was the INR-guided holding of coumadin it could be justified, but this is not applicable in this case and is an inappropriate waste of resources for patients on novel or non-coumadin oral anticoagulants (NOACs).

4. His PTT is 28; hence, he is noncompliant with his apixaban.
    a. True.
    b. False.

The correct answer is b.

Not every patient has an abnormal PT or PTT when taking their NOAC. The test is not even helpful in advising on medication adherence.

5. The surgeon will be using anchoring screws. He needs a urinalysis/urine culture.
    a. True.
    b. False.

The correct answer is b.

As referenced in the discussion, this practice leads to unnecessary antibiotics and to antibiotic resistance.[50]

6. The patient's procedure can be done in your freestanding ambulatory center.
    a. True.
    b. False.

The correct answer is "probably."

He is at increased risk for obstructive sleep apnea (OSA) because of his HTN on two meds, his male sex, age, high BMI, and atrial fibrillation. Severe or untreated OSA may warrant longer monitoring.

7. If the patient handed you his most recent labs done at his primary care physician's office, which of the following could be abnormal and why? Choose all that apply.
    a. Creatinine.
    b. Potassium.
    c. Hemoglobin.
    d. Bicarbonate.
    e. AST/ALT.

The correct answers are a, b, c, d, and e.

CKD increases with age especially in the setting of diabetes. Potassium could be elevated, especially with CKD in the setting of lisinopril. Hemoglobin could be high (polycythemia from hypoxia with OSA events) or low (chronic GI blood loss in setting of aspirin and apixaban).

Bicarbonate could be elevated if he has OSA complicated by obesity hypoventilation syndrome.

Fatty liver is common in the obese population with other components of metabolic syndrome (diabetes/hypertension), so AST/ALT may be abnormal. None of these tests was indicated, and it is unlikely that any management would be changed as a result of them. It is always worth considering what you would look for in lab results related to the particular patient's history and physical.

8. Would any laboratory testing predict his most likely complication?

　a. Yes.
　b. No.

The correct answer is b.

Shoulder arthroscopy is a painful procedure, with the need for opiates in the postoperative period. Opiates have side effects of sedation, PONV, and respiratory depression. If the patient has OSA, he is at risk of increased events at home on night 3, during increased REM episodes (rebound REM sleep). He needs to be educated about this risk and the interventions he should do to decrease it.[56]

REFERENCES

1. Biggerstaff B, Shetty S, Fitzgibbons RJ. Watchful waiting as a treatment strategy in patients with asymptomatic inguinal hernia. *Laparoendoscopic Hernia Surg.* 2018;51–57. https://doi.org/10.1007/978-3-662-55493-7_7
2. HerniaSurge group, International guidelines for groin hernia management. *Hernia.* 2018;**22**(1):1–165.
3. Simons MP, Aufenacker T, Bay-Nielsen M, et al. European Hernia Society guidelines on the treatment of inguinal hernia in adult patients. *Hernia.* 2009;13(4):343–403.
4. Gianetta E, de Cian F, Cuneo S, et al. Hernia repair in elderly patients. *Br J Surg.* 1997;84(7):983–985.
5. Abi-Haidar Y, Sanchez V, Itani KM. Risk factors and outcomes of acute versus elective groin hernia surgery. *J Am Coll Surg.* 2011;213(3):363–369.
6. Bendavid R. New techniques in hernia repair. *World J Surg.* 1989;13(5):522–531.
7. Zanella S, Vassiliadis A, Buccelletti F, et al. Laparoscopic totally extraperitoneal inguinal hernia repair in the elderly: A prospective control study. *Vivo.* 2015;29(4):493–496.
8. Ciftci F. Laparoscopic versus open inguinal hernia repair on patients over 75 years of age. *Int J Clin Exp Med.* 2015;8(6):10016–10020.
9. He Z, Hao X, Li J, et al. Laparoscopic inguinal hernia repair in elderly patients: Single center experience in 12 years. *Ann Laparoscop Endoscop Surg.* 2017;2:88. doi:10.21037/ales.2017.04.04
10. HerniaSurge Group. International guidelines for groin hernia management. *Hernia.* 2018;22(1):1–165. doi:10.1007/s10029-017-1668-x
11. Niebuhr H, Köckerling F. Surgical risk factors for recurrence in inguinal hernia repair: A review of the literature. *Innov Surg Sci.* 2017;2(2):53–59.
12. Hudak KE, Frelich MJ, Rettenmaier CR, et al. Surgery duration predicts urinary retention after inguinal herniorrhaphy: A single institution review. *Surg Endosc.* 2015;29(11):3246–3250.
13. Lundström KJ, Sandblom G, Smedberg S, et al. Risk factors for complications in groin hernia surgery: A national register study. *Ann Surg.* 2012;255(4):784–788.
14. Bay-Nielsen M, Kehlet H. Anaesthesia and post-operative morbidity after elective groin hernia repair: A nation-wide study. *Acta Anaesthesiol Scand.* 2008;52(2):169–174.
15. Turrentine FE, Wang H, Simpson VB, et al. Surgical risk factors, morbidity, and mortality in elderly patients. *J Am Coll Surg.* 2006;203(6):865–877.
16. Mayer F, Lechner M, Adolf D, et al. Is the age of >65 years a risk factor for endoscopic treatment of primary inguinal hernia? Analysis of 24,571 patients from the Herniamed Registry. *Surg Endosc.* 2016;30(1):296–306.
17. Chlebny T, Zelga P, Pryt M, et al. Safe and uncomplicated inguinal hernia surgery in the elderly: Message from anaesthesiologists to general surgeons. *Polski Przeglad Chirurgiczny.* 2017;89(2):5–10.
18. Reinpold W. Risk factors of chronic pain after inguinal hernia repair: A systematic review. *Innovat Surg Sci.* 2017;2(2):61–68.
19. Alfieri S, Amid PK, Campanelli G, et al. *International Guidelines for Prevention and Management of Post-operative Chronic Pain Following Inguinal Hernia Surgery*. Springer; 2011.
20. Kehlet H, Roumen RM, Reinpold W, et al. Invited commentary: Persistent pain after inguinal hernia repair: What do we know and what do we need to know? *Hernia.* 2013;17(3):293–297.
21. Wu JJ, Baldwin BC, Goldwater E, et al. Should we perform elective inguinal hernia repair in the elderly? *Hernia.* 2017;21(1):51–57.
22. McEntee G, O'Carroll A, Mooney B, et al. Timing of strangulation in adult hernias. *Br J Surg.* 1989;76(7):725–726.
23. Jin F, Chung F. Minimizing perioperative adverse events in the elderly. *Br J Anaesth.* 2001;87(4):608–624.
24. Neuman MD, Silber JH, Elkassabany NM, et al. Comparative effectiveness of regional versus general anesthesia for hip fracture surgery in adults. *Anesthesiology.* 2012;117(1):72–92.
25. Memtsoudis SG, Sun X, Chiu Y, et al. Perioperative comparative effectiveness of anesthetic technique in orthopedic patients. *J Am Soc Anesthesiol.* 2013;118(5):1046–1058.
26. Palmer RM. Perioperative care of the elderly patient: An update. *Cleve Clin J Med.* 2009;76(4):S16.
27. Savage GH. Insanity following the use of anæsthetics in operations. *Br Med J.* 1887;2(1405):1199–1200.
28. Evered L, Silbert B, Knopman DS, et al. Recommendations for the nomenclature of cognitive change associated with anaesthesia and surgery-2018. *Br J Anaesth.* 2018;121(5):1005–1012.
29. Rundshagen I. Postoperative cognitive dysfunction. *Dtsch Arztebl Int.* 2014;111(8):119–125.
30. Evered LA, Silbert BS. Postoperative cognitive dysfunction and non-cardiac surgery. *Anesth Analg.* 2018;127(2):496–505.
31. Rundshagen I. Postoperative cognitive dysfunction. *Dtsch Arztebl Int.* 2014;111(8):119.
32. Davis N, Lee M, Lin AY, et al. Post-operative cognitive function following general versus regional anesthesia: A systematic review. *J Neurosurg Anesthesiol.* 2014;26(4):369.
33. Doyle DJ, Hendrix JM, Garmon EH. American society of anesthesiologists classification. Statpearls. 2021. StatPearls Publishing. PMID: 28722969. Bookshelf ID: NBK441940.
34. Godinho P, et al. ASA classification: What is the real impact of the introduction of the new clinical examples? *J Perioper Pract.* 2019;29(7–8):203–209.
35. Nelson SE, Li G, Shi H, et al. The impact of reduction of testing at a Preoperative Evaluation Clinic for elective cases: Value added without adverse outcomes. *J Clin Anesth.* 2019;55:92–99.
36. Knuf KM, Maani CV, Cummings AK. Clinical agreement in the American Society of Anesthesiologists physical status classification. *Perioper Med (Lond).* 2018;7:14.
37. American Society of Anesthesiologists. Practice advisory for preanesthesia evaluation: An updated report by the American Society of Anesthesiologists Task Force on Preanesthesia Evaluation. *Anesthesiology.* 2012;116(3):522–538.

38. Chen CL, Lin GA, Bardach NS, et al. Preoperative medical testing in Medicare patients undergoing cataract surgery. *N Engl J Med.* 2015;372(16):1530–1538.
39. Benarroch-Gampel J, Sheffield KM, Duncan CB, et al. Preoperative laboratory testing in patients undergoing elective, low-risk ambulatory surgery. *Ann Surg.* 2012;256(3):518–528.
40. Feely MA, Collins CS, Daniels PR, et al. Preoperative testing before noncardiac surgery: Guidelines and recommendations. *Am Fam Phys.* 2013;87(6):414–418.
41. Johansson T, Fritsch G, Flamm M, et al. Effectiveness of non-cardiac preoperative testing in non-cardiac elective surgery: A systematic review. *Br J Anaesth.* 2013;110(6):926–939.
42. Kirkham KR, Wijeysundera D, Penarith C, et al. Preoperative testing before low-risk surgical procedures. *CMAJ.* 2015;187(11):E349–E358.
43. O'Neill F, Carter E, Pink N, et al. Routine preoperative tests for elective surgery: Summary of updated NICE guidance. *BMJ.* 2016;354:i3292.
44. Fleisher LA, Fleischmann KE, Auerbach AD, et al. ACC/AHA guideline on perioperative cardiovascular evaluation and management of patients undergoing noncardiac surgery: A report of the American College of Cardiology/American Heart Association Task Force on practice guidelines. *J Am Coll Cardiol.* 2014;64(22):e77–137.
45. Coelho PNMP, Miranda LMRPC, Barros PMP, et al. Quality of life after elective cardiac surgery in elderly patients. *Interact Cardiovasc Thorac Surg.* 2019;28(2):199–205.
46. Schein OD, Katz J, Bass EB, et al. The value of routine preoperative medical testing before cataract surgery. Study of medical testing for cataract surgery. *N Engl J Med.* 2000;342(3):168–175.
47. Chung F, Yuan H, Yin L, et al. Elimination of preoperative testing in ambulatory surgery. *Anesth Analg.* 2009;108(2):467–475.
48. Liu LL, Dzankic S, Leung JM. Preoperative electrocardiogram abnormalities do not predict postoperative cardiac complications in geriatric surgical patients. *J Am Geriatr Soc.* 2002;50(7):1186–1191.
49. Bettelli G. Preoperative evaluation of the elderly surgical patient and anesthesia challenges in the XXI century. *Aging Clin Exp Res.* 2018;30(3):229–235.
50. Salazar JG, O'Brien W, Strymish J, et al. Association of screening and treatment for preoperative asymptomatic bacteriuria with postoperative outcomes among US veterans. *JAMA Surg.* 2019;154(3):241–248.
51. Nicolle LE, Gupta K, Bradley S, et al. Clinical practice guideline for the management of asymptomatic bacteriuria: 2019 update by the Infectious Diseases Society of America. *Clin Infect Dis.* 2019;68(10):1611–1615.
52. Davis KK, Mahishi V, Singal R, et al. Quality improvement in ambulatory surgery centers: A major national effort aimed at reducing infections and other surgical complications. *J Clin Med Res.* 2019;11(1):7–14.
53. Fazeli F, Gooran S, Erfanian M, et al. Evaluating International Prostate Symptom Score (IPSS) in accuracy for predicting postoperative urinary retention after elective cataract surgery: A prospective study. *Global J Health Sci.* 2015 Mar 26;7(7 Spec No):93–96. doi: 10.5539/gjhs.v7n7p93.
54. Mohammadi-Fallah M, Hamedanchi S, Tayyebi-Azar A. Preventive effect of tamsulosin on postoperative urinary retention. *Korean J Urol.* 2012;53(6):419–423.
55. Papageorge CM, Howington B, Leverson G, et al. Preoperative tamsulosin to prevent postoperative urinary retention: A randomized controlled trial. *J Surg Res.* 2021;262:130–139.
56. Chung F, Liao P, Yegneswaran B, et al. Postoperative changes in sleep-disordered breathing and sleep architecture in patients with obstructive sleep apnea. *Anesthesiology.* 2014;120(2):287–298.

5.

MEDICATION MANAGEMENT

DRUG-ELUTING STENT 2 MONTHS AGO

Julio Montejano and Angela Selzer

STEM CASE AND KEY QUESTIONS

A 62-year-old woman with a history of long-standing hip pain presents for preoperative evaluation before elective total hip replacement. She has a past medical history of coronary artery disease, well-controlled hypertension, hyperlipidemia, and type 2 diabetes. Upon further inquiry, the patient describes an episode of sudden-onset nausea and diaphoresis 2 months ago, which led to a diagnosis of ST elevation myocardial infarction (MI). Catheterization was performed during which a stent was placed but the patient does not remember details.

What are the risk factors for ischemic heart disease and signs of a MI? What are indications for coronary intervention versus medical management for patients with acute MI? What coronary interventions are available?

Upon looking at the patient's ECG, Q waves are noted in the II, III, and aVF leads.

Which type of stents are available and in which vessel do you expect a stent was deployed based on the patient's ECG findings? What if the patient presented with Q waves in the lateral leads?

The medical records confirm she received a drug-eluting stent to the right coronary artery, after which she made a full recovery and was discharged home.

Which medications do you expect to have been added to the patient's regimen consisting of amlodipine, atorvastatin, and metformin? What antiplatelet agents are available, and when should they be interrupted prior to elective procedures? How about aspirin?

In addition to her prior medications, the patient is now taking metoprolol, clopidogrel, and aspirin daily. She has been participating in a cardiac rehabilitation program.

Is this patient a candidate for elective surgery at this time? When can she safely proceed with surgery?

You tell the patient that, because of her MI and stent placement 2 months ago, her risk of perioperative MI is elevated but will continue to decrease until a year has passed.

The patient is not happy with this recommendation and is asking you for clarification.

How long after an MI could she safely undergo an elective procedure? Should a patient be prescribed medical management only and no coronary intervention after an MI? How long after a coronary intervention would you recommend the patient wait to have elective surgery? Would that differ based on the kind of intervention (balloon angioplasty vs. different types of stents)? Would your recommendation be different if a coronary intervention was done for stable coronary disease and the patient had not experienced an MI?

The surgeon and patient decide to proceed with nonsurgical management and plan to proceed with the operation once a year has passed.

Would your recommendation be different if the patient were scheduled to undergo a colonoscopy instead? What procedures require interruption of dual antiplatelet therapy (DAPT) or could be performed while continuing therapy?

Over the next 6 weeks, however, the patient begins to experience decreased vision. The ophthalmologist diagnoses the patient with optic atrophy and papilledema and refers the patient to neurology. A head computed tomography (CT) scan reveals a 3.5 cm subfrontal meningioma. The neurosurgeon she is referred to would like to resect the tumor as soon as possible.

What are the indications for surgical resection of brain tumors? What determines the urgency of surgery?

This is determined to be an urgent surgery, which should proceed as soon as possible to avoid permanent loss of vision. The neurosurgeon would like to know how soon she can place the patient on her operating schedule and has referred the patient to the preoperative assessment clinic for evaluation.

In addition to the routine preoperative evaluation, what features of the examination, history, and review of systems should be addressed in patients with brain tumors? Is any specific preoperative laboratory testing indicated? Is there a role for platelet function assays in these patients?

The patient reports occasional palpitations and a constant headache, but no vomiting, seizures, or changes in gait or mental status. Her examination is significant for papilledema.

An ECG, CBC, basic metabolic panel (BMP), HgbA1C, and a type and screen are sent.

The patient has been taking her medications as prescribed and has also been started on prednisone 4 mg four times daily.

Which medications should this patient continue, and which should be held prior to surgery? Should the patient interrupt her DAPT? Should she be bridged with another medication prior to surgery? If so, which one?

The patient stops her DAPT as instructed and proceeds to the operating room for a craniotomy and meningioma resection.

What protective measures can be taken to reduce the likelihood of intraoperative MI? What are the determinants of myocardial oxygen supply and demand? What methods are available for detection of intraoperative MI?

The patient proceeds through the operation without any complication and is transferred to the neurosurgical ICU for postoperative care. On postoperative day 2, she experiences substernal chest pain, similar to her earlier episode. The ICU team obtains a troponin level and a 12-lead ECG. She is diagnosed with a ST-elevation myocardial infarction (STEMI).

What is the most likely diagnosis? What treatment options are now available to this patient? Should she proceed to the catheterization lab?

Because of her recent intracranial surgery, the patient is medically managed.

What is the 30-day mortality rate in patients having an MI following intracranial surgery?

DISCUSSION

RISK FACTORS FOR CORONARY ARTERY DISEASE

There are five major risk factors for coronary heart disease (CHD): dyslipidemia, hypertension, obesity, diabetes, and family history of CHD. Of the 542,008 patients presenting with MI without a prior diagnosis of CHD, 85.6% of them have at least one of the major risk factors.[1] Other risk factors include age, male gender, diet, and sedentary lifestyle. Moderate alcohol intake and regular exercise are protective.[2]

TYPES OF CORONARY HEART DISEASE

CHD is further classified into stable and unstable. Stable ischemic heart disease (SIHD) typically presents with symptoms of exertional angina which lasts for a few minutes. Typical angina meets the following three characteristics: substernal chest discomfort which is provoked by exertion or emotional stress and is relieved by rest or nitroglycerin. It results from an imbalance in myocardial oxygen supply and demand.[3] Women are more likely to report atypical symptoms of angina and are, therefore, less likely to be diagnosed with SIHD. Medical management and lifestyle interventions are the cornerstones of therapy.[4]

Patients with SIHD can progress over time to unstable angina if anginal symptoms occur without an apparent precipitating trigger. The anginal symptoms of unstable angina often last longer and do respond to nitroglycerin. Unstable angina is a subgroup within acute coronary syndrome (ACS), an umbrella term which includes unstable angina and MI. In ACS, a partial rupture or erosion of an atherosclerotic plaque leads to partial or complete occlusion of coronary flow.

Unstable angina and myocardial ischemia are both types of ACS, but they differ in that biomarkers for myocardial injury are not elevated in unstable angina. Unstable angina may result from either a partially occluding thrombus or an atherosclerotic coronary vessel with reduced coronary flow.[5]

DIAGNOSING MYOCARDIAL ISCHEMIA

According to the Fourth Universal Definition of Myocardial Infarction, MI is defined as myocardial injury associated with evidence of acute myocardial ischemia (clinical symptoms, ECG findings, or imaging, angiographic or pathologic evidence).[6] Differentiating the type of MI, type 1 or type 2, has important clinical implications. Type 1 MIs occur as a result of plaque disruption and thrombosis of the coronary arteries.[7] The Fourth Universal Definition defines type 2 MI as infarctions which occur due to an imbalance in myocardial oxygen supply and demand. Type 2 MI is often multifactorial and may occur from respiratory failure, hypoxemia, shock, arrhythmia, or severe anemia especially in the setting of coronary atherosclerosis without plaque rupture. Additionally, coronary vasospasm, coronary embolism, and spontaneous coronary dissection are other forms of type 2 MI.[6]

Type 1 MI patients often have high sensitivity cardiac troponin levels (hs-cTn) several times greater than that of type 2 MI patients, although there is some overlap. In comparison to patients with a type 1 MI, type 2 MI patients are commonly older and often have risk factors for or a known diagnosis of CAD.[8] Therapeutic management also differs. Whereas type 1 MI patients should receive aggressive antithrombotic therapy and urgent coronary revascularization, type 2 patients benefit most from treatments which better balance myocardial oxygen supply to demand.[8] Electrocardiographic changes and symptoms as independent indicators of MI are unreliable of differentiators of MI type unless combined with laboratory values and patient history.

During myocardial ischemia symptoms are often nonspecific and diffuse, and its effects can be self-limited, as in stable angina, or require intervention, as in unstable angina. Any radiating pain "below the nose and above the navel" should trigger a high suspicion for ischemia. Initial ECGs may be normal. Diabetics, women, and elderly patients are more likely to present with dyspnea, weakness, vomiting, palpitations, or syncope than chest discomfort. Early suspicion, laboratory testing, and serial ECG testing may be necessary for diagnosis.[2]

Detection of an elevated cardiac troponin (cTn) level above the 99th percentile upper reference limit (URL) indicates myocardial injury. There are a number of clinical conditions

Table 5.1 CAUSES OF ELEVATED CARDIAC TROPONIN VALUES

Myocardial injury	Myocardial ischemia
Coronary revascularization procedure	Atherosclerotic plaque disruption with thrombosis
Myocarditis	Coronary artery spasm
Cardiomyopathy	Coronary embolism
Takotsubo syndrome	Coronary artery dissection
Heart failure	Sustained bradyarrhythmia
Cardiac procedure	Hypotension or shock
Cardiac contusion	Respiratory failure
Sepsis	Severe anemia
Chronic kidney disease	Sustained tachyarrhythmia
Stroke	Severe hypertension
Pulmonary embolism	
Pulmonary hypertension	
Strenuous exercise	

Adapted from Thygesen K, et al.[6]

which can result in myocardial injury (Table 5.1) The 99th percentile upper reference limit (URL) varies based on the assay system used, and the cutoff can vary from 0.015 to 0.08 ng/mL.[9] hs-cTn testing was introduced in 2010 and is now the global standard of care; it is particularly useful for rapid triage of patients presenting with chest pain.[10] However, the high sensitivity of this test comes at a cost of lowered specificity when compared to traditional cardiac troponin testing.[11] Clinical evidence of myocardial ischemia coupled with a rise and/or fall in troponin values above the 99th percentile URL is considered MI. Serial troponin measurements should be obtained, and some patients may not reach the URL value until 6 hours after initial measurement. Therapeutic decisions should not be delayed until the results of cardiac biomarkers are obtained.[12]

ELECTROCARDIOGRAM FINDINGS DURING MYOCARDIAL ISCHEMIA

There can be a spectrum of ECG findings in patients presenting with clinically concerning chest pain. For non-ST elevation MIs (NSTEMI) ECG findings include ST depression, T wave inversion, and Q waves which are associated with an increased risk of MI. STEMIs are defined as a new ST elevation in two or more anatomically contiguous leads (Table 5.2). The threshold value to define ST-segment elevation is 1 mm or greater except in leads V2 and V3. In normal individuals, the amplitude of the ST junction is highest in these leads so the threshold for considering the ST-segment is higher. For V2 and V3 ST segments to be considered elevated the amplitude must be ≥1.5 mm or greater in women, 2 mm or greater in men 40 years or older, and 2.5 mm or greater in men younger than 40 years.[13]

Infarction in the posterior descending branch territory will result in ST-segment elevation in the inferior leads (II, III, aVF) either from occlusion of the right coronary artery (RCA) or left circumflex coronary artery (LCx), depending on which is the dominant circulation. A traditional 12-lead ECG does not include the right-sided chest leads V3R and V4R. These leads can enable the distinction between an RCA or LCx occlusion. The American College of Cardiology/American Heart Association (ACC/AHA) recommends screening all patients with an inferior STEMI for right ventricular (RV) infarction by recording the right-sided chest leads.[12] If the initial ECG is not diagnostic of STEMI but the patient continues to be symptomatic, serial ECGs at 5- to 10-minute intervals should be obtained.[12]

Table 5.2 ANATOMICALLY CONTIGUOUS ECG LEADS

ANATOMIC CORRELATION OF ST-ELEVATION

ECG LEADS WITH ST ELEVATION	AFFECTED REGION OF MYOCARDIUM	OCCLUDED CORONARY ARTERY	RECIPROCAL ST DEPRESSION
aVR, V1	Septal	LMCA	In ≥8 leads
V1–V4, I, aVL, aVR	Anteroseptal	LAD (proximal)	II, III, aVF, V5
V3–V4	Anterior	LAD (mid)	aVL
V5–V6	Apical	LAD (distal), LCx or RCA	aVL
V7–V9	Inferobasilar	LCx or RCA	V1–V4
V1R–V6R	Right Ventricle	RCA (proximal)	V1–V3
I, aVL	Lateral	LCx	
II, III, avF	Inferior	PDA from LCx	I, aVL
II, III, aVF, V3R–V4R	Inferior	PDA from RCA	I, aVL

Adapted from Wagner GS, et al.[13]

DRUG ELUTING STENT • 55

The presence of a new left bundle branch block (LBBB) in the presence of clinically significant chest pain with elevated cardiac troponins should be considered an acute MI and treated as such; up to 7% of patients may present with a new LBBB.[14] A new LBBB without chest pain and cardiac troponins should not be considered an MI equivalent.

MANAGEMENT OF ST-ELEVATION MYOCARDIAL ISCHEMIA

Initial management of the STEMI patient includes administration of aspirin, morphine sulfate for analgesia (doses of 2–4 mg IV), oxygen to maintain SpO_2 of greater than 90%, discontinuation of non-aspirin NSAIDs, and initiation of beta blocker therapy in hypertensive patients. Patients with signs of heart failure, evidence of a low-output state, or relative contraindications to beta blocker therapy should not receive beta blockers. Non-hypertensive patients without these contraindications should have oral beta blocker therapy initiated within 24 hours of presentation.[15]

As per the 2009 ACC/AHA guidelines, patients with acute STEMIs presenting at hospitals with percutaneous coronary intervention (PCI) capability should be treated with primary PCI (PPCI) within 90 minutes of medical contact.[15]

PERCUTANEOUS CORONARY INTERVENTION CONSIDERATIONS

PCI is superior to coronary reperfusion through fibrinolysis because it results in a higher rate of flow through the coronaries and does not increase the risk of intracranial bleeding.[16] However, this only results in lower in-hospital mortality in institutions which perform the procedure regularly (≥17 PPCIs/year). High-volume institutions performing 49 PPCIs/year or more have the lowest mortality rate (3.4%) compared to low-volume hospitals (6.2%) where PPCI is inferior from a mortality standpoint to fibrinolysis (5.9%).[17]

When the Appropriateness Criteria for Coronary Revascularization were published in 2009, PCI was considered appropriate for patients with one- or two-vessel CAD and proximal LAD stenosis but inappropriate for left main disease.[18] However, the 2009 ACC/AHA update on the management of STEMI stated it was reasonable to consider PCI of the left main coronary in patients considered low risk of PCI complications as an alternative to coronary artery bypass grafting (CABG).[16]

Patients with contraindications for thrombolysis may not be considered candidates for PCI. There are absolute and relative contraindications outlined in Table 5.3.[19] Intracranial hemorrhage is the most feared complication of thrombolysis. However, certain high-risk patients with a thrombolytic contraindication may proceed with coronary revascularization if the benefits outweigh the risk.

Other procedural complications of PCI include failure of stent deployment, coronary dissection, intramural hematoma, coronary perforation, and branch vessel occlusion. Any of these complications can lead to ischemia, infarction, and need for emergency CABG. The incidence of post PCI emergency CABG is 0.1–0.3%.[20] Later complications include restenosis and in-stent thrombosis.

Table 5.3 SELECT CONTRAINDICATIONS TO THROMBOLYSIS

RELATIVE	ABSOLUTE
Severe hypertension (SBP>180, DBP>110 mm Hg)	History of hemorrhagic stroke
Nonhemorrhagic stroke >3 months	Nonhemorrhagic stroke <3 months
Surgery <10 days	Spine/Intracranial Surgery/Trauma <2 months
Pregnancy	Active bleeding

Adapted from Guyyat GH, et al.[19]

CORONARY STENT TYPES

Stents produce and maintain patency in the coronary arteries; however, until the stent becomes endothelialized, they carry a high risk of stent thrombosis. Therefore, DAPT (with a P2Y12 inhibitor and aspirin) should be maintained until endothelialization is complete. Two major types of coronary stents are currently being used: bare metal stents (BMS) and drug-eluting stents (DES). For BMS, endothelialization occurs rapidly—within a month after placement. However, BMS over the long term have a tendency to stenose, and, for this reason, the majority of stents placed are drug-eluting unless cessation is expected to be necessary in the short term, in which case BMS are typically placed. In contrast, DES have a polymer coating combined with an anti-stenotic drug which is released slowly to reduce neointimal proliferation and the development of in-stent stenosis. Because this slows the endothelialization process, the immediate risk of in-stent thrombosis is longer for these stents, and patients with DES require a longer period of DAPT than those with BMS. The first-generation stents contained paclitaxel (PES)[21] or sirolimus (SES)[22] and required 6 months of clopidogrel for thrombosis prophylaxis. These stents are no longer used or available in the United States.

Second-generation stents containing derivatives of sirolimus—everolimus (EES), ridaforolimus (RES), or zotarolimus (ZES)—endothelialize more rapidly, require a minimum of only 3 months of DAPT, and are as effective as their first-generation counterparts.[23,24]

The newest generation of stents focuses not on drug delivery but on the material the stent is made from: these are bioresorbable stents (BRS) and are the fourth revolution in interventional cardiology technology.[25] BRS are drug-eluting stents that act to reduce intimal proliferation and eliminate the risk of late rethrombosis by complete resorption of the scaffold. This theoretically allows the coronary vessel to return to more of a native-state anatomical structure and function. BRS may require shorter DAPT duration than DES, thereby decreasing the risk of post-intervention bleeding. There are, however, several disadvantages to bioresorbable stents including limitations due to stent thickness, tensile strength, and the need for dilation prior to placement of the stent, which increases procedural duration.[26] BioFreedom is a type of BRS which has undergone clinical trials investigating the optimal duration of DAPT and showed that DAPT could be shortened to 1 month with better long-term outcomes when compared to BMS.[27]

OPTIMAL DURATION OF DUAL ANTIPLATELET THERAPY

DAPT reduces but does not eliminate the risk of in-stent thrombus and must be continued for a period of time after myocardial revascularization. In 2016, the ACC/AHA published a focused update on duration of DAPT in patients with CAD.[14] A year and a half later, in 2018, the European Society of Cardiology (ESC) published a focused update on DAPT in CAD in collaboration with the European Association of Cardio-Thoracic Surgery (EACTS).[28] Both of these updates make recommendation on platelet inhibitor selection, management based on different clinical scenarios, and the use of proton pump inhibitors. However, there are important differences, much of which can be attributed to the later publication date of the ESC update and, therefore, inclusion of more clinical trials.[29] The optimal duration of DAPT after insertion of a BMS is 1 month; however, in clinical practice, DES have largely replaced the use of BMS.

Both societies recommend a default duration of DAPT following PCI and DES placement of 6 months for SIHD and 12 months for ACS. Therefore, elective surgery should be postponed ideally for at least 1 year following DES placement for ACS (Class I recommendation). However, when circumstances dictate a more urgent surgery, this interval can be shortened to 6 months (Class IIb recommendations) or even 3 months (Class IIb recommendation) per the recent ESC guidelines for perioperative care.[30]

In very high bleeding risk patients who underwent PCI for SIHD, 3 months of therapy may be acceptable following DES according to ACC/AHA guidelines while the ESC allows for only 1 month of DAPT.[30]

Because of inclusion of additional clinical trials, the recommendation for selection of ticagrelor or prasugrel over clopidogrel for P2Y12 inhibitor therapy in ACS is a Class I recommendation in the ESC update, but Class IIa in the ACC/AHA update.[29] Importantly, both the ACC/AHA and ESC emphasize that all patients, regardless of stent type or age should continue low-dose aspirin indefinitely.[14,28] There are a number of clinical trials currently in progress which will contribute data toward our understanding of optimal aspirin dosing in these patients. An aspirin-free approach to long-term medical therapy is also being studied. One such trial is the ADAPTABLE (Comparative Effectiveness of Aspirin Dosing in Cardiovascular Disease) study which randomized 15,076 patients to receive 81 mg versus 325 mg aspirin and found no significant difference between groups for any of the primary outcomes including mortality and hospitalization for MI or stroke (hazard ratio [HR] 1.02, 95% confidence interval [CI] 0.91–1.14). Based on this study, 81 mg of aspirin appears as efficacious as 325 mg aspirin with a better side-effect profile.[31]

PREOPERATIVE EVALUATION OF PATIENTS WITH ISCHEMIC HEART DISEASE

Patients with a history of MI should have a detailed history taken which includes the date of occurrence, description of symptoms, interventions taken, and medical management. A review of symptoms should include signs of heart failure. Patients with right-sided heart failure can have ascites, edema, and jugular vein distention. Left-sided heart failure can manifest as dyspnea on exertion, nocturnal orthopnea, or rales on examination. Reports from the cardiac catheterization should be obtained and details such as severity of disease, type of stent(s) placed, and location of stent placement noted.

Patients with ischemic heart disease should continue their beta blockers perioperatively. Anti-hypertensives are continued, with the exception of angiotensin-converting enzyme (ACE) inhibitors. ACE inhibitors may be held for 24 hours in patients with well-controlled hypertension having high-risk surgery. Poorly controlled hypertensives and/or patients having low-risk surgery may benefit from continuation. Diuretics are typically withheld on the day of surgery, but exceptions may be made for patients with heart failure either with preserved ejection fraction (HFpEF) or reduced ejection fraction (HFrEF).

Management of antiplatelet medications is discussed in more detail elsewhere in this discussion.

For a highly invasive surgery such as this one, electrolytes, hemoglobin, platelet count, coagulation profile, and type and screen should be obtained. If signs of right heart failure are present, liver function testing may be warranted. In patients with diabetes, HgbA1c is helpful in determining glycemic control.

A post-MI ECG should be obtained preoperatively and is an important baseline to compare postoperative ECGs with. An echocardiogram should be obtained to evaluate left and right heart function and the presence of wall motion abnormalities (WMA) and valvular disease.

These patients should have regular follow-up with a cardiologist, and their cardiologist should be informed of the surgical plan. The cardiologist can comment on whether the patient is currently optimized, compliant with therapy, and an acceptable risk to proceed with the planned surgery.

RISK OF SURGERY AFTER CORONARY STENT PLACEMENT

With approximately 600,000 percutaneous coronary stent procedures performed annually in the United States, 4.4 to 7% of these patients will undergo noncardiac surgery within the first year following stent placement.[32,33] The 7-day incidence of MACE in these postoperative patients is 1.9%, a rate which is 27-fold above the average weekly risk in patients not receiving surgery.[33] Within the first 24 months after coronary stent placement, 22.5% of patients have non-cardiac operations, and 4.7% of these patients experience a major adverse cardiac event (MACE) following surgery.[34] The time spent between stent placement and surgery is inversely related to these events, with a 11.6% incidence of MACE if surgery is performed within 6 weeks of placement, 6.4% within 6 months, 4.2% within 12 months, and 3.5% within 24 months. Other factors which impart a higher risk of MACE include nonelective surgical admission (adjusted odds ratio [AOR] 4.77) and MI within 6 months prior to surgery (AOR 2.63).[34]

When determining if a patient should proceed with surgery within 1 year following MI or DES placement, the urgency of the surgery must be taken into account. The ACC/AHA guideline on Perioperative Cardiovascular Evaluation and Management of Patients Undergoing Noncardiac Surgery defines surgeries as either emergent, urgent, time-sensitive, or elective.[35] Surgeries in which life, limb, or eyesight is threatened if the patient is not in the operating room within 6 hours are considered emergent. Those requiring surgery within 24 hours are considered urgent. Time-sensitive surgeries allow for a delay in the order of weeks to months for optimization without negatively effecting outcomes (oncologic surgeries typically fall into this category). Elective surgeries, on the other hand, can be delayed for up to a year.

Truly elective surgeries should not be undertaken within a year following an MI. While most joint replacements are truly elective, there are situations where impaired joint mobility leads to significant disability and/or loss of income and independence making the surgery somewhat non-elective. In these situations, a detailed risk-benefit discussion with patient, surgeon and cardiologist can inform the decision to proceed prior to a year.

INTERRUPTION OF DUAL ANTIPLATELET THERAPY PRIOR TO SURGERY

Interruption of DAPT during the first 12 months after DES placement is associated with an increased risk of MACE in nonsurgical patients. It must be noted that surgery itself increases the risk of MACE due to the prothrombotic, inflammatory, and physiologically stressful state surgery produces. Therefore, whenever possible, DAPT should be continued during the perioperative period for low bleeding risk procedures. While determination of procedural bleeding risk is an institutionally and departmentally dependent process, there are some procedures which are fairly universally accepted as low-risk. These include endoscopic procedures, dental extractions, ophthalmologic surgeries, and minor orthopedic, plastic, and general surgeries.

However, if periprocedural bleeding risk is high, interruption of DAPT may be necessary. This risk should be balanced by the potentially catastrophic complication of stent thrombosis. The current ACC/AHA guidelines on peri-procedural management of antiplatelet medications recommend continuation of low-dose aspirin (75–100 mg) whenever possible for all patients with coronary stents of any age.[14] Indeed, most surgeries can be performed on low-dose aspirin. However, this always warrants a discussion with the surgeon who ultimately manages surgical bleeding and will, therefore, need to agree with continuation of aspirin. It is also important to inform surgeons that discontinuation of aspirin in patients with coronary stents significantly increases the risk of perioperative cardiac complications, and interruption of therapy is only indicated when the risk of bleeding exceeds the risk of in-stent thrombosis. Principles of preoperative antiplatelet management include assessing and balancing the risk of thrombosis, urgency of surgery, and bleeding risk.[36] Table 5.4 presents these considerations.

Table 5.4 **PRINCIPLES OF PERIOPERATIVE MANAGEMENT OF ANTIPLATELET MEDICATIONS**

	RISK OF THROMBOSIS		**ELECTIVE SURGERY**	**URGENT SURGERY – LOW RISK OF BLEEDING**	**URGENT SURGERY – HIGH RISK OF BLEEDING**
Aspirin and $P2Y_{12}$ inhibitor	High	PTCA within 2 weeks; BMS within 6 weeks; MI without stent within 6 weeks; DES for SIHD within 6 months; DES for ACS within 1 year	Delay until low risk	Continue both medications uninterrupted	Hold $P2Y_{12}$ inhibitor 5–7 days; Continue ASA (70–100 mg)
	Low	Not meeting criteria above	Hold $P2Y_{12}$ inhibitor 5–7 days; Continue ASA (70–100 mg)	Hold $P2Y_{12}$ inhibitor 5–7 days; Continue ASA (70–100 mg)	Hold $P2Y_{12}$ inhibitor 5–7 days; Consider holding ASA (70–100 mg)
Aspirin alone	High	History of ACS, stent, stroke, PAD	Continue ASA (70–100 mg)	Continue ASA (70–100 mg)	Consider holding ASA (70–100 mg)
	Low	Primary prevention	Hold ASA for 7 days	Hold ASA for 7 days	Hold ASA for 7 days

ASA, acetylsalicylic acid; ACS, acute coronary syndrome; BMS, bare metal stent; DES, drug-eluting stent; MI, myocardial infarction; PAD, peripheral artery disease; PTCA, percutaneous transluminal coronary angioplasty.

Adapted from Di Minno MN, et al.[36]

There is some evidence indicating that it may be safe to consider interrupting DAPT after 3–6 months of therapy following a second-generation DES.[37] Studies show that shorter cessation periods did not result in increased stent thrombosis, but these are not generalizable to patients who have had stents placed in the setting of ACS.[36] Our current best available recommendation for those patients is to wait at least 12 months prior to elective surgery.[14]

Regardless of stent type or age, patients with coronary stents should continue aspirin throughout the perioperative period as long as it is not contraindicated for the surgery.[14] The POISE-II trial did show that continuation of aspirin in the perioperative period may result in a significant increase in major surgical bleeding.[38] However, it should be noted that patients in this study were on a relatively high dose of aspirin (200 mg followed by 100 mg daily) and that this study excluded patients with recent coronary stents (<6 months for BMS, <12 months for DES). So we cannot conclude from this trial that patients with coronary stents should discontinue aspirin, especially if continued at a low dose (75–100 mg). The current ACC/AHA guidelines recommend continuation of low-dose aspirin in the perioperative period in patients with stents of any age.[14]

Aspirin is recommended to be stopped for 7–10 days prior to a very high bleeding risk procedures such as posterior chamber of the eye, spine, and intracranial surgery.[39,40] There are circumstances where the risk of stent thrombosis is too high (depending on the location of the stent, history of prior stent thrombosis, stent in a bifurcating lesion), and ophthalmologists or neurosurgeons may be willing to operate on low-dose aspirin. But, again, this decision should be collaborative between the surgeon, interventional cardiologist, and anesthesiologists caring for the patient perioperatively. For P2Y12 inhibitors the length of therapy interruptions varies by the agent used: ticagrelor 3–5 days, clopidogrel 5 days, and prasugrel 7 days.[41] It is important to note that at these cessation intervals platelet function is not fully normalized, and an extra 2 days is necessary to completely achieve this. Surgeries with a high risk of bleeding into a noncompressible anatomic site (e.g., craniotomies) typically require full platelet function to be performed safely. However, urgent and emergent surgeries must proceed regardless of duration of cessation. Utilizing functional assays to assess platelet inhibition in the presence of recent antiplatelet medication can help assess current platelet function. This is discussed in more detail later in the chapter.

SIGNS AND SYMPTOMS OF MENINGIOMAS

In the United States, there are 29,000 estimated new cases of meningioma every year. The median age of diagnosis is 65 years, and the disorder effects women two to three times more frequently as men.[42] Meningiomas represent approximately one-third of all brain tumors; they are typically benign but can cause significant disability if large and compressing important neural structures. Management depends on size, location, symptoms, and patient comorbidities. Small meningiomas (<2 cm) which are asymptomatic are often found incidentally.

Depending on location, surveillance with routine imaging may be the management of choice. Larger or symptomatic tumors may require radiation and/or surgical management. Complete surgical resection is preferred but may be too risky in patients with tumors in locations in close proximity to critical structures. These patients may receive radiation alone. While surgery carries the greatest possibility for cure, our patient should have a detailed risk discussion with the surgeon to determine if surgery is the safest course of action.

PREOPERATIVE EVALUATION OF PATIENTS WITH MENINGIOMAS

Patients with meningiomas may exhibit signs and symptoms secondary to mass effect, cerebral edema, and a hypercoagulable state. Seizures are a frequent symptom (29.2%), and patients are often on antiseizure medications.[43] Headaches are frequent due to cerebral edema and obstructive hydrocephalus; patients may be on corticosteroids to reduce swelling. Patients with elevated intracranial pressure (ICP) can have autonomic dysfunction, bradycardia, arrhythmias, electrolyte abnormalities, hypertension, and ECG changes.

Visual changes may not be detected until formal visual testing is performed. Loss of hearing or smell, mental status changes including apathy or inattention, and extremity weakness are all possible signs and symptoms. Meningiomas can produce a hypercoagulable state, and venous thromboembolism rates in this postoperative population are estimated at 30%.

PERIOPERATIVE MANAGEMENT OF ANTIPLATELET THERAPY IN THE NEUROSURGICAL PATIENT

Intracranial surgeries, with few exceptions, typically require cessation of antiplatelet therapy. Point-of-care assays are available to assess the level of platelet inhibition.[44] These assays are not interchangeable because many test different facets of platelet function. Currently the use of these assays to direct cessation of DAPT and timing of surgery is not recommended as there is not enough data to build a recommendation.[45] Platelet transfusion may be necessary for adequate hemostasis in patients with residual inhibition and has been shown to improve outcomes in patients with intracranial hemorrhage who received clopidogrel; the same is not true for other noncardiac surgeries.[46] Ticagrelor can be potentially reversed by using an experimental monoclonal antibody (PB2452) or through extracorporeal removal via Cytosorb.[47]

Patients with coronary stents will be unprotected from stent thrombosis during this period of DAPT cessation. It has been suggested that glycoprotein (GP) IIb/IIIa inhibitors, which also inhibit platelets and are protective against thrombosis, be considered as a "bridge" during DAPT interruption.

This management has been successfully used in a patient with recent DES placement (<2 months) requiring urgent spinal surgery.[48] However, while the total period during which the patient's stent is "unprotected" may be diminished with this strategy, the GP IIb/IIIa must also be discontinued prior to surgery to reduce perioperative bleeding. Patients are, therefore, not protected during the highest prothrombotic period, the intra- and postoperative state. Indeed, another neurosurgical patient with a recent DES managed with a GP IIb/IIIa bridge prior to her urgent spinal surgery suffered catastrophic stent thrombosis in the morning prior to surgery, approximately 5 hours after her eptifibatide infusion had been discontinued.[49]

A meta-analysis investigated this question in a more rigorous manner and did not find a significant decrease in stent thrombosis in patients with DES receiving GP IIb/IIIa relative to those who did not.[50] Therefore, current best available evidence does not support this management strategy.

When to restart antiplatelet agents postoperatively is another complex management decision which takes into account the type of tumor, findings during surgery, and postoperative course. Aspirin may be restarted as soon as 2 days following surgery, with the P2Y12 inhibitor being restarted 7 or more days postoperatively. There are currently no guidelines or clinical trials addressing this question.

INTRAOPERATIVE MONITORING OF MYOCARDIAL INFARCTION

Continuous ECG monitoring is the easiest, most cost-effective, and least invasive intraoperative monitor for detecting myocardial ischemia. It is also considered an American Society of Anesthesiologists (ASA) standard monitor which should be used during all anesthetics. Using a 5-lead ECG, leads II and V5 can detect myocardial ischemia approximately 80% of the time. The addition of V4 to II and V5 increases sensitivity to 96%.[51] V5 has been traditionally appreciated as the single most sensitive lead for ischemia, with a 75% sensitivity with this lead alone. However, there are more recent 12-lead studies which may challenge this dogma.[52]

If there is an area of known CAD, or stenting, monitoring the lead corresponding to that vessel may improve sensitivity.

In high-risk patients undergoing a general anesthetic, intraoperative transesophageal echocardiography (TEE) should be considered. This method of monitoring is invasive and requires expensive equipment and the presence of a certified examiner. However, it is the most sensitive mode of detecting intraoperative ischemia. Interestingly, in one study of vascular patients with WMAs during preoperative stress echocardiography in whom intraoperative WMAs were noted, there was very poor correlation between the preoperative and intraoperative locations of WMA.[53] There was, however, perfect agreement between postoperative ECG changes and noted locations of intraoperative WMAs.

The high sensitivity of TEE is countered, however, with fairly low specificity.[54] Hemodynamic abnormalities may lead to new WMAs which are transient and do not indicate the presence of ischemia. Hypovolemia or abrupt increases in afterload are some examples of this. This is valuable information for the anesthesiologist in the complex management of these patients.

The pulmonary artery (PA) catheter and use of the pulmonary capillary wedge pressure (PCWP) has been advocated for use in detecting myocardial ischemia. This is an invasive procedure which carries a small but potentially catastrophic risk of PA rupture. For this reason, a PCWP cannot be continuously measured. Other risks include dysrhythmias, complete heart block, valvular injury, and air emboli. PA catheters, however, do not require expensive equipment or a subspecialty-trained anesthesiologist. Like the TEE, an increase in PCWP is sensitive but not specific for ischemia.[54] No studies to date have shown a benefit in outcomes when PCWP are used in noncardiac surgery. The ASA practice guideline on PA catheters state that there is a need for additional research to demonstrate a benefit to PA catheter use but that clinical experience suggests that PA catheter monitoring of select surgical patients can reduce the incidence of perioperative complications.[55]

MECHANISM OF PERIOPERATIVE MYOCARDIAL INFARCTION

Among adults undergoing noncardiac surgery, 8% will suffer myocardial injury and 10% of those patients will die within 30 days.[56] The mortality rates are even higher for patients suffering a perioperative MI, the majority of which occur in the first 3 days following surgery. The pathophysiology of perioperative MIs is not completely understood. The literature is conflicting as to whether supply–demand imbalances (type 2 MIs) or coronary plaque disruptions (type 1 MIs) are the primary etiologies.[7,57,58] Myocardial oxygen demand is determined by left ventricular wall tension (preload and afterload), cardiac contractility, and heart rate. The heart relies almost exclusively on aerobic metabolism to meet its oxygen requirements. Despite constituting 0.5% of body weight, the heart consumes 7% of basal oxygen.

Extraction of oxygen by the myocardium is maximal at baseline, so increases in oxygen demand must be accompanied by increased oxygen supply or an imbalance occurs. Myocardial oxygen supply is determined by blood flow through the coronary arteries and the oxygen-carrying capacity of that blood. Factors which effect oxygen supply include oxygen content, heart rate, diastolic pressure, anemia, left ventricular end-diastolic pressure, coronary artery occlusion, and vascular tone.[59]

All patients experience a hypercoagulable physiology in the postoperative period. In addition, many patients have at least some interruption of antiplatelet therapy as well. In the stented patient, this provides the perfect scenario for the most feared complication, stent thrombosis. Stent thrombosis associated with acute MI is significantly more deadly than other MIs.[60] Up to 5–10% of patients with DES may experience thrombosis.[61] Risk factors include premature discontinuation of DAPT, reduced ejection fraction, diabetes, and renal impairment. Therefore, in patients with coronary stents, aspirin and/or other antiplatelet therapy should be restarted as soon as deemed safe from a surgical perspective.

MANAGEMENT OF POSTOPERATIVE MYOCARDIAL INFARCTION

Regardless of etiology, postoperative MIs frequently go unrecognized. The reasons for this are multifactorial. First, patients on analgesic medication may not experience chest pain. In fact, only 14% of patients experiencing a postoperative MI will report chest pain.[62] Second, those who do report symptoms of an MI (nausea, shortness of breath, radiating pain) have postsurgical reasons to be experiencing them (medication side effect, atelectasis, or surgical pain, for example). Finally, patients may be sedated in the ICU or experience altered mental status postoperatively which can interfere with recognition.

Regardless of symptomatology or lack thereof, perioperative MI is strongly associated with 30-day mortality. Therefore, it may be reasonable to monitor troponin levels and ECGs daily for the first 3 days after surgery in patients with established atherosclerotic disease with a planned inpatient admission following noncardiac surgery.[56,63] A baseline preoperative cTn value can assist in the interpretation of postoperative values.[6] Postoperative patients with coronary stents reporting anginal-type symptoms should be treated as a diagnosis of myocardial ischemia until proved otherwise.[61]

Perioperative stent thrombosis usually manifests as a STEMI in the anatomic location of the stent and is thought to be a far more prevalent cause of perioperative MI than previously thought, particularly in patients with coronary stents.[7] Thrombolysis is a less effective treatment for stent thrombosis than primary MI and is relatively contraindicated in the perioperative period, particularly with craniotomies.

POSTOPERATIVE PERCUTANEOUS CORONARY INTERVENTION

Time to transfer to the interventional cardiac catheterization laboratory is crucial, with mortality increasing after 90 minutes of diagnosis have passed.[61] However, PCI requires anticoagulation and platelet inhibition. While a recent craniotomy is not an absolute contraindication for PCI, the neurosurgical risks of an intracranial hemorrhage would have to be weighed against the potential benefits of coronary revascularization.

Percutaneous transluminal coronary angioplasty (PTCA) is another method of revascularization which does not result in placement of a stent or need for additional thrombolytics. However, anticoagulation is required during the procedure, and PTCA is associated with an increased risk of coronary injury (dissection or perforation), complications this patient is already at increased risk of based on her prior PTCI. With her recent craniotomy, she would not be a candidate for an emergency CABG for repair.

Therefore, medical management may be the safest course of action for the majority of post-craniotomy acute MI patients. Notably, this postoperative complication is associated with the greatest relative risk of mortality in the post-craniotomy patient. The 30-day mortality rate of all patients having a craniotomy is 2.1%. However, 30.4% of post-craniotomy patients experiencing an MI will die within 30 days (odds ratio [OR] 21.5). In fact, MI imparted the highest risk of mortality of all variables, including stroke (16.9%), transfusion (8.1%), and unplanned reoperation (5.8%).[64]

CONCLUSION

- A cardiac troponin level above the 99th percentile indicates myocardial injury.

- MI is defined as myocardial injury associated with evidence of acute myocardial ischemia (symptoms, ECG findings, and/or imaging, angiographic, or pathologic evidence).

- PCI is superior to coronary reperfusion through fibrinolysis in hospitals where 17 PCI procedures or more are performed per year.

- Complications associated with PCI include intracranial hemorrhage, failure, coronary dissection, intramural hematoma, or coronary perforation/branch vessel occlusion.

- Following coronary stent placement, patients should have uninterrupted DAPT with a thienopyridine and aspirin to reduce the risk of stent thrombosis during the period when the stent is becoming endothelialized.

- The decision to interrupt DAPT perioperatively must balance the risk of stent thrombosis with surgical bleeding risk.

- The current recommended duration of uninterrupted DAPT is 1 month for BMS and 6 months for new-generation DES placed in the setting of SIHD. For patients with ACS, a minimal DAPT duration of 3 months should be observed for time-sensitive procedures. Before elective surgeries, a 12-month duration of uninterrupted DAPT should be completed.

- Elective surgery should be postponed for 1 year following MI.

- Patients with coronary stents of any age should continue low-dose aspirin throughout the perioperative period unless absolutely contraindicated.

- One-third of brain tumors are meningiomas, which are typically benign.

- Resection of intracranial tumors typically requires cessation of both P2Y12 inhibitors and aspirin for 1 week prior to surgery.

- Intraoperative monitoring for MI includes ECG, right heart catheterization, and TEE.

- Perioperative MI can occur due to an imbalance in myocardial oxygen supply with demand or plaque disruption and thrombosis.

- The 30-day mortality rate of patients having an MI following craniotomy may be as high as 30%.

- PCI is the preferred treatment for stent thrombosis but may be contraindicated in the immediate postoperative period.

REVIEW QUESTIONS

1. Which of the following is not an established risk factor for coronary artery disease (CAD)?

    a. Obesity.
    b. Family history of CAD.
    c. Moderate alcohol intake.
    d. Diabetes.
    e. Hypertension.

The correct answer is c.

There are five major risk factors for coronary heart disease (CHD): dyslipidemia, hypertension, obesity, diabetes, and family history of CHD. Of the 542,008 patients presenting with MI without a prior diagnosis of CHD, 85.6% of them had at least one of the major risk factors. Other risk factors which are nonmodifiable include age and male gender. Obesity, diet, and sedentary lifestyle impart a lesser risk. Moderate alcohol intake and regular exercise are protective.

2. Which of the following statements is false?

    a. Myocardial injury is defined as a troponin value above the 99th percentile.
    b. Myocardial infarction (MI) is defined as myocardial injury with evidence of myocardial ischemia.
    c. The threshold value defining ST-segment elevation is ≥1 mm in all leads except for V2 and V3.
    d. An MI can be ruled out by a normal or nonspecific ECG.
    e. Women, diabetics, and the elderly more commonly present with nonspecific symptoms such as nausea or diaphoresis than classic chest pain.

The correct answer is d.

Detection of an elevated cardiac troponin (cTn) level above the 99th percentile indicates myocardial injury. MI is defined as myocardial injury associated with evidence of acute myocardial ischemia (clinical symptoms, ECG findings, or imaging, angiographic, or pathologic evidence). Initial ECGs may be normal. Diabetics, women, and elderly patients are more likely to present with dyspnea, weakness, vomiting, palpitations, or syncope than chest discomfort. Early suspicion, laboratory testing, and serial ECG testing may be necessary for diagnosis. The threshold value to define ST-segment elevation is 1 mm or greater except in leads V2 and V3. For V2 and V3 ST segments to be considered elevated, the amplitude must be 1.5 mm or greater in women, 2 mm or greater in men 40 years or older, and, 2.5 mm or greater in men younger than.

3. Which of the following statements about percutaneous coronary interventions (PCI) is true?

    a. PCI is superior to fibrinolysis in centers where the procedure is performed regularly (≥17 PCIs/year).
    b. PCI is never appropriate for left main disease.
    c. The incidence of post-PCI emergency CABG is around 1%.
    d. Dual antiplatelet therapy helps prevent restenosis of the stent.
    e. In patients expecting to have surgery within a year following PCI, drug-eluting stents (DES) are preferred.

The correct answer is a.

PCI is superior to coronary reperfusion through fibrinolysis because it results in a higher rate of flow through the coronaries and does not increase the risk of intracranial bleeding. However, this only results in lower in-hospital mortality in institutions which perform the procedure regularly (≥17 PPCIs/year). High-volume institutions performing 49 PPCIs/year or more have the lowest mortality rate (3.4%) compared to low-volume hospitals (6.2%) where PPCI is inferior from a mortality standpoint to fibrinolysis (5.9%). The 2009 ACC/AHA update on the management of STEMI stated it was reasonable to consider PCI of the left main coronary in patients considered low risk of PCI complications as an alternative to CABG. The incidence of post PCI emergency CABG is 0.1–0.3%. DAPT lowers the risk of in-stent thrombosis while the stent is not yet endothelialized. DES contain medications to reduce neointimal proliferation and lower the risk of stent restenosis.

4. Which of the following statements about postoperative major adverse cardiac events (MACE) in patients with coronary stents is true?

    a. The incidence of MACE is >11% if surgery is performed within 6 weeks of placement.
    b. Nonelective surgery increases the incidence of MACE.
    c. The incidence of MACE continues to decline for 24 months following stent placement.
    d. None of the above statements is true.
    e. All of the above statements are true.

The correct answer is e.

Within the first 24 months after coronary stent placement, 22.5% of patients have noncardiac operations, and 4.7% of these patients experience a MACE following surgery. The time spent between stent placement and surgery is inversely related to these events, with a 11.6% incidence of MACE if surgery is performed within 6 weeks of placement, 6.4% within 6 months, 4.2% within 12 months, and 3.5% within 24 months. Other factors which impart a higher risk of MACE include nonelective surgical admission (adjusted odds ratio [AOR] 4.77) and MI within 6 months prior to surgery (AOR 2.63).

5. A patient with a drug-eluting stent placed 10 months ago for MI was diagnosed with colon cancer and is presenting for total colectomy. Which of the following statements are true?

    a. He should stop his DAPT for 7 days prior to surgery.
    b. DAPT must be continued perioperatively.
    c. Low-dose aspirin should be continued.
    d. Surgery should be postponed for 2 additional months.

e. His 7-day incidence of MACE is increased 10-fold if he proceeds with surgery.

The correct answer is c.

Regardless of stent type or age, patients with coronary stents should continue aspirin throughout the perioperative period as long as it is not contraindicated for the surgery. Interruption of DAPT during the first 12 months after DES placement is associated with an increased risk of MACE in nonsurgical patients. It must be noted that surgery itself increases the risk of MACE due to the prothrombotic, inflammatory, physiologically stressful state surgery produces. Therefore, whenever possible, DAPT should be continued during the perioperative period for low bleeding risk surgeries. However, interruption of DAPT may be necessary based on the relative risk of periprocedural bleeding. Thienopyridines are typically discontinued for 5–7 days prior to major abdominal surgery. Aspirin should be continued. While it is preferable to delay surgery for 1 year following an MI, oncologic surgeries are typically not delayed. The 7-day risk of MACE in a post-MI patient having surgery within 1 year is 1.9%. This is 27-fold above the nonsurgical post-MI patient.

6. Which of the following statements about patients with meningiomas are true?

a. Most experience seizures.
b. Venous thromboembolism rates are high because of a hypercoagulable state.
c. Meningiomas are rarely benign.
d. Patients are often on diuretics to reduce swelling.
e. Surgery is preferred when the tumor is near a critical structure.

The correct answer is b.

Meningiomas can produce a hypercoagulable state, and venous thromboembolism rates in this postoperative population are estimated at 30%. Meningiomas are typically benign. Management depends on size, location, symptoms, and patient comorbidities. Small meningiomas (<2 cm) which are asymptomatic are often found incidentally. Depending on location, surveillance with routine imaging may be the management of choice. Larger or symptomatic tumors may require radiation and/or surgical management. Complete surgical resection is preferred but may be too risky in patients with tumors in locations in close proximity to critical structures. These patients may receive radiation alone. Patients are often on corticosteroids to reduce swelling.

7. Which of the following intraoperative monitors has the highest sensitivity for myocardial ischemia?

a. Transthoracic echocardiography (TTE).
b. Right heart catheterization.
c. Continuous ECG monitoring in leads II and V5.
d. Transesophageal echocardiography (TEE).
e. Cardiac troponin (cTn) levels.

The correct answer is d.

TEE is the gold-standard of sensitivity for intraoperative ischemia detection. However, most new WMAs do not indicate the presence of ischemia. Using a 5-lead ECG, leads II and V5 can detect myocardial ischemia approximately 80% of the time. The addition of V4 to II and V5 increases sensitivity to 96%. TTE is not as sensitive as TEE, and it is difficult during most surgeries to obtain it. cTn is not routinely used as an intraoperative monitor for ischemia. Right heart catheterization is not as sensitive as TEE. Detection of left ventricular ischemia requires a pulmonary capillary wedge pressure, which cannot be continuously monitored due to risks of PA rupture.

8. In regards to duration of DAPT for patients with a history of PCI, all of the following statements are correct, *except*

a. All patients with a history of PCI should continue low-dose aspirin indefinitely.
b. For very high bleeding risk surgeries, DAPT may be interrupted after 3 months of continuous therapy.
c. For patients with PCI for SIHD, 6 months is considered the ideal minimal duration of DAPT.
d. For patients with PCI for ACS, 12 months is considered the ideal minimal duration of DAPT.
e. For patients with PCI for SIHD having high bleeding risk surgery 9 months after DES placement, DAPT should be continued uninterrupted.

The correct answer is e.

The ACC/AHA focused update on duration of DAPT in patients with CAD recommends that periprocedural management of these medications requires an approach which balances the urgency of surgery and bleeding risk with the risk of perioperative thrombosis. In patients with a history of PCI, low-dose aspirin should be continued indefinitely. The ideal minimum duration of DAPT after DES placed for SIHD is 6 months and, after any PCI for ACS, is 12 months. The new ESC guidelines suggest that DAPT interruption for PCI for SIHD can be considered after only 1 month of therapy but at least 3 months after PCI for ACS in patients undergoing time-sensitive noncardiac surgery.

9. What is one key disadvantage for the use of BRS in patients undergoing PCI for ACS when compared to BMS and DES?

a. There are no disadvantages to using BRS.
b. BRS require a longer duration of DAPT.
c. BRS are less effective at reducing intimal proliferation.
d. BRS take longer to place, increasing the time to revascularization.
e. BRS have an increased risk of in-stent thrombosis.

The correct answer is d.

BRS have been called the fourth revolution in interventional cardiology technology. Like DES, they reduce intimal proliferation. Because the stent scaffolding is resorbed, there is a lower risk of in-stent thrombosis and a shorter duration of DAPT is necessary. Because of their greater size, however, angioplasty and vessel dilation is necessary prior to placement, extending the procedural duration and therefore time to coronary revascularization.

10. Which of the following statements about perioperative MI is true?

   a. When perioperative MI occurs in the hospital, it has a lower mortality rate than non-perioperative MI.
   b. When perioperative MI occurs, thrombolysis is preferred rather than PCI.
   c. Only a small minority of perioperative MIs occur due to plaque rupture (type 1 MI).
   d. Postoperative MI is commonly diagnosed when patients are under clinical care in the hospital.
   e. Type 2 MIs in the perioperative period may be a result of anemia, pulmonary complications, hypertension, or sustained tachycardia.

The correct answer is e.

Perioperative MI are frequently unrecognized in the hospital and usually occur in the absence of the classic clinical sign of chest pain.[58] When a perioperative MI is recognized, it confers a higher mortality rate than an MI that occurs in another context. PCI, not fibrinolysis, is the preferred treatment in centers that perform them frequently. Nearly half of all perioperative MIs are a result of plaque rupture. Type 2 MIs can result from a supply–demand imbalance occurring in the perioperative period. Treatment of the underlying cause (anemia, tachycardia, hypertension, decreased oxygenation) is the preferred management.

REFERENCES

1. Canto JG, Kiefe CI, Rogers WJ, et al. Number of coronary heart disease risk factors and mortality in patients with first myocardial infarction. *JAMA*. 2011;306(19):2120–2127. doi:10.1001/jama.2011.1654
2. Miller CD, Lindsell CJ, Khandelwal S, et al. Is the initial diagnostic impression of "noncardiac chest pain" adequate to exclude cardiac disease? *Ann Emerg Med*. 2004;44(6):565–574. doi:10.1016/j.annemergmed.2004.03.021
3. Katz D, Gavin MC. Stable ischemic heart disease. *Ann Intern Med*. 2019 Aug 6;171(3):ITC17–ITC32. doi:10.7326/AITC201908060. PMID: 31382288
4. Mehilli J, Presbitero P. Coronary artery disease and acute coronary syndrome in women. *Heart*. 2020 Apr;106(7):487–492. doi:10.1136/heartjnl-2019-315555. Epub 2020 Jan 13. PMID: 31932287
5. Anderson JL, Morrow DA. Acute myocardial infarction. *N Engl J Med*. 2017 May 25;376(21):2053–2064. doi:10.1056/NEJMra1606915. PMID: 28538121
6. Thygesen K, Alpert JS, Jaffe AS, Chaitman BR, Bax JJ, Morrow DA, White HD; Executive Group on behalf of the Joint European Society of Cardiology (ESC)/American College of Cardiology (ACC)/American Heart Association (AHA)/World Heart Federation (WHF) Task Force for the Universal Definition of Myocardial Infarction. Fourth universal definition of myocardial infarction (2018). *J Am Coll Cardiol*. 2018 Oct 30;72(18):2231–2264. doi:10.1016/j.jacc.2018.08.1038. Epub 2018 Aug 25. PMID: 30153967
7. Gualandro DM, Campos CA, Calderaro D, et al. Coronary plaque rupture in patients with myocardial infarction after noncardiac surgery: Frequent and dangerous. *Atherosclerosis*. 2012;222(1):191–195. doi:10.1016/j.atherosclerosis.2012.02.021
8. Sabatine MS. Differentiating type 1 and type 2 myocardial infarction: Unfortunately, still more art than science. *JAMA Cardiol*. 2021 Jul 1;6(7):781. doi:10.1001/jamacardio.2021.0693. PMID: 33881457
9. Christenson RH, Jacobs E, Uettwiller-Geiger D, et al. Comparison of 13 commercially available cardiac troponin assays in a multicenter North American study. *J Appl Lab Med AACC Publ*. 2017;1(5):544–561. doi:10.1373/jalm.2016.022640
10. Gulati M, Levy PD, Mukherjee D, et al. AHA/ACC/ASE/CHEST/SAEM/SCCT/SCMR guideline for the evaluation and diagnosis of chest pain: A report of the American College of Cardiology/American Heart Association Joint Committee on clinical practice guidelines. *Circulation*. 2021;144(22):e368–e454. doi:10.1161/CIR.0000000000001029
11. Bularga A, Lee KK, Stewart S, et al. High-sensitivity troponin and the application of risk stratification thresholds in patients with suspected acute coronary syndrome. *Circulation*. 2019 Nov 5;140(19):1557–1568. doi:10.1161/CIRCULATIONAHA.119.042866. Epub 2019 Sep 1. PMID: 31475856; PMCID: PMC6831036
12. Antman EM, Anbe DT, Armstrong PW, et al. ACC/AHA guidelines for the management of patients with ST-elevation myocardial infarction: Executive summary. *J Am Coll Cardiol*. 2004;44(3):671–719. doi:10.1016/j.jacc.2004.07.002
13. Wagner GS, Macfarlane P, Wellens H, et al. AHA/ACCF/HRS recommendations for the standardization and interpretation of the electrocardiogram. *J Am Coll Cardiol*. 2009;53(11):1003–1011. doi:10.1016/j.jacc.2008.12.016
14. Levine GN, Bates ER, Bittl JA, et al. 2016 ACC/AHA guideline focused update on duration of dual antiplatelet therapy in patients with coronary artery disease: A report of the American College of Cardiology/American Heart Association Task Force on Clinical Practice Guidelines: An update of the 2011 ACCF/AHA/SCAI guideline for percutaneous coronary intervention, 2011 ACCF/AHA guideline for coronary artery bypass graft surgery, 2012 ACC/AHA/ACP/AATS/PCNA/SCAI/STS guideline for the diagnosis and management of patients with stable ischemic heart disease, 2013 ACCF/AHA guideline for the management of ST-elevation myocardial infarction, 2014 AHA/ACC guideline for the management of patients with non–ST-elevation acute coronary syndromes, and 2014 ACC/AHA guideline on perioperative cardiovascular evaluation and management of patients undergoing noncardiac surgery. *Circulation*. 2016;134(10):e123–e155. doi:10.1161/CIR.0000000000000404
15. Antman EM, Armstrong PW, Green LA, et al. 2007 Focused update of the ACC/AHA 2004 guidelines for the management of patients with ST-elevation myocardial infarction. *J Am Coll Cardiol*. 2008;51(2):210–247. doi:10.1016/j.jacc.2007.10.001
16. Kushner FG, Hand M, Smith SC, et al. 2009 focused updates: ACC/AHA guidelines for the management of patients with ST-elevation myocardial infarction (updating the 2004 guideline and 2007 focused update) and ACC/AHA/SCAI guidelines on percutaneous coronary intervention (updating the 2005 guideline and 2007 focused update): A report of the American College of Cardiology Foundation/American Heart Association Task Force on Practice Guidelines. *Catheter Cardiovasc Interv*. 2009;74(7):E25–E68. doi:10.1002/ccd.22351
17. Magid DJ, Calonge BN, Rumsfeld JS, et al. Relation between hospital primary angioplasty volume and mortality for patients with acute MI treated with primary angioplasty vs thrombolytic therapy. *JAMA*. 2000;284(24):3131–3138. doi:10.1001/jama.284.24.3131
18. Patel MR, Dehmer GJ, Hirshfeld JW, Smith PK, Spertus JA. ACCF/SCAI/STS/AATS/AHA/ASNC 2009 appropriateness criteria for coronary revascularization. *J Am Coll Cardiol*. 2009;53(6):530–553. doi:10.1016/j.jacc.2008.10.005
19. Guyatt GH, Akl EA, Crowther M, Gutterman DD, Schüünemann HJ, American College of Chest Physicians Antithrombotic Therapy and Prevention of Thrombosis Panel. Executive summary: Antithrombotic therapy and prevention of thrombosis, 9th ed: American College of Chest Physicians evidence-based clinical practice guidelines. *Chest*. 2012;141(2 Suppl):7S–47S. doi:10.1378/chest.1412S3

20. Yang EH, Gumina RJ, Lennon RJ, Holmes DR, Rihal CS, Singh M. Emergency coronary artery bypass surgery for percutaneous coronary interventions. *J Am Coll Cardiol*. 2005;46(11):2004–2009. doi:10.1016/j.jacc.2005.06.083
21. Stone GW, O'Shaughnessy C, Greenberg J. A Polymer-based, paclitaxel-eluting stent in patients with coronary artery disease. *N Engl J Med*. 2004;350(3):221–231. doi:10.1056/NEJMoa032441
22. Morice M-C, Hayashi EB, Guagliumi G. A randomized comparison of a sirolimus-eluting stent with a standard stent for coronary revascularization. *N Engl J Med*. 2002;346(23):1773–1780. doi:10.1056/NEJMoa012843
23. Navarese EP, Kowalewski M, Kandzari D, et al. First-generation versus second-generation drug-eluting stents in current clinical practice: Updated evidence from a comprehensive meta-analysis of randomised clinical trials comprising 31 379 patients. *Open Heart*. 2014;1(1):e000064. doi:10.1136/openhrt-2014-000064
24. Kandzari DE, Smits PC, Love MP, et al. Randomized comparison of ridaforolimus- and zotarolimus-eluting coronary stents in patients with coronary artery disease: Primary results from the BIONICS trial (BioNIR Ridaforolimus-Eluting Coronary Stent System in Coronary Stenosis). *Circulation*. 2017;136(14):1304–1314. doi:10.1161/CIRCULATIONAHA.117.028885
25. Lee DH, de la Torre Hernandez JM. The newest generation of drug-eluting stents and beyond. *Eur Cardiol*. 2018;13(1):54–59. doi:10.15420/ecr.2018:8:2
26. Omar WA, Kumbhani DJ. The current literature on bioabsorbable stents: A review. *Curr Atheroscler Rep*. 2019 Nov 25;21(12):54. doi:10.1007/s11883-019-0816-4. PMID: 31768641
27. Garot P, Morice MC, Tresukosol D, et al.; LEADERS FREE Investigators. 2-year outcomes of high bleeding risk patients after polymer-free drug-coated stents. *J Am Coll Cardiol*. 2017 Jan 17;69(2):162–171. doi:10.1016/j.jacc.2016.10.009. Epub 2016 Oct 30. PMID: 27806919
28. Valgimigli M, Bueno H, Byrne RA, et al.; ESC Scientific Document Group; ESC Committee for Practice Guidelines (CPG); ESC National Cardiac Societies. 2017 ESC focused update on dual antiplatelet therapy in coronary artery disease developed in collaboration with EACTS: The task force for dual antiplatelet therapy in coronary artery disease of the European Society of Cardiology (ESC) and of the European Association for Cardio-Thoracic Surgery (EACTS). *Eur Heart J*. 2018 Jan 14;39(3):213–260. doi:10.1093/eurheartj/ehx419. PMID: 28886622
29. Capodanno D, Alfonso F, Levine GN, Valgimigli M, Angiolillo DJ. ACC/AHA versus ESC guidelines on dual antiplatelet therapy: JACC guideline comparison. *J Am Coll Cardiol*. 2018 Dec 11;72(23 Pt A):2915–2931. doi:10.1016/j.jacc.2018.09.057. PMID: 30522654
30. Halvorsen S, Mehilli J, Cassese S, et al. 2022 ESC Guidelines on cardiovascular assessment and management of patients undergoing non-cardiac surgery. *Eur Heart J*. 2022 Oct 14;43(39):3826–3924.
31. Savage P, Cox B, Linden K, Coburn J, Shahmohammadi M, Menown I. Advances in clinical cardiology 2021: A summary of key clinical trials. *Adv Ther*. 2022;39(6):2398–2437. doi:10.1007/s12325-022-02136-y
32. Alshawabkeh LI, Prasad A, Lenkovsky F, et al. Outcomes of a preoperative "bridging" strategy with glycoprotein IIb/IIIa inhibitors to prevent perioperative stent thrombosis in patients with drug-eluting stents who undergo surgery necessitating interruption of thienopyridine administration. *EuroIntervention*. 2013;9(2):204–211. doi:10.4244/EIJV9I2A35
33. Berger PB, Kleiman NS, Pencina MJ, et al. Frequency of major noncardiac surgery and subsequent adverse events in the year after drug-eluting stent placement. *JACC Cardiovasc Interv*. 2010;3(9):920–927. doi:10.1016/j.jcin.2010.03.021
34. Hawn MT, Graham LA, Richman JS, Itani KMF, Henderson WG, Maddox TM. Risk of major adverse cardiac events following noncardiac surgery in patients with coronary stents. *JAMA*. 2013;310(14):1462. doi:10.1001/jama.2013.278787
35. Fleisher LA, Fleischmann KE, Auerbach AD, et al. 2014 ACC/AHA guideline on perioperative cardiovascular evaluation and management of patients undergoing noncardiac surgery: Executive summary: A report of the American College of Cardiology/American Heart Association Task Force on Practice Guidelines. *Circulation*. 2014 Dec 9;130(24):2215–2245. doi:10.1161/CIR.0000000000000105. Epub 2014 Aug 1. PMID: 25085962
36. Di Minno MN, Milone M, Mastronardi P, et al. Perioperative handling of antiplatelet drugs. A critical appraisal. *Curr Drug Targets*. 2013 Jul;14(8):880–888. doi:10.2174/13894501113140800008. PMID: 23627916
37. Wijeysundera DN, Beattie WS, Karkouti K, Neuman MD, Austin PC, Laupacis A. Association of echocardiography before major elective non-cardiac surgery with postoperative survival and length of hospital stay: Population based cohort study. *BMJ*. 2011;342(jun 30 1):d3695–d3695. doi:10.1136/bmj.d3695
38. Devereaux PJ, Mrkobrada M, Sessler DI, et al. Aspirin in patients undergoing noncardiac surgery. *N Engl J Med*. 2014;370(16):1494–1503. doi:10.1056/NEJMoa1401105
39. Oprea AD, Popescu WM. ADP-receptor inhibitors in the perioperative period: The good, the bad, and the ugly. *J Cardiothorac Vasc Anesth*. 2013 Aug;27(4):779–795.
40. Oprea AD, Popescu WM. Perioperative management of antiplatelet therapy. *Br J Anaesth*. 2013 Dec;111 Suppl 1:i3–17.
41. Dimitrova G, Tulman DB, Bergese SD. Perioperative management of antiplatelet therapy in patients with drug-eluting stents. *HSR Proc Intensive Care Cardiovasc Anesth*. 2012;4(3):153–167.
42. Claus EB, Bondy ML, Schildkraut JM, Wiemels JL, Wrensch M, Black PM. Epidemiology of intracranial meningioma. *Neurosurgery*. 2005;57(6):1088–1095; discussion 1088–1095.
43. Englot DJ, Magill ST, Han SJ, Chang EF, Berger MS, McDermott MW. Seizures in supratentorial meningioma: A systematic review and meta-analysis. *J Neurosurg*. 2016;124(6):1552–1561. doi:10.3171/2015.4.JNS142742
44. Pelaez CA, Spilman SK, Bell CT, Eastman DK, Sidwell RA. Not all head injured patients on antiplatelet drugs need platelets: Integrating platelet reactivity testing into platelet transfusion guidelines. *Injury*. 2019;50(1):73–78. doi:10.1016/j.injury.2018.08.020
45. Filipescu DC, Stefan MG, Valeanu L, Popescu WM. Perioperative management of antiplatelet therapy in noncardiac surgery. *Curr Opin Anaesthesiol*. 2020 Jun;33(3):454–462. doi:10.1097/ACO.0000000000000875. PMID: 32371645
46. Baschin M, Selleng S, Zeden JP, et al. Platelet transfusion to reverse antiplatelet therapy before decompressive surgery in patients with intracranial haemorrhage. *Vox Sang*. 2017 Aug;112(6):535–541. doi:10.1111/vox.12542. Epub 2017 Aug 14. PMID: 28809046
47. Ha ACT, Bhatt DL, Rutka JT, Johnston SC, Mazer CD, Verma S. Intracranial hemorrhage during dual antiplatelet therapy: JACC review topic of the week. *J Am Coll Cardiol*. 2021 Sep 28;78(13):1372–1384. doi:10.1016/j.jacc.2021.07.048. PMID: 34556323
48. Roth E, Purnell C, Shabalov O, Moguillansky D, Hernandez CA, Elnicki M. Perioperative management of a patient with recently placed drug-eluting stents requiring urgent spinal surgery. *J Gen Intern Med*. 2012;27(8):1080–1083. doi:10.1007/s11606-012-199-7
49. Singh M, Bolla VH, Berg R. A case of in-stent thrombosis in a patient with drug eluting stents during perioperative management with glycoprotein IIb/IIIa inhibitors: Periprocedural management of patients with DES. *Catheter Cardiovasc Interv*. 2013;82(7):1108–1112. doi:10.1002/ccd.24845
50. Warshauer J, Patel VG, Christopoulos G, Kotsia AP, Banerjee S, Brilakis ES. Outcomes of preoperative bridging therapy for patients undergoing surgery after coronary stent implantation: A weighted meta-analysis of 280 patients from eight studies: Meta-analysis of preoperative bridging therapy for PCI. *Catheter Cardiovasc Interv*. 2015;85(1):25–31. doi:10.1002/ccd.25507
51. London MJ, Hollenberg M, Wong MG, et al. Intraoperative myocardial ischemia: Localization by continuous 12-lead electrocardiography. *Anesthesiology*. 1988;69(2):232–241.

52. Landesberg G, Mosseri M, Wolf Y, Vesselov Y, Weissman C. Perioperative myocardial ischemia and infarction: Identification by continuous 12-lead electrocardiogram with online ST-segment monitoring. *Anesthesiology*. 2002;96(2):264–270.
53. Galal W, Hoeks SE, Flu WJ, et al. Relation between preoperative and intraoperative new wall motion abnormalities in vascular surgery patients: A transesophageal echocardiographic study. *Anesthesiology*. 2010;112(3):557–566. doi:10.1097/ALN.0b013e3181ce9d67
54. Fleisher LA. Real-time intraoperative monitoring of myocardial ischemia in noncardiac surgery. *Anesthesiology*. 2000;92(4):1183–1188.
55. American Society of Anesthesiologists Task Force on Pulmonary Artery Catheterization. Practice guidelines for pulmonary artery catheterization: An updated report by the American Society of Anesthesiologists Task Force on Pulmonary Artery Catheterization. *Anesthesiology*. 2003;99(4):988–1014.
56. Botto F, Alonso-Coello P, Chan MTV, et al. Myocardial injury after noncardiac surgery: A large, international, prospective cohort study establishing diagnostic criteria, characteristics, predictors, and 30-day outcomes. *Anesthesiology*. 2014;120(3):564–578. doi:10.1097/ALN.0000000000000113
57. Duvall WL, Sealove B, Pungoti C, Katz D, Moreno P, Kim M. Angiographic investigation of the pathophysiology of perioperative myocardial infarction. *Catheter Cardiovasc Interv*. 2012;80(5):768–776. doi:10.1002/ccd.23446
58. Landesberg G. Monitoring for myocardial ischemia. *Best Pract Res Clin Anaesthesiol*. 2005;19(1):77–95. doi:10.1016/j.bpa.2004.07.006
59. Braunwald E. Control of myocardial oxygen consumption. *Am J Cardiol*. 1971;27(4):416–432. doi:10.1016/0002-9149(71)90439-5
60. Farb A, Boam AB. Stent thrombosis redux: The FDA perspective. *N Engl J Med*. 2007;356(10):984–987. doi:10.1056/NEJMp068304
61. Barash P, Akhtar S. Coronary stents: Factors contributing to perioperative major adverse cardiovascular events. *Br J Anaesth*. 2010;105:i3–i15. doi:10.1093/bja/aeq318
62. Devereaux PJ. Surveillance and prevention of major perioperative ischemic cardiac events in patients undergoing noncardiac surgery: A review. *Can Med Assoc J*. 2005;173(7):779–788. doi:10.1503/cmaj.050316
63. Biccard BM, Rodseth RN. The pathophysiology of peri-operative myocardial infarction: Pathophysiology of peri-operative myocardial infarction. *Anaesthesia*. 2010;65(7):733–741. doi:10.1111/j.1365-2044.2010.06338.x
64. Goel NJ, Mallela AN, Agarwal P, et al. Complications predicting perioperative mortality in patients undergoing elective craniotomy: A population-based study. *World Neurosurg*. 2018;118:e195–e205. doi:10.1016/j.wneu.2018.06.153

6.

PERIOPERATIVE MANAGEMENT OF MEDICATIONS FOR SUBSTANCE USE DISORDERS

Thomas R. Hickey and Shafik Boyaji

STEM CASE AND KEY QUESTIONS

A 65-year-old man with severe right hip osteoarthritis presents to the preoperative clinic for evaluation before his upcoming total hip arthroplasty. The patient has a history of opioid use disorder (OUD) in sustained remission. His last IV fentanyl use was 3 years ago, and he denies both prescription and nonprescription opioid use since. He is currently on medication for opioid use disorder (MOUD) maintenance therapy with buprenorphine/naloxone 16 mg/4 mg tablet sublingually daily.

What is opioid use disorder?

The 11 diagnostic criteria for OUD described in the *Diagnostic and Statistical Manual of Mental Disorders* (DSM-5)[1] are found in Table 6.1. Severity is established by number of criteria met, ranging from mild (2–3) to severe (6 or more). Two of the criteria, tolerance and withdrawal, are not considered met for those taking opioids under appropriate medical supervision as some degree of these outcomes are physiologically inevitable for anyone taking opioids chronically. While the diagnostic criteria for other use disorders (e.g., alcohol, cannabis) are not detailed in this chapter, they are similar in character to those in Table 6.1. Substance use disorders (SUDs) are increasingly and appropriately seen as chronic, treatable diseases. OUD, for example, has highly effective treatments including buprenorphine.

What is buprenorphine? What forms are available?

Buprenorphine is a US Drug Enforcement Agency (DEA) schedule III drug. It was discovered in the 1960s as a result of a search for an opioid analgesic so safe and effective it could be sold over the counter.[2] Its IV and IM injection formulation (Buprenex) is approved by the US Food and Drug Administration (FDA) for acute pain while the transdermal patch (Butrans) and buccal film (Belbuca) are approved for chronic pain. Sublingual (Subutex), subcutaneous implant (Probuphine), and extended-release subcutaneous (Sublocade) preparations are used for OUD. The most commonly prescribed formulation for OUD is sublingual, typically as a naloxone combination product (Suboxone).

Buprenorphine is best known and widely prescribed as a treatment for OUD, for which it is highly effective. For reference, in a population with angina, the number needed to treat (NNT) with aspirin to prevent fatal myocardial infarction (MI) is 1,357.[3] In a population with OUD, NNT for buprenorphine to prevent death in the year after overdose is 52.6,[4] to decrease risk of relapse 2.9, and to increase retention in treatment 2.6.[5]

Buprenorphine prescribing across the country continues to rise.[6] This trend is expected to further increase after the Consolidated Appropriations Act of 2023[7] eliminated the requirement for clinicians to apply for a waiver to prescribe buprenorphine; as a result, clinicians with schedule III authority on DEA registration may prescribe buprenorphine for OUD.

What are the key pharmacological properties of buprenorphine?

Buprenorphine's partial agonism at the mu opioid receptor (MOR), high affinity for it, long duration of action, and lipophilicity are key pharmacological features.[8] The clinical significance of other pharmacodynamics, including agonism at the opioid receptor-like-1 (ORL1) and antagonism at the kappa and delta opioid receptors,[9,10] and of active metabolites such as norbuprenorphine, is less clear.

Buprenorphine's intrinsic efficacy is low to intermediate,[11] translating to an overall partial MOR response compared to full agonist opioids. However, the degree of agonism for each of the range of typical opioid effects, both desirable (e.g., analgesia, suppression of craving) and undesirable (e.g., nausea, constipation, sedation), varies.

For respiratory depression, buprenorphine is a partial agonist compared to full agonists such as fentanyl. In healthy volunteers, buprenorphine-induced respiratory depression leveled out at approximately 50% of baseline despite increasing doses, whereas escalating doses of fentanyl invariably caused respiratory instability and apnea.[12] Its partial agonism for the endpoint of euphoria is reflected in its low addiction and diversion risk. In a survey of more than 1,600 persons who used drugs, only 17 reported nonprescription buprenorphine use despite their attestation to its widespread availability.[13] And of more than 300 survey respondents who actually were using diverted buprenorphine, the most commonly cited reasons are therapeutic: 80% to prevent withdrawal, two-thirds to maintain abstinence, and over half to self-wean from nonprescription opioids.[14]

Table 6.1 DIAGNOSTIC CRITERIA FOR OPIOID USE DISORDER, VERBATIM FROM DIAGNOSTIC AND STATISTICAL MANUAL OF MENTAL DISORDERS, FIFTH EDITION, PAGE 541. PRINTED WITH PERMISSION FROM THE AMERICAN PSYCHIATRIC ASSOCIATION.

Diagnostic Criteria for Opioid Use Disorder

A. A problematic pattern of opioid use leading to clinically significant impairment or distress, as manifested by at least two of the following, occurring within a 12-month period:

1. Opioids are often taken in larger amounts or over a longer period than was intended.
2. There is a persistent desire or unsuccessful efforts to cut down or control opioid use.
3. A great deal of time is spent in activities necessary to obtain the opioid, use the opioid, or recover from its effects.
4. Craving, or a strong desire or urge to use opioids.
5. Recurrent opioid use resulting in a failure to fulfill major role obligations at work, school, or home.
6. Continued opioid use despite having persistent or recurrent social or interpersonal problems caused or exacerbated by the effects of opioids.
7. Important social, occupational, or recreational activities are given up or reduced because of opioid use.
8. Recurrent opioid use in situations in which it is physically hazardous.
9. Continued opioid use despite knowledge of having a persistent or recurrent physical or psychological problem that is likely to have been caused or exacerbated by the substance.
10. Tolerance, as defined by either of the following:
    a. A need for markedly increased amounts of opioids to achieve intoxication or desired effect.
    b. A markedly diminished effect with continued use of the same amount of an opioid. Note: This criterion is not considered to be met for those taking opioids solely under appropriate medical supervision.
11. Withdrawal, as manifested by either of the following:
    a. The characteristic opioid withdrawal syndrome (refer to Criteria A and B of the criteria set for opioid withdrawal, pp. 547–548).
    b. Opioids (or a closely related substance) are taken to relieve or avoid withdrawal symptoms.
    Note: This criterion is not considered to be met for those individuals taking opioids solely under appropriate medical supervision.

Specify if:
In early remission: After full criteria for opioid use disorder were previously met, none of the criteria for opioid use disorder have been met for at least 3 months but for less than 12 months (with the exception that Criterion A4, "Craving, or a strong desire or urge to use opioids," may be met).
In sustained remission: After full criteria for opioid use disorder were previously met, none of the criteria for opioid use disorder have been met at any time during a period of 12 months or longer (with the exception that Criterion A4, "Craving, or a strong desire or urge to use opioids," may be met).
Specify if:
On maintenance therapy: This additional specifier is used if the individual is taking a prescribed agonist medication such as methadone or buprenorphine and none of the criteria for opioid use disorder have been met for that class of medication (except tolerance to, or withdrawal from, the agonist). This category also applies to those individuals being maintained on a partial agonist, an agonist/antagonist, or a full antagonist such as oral naltrexone or depot naltrexone.
In a controlled environment: This additional specifier is used if the individual is in an environment where access to opioids is restricted.

For the analgesia endpoint, a systematic review and meta-analysis of randomized controlled trials found buprenorphine to be as effective as morphine for acute pain management in the hospital setting in a largely surgical population.[15] They reported on secondary outcomes, finding no difference in nausea/vomiting, dizziness, and hypotension; pruritis was less in the buprenorphine group. In 23 of 24 largely surgical trials comparing buprenorphine to full agonists (morphine, fentanyl, sufentanil, and oxycodone) for the treatment of pain, including severe pain, buprenorphine achieved at least the same analgesic effect.[16] These data demonstrate that buprenorphine is a full agonist for analgesia.

Buprenorphine's affinity for the MOR was second only to sufentanil in a study of 19 opioids.[17] Clinically, it is therefore difficult to displace from the MOR and, as a result, blocks the reinforcing effects (e.g., euphoria) and physiologic effects (e.g., respiratory depression) of other opioids. Buprenorphine's high affinity explains how it can act as an antagonist for individuals on prescribed or nonprescribed opioids, potentially precipitating withdrawal.

Buprenorphine dissociates slowly from the MOR, resulting in a long duration of action. Its serum half-life ranges from 32 to 40 hour after 2 mg and 16 mg sublingual doses, respectively.[18] This facilitates the typical daily dosing regimens in OUD treatment. However, the *analgesic* half-life of buprenorphine suggests that more frequent dosing may be optimal for the treatment of acute pain. An early study comparing morphine versus buprenorphine for treatment of postoperative pain found buprenorphine's duration of analgesia to be 7–8 hours.[19] Other authors found the serum half-life of IV buprenorphine for antinociception to be 155 minutes[20] and for IV and sublingual buprenorphine 177 minutes.[21] Twice (BID) to thrice daily (TID) dosing would be typical for pain and/or OUD with comorbid pain.

Buprenorphine is more lipophilic than most opioids in common use including fentanyl.[22,23] Clinically, higher lipophilicity results in more rapid penetration of the central nervous system (CNS), more rapid onset, and prolonged activity as compared to that predicted by serum half-life.[11] Sublingual administration of a typical MOUD dose results in a peak effect in 30 minutes to 1 hour.[24] Buprenorphine's enteral bioavailability is poor (10%). However, sublingual and buccal administration result in 30% and 46–55% bioavailability, respectively,[25,26] explaining these typical routes of administration.

Why is buprenorphine used as a treatment for OUD? Why does it come in a combination product with naloxone?

The aforementioned pharmacological properties of partial MOR agonism, high affinity for the MOR, and long duration of action make buprenorphine an ideal MOUD.

A typical buprenorphine "induction" is characterized by administration of a small dose then titration of doses over days to weeks until stabilization (e.g., no craving, no withdrawal, and, ideally, no nonprescription opioid use) is achieved. A typical sublingual maintenance dose is approximately 12–20 mg. The most prescribed formulation for OUD treatment is sublingual, typically as a naloxone combination product (Suboxone) in a 4:1 ratio to deter IV misuse. Naloxone is a MOR antagonist. Sublingual naloxone has a very low bioavailability; IV naloxone, however, is 100% bioavailable and would theoretically inhibit buprenorphine MOR agonist effects and possibly precipitate withdrawal.

Is buprenorphine a potential concern in the perioperative period?

Patients maintained on buprenorphine are opioid tolerant with some degree of dependence and will require not only their baseline opioid perioperatively (to maintain both therapy for OUD and prevent withdrawal), but typically require at least 20–30% more than their opioid-naïve counterparts to effectively manage postoperative pain. Moreover, pain in the patient population with OUD is often underrated and inadequately treated, and clinicians may misinterpret increased opioid requirements as misuse.[27,28]

A related concern is that the inherent stress of the perioperative period, pain per se, possible buprenorphine treatment cessation, and the therapeutic exposure to opioids represents a significant period of vulnerability to relapse in the population with OUD.[29] If buprenorphine were stopped and high doses of full agonist opioid were required to treat postoperative pain, the risk of opioid-induced respiratory depression would be expected to increase as the buprenorphine's partial MOR agonism decreases and the full MOR agonism increases.

What are options for managing buprenorphine in the perioperative period?

Up until recently, dogma in the perioperative world was that the presence of buprenorphine would inhibit the effectiveness of other opioids. Therefore, the classic teaching advised at least a 72-hour preoperative dose hold to allow sufficient elimination of buprenorphine and availability of MOR to facilitate full agonist opioid-mediated analgesia. Studies ranging from case reports to prospective randomized controlled trials demonstrate that buprenorphine continuation is not only possible but advantageous.[30-32] These and other studies resulted in the current consensus that buprenorphine should be continued perioperatively.[33-37] There is debate, however, about whether dose adjustments may improve pain management while maintaining therapeutic effects in OUD.

Advocates for a preoperative dose reduction expect that the resulting increased MOR availability will improve full agonist opioid-mediated analgesia while still maintaining enough MOR occupancy to maintain OUD treatment efficacy. Positron emission tomography (PET) imaging demonstrating the gradual increase in MOR occupancy at various time intervals after different maintenance buprenorphine doses, correlated to patient symptoms throughout, are often cited in support of a dose reduction.[38-40] A typical strategy calls for a dose reduction in patients on greater than 16 mg sublingual daily of buprenorphine undergoing surgeries after which more than mild pain is expected; for example, a reduction to 8 mg BID the day prior to surgery and 4 mg BID starting on the day of surgery, to be continued while full agonist opioid is required, after which the prior OUD dose can be resumed. One such strategy is included as Figure 6.1. Presently, there is insufficient evidence to determine whether a dose reduction is appropriate.

Extended-release subcutaneous buprenorphine has a very long half-life. The typical initial 300 mg dose results in a mean plasma half-life of 38 days.[41] Perioperative management of this formulation of buprenorphine is largely informed by case reports, limited clinical experience, and extrapolation from the sublingual evidence base. Current literature suggests performing surgery around the time of the next scheduled dose.[42,43]

What is a reasonable approach in this case—a moderately painful, nonemergent surgery?

The patient should be reassured that buprenorphine will be and should be continued perioperatively. The question of dose reduction is best left to the local subject matter experts including pain specialists, pharmacy, surgery, and addiction clinicians. One recommendation for which there is consensus is that an interdisciplinary team should develop a management strategy for its healthcare system to optimize care coordination and treatment planning for all surgical patients on buprenorphine.[35] A multimodal analgesia strategy including regional techniques should be employed. If full agonist opioids are required, increased doses should be used and titrated to effect. Experimental studies suggest that higher potency opioids such as hydromorphone may be more efficacious.[44]

What if, instead of this surgery, the patient presented for an emergent surgery that is expected to result in moderate to severe pain and usually requires the use of opioids?

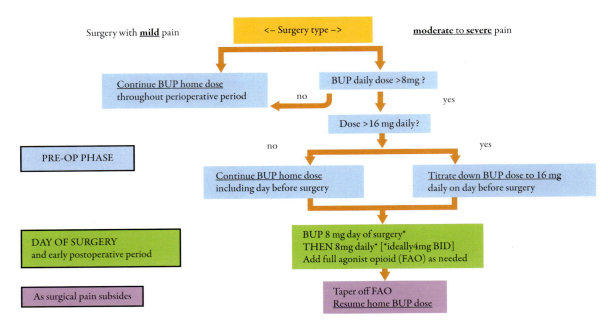

Figure 6.1 Strategy for preoperative dose reduction.
BUP, buprenorphine; BID twice daily.
Used with permission of Dr. Gregory Acampora.

Buprenorphine should still be continued. The same considerations regarding dose reductions apply after emergent surgery. A multimodal analgesia strategy including regional techniques, if appropriate, should be employed.

If the buprenorphine is reduced perioperatively, when should you resume usual buprenorphine maintenance dosing after the surgery?

As mentioned previously, buprenorphine can precipitate withdrawal in patients taking full agonist opioids. Therefore, usual doses of buprenorphine should be resumed once full agonist opioids are no longer necessary. If this occurs after discharge, close follow-up with the buprenorphine prescriber must be arranged and should be arranged in any case. Communication between the inpatient team and the outpatient addiction provider is critical in ensuring an appropriate plan is in place and is executed.

adults with chronic pain, approximately 22% used prescription opioids.[47,48]

Patients on chronic opioids are more likely to have chronic pain, and both are among established risk factors for acute postoperative pain,[49] which itself is a risk factor for persistent postoperative pain.[50] Patients who take opioids chronically (including patients on MOUD) are likely to have abnormal responses to painful stimuli. Two entities that can contribute to these responses are tolerance and opioid-induced hyperalgesia.[51] As mentioned previously, chronic opioid exposure leads to a state where an increased opioid dose is needed to achieve the desired analgesia (e.g., tolerance). Opioid-induced hyperalgesia is a state of increased sensitivity to pain in patients acutely and/or chronically on opioids. Tolerance and opioid-induced hyperalgesia can overlap and be difficult to tease apart. Patients on chronic opioids are also likely to have some degree of dependence and therefore will experience withdrawal if their usual opioid doses are withheld.

DISCUSSION

CONSEQUENCES OF CHRONIC OPIOID USE THAT CONTRIBUTE TO POOR ACUTE PAIN CONTROL

While major national organizations including the Centers for Disease Control and Prevention (CDC) and the US Departments of Veterans Affairs and Defense continue to recommend against the initiation of long-term opioid therapy for chronic noncancer pain,[45,46] a significant number of patients continue to take opioids chronically. Data from the CDC found that of more than 50 million estimated US

PSYCHOSOCIAL BARRIERS TO EFFECTIVE PERIOPERATIVE PAIN MANAGEMENT IN PATIENTS WITH A HISTORY OF OUD

Patients with SUD entering the perioperative environment are likely concerned with fear of withdrawal, fear of discrimination, fear of relapse if in remission, and fear that pain will not be taken seriously and treated effectively.[52] Clinicians on the other hand may mistrust those with SUD, fear respiratory depression from high opioid doses, mistrust claims of pain as fabricated to misuse opioids, fear diversion, and fear the patient interrupting recommended care against medical advice.[52]

METHODS TO OVERCOME THESE BARRIERS

Establishing a good patient–clinician relationship is critical. Clinicians must partner with patients and accept them where they are in recovery. Addressing the patient's concerns up front, setting reasonable expectations, maintaining a matter-of-fact tone, and using nonstigmatizing language will help to establish rapport and trust.[52]

Acute pain should be treated aggressively, including administering both the patient's MOUD (if applicable), multimodal analgesia, and short-acting opioids at higher than usual doses and shorter than usual intervals for breakthrough pain.[53] If pain control is inadequate consultation should be made to the acute pain service and, possibly, an addiction service if these exist in the respective healthcare system.

BUPRENORPHINE AS AN ANALGESIC

Buprenorphine's effectiveness as an analgesic is well established, including the previously referenced systematic review of randomized controlled trials.[15] There is also intriguing evidence supporting its potential in acute postoperative pain management for opioid-naïve patients. A dose of 2 mg sublingual buprenorphine compared to placebo 1 hour before discectomy reduced postoperative pain, analgesic consumption, and nausea.[54] After cholecystectomy, a 400 mcg sublingual dose on arrival to the PACU and again at 6, 12, and 18 hours, compared to fentanyl patient-controlled analgesia (PCA), reduced pain scores and analgesic use, with a trend toward reduced postoperative nausea and vomiting.[55] After mastectomy, 200 mcg sublingual buprenorphine TID versus 100 mg IV tramadol TID within 30 minutes of arrival in PACU resulted in comparable efficacy except for early pain during movement.[56]

In populations post major abdominal surgery, PCA buprenorphine versus morphine resulted in reduced pain, reduced PCA demand, and highest satisfaction.[57] Fentanyl (25 mcg/h) and buprenorphine (10 mcg/h) patches were safe and effective in controlling pain, with less pain in the fentanyl group, less sedation in the buprenorphine group, and 6.7% nausea and vomiting in the buprenorphine group versus 10% in the fentanyl group.[58]

After lower extremity arthroscopy, transdermal buprenorphine (10 mcg/h and 20 mcg/h) versus transdermal fentanyl (25 mcg/h) found pain scores and rescue diclofenac lowest in the 20 mcg/h buprenorphine group, with increased pruritis in the fentanyl group. Transdermal buprenorphine patch (10 mcg/h) resulted in an 11-hour delay to rescue analgesia and more than 300 mg less tramadol compared with transdermal placebo after spine surgery.[59] The patches were applied 12–24 hours preoperatively.

There is considerable enthusiasm for buprenorphine in chronic pain management. It is effective against cancer and neuropathic pain, safe in renal failure and in the elderly, and can be used alongside other opioids.[60] Relative to other opioids it is associated with less tolerance and a milder withdrawal syndrome, is protective against respiratory depression, and results in less cognitive impairment, constipation, immunosuppression, hypogonadism, and drug dependence. Buccal buprenorphine for chronic pain management also resulted in less nausea, vomiting, constipation, somnolence, headache, dizziness, and dry mouth when compared with commonly administered oxymorphone, hydromorphone, and oxycodone.[61] The US Department of Veterans Affairs and the Department of Defense guidelines on the use of opioids in the management of chronic pain includes a new recommendation for buprenorphine in patients receiving daily opioid treatment, citing "a superior safety profile, especially for respiratory depression" and reduced euphoriant effects.[46]

METHADONE

Methadone is also commonly prescribed for OUD. It is a MOR agonist with relatively weak N-methyl-D-aspartate receptor antagonism and some inhibition of serotonin and norepinephrine uptake.[62,63] Typical reported oral bioavailability is 70–80%, with peak plasma concentrations achieved at approximately 3 hours after oral dosing.[64] Like buprenorphine, its duration for suppression of craving (24–36 hours) far exceeds its analgesic duration (4–8 hours), thus for treatment of pain the total dose is typically divided and administered 3–4 times a day.[52] Methadone is notable for highly variable pharmacokinetics; as such, careful titration, particularly during the early stages of treatment, is key given the possibility of accumulation of dangerous levels.[64] Prescribers should also be aware of the potential for numerous drug interactions involving methadone, particularly during the perioperative period where there is a relative polypharmacy.

Patients on methadone maintenance should continue their daily methadone maintenance dose, which should be verified with the maintenance program, and analgesia should be provided with a multimodal regimen including short-acting full agonist opioids as required. As with any chronic opioid, it is important to recognize that the baseline daily methadone dose should not be expected to provide analgesia. If an oral to IV methadone conversion is required, a prudent approach is a 2:1 conversion with recognition that the IV dose may require subsequent titration up toward the 1:1 ratio.[65] Close follow-up with the maintenance program is essential, particularly if postoperative impairments (e.g., inability to ambulate) necessitate an accommodation with take-home doses of methadone.

Methadone can prolong the corrected QT interval (QTc), which may predispose patients to arrhythmias, including torsades de pointes. Polypharmacy and electrolyte abnormalities typical of hospitalized patients can both exacerbate QTc prolongation and predispose to arrhythmia per se. Clinicians should be mindful of these possibilities while managing these patients and monitor for ECG changes.

NALTREXONE

Naltrexone is a MOR antagonist used to treat both opioid and alcohol use disorders. If a need for opioid analgesia is anticipated, naltrexone should be held preoperatively. For oral naloxone (Revia), which has an approximately 10-hour half-life, most recommendations suggest at least a 48-hour abstinence with 72 hours being the commonest approach.[66,67] Extended-release (ER) naltrexone (Vivitrol) is a monthly 380 mg IM injection with a single dose resulting in a three- to four-fold higher exposure than standard the typical 50 mg/d oral maintenance dosing, therapeutic levels at 35 days post-injection, and a 5- to 10-day half-life.[68,69] In an animal antinociceptive study comparing analgesic responses to opioids after ER naltrexone versus placebo, rats required a fentanyl dose 200 times the baseline dose in the placebo group at 19 days and 5 times that baseline dose at 39 days after ER injection.[70] The subjective effects of heroin began to emerge 5 weeks after ER naltrexone injection.[71] While not supported by robust prospective human data, clinical experience and case reports describe the ability to overcome MOR blockade in the fourth week after ER injection.[72] Thus, most recommendations are to schedule elective surgery at least a month after the last ER maintenance dose.

For emergency surgery, multimodal analgesia, including neuraxial or regional techniques, when indicated is appropriate. Effectiveness of opioids will be extremely limited for at least the first day after oral naltrexone administration and first few weeks after ER injection. Particularly if very high doses of opioids are employed, patients should be monitored carefully for sedation and respiratory depression which may arise in the setting of decreasing naltrexone MOR antagonism and increasing MOR agonism. Naltrexone is typically resumed 5–7 days after the last opioid to avoid precipitated withdrawal, though shorter or longer abstinences could be considered for short- and long-acting opioids, respectively.

PERIOPERATIVE ISSUES IN NON-OPIOID SUBSTANCE USE DISORDERS

Overarching Principles

SUD is common, underrecognized, and increases overall perioperative risk.[73,74] Comorbid SUD is common, and, in general, intoxication with multiple substances will worsen the signs and symptoms of intoxication and complicate diagnosis and treatment. Hospitalization of a patient with unrecognized SUD may result in a potentially severe withdrawal syndrome. Widely available screening tools are effective and can be employed at the time of preoperative evaluation.[75] Identification of the SUD prompts a more careful evaluation for diseases occurring as a result of the substance use, recommendations to modify use, and possible referral to treatment.

Stimulants

Amphetamines
Amphetamines stimulate catecholamine release and may be prescribed for attention deficit disorders, narcolepsy, depression, and hyperactivity. Expected effects include alertness, decreased appetite, and decreased sleep. Overdose causes CNS irritability ranging from anxiety to seizure, hypertension, arrhythmia, and tachycardia. Long-term use results in a high degree of dependence and a depletion of catecholamine stores.[76]

Patients taking prescribed amphetamines as instructed should continue these medications perioperatively. These patients may have reduced anesthetic requirements and experience hypotension in the setting of reduced catecholamines; direct-acting vasopressors such as phenylephrine and norepinephrine should be available. Acutely intoxicated patients requiring emergent surgery may present with hypertension, tachycardia, arrhythmia, and hyperthermia and are likely to have increased anesthetic requirements but similar analgetic requirements.[77] Withdrawal symptoms include dysphoria, fatigue, irritability, intense craving for stimulants, increased appetite, and anxiety.

Cocaine
Cocaine blocks presynaptic norepinephrine and dopamine uptake leading to sympathetic stimulation. Duration of action is approximately 45 minutes. Cocaine is associated with vasoconstriction and thrombus formation. It can cause a wide range of organ injury including myocardial ischemia, arrhythmia, aortic dissection, agitation, seizure, hyperthermia, stroke, pulmonary edema, alveolar hemorrhage, bronchospasm, mesenteric ischemia, rhabdomyolysis, and placental abruption. Overdose is characterized by massive sympathetic stimulation. Withdrawal is typically mild and includes fatigue, depression, and increased appetite.

Elective procedures should be delayed in cases of acute cocaine intoxication. Medically necessary procedures, however, should not be delayed simply due to recent use or positive urine drug test. For emergent surgery in the setting of acute intoxication, benzodiazepine premedication may be useful to reduce cardiovascular symptoms, and nitroglycerin and/or nitroprusside should be immediately available to treat severe hypertension. Beta blockers are typically avoided in this scenario due to the possibility of unopposed alpha-adrenergic stimulation resulting in worsening hypertension and, possibly, coronary vasospasm.[78]

Depressants

Alcohol
Alcohol is a CNS depressant with a wide range of molecular sites of action and interactions with a broad range of neurotransmitters. Chronic use increases risk of disease in numerous organ systems, predisposes to multiple cancers, and increases perioperative morbidity and mortality including the consequences of alcohol withdrawal syndrome and delirium tremens (DT).

The chronic depressant exposure causes downregulation of the inhibitory and upregulation of the excitatory neurotransmitter systems, including suppression of the major inhibitory neurotransmitter, gamma aminobutyric acid (GABA). Discontinuation of or marked decrease in alcohol may reveal this imbalance, with excess excitatory influence causing withdrawal syndrome of varying degrees of severity. Symptoms typically arise 6–24 hours after the last drink and peak at 24–36 hours. Tremors, perceptual disturbances, autonomic hyperactivity, agitation, seizure, nausea, and vomiting are characteristic. Risk factors for severe withdrawal syndrome include prior withdrawal syndrome, simultaneous withdrawal from other substance(s), age older than 45, acute illness, and comorbidities. Life-threatening delirium tremens can occur 48–96 hours after the last drink and manifests as a much more severe version of the usual withdrawal syndrome, with hemodynamic changes consistent with excess autonomic tone, more severe mental status change and agitation, and grand mal seizures.[79]

The Clinical Institute Withdrawal Assessment–Alcohol Scale, Revised (CIWA–Ar) is a validated assessment tool widely applied to determine severity of withdrawal and guide treatment, typically with diazepam or lorazepam.[80] Other adjuncts such as beta blockers and/or alpha 2 agonists may be useful in controlling the sympathetic hyperactivity. Vitamin deficiencies should be corrected, including high-dose thiamine followed by glucose infusions to treat presumed Wernicke encephalopathy.[81]

Reductions in alcohol consumption preoperatively are shown to decrease perioperative complications. The three FDA-approved treatments for alcohol use disorder are acamprosate, disulfiram, and naltrexone. Perioperative considerations for naltrexone are described above. Cross-tolerance between alcohol and opioids does not appear to occur. While the acutely intoxicated patient is expected to have decreased anesthetic requirements, the patient with chronic use likely requires increased anesthetic.

Benzodiazepines

Benzodiazepines are the most used anxiolytics. Treatment for benzodiazepine use disorder has risen over the past decades. Acute overdose of benzodiazepines alone is relatively safe compared with barbiturate overdose. However, the presence of benzodiazepines significantly increases the severity of overdose when taken with another substance. Flumazenil, a benzodiazepine receptor antagonist, can be used to both diagnose and reverse benzodiazepine-induced CNS depression; however, flumazenil should not be used indiscriminately as it is associated with seizures, particularly in the patients on long-term benzodiazepines. Baseline benzodiazepines should be continued perioperatively. Withdrawal syndrome can last from days to weeks depending on the half-life of the benzodiazepine used. Symptoms range from anxiety to seizure. Note that symptoms may not begin for 5–7 days for patients on long-acting benzodiazepines. A long taper is often employed for patients desiring to discontinue benzodiazepines.

Barbiturates

Barbiturates are sedative hypnotics which have been largely replaced by benzodiazepines both in clinical practice and in misuse. Tolerance to the reinforcing effects (e.g., euphoria) of barbiturates increases more rapidly than tolerance to their lethal effects, reducing the safety margin considerably. Cross-tolerance to other CNS depressants is expected, potentially resulting in increased anesthetic requirements. Acute overdose manifests as severe CNS depression and ultimately coma. As there is no reversal agent, supportive care, including intubation and mechanical ventilation, may be required.

The withdrawal syndrome can be severe and characterized by tremor, tachycardia, hyperthermia, cardiovascular collapse, and, possibly, grand mal seizures. Benzodiazepines and anti-seizure agents (e.g., phenobarbital) are useful in suppressing withdrawal symptoms.

Hallucinogens

Cannabis

Cannabinol and delta-9-tetrahydrocannabinol are the main cannabinoid type 1 and type 2 receptor agonists.[82] Cannabis use disorder is frequently associated with comorbid SUD. In general, cannabis intake is expected to activate the sympathetic nervous system and inhibit the parasympathetic nervous system. As such there is a dose-dependent increase in both heart rate and blood pressure that persists for 1–2 hour after smoking and possibly longer with chronic use. Cannabis may increase respiratory symptoms including increasing airway reactivity. Its use is associated with increased myocardial infarction, stroke, and arrhythmia. A dose-dependent decrease in cognitive function is seen. Cannabis exposure, particularly in youth, is associated with psychotic disorders. Cannabis hyperemesis syndrome should be suspected in patients using daily cannabis who describe episodic severe nausea and vomiting, classically relieved by a hot bath or shower.

Withdrawal from chronic use presents within 24–72 hours from last use and consists of irritability, insomnia, and depression and resolves within several weeks. Withdrawal from synthetic cannabinoids may manifest with more severe signs and symptoms of autonomic hyperactivity.

Recent guidelines identified a number of recommendations including grades of evidence strength based on the US Preventative Services Task Force grades A–D. Grade A–B recommendations were universal screening including type and frequency of use and last use (A); counseling on potential harms, including to fetus in pregnant patients (B); postponing elective surgery in acute intoxication (A); and discouraging cannabis use in pregnancy (B).[82] While anesthetic requirements are likely decreased in acute cannabis intoxication, they are increased in chronic use. Cannabis users may experience increased postoperative pain and higher opioid requirements compared to nonusers.

Lysergic Acid Diethylamide (LSD)

LSD produces hallucinations and distortions of the environment. There is often increased sympathetic stimulation leading to mydriasis, tachycardia, and hypertension. There is no evidence of physiologic dependence.

Kratom

Kratom is an herbal extract with opioid and stimulant properties; it is as yet not regulated by the DEA.[83] The stimulant properties predominate at low doses and the opioid effects at high doses. It is sold in various forms both online and in smoke shops, where it is typically advertised as a legal, natural cure-all. It has a complicated pharmacology, with agonist effects at the MOR (including some reports of opioid cross tolerance), cyclooxygenase-2 inhibitor, and alpha-2 agonist. Variable person-to-person experience with kratom is at least in part explained by the variability in formulation of this unregulated over-the-counter substance. Chronic self-medication with kratom can lead to dependence, addiction, and withdrawal. Overdose and withdrawal symptoms significantly overlap and are largely neurologic, cardiopulmonary, and gastrointestinal.

Perioperatively, kratom may result in unexpected hemodynamic variability, unexpected drug-drug interactions, unrecognized kidney and liver disease, QTc prolongation, serotonin syndrome, prolonged emergence, postoperative complications, and prolonged length of stay.

CONCLUSION

The perioperative management of patients with SUD can be challenging and requires basic understanding of the disorders themselves, the pharmacology of the substances themselves and medications used to treat the disorders, and perioperative management strategies for these disorders and their treatments. Understanding of MOUDs and their management are of particular importance. Interdisciplinary care planning involving at least the anesthesiologist, surgeon, and SUD clinician is essential to formulate a patient-centered plan.

REVIEW QUESTIONS

1. A 56-year-old man presents for preoperative evaluation for elective total hip arthroplasty. He is maintained on 16 mg/day (8 mg BID) of buprenorphine for opioid use disorder. He is otherwise in generally good health. Which of the following best describes buprenorphine's pharmacologic mechanism?

   a. Full mu agonist, kappa antagonist, partial delta agonist.
   b. Partial mu agonist, kappa antagonist, delta antagonist.
   c. Mu antagonist, full kappa agonist, partial delta agonist.
   d. Full mu agonist, partial kappa agonist, full delta agonist.

   The correct answer is b.

   Buprenorphine is a partial agonist at (and with a very high affinity for) the MOR, a kappa and delta opioid receptor antagonist, and acts as an antagonist in the presence of full agonist opioids.

2. For the above patient, which of the following is the most reasonable perioperative buprenorphine management strategy?

   a. Recommend a 96-hour abstinence.
   b. Recommend doubling the buprenorphine dose starting 72 hours prior to surgery.
   c. Recommend continuing buprenorphine perioperatively at usual dose.

   The correct answer is c.

Buprenorphine is an opioid approved by the FDA for the treatment of pain. It is increasingly prescribed for the treatment of opioid use disorder, which is increasingly prevalent. Its partial agonism at the MOR, long duration of action, and high affinity for the MOR make it very effective for this indication. Historic perioperative practice for surgery expected to result in at least moderate postoperative pain was to recommend at least a 72-hour abstinence from buprenorphine, which was felt to be sufficient time to allow MOR to be available for full agonist opioids. More recent evidence supports both buprenorphine's analgesic effectiveness per se and its effectiveness in combination with full agonists. It is also clear that perioperative outcomes, both in terms of acute pain and for OUD, are worse when buprenorphine is discontinued perioperatively.

3. A 45-year-old man is on buprenorphine/naloxone 32/8 mg sublingually daily for OUD. He presents for cystoscopy having taken his usual dose on the morning of the procedure. The best course of action at this point is

   a. Postpone and reschedule the procedure, proceeding only after a 72-hour abstinence.
   b. Postpone and reschedule the procedure, proceeding only after a dose reduction to 16 mg the day prior to and 8 mg the day of the procedure.
   c. Continue with the cystoscopy.

   The correct answer is c.

   For surgeries expected to result in mild or lesser pain, no change in buprenorphine is required.

4. A 47-year-old woman on transdermal buprenorphine 20 mcg/hour for treatment of chronic lower back pain is scheduled for a nephrectomy and asks for your advice to manage this medication perioperatively. The best course of action is

   a. Continue the buprenorphine patch during the perioperative period.
   b. Stop the buprenorphine patch 12 hours before the surgery.
   c. Stop the buprenorphine patch 72 hours before the surgery.
   d. Stop the buprenorphine patch 1 week before the surgery.

   The correct answer is a.

   It is increasingly recognized that continuation of buprenorphine results in better patient outcomes, particularly for acute pain. Typical doses for treatment of pain are much lower than typical doses for OUD. For example, this patient's transdermal dose is approximately equivalent to a 1 mg sublingual dose. Thus, whereas we might consider reducing the buprenorphine dose for patients on greater than 16 mg/day buprenorphine for OUD, we are well below this threshold in this case. There will be ample MOR available in the likely event that full agonist opioids are required.

5. A 58-year-old man with lung cancer presents to the preoperative clinic for evaluation for his upcoming thoracotomy.

He has a history of OUD and is currently on methadone 50 mg/day for OUD treatment. What is the recommended plan for the methadone?

   a. Stop the methadone for 72 hours before surgery.
   b. Stop the methadone for 1 week before surgery.
   c. Have the patient take the methadone up to and including the day of surgery.
   d. Have the patient transition to buprenorphine and continue that until the day of surgery.

The correct answer is c.

Patients should continue their daily methadone maintenance dose after dose verification with the maintenance program, and analgesia should be provided with short-acting full opioid agonists (as part of a multimodal analgesia strategy, as usual).

6. A 53-year-old man presents to the emergency department following a motor vehicle accident. He is scheduled for urgent repair of a femur fracture. He discloses that he is a heavy alcohol user, last drink was 4 hours ago. In patients with an alcohol use disorder, postoperative opioid requirements are

   a. Increased, because of cross-tolerance between alcohol and opioids.
   b. Decreased, because patients with alcohol use disorder are more resistant to pain.
   c. Unchanged.

The correct answer is c.

There is no cross-tolerance between alcohol and opioids, so there is no need to use higher than standard doses of opioids in alcohol-dependent patients. Acute intoxication will potentiate the respiratory depressant effects of other perioperative medications, notably opioids. It is important to recognize the myriad comorbidities he may have secondary to chronic alcohol use disorder and adjust perioperative management accordingly. It is critical to monitor these patients closely for alcohol withdrawal symptoms in the perioperative period and treat them accordingly.

7. A 61-year-old woman with a history of OUD is scheduled for a total knee replacement in 2.5 weeks. She receives extended-release intramuscular naltrexone every 4 weeks, with the last injection being the day before her preoperative clinic visit. What is the best plan for her surgery at this point?

   a. Continue with the surgery as scheduled in 2.5 weeks.
   b. Postpone the surgery for at least 2 weeks, so that she is about 1 month from her IM naltrexone dose.
   c. Move the surgery up to the next couple days before the naltrexone has a chance to start working.
   d. Postpone the surgery for 4 months, so that she is 4–5 months from her IM naltrexone dose.

The correct answer is b.

Naltrexone is a MOR antagonist. If full agonist opioid use is anticipated, it is generally recommended to delay elective surgery for 72 hours from last oral naltrexone and for 1 month from last extended-release IM injection.

REFERENCES

1. American Psychiatric Association. *Diagnostic and Statistical Manual of Mental Disorders*. 5th ed. American Psychiatric Association; 2013. https://doi.org/10.1176/appi.books.9780890425596
2. Lewis J, Nathan B. Eddy Award lecture: In pursuit of the Holy Grail. The College on Problems of Drug Dependence (CPDD) website. 1998. https://cpdd.org/Media/Index/AwardSpeeches/LewisJ._Eddy1998.pdf
3. NICE. Database of treatment effects. https://www.nice.org.uk
4. Larochelle MR, et al. Medication for opioid use disorder after nonfatal opioid overdose and association with mortality: A cohort study. *Ann Intern Med*. 2018 Aug 7;169(3):137–145.
5. Chou R, Dana T, Blazina I, Grusing S, Fu R, Bougatsos C. Interventions for unhealthy drug use—supplemental report: A systematic review for the U.S. Preventive Services Task Force. Agency for Healthcare Research and Quality (US). 2020 Jun. Report No.: 19-05255-EF-2. PMID: 32550674 Available from: https://www.ncbi.nlm.nih.gov/books/NBK558205/
6. Olfson M, Zhang VS, Schoenbaum M, King M. Trends in buprenorphine treatment in the US, 2009–2018. *JAMA*. 2020 Jan 21;323(3):276–277.
7. H.R.2617. 117th Congress (2021–2022). Consolidated Appropriations Act, 2023. Congress.gov., Library of Congress. 2022, Dec. 29. https://www.congress.gov/bill/117th-congress/house-bill/2617.
8. Coe MA, Lofwall MR, Walsh SL. Buprenorphine pharmacology review: Update on transmucosal and long-acting formulations. *J Addict Med*. 2019;13(2):93–103.
9. Webster L, Gudin J, Raffa RB, et al. Understanding buprenorphine for use in chronic pain: Expert opinion. *Pain Med*. 2020;21(4):714–723.
10. Coe MA, Lofwall MR, Walsh SL. Buprenorphine pharmacology review: Update on transmucosal and long-acting formulations. *J Addict Med*. 2019;13(2):93–103.
11. Greenwald MK, Herring AA, Perrone J, Nelson LS, Azar P. A neuropharmacological model to explain buprenorphine induction challenges. *Ann Emerg Med*. 2022 Dec;80(6):509–524. doi:10.1016/j.annemergmed.2022.05.032.
12. Dahan A. Opioid-induced respiratory effects: New data on buprenorphine. *Palliat Med*. 2006;20(Suppl 1):s3u–8. PMID: 16764215
13. Bach P, Bawa M, Grant C, Milloy MJ, Hayashi K. Availability and use of non-prescribed buprenorphine-naloxone in a Canadian setting, 2014–2020. *Int J Drug Policy*. 2022 Mar;101:103545. doi:10.1016/j.drugpo.2021.103545
14. Cicero TJ, Ellis MS, Chilcoat HD. Understanding the use of diverted buprenorphine. *Drug Alcohol Depend*. 2018 Dec 1;193:117–123. doi:10.1016/j.drugalcdep.2018.09.007
15. White LD, Hodge R, Vlok R, Hurtado G, Eastern K, Melhuish TM. Efficacy and adverse effects of buprenorphine in acute pain management: Systematic review and meta-analysis of randomised controlled trials. *Br J Anaesth*. 2018 Apr;120(4):668–678.
16. Raffa RB, Haidery M, Huang HM, et al. The clinical analgesic efficacy of buprenorphine. *J Clin Pharm Ther*. 2014 Dec;39(6):577–583. doi:10.1111/jcpt.12196
17. Volpe DA, McMahon Tobin GA, Mellon RD, et al. Uniform assessment and ranking of opioid μ receptor binding constants for selected opioid drugs. *Regul Toxicol Pharmacol*. 2011 Apr;59(3):385–390. doi:10.1016/j.yrtph.2010.12.007
18. Subutex [package insert]. 2022 Jun. Invidior Inc., North Chesterfield, VA, USA.
19. Downing JW, Leary WP, White ES. Buprenorphine: A new potent long-acting synthetic analgesic. Comparison with morphine. *Br J Anaesth*. 1977 Mar;49(3):251–255.
20. Yassen A, Olofsen E, Romberg R, Sarton E, Danhof M, Dahan A. Mechanism-based pharmacokinetic-pharmacodynamic modeling of the antinociceptive effect of buprenorphine in healthy volunteers. *Anesthesiology*. 2006 Jun;104(6):1232–1242
21. Koppert W, Ihmsen H, Körber N, Wehrfritz A, Sittl R, Schmelz M, Schüttler J. Different profiles of buprenorphine-induced

analgesia and antihyperalgesia in a human pain model. *Pain.* 2005 Nov;118(1–2):15–22.
22. Avdeef A, Barrett DA, Shaw PN, Knaggs RD, Davis SS. Octanol-, chloroform-, and propylene glycol dipelargonat-water partitioning of morphine-6-glucuronide and other related opiates. *J Med Chem.* 1996 Oct 25;39(22):4377–4381.
23. Peckham EM, Traynor JR. Comparison of the antinociceptive response to morphine and morphine-like compounds in male and female Sprague-Dawley rats. *J Pharmacol Exp Ther.* 2006 Mar;316(3):1195–1201. doi:10.1124/jpet.105.094276
24. Kuhlman JJ Jr, Lalani S, Magluilo J Jr, Levine B, Darwin WD. Human pharmacokinetics of intravenous, sublingual, and buccal buprenorphine. *J Ann Toxicol.* 1996 Oct;20(6):369–378. doi:10.1093/jat/20.6.369
25. Mendelson J, Upton RA, Everhart ET, Jacob P III, Jones RT. Bioavailability of sublingual buprenorphine. *J Clin Pharmacol.* 1997 Jan;37(1):31–37.
26. Belbuca [package insert]. 2019. BioDelivery Sciences International, Inc. Raleigh, NC, USA.
27. Mehta V, Langford RM. Acute pain management for opioid dependent patients. *Anaesthesia.* 2006;61(3):269–276.
28. Rapp SE, Ready BL, Nessly ML. Acute pain management in patients with prior opioid consumption: A case-controlled retrospective review. *Pain.* 1995;61(2):195–201.
29. Wyse JJ, Herreid-O'Neill A, Dougherty J, et al. Perioperative management of buprenorphine/naloxone in a large, national health care system: A retrospective cohort study. *J Gen Intern Med.* 2022 Sep;37(12):2998–3004. doi:10.1007/s11606-021-07118-4
30. Jones HE, O'Grady K, Dahne J, et al. Management of acute postpartum pain in patients maintained on methadone or buprenorphine during pregnancy. *Am J Drug Alcohol Abuse.* 2009;35(3):151–156.
31. Quaye A, Potter K, Roth S, Acampora G, Mao J, Zhang Y. Perioperative continuation of buprenorphine at low-moderate doses was associated with lower postoperative pain scores and decreased outpatient opioid dispensing compared with buprenorphine discontinuation. *Pain Med.* 2020 Sep 1;21(9):1955–1960. doi:10.1093/pm/pnaa020
32. Oifa S, Sydoruk T, White I, et al. Effects of intravenous patient-controlled analgesia with buprenorphine and morphine alone and in combination during the first 12 postoperative hours: A randomized, double-blind, four-arm trial in adults undergoing abdominal surgery. *Clin Ther.* 2009;31(3):527–541.
33. Buresh M, Ratner J, Zgierska A, Gordin V, Alvanzo A. Treating perioperative and acute pain in patients on buprenorphine: Narrative literature review and practice recommendations. *J Gen Intern Med.* 2020 Dec;35(12):3635–3643. doi:10.1007/s11606-020-06115-3
34. Kohan L, Potru S, Barreveld AM, et al. Buprenorphine management in the perioperative period: Educational review and recommendations from a multisociety expert panel. *Reg Anesth Pain Med.* 2021 Oct;46(10):840–859. doi:10.1136/rapm-2021-103007
35. Hickey T, Abelleira A, Acampora G, Becker WC, Falker CG, Nazario M, Weimer MB. Perioperative buprenorphine management: A multidisciplinary approach. *Med Clin North Am.* 2022 Jan;106(1):169–185. doi:10.1016/j.mcna.2021.09.001
36. Acampora GA, Nisavic M, Zhang Y. Perioperative buprenorphine continuous maintenance and administration simultaneous with full opioid agonist: Patient priority at the interface between medical disciplines. *J Clin Psychiatry.* 2020 Jan 7;81(1):19com12810. doi:10.4088/JCP.19com12810
37. Mehta D, Thomas V, Johnson J, Scott B, Cortina S, Berger L. Continuation of buprenorphine to facilitate postoperative pain management for patients on buprenorphine opioid agonist therapy. *Pain Physician.* 2020 Mar;23(2):E163–E174.
38. Greenwald MK, Johanson CE, Moody DE, et al. Effects of buprenorphine maintenance dose on mu-opioid receptor availability, plasma concentrations, and antagonist blockade in heroin-dependent volunteers. *Neuropsychopharmacology.* 2003;28(11):2000–2009.
39. Greenwald M, Johanson C-E, Bueller J, et al. Buprenorphine duration of action: Mu-opioid receptor availability and pharmacokinetic and behavioral indices. *Biol Psychiatry.* 2007;61(1):101–110.
40. Greenwald MK, Comer SD, Fiellin DA. Buprenorphine maintenance and mu opioid receptor availability in the treatment of opioid use disorder: Implications for clinical use and policy. *Drug Alcohol Depend.* 2014;144:1–11.
41. U.S. Food and Drug Administration/Center for Drug Evaluation and Research. FDA Briefing Document on NDA 209819 for RBP-6000 (buprenorphine injectable) for treatment of opioid dependence. 10 31, 2017a. https://www.accessdata.fda.gov/drugsatfda_docs/nda/2017/209819Orig1s000ClinPharmR.pdf
42. Hickey TR, Henry JT, Edens EL, Gordon AJ, Acampora G. Perioperative management of extended-release buprenorphine. *J Addict Med.* 2023 Jan-Feb 01;17(1):e67–e71. doi:10.1097/ADM.0000000000001024
43. Hickey TR, Meeks T, Oxentine H, et al. Perioperative management of extended-release buprenorphine: A narrative review and case series. *Substance Abuse J.* 2023 April 26. https://doi.org/10.1177/08897077231167043
44. De Aquino JP, Parida S, Avila-Quintero VJ, Flores J, Compton P, Hickey T, Gómez O, Sofuoglu M. Opioid-induced analgesia among persons with opioid use disorder receiving methadone or buprenorphine: A systematic review of experimental pain studies. *Drug Alcohol Depend.* 2021 Nov 1;228:109097. doi:10.1016/j.drugalcdep.2021.109097.
45. Dowell D, Ragan KR, Jones CM, et al. CDC clinical practice guideline for prescribing opioids for pain—United States, 2022. *MMWR Recomm Rep.* 2022;71:1–95. doi:10.15585/mmwr.rr7103a1
46. Sandbrink F, Murphy JL, Johansson M, Olson JL, Edens E, Clinton-Lont J, Sall J, Spevak C; VA/DoD Guideline Development Group. The use of opioids in the management of chronic pain: Synopsis of the 2022 updated U.S. Department of Veterans Affairs and U.S. Department of Defense clinical practice guideline. *Ann Intern Med.* 2023 Mar;176(3):388–397. doi:10.7326/M22-2917
47. Zelaya CE, Dahlhamer JM, Lucas JW, Connor EM. Chronic pain and high-impact chronic pain among U.S. adults, 2019. *NCHS Data Brief.* 2020;(390):1–8.
48. Dahlhamer JM, Connor EM, Bose J, Lucas JL, Zelaya CE. Prescription opioid use among adults with chronic pain: United States, 2019. *Natl Health Stat Report.* 2021;(162):1–9. doi:10.15620/cdc:107641
49. Yang MMH, Hartley RL, Leung AA, Ronksley PE, Jetté N, Casha S, Riva-Cambrin J. Preoperative predictors of poor acute postoperative pain control: A systematic review and meta-analysis. *BMJ Open.* 2019 Apr 1;9(4):e025091. doi:10.1136/bmjopen-2018-025091.
50. Kehlet H, Jensen TS, Woolf CJ. Persistent postsurgical pain: Risk factors and prevention. *Lancet.* 2006 May 13;367(9522):1618–1625. doi:10.1016/S0140-6736(06)68700-X
51. Colvin LA, Bull F, Hales TG. Perioperative opioid analgesia: When is enough too much? A review of opioid-induced tolerance and hyperalgesia. *Lancet.* 2019 Apr 13;393(10180):1558–1568.
52. Quinlan J, Cox F. Acute pain management in patients with drug dependence syndrome. *Pain Rep.* 2017;2(4):e611. doi:10.1097/PR9.0000000000000611
53. Calcaterra SL, Bottner R, Martin M, et al. Management of opioid use disorder, opioid withdrawal, and opioid overdose prevention in hospitalized adults: A systematic review of existing guidelines. *J Hosp Med.* 2022 Sep;17(9):679–692. doi:10.1002/jhm.12908
54. Kiabi FH, Emadi SA, Shafizad M, Jelodar AG, Deylami H. The effect of preoperative sublingual buprenorphine on postoperative pain after lumbar discectomy: A randomized controlled trial. *Ann Med Surg (Lond).* 2021 May 1;65:102347. doi:10.1016/j.amsu.2021.102347
55. Norozi V, Ghazi A, Amani F, Bakhshpoori P. Effectiveness of sublingual buprenorphine and fentanyl pump in controlling pain after open cholecystectomy. *Anesth Pain Med.* 2021 Aug 8;11(3):e113909. doi:10.5812/aapm.113909
56. Dokku KS, Nair AS, Prasad Mantha SS, Naik VM, Saifuddin MS, Rayani BK. A randomized controlled study to compare analgesic efficacy of sublingual buprenorphine and intravenous tramadol in patients undergoing mastectomy. *Med Gas Res.* 2023 Jul-Sep;13(3):118–122. doi:10.4103/2045-9912.345170

57. Oifa S, Sydoruk T, White I, et al. Effects of intravenous patient-controlled analgesia with buprenorphine and morphine alone and in combination during the first 12 postoperative hours: A randomized, double-blind, four-arm trial in adults undergoing abdominal surgery. *Clin Ther.* 2009 Mar;31(3):527–541. doi:10.1016/j.clinthera.2009.03.018

58. Arshad Z, Prakash R, Gautam S, Kumar S. Comparison between transdermal buprenorphine and transdermal fentanyl for postoperative pain relief after major abdominal surgeries. *J Clin Diagn Res.* 2015 Dec;9(12):UC01–4. doi:10.7860/JCDR/2015/16327.6917

59. Niyogi S, Bhunia P, Nayak J, Santra S, Acharjee A, Chakraborty I. Efficacy of transdermal buprenorphine patch on post-operative pain relief after elective spinal instrumentation surgery. *Indian J Anaesth.* 2017 Nov;61(11):923–929. doi:10.4103/ija.IJA_118_17

60. Davis MP. Twelve reasons for considering buprenorphine as a frontline analgesic in the management of pain. *J Support Oncol.* 2012 Nov-Dec;10(6):209–219.

61. Hale M, Garofoli M, Raffa RB. Benefit-risk analysis of buprenorphine for pain management. *J Pain Res.* 2021 May 24;14:1359–1369. doi:10.2147/JPR.S305146

62. Gorman AL, Elliott KJ, Inturrisi CE. The d- and l-isomers of methadone bind to the noncompetitive site on the N-methyl-D-aspartate (NMDA) receptor in rat forebrain and spinal cord. *Neurosci Lett.* 1997;223:5–8.

63. Codd E, Shank R, Schupsky J, Raffia R. Serotonin and norepinephrine uptake inhibiting activity of centrally acting analgesics: Structural determinants and role in antinociception. *J Pharmacol Exp Ther.* 1995;274:1263–1270.

64. Lugo RA, Satterfield KL, Kern SE. Pharmacokinetics of methadone. *J Pain Palliat Care Pharmacother.* 2005;19(4):13–24. PMID: 16431829

65. Manfredi PL, Houde RW. Prescribing methadone, a unique analgesic. *J Support Oncol.* 2003 Sep-Oct;1(3):216–220. PMID: 15334878

66. Revia [package insert]. 2013 October. Duramed Pharmaceuticals, Inc., Pomona, NY, USA.

67. Harrison TK, Kornfeld H, Aggarwal AK, Lembke A. Perioperative considerations for the patient with opioid use disorder on buprenorphine, methadone, or naltrexone maintenance therapy. *Anesthesiol Clin.* 2018 Sep;36(3):345–359. doi:10.1016/j.anclin.2018.04.002

68. Turncliff RZ, Dong Q, Silverman B, Ehrich E, Lasseter KC. Single and multiple-dose pharmacokinetics of long-acting injectable naltrexone. *Alcohol Clin Exp Res.* 2006;30:480–490.

69. Vivitrol [package insert]. 2010 Oct. Alkermes, Inc., Waltham, MA, USA.

70. Dean RL, Todtenkopf MS, Deaver DR, et al. Overriding the blockade of antinociceptive actions of opioids in rats treated with extended-release naltrexone. *Pharmacol Biochem Behav.* 2008 Jun;89(4):515–522. doi:10.1016/j.pbb.2008.02.006

71. Comer SD, Collins ED, Kleber HD, Nuwayser ES, Kerrigan JH, Fischman MW. Depot naltrexone: Long-lasting antagonism of the effects of heroin in humans. *Psychopharmacology (Berl).* 2002 Feb;159(4):351–360

72. Sullivan MA, Vosburg SK, Comer SD. Depot naltrexone: Antagonism of the reinforcing, subjective, and physiological effects of heroin. *Psychopharmacology (Berl).* 2006 Nov;189(1):37–46. doi:10.1007/s00213-006-0509-x.

73. Weimer MB, Hines RL. Psychiatric disease, substance use disorders, and drug overdose. In: Hines RL, Jones SB, eds. *Stoelting's Anesthesia and Co-Existing Disease.* 8th ed. Elsevier; 2022:619–644

74. Alford DP, Weinstein ZM. Perioperative management of patients with alcohol- or other drug use. In: Miller SC, Fiellin DA, Rosenthal RN, Saitz R, eds. *The ASAM Principles of Addiction Medicine.* 6th ed. Wolters Kluwer; 2019:1333–1343.

75. National Institute on Drug Abuse. Screening Tools and Prevention. 2023 Jan 6. https://nida.nih.gov/nidamed-medical-health-professionals/screening-tools-prevention

76. Fischer SP, Healzer JM, Brook MW, Brock-Utne JG. General anesthesia in a patient on long-term amphetamine therapy: Is there cause for concern? *Anesth Analg.* 2000;91(3):758–759.

77. Kram B, Kram SJ, Sharpe ML, James ML, Kuchibhatla M, Shapiro ML. Analgesia and sedation requirements in mechanically ventilated trauma patients with acute, preinjury use of cocaine and/or amphetamines. *Anesth Analg.* 2017;124:782–788.

78. Voigt L. Anesthetic management of the cocaine abuse patient. *AANA J.* 1995;63(5):438–443.

79. Kattimani S, Bharadwaj B. Clinical management of alcohol withdrawal: A systematic review. *Ind Psychiatry J.* 2013;22(2):100–108.

80. Sullivan JT, Sykora K, Schneiderman J, Naranjo CA, Sellers EM. Assessment of alcohol withdrawalfhe revised clinical institute withdrawal assessment for alcohol scale (CIWA-Ar). *Br J Addict.* 1989;84(11):1353–1357.

81. Stanley KM, Amabile CM, Simpson KN, Couillard D, Norcross ED, Worrall CL. Impact of an alcohol withdrawal syndrome practice guideline on surgical patient outcomes. *Pharmacotherapy.* 2003;23(7):843–854.

82. Shah S, Schwenk ES, Sondekoppam RV, et al. ASRA Pain Medicine consensus guidelines on the management of the perioperative patient on cannabis and cannabinoids. *Reg Anesth Pain Med.* 2023 Mar;48(3):97–117.

7.

INDICATIONS FOR PREOPERATIVE C-SPINE IMAGING FOR ELECTIVE PROCEDURES

Deborah C. Richman

STEM CASE AND KEY QUESTIONS

A 57-year-old woman presents to your preoperative clinic prior to thyroidectomy for a large goiter. She was asymptomatic until recently, when she noticed occasional difficulty swallowing "dry foods like bread." She has long-standing hypothyroidism on levothyroxine. She was diagnosed with rheumatoid arthritis (RA) 20 years ago and is currently on methotrexate and abatacept.

What is the standard anesthesia management of thyroidectomies? What is surgical positioning for thyroidectomy? What preoperative laboratory testing is indicated?

Physical examination is positive for joint swelling of hands and wrists and bilateral ulnar deviation of the metacarpophalangeal joints. The patient in our case has a body mass index (BMI) of 23. Her Mallampati score is 3. She has a good mouth opening, a large goiter that extends retrosternally, and slightly limited extension of her neck. There is no numbness or tingling of the extremities on movement of her neck. You recommend c-spine imaging, and she expresses concern about the cost and anxiety about more exposure to radiation because she has friend who developed cancer that she ascribes to excessive imaging. Besides, she did not need an x-ray prior to her anesthesia for a knee arthroscopy 6 months earlier.

Does she need any radiology imaging? Would you order plain x-rays, CT, or MRI?

You explain the possibility of ligamentous injury in her neck, as evidenced by the disease process in her hands, and your concern about the neck positioning for the thyroidectomy. She denies any neck symptoms, but she does accede to your request, mentioning that she remembers her nephew with Down syndrome needed neck x-rays for a sports clearance.

Since starting abatacept her disease has been stable and has not required steroids for disease flare in 9 months. Her surgery is in 16 days.

What are the perioperative recommendations for the management of her medications? Does she need a stress dose of steroids?

Her flexion and extension lateral c-spine x-rays reveal a normal atlanto-axial distance but instability between the levels of cervical vertebrae 3 and 4. You contact the surgeon to ask if the procedure can be done in neutral positioning rather than standard marked extension of the neck used for thyroidectomies. He reviews the imaging of her thyroid and concludes that a sternotomy would be needed to safely access and remove the retrosternal part of her thyroid.

How do you proceed?

DISCUSSION

Rheumatoid arthritis (RA) is an autoimmune disease that presents with systemic inflammatory features. Primary presentation is symmetrical progressive arthritis and destruction of small joints, but any synovial joint can be involved. The incidence is about 0.5–1% of the population, with females (possibly due to estrogen effects) being affected more commonly than males in a 2–3:1 ratio. RA presents at any age, with its peak being in the 5th and 6th decades.[1] Pain and disability are hallmark features of the disease but all organ systems can be involved.

The following may be found: constitutional symptoms, anemia of inflammation, subcutaneous nodules, vasculitis, myopathy, pulmonary involvement including restrictive pattern if thoracic joints are involved, pulmonary hypertension, pleural effusions (serositis), and pulmonary fibrosis and/or nodules. Cardiovascular (CV) effects are accelerated atherosclerosis, peripheral vascular disease, stroke, pericardial effusion, fibrosis affecting conduction and causing left ventricular stiffness, vasculitis, valvulopathy (specifically aortic incompetence [AI]), and cardiac amyloid. There is increased CV morbidity and mortality compared with the general population.[2] When applying National Surgical Quality Improvement Program (NSQIP) or other risk calculators the calculated CV risk can be as high as 50% higher in patients with RA.[3] Exercise tolerance may be hard to assess because patients may have limited mobility due to their arthritis. Other organ involvement is found in the renal system (vasculitis, medication side effects, amyloid) and hematological system (anemia, neutropenia, elevated platelets). Ocular effects are the presence of dry eyes. Neurological effects to be aware of are the presence of peripheral neuropathy, vasculitis, nerve entrapment, and

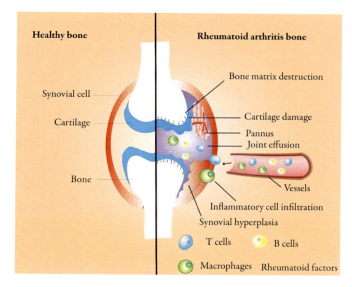

Figure 7.1 Bone microenvironment in healthy (left) and rheumatoid arthritis (RA) (right) bone. Healthy bones have thin and smooth synovium, smooth cartilage tissue, and healthy bone matrix. RA bone shows synovial hyperplasia, pannus formation, inflammatory cell infiltration, cartilage damage, bone matrix destruction, joint effusion, and other symptoms.[6]
From Creative Commons Attribution License (CC BY).

possible spinal cord injury.[4] There is also a higher incidence of lymphoma in this population.[4,5]

Joint involvement starts with synovial inflammation—synovitis, with an associated joint effusion, leading to destruction of cartilage, bony erosions, ligamentous pull-offs, periarticular osteopenia; and ultimately, ankylosis can occur[6] (Figure 7.1).

Goals of treatment are multifactorial and revolve around general health maintenance, symptom control, maintaining function, comorbidity treatment, and decreasing disease activity to prevent permanent joint damage. Therapy is multimodal in nature and includes exercise, adequate nutrition—calcium and vitamin D supplementation, fish oils, risk reduction—weight and lipid control, smoking cessation, being up to date with vaccinations, and physical and occupational therapy. Analgesia is achieved using anti-inflammatory drugs, both nonsteroidal and glucocorticoids. These can be applied locally and/or prescribed systemically. Disease modifying anti-rheumatic drugs (DMARDs) are the mainstay of modern RA control. DMARD treatment has improved outcomes but comes at a cost of medication side effects[7] and poor adherence due to the financial burden. Surgery is offered when needed for joint damage or nerve entrapment.

PERIOPERATIVE CONSIDERATIONS

Organ involvement needs to be considered and managed as it would for any other etiology. Laboratory testing must be tailored to the presence of features of disease—hemoglobin for evaluation of anemia, creatinine if there is concern for kidney disease from long-standing high-dose NSAID use, etc.

One test that could be considered is an early morning cortisol level if there is reason to be concerned about hypothalamic-pituitary-adrenal axis (HPA) suppression. This would guide stress dosing of steroids.[8]

Perioperative medication management is guided by the risk of infection, the treating rheumatologist, and the patient's personal history. Recommendations for perioperative medication management can be found in two recent publications: one is specific for joint replacements from the American College of Rheumatology[9] and the contains other general recommendations from the Society of Perioperative Assessment and Quality Improvement (SPAQI).[10] Goodman and colleagues advise on "conditional" holding for some of the biologics based on low levels of evidence, but they do say to strongly consider holding if there is previous history of joint infection.[9] It is always prudent to involve patients in these decisions because their own personal history can further inform what the best option may be. Many people have missed doses due to insurance issues or other reasons and will have first-hand experience of the ensuing disease flare, or not. If they have had a debilitating flare, they are at risk again and this could impair mobility and successful rehabilitation, possibly requiring high-dose glucocorticoids with all the associated side effects and risks of these rescue medications.

Patients with RA are immunosuppressed due to both the disease and the DMARD treatment. To decrease infection risk, strict hand hygiene, appropriate prophylactic antibiotics, and aseptic techniques are important.

Careful positioning for the procedure is needed, taking into account joint deformities and risk of neuropraxia from preexisting nerve entrapments.

Stress-dose steroids would be given for moderate to higher stress procedures if HPA axis suppression is suspected.

AIRWAY

RA affects the airway in a number of ways, including arthritis of the c-spine, the temporomandibular joints (TMJs), and the arytenoids that can lead to limited neck mobility, limited mouth opening, and obscured glottic opening. Chronic inflammation and associated autoimmune diseases like Sjögren's syndrome can lead to poor dentition. Soft tissue changes from steroid-related body habitus effects and, very rarely, secondary amyloid causing macroglossia can affect airway management, and all of these can lead to a challenging intubation.

Airway evaluation should include assessment for clicking of the TMJs or locking of the jaw, hoarseness, difficulty swallowing, and, of course asking about a history of previous difficult intubation. Imaging for instability is most efficiently done by lateral flexion and extension c-spine x-rays. MRI will show any ligamentous injury including laxity of the transverse ligament (a feature found in 9–27% of patients with Down syndrome[11]). However, this is costly, inconvenient, and a waste of resources because simple x-rays would suffice. MRI is the test of choice if there are long tract signs—features of myelopathy.

C-spine involvement is divided into three main groups:

- *Instability*, either atlanto-axial or subaxial, and also cranial settling. All due to erosions and ligamentous pull-off.
  - More than 50% can be asymptomatic (muscle tone is supportive, but will be abolished in the anesthetized and paralyzed patient under general anesthesia (GA).
  - Most common at the atlantoaxial level (65%), subaxial (20%), and with settling (15%).
  - Seropositive RA and early-onset RA increase the risk for instability.
  - Clinical findings of severe peripheral joint disease suggest similar severity in the c-spine.
  - Subaxial instability is defined as subluxation of one vertebra over another by more than 3.5 mm.
  - Atlanto-axial instability (AAI) is diagnosed by a widening of the anterior atlanto-dens interval (AADI) on flexion by 3 mm or more (Figure 7.2)[12] or a posterior atlanto-dens interval of less than 14 mm. Surgical repair is indicated when the interval is greater than 8 mm.[13]
  - Settling of the occiput on the C1 vertebra with invagination of the odontoid process into the foramen magnum (cord compression with cranial nerve and/or long tract signs) may be present. This is also known as *vertical atlanto-axial subluxation* or *atlanto-axial impaction*.[14]
- *Pannus*, which is inflammatory tissue protruding into the spinal canal at any level (cord compression).
- *Ankylosis*, or late-stage disease, infrequently seen in the era of DMARDs. This fusion of the spine causes immobility but is associated with higher risk of fracture due to osteopenia.

Other diseases and syndromes with c-spine involvement are summarized in Table 7.1.

The American Academy of Pediatrics (AAP) revised their long-standing recommendation for screening c-spine x-rays in individuals with Down syndrome in 2011, changing it to only imaging if there is evidence of symptoms, citing that normal imaging was not predictive of future instability and pathology.[11] This recommendation was validated by Hengartner and colleagues in 2020, who found that AAI in Down syndrome is not a static finding and rarely leads to spinal cord injury.[15] This practice has yet to be widely accepted in the perioperative arena. (AAI in Down syndrome was defined as AADI >4.5 mm; note that the adult AADI is already significant when >3 mm.)

C-spine imaging should be considered in all patients with RA; patients meeting both clinical disease criteria and surgical manipulation criteria should be imaged (see Figure 7.3).

In our patient, the c-spine instability finding led to a neurosurgery referral and plan for fusion prior to her thyroidectomy rather than take on the added risk of a sternotomy. Many other procedures can be done with c-spine precautions as one would proceed with a trauma case. Surgical c-spine

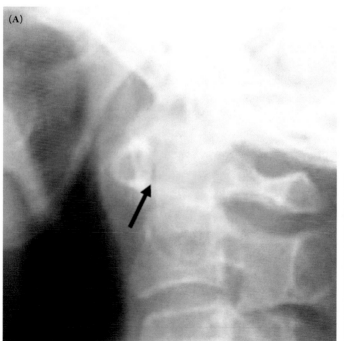
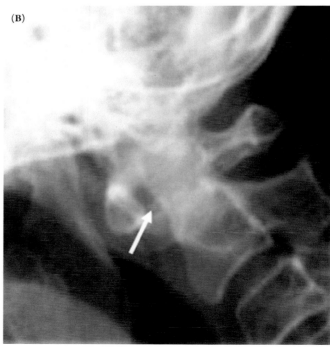

Figure 7.2 Atlanto-axial subluxation (AAS) in neutral position of the neck (A) and anterior flexion (B). Note that, in neutral position, the space between the posterior surface of the anterior arch of the atlas and the anterior aspect of the odontoid process is not well visualized (2 mm) and may be missed (black arrow). Thus, an x-ray of the neck must be done in flexion to reveal the real space between the two anatomical structures (6 mm: white arrow). Reproduced with permission from Springer Nature.[12]

Table 7.1 CONDITIONS WITH C-SPINE ABNORMALITIES

CONDITION	IMAGING	PATHOLOGY	INDICATION	COMMENTS
Down syndrome	Consider lateral flexion/extension cervical spine plain x-rays	Laxity of transverse ligament and AAI	Sports clearance Neck positioning	No longer AAP recommendation (2011)
	MRI	Cervical stenosis	Long tract signs	
RA	Lateral flexion/extension cervical spine plain x-rays	AAI Subaxial instability		
	MRI	Pannus	Long tract signs	
Achondroplasia	Lateral flexion/extension cervical spine plain x-rays			
Mucopolysaccharidoses: I (Hurler/Scheie variants) II (Hunter) IV (Morquio), VI (Maroteaux-Lamy) VII (Sly)	Lateral flexion/extension cervical spine plain x-rays			Morquio commonly has instability and previous fusion

AAP, American Academy of Pediatrics; AAI, atlanto-axial instability; MRI, magnetic resonance imaging.

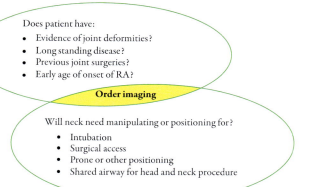

Figure 7.3 Indications for C-spine lateral flexion and extensions X-rays.

stabilization is not necessarily always the best plan. The burden of the treatment also needs to be considered. An elderly patient with Down syndrome complicated by early dementia and AAI, for example, would not be sent for a fusion for routine dental rehabilitation under GA. The surgery, pain, hospitalization in foreign environment, and cervical collar would place undue stress on the patient for limited clinical benefit.

Our patient shared that she was previously on DMARDs and only had mild aches and pain when she held it for her knee arthroscopy procedure; therefore, the plan was to hold her abatacept again for one dosing cycle before and after surgery. As she had had steroids in high doses in the past year and there was concern for HPA suppression, she was prescribed stress-dose steroids for surgery with a moderate risk of stress.

Patients with long-standing large goiters are at risk of tracheomalacia on extubation after thyroidectomy, the goiter having acted as a stent to the trachea. Consider leaving a tube exchanger in place until the patient is awake and evaluate regularly for stridor and signs of airway obstruction.

CONCLUSION

- Rheumatoid arthritis is a systemic inflammatory disease treated in a multimodal fashion, including the use of DMARDs that add risk of infection.
- Biologic and target-specific DMARDs are frequently held for one cycle before and after surgery to decrease this risk.
- Airway involvement in RA is multifactorial, involving joints and soft tissue elements.
- C-spine instability needs to be screened for and treatment plans may need to be altered.
- Other conditions and syndromes have similar c-spine abnormalities.

REVIEW QUESTIONS

1. All patients on chronic oral glucocorticoids should
    a. Continue their usual oral dose on the day of the procedure.
    b. Have an early morning cortisol level ordered.
    c. Receive 100 mg hydrocortisone IV followed by 50 mg every 8 hours after surgery.
    d. Receive 50 mg hydrocortisone IV followed by 25 mg every 8 hours after surgery.

    The correct answer is a.

    Stress dosing depends on maintenance dose and is usually only given when a patient is taking more than 20 mg/day prednisone. Size of stress dose depends of invasiveness of surgery, with only major surgeries needing the higher doses.[16]

2. Check all that apply: diseases associated with RA include
    a. Diabetes mellitus type 1

b. Hashimoto disease
c. Sjögren's syndrome
d. Raynaud's syndrome

The correct answer is a, b, c, and d.

All these are autoimmune diseases and often occur in conjunction with each other.

3. What is the current AAP recommendation for c-spine imaging in patients with Down syndrome?

 a. Lateral flexion extension x-ray of the c-spine at 3 months.
 b. Lateral flexion extension x-ray of the c-spine at 4 years.
 c. MRI of the c-spine.
 d. Imaging only if signs and symptoms that could be attributed to c-spine pathology.

The correct answer is d.

Previous recommendation was to perform a baseline x-ray once mineralization occurred and the cortex was easily visualized (answer b). Since 2011, the recommendation is answer d.[11]

4. Which of the following needs to be held before surgery in an attempt to decrease wound complications?

 a. Abatacept.
 b. Hydroxychloroquine.
 c. Methotrexate.
 d. Prednisone.

The correct answer is a.

Biologics and target-specific DMARDs need to be held where possible. No evidence supports holding the older conventional DMARDs. Holding glucocorticoid would be detrimental and risk adrenal crisis.

5. The imaging of choice to evaluate for c-spine instability in RA is

 a. MRI.
 b. CT scan.
 c. Lateral flexion extension c-spine x-rays.
 d. Series of c-spine x-rays including open mouth view.

The correct answer is c.

Plain dynamic (flexion and extension) imaging is adequate for assessing instability. Cord compression is best assessed on MRI.

6. The patient with long-standing RA presents for a podiatry wound debridement of her left foot. She has no symptoms from her neck. What do you recommend?

 a. Refer to neurosurgery for an evaluation.
 b. Order a c-spine x-ray.
 c. Proceed with planned procedure with c-spine precautions.
 d. Order a CT of her neck.

The correct answer is c.

Because the patient only meets criteria for disease features and not for surgical/positioning features, the procedure would proceed without further workup.

7. Which is incorrect? The c-spine pathology of RA includes

 a. Atlanto-axial instability.
 b. Periarticular erosions and osteopenia.
 c. Settling of the occiput.
 d. Lax transverse ligament.

The correct answer is d.

RA has ligamentous pull-off (Figure 7.4),[12] Down syndrome has an elongated and lax transverse ligament.

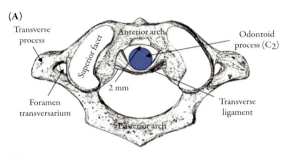

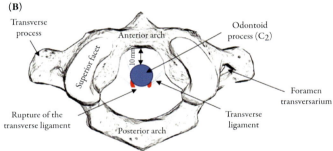

Figure 7.4 A. Schematic representation of the atlanto-axial joint in a healthy individual. Anatomy of the first cervical vertebra (atlas/C_1). Note also the odontoid process of the C_2 vertebra (axis) as well as the synovial membrane that lines the dens anteriorly and posteriorly. The distance between the anterior aspect of the odontoid process and the posterior surface of the anterior arch of the atlas (facet for dens) should measure ≤3 mm. B. Schematic representation of the atlanto-axial subluxation in a patient with rheumatoid arthritis (RA). After rupture of the transverse ligament, there is an anterior translocation of the atlas ring and posterior movement of the odontoid process. Note that the distance between the anterior aspect of the odontoid process and the posterior surface of the anterior arch of the atlas is approximately 10 mm. In this situation, the chance of cord compression is very high and life-threatening.
Reproduced with permission from Springer Nature.[12]

REFERENCES

1. Gravallese EM, Firestein GS. Rheumatoid arthritis: Common origins, divergent mechanisms. *N Engl J Med*. 2023;388:529–542. doi:10.1056/NEJMra2103726
2. Meune C, Touzé E, Trinquart L, Allanore Y. Trends in cardiovascular mortality in patients with rheumatoid arthritis over 50 years: A systematic review and meta-analysis of cohort studies. *Rheumatology (Oxford)*. 2009;48:1309–1313. doi:10.1093/rheumatology/kep252

3. Dijkshoorn B, Raadsen R, Nurmohamed MT. Cardiovascular disease risk in rheumatoid arthritis. *J Clin Med.* 2022;11. doi:10.3390/jcm11102704
4. Smolen JS, Aletaha D, McInnes IB. Rheumatoid arthritis. *Lancet.* 2016;388:2023–2038. doi:10.1016/S0140-6736(16)30173-8
5. Klein A, Polliack A, Gafter-Gvili A. Rheumatoid arthritis and lymphoma: Incidence, pathogenesis, biology, and outcome. *Hematol Oncol.* 2018;36:733–739. doi:10.1002/hon.2525
6. Huang W, Li X, Huang C, et al. LncRNAs and rheumatoid arthritis: From identifying mechanisms to clinical investigation. *Front Immunol.* 2022;12. doi:10.3389/fimmu.2021.807738
7. Aletaha D, Smolen JS. Diagnosis and management of rheumatoid arthritis: A review. *JAMA.* 2018;320:1360–1372. doi:10.1001/jama.2018.13103
8. Deutschbein T, Unger N, Mann K, Petersenn S. Diagnosis of secondary adrenal insufficiency: Unstimulated early morning cortisol in saliva and serum in comparison with the insulin tolerance test. *Horm Metab Res.* 2009;41:834–839. doi:10.1055/s-0029-1225630
9. Goodman SM, Springer BD, Chen AF, et al. American College of Rheumatology/American Association of Hip and Knee Surgeons guideline for the perioperative management of antirheumatic medication in patients with rheumatic diseases undergoing elective total hip or total knee arthroplasty. *Arthritis Rheumatol.* 2022;74:1464–1473. doi:10.1002/art.42140
10. Russell LA, Craig C, Flores EK, et al. Preoperative management of medications for rheumatologic and HIV diseases: Society for Perioperative Assessment and Quality Improvement (SPAQI) consensus statement. *Mayo Clin Proc.* 2022;97:1551–1571. doi:10.1016/j.mayocp.2022.05.002
11. Bull MJ; Committee on Genetics. Health supervision for children with Down syndrome. *Pediatrics.* 2011;128:393–406. doi:10.1542/peds.2011-1605
12. Drosos AA, Pelechas E, Voulgari PV. Radiological findings of the cervical spine in rheumatoid arthritis: What a rheumatologist should know. *Curr Rheumatol Rep.* 2020;22: 19. doi:10.1007/s11926-020-00894-8
13. Mańczak M, Gasik R. Cervical spine instability in the course of rheumatoid arthritis: Imaging methods. *Reumatologia.* 2017;55:201–207. doi:10.5114/reum.2017.69782
14. Jurik AG. Imaging the spine in arthritis: A pictorial review. *Insights Imaging.* 2011;2:177–191. doi:10.1007/s13244-010-0061-4
15. Hengartner AC, Whelan R, Maj R, et al. Evaluation of 2011 AAP cervical spine screening guidelines for children with Down syndrome. *Child Nerv Syst.* 2020;36:2609–2614. doi:10.1007/s00381-020-04855-5
16. Chernow B, Alexander HR, Smallridge RC, et al. Hormonal responses to graded surgical stress. *Arch Intern Med.* 1987;147:1273–1278.

8.

PREHABILITATION BEFORE TOTAL HIP REPLACEMENT

Olivia Belloni, Rashwan Gogue, Luigi Beretta, and Enrico Maria Minnella

STEM CASE AND KEY QUESTIONS

A 70-year-old woman has had chronic osteoarthritis for years, with the hip as the major joint involved. Her chronic pain worsened during the past months, becoming resistant to NSAIDs. Physical therapy no longer benefits her, and she is no longer independent in all daily-life activities.

Her BMI is 28.4 kg/m^2, and she has diabetes, hypertension, and osteoporosis. Her general practitioner prescribed her a hip x-ray, which showed joint space narrowing reflecting cartilage loss and subchondral sclerosis. She was referred to an orthopedic surgeon for possible surgical intervention.

What is the patient's perspective on the surgical outcome?

She was disabled by the continuous pain, and she was becoming very depressed about not being able to enjoy her retirement. She wanted to have surgery to start feeling better, relieve pain, and reduce the daily need for medications. Moreover, her desire was to improve the ability to stand, walk, and climb the stairs. To follow, she wished to regain the capability of performing essential activities such as caring for herself and doing routine daily-life activities. Along with these expectations, she trusts her psychological status would improve as well, which is by itself a desired goal.

What is the surgical risk?

The patient is overweight and has diabetes; she has no history of venous thromboembolism, nor recent major surgery, trauma, malignancy, or use of oral contraceptives. She reports low physical activity level and poor exercise habits even before hip pain. She does not smoke, and she consumes a modest amount of alcohol. Her hemoglobin is 12.7 g/dL. She takes metformin 500 mg two times per day.

How can physical fitness be assessed? Is it needed in this patient?

The first step is initial screening with a 6-minute walk test (6MWT) to assess her physical status. She is asked to walk as fast as she can for 6 minutes. She is advised that rests are permissible, but she never needed to stop. She walked 350 meters in 6 minutes with no desaturation. She is also asked to complete the Duke Activity Status Index (DASI), scoring 15.2. Given these poor results, the nurse navigator referred her to cardiopulmonary exercise testing (CPET), the gold standard for the assessment of physical fitness. As her oxygen uptake at the anaerobic threshold (VO$_2$AT) is 9.9 mL·kg^{-1}·min^{-1}, the physician recommends supervised exercise prehabilitation.

How can nutritional status be assessed? Is it needed in this patient?

Her assessment starts with a careful review of her medical history, including information about food/nutrient intake. She experienced no weight loss or gain during the previous months, but she reports a reduced dietary intake over the most recent months. She has a poor appetite, and she has no longer been enjoying cooking given her limited mobility. She has no nausea, vomiting, dysphagia, or constipation. Her handgrip strength, measured with a dynamometer, is 18.2 kilograms. Given this clinical picture, the physician orders a consult with a dietician.

How can mental health status be assessed? Does this need to be done in this patient?

She reports no history of psychiatric illness, but she feels extremely demotivated and depressed in relation to her joint pain. Her level of anxiety and depression is assessed by the Hospital Anxiety and Depression Scale (HADS), where she scores 8 on the Depression scale and 4 on the Anxiety scale. In consideration of the psychological health status of this patient, the nurse navigator plans for patient education perioperatively and a psychological consult.

How can physical fitness be modified?

Exercise is the key approach to improve and maintain physical fitness. The patient is offered to train three times per week for 8 weeks. One weekly session is directly supervised, and the other two sessions are conducted through tele-prehabilitation programs at home. The exercise program includes progressive resistant training, aerobic training, and walking aid adjustment, aiming to improve aerobic capacity, muscle strength, and daily activity level. A particular focus on the strengthening of skeletal muscle is given. If relevant, comorbidity optimization and smoking cessation would be advised.

How can nutritional status be modified?

The patient is offered a high-intensity nutritional program with weekly follow-ups with a specialist. A balanced meal plan is provided, with a 2:1:2 ratio between starches, meat or fish, and vegetables. Moreover, in consideration of her diabetes, a comprehensive personalized education program is given, including control of carbohydrate and macronutrient content, meal timing, and glycemia control.

How can her mental health status be modified?

In consideration of her psychological assessment, a single session of psychosocial support is proposed to help her cope with mental distress. She is encouraged to disclose personal beliefs and goals about surgery, reframe thoughts and expectations, and reduce maladaptive lifestyle modifications, including physical and dietary aspects. She is prescribed relaxation techniques, such as deep breathing and meditation. Furthermore, specific information is given on the perioperative period, focusing on the importance of early mobilization, discharge planning, and pain control.

Who are the healthcare providers involved in perioperative care?

Throughout the perioperative period, multiple healthcare providers are involved. A nurse navigator planned all functional tests that the patient underwent before surgery and supervised the postoperative period. The kinesiologist/exercise specialist evaluated her physical risk and prescribed and followed her physical training. The nutritionist provided all the nutritional suggestions to be followed both before and after surgery. The psychologist assessed her mental status and started her coping therapy. The orthopedic surgeon and the anesthesiologist overviewed the whole program and follow-up on progression and adherence.

What are the components of optimal perioperative management?

A maltodextrin drink is provided to the patient 2 hours before surgery, and cefazolin 2 g IV is administered in the waiting area. The procedure is performed under neuraxial anesthesia without opioid administration; sedative or anxiolytic drugs are not used. Before surgery, 15 mg/kg of tranexamic acid is administered. A forced-air warming blanket is used during the procedure. A posterolateral approach with standard prosthesis is followed, and no tourniquet is utilized. No drains or urinary catheters are used.

Nonsmoking history and female sex are risk factors for postoperative nausea and vomiting, leading to the administration of ondansetron 4 mg IV and metoclopramide 10 mg IV; dexamethasone is avoided in consideration of her diabetes. Local infiltration analgesia is performed at the end of the procedure for pain control, and regular paracetamol and NSAIDs are prescribed. She is mobilized once she arrives in her room, and low-molecular-weight heparin is initiated at a prophylaxis dose.

What happens after hospital discharge?

The patient has no complications, and she has a rapid recovery. Nonetheless, she felt annoyed by postoperative rehabilitation, although she is aware of the crucial importance of this step.

DISCUSSION

THR is an elective procedure, considered to be one of the most successful medical interventions from a patient-centered perspective.[1] The main indication for THR is severe osteoarthritis,[2] which is one of the largest contributors to global disability.[3] Worldwide, more than 1.4 million THR procedures are performed annually,[4] and the incidence is increasing because of the aging global population.[2] Indeed, the elderly population (>65 years) is the most affected by this condition. It is uncommon before the age of 45. The prevalence is higher among females,[5] who have a higher risk of postoperative complications leading to prolonged hospitalization and an increased risk of morbidity and mortality. The typical clinical picture is of chronic pain, joint stiffness, functional impairment, and deformity in the late stages.[6,7] This clinical scenario frequently leads to anxiety and psychological distress in affected patients.[5,8] Surgical indications for hip arthroplasty are mainly guided by pain and functional impairment refractory to conservative treatments, such as pain killers and/or physiotherapy.[2] Radiographic findings confirm the diagnosis and help with preoperative planning.[2] Success rates are high, with around 95% of patients undergoing THR having adequately functioning prostheses at 10 years after surgery; 85% of them will still be functioning at 20 years.[9,10] Perioperative complications include thromboembolic episodes, cardiovascular events, infections, and structural consequences due to the prosthesis implantation.[11] The association between increased BMI and a higher risk of complications has been shown by multiple studies.[12] In particular, an increased BMI correlates with a higher prevalence of postsurgical thromboembolic events and wound infections.[11,12] Other risk factors are prolonged waiting times that may lead to a worse health status and overall quality of life.[13]

From a patient's perspective, not surprisingly, the common expectation focuses on the reduction of pain. Moreover, a significant portion of patients expect psychosocial benefits, often overlooked by clinicians in the perioperative setting.[14,15] Indeed, recent studies showed that patients' expectations are not always fulfilled.[15,16]

To achieve patient satisfaction, multidisciplinary care featuring tailored communication and coordination may be required; this is facilitated by the current technology and information revolution.[17]

Specific risk factors for delayed recovery and postoperative complications are low physical fitness, poor nutritional status and obesity, anemia, smoking, and alcohol consumption.[18] The enhanced recovery after surgery (ERAS)/prehabilitation model of care aims to develop strategies not only to predict the surgical risk, but also to develop effective strategies to mitigate that risk.

Smoking cessation is a key component of preoperative optimization and is associated with lower morbidity, in particular surgical site infection.[19] Cessation intervention should also be provided in case of high alcohol intake, not only to mitigate surgical risk but also for public health purposes. Preoperative anemia should always be screened for, given the risks associated with allogeneic transfusion, morbidity, length of stay and readmission associated with this condition. A standardized anemia assessment protocol should be implemented to identify the cause and start appropriate therapy.[20] Although patient education and counseling should be provided, its role in accelerating recovery has not been shown. These interventions are strongly recommended from a patient-centered perspective. Moreover, in our clinical scenario, patient education and counseling can help in reducing perioperative anxiety.

A multimodal approach to improve physical, nutritional, and psychological status is the basis of prehabilitation. Its purpose is to attenuate the detrimental effect of surgery on functional status and accelerate recovery. Good results have been achieved in oncologic surgery,[21] but data are still lacking in specific orthopedic procedures.

In the past 5 years, several original trials have been published on prehabilitation before THR (Table 8.1).[23-29] In 2019, there were three different studies on the topic. Denduluri et al.[29] demonstrated how preoperative education and exercise programs can correlate with a shorter length of hospital stay and suggest that increasing exercise intensity is associated with gait independence after THR. Interestingly, the preoperative plan in this study was tailored following a series of online questionnaires, current level of physical function, postoperative goals, and presence of potential high fall risk factors.[29]

In the same year, a randomized controlled trial by Doiron-Cadrin et al.[23] compared usual care for THR candidates with a prehabilitation program performed in the intervention group, either in-person or through tele-prehabilitation. The intervention consisted of exercise training sessions and patients' education focused on pain control for 12 weeks before surgery. Significant differences in certain outcomes were noted in the two intervention groups (tele-rehabilitation vs. control p < 0.001; in-person vs. control p = 0.012). Results suggest that tele-rehabilitation appears to be safe, feasible, and generates high satisfaction for patients; significant improvements were observed on their physical performance outcomes. However, no significant differences between the groups were noted for self-reported outcomes after the intervention. Torisho et al.[24] performed a retrospective analysis on a very large sample of patients undergoing prehabilitation prior to THR. Participants reported either exposure to physiotherapy and/or to patient education conducted in group sessions or individually. Statistically significant differences were found in favor of both physiotherapy and patient education, reporting less pain (p = 0.01), better quality of life outcomes (p = 0.01) in the intervention group.

Another study was conducted by Clode et al.[25] (Table 8.1) analyzing the postsurgery outcomes in patients who followed a physiotherapy and patient education program before THR. Both groups had improved function scores and pain relief after surgery, with a particularly significant difference in the timed up-and-go test from the baseline to the postoperative period (p = 0.01). Results demonstrated that a prehabilitation program is well tolerated by elderly patients with hip osteoarthritis. Patients included in the study reported that patient education prepared them well for surgery, with less fear and more optimism. Beyond improvements in physical status, another study[27] showed how preoperative education encourages patients to assume a central role in their recovery period, which helps achieve sustainable, long-term beneficial postoperative outcomes. In this study as well, the patient education sessions were delivered at home through via digital video discs (DVDs) addressing concepts such as behavior modification, strategies to achieve goals, and relaxation techniques.[27] Moreover, the cost-utility of exercise prior to THR was estimated in a randomized trial that reported that patients allocated to the intervention group had a shorter length of hospital stay and a lower total cost during the follow-up period.[26] Finally, in 2016, Cavill et al. did not show significant differences between their control and intervention groups, although they noted a positive trend in some postoperative outcomes in the prehabilitation group.[28]

In summary, despite a consistent trend toward better clinical outcomes, these trials show significant heterogeneity in study procedures and several weaknesses in their design. Based on our experience in cancer prehabilitation, we can hypotheses that a standardized single-domain intervention, such as preoperative physiotherapy, may be poorly effective in modifying postoperative outcomes.[1] Thus, the approach we propose is to deliver an intervention that focuses on personalization and a multimodal approach fully integrated in an ERAS pathway.[22]

The multidisciplinary team should be composed of the orthopedic surgeon, anesthesiologist, and nurse team, but also, if specific needs are detected, by a geriatrician, physiotherapist/kinesiologist, dietician, and psychologist. Obviously, in some patients, certain professional figures could be more actively present during the prehabilitation pathway than others (Figure 8.1). This approach contributes to an improvement in postoperative outcomes and eases the patient's state of mind.[10] Preoperative care is comprehensive with multiple clinical elements, aimed not only at reducing the morbidity associated with the surgical procedure but also at rapidly restoring the functional capacity of the patient in the postoperative period.[17]

The first step of the preoperative care pathway should include the screening and assessment phase, followed by a selective and personalized intervention. It is important to identify high-risk patients through validated, easy-to-administer, and affordable tools. In this screening phase, aerobic capacity is tested through the 6MWT, with less than 400 meters as a cutoff for high-risk patients.[30] Moreover, the DASI score can be used to check on daily activity level, with a cutoff of 34 for detecting the high-risk category. Valid options are also the timed up-and-go test, the stair climb test, the self-paced walk test, and the sit-to-stand test. Patients with a high nutritional risk may present with any of the following characteristics: involuntary weight loss (>10% in 6 months), reduced dietary intake, nutrition-related symptoms, and low handgrip strength (<20th percentile).[31,32] Last, a validated tool administered to patients during the psychological screening is the HADS, used to determine the level of anxiety and depression.[33] It is a 14-item questionnaire, with each item scored from zero to three. Patients with no impairments may receive usual care with no additional interventions. On the other hand, patients who are screened at higher risk should undergo additional testing to comprehensively assess their functional capacity prior to surgery. CPET is the gold standard to define cardiorespiratory fitness,[34] a registered dietitian performs the nutritional assessment to evaluate their history and clinical examination, and an expert psychologist is in charge of the

Table 8.1 STUDIES OF PREHABILITATION PROGRAMS AND THEIR OUTCOMES

STUDY	DESIGN OF THE	SAMPLE SIZE (N)	MEAN AGE (RANGE), %	JOINT INVOLVED	TYPE OF SURGERY (SUBJECTS)	TYPE OF INTERVENTIONS	DESCRIPTION OF INTERVENTIONS	FREQUENCY & DURATION	OUTCOME VARIABLES	RESULTS	AUTHORS' CONCLUSIONS
Denduluri et al. 2019	PNT	40 subjects (no control group)	65, 57.5%	Hip, Knee	THR (17), TKR (23)	Exercise + Patient education	5 exercise modules on static and dynamic balance, and muscle strengthening (quadriceps, hamstring, gluteus)	Not otherwise specified	Length of stay in hospital, gait independence at 90 days postoperative	Number of preoperative trainings are associated with shorter LOS	Preoperative education and exercise program correlate with decreased LOS and improved gait independence
Doiron-Cadrin et al. 2019	RCT	40 subjects (no control group)	66.1, 73.5%	Hip, Knee	THR (17), TKR (17)	Supervised in-person exercise + patient education vs. tele-prehabilitation vs. usual care	8 educational readings about surgical procedure and hospital care. Education on pain control	12 weeks	Feasibility, functional ability (LEFS, WOMAC), health status (SF-36), patient's perception (GRC), mobility (TUG), physical performance assessment (ST and self-paced walk test)	ST in the tele-prehabilitation group (p=0.018); SPW in both tele-prehabilitation group (p=0.008) and in-person group (p=0.026)	Participants reported excellent satisfaction toward the tele-prehabilitation services and demonstrated excellent compliance with the prehabilitation programs. No significant differences between groups were found for self-reported outcomes after the prehabilitation programs, but significant improvements were observed on physical performance outcomes
Torisho et al. 2019	Retrospective analysis	30,756 subjects (prehabilitation, N=21,716)	68, 55.6%	Hip	THR	Exercise/ physiotherapy or/and patient education	Self-reported exposure to physiotherapy and individually adapted physical exercises, to be carried out in group training sessions or individually. Self-reported exposure to patient education: group sessions about their disease, how to manage and cope with OA symptoms	Not otherwise specified	Quality of life (EQ-5D), hip pain (VAS, EQ-VAS), self-reported Charnley classification	Physiotherapy: less pain VAS (p=0.01), better EQ-5D index (p=0.01) and better E-VAS (p=0.01). Patient education: better EQ-5D index and EQVAS	Statistically significant differences in favour of physiotherapy and patient education were found, but the magnitude of those were too small and inconsistent to conclude a truly positive influence. Further research is needed with more specific and demarcated physiotherapy interventions
Clode et al. 2018	PNT	75 subjects (prehabilitation, N=52)	66, 49.3%	Hip, Knee	THR, TKR	Exercise + Patient education	45 mins of strengthening and stretching class (13 exercise stations with 2 mins spent at each station)	Twice a week for 8 weeks	Pain (10-points NRS), functional ability (WOMAC), mobility (TUG, 5xSTS),	5XSTS improved by a mean score of 5.55s (p=0.00). Both groups improved in pain and function scores post-op,	Participants felt prehabilitation prepared them well for surgery and influenced expectations post-operatively. Overall, prehabilitation may improve post-op outcome

(continued)

Table 8.1 CONTINUED

STUDY	DESIGN OF THE	SAMPLE SIZE (N)	MEAN AGE (RANGE), %	JOINT INVOLVED	TYPE OF SURGERY (SUBJECTS)	TYPE OF INTERVENTIONS	DESCRIPTION OF INTERVENTIONS	FREQUENCY & DURATION	OUTCOME VARIABLES	RESULTS	AUTHORS' CONCLUSIONS
							15 mins of education sessions based on talks and addressed concepts (early mobilisation, discharge planning, pain control, benefits of exercise for arthritis, dietary education and post-operative rehabilitation)		quality of life (EQ-5D), length of stay in hospital	in particular a significant difference in TUG from baseline to post-op was observed (p= 0.01) in the prehab group. No other statistically significant changes were found	
Fernandes et al. 2017	RCT	165 subjects (prehabilitation, N=84)	67.4, 55.7%	Hip, Knee	THR (43), TKR (41)	Exercise	Preoperative neuromuscular exercise focused on lower extremity muscular control and quality of movement, consisted of three parts: warm-up, circuit programme and cool-down (1 hour)	Twice a week for 8 weeks	Clinical effect (HOOS), Cost effective analysis (QALYs)	HOOS were statistically significantly improved	One-year clinical effects were small to moderate and favoured the intervention group, but only statistically significant for quality of life measures. Prehabilitation found to be cost-effective in patients
Cooke et al. 2016	RCT	82 subjects (prehabilitation, N=40)	67, 63.4%	Hip, Knee	THR, TKR	Patient education	Self-efficacy-based education: behaviour modification, improve self-confidence, problem solving, strategies to achieve goals and relaxation techniques. Sessions last of around 20–30 minutes delivered via a DVD	Participants were asked to review a DVD within 72 hours and work through the activities at home 4 times before admission for surgery	Pain (11-points NRS), anxiety (STAI), self-efficacy (10-item GSE), pain management (TQPM)	No significant differences between groups were noted in pain, anxiety or self-efficacy. Almost all patients (91%) expressed satisfaction with postoperative pain management.	This study provides preliminary evidence for the physical and psychological benefits that the pre-operative education can provide to patients undergoing hip or knee replacement. Importantly, pre-operative education encourages patients to take a central role in their recovery promoting long-term positive outcomes
Cavill et al. 2016	RCT	20 Subjects (prehabilitation, N=9)	64.4, 47.9%	Hip	THR	Exercise	Self-efficacy-based education: behaviour modification, improve self-confidence, problem solving, strategies to achieve goals and relaxation techniques. Sessions last of around 20–30 minutes delivered via a DVD	Twice a week for at least 3-4 weeks	Pain (VAS), quality of life (EQ-5D), mobility (TUG), activity limitation (PSFS), length of stay in the hospital	Health utility (p= 0.50); PSFS (p= 0.73); TUG (p= 0.08); EQ-5D VAS (p=0.11)	No between-group differences. There was a trend to post-operative improvement in VAS and TUG times in the prehabilitation group. The trial was conducted to generate evidence that would allow a larger and appropriately powered study

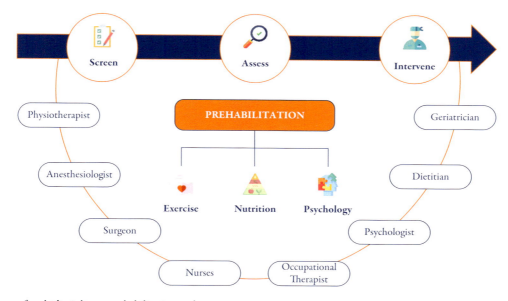

Figure 8.1 Components of multidisciplinary prehabilitation pathway.

assessment of mental health status. This phase is useful not only to have a more objective picture of the patient's functional level, but also to detect specific impairments so that a proper prehabilitation program can be planned.

Exercise is the key intervention to improve fitness, aimed at improving the endurance and strength of patients. To improve nutritional status, it is important that the patient follows a dietary program that is extended into the postoperative phase. Patient education about clinical condition, surgical procedure, pain management, and psychological aspects is also needed.

Since exercise capacity is associated with substantial benefits in perioperative outcomes, improving physical fitness during the prehabilitation pathway may have a role in achieving better postoperative outcomes. This is particularly useful in those patients with poor physical/health status who are at higher risk for complications and prolonged or incomplete recovery.[35] Improving physical fitness is done through exercise, defined as a planned physical activity that is purposeful to improve or maintain a patient's physical fitness. A similar role may be played by diet therapy because malnutrition in patients undergoing total joint arthroplasty is associated with postoperative renal and cardiac complications and longer hospital stay.[36,37] Psychological variables appear to directly affect emotional and functional capacities and early surgical recovery.[38,39] Results suggest that guiding patients' expectations within the perioperative period is a fundamental part of a successful discharge.[40]

Compared to prehabilitation in oncological surgery,[41] the joint replacement preoperative period available for patient optimization is longer. Indeed, in the setting of orthopedic surgery, physical status plays a more relevant role and needs more time to be assessed and subsequently modified.

Finally, strict adherence to ERAS milestones is mandatory to enable patients to achieve successful outcomes. Progress in pain management techniques in recent years had a great impact on the practice of THR.[42] Analgesia should be multimodal, intervening at multiple sites in the pain pathways, and include local and IV anesthetics.[43] Poorly managed pain exacerbates surgical stress and leads to unfavorable outcomes such as poor mobilization, prolonged bed rest, and increased length of hospital stay.[44] It is crucial that the surgeon and the anesthesiologist discuss personalized programs and share consistent objectives to provide patients with a positive and safe experience. Likewise, smoking and alcohol cessation planned within an ERAS protocol will improve the physical fitness of the patient in the preoperative period. Interesting data may be drawn from an ongoing study on preoperative nutrition optimization.[45] Since patient discharge after THR depends on a variety of factors such as pain control, management of comorbidities, and progress with physical therapy, ameliorating these aspects will lead to a reduction in the length of hospital stay and will have an impact on the total cost of care.[46–48]

Despite advancements in surgical techniques and hospital care, patient-centered outcomes are still poorly recognized. The detrimental effects on quality of life, physical functioning, and psychosocial outcome still need to be quantified. Prospective high-quality trials are needed to investigate the role and effectiveness of prehabilitation and to develop and evaluate the optimal approach of new programs.

CONCLUSION

- The results from the limited number of recent trials about prehabilitation are promising.
- Postoperative outcomes are shown to be positively influenced by the prehabilitation program.
- A multidisciplinary team is fundamental in the management of the patient.
- Prehabilitation is shown to be cost-effective, and it reduced the length of stay in the hospital.

- The preoperative program must be implemented to include the postoperative follow-up period.
- Further studies are needed, especially with a specific focus on patient nutritional and psychological status.

REVIEW QUESTIONS

1. What role does surgery play in the management of osteoarthritis?

    a. It is the first-line treatment for osteoarthritis.
    b. It is indicated for patients who failed conservative treatment or previous surgical options.
    c. It is indicated for every patient affected by osteoarthritis.
    d. It is the only treatment available for this disease.

    The correct answer is b.
    Conservative treatment should always be used as first-line therapy.

2. The prehabilitation program

    a. Includes only the interventions on physical status because this is the most important aspect for a patient.
    b. Includes interventions such as preoperative glycemic control with insulin administration.
    c. Includes interventions for physical, nutritional, and psychological status.
    d. Is the postoperative process for patients undergoing THR.

    The correct answer is c.
    Prehabilitation is a multimodal intervention.

3. Which healthcare provider is not usually involved in the perioperative care of these patients?

    a. The anesthesiologist.
    b. The nurse.
    c. The psychologist.
    d. The microbiologist.

    The correct answer is d.
    A team approach is vital to the success of a prehabilitation program.

4. Which is a common tool used to assess the physical status of a patient undergoing THR?

    a. A total body x-ray.
    b. The total body surface area.
    c. The BMI and total body surface area.
    d. The 6MWT together with CPET.

    The correct answer is d.
    CPET is indicated after a poor result in the 6MWT. A healthy patient can do 400–700 meters in the 6MWT.

5. Which is not a common tool to assess the psychological status of the patient?

    a. A visit with the surgeon and the anesthesiologist.
    b. The Hospital Anxiety and Depression Scale (HADS).
    c. The State-Trait Anxiety Inventory (STAI).
    d. The psychological consult.

    The correct answer is a.
    Validated tools are far superior to a hurried, surgically focused history.

6. Which is *not* a tool used to assess the nutritional status of the patient?

    a. BMI.
    b. Laboratory exams, such as albumin or A1C.
    c. The weight loss of the patient in the previous 6 months.
    d. The history of a patient's allergies.

    The correct answer is d.
    BMI, laboratory exams, and weight loss within the previous 6 months are used to assess nutritional status. Assessment of a patient's allergies is important when treating, but not to assess current nutritional status.

7. The anesthesiology perioperative program

    a. Is not relevant in the context of THR.
    b. Includes only the anesthesiologist as a professional figure.
    c. Is based on a multimodal approach and needs the cooperation of the multidisciplinary team.
    d. Does not play a role in the patient's pain management perioperatively.

    The correct answer is c.
    Anesthesiologists play a vital role in understanding perioperative needs and, as such, are well placed to coordinate multidisciplinary care.

REFERENCES

1. Wang L, Lee M, Zhang Z, et al. Does preoperative rehabilitation for patients planning to undergo joint replacement surgery improve outcomes? A systematic review and meta-analysis of randomised controlled trials. *BMJ Open*. 2016;6:e009857. doi:10.1136/bmjopen-2015-009857
2. Pivec R, Johnson AJ, Mears SC, Mont MA. Hip arthroplasty. *Lancet*. 2012;380(9855):1768–1777. doi:10.1016/S0140-6736(12)60607-2
3. Cross M, Smith E, Hoy D, et al. The global burden of hip and knee osteoarthritis: Estimates from the global burden of disease 2010 study. *Ann Rheum Dis*. 2014;73(7):1323–1330. doi:10.1136/annrheumdis-2013-204763
4. de Fatima de Pina M, Ribeiro AI, Santos C. Epidemiology and variability of orthopaedic procedures worldwide. In: Bentley G, ed. *European Instructional Lectures*. Springer Berlin Heidelberg; 2011:9–19. doi:10.1007/978-3-642-18321-8_2
5. Australian Institute of Health and Welfare. A picture of osteoarthritis in Australia, Table of contents. https://www.aihw.gov.au/reports/

chronic-musculoskeletal-conditions/picture-osteoarthritis-australia/contents/table-of-contents

6. Hawker GA, Stewart L, French MR, et al. Understanding the pain experience in hip and knee osteoarthritis: An OARSI/OMERACT initiative. *Osteoarthritis Cartilage*. 2008;16(4):415–422. doi:10.1016/j.joca.2007.12.017

7. Sale JEM, Gignac M, Hawker G. The relationship between disease symptoms, life events, coping and treatment, and depression among older adults with osteoarthritis. *J Rheumatol*. 2008;35(2):335–342.

8. Archer KR, Castillo RC, Wegener ST, Abraham CM, Obremskey WT. Pain and satisfaction in hospitalized trauma patients: The importance of self-efficacy and psychological distress. *J Trauma Acute Care Surg*. 2012;72(4):1068–1077. doi:10.1097/TA.0b013e3182452df5

9. Evans JT, Evans JP, Walker RW, Blom AW, Whitehouse MR, Sayers A. How long does a hip replacement last? A systematic review and meta-analysis of case series and national registry reports with more than 15 years of follow-up. *Lancet*. 2019;393(10172):647–654. doi:10.1016/S0140-6736(18)31665-9

10. Crawford RW, Murray DW. Total hip replacement: Indications for surgery and risk factors for failure. *Ann Rheum Dis*. 1997;56(8):455–457. doi:10.1136/ard.56.8.455

11. Wallace G, Judge A, Prieto-Alhambra D, de Vries F, Arden NK, Cooper C. The effect of body mass index on the risk of post-operative complications during the 6 months following total hip replacement or total knee replacement surgery. *Osteoarthritis Cartilage*. 2014;22(7):918–927. doi:10.1016/j.joca.2014.04.013

12. Pozzobon D, Ferreira PH, Blyth FM, Machado GC, Ferreira ML. Can obesity and physical activity predict outcomes of elective knee or hip surgery due to osteoarthritis? A meta-analysis of cohort studies. *BMJ Open*. 2018;8(2):e017689. doi:10.1136/bmjopen-2017-017689

13. Derrett S, Paul C, Morris J. Waiting for elective surgery: Effects on health-related quality of life. *Int J Qual Health Care*. 1999;11(1):47–57. doi:10.1093/intqhc/11.1.47

14. Mancuso CA, Salvati EA, Johanson NA, Peterson MGE, Charlson ME. Patients' expectations and satisfaction with total hip arthroplasty. *J Arthroplasty*. 1997;12(4):387–396. doi:10.1016/S0883-5403(97)90194-7

15. Nilsdotter AK, Toksvig-Larsen S, Roos EM. Knee arthroplasty: Are patients' expectations fulfilled? A prospective study of pain and function in 102 patients with 5-year follow-up. *Acta Orthop*. 2009;80(1):55–61. doi:10.1080/17453670902805007

16. Scott CEH, Bugler KE, Clement ND, MacDonald D, Howie CR, Biant LC. Patient expectations of arthroplasty of the hip and knee. *J Bone Joint Surg Br*. 2012;94(7):974–981. doi:10.1302/0301-620X.94B7.28219

17. Tan K-Y, Tan PX-Z. Transdisciplinary care for elderly surgical patients. In: Tan K-Y, ed. *Colorectal Cancer in the Elderly*. Springer Berlin Heidelberg; 2013:83–92. doi:10.1007/978-3-642-29883-7_8

18. Hansen TB, Bredtoft HK, Larsen K. Preoperative physical optimization in fast-track hip and knee arthroplasty. *Dan Med J*. 2012;59(2):A4381.

19. Thomsen T, Villebro N, Møller AM. Interventions for preoperative smoking cessation. *Cochrane Database Syst Rev*. 2014;(3):CD002294. doi:10.1002/14651858.CD002294.pub4

20. Muñoz M, Gómez-Ramírez S, Cuenca J, et al. Very-short-term perioperative intravenous iron administration and postoperative outcome in major orthopedic surgery: A pooled analysis of observational data from 2547 patients. *Transfusion*. 2014;54(2):289–299. doi:10.1111/trf.12195

21. Minnella EM, Bousquet-Dion G, Awasthi R, Scheede-Bergdahl C, Carli F. Multimodal prehabilitation improves functional capacity before and after colorectal surgery for cancer: A five-year research experience. *Acta Oncol*. 2017;56(2):295–300. doi:10.1080/0284186X.2016.1268268

22. Minnella EM, Coca-Martinez M, Carli F. Prehabilitation: The anesthesiologist's role and what is the evidence? *Curr Opin Anaesthesiol*. 2020;33(3):411–416. doi:10.1097/ACO.0000000000000854

23. Doiron-Cadrin P, Kairy D, Vendittoli P-A, Lowry V, Poitras S, Desmeules F. Feasibility and preliminary effects of a tele-prehabilitation program and an in-person prehablitation program compared to usual care for total hip or knee arthroplasty candidates: A pilot randomized controlled trial. *Disabil Rehabil*. 2020;42(7):989–998. doi:10.1080/09638288.2018.1515992

24. Torisho C, Mohaddes M, Gustafsson K, Rolfson O. Minor influence of patient education and physiotherapy interventions before total hip replacement on patient-reported outcomes: An observational study of 30,756 patients in the Swedish Hip Arthroplasty Register. *Acta Orthopaedica*. 2019;90(4):306–311. doi:10.1080/17453674.2019.1605669

25. Clode NJ, Perry MA, Wulff L. Does physiotherapy prehabilitation improve pre-surgical outcomes and influence patient expectations prior to knee and hip joint arthroplasty? *Int J Orthop Trauma Nurs*. 2018;30:14–19. doi:10.1016/j.ijotn.2018.05.004

26. Fernandes L, Roos EM, Overgaard S, Villadsen A, Søgaard R. Supervised neuromuscular exercise prior to hip and knee replacement: 12-month clinical effect and cost-utility analysis alongside a randomised controlled trial. *BMC Musculoskelet Disord*. 2017;18(1):5. doi:10.1186/s12891-016-1369-0

27. Cooke M, Walker R, Aitken LM, et al. Pre-operative self-efficacy education vs. usual care for patients undergoing joint replacement surgery: A pilot randomised controlled trial. *Scand J Caring Sci*. 2016;30(1):74–82. doi:10.1111/scs.12223

28. Cavill S. The effect of prehabilitation on the range of motion and functional outcomes in patients following the total knee or hip arthroplasty: A pilot randomized trial. *Physiother Theory Pract*. 2016 May;32(4):262–270.

29. Denduluri SK, Huddleston JI, Amanatullah DF. Preoperative exercise participation reflects patient engagement and predicts earlier hospital discharge and less gait aid dependence after total joint arthroplasty. *Orthopedics*. 2020;43(5):e364–e368. doi:10.3928/01477447-20200619-04

30. ATS Committee on Proficiency Standards for Clinical Pulmonary Function Laboratories. ATS statement: Guidelines for the six-minute walk test. *Am J Respir Crit Care Med*. 2002;166(1):111–117. doi:10.1164/ajrccm.166.1.at1102

31. Gabrielson DK, Scaffidi D, Leung E, et al. Use of an abridged scored Patient-Generated Subjective Global Assessment (abPG-SGA) as a nutritional screening tool for cancer patients in an outpatient setting. *Nutr Cancer*. 2013;65(2):234–239. doi:10.1080/01635581.2013.755554

32. Flood A, Chung A, Parker H, Kearns V, O'Sullivan TA. The use of hand grip strength as a predictor of nutrition status in hospital patients. *Clin Nutr*. 2014;33(1):106–114. doi:10.1016/j.clnu.2013.03.003

33. Singer S, Kuhnt S, Götze H, et al. Hospital anxiety and depression scale cutoff scores for cancer patients in acute care. *Br J Cancer*. 2009;100(6):908–912. doi:10.1038/sj.bjc.6604952

34. Levett DZH, Jack S, Swart M, et al. Perioperative cardiopulmonary exercise testing (CPET): Consensus clinical guidelines on indications, organization, conduct, and physiological interpretation. *Br J Anaesth*. 2018;120(3):484–500. doi:10.1016/j.bja.2017.10.020

35. Moran J, Wilson F, Guinan E, McCormick P, Hussey J, Moriarty J. Role of cardiopulmonary exercise testing as a risk-assessment method in patients undergoing intra-abdominal surgery: A systematic review. *Br J Anaesth*. 2016;116(2):177–191. doi:10.1093/bja/aev454

36. Huang R, Greenky M, Kerr GJ, Austin MS, Parvizi J. The effect of malnutrition on patients undergoing elective joint arthroplasty. *J Arthroplasty*. 2013;28(8 Suppl):21–24. doi:10.1016/j.arth.2013.05.038

37. Bohl DD, Shen MR, Kayupov E, Della Valle CJ. Hypoalbuminemia independently predicts surgical site infection, pneumonia, length of stay, and readmission after total joint arthroplasty. *J Arthroplasty*. 2016;31(1):15–21. doi:10.1016/j.arth.2015.08.028

38. Bandura A, Freeman WH, Lightsey R. Self-efficacy: The exercise of control. *J Cogn Psychother*. 1999;13(2):158–166. doi:10.1891/0889-8391.13.2.158

39. Mavros MN, Athanasiou S, Gkegkes ID, Polyzos KA, Peppas G, Falagas ME. Do psychological variables affect early surgical recovery? *PLoS One*. 2011;6(5):e20306. doi:10.1371/journal.pone.0020306

40. Padilla JA, Feng JE, Anoushiravani AA, Hozack WJ, Schwarzkopf R, Macaulay WB. Modifying patient expectations can enhance total hip arthroplasty postoperative satisfaction. *J Arthroplasty*. 2019;34(7):S209–S214. doi:10.1016/j.arth.2018.12.038

41. Ljungqvist O, Francis NK, Urman RD, eds. *Enhanced Recovery After Surgery: A Complete Guide to Optimizing Outcomes*. Springer International Publishing; 2020. doi:10.1007/978-3-030-33443-7

42. Maheshwari AV, Blum YC, Shekhar L, Ranawat AS, Ranawat CS. Multimodal pain management after total hip and knee arthroplasty at the Ranawat Orthopaedic Center. *Clin Orthop Relat Res*. 2009;467(6):1418–1423. doi:10.1007/s11999-009-0728-7

43. Gandhi K, Viscusi E. Multimodal pain management techniques in hip and knee arthroplasty. *Knee Arthroplasty*. 2009;13:10.

44. Desborough JP. The stress response to trauma and surgery. *Br J Anaesth*. 2000;85(1):109–117. doi:10.1093/bja/85.1.109

45. Morrison RJM, Bunn D, Gray WK, et al. VASO (Vitamin D and Arthroplasty Surgery Outcomes) study: Supplementation of vitamin D deficiency to improve outcomes after total hip or knee replacement: Study protocol for a randomised controlled feasibility trial. *Trials*. 2017;18(1):514. doi:10.1186/s13063-017-2255-2

46. Sikora-Klak J, Zarling B, Bergum C, Flynn JC, Markel DC. The effect of comorbidities on discharge disposition and readmission for total joint arthroplasty patients. *J Arthroplasty*. 2017;32(5):1414–1417. doi:10.1016/j.arth.2016.11.035

47. Sharareh B, Le NB, Hoang MT, Schwarzkopf R. Factors determining discharge destination for patients undergoing total joint arthroplasty. *J Arthroplasty*. 2014;29(7):1355–1358.e1. doi:10.1016/j.arth.2014.02.001

48. Regenbogen SE, Cain-Nielsen AH, Norton EC, Chen LM, Birkmeyer JD, Skinner JS. Costs and consequences of early hospital discharge after major inpatient surgery in older adults. *JAMA Surg*. 2017;152(5):e170123. doi:10.1001/jamasurg.2017.0123

9.

CARDIOPULMONARY EXERCISE TESTING

Paris Dove, Emily Traer, Hilmy Ismail, and Bernhard Riedel

STEM CASE 1 AND KEY QUESTIONS

A 60-year-old patient with a past medical history of ischemic heart disease (IHD), hypertension, and dyslipidemia is referred for cardiopulmonary exercise testing (CPET) for workup prior to esophagectomy. The patient underwent percutaneous coronary intervention 10 years earlier. Current medications include clopidogrel, telmisartan, ramipril, aspirin, and a statin. The patient has not had a recent cardiology review and currently smokes 20 cigarettes per day with a calculated 40-pack year history. Subjectively, the patient reports excellent exercise tolerance with no episodes of angina.

CPET is conducted on an upright cycle ergometer on a 20 watt/min ramp protocol. Anaerobic threshold (AT) is reached in 9.5 minutes, and the test concluded at peak exercise after 13.5 minutes due to dyspnea and fatigue. Of note, there is a plateau in oxygen pulse at peak exercise. The 12-lead ECG trace shows sinus rhythm throughout but develops 3 mm of ST-segment depression in leads V3 to V6 at peak exercise in the absence of chest pain (Figure 9.1a). The ST segments normalize in recovery. The test results are provided in Table 9.1 and Figure 9.1b. The patient has a BMI of 32 kg/m² and a body surface area (BSA) of 2.0 m².

Is this a maximal exercise test that allows for objective interpretation? List the findings to back your conclusion.

This is a maximal exercise test supported by the following findings:

- Respiratory exchange rate (RER) of 1.3 at peak exercise; see panel 8.
  - A peak RER of 1.10 or greater is widely accepted as an indication of satisfactory patient effort during CPET.[1,2]
- Heart rate (HR) 156 beats per minute (bpm) at peak (98% of predicted maximal heart rate); see panel 2.
- $\dot{V}O_{2peak}$ (oxygen consumption at peak exercise) 19.4 mL/kg/min (82% of predicted); see panels 3 and 5 (x-axis).
- Peak WR 122 watts (W) (100% predicted); see panels 1 and 3:
- Normal breathing reserve (MVV – $\dot{V}E_{peak}$ / MVV = 123 – 95 / 123 = 23%); see panels 4 and 7.

- Maximal voluntary ventilation (MVV) is the theoretical ventilatory limit of the respiratory system.[3] MVV can be estimated indirectly, by the calculation of forced expiratory volume within 1 second (FEV_1) × 35 – 40, or directly, measuring minute ventilation ($\dot{V}E$) over 10–15 seconds of breathing at maximal effort using a spirometer.[3,4]

- In healthy subjects, ventilatory demand does not normally encroach on ventilatory capacity during exercise and, as such, respiratory reserve is greater than 15%.[3] It is important to note that breathing reserve demonstrates significant variability among the normal population and that $\dot{V}E_{peak}$ (minute ventilation at peak exercise) may approach MVV in fit individuals and in the elderly in the absence of disease.[3]

What is the anaerobic threshold, and how do you determine this on the nine-panel plot?

In an incremental exercise test, the anaerobic threshold (AT) is defined as the oxygen uptake value at which aerobic metabolism is supplemented by anaerobic glycolysis.[1,3,5] The measurable metabolic changes occurring after AT are a systematic increase in CO_2 production ($\dot{V}CO_2$), an increase in the respiratory exchange ratio (RER; or ratio of $\dot{V}CO_2/\dot{V}O_2$), a rise in blood lactate levels, a fall in blood bicarbonate levels, and a decrease in blood pH.[1,3,5] For this reason, AT may also be described as the "lactate threshold."[5] AT is determined by interpreting the nine-panel plot according to three set criteria outlined in the CPET consensus clinical guidelines[5]:

- *Criterion 1*: Identify excess $\dot{V}CO_2$ relative to $\dot{V}O_2$ (i.e., use the V-slope or modified V-slope method; see panel 5). The inflection observed in the $\dot{V}CO_2 - \dot{V}O_2$ relationship here is secondary to the buffering of anaerobic lactate *after* AT with consequent generation of more CO_2 (i.e., H^+ + $HCO_3^- \leftrightarrow H_2CO_3 \leftrightarrow H_2O + CO_2$).

- *Criterion 2*: Identify hyperventilation with respect to O_2 uptake (i.e., by the nadir of the slope for the ventilatory equivalents of oxygen [$\dot{V}E/\dot{V}O_2$] see panel 6) or the rise in the end tidal oxygen ($P_{ET}O_2$) slope (see panel 9). At this point, $\dot{V}E$ increases and is driven by the excess CO_2 of anaerobic glycolysis without a corresponding increase in $\dot{V}O_2$.

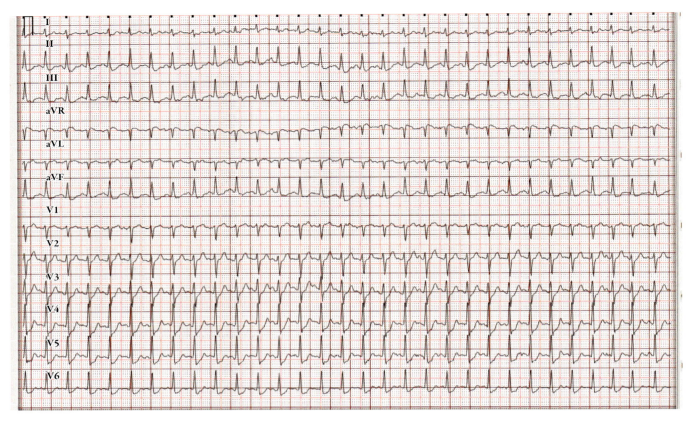

Figure 9.1a Case 1 ECG.

Table 9.1 CASE 1 CPET DATA REFLECTING PARAMETERS AT BASELINE (REST) AND DURING EXERCISE AT ANAEROBIC THRESHOLD (AT) AND AT PEAK EXERCISE (PEAK)

DATA	REST	AT	PEAK	% PREDICTED MAXIMUM AT PEAK EXERCISE
FEV_1 [L]	3.1			131
MVV [L/min]	123			93
Breathing reserve [%]	23			
DLCO [mL/min/mm Hg]	23.5			83
$\dot{V}E/\dot{V}CO_2$	39.5	29.7	35.0	
$\dot{V}E$ [L/min]	11	30	95	
SpO_2 [%]	100	100	100	
HR [bpm]	83	117	156	98
BP [mm Hg]	119/65	145/70	160/80	Recovery 155/72
$\dot{V}O_2$ [mL/kg/min]	4.0	13.0	19.4	82
O_2 pulse [mL/beat]	4.5	10.3	11.6	84
RER	0.78	0.94	1.3	
Load [W]	0	69	122	100
Blood results	Hb g/L 142	Albumin g/L 38	CRP mg/L 4	Transferrin saturation % 28

FEV_1, forced expiratory volume in the first second of forced expiration; MVV, maximum voluntary ventilation; DLCO, lung diffusing capacity for carbon monoxide; E, minute ventilation; CO_2, carbon dioxide output; SpO_2, peripheral oxygen saturation; HR, heart rate in beats per minute (bpm); BP, blood pressure; O_2, oxygen uptake; O_2 pulse, oxygen pulse; RER, respiratory exchange ratio; Hb, hemoglobin; CRP, C-reactive protein

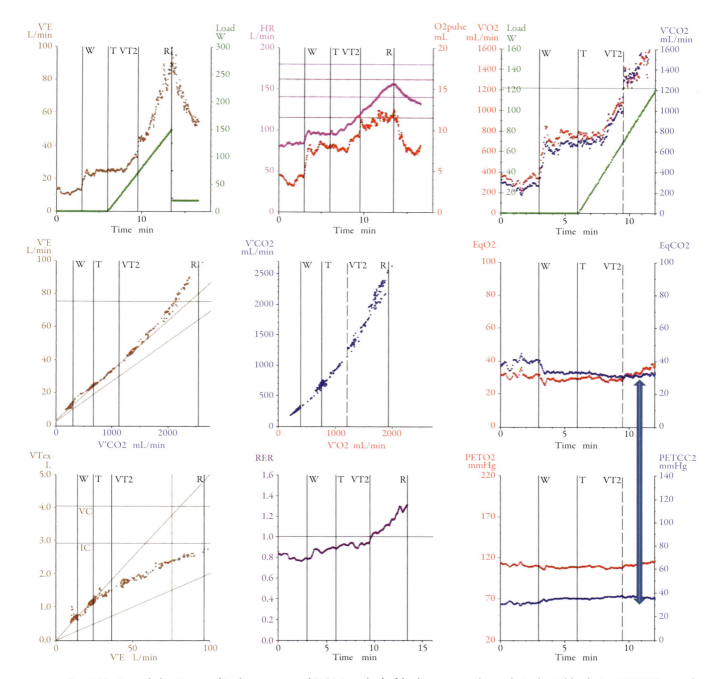

Figure 9.1b Case 1 The 9-panel plot: Presented in the conventional UCLA method of displaying gas-exchange derived variables during CPET. The panels are numbered sequentially 1–9, from left to right, top row to bottom row.
W, unloaded cycling; T, loaded cycling; VT2, anaerobic threshold; R, recovery; $\dot{V}E$, minute ventilation; HR, heart rate; $\dot{V}O_2$, oxygen uptake; $V'CO_2$, carbon dioxide output; EqO_2, ventilatory equivalents for oxygen; $EqCO_2$, ventilatory equivalents for carbon dioxide; VTex, tidal volume expired; RER, respiratory exchange ratio; $PETO_2$, end tidal pressure of oxygen; $PETCO_2$, end tidal pressure of carbon dioxide.

- *Criterion 3*: Exclude hyperventilation with respect to the production of CO_2 (i.e., confirm a plateau or decrease in the ventilatory equivalents for carbon dioxide [$\dot{V}E/\dot{V}CO_2$], occurring at the point determined by criteria 1 and 2 above; see panels 6 and 9).

It is worth noting that the rise in $\dot{V}E/\dot{V}CO_2$ and decline in end tidal carbon dioxide ($P_{ET}CO_2$), as represented by divergent curves and depicted by the arrow in panels 6 and 9 (Figure 9.1b),

is defined as the respiratory compensation point, and AT should occur before this point.

This patient achieved AT at $\dot{V}O_2$ of 13 mL/kg/min.

What is the difference between $\dot{V}O_{2max}$ (maximal) and $\dot{V}O_{2peak}$ (at peak exercise)?

$\dot{V}O_{2max}$ is an end point where oxygen uptake cannot be increased further despite increasing workload[5] and may be derived by the Fick equation[1]: $\dot{V}O_{2max} = (HR \times SV) \times [C(\text{a-v})$

O_2] where HR is heart rate, SV is stroke volume, and $C(a-v)O_2$ is the arterial-venous difference in oxygen content. $\dot{V}O_{2max}$ is representative of the upper limit of an individual's functional capacity. This is the sum of their cardiorespiratory, vascular, hematologic, musculoskeletal, and metabolic systems working at their physiological maximum.[1,3,5] In athletes, $\dot{V}O_{2max}$ may be observed as a plateau in the $\dot{V}O_2$ at peak, though in practice this is rarely seen in the typical patient who presents to CPET for perioperative evaluation.[1,3,5]

The $\dot{V}O_{2peak}$ is the highest oxygen uptake value achieved during an incremental exercise test.[1-3] It is averaged over 20–30 seconds or 3–5 breaths during the final portion of incremental work.[5] $\dot{V}O_{2peak}$ is influenced by age and gender and is typically indexed to weight in kilograms (mL/kg/min). Occasionally, $\dot{V}O_{2peak}$ is indexed to body surface area (mL/m²), and this may help overcome artificially high or low $\dot{V}O_{2peak}$ measures at extremes of body weight.[6,7] Nonathletes typically achieve $\dot{V}O_{2peak}$ and not $\dot{V}O_{2max}$. The advantages of the $\dot{V}O_{2peak}$ are that it is easy to identify on the nine-panel plot and it is reproducible on repeat testing.[5] The limitations of $\dot{V}O_{2peak}$ are that it is related to a patient's volitional effort and the provision of subject encouragement to reach a maximum effort.[5] Despite these limitations, there remains merit in evaluating $\dot{V}O_{2peak}$ given the increasing body of evidence correlating $\dot{V}O_{2peak}$ to perioperative outcomes.[5,6,8–10] Other useful metrics derived at peak exercise include HR_{peak} relative to age-predicted maximum heart rate and RER_{peak} of greater than 1.1.[2,5]

Identify the CPET results that indicate the presence of myocardial ischemia during exercise.

This patient has 3 mm of ST depression in leads V3 to V6 at peak exercise that could suggest lateral territory myocardial ischemia, without chest pain. Heart rate and blood pressure remained stable throughout exercise, and the patient was permitted to continue the test to their peak effort. According to guidelines,[3,5] the ECG criteria for premature CPET termination are greater than 2 mm ST depression if the patient is symptomatic, or 4 mm ST depression if the patient is asymptomatic, or greater than 1 mm ST elevation.

Another useful CPET derivative of the Fick equation is the oxygen pulse: $\dot{V}O_2/HR = SV \times [C(a-v)O_2]$. It is a surrogate marker for stroke volume that provides dynamic information about myocardial function.[1,3] The oxygen pulse describes the oxygen uptake per heartbeat[1,3,11] assuming no impairments to oxygen extraction and normal chronotropic activity.[1] The normal shape of the $\dot{V}O_2/HR$ relationship (also known as $\dot{V}O_2$ pulse) is hyperbolic with a linear increase observed early in exercise as stroke volume makes a significant contribution to increased cardiac output.[1,3,11] In late exercise, this reaches a plateau because further increase in cardiac output is supplemented by a rise in heart rate at high WRs.[3] A premature asymptote, described as a "flattened" oxygen pulse, is indicative of cardiogenic limitation to exercise.[1,2,12] and, as seen in this case (panel 2), myocardial ischemia. A low peak oxygen pulse may also be observed in deconditioning if the patient has an arrhythmia such as atrial fibrillation, is on beta blockers, or if exercise is terminated early for any cause.[3]

DISCUSSION

One of the first considerations when interpreting CPET results is to determine the adequacy of patient effort. Several objective CPET variables are used for this purpose including HR, RER, and $\dot{V}O_2$ at peak exercise.[5] Subjective information from the patient can be obtained using the Borg score, representing perceived exertional effort and their reason for stopping the test (e.g., breathlessness, muscle fatigue). Comments and observations made by the CPET scientist and attending clinician may also aid in interpreting CPET data.

In the absence of a plateau in $\dot{V}O_2$, other CPET criteria are used to assess whether the patient pushed themselves to their physiological maximum.[3,5] The maximum heart rate response to exercise is estimated by the equation 220 − age, though the standard deviation is large (± 15 bpm).[3] Achieving a maximum heart rate 85% or better of predicted is regarded as excellent patient effort and may be taken as an indicator of a maximal test.[1,3] In practice, case-by-case interpretation of maximum heart rate is necessary as resting tachycardia, atrial fibrillation, and prescribed beta blockers are frequently seen among the clinical cohort of patients referred for perioperative assessment.

The RER is the ratio of $\dot{V}CO_2$ to $\dot{V}O_2$ measured from expired gas at the mouthpiece during exercise.[1,3] With increasing WR and the evolution of anaerobic metabolism, the consequent bicarbonate buffering of hydrogen ions generated from lactic acidosis liberates more CO_2, leading to an increase in the RER.[1] A peak RER of 1.1 or higher is widely accepted as an indication of satisfactory patient effort during CPET.[1,2] The AT occurs at an RER somewhere between 0.8 and 0.99; therefore, when RER = 1.0, AT has already passed.[1] Cessation of exercise at an RER of less than 1.0, in the absence of patient symptoms and cardiac abnormalities, generally signifies inadequate patient effort, though this may also be seen in patients limited secondarily by respiratory disease or metabolic impairment.[1,5]

External work is most accurately measured during CPET using an electronically braked cycle ergometer,[3] where exercise is performed by large muscle groups with limited reliance on balance or cadence. In the setting of a steadily increasing WR, oxygen consumption should increase in a linear fashion.[3] The correlation of $\dot{V}O_2$ to WR, or the $\Delta\dot{V}O_2/\Delta WR$ slope (also called the $\dot{V}O_2$/Work rate slope), has been found to be remarkably constant, with a value of approximately 10 mL/W independent of age, gender, height, or training.[3] As such, the $\Delta\dot{V}O_2/\Delta WR$ relationship represents the gain of the system, and any reduction in this metric indicates pathology affecting the heart, lungs, circulation, muscles, or mitochondrial function.[3]

Lactate production results through any or a combination of the following[3]:

- Exhaustion of oxygen delivery DO_2 mechanisms, where $DO_2 = CO \times [(Hb \times SaO2 \times 1.34) + (PaO_2 \times 0.003)]$.
- Relative use of glycolytic type II muscle fibers (high-intensity work) over oxidative type I muscle fibers (low-intensity work).

- Insufficiency of oxidative respiration at the cellular level (i.e., reduced number or enzymatic function of mitochondria).

While AT has become an important metric in CPET it is only useful when interpreted together with the other derived variables including baseline fitness, patient subjective effort, RER, $\dot{V}O_{2peak}$, oxygen pulse, chronotropic response to exercise, heart rate recovery, ECG changes, lung function, ventilatory efficiency, and $\Delta\dot{V}O_2/\Delta WR$. The point at which AT rises varies across populations and occurs between 35% and 80% of peak $\dot{V}O_2$.[3] AT is influenced by the type of activity undertaken because of differences in muscle mass and fiber type used, with increasing values seen in arm crank, cycle ergometry, and treadmill exercises, respectively.[3] AT is higher in athletes, who have greater cardiorespiratory fitness compared to the deconditioned population.[1] AT is reached earlier in disease states.[5] In the elderly, AT occurs later in exercise as a proportion of a lower $\dot{V}O_{2peak}$.[3] Unlike $\dot{V}O_{2peak}$, AT is nonvolitional[5] and is easily reproduced with minimal effort for most patients,[1] hence AT is widely referenced in perioperative assessment.

Determination of AT may assist the perioperative physician in several ways. Knowing AT enables assessment of a patient's baseline fitness and therefore can guide the prescription of an individualized exercise-training program[2,3,11] based on Borg Scale, heart rate, or watts measured at AT (e.g., moderate to high-intensity interval training [HIIT]). Inactive subjects have been shown to improve their AT and $\dot{V}O_{2peak}$ by 10–25% with exercise training.[1] AT can be utilized to predict perioperative risk for specific surgical cohorts[5,6,8,9] and to resourcefully triage postoperative disposition to the surgical ward, to an enhanced care area, or to a high-dependency unit (HDU).[6,8,9] That is, CPET has a role in preoperative risk stratification, prehabilitation, and postoperative care planning. After completion of CPET the patient in this case study was referred to a cardiologist for optimization of cardiac risk factors, with the recommendation of high-dependency level care postoperatively.

STEM CASE 2 AND KEY QUESTIONS

The colorectal surgical team referred a 70-year-old patient to your CPET clinic for assessment prior to a major open abdominal cancer resection. They request your assessment in anticipation of a multidisciplinary team meeting. The patient is currently being worked up for exertional dyspnea and desaturation during a 6-minute walk test (6MWT). Arterial blood gas demonstrates hypoxemia on room air with a P_aO_2 of 55 mm Hg and an alveolar-arterial gradient of 50 mm Hg.

Clinical information includes a 90-pack year ex-smoking history, ischemic heart disease with distal left anterior descending coronary artery stenosis not amenable to coronary stenting, paroxysmal atrial fibrillation, and non–insulin dependent diabetes mellitus with renal impairment. The patient has a BMI of 33 kg/m² and a BSA 2.2 m².

You conduct a symptom-limited CPET with gas-exchange analysis on an upright cycle ergometer using a 15 watt/min ramp exercise protocol. The test is stopped by the patient after 12.5 minutes of cycling due to dyspnea and fatigue. The test results are provided in Table 9.2 and Figure 9.2.

Identify the CPET-derived data in support of a respiratory etiology to explain this patient's exercise limitation. Ensure that you distinguish between indices of ventilatory inefficiency and mechanical ventilatory limitation.

- The absence of cardiac limitation as seen by a normal $\Delta\dot{V}O_2/\Delta WR$ slope and oxygen pulse (see panel 2) and no ischemic symptoms or ECG changes during exercise.
- Desaturation during exercise.
- Reduced FEV_1 and DLCO (lung diffusing capacity for carbon monoxide).
- Low $\dot{V}O_{2peak}$ 12.9 mL/kg/min (63% of predicted); see panel 3.
- Elevated $\dot{V}E/\dot{V}CO_2$ of 39.3 at AT (normal <35 at AT); see panel 6.
- Low breathing reserve (MVV – $\dot{V}E_{peak}$/ MVV = 92.4 – 80/92.4 = 13%; normal >15%); see panels 4 and 7.

A low breathing reserve (<15%) indicates mechanical ventilatory limitation[3] and a $\dot{V}E/\dot{V}CO_2$ slope of greater than 30[1,2] or a $\dot{V}E/\dot{V}CO_2$ at AT of greater than 35 (see panels 4 and 6, respectively) indicates ventilatory inefficiency.[3,5]

What additional tests might you consider after analyzing the CPET results and why?

- Computed tomography (CT) pulmonary angiogram (CTPA) to investigate for pulmonary embolism.
- High-resolution CT scan to assess for pulmonary fibrosis.
- Transthoracic echocardiogram to assess for pulmonary hypertension.
- Arterial blood gas on room air and on 100% oxygen to assess for right to left anatomical shunt.

Explain the mechanism of increased $\dot{V}E/\dot{V}CO_2$ in patients with chronic lung disease.

Increased $\dot{V}E/\dot{V}CO_2$ represents a ventilation-perfusion (V/Q) mismatch. This may be related to increased physiologic dead space in patients with chronic lung disease.[1,3,8,9] Differential diagnoses include chronic obstructive pulmonary disease (COPD), congestive cardiac failure (CCF), pulmonary embolism, and pulmonary hypertension. As $\dot{V}E/\dot{V}CO_2$ deviates further from normal, the likelihood of secondary pulmonary hypertension increases.[2] $\dot{V}E/\dot{V}CO_2$ may also be increased in voluntary hyperventilation or states of increased ventilatory drive.[3,8,9]

Explain the importance of the observed desaturation during exercise.

Table 9.2 CASE 2 CPET DATA REFLECTING PARAMETERS AT BASELINE (REST) AND DURING EXERCISE AT ANAEROBIC THRESHOLD (AT) AND AT PEAK EXERCISE (PEAK)

DATA	REST	AT	PEAK	% PREDICTED MAXIMUM AT PEAK EXERCISE
FEV_1 [L]	2.3			79 No reversibility with bronchodilator
FVC [L]	3.5			71
FEV_1 / FVC ratio [%]	65			
MVV [L/min]	92.4			78
Breathing reserve [%]	13			
DLCO [mL/min/mm Hg]	15.1			47
$\dot{V}E/\dot{V}CO_2$	45.2	39.3	41.9	
$\dot{V}E$ [L/min]	11	40	80	
SpO_2 [%]	96	93	94	
HR [bpm]	82	114	122	81
BP [mm Hg]	144/49	159/85	182/72	Recovery 176/70
$\dot{V}O_2$ [mL/kg/min]	3.3	10.5	12.9	63
O_2 pulse [mL/beat]	4.1	9.6	11.0	78
RER	0.79	0.98	1.15	
Load [W]	0	71	94	71
Blood results	Hb g/L 156	Albumin g/L 37	CRP mg/L 10	Transferrin saturation % 31

FEV_1, forced expiratory volume in the first second of forced expiration; FVC, forced vital capacity; MVV, maximum voluntary ventilation; DLCO, lung diffusing capacity for carbon monoxide; E, minute ventilation; CO_2, carbon dioxide output; SpO_2, peripheral oxygen saturation; HR, heart rate in beats per minute (bpm); BP, blood pressure; O_2, oxygen uptake; O_2 pulse, oxygen pulse; RER, respiratory exchange ratio; Hb, hemoglobin; CRP, C-reactive protein.

Desaturation by 5% or more is considered abnormal during CPET[1–3] and warrants further investigation into the underlying etiology.[1–3] Laboratories do vary in practice, and many will use thresholds of less than 80–85% desaturation for exercise termination.[1,3] Exercise-induced desaturation is observed in COPD, interstitial lung disease, and pulmonary hypertension,[2] and its presence is indicative of advanced pathology.[2]

DISCUSSION

CPET is frequently utilized to determine the cause of exertional dyspnea.[1–3] In this case, it is apparent that respiratory pathology is the major underlying disease process responsible for the patient's exercise limitation. As the patient's heart rate did not reach their age-predicted maximum and peak WR was low, maximal myocardial work was not reached. Therefore, cardiac limitation cannot be assumed despite the patient's history of coronary artery disease. Resting pulmonary function tests do not give information about a patient's functional status, nor do they provide guidance about the patient's physiological reserve. Research supports the objectivity of CPET in this field.[3,13] In one study, marked variability was observed between the measured peak $\dot{V}O_2$ during exercise testing and the degree of airflow obstruction on pulmonary function testing.[13] This illustrates how CPET may outperform spirometry for the assessment of functional capacity in respiratory disease. CPET has also been shown to be more sensitive than a 6MWT in measuring exercise capacity in COPD after bronchodilator therapy.[3]

The $\dot{V}E/\dot{V}CO_2$ relationship provides information about the effectiveness of V/Q matching in the lungs.[2,5,6] A normal $\dot{V}E/\dot{V}CO_2$ is described as being less than 32–34 at AT,[3] and, in healthy young individuals, it is usually less than 30.[2,3] The $\dot{V}E/\dot{V}CO_2$ slope value is independent of the test protocol used and the type of exercise conducted, with reported demonstrable re-test accuracy.[1] Reduced ventilatory efficiency, as shown here by the high $\dot{V}E/\dot{V}CO_2$ ratio, suggests either a low arterial P_aCO_2 (seen in acute hyperventilation or in states of increased ventilatory drive) or increased physiologic dead space.[3,5,8,9] An elevated $\dot{V}E/\dot{V}CO_2$ is commonly seen in patients with COPD, interstitial lung disease, heart failure, and pulmonary hypertension.[1,2,5,8,9] Disease severity and prognosis correlate with the degree of deviation from

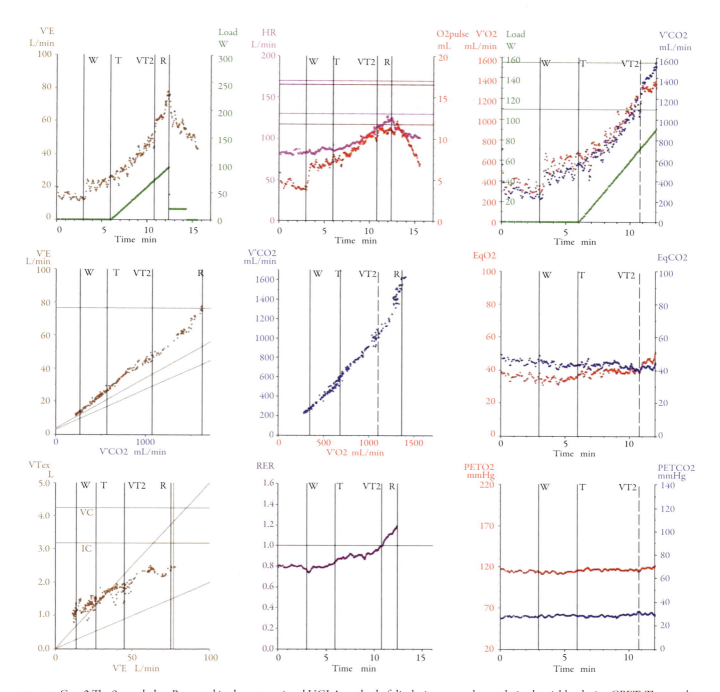

Figure 9.2 Case 2 The 9-panel plot: Presented in the conventional UCLA method of displaying gas-exchange derived variables during CPET. The panels are numbered sequentially 1–9, from left to right, top row to bottom row.
W, unloaded cycling; T, loaded cycling; VT2, anaerobic threshold; R, recovery; V'E, minute ventilation; HR, heart rate; $\dot{V}O_2$, oxygen uptake; $\dot{V}CO_2$, carbon dioxide output; EqO$_2$, ventilatory equivalents for oxygen; EqCO$_2$, ventilatory equivalents for carbon dioxide; VTex, tidal volume expired; RER, respiratory exchange ratio; PETO$_2$, end tidal pressure of oxygen; PETCO$_2$, end tidal pressure of carbon dioxide.

normal.[1,2,5] As such, $\dot{V}E/\dot{V}CO_2$ is a powerful tool in perioperative risk stratification[2,5] and acts as a risk predictor for postoperative morbidity and mortality for a number of surgical procedures.[6,14–17]

Best practice management of chronic respiratory disease includes pulmonary prehabilitation and exercise training, which has been associated with improved lung function.[18,19] CPET can be utilized to evaluate the impact of such therapeutic interventions.[3] The foundations of pulmonary prehabilitation have since been adopted in perioperative medicine with the aim of reducing the incidence of postoperative pulmonary complications such as pneumonia.[20–23] Pulmonary prehabilitation before surgery for lung cancer has been associated with reduced postoperative pulmonary complications in observational studies.[24] Prospective studies have also shown improved postoperative recovery through decreased duration of intubation and length of hospital stay.[25] Pulmonary bundles of care (e.g., iCOUGH[21]) demonstrate a reduction in postoperative pneumonia and other respiratory complications in surgical ward patients.[20,21] In patients scheduled for elective upper abdominal surgery, prehabilitation with a 30-minute physiotherapy session halved the incidence of postoperative pulmonary complications (number needed to treat = 7 and 95% confidence interval 5–14).[25]

The principles of pulmonary prehabilitation can be introduced on the day of CPET by teaching patients deep breathing and coughing exercises. Written educational material may be provided allowing patients to practice cycles of deep breathing exercises at home. Such education was given to the patient in this case, as well as a referral to a respiratory physician for optimization. After 3 weeks of inhaled corticosteroid therapy and deep breathing exercises, the patient re-presented to CPET. Between tests, the patient did not engage in a prescribed exercise program due to knee pain but did perform the breathing exercises. Subsequent oxygen saturations at rest and on room air improved to 98% with a nadir of 94% when exercising. Despite this improvement, as well as an increase in ventilatory efficiency of 5% from baseline, it was concluded at shared decision-making that nonoperative management was more suited to the patient's personal goals and preferences. Despite not choosing to have surgery, the patient's quality of life was improved through this respiratory optimization and improved symptom control.

STEM CASE 3 AND KEY QUESTIONS

A 75-year-old patient diagnosed with distal esophageal adenocarcinoma is referred for CPET to assess baseline functional capacity prior to commencement of neoadjuvant chemoradiotherapy and to undertake risk stratification in anticipation of surgical resection. The patient lives independently at home and currently takes medication for hypercholesterolemia and gastroesophageal reflux disease.

CPET with gas-exchange analysis is conducted on an upright cycle ergometer with a 20 watt/min ramp protocol. The patient terminates the test after 12 minutes of cycling due to exhaustion. The patient has a BMI of 25 kg/m² and BSA 1.65 m².

Summarize and interpret the results of the CPET shown in Table 9.3a and Figure 9.3a

This is a maximal exercise test as evidenced by a $\dot{V}O_{2peak}$ of 20.6 mL/kg/min, RER_{peak} 1.35, HR_{peak} at 154 bpm, and peak WR of 120 W, all of which exceed the age-predicted maximum values. CPET provides objective evidence of favorable physiological reserve in this patient. The AT value of 15.1 mL/kg/min, $\dot{V}O_{2peak}$ of 20.6 mL/kg/min, and $\dot{V}E/\dot{V}CO_2$ of 29.2 at AT place patient in the low-risk category for postoperative complications.[11] Therefore, it is reasonable to consider surgery as a viable treatment option. The patient is advised to sustain

Table 9.3a CASE 3 CPET DATA, PRIOR TO NEOADJUVANT THERAPY, REFLECTING PARAMETERS AT BASELINE (REST) AND DURING EXERCISE AT ANAEROBIC THRESHOLD (AT) AND AT PEAK EXERCISE (PEAK)

DATA	REST	AT	PEAK	% PREDICTED MAXIMUM AT PEAK EXERCISE
FEV_1 [L]	2.5			125
MVV [L/min]	100			128
Breathing reserve [%]	21			
DLCO [mL/min/mm Hg]	22.3			101
$\dot{V}E/\dot{V}CO_2$	33.7	29.2	36.7	
$\dot{V}E$ [L/min]	7	27	79	
SpO_2 [%]	100	99	100	
HR [bpm]	90	125	154	106
HRR_1 [bpm]				Recovery 135
BP [mm Hg]	130/85	155/83	172/80	Recovery 150/90
$\dot{V}O_2$ [mL/kg/min]	4.2	15.1	20.6	122
O_2 pulse [mL/beat]	2.8	7.6	8.5	109
RER	0.84	0.94	1.35	
Load [W]	0	72	120	222
Blood results	Hb g/L 139	Albumin g/L 36	CRP mg/L 2.0	Transferrin saturation % 18

FEV_1, forced expiratory volume in the first second of forced expiration; MVV, maximum voluntary ventilation; DLCO, lung diffusing capacity for carbon monoxide; E, minute ventilation; CO_2, carbon dioxide output; SpO_2, peripheral oxygen saturation; HR, heart rate in beats per minute (bpm); HRR_1, heart rate at 1 minute recovery; BP, blood pressure; O_2, oxygen uptake; O_2 pulse, oxygen pulse; RER, respiratory exchange ratio; Hb, hemoglobin; CRP, C-reactive protein.

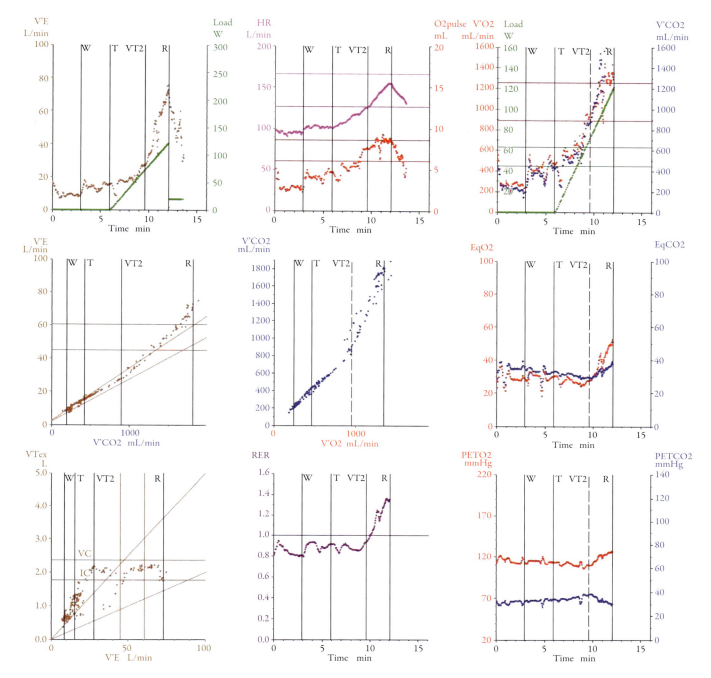

Figure 9.3a Case 3. The 9-panel plot: Presented using the conventional UCLA method of displaying gas-exchange derived variables during CPET. The panels are numbered sequentially 1–9, from left to right, top row to bottom row. W, unloaded cycling; T, loaded cycling; VT2, anaerobic threshold. R, recovery; V̇E, minute ventilation; HR, heart rate; V̇O2, oxygen uptake; V̇CO2, carbon dioxide output; EqO2, ventilatory equivalents for oxygen; EqCO2, ventilatory equivalents for carbon dioxide; VTex, tidal volume expired; RER, respiratory exchange ratio; PETO2, end tidal pressure of oxygen; PETCO2, end tidal pressure of carbon dioxide.

an exercise regime during neoadjuvant chemoradiotherapy, as deconditioning with a 15–20% decline in AT and $\dot{V}O_{2peak}$ from baseline values, can be observed.[26–29]

You see this patient again in CPET clinic after neoadjuvant therapy is completed. Side effects of treatment include reduced energy levels and poor appetite. Their BMI and BSA, however, have remained unchanged. List the CPET variables that indicate that the patient is now at a higher risk of postoperative complications (Table 9.3b and Figure 9.3b below) compared to the baseline CPET.

- Reduced AT = 10.1 mL/kg/min; see panels 5, 6, and 9 using the three criteria for AT determination.

- Reduced $\dot{V}O_{2peak}$ = 16.5 mL/kg/min (95% predicted); see panel 3.

- Increase in $\dot{V}E/\dot{V}CO_2$ to 31.3 at AT; see panel 6.

- Resting tachycardia with HR 120 bpm; see panel 2.

  - The normal chronotropic response to exercise should be greater than 25 bpm from baseline to AT and a greater

Table 9.3b **CASE 3 CPET DATA, AFTER NEOADJUVANT THERAPY, REFLECTING PARAMETERS AT BASELINE (REST) AND DURING EXERCISE AT ANAEROBIC THRESHOLD (AT) AND AT PEAK EXERCISE (PEAK)**

DATA	REST	AT	PEAK	% PREDICTED MAXIMUM AT PEAK EXERCISE
$\dot{V}E/\dot{V}CO_2$	36.9	31.3	37.9	
$\dot{V}E$ [L/min]	10	22	60	
SpO_2 [%]	99	98	99	
HR [bpm] HRR$_1$ [bpm]	120	127	147	101 Recovery 140
BP [mm Hg]	135/90	156/85	166/80	Recovery 145/95
$\dot{V}O_2$ [mL/kg/min]	4.4	10.1	16.5	95
O_2 pulse [mL/beat]	2.3	5.3	7.3	99
RER	0.87	0.88	1.20	
Load [W]	0	38	82	152
Blood results	Hb g/L 112	Albumin g/L 23	CRP mg/L 18	Transferrin saturation % 12

$\dot{V}E$, minute ventilation; CO_2, carbon dioxide output; SpO_2, peripheral oxygen saturation; HR, heart rate; HRR$_1$, heart rate at 1 minute recovery; BP, blood pressure; O_2, oxygen uptake; O_2 pulse, oxygen pulse; RER, respiratory exchange ratio; Hb, hemoglobin; CRP, C-reactive protein.

than 40 bpm rise in HR from baseline to peak exercise, respectively.

- Poor heart rate decline in the recovery phase (low risk is depicted by >12 bpm reduction in HR after 1-minute recovery); see panel 2 (147 – 140 = 7 bpm).
- Flatter profile of the oxygen pulse (slope and at peak exercise); see panel 2.
- Hypoalbuminemia and anemia, likely due to raised inflammatory markers on blood test results.

What strategies can you implement to optimize this patient's fitness for surgery?

- The following multidisciplinary approach may be considered:
  - To improve functional status, refer to a physiotherapist for guidance on a structured exercise prescription and pulmonary prehabilitation in the period prior to surgery. Schedule a repeat CPET test in 4 weeks.
  - Do a complete hematinic evaluation for possible iron deficiency and consider a hematology consult for further anemia management.
  - Refer to a dietician for nutritional education and supplementation to manage the self-reported reduced appetite and low albumin level.
  - Consider a psychology referral if the patient exhibits signs of anxiety and/or depression.
  - Consider a group education session (e.g., Surgery School) to prepare the patient for an enhanced recovery after surgery (ERAS) program.

After 4 weeks of prehabilitation and a dedicated exercise program the patient undergoes repeat CPET. Summarize and interpret your findings from the CPET results shown in Table 9.3c and Figure 9.3c).

This is a maximal exercise test as evidenced by a $\dot{V}O_{2peak}$ of 19.7 mL/kg/min, RER$_{peak}$ 1.24, HR$_{peak}$ 170 bpm (117% predicted maximal heart rate), and peak WR of 95 W, all of which show an improvement after prehabilitation. An AT of 14.9 mL/kg/min and $\dot{V}E/\dot{V}CO_2$ of 30.0 at AT indicate that this patient is now in a low-risk perioperative category. The tachycardia seen at rest is still present but is improved compared to the previous test.

Optimization of modifiable risk factors after neoadjuvant therapy has increased the physiological capacity of this patient. While CPET provides objective evidence of accrued homeostatic reserve, high-dependency care should be planned postoperatively because of the procedural risk involved. Surgical options should only proceed once the patient is fully informed of the risks of having major surgery with curative intent while also being given the opportunity to express their life values and goals in the context of their disease and treatment options. This process of shared decision-making (SDM), discussing whether to proceed with major curative surgery, palliative surgery, or nonsurgical management, is complex. In this case, the CPET results before and after prehabilitation were instrumental in guiding the multidisciplinary discussion of risk versus benefit. The patient opted for operative intervention, which was successful, and they made a full recovery.

DISCUSSION

Clinician-based subjective assessment of patient functional status and surgical risk is notoriously poor at forecasting

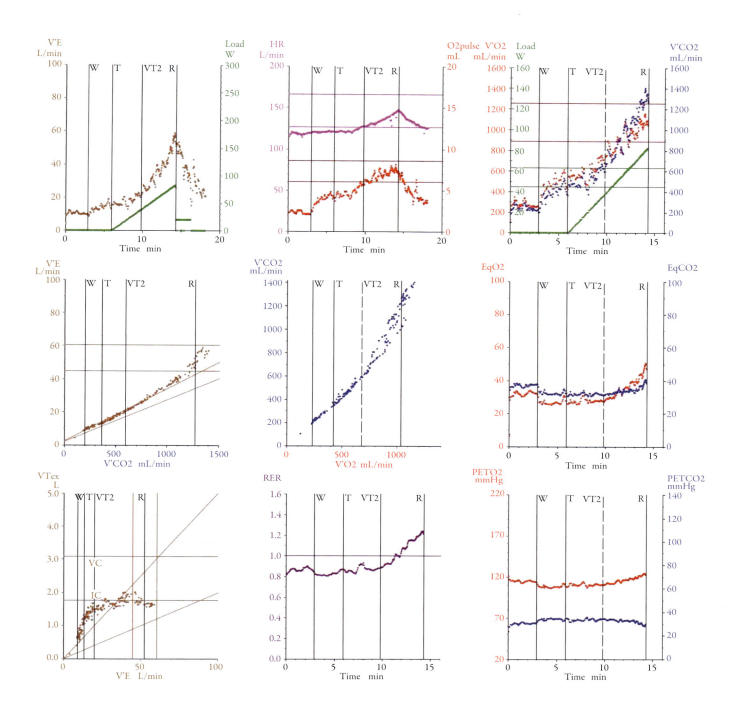

Figure 9.3b Case 3 (after neoadjuvant therapy) The 9-panel plot: Presented using the conventional UCLA method of displaying gas-exchange derived variables during CPET. The panels are numbered sequentially 1–9, from left to right, top row to bottom row.
W, unloaded cycling; T, loaded cycling; VT2, anaerobic threshold; R, recovery; $\dot{V}$E, minute ventilation; HR, heart rate; $\dot{V}O_2$, oxygen uptake; $\dot{V}CO_2$, carbon dioxide output; EqO$_2$, ventilatory equivalents for oxygen; EqCO$_2$, ventilatory equivalents for carbon dioxide; VTex, tidal volume expired; RER, respiratory exchange ratio; PETO$_2$, end tidal pressure of oxygen; PETCO$_2$, end tidal pressure of carbon dioxide.

postoperative morbidity and mortality.[10] Objective, evidence-based, and resourceful means of risk stratifying preoperative patients prior to major surgery are necessary to mitigate modifiable risks, plan prehabilitation, guide intra- and postoperative management, and inform SDM discussions for complex patients.[30] A recent multicenter, prospective, cohort study found CPET improved predictions of moderate or severe postoperative complications.[10] CPET, however, is resource-intensive, and, as such, we need to identify the cohort of patients for whom CPET will provide the greatest benefit. It is recommended that tools such as the Duke Activity Score Index (DASI), the American College of Surgeons National Quality Improvement Program (NSQIP) risk calculator, and biomarkers such as B-type natriuretic peptide (BNP) and

Table 9.3c CASE 3 CPET DATA AFTER PREHABILITATION, REFLECTING PARAMETERS AT BASELINE (REST) AND DURING EXERCISE AT ANAEROBIC THRESHOLD (AT) AND AT PEAK EXERCISE (PEAK)

DATA	REST	AT	PEAK	% PREDICTED MAXIMUM AT PEAK EXERCISE
$\dot{V}E/\dot{V}CO_2$	37.8	30.0	38.1	
$\dot{V}E$ [L/min]	8	30	75	
SpO_2 [%]	99	98	100	
HR [bpm]	108	155	170	117
HRR_1 [bpm]				Recovery 160
BP [mm Hg]	128/82	150/83	175/80	Recovery 158/95
$\dot{V}O_2$ [mL/kg/min]	4.2	14.9	19.7	117
O_2 pulse [mL/beat]	2.3	5.9	7.3	100
RER	0.88	0.99	1.24	
Load [W]	0	62	95	169
Blood results	Hb g/L 124	Albumin g/L 33	CRP mg/L 3.0	Transferrin saturation % 15

E, minute ventilation; CO_2, carbon dioxide output; SpO_2, peripheral oxygen saturation; HR, heart rate in beats per minute (bpm); HRR_1, heart rate at 1 minute recovery; BP, blood pressure; O_2, oxygen uptake; O_2 pulse, oxygen pulse; RER, respiratory exchange ratio; Hb, hemoglobin; CRP, C-reactive protein.

troponin are utilized for this purpose.[6,10,30] Research suggests that patients embarking upon neoadjuvant therapy and high-risk surgery, as in this case, should undergo CPET triaging irrespective of their underlying burden of comorbid disease because of the deconditioning of chemoradiotherapy treatment.[5,6] The association between CPET-derived indices of physical fitness and postoperative outcomes have been summarized in multiple systematic reviews.[6,8,9,31]

The association between oxygen utility and mortality has been clearly established with data from the US veteran population linking a 15% increase in all-cause mortality with each decrease of peak $\dot{V}O_2$ by 3.5 mL/kg/min[32] (i.e., one metabolic equivalent [MET]). Greater functional capacity measured as $\dot{V}O_2$ has been shown to be specifically associated with cancer survival[33] and better postoperative outcomes, measured in length of stay, quality of life, and reductions in complications.[34,35]

AT, peak $\dot{V}O_2$, and $\dot{V}E/\dot{V}CO_2$ have consistently shown prognostic value.[5,6,8,9,17,36,37] These CPET-derived variables have been studied over a wide range of major surgical procedures including abdominal aortic aneurysm surgery, hepatobiliary surgery, liver and cardiac transplant surgery, upper gastrointestinal surgery, colorectal surgery, urological surgery, and thoracic surgery.[1,6,7,11,14–17,36,38,39] Different surgical approaches, institutional variations, and patient cohorts may impact the external validity of CPET data.[6] As perioperative care pathways evolve, current research aims to identify individualized CPET thresholds for different types of procedures.[6] However, broadly speaking, patients at increased risk of postoperative morbidity and mortality are seen to have an AT of less than 10–11 mL/kg/min and peak $\dot{V}O_2$ of less than 15–16 mL/kg/min.[6,14–17,36–38]

The stress of major surgery and recovery can compromise the homeostatic reserve of our high-risk patients, leading to postoperative morbidity and mortality.[40] CPET data empower the perioperative physician at preoperative counseling to inform on strategies for prehabilitation, medical optimization, and SDM. The data also aid forward planning of intraoperative management and postoperative disposition or consideration of palliative care.[5,6,8,9,17] This consequently allows for better utilization of our healthcare resources, but, more importantly, better patient outcomes.[5,6,8,9,17]

As postoperative complications, including minor complications (Clavien-Dindo Grade I–II) are associated with a significant increase in hospital costs, reducing complications is a key target for cost containment strategies.[41] Conversely, low-risk patients identified via CPET can be safely cared for in the general surgical ward postoperatively at lower costs than in the HDU/ICU.[9] Both categories of patients should receive treatment within the framework of institutional ERAS pathways to reduce variability in perioperative management.

So that each patient can better withstand the homeostatic disturbance of surgery, evidence directs us toward a holistic approach to encourage physical and mental resilience in our patients.[42,43] Prehabilitation encompasses this multimodal ideology, with a focus on preoperative exercise training, nutritional supplementation, anemia optimization, medical optimization, smoking cessation, psychosocial well-being, and education. Preoperative risk predictors found to correlate with postoperative complications include anemia, low albumin, high neutrophil count, and low functional capacity.[44] Successful modification of these factors through multimodal prehabilitation is enhanced by patient education and participation in their perioperative care (see Figure 9.4).[42–45]

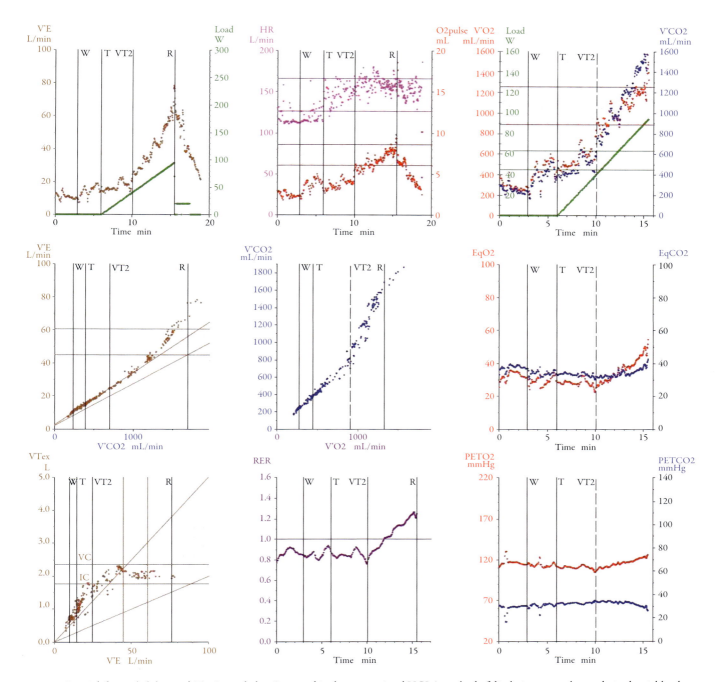

Figure 9.3c Case 3 (after prehabilitation) The 9-panel plot: Presented in the conventional UCLA method of displaying gas-exchange derived variables during CPET. The panels are numbered sequentially 1–9, from left to right, top row to bottom row.
W, unloaded cycling; T, loaded cycling; VT2, anaerobic threshold; R, recovery; $\dot{V}E$, minute ventilation; HR, heart rate; $\dot{V}O_2$, oxygen uptake; $\dot{V}CO_2$, carbon dioxide output; EqO_2, ventilatory equivalents for oxygen; $EqCO_2$, ventilatory equivalents for carbon dioxide; VTex, tidal volume expired; RER, respiratory exchange ratio; $PETO_2$, end tidal pressure of oxygen; $PETCO_2$, end tidal pressure of carbon dioxide.

As an example, "Surgery School" utilizes the multidisciplinary team to deliver patient education about each of these elements of prehabilitation in an interactive, classroom-based environment.[30,46] Comradery is built through empathy as the patients learn together about the expectations for their surgical journey.[30,46] In addition, patient-centered education improves compliance, as they feel a sense of ownership over their care and responsibility toward outcomes.[46] Encouraging a patient to attend Surgery School with a relative or friend also brings motivation into prehabilitation within the framework of an external person providing support, encouragement, and accountability for prehabilitation. The process of prehabilitation can be either initiated or otherwise facilitated at a patient's CPET appointment, as this is an opportunity to target all these modifiable risk factors.

CPET helps tailor an individualized, responsive exercise prescription to the patient's baseline functional capacity, aiming to increase physiological reserve before surgery and reduce

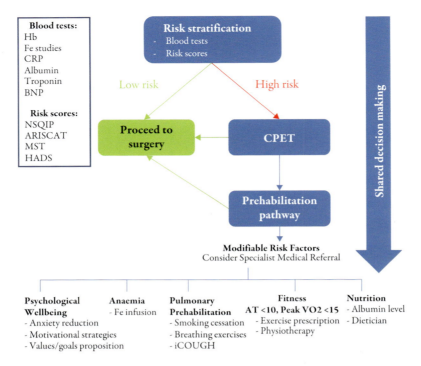

Figure 9.4 Prehabilitation.
Hb, hemoglobin; CRP, C-reactive protein; BNP, B-type natriuretic peptide; NSQIP, National Surgical Quality Improvement Program risk calculator; ARISCAT, Assess Respiratory Risk in Surgical Patients in Catalonia study—score for postoperative pulmonary complications; MST, malnutrition screening tool; HADS, Hospital Anxiety and Depression Scale; Fe, iron; iCOUGH, *i*ncentive spirometry; *c*oughing and deep breathing; *o*ral care; *u*nderstanding; *g*etting out of bed; *h*ead of bed elevation.

perioperative risk. Exercise training has been proved to be beneficial among many patient populations including those with COPD, stroke, heart failure, and claudication.[8,9,39] Exercise training is safe, feasible, and improves health-related quality of life.[26,39] While more robust research is required to demonstrate a clear link between exercise training and clinically relevant postoperative outcomes,[42] CPET provides an objective method to interrogate the efficacy of exercise training and the whole package of prehabilitation.[8]

In this case study, the patient received neoadjuvant chemoradiotherapy, and CPET highlights the decremental impact of such treatment on functional status. A blinded interventional pilot study demonstrated a significant reduction in AT and $\dot{V}O_{2peak}$ in consecutive rectal cancer patients after neoadjuvant chemoradiotherapy.[26] Those patients who underwent a 6-week structured exercise training program showed a return of AT and $\dot{V}O_{2peak}$ back to baseline, while the control group continued to demonstrate a decline in functional capacity from baseline.[26] Similar treatment-related deconditioning has been observed in patients with gastroesophageal cancer receiving neoadjuvant chemotherapy.[27–29] A number of clinical trials will further examine the effect of exercise programs implemented during neoadjuvant therapy and their impact on fitness, symptoms, recovery, and surgical and cancer outcomes,[47–49] while others have found multimodal prehabilitation to demonstrably reduce postoperative complications, length of stay, recovery, and quality of life.[34,35] As perioperative clinicians, we should strive to better quantify and qualify our prehabilitation programs[9] to best serve high-risk patients, particularly at the 6–12 week window of opportunity between neoadjuvant treatment and surgery.[8,9]

Multimodal prehabilitation centered around CPET allows practitioners to deliver on the value-based proposition of healthcare (value = outcomes / cost) through optimization of modifiable risk factors (e.g., anemia, nutrition, physical activity, smoking, alcohol, mental well-being) by targeting health promotion and patient education.[50] A recent review suggested that two out of three patients are malnourished prior to gastrointestinal surgery with an associated three-fold increased morbidity and five-fold increased mortality.[51] Despite this, only 1 in 5 hospitals surveyed in the United States provided nutritional screening, and only 1 in 5 patients received nutritional optimization preoperatively.[51] Health economic data indicate that for every $1 invested in nutritional optimization, there are an estimated $52 in hospital savings.[51] Early identification and treatment of preoperative anemia with the adoption of a system-wide patient blood management program resulted in reduced blood transfusions, reduced hospital length of stay, reduced patient mortality, and considerable healthcare savings in Australia.[52] Physiotherapist-led preoperative breathing exercise training for patients receiving upper abdominal surgery has shown to decrease postoperative pulmonary complications rates by half.[25] Similarly, small randomized controlled trials utilizing multimodal prehabilitation have demonstrated a reduction in postoperative complications by 50%.[53]

Prehabilitation is an evolving a risk-adapted approach to perioperative medicine[54] balanced against our finite health resources, and perioperative physicians are at the cornerstone of opportunity for ensuring improved patient outcomes after surgery and reduced healthcare costs through CPET.

STEM CASE 4 AND KEY QUESTIONS

A 31-year-old patient is booked for laparotomy and resection of a retroperitoneal sarcoma. An acute-onset cardiomyopathy secondary to neoadjuvant anthracycline chemotherapy was diagnosed prior to presenting for CPET. The patient is managed medically with an ACE inhibitor, diuretics including spironolactone, ivabradine, digoxin, and amiodarone. The most recent transthoracic echocardiogram reports an ejection fraction of 20% and grade 4 global systolic dysfunction. The CPET referral form asks you to risk-stratify this patient and triage their postoperative disposition. You begin exercise on a 10 watt/min ramp protocol. The test is stopped after 8.1 minutes of cycling on an upright cycle ergometer when the patient complains of feeling lightheaded. The test results are provided in Table 9.4 and Figure 9.5. The patient has a BMI of 28 kg/m² and BSA 1.8 m².

Is this a maximal exercise test? List the findings to back your conclusion.

This is a submaximal test.

- AT is not achieved; see panels 5, 6, and 9 using the three criteria for AT determination.
- RER is less than 1.0 at peak; see panel 8.
- Low peak $\dot{V}O_2$ of 7.0 mL/kg/min (30% of predicted); see panel 3.

A low maximal HR of 90 (45% of predicted) is observed (see panel 2). Ivabradine selectively inhibits the sinoatrial node and may be responsible for the patient's poor chronotropic response to exercise.

Identify the CPET data that support a cardiac etiology to explain this patient's exercise limitation.

- Symptom-limited test secondary to lightheadedness.
- Exercise-induced decrease in systolic blood pressure.
- AT not achieved; see panels 5, 6, and 9 using the three criteria for AT determination.
- Low oxygen pulse at peak exercise; see panel 2.
- $\dot{V}O_2$/WR less than 10 mL/W; see panel 3.
- Oscillatory breathing during exercise suggestive of heart failure; see panels 1, 3, 6, and 9.

Table 9.4 CASE 4 CPET DATA, REFLECTING PARAMETERS AT BASELINE (REST) AND DURING EXERCISE AT ANAEROBIC THRESHOLD (AT) AND AT PEAK EXERCISE (PEAK)

DATA	REST	AT	PEAK	% PREDICTED MAXIMUM AT PEAK EXERCISE
FEV₁ [L]	3.0			58.5
MVV [L/min]	110			90
Breathing reserve [%]	82			
DLCO [mL/min/mm Hg]	15			62
$\dot{V}E/\dot{V}CO_2$	39.8	35.7	37.5	
$\dot{V}E$ [L/min]	8	13	20	
SpO₂ [%]	100	96	98	
HR [bpm]	76	85	89	47
HRR₁ [bpm]				Recovery 85
BP	95/50	70/45	70/48	Recovery 90/60
$\dot{V}O_2$ [mL/kg/min]	2.8	6.1	7.0	27
O₂ pulse [mL/beat]	2.7	5.3	5.9	58
RER	0.89	0.78	0.88	
Load [W]	0	3	34	26
Blood results	Hb g/L 95	Albumin g/L 35	CRP mg/L 45	Transferrin saturation % 21

FEV₁, forced expiratory volume in the first second of forced expiration; MVV, maximum voluntary ventilation; DLCO, lung diffusing capacity for carbon monoxide; E, minute ventilation; CO₂, carbon dioxide output; SpO₂, peripheral oxygen saturation; HR, heart rate in beats per minute (bpm); HRR₁, heart rate at 1 minute recovery; BP, blood pressure; O₂, oxygen uptake; O₂ pulse, oxygen pulse; RER, respiratory exchange ratio; Hb, hemoglobin; CRP, C-reactive protein.

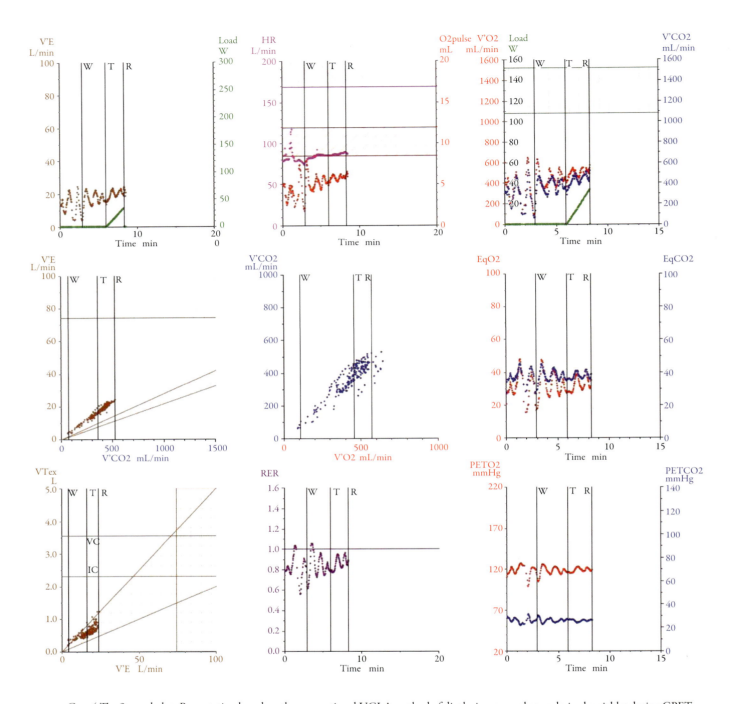

Figure 9.5 Case 4 The 9-panel plot: Presentation based on the conventional UCLA method of displaying gas-exchange derived variables during CPET. The panels are numbered sequentially 1–9, from left to right, top row to bottom row.
W, unloaded cycling; T, loaded cycling; VT2, anaerobic threshold; R, recovery; $\dot{V}E$, minute ventilation; HR, heart rate; $\dot{V}O_2$, oxygen uptake; $\dot{V}CO_2$, carbon dioxide output; EqO_2, ventilatory equivalents for oxygen; $EqCO_2$, ventilatory equivalents for carbon dioxide; VTex, tidal volume expired; RER, respiratory exchange ratio; $PETO_2$, end tidal pressure of oxygen; $PETCO_2$, end tidal pressure of carbon dioxide.

- Poor heart rate recovery at 1 minute after cessation of exercise (<12 bpm difference in HR from peak exercise to 1 minute recovery; 89 − 85 = 4 bpm); see panel 2.
- Normal breathing reserve (MVV − $\dot{V}E_{peak}$/ MVV >15%; 110 − 20/110 = 82%); see panels 4 and 7.

What is your interpretation of the patient's blood pressure response to exercise and during recovery?

In health, systolic blood pressure increases with workload and diastolic blood pressure remains unchanged or may slightly decrease.[3] A reduction in systolic blood pressure should raise concern of significant cardiac pathology including myocardial ischemia, ventricular dysfunction, or ventricular outflow tract obstruction.[1,3] Hypotension during exercise may also be caused by medications (e.g., diuretics, ACE inhibitors), autonomic dysregulation (e.g., diabetes), or hypovolemia.[3] This patient has a low blood pressure prior to CPET in the context of heart failure. The symptomatic reduction in blood pressure with exercise is demonstrative of heart failure severity and is compounded by medical therapy. This is an absolute indication to stop the test and continue monitoring during the recovery phase until baseline status has returned.[3] The blood pressure returned to the pre-test level with recovery in this patient.

What is your interpretation of the patient's heart rate response during the exercise and recovery phase of CPET?

Heart rate normally increases in proportion to WR during incremental exercise. This is a result of increased sympathetic and decreased parasympathetic nervous system activity.[55] The rate of change in heart rate, or chronotropic response, can be affected by a number of factors such as age, fitness, type of exercise, body posture, medications (e.g., beta blockers), and heart transplantation.[56] In this case, selective inhibition of the sinoatrial node with ivabradine may have contributed to the chronotropic incompetence that was observed (<80–85% predicted maximum heart rate for age at peak exercise).[57] The heart rate at 1 minute into the recovery phase (85 bpm) is within 12 bpm of the heart rate value at peak (89 bpm), and this suggests a lack of parasympathetic reactivation normally observed in healthy individuals.[1,55]

DISCUSSION

Heart failure is the predominant pathology responsible for this patient's exercise limitation, although an element of global deconditioning is also likely to be contributing to the overall functional impairment. Cardiac output cannot be increased sufficiently to meet the metabolic demands of exercising skeletal muscle and end-organ perfusion is compromised, leading to presyncope and test termination. This occurs before sufficient anaerobic metabolism takes place such that AT is not achieved.

CPET provides important prognostic information for patients with heart failure.[1,2] It is used to prescribe exercise for cardiac rehabilitation,[1] assess the efficacy of heart failure treatment,[1,2] and guide patient selection for advanced heart failure therapies such as placement of ventricular assist devices and heart transplantation.[1,2,12,58] Peak oxygen consumption is predictive of death in patients with heart failure regardless of beta blocker status or whether patients have reduced or preserved ejection fraction.[59] Weber Classes A, B, C, and D corresponding to peak $\dot{V}O_2$ >20, 16–20, 10–15.9, and less than 10 mL/kg/min, respectively, are used for risk stratification in patients with cardiac failure and also for presurgical assessment.[2,11] This patient's exercise test was used to assess heart failure severity and monitor for reversibility of cardiac toxicity caused by anthracycline chemotherapy before surgery.

Valuable information about functional status, disease severity, and prognosis can be gained even from this submaximal CPET.[12] As discussed earlier, the oxygen pulse ($\dot{V}O_2$/HR ratio) provides dynamic information about cardiac function[12] and corresponds to stroke volume changes during exercise.[1,2,60] In this example, a low oxygen pulse suggests an inability of the heart to augment stroke volume in response to increasing workload.[1,2] Thus, a flat oxygen pulse may be an early warning of evolving myocardial ischemia[1,2,12] and, in some patients, will be corroborated by ECG changes during exercise.

The ventilatory efficiency ($\dot{V}E/\dot{V}CO_2$ relationship) can also provide useful data in the submaximal exercise test. In fact, $\dot{V}E/\dot{V}CO_2$ is superior to peak $\dot{V}O_2$ at predicting outcomes and prognosis in heart failure[1,2] with a value of greater than 34 pertaining to high risk.[1] As the $\dot{V}E/\dot{V}CO_2$ slope deviates further from normal, the risk of cardiac-related adverse events proportionately increases, as demonstrated in the Ventilatory Classification System (Class I <30, Class II 30–35.9, Class III 36–44.9, Class IV ≥45).[1,2,61]

The exercise-associated pattern of oscillatory breathing seen in this case is pathognomonic of heart failure and independently conveys a poor prognosis, irrespective of reduced or preserved ejection fraction.[2,62] This breathing pattern is characterized by a cyclical pattern of hyperpnea and hypopnea, with an amplitude of 15% or more of the average resting value for 60% or more of exercise.[1,2] Oscillatory breathing has been shown to strengthen the predictive value of $\dot{V}E/\dot{V}CO_2$ and peak $\dot{V}O_2$ for morbidity and mortality.[63]

Chronotropic incompetence is quoted in the literature as an attenuated heart rate response to exercise and is referenced as less than 80–85% of the age-predicted maximum.[1,55–57] It has been associated with increased mortality in patients presenting for surgery with coronary artery disease.[1,55–57] However, medications (e.g., beta blockers) may confound its interpretation.[1,55–57] Heart rate recovery, a manifestation of returning parasympathetic nervous system tone,[55] is defined as the difference between the HR at peak exercise and the HR recovery at 1 minute (HRR$_1$) after peak exercise, and it is normally greater than 12 bpm.[2] It is a powerful, independent predictor of all-cause mortality when adjusted for age; gender; exercise capacity; the presence or absence of comorbidities such as hypertension, IHD, or chronic lung disease; and the use of beta blockers.[1,55] Subject effort does not impact HRR$_1$ and, as such, it remains valuable even in submaximal tests as illustrated in this case discussion.[55] HRR$_1$ adds value to $\dot{V}E/\dot{V}CO_2$ in predicting risk of death or hospitalization in patients with heart failure.[64] The analysis of HR during CPET may have even broader applications. In one study, CPET was found to be superior to stress ECG for identifying inadequately treated coronary heart disease by investigation of the change in HR to WR relationship (e.g., ΔHR-WR slope).[65]

In this case study, the process of SDM resulted in a patient-led decision for a nonsurgical approach, and further cardiac prehabilitation was pursued. Myocardial function somewhat recovered to an EF of 35% and grade 3 global systolic dysfunction. Over time, the patient reported feeling better, with improved exercise tolerance. Although routine transthoracic echocardiogram is not recommended for preoperative risk assessment in the absence of specific cardiac lesions (e.g., obstructive heart abnormality, severe pulmonary hypertension, undiagnosed cardiomyopathy),[66] echocardiographic findings may influence anesthetic technique and intraoperative management. For this patient, demonstrating reversibility of the cardiomyopathy broadened the spectrum of chemotherapeutic agents available for cancer treatment. It was the full integration of cardiovascular, respiratory, hematologic, and metabolic assessment offered by CPET, however, that helped this patient and their treating team make an informed decision about the risk-benefit profile related to surgical intervention.

CONCLUSION

- CPET is traditionally performed as a diagnostic test, however, its utility is far more extensive. It offers a means to identify and optimize modifiable risk factors, educate and motivate our patients, and guide exercise prescriptions and assess the results of prehabilitation. Used within a multidisciplinary context and in SDM, CPET can help the patient to understand their choices framed in the context of their health, disease status, and quality of life. In this role, CPET aligns with the evidence base for major surgery and is essential in the armamentarium of the perioperative medicine clinician.[8,9,16]

- CPET is an objective clinical test which interrogates functional capacity to assess perioperative risk.

- The results of CPET can help elucidate the underlying etiology of functional decline, including deconditioning and cardiac and respiratory pathology, thus representing an opportunity to optimize modifiable risk factors.

- A growing body of evidence supports the role of CPET in preoperative risk stratification to guide prehabilitation strategies, multidisciplinary management, postoperative care planning, patient-centered education, and SDM.

REVIEW QUESTIONS

1. Which feature of the 9-panel plot is used to determine AT?

    a. The $\dot{V}O_2$ value when RER greater than 1.1.
    b. The $\dot{V}O_2$ value when HR is greater than 85% of age-predicted maximum.
    c. The modified V-slope method, which detects the inflection point of CO_2 from a tangent of $\Delta \dot{V}CO_2 / \Delta \dot{V}O_2 = 1.0$.
    d. Identification of hyperventilation relative to CO_2 production.

The correct answer is c.

AT is defined as the oxygen uptake value at which aerobic metabolism is supplemented by anaerobic glycolysis.[1,3,5] The measurable metabolic changes occurring after AT are a systematic increase in CO_2 production, an increase in the respiratory exchange ratio (RER; or ratio of $\dot{V}CO_2/\dot{V}O_2$), a rise in blood lactate levels with a fall in blood bicarbonate levels, and a decrease in blood pH.[1,3,5] RER does not define the detection of AT; however, an AT greater than 1.0 indicates AT has already been reached.[1] The criterion used to identify AT are:

Criterion 1: Identify excess $\dot{V}CO_2$ relative to $\dot{V}O_2$ (i.e., use the V-slope or modified V-slope method). The inflection observed in the $\dot{V}CO_2 - \dot{V}O_2$ relationship here is secondary to the buffering of anaerobic lactate after AT with consequent generation of more CO_2 (i.e., $H^+ + HCO_3^- \leftrightarrow H_2CO_3 \leftrightarrow H_2O + CO_2$).

Criterion 2: Identify hyperventilation with respect to O_2 uptake (i.e., locate the nadir of the ventilatory equivalents for oxygen ($\dot{V}E/\dot{V}O_2$) slope and a rise in the end tidal oxygen ($P_{ET}O_2$) slope. At this point, $\dot{V}E$ increases and is driven by the excess CO_2 of anaerobic glycolysis without a corresponding increase in $\dot{V}O_2$.

Criterion 3: Exclude hyperventilation with respect to CO_2 production (i.e., confirm a plateau or decrease in the ventilatory equivalents for carbon dioxide ($\dot{V}E/\dot{V}CO_2$) occurring at the point determined by criteria 1 and 2 above.

2. AT is seen as an inflection on the V-slope where the production of CO_2 increases in relation to O_2 uptake. What other CPET variables assist in the determination of AT?

    a. $\dot{V}E/\dot{V}CO_2$ remains constant or continues to decrease while $\dot{V}E/\dot{V}O_2$ rises.
    b. There is a fall in $P_{ET}O_2$.
    c. There is enhanced isocapnic buffering.
    d. There is a fall in $P_{ET}CO_2$.

The correct answer is a.

AT is the point at which anaerobic glycolysis is required to sustain adenosine triphosphate (ATP) production.[1,3,5] The consequent metabolic acidosis leads to an increase in P_aCO_2 matched with a proportional increase in $\dot{V}E$.[1,3,5] Therefore, at AT, the $\dot{V}E/\dot{V}CO_2$ relationship remains constant or decreases as $\dot{V}E/\dot{V}O_2$ starts to rise.[5] The phase during CPET when $P_{ET}O_2$ begins to rise and $P_{ET}CO_2$ remains stable is termed *isocapnic buffering*.[3] A fall in $P_{ET}CO_2$ at AT would indicate there was nonspecific hyperventilation. The absence of a fall in $P_{ET}CO_2$ at AT excludes hyperventilation because the increase in $\dot{V}E$ is proportional to $\dot{V}CO_2$.[5]

3. Select the statement(s) which are true:

    a. Cardiac output normally increases linearly with respect to $\dot{V}O_2$.
    b. $\dot{V}O_2$ and WR should increase linearly.
    c. $\dot{V}O_{2peak}$ is independent of volition.
    d. $\dot{V}O_{2peak}$ is reproducible and is largely independent of ramp gradient.

The correct answers are a, b, d.

In the setting of a steadily increasing WR, oxygen consumption increases at a constant rate of approximately 10 mL/W and is independent of age, gender, BSA, or training.[3]

$\dot{V}O_{2peak}$ is reported as an absolute value in mL/min or L/min indexed to bodyweight (mL/kg/min or L/kg/min) or body surface area (mL/m²/min) and can be affected by the subject's sex, volition, or willingness to engage; too steep a ramp gradient and the patient may elect to "give up" when they may have been encouraged to continue on a lesser gradient to a higher $\dot{V}O_{2peak}$.

4. Are the following statements true or false: $\dot{V}O_{2max}$
   a. Is the highest oxygen uptake value measured during an incremental exercise test and can be determined in most patients.
   b. Is a physiological end point where oxygen uptake cannot be increased further despite an increase in work and is often seen in highly trained athletes.
   c. Is represented by $\dot{V}O_{2max} = (HR \times SV) \times [C(a\text{-}v)O_2]$.
   d. Is rarely seen in the typical patient presenting to CPET.

The correct answers are a, false; b, true; c, true; and d, true.
$\dot{V}O_{2max} = (HR \times SV) \times [C(a\text{-}v)O_2]$ is representative of the maximal limit of an individual's functional capacity and is independent of volition and effort and is rarely measured in nonathletes. $\dot{V}O_{2max}$ is an end point where oxygen uptake cannot be increased further despite increasing workload[5]; thus it is the sum total of their cardiorespiratory, vascular, hematological, musculoskeletal, and metabolic systems working at their physiological maximum.[1,3,5]

5. Are the following statements true or false? $\dot{V}O_{2peak}$
   a. Is the highest $\dot{V}O_2$ recorded during the test.
   b. Provides an accurate representation of a patient's exercise limitation as shown by a plateauing of the O_2-WR relationship.
   c. Can be used to calculate metabolic equivalents of task (MET).
   d. Has be shown to be directly correlated with mortality in the general population.

The correct answers are a, false; b, true; c, true; and d, true.
$\dot{V}O_{2peak}$ is the highest averaged over 20 seconds (or 3–5 breaths) during the final period of incremental work. $\dot{V}O_{2peak}$ may be altered by a patient's volition or with encouragement.[5] However, this does not mean it is not a useful CPET measurement.
$\dot{V}O_{2peak}$ increasing is used as risk indicator for mortality risk postoperatively; it is referenced to the patient's age-predicted maximum or BSA and is increasingly being used to describe exercise limitation.[6]
One MET equals 3.5 mLO_2/kg/min. An increase in $\dot{V}O_{2peak}$ of just one MET has been shown to decrease mortality by 15%.[67,68]

6. Premature termination of CPET testing is advised
   a. In the setting of dyspnea and chronic atrial fibrillation.
   b. In the setting of multiple premature ventricular complexes.
   c. In the setting of ST depression of 3 mm and the patient is asymptomatic.
   d. None of the above.

The correct answer is d.
According to guidelines the ECG criteria for premature CPET termination are greater than 2 mm ST depression if the patient is symptomatic, or 4 mm ST depression if the patient is asymptomatic, or greater than 1 mm ST elevation.[3,5] Dyspnea alone is not a reason to limit a test unless saturations fall markedly.[3] AF is not a reason to limit a test unless a lack of rate control leads to a fall in blood pressure.[5] Atrial and ventricular ectopic beats are not uncommon.

7. Select which of the following statements are true.
   a. RER is a ratio of $\dot{V}CO_2$ to $\dot{V}O_2$ measured at the mouthpiece.
   b. RER is affected by diet.
   c. A peak RER of greater than 1.1 is reassurance the patient worked hard during CPET.
   d. RER of less than 0.6 is physiologically implausible.

The correct answers are a, b, c, and d.
The respiratory exchange ratio (RER) is the ratio of $\dot{V}CO_2$ to $\dot{V}O_2$ measured from expired gases at the mouthpiece during exercise.[1,3] This differs from the respiratory quotient (RQ), which is the ratio of CO_2 produced to O_2 consumed at the cellular level.[3] During steady-state conditions, RER approximates to RQ and therefore RER may be used to determine whether carbohydrate or fat is the predominant fuel source for the production of CO_2.[3] At rest, with a balanced diet, this ratio is normally about 0.8.[3] This increases with exercise as $P_{ET}CO_2$ increases in response to aerobic and anaerobic respiration and $P_{ET}O_2$ decreases with greater O_2 uptake by working muscles.[3] To standardize CPET results, patients are asked to fast for 2 hours before CPET.[3] A peak RER of greater than 1.1 is widely accepted as an indication of satisfactory patient effort.[1,2]

8. Select which of the following statements are true.
   a. The $\dot{V}E/\dot{V}CO_2$ relationship provides information on dead space and V/Q matching.
   b. Normal $\dot{V}E/\dot{V}CO_2$ is described as greater than 35 at AT.
   c. Elevated $\dot{V}E/\dot{V}CO_2$ is commonly seen in patients with COPD, interstitial lung disease, heart failure, and pulmonary hypertension.
   d. Patients with cardiac failure do not generally exhibit oxygen desaturation.

The correct answers are a, c, and d.
Normal $\dot{V}E/\dot{V}CO_2$ is less than 32–34 at AT and often less than 30 in healthy young individuals.[2,3] A high $\dot{V}E/\dot{V}CO_2$ ratio suggests either a low arterial P_aCO_2 (seen in acute hyperventilation or in states of increased ventilatory drive) or increased physiologic dead space.[3,5,8,9] An elevated $\dot{V}E/\dot{V}CO_2$ is commonly seen in patients with COPD, interstitial lung disease, heart failure, and pulmonary hypertension.[1,2,5,8,9] Unlike patients with lung disease, desaturation is less common in isolated cardiac disease.[2]

9. Which of the following statements are correct with respect to the maximal voluntary ventilation (MVV)?
   a. MVV may be estimated as: $FEV_1 \times 40$.

b. It is the volume of gas inhaled and exhaled per minute.
c. It is the maximal minute ventilation possible.
d. It guides measurement of peak performance of lung and respiratory muscles.

The correct answers are a, c, and d.

MVV is maximal voluntary ventilation and it is the theoretical ventilatory limit of the respiratory system.[3] It is estimated indirectly by multiplying $FEV_1 \times 35$ or 40, or it can be measured directly with spirometry.[3]

10. The following statements about breathing reserve are true:

    a. Breathing reserve is $MVV - \dot{V}E_{peak}$
    b. Normal breathing reserve is normally greater than 15% of the MVV.
    c. $\dot{V}E_{peak}$ may approach MVV in fit individuals and in the elderly in the absence of disease.
    d. Breathing reserve shows an age-related decline related to an increase in dead space.

The correct answers are b and c.

Normal breathing reserve = $MVV - \dot{V}E_{peak}/ MVV$. In healthy subjects, ventilatory demand does not encroach upon ventilatory capacity during exercise, and, as such, respiratory reserve is greater than 15%.[3]

Breathing reserve will be affected by pulmonary pathology, hence it shows a strong correlation; however, it is important to note that breathing reserve demonstrates significant variability among the normal population and that $\dot{V}E_{peak}$ may approach MVV in fit individuals and in the elderly in the absence of disease.[3] Breathing reserve is related to the volume of expired air and not dead space.[3]

REFERENCES

1. Balady GJ, Arena R, Sietsema K, et al. Clinician's guide to cardiopulmonary exercise testing in adults: A scientific statement from the American Heart Association. *Circulation.* 2010;122(2):191–225. doi:10.1161/CIR.0b013e3181e52e69
2. Guazzi M, Adams V, Conraads V, et al. EACPR/AHA Scientific Statement: Clinical recommendations for cardiopulmonary exercise testing data assessment in specific patient populations. *Circulation.* 2012;126(18):2261–2274. doi:10.1161/CIR.0b013e31826fb946
3. ATS/ACCP Statement on cardiopulmonary exercise testing. *Am J Respir Crit Care Med.* 2003;167(2):211–277. doi:10.1164/rccm.167.2.211
4. Lumb A. *Nunn's Applied Respiratory Physiology.* 8th ed. Elsevier; 2016.
5. Levett DZH, Jack S, Swart M, et al. Perioperative cardiopulmonary exercise testing (CPET): Consensus clinical guidelines on indications, organization, conduct, and physiological interpretation. *Br J Anaesth.* 2018;120(3):484–500. doi:10.1016/j.bja.2017.10.020
6. Older PO, Levett DZH. Cardiopulmonary exercise testing and surgery. *Ann Am Thoracic Soc.* 2017;14(Supplement_1):S74–s83. doi:10.1513/AnnalsATS.201610-780FR
7. Nagamatsu Y, Shima I, Yamana H, Fujita H, Shirouzu K, Ishitake T. Preoperative evaluation of cardiopulmonary reserve with the use of expired gas analysis during exercise testing in patients with squamous cell carcinoma of the thoracic esophagus. *J Thoracic Cardiovasc Surg.* 2001;121(6):1064–1068. doi:10.1067/mtc.2001.113596
8. Levett DZ, Grocott MP. Cardiopulmonary exercise testing, prehabilitation, and Enhanced Recovery After Surgery (ERAS). *Can J Anaesth/J canadien d'anesthesie.* 2015;62(2):131–142. doi:10.1007/s12630-014-0307-6
9. Levett DZ, Grocott MP. Cardiopulmonary exercise testing for risk prediction in major abdominal surgery. *Anesthesiol Clin.* 2015;33(1):1–16. doi:10.1016/j.anclin.2014.11.001
10. Wijeysundera DN, Pearse RM, Shulman MA, et al. Assessment of functional capacity before major non-cardiac surgery: An international, prospective cohort study. *Lancet.* 2018;391(10140):2631–2640. doi:10.1016/s0140-6736(18)31131-0
11. Guazzi M, Arena R, Halle M, Piepoli MF, Myers J, Lavie CJ. 2016 Focused update: Clinical recommendations for cardiopulmonary exercise testing data assessment in specific patient populations. *Circulation.* 2016;133(24):e694–711. doi:10.1161/cir.0000000000000406
12. Malhotra R, Bakken K, D'Elia E, Lewis GD. Cardiopulmonary Exercise Testing in Heart Failure. *JACC. Heart failure* 2016;4(8):607–616 doi:10.1016/j.jchf.2016.03.022
13. Ganju AA, Fuladi AB, Tayade BO, Ganju NA. Cardiopulmonary exercise testing in evaluation of patients of chronic obstructive pulmonary disease. *Indian j chest dis allied sci.* 2011;53(2):87–91.
14. Kasivisvanathan R, Abbassi-Ghadi N, McLeod AD, et al. Cardiopulmonary exercise testing for predicting postoperative morbidity in patients undergoing hepatic resection surgery. *HPB.* 2015;17(7):637–643. doi:10.1111/hpb.12420
15. Moran J, Wilson F, Guinan E, McCormick P, Hussey J, Moriarty J. Role of cardiopulmonary exercise testing as a risk-assessment method in patients undergoing intra-abdominal surgery: A systematic review. *Br J Anaesth.* 2016;116(2):177–191. doi:10.1093/bja/aev454
16. Tolchard S, Angell J, Pyke M, et al. Cardiopulmonary reserve as determined by cardiopulmonary exercise testing correlates with length of stay and predicts complications after radical cystectomy. *BJU Int.* 2015;115(4):554–561. doi:10.1111/bju.12895
17. Wilson RJ, Davies S, Yates D, Redman J, Stone M. Impaired functional capacity is associated with all-cause mortality after major elective intra-abdominal surgery. *Br J Anaesth.* 2010;105(3):297–303. doi:10.1093/bja/aeq128
18. Nici L, Donner C, Wouters E, et al. American Thoracic Society/European Respiratory Society statement on pulmonary rehabilitation. *Am J Respir Crit Care Med.* 2006;173(12):1390–1413. doi:10.1164/rccm.200508-1211ST
19. Ries AL, Bauldoff GS, Carlin BW, et al. Pulmonary rehabilitation: Joint ACCP/AACVPR evidence-based clinical practice guidelines. *Chest.* 2007;131(5 Suppl):4s–42s. doi:10.1378/chest.06-2418
20. Wren SM, Martin M, Yoon JK, Bech F. Postoperative pneumonia-prevention program for the inpatient surgical ward. *J Am Coll Surg.* 2010;210(4):491–495. doi:10.1016/j.jamcollsurg.2010.01.009
21. Cassidy MR, Rosenkranz P, McCabe K, Rosen JE, McAneny D. I COUGH: Reducing postoperative pulmonary complications with a multidisciplinary patient care program. *JAMA Sur.* 2013;148(8):740–745. doi:10.1001/jamasurg.2013.358
22. Boston University School of Medicine –Surgery. I COUGH. Secondary I COUGH. n.d. https://www.bumc.bu.edu/surgery/quality-safety/i-cough/
23. Central Manchester University Hospitals – NHS Foundation Trust. I COUGH UK. *Secondary I COUGH UK.* 2018. http://www.cmft.nhs.uk/information-for-patients-visitors-and-carers/enhanced-recovery-programme/icoughuk
24. Saito H, Hatakeyama K, Konno H, Matsunaga T, Shimada Y, Minamiya Y. Impact of pulmonary rehabilitation on postoperative complications in patients with lung cancer and chronic obstructive pulmonary disease. *Thoracic Cancer.* 2017;8(5):451–460. doi:10.1111/1759-7714.12466
25. Boden I, Skinner EH, Browning L, Reeve J, Anderson L, Hill C, Robertson IK, Story D, Denehy L. Preoperative physiotherapy for the prevention of respiratory complications after upper abdominal surgery: Pragmatic, double blinded, multicentre randomised controlled trial. *BMJ.* 2018;360:j5916. *AORN J* 2018;108(4):461–467. doi:10.1002/aorn.12369

26. West MA, Loughney L, Lythgoe D, et al. Effect of prehabilitation on objectively measured physical fitness after neoadjuvant treatment in preoperative rectal cancer patients: A blinded interventional pilot study. *Br J Anaesth.* 2015;114(2):244–251. doi:10.1093/bja/aeu318
27. Jack S, West MA, Raw D, et al. The effect of neoadjuvant chemotherapy on physical fitness and survival in patients undergoing oesophagogastric cancer surgery. *Eur J Surg Oncol.* 2014;40(10):1313–1320. doi:10.1016/j.ejso.2014.03.010
28. Navidi M, Phillips AW, Griffin SM, et al. Cardiopulmonary fitness before and after neoadjuvant chemotherapy in patients with oesophagogastric cancer. *Br J Surg.* 2018;105(7):900–906. doi:10.1002/bjs.10802
29. Sinclair R, Navidi M, Griffin SM, Sumpter K. The impact of neoadjuvant chemotherapy on cardiopulmonary physical fitness in gastro-oesophageal adenocarcinoma. *Ann R Coll Surg Engl.* 2016;98(6):396–400. doi:10.1308/rcsann.2016.0135
30. Grocott MPW, Plumb JOM, Edwards M, Fecher-Jones I, Levett DZH. Re-designing the pathway to surgery: Better care and added value. *Periop Med (London, England).* 2017;6:9. doi:10.1186/s13741-017-0065-4
31. Lee CHA, Kong JC, Ismail H, Riedel B, Heriot A. Systematic review and meta-analysis of objective assessment of physical fitness in patients undergoing colorectal cancer surgery. *Dis Colon Rectum.* 2018;61(3):400–409. doi:10.1097/dcr.0000000000001017
32. Kokkinos P, Myers J, Kokkinos JP, et al. Exercise capacity and mortality in black and white men *Circulation.* 2008 Feb 5;117(5):614–622. doi:10.1161/CIRCULATIONAHA.107.734764
33. Imboden MT, Harber MP, Whaley MH, Finch WH, Bishop DL, Kaminsky LA. Cardiorespiratory fitness and mortality in healthy men and women. *J Am Coll Cardiol.* 2018 Nov 6;72(19):2283–2292. PMID: 30384883. doi:10.1016/j.jacc.2018.08.2166
34. Steffens D, Ismail H, Denehy L, et al. Preoperative cardiopulmonary exercise test associated with postoperative outcomes in patients undergoing cancer surgery: A systematic review and meta-analyses. *Ann Surg Oncol.* 2021 Nov;28(12):7120–7146. doi:10.1245/s10434-021-10251-3. PMID: 34101066
35. Molenaar CJL, Minnella EM, Coca-Martinez M, Ten Cate DWG, Regis M, Awasthi R, Martínez-Palli G, López-Baamonde M, Sebio-Garcia R, Feo CV, van Rooijen SJ, Schreinemakers JMJ, Bojesen RD, Gögenur I, van den Heuvel ER, Carli F, Slooter GD. PREHAB study group effect of multimodal prehabilitation on reducing postoperative complications and enhancing functional capacity following colorectal cancer surgery: The PREHAB randomized clinical trial. *JAMA Surg.* 2023 Mar 29;e230198. PMID: 36988937. PMCID. doi:10.1001/jamasurg.2023.0198
36. Fleisher LA, Fleischmann KE, Auerbach AD, et al. 2014 ACC/AHA guideline on perioperative cardiovascular evaluation and management of patients undergoing noncardiac surgery: A report of the American College of Cardiology/American Heart Association Task Force on practice guidelines. *J Am Coll Cardiol.* 2014;64(22):e77–137. doi:10.1016/j.jacc.2014.07.944
37. Hennis PJ, Meale PM, Grocott MP. Cardiopulmonary exercise testing for the evaluation of perioperative risk in non-cardiopulmonary surgery. *Postgrad Med J.* 2011;87(1030):550–557. doi:10.1136/pgmj.2010.107185
38. Goodyear SJ, Yow H, Saedon M, et al. Risk stratification by preoperative cardiopulmonary exercise testing improves outcomes following elective abdominal aortic aneurysm surgery: A cohort study. *Periop Med (London, England).* 2013;2(1):10. doi:10.1186/2047-0525-2-10
39. O'Doherty AF, West M, Jack S, Grocott MP. Preoperative aerobic exercise training in elective intra-cavity surgery: A systematic review. *Br J Anaesth.* 2013;110(5):679–689. doi:10.1093/bja/aes514
40. Sankar A, Beattie WS, Wijeysundera DN. How can we identify the high-risk patient? *Curr Opin Crit Care.* 2015;21(4):328–335. doi:10.1097/mcc.0000000000000216
41. Ludbrook GL. The hidden pandemic: The cost of postoperative complications. *Curr Anesthesiol Rep.* 2022;12:1–9. https://doi.org/10.1007/s40140-021-00493
42. Levett DZ, Edwards M, Grocott M, Mythen M. Preparing the patient for surgery to improve outcomes: Best practice and research. *Clin Anaesthesiol.* 2016;30(2):145–157. doi:10.1016/j.bpa.2016.04.002
43. Wynter-Blyth V, Moorthy K. Prehabilitation: Preparing patients for surgery. *BMJ (Clinical research ed.)* 2017;358:j3702. doi:10.1136/bmj.j3702
44. Bolshinsky V, Ismail H, Li M, et al. Clinical covariates that improve surgical risk prediction and guide targeted prehabilitation: An exploratory, retrospective cohort study of major colorectal cancer surgery patients evaluated with preoperative cardiopulmonary exercise testing. *Periop Med.* 2022;11:20. https://doi.org/10.1186/s13741-022-00246-
45. Gillis C, Li C, Lee L, et al. Prehabilitation versus rehabilitation: A randomized control trial in patients undergoing colorectal resection for cancer. *Anesthesiology.* 2014;121(5):937–947. doi:10.1097/aln.0000000000000393
46. University Hospital Southampton – NHS Foundation Trust. Press release: Hospital's innovative 'surgery school' transforming fitness of patients. 2018. http://www.uhs.nhs.uk/AboutTheTrust/Newsandpublications/Latestnews/2018/October-2018/Press-release-Hospital's-innovative-'surgery-school'-transforming-fitness-of-patients.aspx
47. NIH U.S. National Library of Medicine – ClinicalTrials.gov. Exercise During and After Neoadjuvant Rectal Cancer Treatment (EXERT). 2018. https://clinicaltrials.gov/ct2/show/NCT03082495
48. NIH U.S. National Library of Medicine – ClinicalTrials.gov. The effects of a 9 week exercise programme on fitness and quality of life in rectal cancer patients after chemoradiotherapy and before surgery (SRETP). 2016. https://clinicaltrials.gov/ct2/show/NCT01914068
49. Steffens D, Young J, Riedel B, et al. PRehabIlitatiOn with pReoperatIve exercise and educaTion for patients undergoing major abdominal cancer surgery: Protocol for a multicentre randomised controlled TRIAL (PRIORITY trial) BMC CANCER | BMC. 2022. doi:10.1186/s12885-022-09492-6
50. Scheede-Bergdahl C, Minnella EM, Carli F. Multi-modal prehabilitation: Addressing the why, when, what, how, who and where next? *Anaesthesia.* 2019;74 Suppl 1:20–26. doi:10.1111/anae.14505
51. Williams JD, Wischmeyer PE. Assessment of perioperative nutrition practices and attitudes: A national survey of colorectal and GI surgical oncology programs. *Am J Surg.* 2017;213(6):1010–1018. doi:10.1016/j.amjsurg.2016.10.008
52. Leahy MF, Hofmann A, Towler S, et al. Improved outcomes and reduced costs associated with a health-system-wide patient blood management program: A retrospective observational study in four major adult tertiary-care hospitals. *Transfusion.* 2017;57(6):1347–1358. doi:10.1111/trf.14006
53. Barberan-Garcia A, Ubre M, Roca J, et al. Personalised prehabilitation in high-risk patients undergoing elective major abdominal surgery: A randomized blinded controlled trial. *Ann Surg.* 2018;267(1):50–56. doi:10.1097/sla.0000000000002293
54. Grocott MPW, Edwards M, Mythen MG, Aronson S. Peri-operative care pathways: Re-engineering care to achieve the "triple aim." *Anaesthesia.* 2019;74 Suppl 1:90–99. doi:10.1111/anae.14513
55. Cole CR, Blackstone EH, Pashkow FJ, Snader CE, Lauer MS. Heart-rate recovery immediately after exercise as a predictor of mortality. *N Engl J Med.* 1999;341(18):1351–1357. doi:10.1056/nejm199910283411804
56. Lauer MS, Okin PM, Larson MG, Evans JC, Levy D. Impaired heart rate response to graded exercise. Prognostic implications of chronotropic incompetence in the Framingham Heart Study. *Circulation.* 1996;93(8):1520–1526.
57. Gibbons RJ, Balady GJ, Bricker JT, et al. ACC/AHA 2002 guideline update for exercise testing: Summary article. A report of the American College of Cardiology/American Heart Association Task Force on Practice Guidelines (Committee to Update the 1997 Exercise Testing Guidelines). *J Am Coll Cardiol.* 2002;40(8):1531–1540.
58. Mancini DM, Eisen H, Kussmaul W, Mull R, Edmunds LH, Jr., Wilson JR. Value of peak exercise oxygen consumption for optimal

timing of cardiac transplantation in ambulatory patients with heart failure. *Circulation*. 1991;83(3):778–786.
59. Peterson LR, Schechtman KB, Ewald GA, et al. The effect of beta-adrenergic blockers on the prognostic value of peak exercise oxygen uptake in patients with heart failure. *J Heart Lung Transplant*. 2003;22(1):70–77.
60. Abbott TEF, Minto G, Lee AM, Pearse RM, Ackland GL. Elevated preoperative heart rate is associated with cardiopulmonary and autonomic impairment in high-risk surgical patients. *Br J Anaesth*.2017;119(1):87–94 doi:10.1093/bja/aex164
61. Arena R, Myers J, Abella J, et al. Development of a ventilatory classification system in patients with heart failure. *Circulation*. 2007;115(18):2410–2417. doi:10.1161/circulationaha.107.686576
62. Dhakal BP, Lewis GD. Exercise oscillatory ventilation: Mechanisms and prognostic significance. *World J Cardiol*. 2016;8(3):258–266. doi:10.4330/wjc.v8.i3.258
63. Sun XG, Hansen JE, Beshai JF, Wasserman K. Oscillatory breathing and exercise gas exchange abnormalities prognosticate early mortality and morbidity in heart failure. *J Am Coll Cardiol*. 2010;55(17):1814–1823. doi:10.1016/j.jacc.2009.10.075
64. Arena R, Guazzi M, Myers J, Peberdy MA. Prognostic value of heart rate recovery in patients with heart failure. *Am Heart J*. 2006;151(4):851.e7–13. doi:10.1016/j.ahj.2005.09.012
65. Chaudhry S, Kumar N, Behbahani H, et al. Abnormal heart-rate response during cardiopulmonary exercise testing identifies cardiac dysfunction in symptomatic patients with non-obstructive coronary artery disease. *Int J Cardiol*. 2017;228:114–121. doi:10.1016/j.ijcard.2016.11.235
66. Duceppe E, Parlow J, MacDonald P, et al. Canadian Cardiovascular Society Guidelines on perioperative cardiac risk assessment and management for patients who undergo noncardiac surgery. *Can J Cardiol*. 2017;33(1):17–32. doi:10.1016/j.cjca.2016.09.008
67. Blair SN, Kohl HW, III, Barlow CE, Paffenbarger RS, Jr., Gibbons LW, Macera CA. Changes in physical fitness and all-cause mortality. A prospective study of healthy and unhealthy men. *JAMA*. 1995;273(14):1093–1098.
68. Lee D-c, Artero EG, Sui X, Blair SN. Mortality trends in the general population: The importance of cardiorespiratory fitness. *J Psychopharmacol*. 2010;24(4 Suppl):27–35. doi:10.1177/1359786810382057

PART II

AGE

10.

EX-PREMIE FOR INTERVAL HERNIA REPAIR AT 11 WEEKS

Joseph P. Resti and Bettina Smallman

STEM CASE AND KEY QUESTIONS

A 11-week-old female infant, born at 27 weeks of gestational age, presents for bilateral inguinal hernia repair. Birthweight was 1.1 kg, and she spent 9 weeks in the neonatal ICU (NICU) before discharge to home 2 weeks ago. She now weighs 2.3 kg and has been on nasal cannula oxygen at home since discharge (0.25 L/min).

How severe is this patient's prematurity?

This patient would be categorized as "extremely preterm" because she was born at less than 28 weeks. Furthermore, her oxygen requirement would suggest she suffers from significant bronchopulmonary dysplasia (BPD), the chronic lung disease of prematurity. A thorough history of the patient's course in the NICU, such as length of mechanical ventilation and any central nervous system issues would also be helpful in understanding the patient's disease severity.

What types of preoperative questions should be asked of the patient's family before her anesthetic?

General questions related to her course in the NICU and development and growth since discharge should be covered. Specific focus on the respiratory system is particularly important, with questions regarding sick exposures at home, changes in oxygen requirement, and adherence to the pulmonary medication regimen.

Is any cardiac preoperative evaluation warranted in this patient?

One of the most serious and high-risk complications of prematurity and BPD is persistent pulmonary hypertension (PPH). Either a cardiac catheterization with direct measurement of pulmonary vascular resistance (PVR) or an echocardiogram with estimate of PVR and right-sided heart pressure are important to review in any patient with significant BPD, especially if oxygen dependent. Concurrent PPH along with BPD significantly increases the perioperative risk for this subset of patients.[1]

In addition, evaluation for murmurs and other features of congenital cardiac abnormalities should be performed. Any positive findings should be confirmed and quantitated by echocardiography.

What are the fasting recommendations for this infant?

Standard fasting guidelines should be followed with these patients (2 hours for clear liquids, 4 hours for breast milk, and 6 hours for formula). Every effort should be made to minimize the fasting times in these patients, not only for concerns of hypovolemia but also hypoglycemia. Strategies to minimize fasting times include scheduling the surgery for early in the day (to reduce the possibilities of delay from other surgeries) and being very explicit with families about precise times of stopping each type of feed. In times of prolonged fasting, consider establishing IV access preoperatively for dextrose and IV fluid administration for maintenance of normovolemia and avoidance of hypoglycemia.

What types of anesthetic options are available for this patient?

The most common anesthetic plan for this patient population is general anesthesia (GA). An adjunct along with GA often chosen by anesthesiologists is a single-shot caudal block allowing for reliable analgesia and minimization or elimination of perioperative opiate administration. Opioids put these patients at higher risk of respiratory complications. Another option would be spinal anesthesia, which has the upside of not instrumenting or significantly altering the patient's respiratory system. However, this is limited by a short duration of block and is best performed in institutions familiar with this practice.

Should any medications be administered to this patient preoperatively?

Patients who suffer from BPD benefit from short-acting beta agonists administered preoperatively, 1–2 hours prior to induction of anesthesia. A patient on continued oral steroid therapy for BPD may need a stress-dose steroid administered preoperatively. It is very important that these patients continue their home medication regimen, which often consists of short-acting beta agonists and inhaled steroids. Gastroesophageal reflux disease (GERD) is more prevalent in this population,[2] and patients should continue any home medications if applicable. When patients are quite young, anxiolytic premedications are not needed. As children age into older infancy and toddlerhood, anxiolytics can be considered as premedication.

Is the use of a laryngeal mask airway (LMA) an option in this patient?

Although LMAs are commonly utilized in pediatric anesthesiology, even in very young patients, there is considerable risk in this patient population. The premature infant is already at high risk of respiratory complications and, due to high closing capacity, is at a very high risk for atelectasis related to spontaneous ventilation under GA. Mechanical ventilation with an endotracheal tube allows for minimization of intraoperative and postoperative atelectasis and optimizes oxygenation postoperatively.

Does the patient have to be observed overnight after her anesthetic?

Because of the higher risk of apnea in ex-premature infants, overnight observation after anesthesia is essential in maintaining safety for these patients.[3] Although policies differ between institutions, many children's hospitals observe patients born prematurely overnight who are less than 60 weeks postconceptual age.

Does the patient need a higher level of care (such as ICU) postoperatively?

An intensive care bed is not automatically necessary postoperatively, although it is prudent to have this discussion preoperatively with the family and involved services because these patients have a higher risk of respiratory complications, including the need for postoperative intubation and mechanical ventilation.

Should this surgery be delayed until the patient is larger and older?

This discussion needs to occur with our surgical colleagues as waiting may carry increased surgical risk. There is no "magic" age where the anesthetic risk to this patient dissipates, and the timing of surgery must be a conversation between the family, the pediatric surgeon, and the pediatric anesthesiologist.

DISCUSSION

DEFINITIONS AND EPIDEMIOLOGY

Preterm birth is defined as an infant born before 37 weeks of gestational age. This is further divided into late preterm (32–<37 weeks), very preterm (28–<32 weeks), and extremely preterm (<28 weeks).[4] Separate, but related, are different categories related to birth weight. These are low birth weight (LBW, <2,500 g), very low birth weight (VLBW, <1,500 g), and extremely low birth weight (ELBW, <1,000 g).[5]

15 million infants globally are born prematurely each year.[4] This disproportionally affects lower- and middle-income countries. Within the United States, approximately 500,000 infants are born prematurely each year, which represents 1 out of 10 births. Women of color are more likely to have a premature birth, with a rate of 14.4% in the Black population versus 9.3% and 10% in White women and Hispanic women, respectively. 6% of preterm births are characterized by gestational age at delivery of less than 28 weeks (extremely preterm).

HISTORICAL PERSPECTIVE

Prior to 1990, outcomes for extremely preterm infants (<28 weeks gestational age) were very poor, especially less than 25 weeks. However, due to significant advances in the care of these infants, mortality has steadily improved over the past two and half decades (see Figure 10.1). These advances include antenatal maternal steroid administration, the introduction of artificial surfactant, improvements in ventilator technology, targeted oxygen therapy, and focusing of care at high-level NICUs. However, with an improvement in mortality comes an increased burden of morbidity in these patients. These patients often present for various surgical procedures requiring anesthesia, which include inguinal hernia repair, ligation of a patent ductus arteriosus (PDA), laparotomy for necrotizing enterocolitis (NEC), and neurosurgical procedures for intraventricular hemorrhage and hydrocephalus.

NEURODEVELOPMENT

The brain is developing rapidly in the fetus and continues to do so throughout infancy. The insult of prematurity to the developing brain can be profound and carry lifelong neurodevelopmental sequelae. Neurologic insults to the premature brain are complex and involve both hypoxic/ischemic insults as well as reperfusion injuries. Not surprisingly, both gestational age and birth weight are the strongest predictors of neurologic outcomes. Other risk factors for poor neurodevelopmental

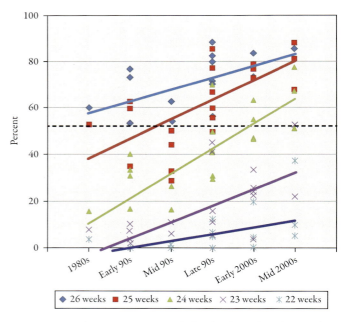

Figure 10.1 Survival rates among extremely-low-birth weight infants in the United States.
From Glass HC, Costarino AT, Stayer SA, Brett CM, Cladis F, Davis PJ. Outcomes for extremely premature infants. *Anesth Analg*. 2015;120(6): 1337–1351.

outcomes include congenital heart disease needing surgery, extracorporeal membrane oxygenation (ECMO) use, the presence of other congenital defects, and postnatal cardiac arrest.

White matter injury is most common and involves two related processes, periventricular hemorrhagic infarction (PVHI) and periventricular leukomalacia. The periventricular white matter is undergoing its fastest development during the late second trimester (24–28 weeks gestation), and this critical time makes it most susceptible to injury in these individuals.[6] Gray matter injury also is common and is strongly associated with concurrent white matter injury. Approximately 50% of VLBW infants have been found to have brain injury based on MRI findings.

Long-term outcomes of these patients are variable. They can range from devastating cerebral palsy with significant neurosensory deficits, such as cortical blindness and hearing loss, to more subtle findings that can only be found on sensitive neurocognitive testing. A higher incidence of depression and anxiety has been found in ex-premature infants. Interestingly, deficits in executive function and decision-making have been noted in ex-premature infants who are now adolescents or young adults. When ELBW infants (<1,000 g at birth) were evaluated for neurocognitive function at age 3, 67% had impairment and the remaining 33% skewed toward the low end of normal.[7]

The anesthetic implications of these neurologic issues are multiple. First, decreased cough reflex and other bulbar dysfunction in severely impacted patients can result in poor airway clearance, putting these patients at higher risk for extubation failure. Second, patients who experience these neurologic insults are at higher risk of hydrocephalus from intraventricular hemorrhage, necessitating placement of a cerebrospinal fluid (CSF) reservoir and ventricular shunting procedures, requiring anesthesia care. Finally, patients with severe neurocognitive outcomes often need related procedures in the future, such as botulinum toxin injection and orthopedic procedures, and will often frequently need anesthesia care.

A related topic is the issue of potential anesthetic neurotoxicity. Although not clearly linked to poor outcomes in humans, there is evidence in animal studies that many anesthetics (including volatile anesthetics, benzodiazepines, ketamine, propofol, among others) could impact neurodevelopment. This is most impactful in younger infants, when neurodevelopment is rapid, and it is likely that the ex-premature infant at a young post-conceptual age would be at the highest risk. Although it is very difficult to isolate the effects on anesthetic compared to general neurologic insult of prematurity on the developing brain, there is some encouraging data from the General Anesthesia Versus Spinal (GAS) study. The study, which randomized infants to GA versus spinal anesthesia for inguinal hernia repair, while not looking specifically at premature infants (although 55% of enrollees were born prematurely), did not show any difference in neurodevelopmental outcomes when comparing the two groups at age 3 or age 5.[8] It should be noted, however, that patients with known neurodevelopmental injury such as PVCI or intraventricular hemorrhage were excluded from the study, and the study only looks at patients having one single anesthetic episode about 1 hour in length.

Although the data do not show a clear relationship in humans between anesthetic agents and neurotoxicity, a reasonable approach to these patients in preventing any potential neurotoxicity is to use opiates as a balanced anesthetic with lower concentrations of volatile anesthetics and utilize regional anesthesia when appropriate.

RETINOPATHY OF PREMATURITY

Another condition associated with premature birth is retinopathy of prematurity (ROP). Again, extremes of prematurity put the patient at high risk for development of ROP; 70% of infants with a birth weight of less than 1,000 g develop ROP. Other risk factors include oxygen exposure, mechanical ventilation, neonatal sepsis, and history of transfusions.[9] Earlier exposure to oxygen results in worsening outcomes for these patients. Goal oxygen saturation in these at-risk patients is quite low when compared to goal saturation of other patients, often between 85% and 93% depending on the institution.

The pathogenesis of ROP is complex and multifactorial but is commonly described as having two stages. First is the initial phase (30–32 weeks of gestational age). which is represented by inhibition of retinal growth along with loss of vessels. The second stage is represented by neovascularization and occurs between 32 and 34 weeks of gestational age. This new blood vessel formation, which is formed in areas where vasculature is often not present, can result in retinal detachment, which is the most severe form of ROP.[10]

The mainstay treatment of ROP is laser photocoagulation, which functions to reduce the abnormal growth of blood vessels within the retina. Although it is very institution-dependent, these procedures can be done at the bedside in the NICU under local anesthesia and sedation or in the operating room under GA. This is usually decided by the preference of the ophthalmologist.

Our care of these patients, especially ones still in the early weeks after birth, can affect their outcomes when it comes to ROP. Oxygen limitation is important during these key stages of retinal development, and prolonged hyperoxia, even during a few hours of anesthesia, may impact the development of disease. Therefore, the anesthesiologist caring for these patients must always be prudent to keep the FiO_2 as low as possible to reduce the incidence of ROP in our youngest, most vulnerable patients.

GASTROINTESTINAL ABNORMALITIES

The premature infant may present with feeding difficulties and oral aversion. For patients who had prolonged respiratory support and associated enteral feeding, transitioning to oral eating can be difficult, especially in a patient who suffered a neurological insult during their first few months of life. These patients may need long-term enteral access in the form of a gastrostomy tube before discharge from the NICU.

GERD is more common in the ex-premature infant.[2] Management includes H2 blockers and, more rarely, proton pump inhibitors. Poorly controlled GERD can worsen preexisting lung disease, especially in infants with concurrent neurodevelopmental abnormalities.

NEC is the most common intra-abdominal pathology requiring surgery in the newborn and is the leading cause of short bowel syndrome, a disease where total parenteral nutrition (TPN) dependency and its complications leads to significant morbidity and mortality later in childhood. There are many risk factors to developing NEC, but the most major are extremes of prematurity and birth weight. The average gestational age for an infant who develops NEC is 29 weeks, and 65% of cases occur in patients with birth weights of less than 1,500 g. Other risk factors include presence of PDA, neonatal hypoxemia, and umbilical artery catheterization.[11]

The patient who suffered from NEC during their NICU course may present for various procedures as a young infant. These include central line placement for TPN administration and ostomy reversal as an older child.

CARDIOPULMONARY ABNORMALITIES

Infants born prematurely are at a considerably high risk for PDA. This risk increases inversely with gestational age at birth. PDA has multiple physiologic consequences for the infant and is treated surgically if medical management fails.

In extrauterine life, when patent, the ductus arteriosus allows left to right shunting from the distal aortic arch to the pulmonary artery. This results in extra right heart strain and possible right-sided volume overload and heart failure. The extra flow and pressure through the pulmonary vasculature has the consequence of causing pulmonary edema, making oxygenation and ventilation of a patient with significant BPD even more challenging. Diuretics are a mainstay therapy in these patients to reduce the burden of pulmonary edema on lung parenchyma that has reduced oxygen diffusion capacity. Fluid restriction and positive end-expiratory pressure also is used to medically manage the extra right ventricular volume.

Left to right shunting through a PDA in the premature infant also puts the patient at higher risk for NEC. This is due to "diastolic runoff" or "steal" phenomenon where blood runs from the aorta to the pulmonary artery during diastole, resulting in a lower diastolic blood pressure, lower mean arterial pressure, and wider pulse pressures. Because small infants have heart rate–dependent cardiac output (due to a fixed stroke volume from immature myocytes) this runoff results in hypoperfusion of organ systems distal to the ductus arteriosus, including the mesenteric circulation. Renal injury can also occur from the "runoff" phenomenon.

Most concerning, the pulmonary overcirculation from PDA (or any lesion with left to right shunting, such as a ventricular or atrial septal defect) can result in pulmonary vascular remodeling. The prolonged increased pressure and volume results in pulmonary arterial hypertension, which can lead to worsening outcomes especially in patients with significant BPD. It is important for the anesthesiologist to have an understanding of the degree of pulmonary hypertension in the ex-premature infants because this is one of the biggest predictors of morbidity in the perianesthetic period. Patients with severe pulmonary hypertension from prematurity (also termed *persistent pulmonary hypertension*) will often be on agents to reduce pulmonary vascular resistance. Agents include phosphodiesterase inhibitors (e.g., sildenafil), endothelin-receptor antagonists (e.g., bosentan), continued IV prostacyclin, and inhaled nitric oxide. These patients will almost always be on supplemental oxygen, which has the benefits of decreasing pulmonary vascular resistance. Patients with Down syndrome are at higher risk for developing persistent pulmonary hypertension.[12]

Management of these patients can be quite challenging as small changes in their physiology can result in dangerously high pulmonary vascular resistance, resulting in right heart failure and systemic hypotension and cardiovascular collapse. When taking care of patients with PPH, there are a number of key clinical pearls. First, ensure there is adequate depth of anesthesia during stimulating parts of the anesthetic, such as intubation or incision. Second, precise control of both ventilation and oxygenation is essential to ensure PVR does not become elevated. Third, avoid hypothermia and acidosis, as these will increase PVR. Finally, be prepared to treat a pulmonary hypertensive crisis with inhaled nitric oxide readily available along with vasoactive agents.

PULMONARY ABNORMALITIES

Perhaps the most profound problems in the ex-premature infant for the pediatric anesthesiologist are related to the respiratory system and the issues the evolve during the first few months of life after premature birth. These problems are most responsible for the increased risk carried by the premature infant during anesthesia care, and intimate knowledge of these issues is key to managing these risks when caring for these patients.

RESPIRATORY SYSTEM DEVELOPMENT

Knowledge of fetal lung development is essential to understanding the disease that affects the respiratory system of the premature infant. It is the arrest and maldevelopment during the insult of premature birth that causes both the acute and chronic lung disease of prematurity.

Pulmonary development is divided into five stages (see Table 10.1). The respiratory system develops proximally to distally, starting with the upper airway in the embryonic stage and ending with alveolar development, which continues after birth until around 18 months of age.[13] Although problems with development in the first two stages (up until 16 weeks of gestational age) can result in airway anomalies, these stages are not as important to the discussion regarding the premature infant because birth during these early development stages is not compatible with life.

The canalicular stage of development, between 16 and 26 weeks of gestation, is marked by acini development. By this point, the main stem bronchi and conducting bronchioles have formed. The acini are the most distal part of the respiratory tree and contain respiratory bronchioles and alveoli. However, during this stage (especially in the early part of the

Table 10.1 THE STAGES OF FETAL LUNG DEVELOPMENT

STAGE	GESTATION	EVENTS
Embryonic	4–7 weeks	Formation of primitive lung tissue and vascular connections.
Pseudoglandular	5–17 weeks	Development of a bronchial tree that begins to form lumens.
Canalicular	16–26 weeks	Alveoli begin to form. Vascular and lymphatic systems develop alongside the bronchial tree. Differentiation of type 1 and type 2 pneumocytes with beginning of surfactant production. Extrauterine life possible at later weeks.
Saccular	24 weeks–birth	Peripheral bronchiole branching. Maturation of surfactant system. Breathing efforts begin. 30 to 50 million alveoli at birth.
Alveolarization	Birth–3+ years	Continued alveolar growth to adult level of approximately 500 million. Reduction of interstitial tissues.

Adapted from Schittny JC.[13]

stage), no terminal air sacs have formed, nor have the capillary units around them. This underdevelopment is why extrauterine viability is so poor before 26 weeks—there is simply not enough development of the respiratory units for gas exchange to be adequate for extrauterine life.

One intervention that is common to assist in the acceleration of fetal lung development is antenatal maternal steroid administration. If there are any signs of potential premature birth, the expectant mother receives a corticosteroid, ideally between 2 and 7 days before delivery. Administration of corticosteroids accelerates development of both type 1 and type 2 pneumocytes,[14] resulting in improved surfactant production and gas exchange.

SURFACTANT AND RESPIRATORY DISTRESS SYNDROME

Surfactant (also known as surface active material [SAM]) is responsible for decreasing surface tension in the lung, resulting in the maintenance of open alveoli throughout the respiratory cycle and improved compliance due to less surface tension. The absence of this lipid-rich molecule, formed and stored by type 2 pneumocytes, was discovered in 1950s to be the cause of respiratory distress syndrome (RDS). Prior to the development of exogenous surfactant, RDS was characterized by respiratory distress, poor oxygenation, respiratory acidosis, and death. This often occurred in the first few days of life. Along with poor lung development and absence of surfactant, barotrauma from high pressures of mechanical ventilation often contributed to the lung damage and poor outcomes seen in these patients. Although premature infants are at higher risk for RDS (with risk strongly correlated with an earlier gestational age), it can also occur in term infants, representing about 5% of cases of RDS. Infants of diabetic mothers are at higher risk for development of RDS.

In 1990, the first commercially produced surfactant was introduced to clinical practice in the United States. The benefits of this drug, by improving end-expiratory volumes and distensibility, significantly decreased the incidence and severity of RDS.[15]

BRONCHOPULMONARY DYSPLASIA

The chronic lung disease of prematurity is termed "bronchopulmonary dysplasia." Development of BPD occurs not only from the insult of maldevelopment after premature birth, but also from the supportive care of these infants during the first few months of life. This includes damage from oxygen administration and mechanical ventilation, such as barotrauma and volutrauma. Although the introduction of surfactant greatly improved the survival and severity of BPD, it is still a major contributor of morbidity and mortality in infants even after discharge from the NICU.

The terminology and diagnostic criteria for chronic lung disease of prematurity is constantly evolving.[16] This is partially caused by the "changing" of the disease after introduction of exogenous surfactant. Before 1990 (what is commonly termed as "old"), BPD was a fibroproliferative process, one characterized significant fibrosis from lung inflammation and epithelial injury, which would result in loss of airway space and heterogeneity of lung disease on chest radiograph. However, with surfactant treatment, "new" BPD is instead characterized by arrested development of the lungs in the canicular stage. Fibrosis is not often seen in "new" BPD. "New" BPD is often seen in only the most premature infants, whereas "old" BPD was more widespread among gestational ages. The arrested development is from a variety of insults during the first few months of life, including hyperoxia, mechanical ventilation, and steroid administration among others.

Patients who meet criteria from BPD (see Table 10.2) are at higher risk of respiratory morbidity even after discharge from the NICU, particularly in the first years of life. Pulmonary function is compromised well into childhood and beyond. During the first years of life, hospitalization for respiratory illness is common. Respiratory syncytial virus (RSV) is particularly devastating for the patient with BPD; because of this, these patients are often selected to receive palivizumab, an antibody therapy administered to high-risk patients to reduce the severity of illness from RSV. Even into older childhood and young adulthood, pulmonary dysfunction continues to be present, albeit with reduced symptomatology and morbidity. There is also a higher incidence of reduced exercise tolerance as well as long-term inhaler use into older ages.

This abnormal pulmonary physiology increases the respiratory risk in the perioperative period. Assessment of these patients begins with thorough preoperative evaluation.

Table 10.2 DIAGNOSTIC CRITERIA FOR BRONCHOPULMONARY DYSPLASIA

	GESTATIONAL AGE	
	< 32 WEEKS	≥32 WEEKS
Time of assessment	36 weeks PMA or discharge	>28 days and <56 days postnasal age or discharge
	TREATMENT WITH OXYGEN >21% FOR 28 DAYS	
Mild BPD	Room air at 36 weeks PMA/discharge	Room air at 56 days postnatal age/discharge
Moderate BPD	Need <30% O_2 at 36 weeks PMA/discharge	Need <30% O_2 at 56 days postnatal age/discharge
Severe BPD	Need ≥30% O_2 and/or positive pressure ventilation at 36 weeks PMA/discharge	Need ≥30% O_2 and/or positive pressure ventilation at 56 days postnatal age/discharge

Adapted from NIH/NICHD Criteria of Bronchopulmonary Dysplasia.
PMA, post menstrual age; BPD, bronchopulmonary dysplasia.

Management involves continued use of bronchodilators throughout the perioperative period, including administration of a short-acting beta agonist 1–2 hours before the anesthetic. The absence of wheezing is quite common; these patients exhibit more obstructed exhalation from airway trapping than bronchial constriction. Be very cautious about any concurrent or recent respiratory illnesses; even the most innocuous of viruses can have serious implications on the respiratory system of a patient with significant BPD. Patients on diuretics for management of BPD can be hypovolemic and have metabolic derangements.

Anesthetic considerations include the potential of air trapping in these patients. This has multiple consequences. First, nitrous oxide should be used cautiously as a closed space can be expanded by administration of this drug. Second, a longer expiration time may be needed during mechanical ventilation. Another consideration is that many of these patients have some degree of subglottic stenosis, so a smaller endotracheal tube may be necessary when intubating these patients.

APNEA OF PREMATURITY

A common clinical problem encountered with premature infants is apnea. This apnea is defined as a pause in breathing (>15 seconds in length) or an apneic spell associated with desaturation and bradycardia. Although this can be both central and obstructive apnea, the patients with more extremes of prematurity tend to have a higher incidence of central apnea. Risk factors for apnea of prematurity include extremes of gestational age (and, as they age, post-conceptual age), anemia, history of apnea and bradycardia, and history of mechanical ventilation.[17]

Premature infants have an abnormal, immature response to hypoxia termed the *biphasic response*. In older children and adults with fully developed respiratory centers, hypoxia is associated with an increased drive to breathe, although carbon dioxide and hypercapnia are still the strongest contributor to respiratory drive. However, premature infants will often have an initial increase in ventilation in response to hypoxia, then followed by apnea is response to prolonged hypoxemia. This propensity to apnea is worsened by exposure to anesthetic agents. If apneic episodes are frequent and not self-resolving, options for treatment included continuous positive airway pressure (CPAP) or high-flow nasal cannula and, if those measures fail, intubation and mechanical ventilation.

REGIONAL ANESTHESIA, POSTOPERATIVE APNEA, AND OTHER ANALGESIC CONSIDERATIONS

A common anesthetic option selected in these patients, in conjunction with GA or by itself, is neuraxial anesthesia. These techniques have some unique advantages in the ex-premature population when compared to the older population. It is important to note that use of neuraxial anesthesia without GA or sedation is very institution-dependent and requires collaboration with surgical colleagues to ensure the success of these techniques.

Many of the surgeries the premature infant experiences are infraumbilical (e.g., inguinal hernia repair, circumcision, hydrocelectomy) and particularly amenable to spinal anesthesia or caudal anesthesia, by itself or as an adjunct to GA. In the United States, GA is the much more common choice in these patients; however, a number of institutions prefer neuraxial anesthesia as the primary anesthetic techniques for infants having infraumbilical surgeries. There are multiple reasons why an institution may make this choice. First, there is a lower incidence of postoperative apnea in patients who received isolated neuraxial anesthesia with no agents given systemically. Second, with concerns for neurotoxicity from GA, there may be an advantage to neurodevelopment (although, as previously discussed, there was no difference in neurodevelopmental outcomes between these patient groups from the GAS study). Last, respiratory complications related to induction, intubation, mechanical ventilation, and extubation are avoided in patients who receive a successful neuraxial block. Neuroaxial blocks can be technically challenging and have a higher rate of failure when compared to older children and adults. Higher rates of CSF production and absorption affect duration of spinal anesthesia. Blocks last one-third to one-half the time of those in adults, even when doses are adjusted for a higher CSF volume. A continuous epidural catheter can be used to prolong a block for longer procedures.

Postoperative apnea is an important consideration when taking care of the premature infant. Postoperative apnea can occur after all types of anesthetics, although it is more common after general anesthetics or regional anesthesia with systemic sedation (such as ketamine). Despite anesthetic agents being shorter acting than in the past (sevoflurane or desflurane vs. halothane) postoperative apnea continues to be a safety concern. A recent evaluation of this was done using the GAS study population, where one study group had spinal anesthesia with no sedation and the other had GA with a regional anesthesia adjunct (caudal or ilioinguinal block) and no opioids.[18] The overall apnea rate was similar between the group; however, the incidence of early postoperative apnea (<30 minutes postanesthetic) was lower in the spinal anesthesia group than the regional group, although there was no difference in late apnea between the two groups. This suggests that the difference between the anesthetic techniques in preventing apnea is short lived and may not have any clinical impact past PACU discharge.

Regardless of the GAS study finding that late postoperative apnea is not as prevalent as it has been in the past (likely due to shorter-acting anesthetic agents), hospital policies are still very conservative in the postoperative monitoring of these patients. These policies reflect the higher risk that premature infants carry versus term infants. For premature infants, most hospitals require 24-hour observation after anesthesia anywhere from 50 to 60 weeks post-conceptual age. Term infants are rarely admitted for observation past 44 weeks post-conceptual age. Recent trends are to be more selective in who needs observation and promote sending these older infants home on the day of surgery. At our institution, we have chosen to be conservative and require observation up to 60 weeks post-conceptual age in preterm infants and 44 weeks post-conceptual age for term infants.

Even if GA is chosen, neuraxial blocks offer reliable postoperative analgesia in many procedures. The single-shot caudal is a frequently chosen block for these circumstances. Caudal anesthesia has many advantages as an adjunct to GA. First, it is technically a simple, reliable, and safe way to provide regional analgesia for infraumbilical surgeries. Second, it reduces or eliminates the need for opioid analgesics, which increase the risk of respiratory events in the perioperative period in the premature infant with an abnormal respiratory control center. Finally, it allows for reducing the amount of drug needed for GA, resulting in a quicker emergence and recovery. This technique should be strongly considered in the ex-premature infant requiring any surgery below the umbilicus.

CONCLUSION

- The ex-premature infant is one of the most challenging patient populations for pediatric anesthesiologists.
- Prematurity is common in the United States, representing 10% of live births, with an even higher incidence globally.
- Improvement in survival of the most premature infants results in higher chance that these patients will require surgery and anesthesia later in life.
- Neurodevelopment outcomes in the premature infant are multifactorial and vary greatly.
- PPH is common in these patients and must be recognized preoperatively.
- BPD is the chronic lung disease of prematurity and has the highest impact of perianesthetic morbidity.
- Apnea of prematurity and postoperative apnea have significant clinical implications to safety after anesthesia, and familiarity with institutional policies is key.
- Regional anesthesia has specific advantages in the ex-premature infant population and should be considered strongly during the preoperative planning process.

REVIEW QUESTIONS

1. What is the rate in the United States for premature birth?

   a. 4%.
   b. 7%.
   c. 10%.
   d. 18%.

   The correct answer is c.
   10% of births in the United States are considered premature, meaning less than 37 weeks of gestational age.

2. Which of the following is *not* responsible for improved mortality over the past 30 years in extremely low-birth-weight infants?

   a. Introduction of surfactant.
   b. Focusing of cares at higher-level NICUs.
   c. Improved ventilation technology.
   d. Better neurologic outcomes.

   The correct answer is d.
   Mortality has improved for VLBW infants due to many factors. However, neurologic outcomes have not improved and have become a larger burden as the VLBW infants have improved mortality.

3. Which of the following does *not* impact pulmonary vascular resistance?

   a. Carbon dioxide levels.
   b. Anemia.
   c. Body temperature,
   d. Acid/base status.

   The correct answer is b.
   Anemia has no impact on PVR.

4. True or false? The incidence of BPD is decreasing over time, with improvements in mortality.

   The correct answer is false.
   BPD continues to be a concern for ex-premature infants, with clinical significance for the anesthesiologist caring for these children.

5. Which of the following is *not* a risk factor for apnea of prematurity?

   a. Post-conceptual age.
   b. Anemia.
   c. Previous history of apnea.
   d. Small for gestational age (SGA).

The correct answer is d.

SGA has not been categorized as a risk factor for apnea of prematurity.

6. True or false? Spinal anesthesia without sedation eliminates the risk of postoperative apnea in the premature infant.

The correct answer is false.

Although apnea is less when systemic anesthetics and sedatives are avoided, it is still a risk even with neuraxial anesthesia by itself.

7. Spinal anesthesia in infants, when compared to adults, has a duration of action of

   a. One-sixth.
   b. One-third
   c. Three-quarters.
   d. Two times.

The correct answer is b.

There is a significantly shorter duration of action for spinal anesthesia in infants due to rapid production and turnover of CSF in this age group.

REFERENCES

1. Schmidt AR, Ramamoorthy C. Bronchopulmonary dysplasia. *Pediatr Anesth*. 2022;32:174–180. doi:10.1111/pan.14365
2. Gulati IK, Jadcherla SR. Gastroesophageal reflux disease in the neonatal intensive care unit infant: Who needs to be treated and what approach is beneficial? *Pediatr Clin North Am*. 2019 Apr;66(2):461–473. doi:10.1016/j.pcl.2018.12.012. Epub 2019 Feb 1. PMID: 30819348;PMCID: PMC6400306
3. Coté CJ, Zaslavsky A, Downes JJ, Kurth CD, Welborn LG, Warner LO, Malviya SV. Postoperative apnea in former preterm infants after inguinal herniorrhaphy: A combined analysis. *Anesthesiology*. 1995 Apr;82(4):809–822. PubMed PMID: 7717551
4. World Health Organization. Preterm birth factsheet. 2023, May 10. https://www.who.int/news-room/fact-sheets/detail/preterm-birth
5. World Health Organization. ICD-10, P07. 10th Revision Fifth Edition, 2016. https://icd.who.int/browse10/2010/en#/P07
6. Jarjour IT. Neurodevelopmental outcome after extreme prematurity: A review of the literature. *Pediatr Neurol*. 2015;52(2):143–152.
7. Glass HC, Costarino AT, Stayer SA, Brett CM, Cladis F, Davis PJ. Outcomes for extremely premature infants. *Anesth Analg*. 2015;120(6):1337–1351.
8. McCann ME, de Graaff JC, Dorris L, et al.; GAS Consortium. Neurodevelopmental outcome at 5 years of age after general anaesthesia or awake-regional anaesthesia in infancy (GAS): An international, multicentre, randomised, controlled equivalence trial. *Lancet*. 2019;393(10172):664–677.
9. Peiris K, Fell D. The prematurely born infant and anaesthesia. *Cont Educ Anaesthes Crit Care Pain*. 2009;9(3):73–77.
10. Molinari A, Weaver D, Jalali S. Classifying retinopathy of prematurity. *Community Eye Health*. 2017;30(99):5–56. PMID: 29434438;PMCID: PMC5806220
11. Fox TP, Godavitarne C. What really causes necrotising enterocolitis? *ISRN Gastroenterol*. 2012;2012:628317. doi:10.5402/2012/628317
12. Stayer SA, Liu Y. Pulmonary hypertension of the newborn. *Best Pract Res Clin Anaesthesiol*. 2010;24(3):375–386.
13. Schittny JC. Development of the lung. *Cell Tissue Res*. 2017 Mar;367(3):427–444. doi:10.1007/s00441-016-2545-0. Epub 2017 Jan 31. PMID: 28144783;PMCID: PMC5320013
14. Roberts D, Brown J, Medley N, Dalziel SR. Antenatal corticosteroids for accelerating fetal lung maturation for women at risk of preterm birth. *Cochrane Database Syst Rev*. 2017 Mar 21;3(3):CD004454. doi:10.1002/14651858.CD004454.pub3. Update in: *Cochrane Database Syst Rev*. 2020 Dec 25;12:CD004454. PMID: 28321847;PMCID: PMC6464568
15. Ma CC, Ma S. The role of surfactant in respiratory distress syndrome. *Open Respir Med J*. 2012;6:44–53. doi:10.2174/1874306401206010044. Epub 2012 Jul 13. PMID: 22859930;PMCID: PMC3409350
16. Mosca F, Colnaghi M, Fumagalli M. BPD: Old and new problems. *J Matern Fetal Neonatal Med*. 2011 Oct;24 Suppl 1:80–82. doi:10.3109/14767058.2011.607675. Epub 2011 Sep 5. PMID: 21892878
17. Eichenwald EC, Watterberg KL, Aucott S, et al. Committee on Fetus and Newborn. Apnea of prematurity. *Pediatrics*. 2016 Jan;137(1):e20153757. 10.1542/peds.2015-3757
18. Davidson AJ, Morton NS, Arnup SJ, et al. General Anesthesia Compared to Spinal Anesthesia (GAS) Consortium. Apnea after awake regional and general anesthesia in infants: The General Anesthesia Compared to Spinal Anesthesia Study: Comparing apnea and neurodevelopmental outcomes, a randomized controlled trial. *Anesthesiology*. 2015 Jul;123(1):38–54.

11.

GERIATRIC ASSESSMENT

"THE GET UP AND GO, GOT UP AND LEFT"

Kaitlin Willham and Heather E. Nye

STEM CASE AND KEY QUESTIONS

A 90-year-old man with a history of coronary artery disease (CAD) and remote coronary artery bypass surgery, hypertension, heart failure with preserved ejection fraction, and atrial fibrillation on anticoagulation lives independently at baseline. He experiences a mechanical fall that results in a complete quadriceps tendon rupture of the left leg.

The patient is admitted to a hospital. Laboratory data and cardiac and pulmonary evaluations yield no overt concerns to warrant delay of recommended expedient surgical repair. Anticoagulation is held in anticipation of a procedure. The patient, however, expresses great worry and believes he may be "too old for surgery." He decides against surgery and is discharged to a skilled nursing facility (SNF) after 1–2 days. He may bear weight but is told to keep his leg in an immobilizer indefinitely. After 6 weeks, he returns home and shortly thereafter presents to his primary care physician's (PCP) office for a follow-up visit.

In addition to usual medical considerations, what are important components of the preoperative evaluation of an older adult?

Since discharge from the SNF 6 weeks ago, the patient has lost 15 pounds and become increasingly fatigued. Due to limited mobility and weakness, he is no longer able to perform with his local marching band. Moreover, he now requires assistance with getting groceries, bathing, and dressing. He denies pain but a few weeks ago he experienced dizziness with standing and "blacked out." Though the inpatient physicians strongly recommended surgery, he did not fully appreciate how impaired mobility would affect his daily life. His PCP learns from her orthopedic colleagues that without surgical repair, the patient will not walk normally again, and the longer surgery is delayed, the more likely scarring and retraction will affect the outcome. The surgery itself comes with similar risks to nonoperative management—immobility, pain, and deep vein thrombosis, but also incurs risks of infection, blood loss, and anesthesia.

How does functional status differ from frailty, and how can each be assessed?

What are effective ways to determine nutrition prior to surgery?

How do these factors relate to surgical outcomes?

The patient also notes that he was very confused during his hospitalization and still feels less mentally sharp than usual. His niece, present for the encounter, agrees. He is hearing-impaired but does not regularly wear hearing aids. His urinary retention due to prostatic hypertrophy has worsened somewhat in recent weeks. Vital signs are within normal limits and physical exam is remarkable for a thin, pale, stooped over older man who is unable to complete a Timed Up and Go test due to immobility. A Mini-Cog is suggestive of cognitive impairment.

What cognitive screening tools can be used to detect cognitive impairment before surgery?

What factors increase the risk of postoperative delirium?

What is unique to the conversation with an older adult about surgery?

During the conversation, the patient says he understands the risks of surgery and that he has a greater likelihood of walking again with it than without it. Without walking, he anticipates limited quality of life and chooses to move ahead with surgical planning. An echocardiogram, myocardial perfusion scan, and cardiac event monitoring are ordered to better assess known CAD and recent syncope. He is also referred to physical and occupational therapy for education and strengthening and asked to return for another visit with his PCP for further preoperative evaluation.

What interventions can address delirium risk and function prior to surgery?

On his return visit, the patient's medications are reviewed. They include stable doses of rivaroxaban 20 mg/day, furosemide 20 mg/day, acetaminophen 650 mg TID, metoprolol 12.5 mg BID, tamsulosin 0.4 mg/day, simvastatin 20 mg/day, and multiple herbal supplements. In addition, during his recent hospitalization he was started on docusate 100 mg BID, hydrocodone/acetaminophen 1 tab TID as needed, and trazodone 25 mg nightly. Laboratory data are remarkable for normal electrolytes, BUN of 30 mg/dL, creatinine of 1.2 (estimated glomerular filtration rate [eGFR] = 40 cc/min), and hemoglobin of 12.5 g/dL. Perfusion study reveals normal ejection fraction and no areas of cardiac ischemia. Event monitor shows paroxysmal atrial fibrillation with rates from 50 to 130.

What are the components of a preoperative medication review in older adults?

The patient's record does not include an advance directive. During the visit, he completes one identifying his niece as his durable power of attorney for medical decisions. He meets with a social worker who verifies eligibility for SNF care under Medicare, should it be needed. Several weeks later, he is admitted for his planned surgical procedure and undergoes quadriceps tendon reconstruction with Achilles tendon allograft.

What components of advance care planning are critical prior to surgery?

Postoperatively, the patient is followed by an orthopedist, a hospitalist, and a geriatrician. He is seen promptly by physical and occupational therapists. Standard interventions are employed to reduce delirium; however, confusion develops on postoperative day 2, likely due to urinary retention, disrupted sleep, and pain. As a result, he has inadequate oral intake and does not participate well in rehabilitation. His niece is involved in discussions around disposition, and he is ultimately discharged to SNF. His rehabilitation progresses slowly due to clearing delirium and deconditioning but, after 3 months, he returns home.

What models of care have been shown to improve outcomes before and after surgery in older adults?

DISCUSSION

INTRODUCTION

The number of surgeries in older adults continues to rise as the population of adults 65 years and older increases. More than one in three surgical procedures in the United States is performed on a patient 65 years or older.[1] Advanced age is frequently associated with increases in postoperative morbidity and mortality[2]; and when older adults experience complications after surgery, they are less likely to survive.[3] It has been hypothesized that the association between geriatric syndromes and worsening health status, rather than age itself, underlies this increase in perioperative risk. Patients with cognitive impairment, functional dependence, frailty, and depression experience higher rates of death, delirium, disability, and discharge to an institution following major surgery.[4–8] These findings underscore the need for an enhanced preoperative evaluation for older adults. Partnership between the American College of Surgeons National Surgical Quality Improvement Program (ACS-NSQIP) and the American Geriatrics Society (AGS) yielded publications in 2012 and 2016 outlining best practices in preoperative assessment and perioperative management of older adults.[1,9] In addition, the American College of Surgeons created the Geriatric Surgery Verification (ACS GSV) Quality Improvement Program in 2019; the program provides a blueprint of institutional and clinical standards for geriatric surgery. The standards encompass preoperative evaluation and decision-making. Each of these guides recommends a multidomain assessment that identifies vulnerabilities known to be associated with poor surgical outcomes in older adults in addition to standard preoperative risk assessments (i.e., cardiovascular and pulmonary). There are several benefits to an enhanced assessment: modifiable risk factors can be identified and intervened upon, clinicians may better project and communicate risks to the patient and other surgical team members, and the patient's healthcare goals, priorities, and expectations can be incorporated into a shared decision about treatment options.

APPROACH TO PREOPERATIVE ASSESSMENT IN OLDER ADULTS

The comprehensive geriatric assessment (CGA) is a traditional method for identifying medical, psychosocial, and functional limitations and creating a multi-professional treatment plan that incorporates the older adult's preferences. Benefits in both outpatient and inpatient settings include improved mortality, independence, and positive effects on physical and cognitive function.[10,11] In the surgical setting, problems identified in the CGA correlate with an increase in postoperative complications such as pneumonia, delirium, pressure injuries, urinary tract infections, and prolonged length of stay.[12] Performance of a CGA has been shown to correlate with fewer complications and more frequent return to home rather than an institution upon hospital discharge.[13]

Despite its potential benefits, time and resource constraints often limit a formal CGA to the highest-risk surgical candidates with ample lead time before their procedure. A more feasible approach for other geriatric patients includes preoperative use of targeted screening tools and assessments. These assessments can inform decision-making, patient expectations, and risk reduction strategies throughout the perioperative period.

COMPONENTS OF THE PREOPERATIVE ASSESSMENT

In addition to a standard medical evaluation, assessment of the older adult prior to surgery must encompass geriatric-specific vulnerabilities. The ACS-NSQIP/AGS guidelines recommend screening for cognitive impairment, depression, alcohol and substance use, frailty, and assessing risk of postoperative delirium, functional status, nutrition, polypharmacy, and social support.[1] Depending on the instrument used, a frailty screen may survey a number of these domains simultaneously. ACS GSV outlines screening for high-risk characteristics such as advanced age (85+), functional impairment, mobility impairment, cognitive impairment, malnutrition, difficulty swallowing, delirium risk, and need for palliative care assessment. Surgical decision-making should be reaffirmed, including treatment goals, expectations, and reasoning, and be grounded in the patient's overall goals of care. Another important part of the conversation is confirming the patient's preferred surrogate decision-maker. Preoperative assessment and risk reduction strategies may involve variety of professionals—from the surgeon, anesthesiologist, internist/family physician, specialist, hospitalist, or geriatrician to the physical therapist (PT), occupational therapist (OT), social worker (SW) and registered dietician (RD). Whether involvement and communication between professionals is triggered on an as-needed basis or roles are formalized into a model of care, it is critical that there are clear and timely paths for communicating findings, concerns, and recommendations.

Function

Function, or a person's ability to carry out activities of independent living, is an important predictor of short- and long-term surgical outcomes. Dependence in an activity of daily living 30 days before surgery is an independent risk factor for loss of function after surgery and death within a year of major surgery.[2,4] The basic activities of daily living are outlined in the Katz Activities of Daily Living (ADL) Index (bathing, dressing, toileting, transferring, continence and eating).[14] More complex activities are outlined in the Lawton Instrumental Activities of Daily Living (IADL) Scale (using the telephone, shopping, cooking, laundry, housekeeping, medications, managing finances, and transportation).[15] A person is considered to have impairment in a task when they require the help of another person to complete it. When assessing function, it is important to consider the ability of any given reporter to provide accurate information. If there is known or suspected cognitive impairment, seeking permission to obtain collateral information is prudent.

Detection of functional impairments can guide specific interventions. For example, difficulty with ADLs may warrant a referral to physical and occupational therapy for education on exercises, equipment, and home modifications that may be necessary after surgery. Impairments in IADLs may trigger supportive strategies such as increased family/caregiver involvement, transportation support, or meal delivery services, especially in the postoperative period. Patients and families should be made aware of the likely impact of surgery on function and the potential need for nursing home–level care, either temporary or permanent. A social worker can help determine eligibility for nursing home care or discuss options for increased caregiver support.

Even functionally independent individuals will likely experience functional decline after surgery. Education from a PT or OT on expected limitations as well as strategies to mitigate these may help individuals prepare for recovery.

Cognition, Mental Health, and Delirium

Before elective surgery, cognitive impairment is detected in up to one-quarter of older adults.[16] Cognitive impairment is the strongest risk factor for postoperative delirium and is associated with longer hospital length of stay and discharge to a place other than home.[5] Multiple screening tools are available to assess cognition. Common examples include the Mini-Mental State Exam (MMSE), Montreal Cognitive Assessment (MoCA), and Mini-Cog. The Mini-Cog is recommended as a screen by the ACS-NSQIP/AGS guidelines for older adults *without* known impairment.[1] It is an appealing tool because it is brief, has similar sensitivity and specificity for cognitive impairment as the MMSE, and is less biased by low education and literacy.[17] A positive screen should be followed by a longer tool such as the MMSE or MoCA. This will reduce the rate of false positives and provide a cognitive baseline. MMSE or MoCA should also be performed in patients with known cognitive impairment to obtain a presurgery benchmark. When administering any cognitive screen, it is important to consider the impact of communication barriers, language incongruence, and mood on the results.

The presence of cognitive impairment may prompt a review of the individual's understanding of the surgery and elevate the importance of involving a family member or friend in the conversation. Except in rare circumstances, a full cognitive evaluation by specialist is unlikely to be helpful prior to surgery, but an evaluation after surgery should be encouraged.

Depression is also independently associated with postoperative delirium, impaired recovery, and increased risk of death 1 year following major surgery surgery.[4,18,19] Multiple tools are available to screen for depression. ACS-NSQIP/AGS recommends using the Patient Health Questionnaire-2 (PHQ-2) as a rapid screen for depression in the preoperative setting.[1] In the event of a positive screen, further evaluation of mood along with review of patient expectations and anticipated ability to participate in postoperative care is warranted.

Whether or not cognitive impairment or depression are suspected, additional risk factors for delirium should be carefully elicited. Patients and caregivers should be educated about the potential for delirium, and modifiable risk factors should be addressed. See Table 11.1 for delirium risk factors and prevention strategies.

Medication Review

During any preoperative assessment, a full review of medications and herbal supplements should be performed with an eye to overall safety of each drug in the perioperative period. Medication review in older adults additionally requires identification of potentially harmful drugs due to delirium risk, drug-drug interactions, or drug-disease interactions, and cessation of medications that are unnecessary.

The AGS "Beers List" is a comprehensive list of potentially inappropriate medications (PIMs) in older patients.[20] Such medications may negatively impact cognition or renal function, and efforts should be made to taper or eliminate them. The clinician should be mindful of deliriogenic medications—medications that may lower the delirium threshold—such as anticholinergics, benzodiazepines, and antihistamines. If these cannot be safely discontinued, patients and families should be educated on the possibility of delirium. When reviewing all medications of an older adult undergoing major surgery, one must consider postoperative renal function, drug clearance, drug-drug interactions, and potential administration of concomitant nephro- or hepatotoxic agents.[1]

Table 11.1 DELIRIUM RISK FACTORS

	PREVENTION STRATEGIES
Preoperative • Age ≥70 • Cognitive impairment • Depression • Sensory impairment • Alcohol use • Polypharmacy • Renal insufficiency • Poor nutrition	• Reduce or eliminate alcohol intake • Stop unnecessary medications • Address depression
Intraoperative • Type of surgery • Duration of surgery • Type of anesthesia	• Avoid medications on Beers list • Regional over general anesthesia when appropriate
Postoperative • Sleep deprivation • Inadequately controlled pain • More than three new medications • Bladder catheters • Complications of surgery	• Remove bladder catheters/tethers • Use of visual and communication aids • Adequate pain control • Limit overnight disturbances • Prevent constipation, dehydration and urinary retention • Promote physical activity • Frequent orienting communication • Nutritional assistance • Encourage presence of family

Polypharmacy is common in older adults. In a cohort study of older adults in the community, the average number of medications and dietary supplements was 8.4.[21] One out of six individuals were on 10 or more medications, and one-third were taking a PIM.[21] Higher numbers of medications correlated with increased incidence of hospitalization and death in a 2- to 3-year follow-up period.[21] Polypharmacy is associated with adverse events such as drug-drug interactions, falls, and worse outcomes postoperatively.[22] As such, it is prudent to consider stopping medications that may not be necessary. Medications that may have been indicated earlier in a person's life may now be unnecessary because a condition or symptom has resolved; because treatment goals for certain diseases, like diabetes, become more lenient; or because of limited life expectancy.

Frailty

Frailty is generally characterized as a dynamic state of reduced reserve that results in increased vulnerability to stressors. Frailty is associated with death and disability and has prognostic value in the preoperative setting.[23–25] Studies relating various measures of frailty to surgical outcomes have found that frailty is associated with increased risk of complications, length of stay, new admission to a skilled or assisted living facility, and death.[25–29] A systematic review of 23 studies found a strong association between frailty and 30-day mortality in a variety of surgical types—cardiac, oncologic, general, hip fracture, and vascular.[30] However, this review highlighted a limitation to the integration of frailty into the surgical risk assessment: tools used to detect frailty are highly variable and tend to focus on short-term outcomes rather than long-term disability or quality of life.

Though most agree on the general description of frailty, there is no consensus on an operational definition of frailty. Two early models of frailty were based on the concept of either phenotypic frailty or the accumulation of deficits.[23,24] Phenotypic or "physical" frailty, defined by Fried et al., includes measurement of weight loss, strength, exhaustion, slowness, and low physical activity.[23] The Frailty Index, also called Deficit Accumulation Index, measures the accumulation of symptoms, signs, laboratory values, diseases, and disabilities.[24] Both methods are highly cited in frailty literature; however, they are time-consuming and at times require specialized expertise or equipment. Therefore, simpler tools have been developed that can be incorporated into the preoperative visit.

Though grounded in one of the two early concepts of frailty, these tools each tend to measure different aspects of health, disability, and cognition. Examples include the Clinical Risk Analysis Index (RAI-C), Clinical Frailty Scale (CFS), Edmonton Frail Scale (EFS), the modified Frailty Index, modified Fried Index, Vulnerable Elders Survey (VES-13), and frailty as defined by Robinson et al.[28,29] Single variable tools that assess mobility and gait speed such as the Timed Up and Go (TUG) have also been studied preoperatively.[27]

Few studies have compared frailty screening tools; however, the comparisons that have been made are included in Table 11.2.[23,25–27,31–34] While the ACS-NSQIP/AGS suggests using the Fried Index to screen for frailty, due to lack of standardization in the field, the Society for Perioperative Assessment and Quality Improvement (SPAQI) recommends that the demands of the institution, healthcare setting, availability of multiprofessional team members, the patient population, and the goals of screening all weigh into the decision to integrate frailty screening into the preoperative assessment.[1,35] Any tool that is deemed to fit the specific clinical setting should first be piloted to determine how well it performs in the patient population, and it should be followed by appropriate interventions to address the needs of patients who have positive screening tests. One potential method is for the surgeon or anesthesiologist to administer a frailty screen at the preoperative visit and, if frailty is identified, then the individual may be referred for comprehensive assessment by a geriatrician and other pertinent professionals. Alternatively, some centers may refer adults according to age and/or surgical type for a comprehensive assessment in which a frailty assessment is embedded.

Nutrition

Stress and inflammation from surgery induce a catabolic state in which the body's focus is to mobilize factors for tissue repair rather than to build protein.[36] Adequate nutritional stores are critical to respond to surgery, and their absence may compromise surgical outcomes. Numerous studies have shown increased complications (surgical site infection, pneumonia, urinary tract infection, wound dehiscence, and mortality) following surgery in individuals with poor nutritional status.[37–39] The prevalence of malnourishment or nutritional risk has been estimated to be as high as 66% in older adults in the hospital, nursing home, and community.[40] This can be

Table 11.2 **FRAILTY SCREENING TOOLS IN THE PREOPERATIVE SETTING**

PHENOTYPIC (PHYSICAL) MODEL		ACCUMULATED DEFICITS MODEL
Multicomponent Frailty Phenotype (Fried Index) 5-item survey: - Weight loss - Weakness (grip strength) - Self-report of exhaustion - Low physical activity - Slow walking (15 feet walking speed) Associated with postoperative complications, length of stay and discharge to institution.[23,25] Clinical Frailty Scale 7-point scale: - Rating of frailty by clinician's judgment In elective noncardiac surgery, CFS had similar performance to the Frailty Phenotype in predicting death or disability and was rated as easier to use by clinicians.[31]	**Single-component** Timed Up and Go - Rise from chair, walk 10 feet, turn around, return to chair, and sit down - >15 seconds associated with increased discharge to institution after surgery[27]	**Multicomponent** Edmonton Frail Scale 15-item survey: - Functional status - Mood - Social support - Medications - Clock draw - Timed Up and Go Higher scores associated with postoperative complications, increased length of stay and inability to be discharged home.[26] Clinical Risk Assessment Index (RAI-C) Brief, self-report survey: - Age - Comorbidities - Weight loss - Place of residence - Function - Cognitive decline Validated in older, male surgical populations and predictive of complications and death.[32-34]

due to either poor overall caloric intake or to chronic disease that predisposes to malnutrition. Additionally, in the postoperative period, many factors can lead to inadequate caloric intake and further compound impaired healing and immune response.

Indicators of malnutrition may include loss of 10% or more body weight over 6 months, a BMI of less than 22, and albumin levels of less than 3.0.[41] However, malnutrition may also occur in the absence of weight loss or low BMI. The Geriatric Nutritional Risk Index (GNRI) and Nutrition Risk Screen (NRS 2002) are suggested multifactor screening tools effective in identifying patient at risk for malnutrition.[42,43] The GNRI is shown to have predictive power for postoperative outcomes in several types of surgeries.[37]

When individuals with malnutrition or nutritional risk are identified, dietary interventions are often recommended prior to or after surgery.[1,41] Interventions may include referral to a registered dietician, oral nutrition supplementation (ONS), reduced duration of preoperative fasting, and early postoperative feeding.[1,41] ONS formulations are often high in protein and have been studied both independently prior to surgery and as part of multimodal prehabilitation interventions.[44] Overall, evidence supporting this practice is conflicting and often of poor quality. However, one meta-analysis found that, after hip fracture surgery, patients receiving ONS had decreased wound, respiratory, and urinary tract infections.[45] Other studies, though, show limited benefit for ONS in variety of surgeries.

SHARED DECISION-MAKING

One major purpose of the multidomain assessment of older adults is to gather the information necessary to communicate a realistic projection of short- and long-term impacts of surgery so that an individual can make an informed decision. When different aspects of the assessment are carried out by different clinicians, it is critical that there is effective communication among clinicians about perceived risks, benefits, concerns, and patient goals. It is the responsibility of the clinician engaging the patient in shared decision-making (SDM), be it the surgeon, internist/family physician, geriatrician, or anesthesiologist, to consolidate the input of the other team members.

Presenting an informed projection of surgical expectations and outcomes is one component of SDM. The second is eliciting the patient's overall healthcare goals. The success of either endeavor depends on optimal communication with the individual. Addressing hearing impairment with a voice amplifier or a speech impairment through written or visual aids are examples of simple interventions that greatly improve communication. Communication should be directed toward the individual, but family or caregivers should also be involved if appropriate. Extra time should be allotted when necessary.

The clinician engaging in SDM assists the patient in determining if expected outcomes are aligned with their own healthcare goals. The ACS NSQIP Surgical Risk Calculator is a web-based tool which projects postoperative complications, including those pertinent to older adults.[46] This type of data and questions in Table 11.3 can be helpful in guiding conversations around goals, understanding, and expectations to determine if these align with anticipated outcomes. There are also patient-facing resources, such as the Question Prompt List, that can help guide the preoperative discussion.[47] While older adults may take a variety of factors into account when making a serious medical decision, survival and self-sufficiency tend to be most highly valued.[48] In terms of specific communication techniques in exploratory discussions, best- and worst-case

Table 11.3 **KEY QUESTIONS FOR THE OLDER ADULT BEFORE SURGERY**

Understanding	Goals	Expectations and plans
What have you been told are the risks of surgery?	What are you hoping this surgery will do for you?	Where do you plan on going when you are ready to leave the hospital after surgery?
What are the likely benefits?	How would you feel about this surgery if it resulted in you no longer being able to live independently?	If you go directly home, what help would be available to you at home?
What is most likely to happen to you if you have this surgery?		
What is most likely to happen if you do not have this surgery?	How would you feel about this surgery if it didn't help you live longer?	

scenarios can help paint a picture of risks and benefits. In the setting of limited life expectancy, an individual may choose not to pursue a major surgery that could result in a complicated or prolonged recovery. Prognostic indices, such as those available on the online resource, ePrognosis, can help the clinician estimate and—if the patient desires—communicate average life expectancy.[49]

Illuminating healthcare goals and expectations may reveal that surgery is not likely to help an individual reach their goals. In this case, it is important that a decision *for or against* surgery is not the focus, but rather a decision between treatment options—each one with its own risks and benefits. If desired, the physician may share a recommendation, grounded in likely surgical outcomes and the individual's goals. Alternatives to surgery may include watchful waiting, less-invasive procedures, or rehabilitative therapy. Palliative care may be utilized both as an alternative or as an adjunct to surgery, particularly if life expectancy is limited.

ADVANCE CARE PLANNING

Advance care planning is a process that supports adults in making and sharing preferences for future medical care.[50] The prospect of surgery can serve as a reminder of the importance of such planning and the time leading up to surgery is an appropriate time to have a focused discussion about preferences and decision-making.

If they have not done so already, individuals should be asked to identify their preferred healthcare surrogate should they experience complications that render then unable to communicate after surgery. Clinicians should be aware of local state laws regarding surrogate designation. Many, but not all, states designate a default hierarchy of surrogates, which may or may not mirror the individual's preferences. In general, a written appointment of a durable power of attorney is required to override the default hierarchy. Completing advance directive paperwork is the most reliable way to appoint a surrogate decision maker. Advance directive forms must meet state-specific criteria to be valid and free and low-cost forms and patient-oriented materials are available from online resources.[51]

Depending on the perceived likelihood of adverse outcomes after surgery, the clinician may elicit the patient's preferences for care in certain circumstances and document these preferences in the medical record or advance directive and

Box 11.1 **QUESTIONS TO ASK ABOUT ADVANCE CARE PLANNING PRIOR TO SURGERY**

If you were too sick to make a medical decision for yourself after surgery, who would you trust to decide for you?

Have you told this person enough about your preferences so that they could make the decisions you would want them to make?

If you haven't already, would you like to fill out an advance directive naming _____ as your preferred decision-maker?

facilitate communication of those preferences with the individual's preferred surrogate decision-maker (see Box 11.1).

PREHABILITATION

Prehabilitation generally refers to an intervention that is aimed at improving health and fitness in advance of a stressor such as surgery. Prehabilitation may include cardiopulmonary exercises, balance and strengthening movements, nutritional supplements, cognitive exercises, and other interventions. To date, studies demonstrating positive effects of prehabilitation have been limited to a few surgical types. The strongest evidence for benefit is prior to joint replacement surgery. A 2016 meta-analysis summarized the findings of 22 studies, the majority of which evaluated physiotherapist-supervised exercise.[52] The studies suggested that prehabilitation may improve early postoperative pain and function. A 2023 meta-analysis included 48 studies for hip replacement, knee replacement, or lumbar surgery and included various exercise interventions prior to surgery.[53] The study suggested that prehabilitation interventions were associated with improved function 6 weeks after knee replacement and improved function 6 months after lumbar surgery.[53]

For other surgical types, evidence is more limited. A meta-analysis of prehabilitation interventions prior to abdominal surgery demonstrated that prehabilitation may reduce postoperative complications, particularly pulmonary complications, but not length of stay.[54] Before colorectal surgery, lower-intensity regimens may be more beneficial or have increased adherence, than higher-intensity regimens.[55] Also in this setting, resistance exercises, nutritional counseling, protein supplementation, and relaxation exercises were associated with improved 6-minute walk tests at four and eight weeks with low certainty of evidence.[56] Preoperative PT has been evaluated in a few studies prior to elective cardiac surgery.

The majority included inspiratory muscle training and found reduced pulmonary complications and length of stay.[57]

Before prehabilitation is widely prescribed in the preoperative setting, further research is required to outline the ideal components, timing and patient selection.[58] Preoperatively, the American Heart Association and Centers for Disease Control and Prevention recommendation of 150 minutes per week of moderate physical activity such as brisk walking may be reinforced—if this would represent a marked increase in activity for the individual, they may be counseled to gradually increase physical activity within the context of their comorbidities and physical ability. Referral to a PT and/or OT for optimization of specific impairments or education on anticipated physical decline after surgery may also be helpful.

MODELS OF PERIOPERATIVE CARE

Several care models have been specifically designed to meet the needs of high-risk older adults undergoing surgery. The Perioperative Optimization of Senior Health (POSH) includes a one-time interprofessional presurgical evaluation for high-risk older adults prior to elective surgery paired with postoperative geriatrics consultation. It has been shown to reduce complications and length of hospital stay and increase frequency of discharge to home.[13] Proactive care of older people undergoing surgery (POPS) is another model that pairs a preoperative, multiprofessional CGA with postoperative geriatric consultation.[59] It has been shown to reduce postoperative medical complications and length of hospital stay.[59] Given that these care models are not widely available, the ACS GSV recommends for any person who is identified as high risk based on the geriatric preoperative assessment that a case conference including a surgeon, anesthesiologist, geriatrician, nurse, and a case manager or social worker is held, an interdisciplinary treatment plan is created, and recommendations are communicated to the patient.

While POSH and POPS involve preoperative and postoperative interventions, there are other care models limited to the postoperative period. After hip fracture surgery, the geriatric co-management model has been shown to reduce length of hospital stay, postoperative complications, and mortality.[60–62] The Hospital Elder Life Program (HELP) is a multifaceted program that usually involves geriatric expertise and nursing interventions to reduce incidence of delirium in hospitalized adults. It the postoperative setting, a HELP that included daily orienting communication, oral and nutritional assistance, and early mobilization resulted in reduced delirium incidence and shorter length of hospital stay.[63]

Perioperative assessment of older adults is complex and requires a team-based approach. It is most likely to be effective when coupled with interventions in the pre-, intra-, and postoperative period to optimize outcomes. Implementation of tailored surgical care for older adults depends on the resources of a particular setting. While all older adults should receive the recommended assessments and focused interventions, when and from whom they receive such care will vary according to the institution.

CASE SUMMARY

Ideally, the patient in the case and his niece would have been provided with information necessary to make an informed decision immediately after his initial injury. The delay in surgery led to loss of function and was not in line with his goals. Fortunately, he was able to undergo the surgery later. Despite key interventions, he suffered delirium and resultant prolonged recovery. This emphasizes the importance of proactive discussions before surgery with patients, family, and/or caregivers. In the realm of elective surgery, it is easy to conceive of examples that would not so strongly favor surgery—such as limited life expectancy, high-risk surgery, and unclear benefit. Balancing the risks, which may include death, disability and institutionalization, with the most likely outcomes and the individuals' goals is key when coming to a shared decision about treatment.

CONCLUSION

- Older adults are more likely to have medical, functional, and psychosocial limitations that increase perioperative risk.

- Prior to elective surgery, national guidelines recommend a multidomain assessment of all older adults in addition to the standard preoperative evaluation.

- The evaluation should be tailored to the individual and to the surgery; in addition to a standard assessment, function, cognition, depressive symptoms, delirium risk, nutritional status and medications should be assessed

- Integration of frailty screening into the preoperative assessment may refine risk stratification and identify older adults who would benefit from a comprehensive geriatric assessment and/or prehabilitation strategies prior to surgery.

- Effective communication between clinicians involved in preoperative care is crucial.

- The clinician engaging in shared decision making must guide the patient in determining whether the surgery's likely outcomes are in line with the patient's healthcare goals.

- The preoperative setting provides an excellent opportunity for individuals to identify surrogate decision-makers and share their preferences for future care.

- For the average-risk older adult, risk reduction strategies may include physical and occupational therapy, delirium reduction techniques, medication adjustments, and anticipatory guidance.

- For high-risk older adults, perioperative care models shown to improve outcomes pair preoperative comprehensive geriatric assessment with postoperative geriatric consultation.

REVIEW QUESTIONS

1. A 65-year-old man with CAD, diabetes mellitus, OA, chronic pain, and hypertension is scheduled to undergo laparoscopic cholecystectomy. He smokes two packs per day and has three beers each night with dinner. What modifiable factors place him at higher risk for delirium in the perioperative period?

   a. Ongoing EtOH use.
   b. Tobacco use.
   c. Chronic opiate use.
   d. a and c.

   The correct answer is d.

   A focus on modifiable risk factors for delirium is critical to implement risk reduction strategies. Older patients who regularly drink alcohol or use opiates are at higher risk for delirium and, with ample time and encouragement, can convinced to reduce or eliminate use of both agents safely. While tobacco use places patients at higher risk for pulmonary complications and poor wound healing and should be reduced, it has no impact on delirium.

2. A 67-year-old woman with minimal past medical history is seen for preoperative evaluation prior to total hip replacement. During the evaluation, family members present describe worsening memory in the past 7 months, although she still performs all ADLs and IADLs independently. Following your exam, you perform a Mini-Cog where the patient draws a clock appropriately but is unable to recall any of the three words you gave her after 3 minutes. When a positive Mini-Cog screen is obtained at a perioperative visit, it should prompt *all* the following, *except*:

   a. Thorough review for unnecessary medications or those related to delirium risk.
   b. Delay of surgery.
   c. Longer cognitive screening tool (i.e., MMSE or MoCA).
   d. Discussion and education about postoperative delirium.

   The correct answer is b.

   This patient is undergoing an elective procedure and has a positive screen for possible cognitive impairment. While she is otherwise functional and living independently, cognitive impairment may place her at higher risk for postoperative complications such as delirium. In a multiethnic sample, it had a false positive rate of 17%.[17] Administration of a MMSE or MoCA may gather a more comprehensive picture of deficits. A delay in surgery is not necessary given that it would not be likely to change the risk of delirium. However, an individual and/or family may opt to forego surgery after learning about possible untoward postoperative outcomes.

3. An 82-year-old man with rheumatoid arthritis, mild cognitive impairment, COPD, and benign prostatic hypertrophy has severe urinary retention despite medical treatment. He performs intermittent clean catheterization four times daily, but this has become increasingly difficult with poor upper arm mobility. He is offered a chronic Foley, which will severely limit his mobility or to undergo an intermediate-risk transurethral prostate resection. In assessing his risk for the procedure, SDM is best represented by a discussion on

   a. Holding of immunomodulatory meds prior to surgery.
   b. Likelihood of major adverse cardiac events.
   c. Preferences around resuscitation and post-resuscitation measures.
   d. Best- and worst-case scenarios for procedure outcomes.

   The correct answer is d.

   This patient will need information to assist him in deciding about whether to continue nonoperative management for his urinary retention or have surgery. While instructions about his RA medication management and the absolute risk of cardiac events are important information, they are less likely to address whether his stated healthcare goals will be met with the given procedure. SDM can utilize best-/worst-case scenarios and should discuss preferences around healthcare surrogates and resuscitation preference. For this patient, discussion of benefits of being without a Foley and improved mobility versus postoperative course complicated by delirium, RA flare, and prolonged functional and/or cognitive decline would be an example of best- and worst-case scenarios. This would help delineate the importance of mobility in the patient's quality of life.

4. A 90-year-old woman with hypertension, chronic kidney disease stage 3, and diabetes mellitus is seen 2 days after an uncomplicated hemiarthroplasty following hip fracture. Her daughter, at the bedside, is concerned that she doesn't seem to be herself; she appears uninterested in lunch and appears drowsy. The nurse states that overnight she was awake and frequently calling for help. Which of the following is *not* a feature of delirium?

   a. Acute onset and fluctuating course.
   b. Altered level of consciousness.
   c. Inability to say the months of the year backward.
   d. Being unable to state the date.

   The correct answer is d.

   The Confusion Assessment Method (CAM) is validated tool for detecting delirium.[64] The key features are acute onset/fluctuating course and inattention plus either disorganized thinking or altered level of consciousness. Inattention can be detected if the individual is unable to say the months of the year backward. Inability to state the year or day of the week may be a sign of delirium if it represents a deviation from the individual's baseline; however, the date is generally not included in operational definitions.[65]

5. A 78-year-old man with end-stage renal disease on hemodialysis, diabetes mellitus on insulin, CAD s/p coronary artery bypass graft, alcohol use, frequent falls with limited mobility, and insecure housing is considering a lumbar decompression surgery for chronic sciatica. Which would be the best option for detecting frailty in this individual?

a. Comprehensive geriatric assessment.
   b. Frailty Index (Deficit Accumulation Index).
   c. Frailty Phenotype (Fried Index).
   d. Timed Up and Go.

The correct answer is a.

There is no gold standard for detecting frailty. Many frailty detection tools exist and are generally based on one of two conceptualizations of frailty: physical phenotype versus an accumulation of deficits. Some frailty detection tools, such as the Edmonton Frail Scale, draw directly from domains that would be assessed in a comprehensive geriatric assessment. The patient in question is clearly high risk for this elective surgery. The advantage of a comprehensive geriatric assessment is that it pairs an assessment with an integrated plan to optimize functioning and gives an opportunity to clarify goals of care.

6. A 74-year-old man with history of obesity, heart failure, chronic kidney disease stage 3, orthostatic hypotension, diabetes mellitus on insulin, insomnia and prostate cancer presents for evaluation prior to prostate resection. Which of the following is *least* important to consider when reviewing the medication list?

   a. Potentially inappropriate mediations (e.g., Beers list).
   b. Number of medications.
   c. Indication for each drug.
   d. Medications that are associated with delirium.

The correct answer is b.

While polypharmacy may trigger the clinician to be extra vigilant when reviewing the medication list, the number of medications is less important than each medication's potential harm given the individual's age (e.g., Beers list), interactions with other medications the individual is taking or will likely take perioperatively, delirium risk, and the necessity for each medication or supplement.

7. Following chemotherapy and radiation for pharyngeal squamous cell carcinoma, a 72-year-old man prepares for his upcoming surgical resection of tumor. Since his diagnosis 3 months ago, he has had a poor appetite, difficulty swallowing, and nausea due to pain medications. Which measures may indicate a state of malnutrition, and which evidence-based interventions should be recommended to improve outcomes?

   a. Weight loss of more than 5 lbs; high-fiber, low-fat diet in weeks prior to surgery.
   b. Albumin less than 4.0; high-caloric intake in weeks prior to surgery.
   c. Weight loss of greater than 15% over 3 months, albumin less than 3.0; protein-enriched diet in weeks prior to surgery.
   d. Geriatric Nutritional Risk Index (GNRI); preoperative carbohydrate load.

The correct answer is c.

Important indicators of malnutrition include weight loss of greater than 10–15%, albumin of less than 3.0, and BMI of less than 22 in older adults. These items are incorporated into several screening tools, including the GNRI. The data on preoperative dietary interventions that improve outcomes are mixed. However, a consensus exists for recommending high-protein diets 10–14 days prior to surgery for undernourished patients. Preoperative carbohydrate loads have been studied with variable success through the Enhanced Recovery After Surgery protocol, but a Cochrane review did not demonstrate improved postoperative outcomes.[66]

8. Which of the following is true for prehabilitation?

   a. It refers to a standard set of interventions prior to surgery.
   b. Rigorous physical activity is likely better than moderate.
   c. It has primarily been studied before colorectal and orthopedic surgeries.
   d. It is currently recommended for all high-risk patients before elective surgery.

The correct answer is c.

Prehabilitation refers to a variety of different interventions that usually include a component of physical activity. It has largely been studied prior to colorectal and orthopedic surgeries. While some evidence supports the role of prehabilitation in enhanced recovery of physical function, further evidence is needed before it is widely recommended.

REFERENCES

1. Chow WB, Rosenthal RA, Merkow RP, et al. Optimal preoperative assessment of the geriatric surgical patient: A best practices guideline from the American College of Surgeons National Surgical Quality Improvement Program and the American Geriatrics Society. *J Am Coll Surg.* 2012;215:453–466. doi:10.1016/j.jamcollsurg.2012.06.017
2. Turrentine FE, Wang H, Simpson VB, Jones RS. Surgical risk factors, morbidity, and mortality in elderly patients. *J Am Coll Surg.* 2006;203:865–877. doi:10.1016/j.jamcollsurg.2006.08.026
3. Gajdos C, Kile D, Hawn MT, et al. Advancing age and 30-day adverse outcomes after nonemergent general surgeries. *J Am Geriatri Soc.* 2013;61:1608–1614. doi:10.1111/jgs.12401
4. Tang VL, Jing, B, Boscardin J, et al. Association of functional, cognitive and psychological measures with 1-year mortality in patients undergoing major surgery. *JAMA Surg.* 2020;155:412–418. doi:10.1001/jamasurg.2020.00915
5. Culley DJ, Flaherty D, Fahey MC, et al. Poor performance on a preoperative cognitive screening test predicts postoperative complications in older orthopedic surgical patients. *Anesthesiology.* 2017;127:765–774. doi:10.1097/ALN.0000000000001859
6. Mahanna-Gabrielli E, Zhang K, Sieber FE, et al. Frailty is associated with postoperative delirium but not with postoperative cognitive decline in noncardiac surgery patients. *Anesth Analg.* 2020;130:1516–1523. doi:10.1213/ANE.0000000000004773
7. Tang VL, Cenzer I, McCulloch CE, et al. Preoperative depressive symptoms associated with poor functional recovery after surgery. *J Am Geriatri Soc.* 2020;68:2814–2821. doi:https://doi.org/10.1111/jgs.16781
8. Gill TM, Vander Wyk B, Leo-Summers L, et al. Population-based estimates of 1-year mortality after major surgery among community-living older US adults. *JAMA Surg.* 2022;157:e225155. doi:10.1001/jamasurg.2022.5155
9. Mohanty S, Rosenthal RA, Russell MM, et al. Optimal perioperative management of the geriatric patient: A best practices guideline from the American College of Surgeons NSQIP and the American

Geriatrics Society. *J Am Coll Surg*. 2016;222:930–947. doi:10.1016/j.jamcollsurg.2015.12.026

10. Stuck AE, Siu AL, Wieland GD, et al. Comprehensive geriatric assessment: A meta-analysis of controlled trials. *Lancet*. 1993;342:1032–1036. doi:10.1016/0140-6736(93)92884-v

11. Ellis G, Gardner M, Tsiachristas, et al. Comprehensive geriatric assessment for older adults admitted to the hospital. *Cochrane Database Syst Rev*. 2017;9:CD006211. doi:10.1002/14651858.CD006211.pub3

12. Kim KI, Park KH, Koo KH, et al. Comprehensive geriatric assessment can predict postoperative morbidity and mortality in elderly patients undergoing elective surgery. *Arch Gerontol Geriatr*. 2013;56:507–512. doi:10.1016/j.archger.2012.09.002

13. McDonald SR, Heflin MT, Whitson HE, et al. Association of integrated care coordination with postsurgical outcomes in high-risk older adults the Perioperative Optimization of Senior Health (POSH) initiative. *JAMA Surg*. 2018;153:454–462. doi:10.1001/jamasurg.2017.5513

14. Katz S, Ford AB, Moskowitz RW, et al. Studies of illness in the aged: The index of ADL: A standardized measure of biological and psychosocial function. *JAMA*. 1963;185:914–919. doi:10.1001/jama.1963.03060120024016

15. Lawton MP, Brody EM. Assessment of older people: Self-maintaining and instrumental activities of daily living. *Gerontologist*. 1969;9:179–186. doi:10.1093/geront/9.3_Part_1.179

16. Culley DJ, F. D., Reddy S, et al. Preoperative cognitive stratification of older elective surgical patients: A cross-sectional study. *Anesth Analg*. 2016;123:186–192, doi:10.1213/ANE.0000000000001277

17. Borson S, Scanlan J, Brush M, et al. The Mini-Cog: A cognitive "vital signs" measure for dementia screening in multi-lingual elderly. *Int J Geriatri Psychiatry*. 2000;15:1021–1027, doi:10.1002/1099-1166(200011)15:11<1021::aid-gps234>3.0.co;2-6

18. Doering LV, Moser DK, Lemankiewicz W, et al. Depression, healing and recovery from coronary artery bypass surgery. *Am J Crit Care*. 2005;14:316–324. doi:https://doi.org/10.4037/ajcc2005.14.4.316

19. Falk A, Kåhlin J, Nymark C, et al. Depression as a predictor of postoperative delirium after cardiac surgery: A systematic review and meta-analysis. *Interactive Cardiovasc Thorac Surg*. 2021;32:371–379. doi:https://doi.org/10.1093/icvts/ivaa277

20. American Geriatrics Society. 2023 updated AGS Beers Criteria® for potentially inappropriate medication use in older adults. *J Am Geriatri Soc*. 2023. doi:https://doi.org/10.1111/jgs.18372

21. Secora A, Alexander GC, Ballew SH, et al. Kidney function, polypharmacy, and potentially inappropriate medication use in a community-based cohort of older adults. *Drugs Aging*. 2018;35(8):735–750. doi:30039344; PMCID: PMC6093216

22. Nightingale G, Skonecki E, Boparai MK. The impact of polypharmacy on patient outcomes in older adults with cancer. *Cancer J*. 2017;23:211–218. doi:10.1097/PPO.0000000000000277

23. Fried LP, Tangen CM, Walston J. Frailty in older adults: Evidence for a phenotype. *J Gerontol A Biol Sci Med Sci*. 2001;56:146–156. doi:10.1093/gerona/56.3.m146

24. Mitnitski AB, Mogilner AJ, Rockwood K. Accumulation of deficits as a proxy measure of aging. *Sci World J*. 2001;1:323–336. doi:10.1100/tsw.2001.58

25. Makary MA, Segev DL, Pronovost PJ. Frailty as a predictor of surgical outcomes in older patients. *J Am Coll Surg*. 2010;219:901–908. doi:10.1016/j.jamcollsurg.2010.01.028

26. Dasgupta M, Rolfson D, Stolee P. Frailty is associated with postoperative complications in older adults with medical problems. *Arch Gerontol Geriatr*. 2009;48:78–83. doi:10.1016/j.archger.2007.10.007

27. Robinson TN, Wu DS, Sauaia A, et al. Slower walking speed forecasts increased postoperative morbidity and 1-year mortality across surgical specialties. *Ann Surg*. 2013;258:582–588. doi:10.1097/SLA.0b013e3182a4e96c

28. Robinson TN, Eiseman B, Wallace JI, et al. Redefining geriatric preoperative assessment using frailty, disability and co-morbidity. *Ann Surg*. 2009;250:449–455. doi:10.1097/SLA.0b013e3181b45598

29. Robinson TN, Wallace JI, Wu DS, et al. Accumulated frailty characteristics predict postoperative discharge institutionalization in the geriatric patient. *J Amm Coll Sug*. 2011;213:37–42. doi:10.1016/j.jamcollsurg.2011.01.056

30. Lin HS, Watts JN, Peel NM, Hubbard RE. Frailty and post-operative outcomes in older surgical patients: A systematic review. *BMC Geriatr*. 2016;16:157. doi:10.1186/s12877-016-0329-8

31. McIsaac DI, Taljaard M, Bryson GL, et al. Frailty as a predictor of death or new disability after surgery: A prospective cohort study. *Ann Surg*. 2020;271:283–289. doi:10.1097/SLA.0000000000002967

32. Shah R, Attwood K, Arya S, et al. Association of frailty with failure to rescue after low-risk and high-risk inpatient surgery. *JAMA Surg*. 2018;153:e180214. doi:10.1001/jamasurg.2018.0214

33. Hall DE, Arya S, Schmid KK, et al. Development and initial validation of the Risk Analysis Index for measuring frailty in surgical populations. *JAMA Surg*. 2017;152:175–182. doi:10.1001/jamasurg.2016.4202

34. George EL, Hall DE, You A, et al. Association between patient frailty and postoperative mortality across multiple noncardiac surgical specialties. *JAMA Surg*. 2021;156:e20512. doi:10.1001/jamasurg.2020.5152

35. Alvarez-Nebreda ML, Bentov N, Urman RD, et al. Recommendations for preoperative management of frailty from the Society for Perioperative Assessment and Quality Improvement (SPAQI). *J Clin Anesth*. 2018;47:33–42. doi:10.1016/j.jclinane.2018.02.011

36. Alazawi W, Pirmadjid N, Lahiri R, et al. Inflammatory and immune response to surgery and their clinical impact. *Ann Surg*. 2016;264:73–80. doi:10.1097/SLA.0000000000001691

37. Kushiyama S, Sakurai K, Kubo N, et al. The preoperative Geriatric Nutritional Risk Index predicts postoperative complications in elderly patients with gastric cancer undergoing gastrectomy. *In Vivo*. 2018;32:1667–1672. doi:10.21873/invivo.11430

38. Yeh DD, Fuentes E, Quraishi SA, et al. Adequate nutrition may get you home: Effect of caloric/protein deficits on the discharge destination of critically ill surgical patients. *J Parenter Enteral Nutr*. 2016;40(1):37–44. doi:10.1177/0148607115585142.

39. Bachrach-Lindström M, Johansson T, Unosson M, Ek AC, et al. Nutritional status and functional capacity after femoral neck fractures: A prospective randomized one-year follow-up study. *Aging*. 2000;12:366–374. doi:10.1007/BF03339862

40. Kaiser MJ, Bauer JM, Rämsch C, et al. Mini Nutritional Assessment International Group. Frequency of malnutrition in older adults: A multinational perspective using the mini nutritional assessment. *J Am Geriatri Soc*. 2010;58:1734–1738. doi:10.1111/j.1532-5415.2010.03016

41. Weimann A, Braga M, Carli F, et al. ESPEN guideline: Clinical nutrition in surgery. *Clin Nutr*. 2017;36:623–650. doi:10.1016/j.clnu.2017.02.013

42. Bouillanne O, Morineau G, Dupont C, et al. Geriatric Nutritional Risk Index: A new index for evaluating at-risk elderly medical patients. *Am J Clin Nutr*. 2005;82:777–783. doi:10.1093/ajcn/82.4.777

43. Kondrup J, Rasmussen HH, Hamberg O, et al. Nutritional risk screening (NRS 2002): A new method based on an analysis of controlled clinical trials. *Clin Nutr*. 2003;22:321–336. doi:10.1016/s0261-5614(02)00214-5

44. Gillis C, Li C, Lee L, et al. Prehabilitation versus rehabilitation: A randomized control trial in patients undergoing colorectal resection for cancer. *Anesthesiology*. 2014;121:9370947. doi:10.1097/ALN.0000000000000393

45. Liu M, Yang J, Yu X, et al. The role of perioperative oral nutritional supplementation in elderly patients after hip surgery. *Clin Interv Aging*. 2015;19:849–858. doi:10.2147/CIA.S74951

46. Hornor MA, Meixi M, Zhou L, et al. Enhancing the American College of Surgeons NSQIP surgical risk calculator to predict geriatric outcomes. *J Am Coll Surg*. 2020;230:88. doi:10.1016/j.jamcollsurg.2019.09017

47. Steffens NM, Tulchoka J, Nabozny MJ, et al. Engaging patients, health care professionals, and community members to improve preoperative

decision making for older adults facing high-risk surgery. *JAMA Surg.* 2016;151:938–945. doi:10.1001/jamasurg.2016.1308

48. Petrillo LA, McMahan R, Tang V, et al. Older adult and surrogate perspectives on serious, difficult, and important medical decisions. *J Am Geriatri Soc.* 2018;66:1515–1523. doi:10.1111/jgs.15426

49. Yourman LC, Lee SJ, Schonberg MA, et al. Prognostic indices for older adults: A systematic review. *JAMA.* 2012;307(2):182–192. doi:10.1001/jama.2011.1966

50. Sudore RL, Lum HD, You JJ, et al. Defining advance care planning for adults: A consensus definition from a multidisciplinary delphi panel. *Pain Symptom Manage.* 2017;54:821–832.e821. doi:10.1016/j.jpainsymman.2016.12.331

51. Freytag J, Street RL, Barnes DE, et al. Empowering older adults to discuss advance care planning during clinical visits: The PREPARE randomized trial. *J Am Geriatr Soc.* 2020;68:1210–1217. doi:10.1111/jgs.16405

52. Wang L, Lee M, Zhang Z, et al. Does preoperative rehabilitation for patients planning to undergo joint replacement surgery improve outcomes? A systematic review and meta-analysis of randomised controlled trials. *BMJ Open.* 2016;e009857. doi:10.1136/bmjopen-2015-009857

53. Punnoose A, Claydon-Mueller LS, Weiss O, et al. Prehabilitation for patients undergoing orthopedic surgery: A systematic review and meta-analysis. *JAMA Netw Open.* 2023;6. doi:10.1001/jamanetworkopen.2023.8050

54. Moran J, Guinan E, McCormick P, et al. The ability of prehabilitation to influence postoperative outcome after intra-abdominal operation: A systematic review and meta-analysis. *Surgery.* 2016;160:1189–1201. doi:10.1016/j.surg.2016.05.014

55. Carli F, Charlebois P, Stein B, et al. Randomized clinical trial of prehabilitation in colorectal surgery. *Br J Surg.* 2010;97:1187–1197. doi:10.1002/bjs.7102

56. Molenaar CJL, van Rooijen SJ, Fokkenrood JHP, et al. Prehabilitation versus no prehabilitation to improve functional capacity, reduce postoperative complications and improve quality of life in colorectal cancer surgery. *Cochrane Database Syst Rev.* 2022;5:CD013259. doi:10.1002/14651858.CD013259.pub2

57. Hulzebos EH, Smit Y, Helders PP, van Meeteren NL. Preoperative physical therapy for elective cardiac surgery patients. *Cochrane Database Syst Rev.* 2012;11:CD010118. doi:10.1002/14651858.CD010118.pub2

58. McIsaac DI, Gill M, Boland L, et al. Prehabilitation in adult patients undergoing surgery: An umbrella review of systematic reviews. *Br J Anaesth.* 2022;128:244–257. doi: 10.1016/j.bja.2021.11.014

59. Harari D, Hopper A, Dhesi J, et al. Proactive care of older people undergoing surgery ("POPS"): Designing, embedding, evaluating and funding a comprehensive geriatric assessment service for older elective surgical patients. *Age Ageing.* 2007;36(2):190–196. doi:10.1093/ageing/afl163

60. Friedman SM, Mendelson DA, Bingham KW, Kates SL. Impact of a comanaged geriatric fracture center on short-term hip fracture outcomes. *Arch Intern Med.* 2009;169:1712–1717. doi:10.1001/archinternmed.2009.321

61. Vidán M, Serra JA, Moreno C, Riquelme G, Ortiz J. Efficacy of a comprehensive geriatric intervention in older patients hospitalized for hip fracture: A randomized, controlled trial. *J Am Geriatri Soc.* 2005;53:1476–1482. doi:10.1111/j.1532-5415.2005.53466.x

62. Grigoryan KV, Javedan H, Rudolph JL. Orthogeriatric care models and outcomes in hip fracture patients: A systematic review and meta-analysis. *J Orthop Trauma.* 2014;28:e49–55. doi:10.1097/BOT.0b013e3182a5a045

63. Chen CC, Li H-C, Liang JT, et al. Effect of a modified hospital elder life program on delirium and length of hospital stay in patients undergoing abdominal surgery: A cluster randomized clinical trial. *JAMA Surg.* 2017;152:827–834. doi:10.1001/jamasurg.2017.1083

64. Inouye SK, van Dyck. C, Alessi CA, et al. Clarifying confusion: The confusion assessment method. A new method for detection of delirium. *Ann Intern Med.* 1990;113:941–948. doi:10.7326/0003-4819-113-12-941

65. Marcantonio ER, Ngo LH, O'Connor M, et al. 3D-CAM: Derivation and validation of a 3-minute diagnostic interview for CAM-defined delirium: A cross-sectional diagnostic test study. *Ann Intern Med.* 2014;161:554–561. doi:10.7326/M14-0865

66. Smith MD, McCall J, Plank L, et al. Preoperative carbohydrate treatment for enhancing recovery after elective surgery. *Cochrane Database Syst Rev.* 2014;8. doi:10.1002/14651858.CD009161.pub2

PART III

ORGAN SYSTEMS

CARDIAC

12.

AHA GUIDELINES APPLICATION

Samuel Papke, Michael Benson, and Joshua Zimmerman

STEM CASE AND KEY QUESTIONS

A 75-year-old man presents for evaluation in the preoperative clinic 1 week before a radical prostatectomy for prostate cancer. He has a history of hypertension, hyperlipidemia, and coronary artery disease (CAD). He had a drug-eluting stent (DES) placed 7 months ago after a positive stress test and cardiac catheterization. He has no allergies and is currently on metoprolol, lisinopril, atorvastatin, aspirin, and clopidogrel. While you are preparing to see the patient, the surgeon calls to ask whether the patient is "cleared" for prostatectomy or whether additional evaluation is needed.

Should the patient proceed with prostatectomy? What are the decision-making steps in assessing perioperative cardiac risk and need for further testing?

The surgeon states that the patient should proceed with the prostatectomy as soon as possible.

What is the distinction between emergent, urgent, time-sensitive, and elective cases? What type of procedure is this patient's prostatectomy?

You clarify that his procedure is not urgent, and, if you discover any concerning findings, his surgery may need to be postponed.

How would you quantify this patient's cardiac risk for the prostatectomy? Are there any tools to help decide risk? How is functional capacity quantified?

You tell the surgeon that, assuming there are no new symptoms and the patient reports "good" functional capacity, you recommend proceeding. The surgeon asks whether the patient should have another stress test prior to the procedure.

What are indications for preoperative cardiac testing, and how would you decide what test and when is it indicated?

As a last question, the surgeon asks for your recommendations regarding the patient's clopidogrel and aspirin.

What are the current guidelines regarding cessation of dual antiplatelet therapy (DAPT) for patients with cardiac stents undergoing noncardiac surgery? Do the recommendations differ if stents were placed in the setting of an acute coronary syndrome versus stable ischemic heart disease (SIHD)?

As you interview the patient, he reports significant dyspnea on exertion and lightheadedness while walking across his living room. He states that he passed out last week while walking his dog. He says that 3 months ago, he could slowly walk up a flight of stairs, but now he is no longer able to do this. He denies orthopnea.

During the physical examination, you discover a harsh, holosystolic murmur best heard at the right upper sternal border that radiates to his carotid arteries bilaterally and which decreases in intensity with Valsalva maneuver. The carotid pulse has a slow sustained upstroke. His lungs are clear to auscultation, and he has no lower extremity edema.

You are concerned about these findings and discuss them with the surgeon. The surgeon shares your concern, particularly given the magnitude of the case and the potential for significant blood loss. You suggest further evaluation prior to proceeding with the surgery and that the case be delayed until the evaluation is complete. Given the nonemergent nature of the case, the surgeon agrees.

You proceed to perform a point-of-care ultrasound (POCUS). Your imaging reveals normal biventricular systolic function, severe concentric left ventricular hypertrophy, significant aortic valve calcification, and limited excursion of the aortic valve leaflets. There are no other significant valvular abnormalities (Figure 12.1).

What are the signs and symptoms of aortic stenosis? What is the gold standard for diagnosis of aortic stenosis?

After your POCUS exam, you refer the patient for a formal transthoracic echocardiogram. The results of the echocardiogram show that the mean gradient across the aortic valve is 46 mm Hg and the aortic valve area is calculated to be 0.89 cm^2.

What are the echocardiographic criteria for severe aortic stenosis?

You discuss with the patient and the surgeon his diagnosis of severe aortic stenosis and review his options.

According to the ACC/AHA guidelines, what are the options prior to this surgery for a patient with severe aortic stenosis?

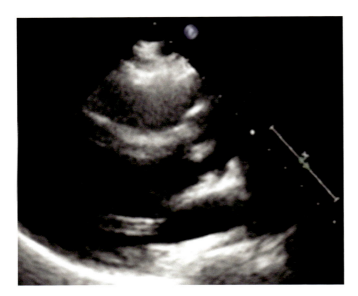

Figure 12.1 Representative transthoracic echocardiographic image of a patient with severe aortic stenosis. Sclero-calcification of the aortic valve in the parasternal long axis view.

The patient discusses the risks, benefits, and alternatives with his family, the surgeon, and his oncologist. He decides that he will delay the surgery for an aortic valve replacement. You discuss this with the surgeon and consult the cardiology and cardiothoracic surgical teams.

Given his surgical risk and the time constraint for his prostatectomy, he is scheduled for transcatheter aortic valve replacement (TAVR) later that week. Fortunately, you are scheduled to care for the patient on the day of his TAVR.

What are the hemodynamic goals during induction and maintenance of anesthesia for this patient?

The TAVR procedure goes well. The patient spends 1 night in the ICU for additional monitoring and is discharged to home on postoperative day 2.

He returns for prostatectomy 4 weeks later. Again, you are scheduled to take care of him. His exercise tolerance has significantly improved, and a repeat echocardiogram reveals a transcatheter valve in the aortic position that is well seated with normal opening and no evidence of paravalvular leak or stenosis. He is pleased with his decision and is now ready to undergo his prostatectomy.

What are the indications for subacute bacterial endocarditis prophylaxis in a patient with a bioprosthetic valve?

The prostatectomy proceeds without incident and the patient tolerates it well. He spends 2 nights in the ICU and is discharged home on postoperative day 5.

DISCUSSION

The American College of Cardiology and the American Heart Association (ACC/AHA) have published numerous guidelines, several of which apply to patients undergoing major noncardiac surgery. This discussion focuses on the application of these guidelines in the perioperative period.

CORONARY ARTERY DISEASE

CAD is commonly seen in our surgical population. Annually, up to 40% of surgical patients in the United States will either have or be at risk for CAD.[1] Myocardial ischemia is caused by an imbalance of oxygen supply and oxygen demand, which can result from CAD. Heart rate (HR), wall tension, and contractility are the primary determinants of myocardial oxygen demand, of which HR is the principal consideration. As HR increases, there is increased oxygen demand and a decrease in oxygen delivery secondary to decreased diastolic perfusion time of the diseased coronary arteries which have decreased flow.[2]

PERIOPERATIVE TESTING ALGORITHM FOR PATIENTS UNDERGOING NONCARDIAC SURGERY

According to the 2014 ACC/AHA guideline on perioperative cardiovascular evaluation and management of patients undergoing non-cardiac surgery, the steps to determine if further testing is indicated are[3]:

1. Is the surgery emergent?
2. Does the patient have an acute coronary syndrome (ACS)?
3. What is the patient's risk of major adverse cardiac event (MACE) for the proposed procedure (low <1% vs. elevated >1%)?
4. What is the patient's functional capacity?
5. Is there additional cardiac testing indicated?

DEFINITION OF SURGICAL URGENCY

An emergent case is defined as life- or limb-threatening if not in the operating room within less than 6 hours. There is limited or no time for preoperative evaluation. An urgent case is defined as life- or limb-threatening if not in the operating room within 6–24 hours. There is typically time for a limited preoperative evaluation. A time-sensitive case is defined as one in which a delay of up to 6 weeks will not negatively affect the outcome. Oncologic procedures typically to fall into this category. An elective case is one that could be delayed up to 1 year without negatively affecting outcomes.[3]

DEFINITION OF COMBINED MEDICAL/SURGICAL RISK FOR A PROPOSED PROCEDURE

In the previous version of the ACC/AHA guidelines (2007) as well as in the current European Society of Cardiology[4] guidelines, surgical risk is assessed separately from medical risk. Traditionally, low-risk procedures have a less than 1% risk of MACE (which is defined as non-fatal stroke, non-fatal MI or death), while procedures such as open aortic aneurysm replacement, esophagectomy, lung transplant, and high fluid shift procedures portend a high risk (>5%). Most procedures have an intermediate risk of 1–5%.[5]

Historically, patient's medical risk has been quantified using the Revised Cardiac Risk Index (RCRI), which includes five comorbidities: CAD, congestive heart failure (CHF), cerebrovascular disease (CVD), chronic renal failure (CRF) with a creatinine level of greater than 2 mg/dL, and diabetes on insulin treatment. It also considers elevated risk surgery such as an intraperitoneal, intrathoracic, or suprainguinal vascular surgery.[6]

The current 2014 ACC/AHA guidelines endorse assessing a combined medical and surgical risk of MACE (low <1% vs. elevated >1%). This could be derived either by multiplying the surgical risk with the medical one or using a separate, comprehensive tool such as the American College of Surgeons National Surgical Quality Improvement (ACS-NSQIP) calculator.[7]

Regardless of approach, a validated risk prediction tool should be used to predict the risk of perioperative MACE in patients undergoing non-cardiac surgery.[7] In addition to the RCRI and the ACS-NSQIP calculator, the NSQIP-Myocardial Infarction or Cardiac Arrest (MICA) calculator can be used. Finally, the newest risk calculator, published in 2019, is the American University of Beirut (AUB)-HAS2 Cardiovascular Risk index, which predicts 30-day stroke, myocardial infarction (MI) or death of patients undergoing non-cardiac surgery. It incorporates six elements: age older than 75, anemia with hemoglobin of less than 12, history of heart disease, active angina or dyspnea, vascular surgery, and surgical urgency (elective vs. emergency).[8] Each calculator has been validated, though they vary and have their own limitations.[9] Ongoing studies continue to validate these tools and consider other components such as monitoring of biomarkers like N-terminal pro-B-type natriuretic peptide (NT-proBNP) or troponins to further refine their predictive value in identifying high-risk patients.[10] In the most recent 2022 ESC guidelines, they recommend (Class I) obtaining troponins and NT-proBNP for high-risk patients or consider (Class IIa) obtaining in those undergoing intermediate- or high-risk surgery both preoperatively and trending at 24 and 48 hours. This improves the diagnosis of unrecognized heart failure and allows for more accurate diagnosis of perioperative MI.[5]

FUNCTIONAL CAPACITY

Functional capacity is an independent predictor of perioperative cardiac events and is described in terms of metabolic equivalents (METs).[11] One MET is the basal oxygen consumption of a 40-year-old, 70 kg male. When patients are unable to achieve 4 METs of work, perioperative morbidity and mortality are increased.[3]

Traditionally, functional capacity has been assessed by subjective estimates based on activities of daily living.[12] Activities that are associated with more than 4 METS include climbing one flight of stairs, walking up a hill, walking on level ground at 4 miles per hour, or performing "heavy work" around the house.[3]

More recently, studies demonstrated that subjective assessment of functional capacity does not accurately identify patients at risk for perioperative morbidity and mortality.[11–3] A recent multicenter prospective cohort study examined death or other complications following major elective non-cardiac surgery. It compared preoperative subjective assessment with alternative markers of fitness including cardiopulmonary exercise testing (CPET), scores on the Duke Activity Status Index (DASI) questionnaire, and NT pro-BNP. It was found that only the DASI scores were associated with predicting death or MI within 30 days after surgery. Consequently, physicians should consider validated objective measures, including DASI scores, when assessing functional capacity for the purpose of predicting perioperative risk.[4,11]

PREOPERATIVE CARDIAC TESTING

Preoperative cardiac testing can include 12-lead ECG, the assessment of left ventricular (LV) systolic function via echocardiography, exercise or pharmacologic stress testing, and coronary angiography. The recommendations and level of evidence for each recommendation differ depending on the specific clinical scenario. There is no benefit (Class III recommendation) for the *routine* use of any of these tests.[3]

Per the 2014 ACC/AHA algorithm, if a patient is identified with elevated risk of MACE and has unknown or poor functional capacity (<4 METS), then further cardiac testing is warranted. However, it should be determined with the patient and surgical team whether further testing will change perioperative management and if the patient would be willing to undergo coronary artery bypass graft (CABG) surgery or percutaneous coronary intervention (PCI) if CAD is identified. At minimum, in those with known cardiac disease, it is reasonable (Class IIa) to obtain a 12-lead ECG to establish a baseline against which to monitor changes.[3]

Second, it is reasonable (Class IIa) to evaluate patients with dyspnea on exertion of unknown origin or those with heart failure with any change in clinical status by transthoracic echocardiography (TTE) to evaluate their LV function. It should be considered (Class IIb) to reassess those with established LV dysfunction if there is no echocardiographic evaluation in the past year.[3] Diminished LV function of less than 30% is an independent risk factor for perioperative cardiac events and long-term mortality.[14]

Additionally, exercise testing should be considered in those with unknown or poor (<4 METs) functional status. Simple ECG stress testing can identify ischemic changes and provide an understanding of functional status in ambulatory patients. In most patients, stress echocardiography is the preferred modality, especially those with resting ECG characteristics that impair diagnostic interpretation (e.g., left bundle branch block), with concomitant valvular abnormalities, or concern for LV dysfunction.[3] If patients are indicated for stress testing and unable to achieve their maximal cardiopulmonary effort secondary to physical limitations (e.g., severe hip osteoarthritis), then dobutamine stress echo (DSE) or myocardial perfusion imaging (MPI) is the alternative in risk assessment.[3]

The goal is to identify inducible ischemia which could be revascularized or, at minimum, to risk stratify patients with at-risk myocardium and help to modify anesthetic plans. Dobutamine should be avoided in patients with uncontrolled severe hypertension, recent MI (<48 hours), severe symptomatic arrhythmias, hypertrophic obstructive cardiomyopathy (HOCM), unstable angina, and aortic dissection. MPI should be avoided in patients with severe bronchospasm, caffeine intake in prior 24 hours, hypotension (SBP <90 mmHg), and pregnancy. Coronary computed tomography angiography (CCTA) seems to be excellent noninvasive alternative to coronary angiography, and it is recommended in the 2022 ESC guidelines.[5] CCTA should be considered to rule out CAD in patients with suspected chronic coronary syndrome or biomarker-negative ACS in cases of low to intermediate clinical likelihood of CAD, or in patients unsuitable for noninvasive functional testing undergoing non-urgent, intermediate-, and high-risk non-cardiac surgery.[5]

Last, if inducible ischemia is discovered, coronary angiography and revascularization can be considered. The decision for this depends on risks of revascularization, risk of delaying the surgery, and risks of proceeding with surgery without revascularization. Careful consideration should be paid to PCI, placement of stents, and the need for DAPT and its interaction with the intended non-cardiac surgery. Routine revascularization of stable CAD is not recommended (Class III) prior to non-cardiac surgery to reduce perioperative events.[15]

DUAL ANTIPLATELET THERAPY

The 2016 ACC/AHA guidelines first differentiate between patients that underwent PCI for SIHD or for an ACS.[16,17] ACS are defined as ST elevation myocardial infarction (STEMI), non-ST elevation myocardial infarction (NSTEMI), and unstable angina.[18]

Multiple randomized controlled trials have compared a shorter duration (3–6 months) of DAPT with 12 months of DAPT.[19-22] These trials mainly enrolled non-ACS patients. The shorter duration DAPT had no increased risk of in-stent thrombosis and fewer bleeding complications when using newer-generation DES.[16,17,23,24]

Per ACC/AHA guideline, it is indicated (Class I) that DAPT should be continued for 6 months for a DES placed for SIHD. It should be discontinued if there is a high risk of bleeding. If the DES was placed for a STEMI, DAPT should (Class I) be continued for 12 months; however, it may be reasonable (Class IIb) to discontinue DAPT after 6 months if there is a high risk of bleeding. All elective non-cardiac surgery should optimally be delayed 12 months from the implantation of a DES.[16,17]

In the case of time-sensitive non-cardiac surgery, placement of a DES and compliance with DAPT could pose problems. Alternatives include balloon angioplasty and bare metal stent (BMS) placement. Those who undergo balloon angioplasty should have their non-cardiac surgery delayed a minimum of 14 days after their PCI. DES is preferred over BMS due to their decreased re-thrombosis risk. Historically, the advantage of BMS is that DAPT may be discontinued at 1 month compared to 6 months for DES.[16,17] However, with newer-generation DES, the current ESC guidelines only recommend (Class I) a minimum of 1-month delay for time-sensitive non-cardiac surgery. In high-risk patients (e.g., proximal left anterior descending [LAD] or left main (LM) bifurcated stent) with recent DES, the ECS advises considering a 3-month delay (Class IIa) before time-sensitive non-cardiac surgery.[5] In the setting of cardiac stents, except in cases of extremely high-risk bleeding—that is, major intracranial surgery—aspirin is typically continued through the perioperative period while the $P2Y_{12}$ inhibitor is held.[25]

Careful risk-benefit analysis of the risk of ischemia, bleeding risk, complications of delay, and other patient comorbidities must be accounted for when deciding plans for revascularization as well as continuation or discontinuation of DAPT.

AORTIC STENOSIS

A systolic murmur can be indicative of aortic stenosis, mitral regurgitation, pulmonic stenosis, tricuspid regurgitation, an innocent murmur, a flow murmur, an atrial septal defect (ASD), a dynamic outflow tract obstruction, or a ventricular septal defect (VSD). Historically, severe aortic stenosis was associated with a perioperative mortality of up to 13%.[26] However, today, the 30-day mortality rate for patients with moderate to severe aortic stenosis undergoing surgery is 2.1% compared to 1.0% in propensity-matched patients without aortic stenosis.[27] In emergency surgery, mortality was significantly increased in patients with aortic stenosis, especially if these patients were symptomatic.[28]

The classic triad of symptoms associated with aortic stenosis includes dyspnea on exertion, syncope, and angina.[29] Many patients who meet criteria for severe aortic stenosis remain asymptomatic given that the criteria are highly sensitive to identify patients who may benefit from intervention.

On physical exam, you will find a low volume and slow-rising carotid pulse and a loud mid- to late-peaking harsh systolic murmur heard best in the in the right second intercostal space that radiates to the carotid arteries.[29]

DIAGNOSIS OF VALVULAR DISEASE

TTE is the standard diagnostic test in the initial evaluation of known or suspected valvular heart disease (VHD), including aortic stenosis. TTE confirms the diagnosis, establishes the etiology, determines the severity of the lesion, assesses the hemodynamic consequences, and evaluates for the timing of interventions. Cardiac catheterization for hemodynamic assessment is recommended for symptomatic patients when TTE is inconclusive or when there is a discrepancy in findings between noninvasive testing and physical exam with regard to the severity of the disease.[30] In this patient's case, the echocardiographic diagnostic criteria for severe aortic stenosis are as

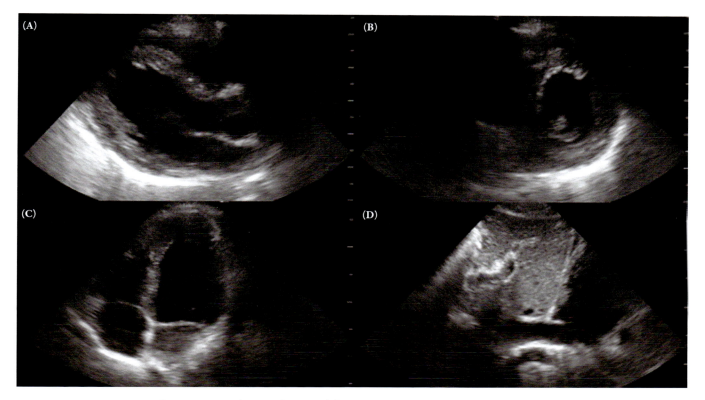

Figure 12.2 Representative point-of-care ultrasound (POCUS) images. (A) Parasternal long axis view. (B) Parasternal short axis view. (C) Apical four-chamber view. (D) Subcostal inferior vena cava (IVC) long axis view.

follows: mean gradient greater than 40 mm Hg, AVA of less than 1 cm², indexed AVA of less than 0.60 cm², velocity ratio less than 0.25, and peak velocity greater than 4.0 m/s.[31]

POCUS is a simplified, clinician-performed application of echocardiography that aims to provide timely data to answer specific clinical questions often relating to signs of heart failure or hemodynamic instability.[32-34] Previously, ultrasound studies were performed by sonographers and interpreted by cardiologists or radiologists, given their technical skills and specific content knowledge. However, there is an increasing body of literature describing the scope of practice of bedside ultrasound by practicing physicians, including anesthesiologists.[32] This is a tool that can provide vital information prior to and during surgery and, given its wide availability, should be employed perioperatively by anesthesiologists with adequate training and an understanding of its limitations.[32]

POCUS typically involves the acquisition of four basic images: parasternal long axis (PLAX), parasternal short axis (PSAX), apical four-chamber (A4), and subcostal inferior vena cava (IVC) long axis (Figure 12.2).

POCUS involves the qualitative assessment of biventricular systolic function, valvular function, pericardial effusion, and volume status.[34] Typically, an anesthesiologist is answering binary questions such as normal or abnormal LV systolic function to inform their anesthetic considerations. In the setting of our patient, high clinical suspicion for a valvular lesion is confirmed by visualizing a calcified, sclerotic, poorly mobilizing aortic valve. Quantifying the specific mean gradient and classifying the severity of aortic stenosis is less important compared to identifying the pathology which informs the next step in the clinical pathway, to delay surgery and obtain a formal echo.

PERIOPERATIVE OPTIONS FOR PATIENTS WITH SEVERE AORTIC STENOSIS

In 2020, the ACC/AHA updated clinical practice guideline for the Management of Patients with Valvular Heart Disease which includes classification and management options. The prior classification system of A (at risk), B (progressive), C (asymptomatic severe), and D (symptomatic severe) with various subgroups is still preserved. Based on these criteria, the interventions for aortic stenosis include no intervention, balloon aortic valvuloplasty (BAV), or aortic valve replacement (AVR). AVR includes both surgical AVR (SAVR) and transcatheter AVR (TAVR) depending on patient risk and the urgency and type of the upcoming surgery. Choice of valve material, bioprosthetic versus mechanical, and timing of these procedures is also important, and recommendations are provided.[35]

Timing of AVR, whether it be SAVR or TAVR is an important consideration. AVR is recommended (Class I) for any patient with Stage D1–3 aortic stenosis (severe symptomatic). It is recommended (Class I) for patients with

Stage C2 aortic stenosis (severe asymptomatic with LVEF <50%). It is also recommended (Class I) for patients with Stage C1 (severe asymptomatic with preserved ejection fraction) who are undergoing another indicated cardiac procedure.[35]

Last, the decision between TAVR and SAVR, as well as the choice of bioprosthetic versus mechanical valve, is nuanced. The ACC/AHA offers guidelines but ultimately acknowledge that this is a complicated decision. Factors such as valve durability, time to re-intervention, need for long-term anticoagulation, patient risk during open procedure, and patient preferences are at play. For a more detailed description of management of aortic stenosis, refer to the 2020 ACC/AHA Guideline for the Management of Patients with Valvular Heart Disease.[35]

HEMODYNAMIC CONSIDERATIONS

Valvular disease is commonly seen in our surgical population and either produces pressure overload (mitral stenosis, aortic stenosis) or volume overload (mitral regurgitation, aortic insufficiency).[36] Patients with severe cardiac disease often have limited cardiac reserve, and induction and maintenance of anesthesia requires careful selection of medications. Invasive and noninvasive monitoring including standard ASA monitors and consideration of an intra-arterial pressure monitor, a pulmonary artery catheter (PAC), and a transesophageal echocardiography (TEE) should be considered.

Optimal hemodynamic parameters and vasoactive medications should be thoughtfully considered to maintain forward flow in patients with severe cardiac disease. The primary parameters to consider are HR, preload, afterload, contractility, and the maintenance of sinus rhythm.

As an example, aortic stenosis is a fixed obstruction causing chronic pressure overload and hypertrophy of the left ventricle. This leads to increased myocardial oxygen demand and decreased compliance.[37,38] In late stages, it can result in reduced LV systolic function. In aortic stenosis, HR should remain low-normal (60–80 beats per minute [bpm]) to allow for adequate diastolic filling and coronary perfusion. Preload should be maintained to have adequate volume fill the hypertrophied and noncompliant ventricle. Afterload, specifically the diastolic blood pressure, should be preserved to maintain coronary perfusion pressure. Contractility should also be maintained, given that the LV is ejecting against a high fixed afterload to maintain forward flow. Sinus rhythm is important to maintain as the atrial kick can be responsible for up to 20% of cardiac output in these patients. The alpha-1 agonist phenylephrine is an optimal vasoactive medication in patients with aortic stenosis given its ability to increase SVR and cause a reduction in HR secondary to the baroreceptor reflex.

Hemodynamic goals can be complex and even competing in patients with cardiac disease. For these patients, it is important to take all lesions into consideration and stratify their importance and severity.

INDICATIONS FOR SUBACUTE BACTERIAL ENDOCARDITIS PROPHYLAXIS

Subacute bacterial endocarditis (SBE)[8] antibiotic prophylaxis is recommended for moderate- and high-risk lesions. These lesions include[39]

- Prosthetic cardiac valve or prosthetic material used for cardiac valve repair
- Previous infective endocarditis (IE).
- Congenital heart disease
  - Unrepaired cyanotic CHD, including palliative shunts and conduits
  - Completely repaired congenital heart defect with prosthetic material or device during the first 6 months after the procedure.
  - Repaired CHD with residual defects
- Cardiac transplantation recipients with concomitant valvulopathy

SBE antibiotic prophylaxis is only recommended for the above patients receiving the following procedures[39]:

- All dental procedures that involve manipulation of gingival tissue or the periapical region of teeth or perforation of the oral mucosa
- It is reasonable for procedures on respiratory tract or infected skin, skin structures, or musculoskeletal tissue

Antibiotic prophylaxis solely to prevent IE is not recommended for GU or GI tract procedures.

SUBACUTE BACTERIAL ENDOCARDITIS PROPHYLAXIS REGIMENS

The recommended SBE prophylaxis regimen for adults is 2 g of oral amoxicillin, 30–60 minutes prior to the procedure. If patients are allergic to penicillin, 2 g cephalexin, 600 mg clindamycin, or 500 mg of azithromycin or clarithromycin may be substituted.[39]

For patients who are unable to take oral medications, 2 g of ampicillin or 1 g of cefazolin or ceftriaxone IV or IM may be substituted. If these patients are allergic to penicillin or ampicillin, 600 mg of clindamycin, 1 g of cefazolin, or 1 g of ceftriaxone IV or IM may be substituted.[39]

CONCLUSION

- A low-risk procedure is one in which the risk of MACE (including non-fatal stroke, non-fatal MI or death) is less than 1%.

- A procedure with a risk of MACE of greater than 1% is considered elevated risk.
- A validated risk prediction tool should be used to predict the risk of perioperative MACE in patients undergoing noncardiac surgery.
- When patients are unable to achieve 4 METs of work, perioperative risks are increased, and further testing should be considered.
- Subjective assessment of functional capacity does not accurately identify patients at risk for perioperative morbidity and mortality; consider validated objective measures, such as the Duke Activity Status Index (DASI)
- TTE is the standard diagnostic test in the initial evaluation of known or suspected valvular heart disease.
- DAPT in patients with PCI should be continued for at least 6 months in patients who underwent PCI for SIHD and for at least 12 months in patients who underwent PCI for ACS.
- POCUS is a simplified, clinician-performed point-of-care application of echocardiography that anesthesiologists should use, with adequate training.
- SBE[8] antibiotic prophylaxis is recommended for patients with moderate- and high-risk lesions undergoing specific procedures.

REVIEW QUESTIONS

1. You are seeing a 65-year-old woman in the preoperative clinic. She is undergoing a total knee arthroplasty for worsening osteoarthritis in 2 weeks and was sent by her orthopedic surgeon for surgical clearance. She had an MI 5 months prior and had a DES placed. She is currently on aspirin, clopidogrel, simvastatin, and metoprolol. When can she discontinue her clopidogrel and undergo surgery?

    a. She is cleared to proceed with surgery in 2 weeks.
    b. She should wait at least 1 more month before undergoing surgery.
    c. She should wait at least 7 more months before undergoing surgery.
    d. She should wait at least 19 more months before undergoing surgery.

The correct answer is c.

A total knee arthroplasty is an elective procedure, and the patient underwent a PCI for ACS. As a result, it is recommended that DAPT be continued for at least 12 months. In patients who underwent PCI for SIHD, DAPT should be continued for at least 6 months. She should continue aspirin at the time of surgery while likely holding clopidogrel.

2. You are seeing a 65-year-old woman in the preoperative clinic. She is undergoing a hysterectomy for endometrial cancer in 2 weeks and was sent by her surgeon for surgical clearance. She had an MI 5 months prior and had a DES placed. She is currently on aspirin, clopidogrel, simvastatin, and metoprolol. When can she discontinue her clopidogrel and undergo surgery?

    a. She is cleared to proceed with surgery in two weeks.
    b. She should wait at least 1 month before undergoing surgery.
    c. She should wait at least 7 months before undergoing surgery.
    d. She should wait at least 19 months before undergoing surgery.

The correct answer is b.

This is a complicated question and depends on the extent and likelihood of spread for her cancer. However, an oncologic procedure is time-sensitive and the patient underwent a PCI for ACS. As a result, it is recommended that DAPT be continued for at least 12 months. However, it is reasonable to discontinue the clopidogrel at 6 months if there is a high risk of bleeding, which this surgery has.

3. A 64-year-old man who underwent cardiac transplantation for nonischemic cardiomyopathy presents to the dentist for a tooth cleaning. His transplant is functioning well with a normal ejection fraction and no valvular abnormalities. Is SBE prophylaxis required?

    a. Yes.
    b. No.
    c. Yes, only if cavities are being filled.

The correct answer is b.

While dental procedures that involve manipulation of gingival tissue can require SBE prophylaxis, only cardiac transplantation recipients with concomitant valvulopathy need it. Because this patient has no valvular abnormalities, SBE prophylaxis is not required.

4. You are caring for a 34-year-old man undergoing hernia repair. He is a former IV drug user with a history of IE. The surgeon states that antibiotics are not required for this procedure. Should he receive additional SBE prophylaxis.

    a. Yes
    b. No

The correct answer is b.

Although patients with a prior history of IE do require SBE prophylaxis for certain procedures, a hernia repair is not one of them. Antibiotic prophylaxis solely to prevent IE is not recommended for GU or GI tract procedures.

5. During induction of general anesthesia on a patient with severe aortic stenosis, the patient becomes tachycardic and hypotensive. The vasoactive medication most suited for this situation is

    a. Epinephrine.
    b. Ephedrine.
    c. Phenylephrine.
    d. None of the above.

The correct answer is c.

Epinephrine and ephedrine both have beta-1 agonist properties, which can increase HR and contractility, which could worsen the situation. Phenylephrine is an alpha-1 agonist, which will increase SVR and cause a reflex decrease in HR. For aortic stenosis, HR should remain low-normal (60–80 bpm) to allow for adequate diastolic filling and coronary perfusion of the hypertrophied ventricle. In addition, the SVR, especially diastolic blood pressure, must be maintained to allow for adequate perfusion of the hypertrophied left ventricle during diastole.

6. A 34-year-old otherwise healthy woman is undergoing a lumpectomy. This surgery is defined as a

   a. Low-risk surgery.
   b. Intermediate-risk surgery.
   c. High-risk surgery.

   The correct answer is a.

   Breast surgery in an otherwise healthy female is considered a low-risk surgery, defined as a procedure in which the risk of a MACE is less than 1%.

7. A 68 year-old man with a medical history of well-controlled hypertension and type 2 diabetes is undergoing a carotid endarterectomy. This surgery is defined as a

   a. Low risk surgery.
   b. Intermediate risk surgery.
   c. High risk surgery.

   The correct answer is b.

   Carotid endarterectomy is considered an intermediate-risk surgery in a patient with otherwise well-controlled comorbidities. An intermediate-risk surgery is defined as a procedure in which the risk of a MACE is 1–5%. Interestingly, other major vascular surgery is defined as high-risk surgery, but a carotid endarterectomy does not fall into this category.

8. A 54-year-old man with no known medical history is undergoing an emergent exploratory laparotomy for a splenic laceration and hemorrhage sustained during a car accident. He is tachycardic and hypotensive. This surgery is defined as a

   a. Low-risk surgery.
   b. Intermediate-risk surgery.
   c. High-risk surgery.

   The correct answer is c.

   An emergent major surgery with large fluid shifts and/or blood loss is a high-risk surgery, defined as a procedure in which the risk of a MACE, is greater than 5%.

9. A 78 year-old man with a medical history of hypertension, coronary artery disease with a remote MI without intervention, type 2 diabetes on insulin, and peripheral vascular disease is undergoing a total hip arthroplasty for severe osteoarthritis. The patient is unable to assess his exercise capacity because his hip pain limits him. He has a new-onset systolic murmur on physical exam. What is the next step?

   a. Proceed with surgery because this is only an intermediate-risk surgery.
   b. Delay surgery for further assessment.
   c. Delay surgery until an ICU bed can be arranged for the patient for recovery.
   d. Tell the patient he cannot receive this surgery because of his poor exercise capacity.

   The correct answer is b.

   According to ACC/AHA guidelines, the steps (and answers to each step) to determine if further testing is indicated are as follows:

   1. Is the surgery emergent? *No.*
   2. Does the patient have an ACS? *No.*
   3. What is the patient's risk of MACE for the proposed procedure? Is it low less than 1% or elevated greater than 1%? *Elevated (>1%) because he has several comorbidities (CAD, diabetes) as well as unquantified valvular disease and is undergoing an intermediate-risk orthopedic procedure (1–5%).*
   4. Can the patient achieve more than 4 METs? *Unknown.*
   5. Will further testing impact clinical decision-making? *Yes, it certainly could if he were found to have severe CAD or a severe valvular lesion.*

REFERENCES

1. Mangano DT, Goldman L. Preoperative assessment of patients with known or suspected coronary disease. *N Engl J Med.* 1995;333(26):1750–1756.
2. Barash PG. *Clinical Anesthesia.* 7th ed. Wolters Kluwer/Lippincott Williams and Wilkins; 2013.
3. Fleisher LA, Fleischmann KE, Auerbach AD, et al. ACC/AHA guideline on perioperative cardiovascular evaluation and management of patients undergoing noncardiac surgery: A report of the American College of Cardiology/American Heart Association Task Force on Practice Guidelines. *Circulation.* 2014;130(24):e278–333.
4. Lurati Buse GA, Mauermann E, Ionescu D, et al. Risk assessment for major adverse cardiovascular events after noncardiac surgery using self-reported functional capacity: International prospective cohort study. *Br J Anaesth.* 2023;130(6):655–665.
5. Halvorsen S, Mehilli J, Cassese S, et al. ESC Guidelines on cardiovascular assessment and management of patients undergoing non-cardiac surgery developed by the task force for cardiovascular assessment and management of patients undergoing non-cardiac surgery of the European Society of Cardiology (ESC). Endorsed by the European Society of Anaesthesiology and Intensive Care (ESAIC)]. *G Ital Cardiol (Rome).* 2023;24(1 Suppl 1):e1–e102.
6. Ford MK, Beattie WS, Wijeysundera DN. Systematic review: Prediction of perioperative cardiac complications and mortality by the revised cardiac risk index. *Ann Intern Med.* 2010;152(1):26–35.
7. Cohen ME, Ko CY, Bilimoria KY, et al. Optimizing ACS NSQIP modeling for evaluation of surgical quality and risk: Patient risk adjustment, procedure mix adjustment, shrinkage adjustment, and surgical focus. *J Am Coll Surg.* 2013;217(2):336–346 e1.
8. Dakik HA, Chehab O, Eldirani M, et al. A new index for pre-operative cardiovascular evaluation. *J Am Coll Cardiol.* 2019;73(24):3067–3078.
9. Glance LG, Faden E, Dutton RP, et al. Impact of the choice of risk model for identifying low-risk patients using the 2014 American College of Cardiology/American Heart Association perioperative guidelines. *Anesthesiology.* 2018;129(5):889–900.

10. Vernooij LM, van Klei WA, Moons KG, et al. The comparative and added prognostic value of biomarkers to the Revised Cardiac Risk Index for preoperative prediction of major adverse cardiac events and all-cause mortality in patients who undergo noncardiac surgery. *Cochrane Database Syst Rev*. 2021;12(12):CD013139.
11. Wijeysundera DN, Pearse RM, Shulman MA, et al. Assessment of functional capacity before major non-cardiac surgery: An international, prospective cohort study. *Lancet*. 2018;391(10140):2631–2640.
12. Reilly DF, McNeely MJ, Doerner D, et al. Self-reported exercise tolerance and the risk of serious perioperative complications. *Arch Intern Med*. 1999;159(18):2185–2192.
13. Melon CC, Eshtiaghi P, Luksun WJ, et al. Validated questionnaire vs physicians' judgment to estimate preoperative exercise capacity. *JAMA Intern Med*. 2014;174(9):1507–1508.
14. Healy KO, Waksmonski CA, Altman RK, et al. Perioperative outcome and long-term mortality for heart failure patients undergoing intermediate- and high-risk noncardiac surgery: Impact of left ventricular ejection fraction. *Congest Heart Fail*. 2010;16(2):45–49.
15. McFalls EO, Ward HB, Moritz TE, et al. Coronary-artery revascularization before elective major vascular surgery. *N Engl J Med*. 2004;351(27):2795–2804.
16. Levine GN, et al. 2016 ACC/AHA guideline focused update on duration of dual antiplatelet therapy in patients with coronary artery disease: A report of the American College of Cardiology/American Heart Association Task Force on clinical practice guidelines. *J Am Coll Cardiol*. 2016;68(10):1082–1115.
17. Mauri L, Smith SC Jr. Focused update on duration of dual antiplatelet therapy for patients with coronary artery disease. *JAMA Cardiol*. 2016;1(6):733–734.
18. Switaj TL, Christensen SR, Brewer DM. Acute coronary syndrome: Current treatment. *Am Fam Physician*. 2017;95(4):232–240.
19. Colombo A, Chieffo A, Frasheri A, et al. Second-generation drug-eluting stent implantation followed by 6- versus 12-month dual antiplatelet therapy: The SECURITY randomized clinical trial. *J Am Coll Cardiol*. 2014;64(20):2086–2097.
20. Feres F, Costa RA, Abizaid A, et al. Three vs twelve months of dual antiplatelet therapy after zotarolimus-eluting stents: The OPTIMIZE randomized trial. *JAMA*. 2013;310(23):2510–2522.
21. Gwon HC, Hahn JY, Park KW, et al. Six-month versus 12-month dual antiplatelet therapy after implantation of drug-eluting stents: The Efficacy of Xience/Promus Versus Cypher to Reduce Late Loss After Stenting (EXCELLENT) randomized, multicenter study. *Circulation*. 2012;125(3):505–513.
22. Kim BK, Hong MK, Shin DH, et al. A new strategy for discontinuation of dual antiplatelet therapy: The RESET Trial (REal Safety and Efficacy of 3-month dual antiplatelet Therapy following Endeavor zotarolimus-eluting stent implantation). *J Am Coll Cardiol*. 2012;60(15):1340–1348.
23. Bonow RO, Brown AS, Gillam LD, et al.; ACC/AATS/AHA/ASE/EACTS/HVS/SCA/SCAI/SCCT/SCMR/STS. 2017 Appropriate use criteria for the treatment of patients with severe aortic stenosis. *Eur J Cardio-Thorac Surg*. 2018;53(2):306.
24. Navarese EP, Tandjung K, Claessen B, et al. Safety and efficacy outcomes of first and second generation durable polymer drug eluting stents and biodegradable polymer biolimus eluting stents in clinical practice: Comprehensive network meta-analysis. *BMJ*. 2013;347:f6530.
25. Biccard BM, Sigamani A, Chan MTV, et al. Effect of aspirin in vascular surgery in patients from a randomized clinical trial (POISE-2). *Br J Surg*. 2018;105(12):1591–1597.
26. Goldman L, Caldera DL, Nussbaum SR, et al. Multifactorial index of cardiac risk in noncardiac surgical procedures. *N Engl J Med*. 1977;297(16):845–850.
27. Agarwal S, Rajamanickam A, Bajaj NS, et al. Impact of aortic stenosis on postoperative outcomes after noncardiac surgeries. *Circ Cardiovasc Qual Outcomes*. 2013;6(2):193–200.
28. Andersson C, Jorgensen ME, Martinsson A, et al. Noncardiac surgery in patients with aortic stenosis: A contemporary study on outcomes in a matched sample from the Danish health care system. *Clin Cardiol*. 2014;37(11):680–686.
29. Grimard BH, Larson JM. Aortic stenosis: Diagnosis and treatment. *Am Fam Physician*. 2008;78(6):717–724.
30. Nishimura RA, Otto CM, Bonow RO, et al. *2014 AHA/ACC guideline for the management of patients with valvular heart disease: A report of the American College of Cardiology/American Heart Association Task Force on Practice Guidelines. Circulation*. 2014;129(23):e521–643.
31. Baumgartner H, Hung J, Bermejo J, et al. Echocardiographic assessment of valve stenosis: EAE/ASE recommendations for clinical practice. *J Am Soc Echocardiogr*. 2009;22(1):1–23; quiz 101–102.
32. Coker BJ, Zimmerman JM. Why anesthesiologists must incorporate focused cardiac ultrasound into daily practice. *Anesth Analg*. 2017;124(3):761–765.
33. Via G, Hussain A, Wells M, et al. International evidence-based recommendations for focused cardiac ultrasound. *J Am Soc Echocardiogr*. 2014;27(7):683 e1–683 e33.
34. Zimmerman JM, Coker BJ. The nuts and bolts of performing Focused Cardiovascular Ultrasound (FoCUS). *Anesth Analg*. 2017;124(3):753–760.
35. Otto CM, Nishimura RA, Bonow RO, et al. 2020 ACC/AHA guideline for the management of patients with valvular heart disease: Executive summary: A report of the American College of Cardiology/American Heart Association Joint Committee on clinical practice guidelines. *Circulation*. 2021;143(5):e35–e71.
36. Carabello BA, Crawford FA Jr. Valvular heart disease. *N Engl J Med*. 1997;337(1):32–41.
37. Hess OM, Ritter M, Schneider J, et al. Diastolic stiffness and myocardial structure in aortic valve disease before and after valve replacement. *Circulation*. 1984;69(5):855–865.
38. Johnson LL, Sciacca RR, Ellis K, et al. Reduced left ventricular myocardial blood flow per unit mass in aortic stenosis. *Circulation*. 1978;57(3):582–590.
39. Wilson W, Taubert KA, Gewitz M, et al. Prevention of infective endocarditis: Guidelines from the American Heart Association: A guideline from the American Heart Association Rheumatic Fever, Endocarditis, and Kawasaki Disease Committee, Council on Cardiovascular Disease in the Young, and the Council on Clinical Cardiology, Council on Cardiovascular Surgery and Anesthesia, and the Quality of Care and Outcomes Research Interdisciplinary Working Group. *Circulation*. 2007;116(15):1736–1754.

13.

PERIOPERATIVE ATRIAL FIBRILLATION AND ANTICOAGULATION MANAGEMENT

Jing Tao and Adriana D. Oprea

STEM CASE AND KEY QUESTIONS

75-year-old man is evaluated in the preadmission testing center for an inguinal hernia repair. History and physical examination are unremarkable except he is found to have an irregular pulse at a rate of 121 beats per minute (bpm). He denies ever hearing the term "atrial fibrillation" or "irregular heart rate." An ECG is obtained in the clinic, which confirms the diagnosis of atrial fibrillation.

What is atrial fibrillation, and how is it diagnosed?

The patient states that he has not seen a physician in many years because he "feels fine." On further evaluation, he admits to smoking a half pack a day since he was 18 years old. He is able to walk and climb stairs without chest pressure, but endorses fatigue and shortness of breath at times.

What risk factors and comorbidities are associated with atrial fibrillation (AF)? What are the sequelae if left untreated?

The patient has a blood pressure of 160/90 in the preadmission clinic. His other labs appear within normal limits. He also denies any history of stroke/transient ischemic attack (TIA) or heart failure.

What other work-up is necessary in a patient with recently detected AF?

His basic metabolic panel appears within normal limits except for an elevated creatinine of 1.5. Further laboratory work, including a magnesium level and thyroid function test, are normal. A cardiology evaluation is requested, and a transthoracic echocardiogram (TTE) shows global hypokinesis with an ejection fraction (EF) of 40–45%, but no other abnormalities.

Why is anticoagulation needed in AF? How do you determine which patient will need chronic anticoagulation? In addition, what other treatment modalities are recommended for patients with AF?

The cardiologist recommends starting metoprolol for rate control and advises the patient on lifelong chronic anticoagulation to decrease complications associated with AF. The patient would like to know what oral anticoagulants are available to him and what the benefits and risks are of these medications.

What types of oral anticoagulation are available? Describe their pharmacokinetics.

The patient's cardiologist prescribes warfarin. He is told that he will require regular blood draws for drug monitoring as well as maintain a stricter diet. The patient asks, now that he is properly treated for AF, when he will be able to have his hernia repaired.

How long prior to an invasive procedure should warfarin be stopped? Are there any lab tests to get prior to surgery?

The patient is told that he will need to stop his warfarin 5 days before his surgery. The patient is concerned that he will be at risk for stroke or systemic embolism if his blood thinners are temporarily interrupted.

Which patients are at high risk for thromboembolic complications during warfarin interruption? What is bridging therapy, and how do you determine if the patient will require bridging therapy?

The patient understands that bridging therapy is not necessary for him, but would like a clear understanding of what the process would entail.

What is bridging therapy? What drugs are available for bridging therapy? What are the considerations when choosing a specific bridging agent and their dose?

Assume the cardiologist prescribes a direct oral anticoagulant (DOAC) instead of warfarin.

How long prior to an invasive procedure should apixaban be stopped? Is this different from other direct oral anticoagulants like rivaroxaban, endoxaban, and dabigatran? Are there any laboratory tests to obtain prior to proceeding with surgery?

The patient is very concerned about his risk of stroke while off anticoagulation. He would like to know if being off apixaban for 2 days will put him at increased risk. He would also like to know how soon after surgery will he be able to restart apixaban.

Is bridging therapy required for DOACs before surgery? When can anticoagulation be restarted postoperatively?

What are considerations for perioperative interruption of oral anticoagulation in patients undergoing regional anesthesia? Are there any guidelines?

DISCUSSION

ATRIAL FIBRILLATION DEFINITION AND RISK FACTORS

AF is characterized by irregular and often rapid atrial discharges. It is the most commonly encountered cardiac arrhythmia, afflicting approximately 3–6 million people in the United States alone, with an increasing prevalence in the elderly population.[1] It is characterized by an irregular rhythm with a lack of distinct p waves on the ECG. Atrial activity is poorly defined (usual rates at ~300/min) or absent. Ventricular activity is mostly irregular.

Multiple risk factors have been identified in AF development. Data from the 1994 Framingham Heart Study found age, hypertension, congestive heart failure (CHF), coronary heart disease (CAD), valvular heart disease, and diabetes mellitus (DM) to be independent predictors.[2] CHF and valvular heart disease present the two strongest risk factors for AF development, while hypertension has the highest prevalence in AF patients given its pervasiveness.[3,4] In addition, more recent studies also found left ventricular hypertrophy (LVH), obesity, obstructive sleep apnea (OSA) with or without the presence of obesity, physical inactivity, smoking, and excessive alcohol use to be associated with AF[5–7] (Table 13.1). Lone AF, defined as AF without an identifiable risk factor, appears to be quite rare.[8]

DIAGNOSIS AND TREATMENT

Diagnosis of AF is primarily by ECG. Patients with AF will show an absence of P waves and irregularly irregular QRS intervals on ECG. In patients with intermittent symptoms consistent with paroxysmal AF, continuous ECG monitoring with a Holter device may be helpful at capturing the arrhythmia.[9]

Once AF is diagnosed, etiology and associated comorbidities should be identified to ensure appropriate therapy. Follow-up TTE is recommended in all patients with newly diagnosed AF to evaluate for possible structural or functional heart disease, establish a baseline cardiac status, and identify patients in whom rhythm control with cardioversion should be utilized.[9] If TTE does not provide adequate information or finds structural abnormalities like valvular disease, transesophageal echocardiogram (TEE) may be warranted.

Therapeutic options for AF include controlling the ventricular rate to prevent tachycardia-mediated cardiomyopathy and preventing stroke with systemic anticoagulation.

Control of the ventricular rate can be achieved using either a rhythm control or a rate control strategy with a goal of achieving heart rates in the normal range (<80 bpm at rest and <110 during physical activity). While a rhythm control strategy used to be the preferred therapeutic option, there is no difference in outcome when adopting a rate control modality (such as calcium channel blocker or beta blocker treatment) in a majority of patients.[10] Rhythm control is generally reserved for symptomatic patients and may be preferred in elderly (>75 years old), high cardiovascular risk patients where this strategy may confer a survival benefit at 12 months after diagnosis.[11] In certain situations (i.e., unstable hemodynamics), immediate cardioversion is required. Cardioversion, in the absence of therapeutic anticoagulation, is only safe when it is certain that the episode of AF is less than 48 hours. Otherwise, immediate cardioversion should be attempted only after a TEE confirms a lack of clot in the left atrial appendage. When time and the clinical scenario allows (stable hemodynamics but a rhythm control strategy is desired), cardioversion should be attempted after a 21-day therapeutic anticoagulation window to decrease the risk of embolic stroke. Cardioversion can be either electrical or chemical. Class IC antiarrhythmics (i.e., propafenone, mexiletine, ibutilide dofetilide) or class III antiarrhythmics (i.e., amiodarone) are the preferred agents for cardioversion with agents like sotalol. Maintenance of sinus rhythm is usually not necessary after the first cardioversion especially if there is no structural heart disease or there is a precipitating factor.[1]

Most of the time, a rate control strategy is adopted using calcium channel or beta blockade therapy. Digoxin is reserved for patients where calcium channel and beta blockers failed or for patients with associated systolic heart failure.

COMPLICATIONS

Untreated AF can lead to several complications. Risk of dementia, myocardial infarction, heart failure, and early death are increased in patients with poorly managed AF[12] (Table 13.1).

The most common sequelae of AF continue to be cerebral vascular accident (CVA) and TIA. Reduced left atrial contraction leads to blood stasis and increased risk of clot formation, especially in the left atrial appendage.

Table 13.1 ATRIAL FIBRILLATION RISK FACTORS AND COMPLICATIONS

RISK FACTORS	COMPLICATIONS
Age	Stroke
Hypertension	Venous thromboembolisms
Congestive heart failure	Myocardial infarction
Coronary artery disease	Heart failure
Valvular heart disease	Dementia
Diabetes mellitus	Early death
Left ventricular hyperplasia	
Obesity	
Obstructive sleep apnea	
Physical inactivity	
Smoking	
Excessive alcohol use	

Stroke risk as a result AF has traditionally been assessed using the CHADS$_2$ score. Comorbidities including CHF, hypertension, age 75 or older, DM, and previous CVA/TIA are graded to predict an annual risk (Table 13.2). Patients with a CHADS$_2$ score of 0–1 are considered low risk (annual risk 1.9–2.8%). Those who score 2 or higher are considered high risk (annual risk 4–18.2%).[13]

More recently, the CHA$_2$D$_2$-VASc score was developed to better identify CVA risk in patients with CHADS$_2$ score 0–1.[14] Presence of vascular disease, age 65–74, and female sex are included as additional risk factors. Due to a greater severity of strokes in the setting of AF as compared to patients with no AF, it is imperative to accurately risk-stratify these patients.[15] Patients who score 2 points or higher on the CHA$_2$D$_2$-VASc scale incur an annual stroke risk of 2.2–15.2% and may benefit from long-term systemic oral anticoagulation[1] (Table 13.2).

Currently, the 2014 American Heart Association/American College of Cardiology/Heart Rhythm Society (AHA/ACC/HRS) Guideline for the Management of Patients with Atrial Fibrillation recommends using the CHA$_2$D$_2$-VASc scoring system over CHADS$_2$ when determining if oral anticoagulation is necessary for patients with AF.[1]

POSTOPERATIVE ATRIAL FIBRILLATION

Postoperative AF occurs in 3% of unselected patients but is much more frequent after thoracic (30%) and cardiac surgery. Factors such as the activation of the sympathetic system, as well as hypovolemia, electrolyte imbalances, hemodynamic instability, anemia, and pain can contribute to its onset. Volume overload leads to distension of the right atrial myocytes and development of AF. While usually the episodes of postoperative AF are self-limited, there is a higher risk of stroke within 30 days of the surgical procedures. Similar to preoperative AF, persistent postoperative AF mandates rhythm versus rate control strategies as well as anticoagulation.[16]

ORAL ANTICOAGULATION

Stroke Risk Reduction

There are two classes of oral anticoagulants available for chronic outpatient therapy: vitamin K antagonists (VKA) and DOACs. Warfarin is the most commonly used VKA and has been the cornerstone of chronic anticoagulation for the past 5 decades. Its anticoagulant effect is due to decreasing the synthesis of vitamin K-dependent clotting factors II, VII, IX, and X. Because warfarin also inhibits protein C and S, there is an initial pro-thrombotic state before the anticoagulant effect takes effect.[17] Warfarin is metabolized by the P450 system in the liver and excreted through urine. Half-life is approximately 36–40 hours.[18]

In addition to stroke prevention in the setting of AF, other indications for warfarin use include treatment and prevention of systemic venous thromboembolisms (VTE) and prevention of thrombus formation after mechanical and bioprosthetic heart valve replacement.[19–21]

Because warfarin mainly affects vitamin K-dependent clotting factors, the anticoagulant effect will be monitored and tailored using a prothrombin time (PT) or international normalizing ratio (INR).[22] For most hypercoagulable states like AF, goal INR is 2–3.[1] Exceptions are patients with mechanical mitral heart valves, older aortic valves, and new-generation aortic valves in the presence of risk factors for stroke or in patients with ventricular assist device (VAD), where a higher target INR (2.5–3.5) is recommended.[1]

The DOACs are a second, more recently developed class of oral anticoagulants with two subgroups: direct thrombin

Table 13.2 CHADS$_2$ AND CHA$_2$D$_2$-VASC SCORE AND ANNUAL RISK OF STROKE

	CHADS$_2$ SCORE				CHA$_2$D$_2$-VASC SCORE	
ANNUAL RISK OF STROKE (%)	CHADS$_2$ SCORE	POINTS	RISK FACTORS	POINTS	CHA$_2$DS$_2$-VASC SCORE	ANNUAL RISK OF STROKE (%)
0.6	0	1	Congestive heart failure	1	0	0.2
3.0	1	1	Hypertension	1	1	0.6
4.2	2	1	Age ≥75	2	2	2.2
7.1	3	1	Diabetes mellitus	1	3	3.2
11.1	4	2	Prior cerebrovascular accident/transient ischemic attack	2	4	4.8
12.5	5		Vascular disease	1	5	7.2
13	6		Age 65–74	1	6	9.7
			Female sex	1	7	11.2
					8	10.8
					9	12.2

inhibitors and factor Xa inhibitors. Dabigatran, a direct thrombin inhibitor, was the first DOAC to be approved by the US Food and Drug Administration (FDA) for the prevention of stroke associated with AF.[23] Since then, its indications have expanded to include treatment and prevention of systemic VTE and prophylaxis against VTE after hip and knee replacement surgery.[23]

Dabigatran works to inhibit formation by directly inhibiting thrombin. It has a quick onset of action, reaching peak plasma concentration in 2 hours. Drug metabolism occurs in the liver, but excretion is 80% unchanged in the urine. As a result, its anticoagulant effect may be prolonged in patients with renal impairment. Dabigatran's half-life is approximately 9 hours in patients with normal kidney function, 12–17 hours in elderly patients and patients with moderate kidney disease, and up to 26–34 hours in patients with severe kidney disease.[24,25]

Dabigatran demonstrates multiple benefits over warfarin. The RE-LY trial found it not only reduced stroke risk in patients with AF better than warfarin, but also decreased episodes of major bleeding.[26] Furthermore, dabigatran is not affected by diet or nutritional status, and does not require regular blood draws for drug monitoring.

The second class of DOACs is the factor Xa inhibitors: rivaroxaban, apixaban, and edoxaban. Indications for use also include prevention of stroke as a result of AF, treatment and prevention of systemic VTE, and prophylaxis against VTE after hip and knee replacement surgeries.[27,28] Betrixaban is the last FDA-approved anti-Xa anticoagulant used for prophylaxis of VTE in adult patients hospitalized for an acute medical illness who are at risk for thromboembolic complications due to moderate or severe restricted mobility and other risk factors for VTE.[29]

Factor Xa inhibitors directly inhibit factor Xa to reduce thrombin formation. Much like dabigatran, this subgroup of DOACs also reaches peak plasma concentration quickly after ingestion: rivaroxaban in 2–4 hours, apixaban in 1–3 hours, and edoxaban in 1–1.5 hours. Metabolism is primarily through the liver, but, compared to dabigatran, factor Xa inhibitors depend much less on the kidneys for excretion.[30,31] Rivaroxaban is excreted 35% unchanged in urine, edoxaban 50%, and apixaban 25%, making these anticoagulants a better choice for patients with renal impairment.[31] Rivaroxaban has a half-life of 9 hours in young healthy patients, but increases to 11–13 hours in elderly patients and those with severe kidney disease. Half-life of apixaban is 10–14 hours and edoxaban is 8–10 hours[30,31] (Table 13.3).

Table 13.3 **ORAL ANTICOAGULATION INDICATIONS AND PHARMACOKINETICS**

	DRUG GROUP	INDICATIONS	TIME TO C_{MAX} (H)	CYP 450 METABOLISM	EXCRETION	HALF-LIFE (H)
Warfarin	Vitamin K antagonist	Venous thromboembolism (VTE) treatment and prevention Stroke reduction in nonvalvular atrial fibrillation (AF) Post mechanical and prosthetic heart valve replacement Prevention of recurrent and death after myocardial infarction	72–96 h	Yes	Urine (90% unchanged)	36–40 h
Dabigatran	Direct thrombin inhibitor	VTE treatment and prevention Stroke reduction in non-valvular AF VTE prophylaxis after hip replacement surgery	2 h	No	Urine (80% unchanged)	9 h (normal renal function) 12–17 h (elderly) 34 h (severe renal impairment)
Rivaroxaban	Factor Xa inhibitor	VTE treatment VTE prevention after hip/knee surgery Stroke reduction in non-valvular AF Stroke, myocardial infarction, and death prevention in patients with coronary artery disease and PVD (with low-dose aspirin)	2–4 h	Liver (CYP450)	Urine (35% unchanged)	5–9 h (normal renal function) 11–13 h (elderly/severe renal impairment)
Apixaban	Factor Xa inhibitor	VTE prophylaxis after hip and knee replacement surgery VTE treatment Stroke reduction in non-valvular AF	1–3 h	Liver (CYP450)	Urine (27% unchanged)	10–14 h
Edoxaban	Factor Xa inhibitor	VTE treatment and prevention Stroke reduction in non-valvular atrial fibrillation	1–2 h	No	Urine (50% unchanged)	8–10 h
Betrixaban	Factor Xa inhibitor	VTE treatment and prevention in medical patients	3–4 h	No	Urine (18%)	19–27 h

Adapted with permission from Huisman MV, Klok FA. Pharmacological properties of betrixaban. *Eur Heart J.* 2018 May;20(Suppl E):E12–E15.

The use of rivaroxaban and apixaban for reduction of stroke risk associated with AF has significantly increased in recent years due to their improved efficacy, ease of use, and favorable pharmacokinetics. The ROCKET AF trial found rivaroxaban to be noninferior at stroke prevention and incur lower rates of intracranial and fatal bleed when compared to warfarin.[32] Similarly, the ARISTOLE trial found apixaban to be superior to warfarin at reducing stroke, systemic thromboembolism, and overall morality in patients with AF.[33] Factor Xa inhibitors have minimal interactions with medications and diet and do not require regular blood test monitoring.

Preoperative Management

Management of oral anticoagulation before invasive procedures will depend on several factors, including patient's risk of thromboembolism, procedural risk of bleeding, and the specific anticoagulant drug.

The patient's thromboembolic risk depends on the indication for the anticoagulant therapy. As stated above, patients with AF are risk-stratified based on their $CHADS_2$ or CHA_2D_2-VASc scores. As such, patients considered at low risk of thrombosis include those with a CHA_2D_2-VASc score of 0–4 or a $CHADS_2$ score of 0–2. Patients at moderate risk of stroke are patients with CHA_2D_2-VASc score of 5–6 or a $CHADS_2$ score of 3–4. Patients at high risk of stroke include those with a history of recent stroke (within 3 months) and patients with high CHA_2D_2-VASc score (7–9) or $CHADS_2$ score of 5–6.[34–36]

For patients with a history of deep vein thrombosis (DVT)/pulmonary embolism (PE) the most important predictor of event recurrence and therefore driving the risk is the length of time passed from the previous DVT/PE episode. As such, patients with an episode of VTE greater than 12 months ago are considered at low risk of recurrence; patients with a prior episode of VTE 3–12 months before or with active cancer are considered intermediate risk; and patients at high risk have had a VTE less than 3 months prior, have severe or multiple thrombophilias, or have certain active cancers (e.g., pancreatic cancer).[34,35]

Similarly, patients with mechanical valves are risk-stratified based on the type of valve as well as the presence of other thrombophilia. Patients with bicuspid aortic valves without the presence of other risk factors are considered at low risk of thromboembolism while patients with the same valves in the presence of AF or other risk factors such as history of prior CVA/TIA, hypertension, diabetes, CHF, or older than 75 years are considered at intermediate risk.

Patients with mitral mechanical valves or older-model aortic valves (e.g., disk tilting or ball-in-cage) are considered at very high risk of thromboembolism.[34,35]

To estimate the surgical bleeding risk, several tools have been proposed, such as the HAS BLED score. The HAS BLED score takes into account several comorbidities such as *h*ypertension, *a*bnormal liver or kidney function, *s*troke, *b*leeding, *l*abile INR, *e*lderly, *d*rug or alcohol use, with each comorbidity counting for 1 point (patients with HAS BLED scores greater than 3 are considered to be at high risk).[37] Other modalities of quantifying the bleeding risk have been proposed: procedures that incur a greater than 2% risk of major bleeding within 2 days of surgery generally are considered high risk, while procedures with a less than 2% rate of bleeding are low risk.[38,39]

Most minimally invasive procedures such as dental extraction, cataract surgery, diagnostic GI endoscopy (without disrupting the mucosa), and bedside diagnostic or therapeutic procedures (thoracentesis, paracentesis) are considered low risk for bleeding[39–41] (Table 13.4).

Procedures considered high risk for bleeding include those with major tissue interruption or are performed near highly vascularized areas, where access to site of bleeding is limited and consequences of bleeding are devastating.[40–42] Major orthopedic, cardiac, vascular, neurosurgical, and neuraxial anesthesia procedures are all considered high risk[38] (Table 13.4).

PERIOPERATIVE MANAGEMENT OF WARFARIN

For patients on warfarin, advanced planning before invasive procedures is required due to its long half-life, and more so patients for at high risk of thromboembolism. Although each patient should be assessed on an individual basis, those undergoing low bleeding risk procedures will usually not require complete drug cessation. In some instances, such as dental extractions, minor skin lesion excision, or cataract surgery, warfarin can be continued throughout the perioperative period. Multiple studies found that bleeding from these procedures even while fully anticoagulated is often minor and self-limiting.[43–45]

For low bleeding risk procedures (<2% 48-hour perioperative risk), warfarin can be held for 2–3 days so that the anticoagulant level becomes subtherapeutic but the drug is not completely metabolized.[34] This would allow for some degree of protection against a hypercoagulable state but also decrease the risk of clinical bleeding.[38]

Warfarin management before surgeries with moderate to high risks of bleeding becomes much more complex. For these procedures, warfarin will need to be stopped long enough to allow for complete regeneration of vitamin K-dependent clotting factors.[36] To determine the exact length of drug interruption, the American College of Cardiologists (ACA) recommends that patients have their INR checked 5–7 days before surgery.[36] Those with supratherapeutic INR should have their warfarin held for at least 5 days. Those with therapeutic INR should hold it for 5 days, and those with subtherapeutic INR for 3–4 days.[36] In addition, INR should be rechecked 24 hours before the procedure date to ensure that it is below 1.5.[36,42]

BRIDGING THERAPY

While for certain patients the risk of thrombosis is low when anticoagulation is interrupted perioperatively, patients at high risk of thrombosis require bridging therapy to mitigate this risk.[34] Bridging therapy consists of replacing oral anticoagulants with a parenteral anticoagulant such as unfractionated

Table 13.4 COMMON SURGICAL PROCEDURES AND RISK OF BLEEDING

MINIMAL BLEEDING RISK	LOW BLEEDING RISK (<2%)	HIGH BLEEDING RISK (>2%)
Dental procedures - Up to two teeth extractions - Subgingival scaling - Gingival biopsy - Periodontal surgery - Root canal	Laparoscopic cholecystectomy	Any procedure involving neuraxial anesthesia
Minor skin procedures - Skin biopsy/excision	Laparoscopic inguinal hernia repair	Cardiac surgery
Endoscopic procedures without biopsy	Other dermatologic procedures	Neurosurgery (intracranial or spinal surgery)
Cataract surgery	Noncataract ophthalmologic procedures	Major vascular surgery (e.g., aortic aneurysm repair, aortofemoral bypass)
Pacemaker/defibrillator implant	Other intra-abdominal, intrathoracic, orthopedic, or vascular surgery	Major urologic surgery (e.g., prostatectomy, bladder tumor resection)
	Coronary angiography	Major lower limb orthopedic surgery (e.g., hip/knee joint replacement surgery)
		Lung resection surgery
		Intestinal anastomosis
		Major open vascular or endovascular surgery
		Selected procedures (e.g., kidney biopsy, prostate biopsy, cervical cone biopsy, pericardiocentesis, colonic polypectomy)

Adapted with permission from Bell BR, Spyropoulos AC, Douketis JD. Perioperative management of the direct oral anticoagulants: A case-based review. *Hematol Oncol Clin North Am.* 2016;30(5):1073–1084.

heparin (UFH) or low-molecular-weight heparin (LMWH). Because half-lives of UFH and LMWH are short, they can be stopped in proximity to the surgical procedure. This allows for minimal anticoagulation interruption while also reducing the risk of procedural bleeding.

The benefit of bridging therapy depends on balancing the risk of thrombosis while off anticoagulation with the risk of periprocedural bleeding. Factors that determine the risk of perioperative thrombosis are the $CHADS_2$ or CHA_2D_2-VASc scores for patients with AF, timing since a prior episode of VTE, and type of mechanical heart valve replacement. Similarly, factors that increase the patient's risk of bleeding while on bridging therapy include platelet abnormalities, aspirin use, history of bleeding while on bridging therapy, or history of major systemic or intracranial hemorrhage (ICH) within the past 3 months.[36]

It is currently accepted that patients at low risk of thrombosis will not need to be bridged. Patients at high risk of thrombosis who possess no other risk factors for bleeding, or whose risk factors for bleeding are reversible, will likely benefit from bridging therapy. However, in high-risk patients who suffered a major bleeding event or ICH within the past 3 months, risk of bleeding with bridging may outweigh its benefits[36] (Table 13.5).

In patients at moderate risks of thrombosis, the benefit of bridging therapy is unclear and the decision to bridge is usually left at the discretion of the treating physician.

Traditionally, patients with AF and a $CHADS_2$ score or 3–4 have been considered at intermediate risk of thrombosis. However, the BRIDGE trial, which assessed bridging therapy in patients with AF and a mean $CHADS_2$ score of 2.3, concluded that foregoing bridging in patients requiring warfarin interruption decreased the risk of bleeding and was found to be noninferior in terms of stroke protection when compared with no bridging.[46] Moreover, recent literature challenged the antithrombotic benefit of bridging.[47] A meta-analysis involving 34 studies described a 13–15% risk for perioperative bleeding and a 3–4% increased risk of major bleeding with no evidence of decreased risk for thrombosis with bridging as compared with stopping warfarin alone.[48] Currently, the 2017 ACC Expert Consensus Decision Pathway for Periprocedural Management of Anticoagulation in Patients with Nonvalvular Atrial Fibrillation recommends that, in intermediate thrombotic risk patients, bridging will only likely benefit those without risk factors for bleeding but who also suffered a CVA/TIA in the past.[36]

A summary of recommendations for bridging therapy based on the indication for oral anticoagulant can be found in Table 13.5.[34]

Once a patient is deemed appropriate for bridging, either UFH or LMWH can be used. UFH prevents clot formation by activating antithrombin III, and it has an extremely short half-life of 1–1.5 hours. Because drug metabolism at therapeutic doses is through endothelial cells, UFH can be safely

Table 13.5 RECOMMENDATIONS FOR BRIDGING THERAPY

THROMBOTIC RISK	ATRIAL FIBRILLATION	MECHANICAL HEART VALVE	VENOUS THROMBOEMBOLISM (VTE)	BRIDGING
High (>10%/yr)	CHADS$_2$ score 5–6 CHA$_2$DS$_2$-VAS$_C$ score 7–9 (No history of intracranial hemorrhage or major bleed within 3 months) Recent embolic stroke <3 months	Mechanical mitral valve replacement (MVR) Old mechanical aortic valve replacement (AVR)	VTE <3 months Severe thrombophilia Multiple thrombophilias Active cancer with high VTE risk	Yes
Moderate (5–10%/yr)	CHA$_2$DS$_2$-VAS$_C$ 5–6 CHADS$_2$ 3–4	Bileaflet mechanical AVR *with* risk factors for stroke[a]	VTE 3–12 months Recurrent VTE Thrombophilia Active cancer	Clinician discretion
Low (<5%/yr)	CHADS$_2$ 0–2 CHA$_2$DS$_2$-VAS$_C$ 1–4	Bileaflet mechanical AVR *without* risk factors for stroke[a]	VTE >12 months	No

[a]Risk factors for stroke: AF, prior CVA/TIA, hypertension, DM, CHF, ≥75 years old.

used in patients with renal impairment. The level of anticoagulation is measured through activated partial thromboplastin time (aPTT), which must be drawn every 6 hours until UFH reaches therapeutic levels.[49] Unfortunately, UFH can only be administrated parenterally and requires an inpatient admission.

LMWH also exerts its anticoagulant effect by activating antithrombin III and subsequently inhibiting factor Xa. It offers similar thromboembolic protection as UFH, but it has several advantages over UFH, such as use in an outpatient setting because of its subcutaneous delivery, more predictable anticoagulant effect, and dose-independent clearance. Enoxaparin, the most commonly used LMWH, is prescribed at 1 mg twice a day or 1.5 mg/day.[47,50]

Metabolism is primarily through the liver, with 40% of the drug excreted through the urine.[51–53] Given its high degree of renal excretion, the anticoagulant effect will accumulate in patients with kidney disease.[51,52,54] As a result, treatment dose is reduced from 1 mg every 12 to 1 mg every 24 hours in patients with a creatinine clearance (CrCl) of less than 30 mL/min.[49] The half-life of LMWH is approximately 4 hours in patients with normal renal function. Routine laboratory monitoring is not necessary for LMWH because of its predictable pharmacokinetics. However, anti-Xa levels may be useful to monitor drug plasma levels in patients with moderate to severe renal impairment.[55]

Bridging therapy should generally be initiated when the INR is lower than 2 (with the exception of mechanical mitral valves when bridging is started at a higher INR of 2.5). UFH should be stopped at least 4 hours before surgery. For patients on LMWH, the last dose should be administered at half the daily dose at least 24 hours prior to the procedure.[36,56]

MANAGEMENT OF DOACS

With the advent of the DOACs, perioperative management of chronic anticoagulation has become much more simplified. Due to the DOACs' short half-lives and predictable pharmacokinetics, patients are usually able to remain on their home regimen until shortly before surgery.

As with warfarin, certain procedures at minimal bleeding risk (i.e., dental, skin, cataract surgery) do not require interruption of DOACs.[47]

For majority of procedures, however, temporary interruption of anticoagulation is required. Determining the precise time for DOAC cessation depends on the periprocedural risk of bleeding (low vs. high risk) and on the patient's renal function, which determines the drug's half-life. The National Kidney Foundation recommends calculating the CrCl using the Cockcroft-Gault equation to best manage drugs dependent on renal excretion. Serum creatinine should not be used since it is affected by multiple factors such as age, race, muscle mass, and protein intake.[57]

Dabigatran, excreted 80% unchanged in the urine, is the DOAC most heavily influenced by kidney function. As a result, a small decrease in CrCl may lead to a significant increase in residual anticoagulant effect.

In patients with normal kidney function, dabigatran should be stopped at least 24 hours before surgery for low-risk bleeding procedures and at least 48 hours prior to high-risk procedures. Discontinuation of dabigatran prior to surgical procedures is detailed in Table 13.6.[36,56]

Factors Xa inhibitors, on the other hand, depend much less on renal excretion. As a result, interruption time will be shorter in patients with moderate kidney dysfunction, but it may still be prolonged in patients with severe impairment. For low-risk bleeding procedures, the 2017 ACC Expert Consensus Decision Pathway for Periprocedural Management of Anticoagulation in Patients with Nonvalvular Atrial Fibrillation recommends that rivaroxaban, apixaban, and edoxaban be held for 24 hours in patients with a CrCl of 30 mL/min or more, 36 hours if CrCl is 15–29 mL/min, and 48 hours if the CrCl is less than 15 mL/min. For high-risk procedures, factor Xa inhibitors should be stopped for at least 48 hours if the CrCl is 30 mL/min or more and 72 hours in patients

Table 13.6 DABIGATRAN INTERRUPTION TIME

CrCl mL/min	PROCEDURAL BLEEDING RISK Low	High
≥80	24 h (1 day)	48 h (2 days)
50–79	36 h (1.5 days)	72 h (3 days)
30–49	48 h (2 days)	96 h (4 days)
15–29	72 h (3 days)	120 h (5 days)
<15	No data At least 96 h (4 days) Consider measuring diluted thrombin time (dTT)	No data Consider measuring dTT

Table 13.7 RIVAROXABAN, EDOXABAN, APIXABAN INTERRUPTION TIMES

CRCL ML/MIN	PROCEDURAL BLEEDING RISK LOW	HIGH
≥30	24 h (1 day)	48 h (2 days)
15–29	36 h (1.5 days)	No data. At least 72 h (3 days) Consider measuring anti-Xa levels
<15	No data At least 48 h (2 days) Consider measuring anti-Xa level	

with a CrCl of less than 30 mL/min[36] (Table 13.7). Similar recommendations are suggested by the 2022 "Perioperative Management of Antithrombotics: An American College of Chest Physicians Clinical Practice Guideline."[35]

Because DOACs possess short half-lives, bridging therapy is generally not required. Two large prospective trials actually found that bridging therapy significantly increases the risk of major bleeding events without decreasing the risk of cardiovascular or thromboembolic events.[58,59]

Bridging of DOACs with LMWH is not recommended for patients with AF. The decision is informed by the results of the PAUSE study. The PAUSE study investigated 3,008 patients with AF on rivaroxaban and apixaban who had their DOAC stopped preoperatively based on a standardized approach (1 day prior to surgery for low-risk bleeding procedures and 2 days prior to surgery for high-risk bleeding procedures). The study detected a low risk of thromboembolism with a risk of bleeding of less than 2%.[60]

Similarly, bridging for DOACs in patients with a VTE indication is generally not needed. However, the recently published European Society of Cardiology Guidelines on cardiovascular assessment and management of patients undergoing noncardiac surgery suggest a case-by-case decision when bridging a DOAC especially in patients with a history of recent stroke as well as those who experienced a thromboembolic event in the setting of DOAC interruption previously.[61]

MANAGEMENT OF DOACS BEFORE REGIONAL ANESTHESIA

For surgeries where regional anesthesia may be beneficial to the patient, the American Society of Regional Anesthesiologists (ASRA) updated its recommendations in 2018.[42] In addition to neuraxial anesthesia, high-risk regional procedures are narrowed to peri-neuraxial (paravertebral block), deep plexus (lumbar plexus block), and deep peripheral nerve blocks (sciatic and infraclavicular block).[42]

Factor Xa inhibitors taken at prophylactic doses in patients with normal renal function will only require 1 day of cessation before high-risk regional procedures can be done. However, patients taking a full treatment dose or who have moderate renal dysfunction will need to hold their anticoagulation for at least 3 days.[42]

As described in detail above, optimal interruption time for dabigatran interruption is recommended mainly based on CrCl, and the 2018 ASRA guidelines for dabigatran management before high-risk regional anesthesia procedures recommend interruption times similar to those observed for high-risk bleeding surgical procedures (stopping at least 72 hours prior). High-risk bleeding regional anesthesia procedures are not recommended in patients on dabigatran who have a CrCl of less than 30 mL/min because severe kidney disease renders its excretion slow and unpredictable.[42]

Finally, a first dose of all DOACs can be restarted 6 hours after procedure puncture or catheter withdrawal with the exception of betrixaban, which can be started 5 hours after.[42,62] A summary of ASRA recommendation in patients taking oral anticoagulation can be found in Table 13.8.

Newer literature suggests that low-risk regional techniques (such as tap blocks) can be done while continuing oral anticoagulation per the European Society of Regional Anesthesia (while not clearly recommended by ASRA).[63,64] ASRA suggests management of anticoagulation before these procedures be guided by compressibility, vascularity, and consequences of bleeding but does not clearly endorse continuation of anticoagulation.[42,62]

DOACS LABORATORY MONITORING

Laboratory testing to monitor DOAC levels has proved difficult and is not recommended prior to surgical procedures.[65] Conventional laboratory tests such as aPTT and PT have poor sensitivity and specificity when testing the anticoagulant effects of DOACs (Table 13.9). For direct thrombin inhibitors, aPTT can detect that drug level in the therapeutic and supratherapeutic range. However, it is only linear with dabigatran level in the therapeutic range and becomes unreliable when dabigatran is supratherapeutic. A normal aPTT excludes dabigatran as a source of bleeding.[66] While an aPTT can be sensitive in detecting low dabigatran levels when interrupted prior to surgical procedures, a diluted thrombin time or an ecarin clotting test (which are not readily available) are specific tests for dabigatran.[67]

Table 13.8 AMERICAN SOCIETY OF REGIONAL ANESTHESIOLOGISTS GUIDELINES ON DIRECT ORAL ANTICOAGULANT INTERRUPTION TIMES BEFORE HIGH-RISK REGIONAL ANESTHESIA PROCEDURES

RIVAROXABAN	INTERRUPTION TIME	APIXABAN	INTERRUPTION TIME	EDOXABAN	INTERRUPTION TIME	BETRIXABAN	INTERRUPTION TIME
Dose ≤10 mg/day	22–26 h (1 day)	Dose ≤2.5 mg/day	26–30 h (1 day)	Dose ≤30 mg/day	20–28 h (1 day)		72 h
Dose >10 mg/day CrCl <50 mL/min	44–65 h (2–3 days)	Dose 5 mg/day Cr 1.5 and >80 y/o or ≤60 kg	40–75 h (2–3 days)	Dose >30 mg/day CrCl 15–50 mL/min ≤60 kg On P-GP inhibitors (clarithromycin, erythromycin, ritonavir, verapamil)	40–70 h (2–3 days)	CrCl 15–29 mL/min On P-GP inhibitors (clarithromycin, erythromycin, ritonavir, verapamil)	76–135 h
1st dose after block placement or catheter withdraw	6 h	1st dose after block placement or catheter withdraw	6 h	1st dose after block placement or catheter withdraw	6 h	1st dose after block placement or catheter withdraw	5 h

Table 13.9 LABORATORY TESTS FOR DIRECT ORAL ANTICOAGULANT (DOAC) MONITORING

		LABORATORY MEASUREMENTS			
DRUG	PREFERRED TEST	APTT	PT/INR	TEG	ROTEM
Dabigatran	Dilute thrombin time or ecarin clotting time	Linear relationship in therapeutic range Normal aPTT excludes bleeding from dabigatran	Does not correlate with dabigatran level	Quantifies but cannot reliably qualify drug level Increases R time	Quantifies but cannot reliably qualify drug level Increases clotting time
Rivaroxaban	Anti-Xa calibrated for rivaroxaban	Nonspecific and not reliable	Linear relationship in therapeutic and supratherapeutic range Normal PT excludes bleeding from rivaroxaban		
Edoxaban	Anti-Xa calibrated for edoxaban	Nonspecific and not reliable	Linear relationship in therapeutic and supratherapeutic range Normal PT excludes bleeding from edoxaban		
Apixaban	Anti-Xa calibrated for apixaban	Nonspecific and not reliable	Nonspecific and not reliable		

aPTT, activated partial thromboplastin time; PT, prothrombin time; ROTEM, rotational thromboelastometry; TEG, thromboelastography.

For factor Xa inhibitors, anti-Xa level is the most useful test to monitor drug concentration. Anti-Xa calibrated to a specific factor Xa inhibitor shows a linear relationship with drug plasma level in the subtherapeutic, therapeutic and supratherapeutic range. A normal anti-Xa excludes clinically relevant levels of rivaroxaban, apixaban, and edoxaban.[66,68]

Despite lack of specificity, conventional coagulation testing can also provide some information, although these tests are much less useful. PT demonstrates a linear relationship with rivaroxaban and edoxaban in the therapeutic and, up to a certain degree, supratherapeutic ranges. However, the aPTT is not a reliable test for either rivaroxaban or edoxaban. Unfortunately, both aPTT and PT are unreliable tests for apixaban.[66,68]

Thromboelastography (TEG) can also be employed for DOAC monitoring but is also nonspecific. Kaolin reaction time can detect the presence of dabigatran, rivaroxaban, and apixaban but cannot accurately quantify drug level as therapeutic or supratherapeutic.[69]

Table 13.10 **ANTICOAGULATION REINITIATION**

	SURGICAL RISK OF BLEEDING			
	LOW		HIGH	
PATIENT THROMBOTIC RISK	WARFARIN	DOAC	WARFARIN	DOAC
Low	Within 24 h	POD 1	POD 2–3	POD 2–3
High	Warfarin + bridging therapy when INR <2 within 24 h	POD 1	Start UFH without bolus dose *or* Start UFH or LMWH at the prophylactic dose for VTE *or* Start VKA without bridging	POD 2–3

DOAC, direct oral anticoagulant; LMWH, low-molecular-weight heparin; UFH, unfractionated heparin; VKA, vitamin K antagonists; VTE, venous thromboembolism.

REINITIATION OF ORAL ANTICOAGULATION AFTER INVASIVE PROCEDURE

Oral anticoagulation after invasive procedures should only be reinitiated after close communication with the surgical and anesthesia teams (Table 13.10). Factors to take into consideration include adequacy of surgical site hemostasis, risk of postoperative bleeding, consequences of potential bleeding events, and the patient's risk of thrombosis.

In most cases, patients can resume warfarin within 24 hours of surgery. Because warfarin requires 2–3 days to exert anticoagulant effect and 5–7 days to reach peak effect, it will not increase the risk of early postoperative bleeding. However, if the patient is at low risk of thrombosis and the surgical procedure has a high risk of bleeding, reinitiation of therapeutic anticoagulation may need to be delayed.

When perioperative bridging was administered preoperatively, LMWH can be restarted 24 hours after surgery for procedures with a low bleeding risk and 48–72 hours following surgery for patients with a high bleeding risk.[36,47]

In circumstances where the surgical risk of postoperative bleeding is high and the patient's risk of thromboembolism is also high, the 2017 ACC Expert Consensus Decision Pathway for Periprocedural Management of Anticoagulation in Patients with Nonvalvular Atrial Fibrillation recommends considering the following strategies: starting UFH without a bolus dose, starting UFH or LMWH at the prophylactic dose for VTE, or starting VKA without bridging. No matter the technique, when bridging therapy and/or warfarin are used postoperatively, INR should be closely monitored to avoid over anticoagulation.[36] Perioperative bridging therapy can be discontinued after surgery as long as INR levels have been in the desired therapeutic range for at least 48 hours.[47]

Reinitiating DOACs after surgery involves a slightly different set of considerations. Because DOACs reach peak plasma level within a few hours, patients will be considered fully anticoagulated soon after restarting their medication. As a result, DOACs should be held postoperatively for 2–3 days in patients with questionable hemostasis and in patients or after surgeries with high risks for bleeding. If effective surgical hemostasis has been reached and the procedural risk of bleeding is low, DOACs may be restarted the day after surgery.[36]

When restarting DOACs, dosing should not automatically default to the preoperative state. Postoperative CrCl should be calculated so that potential postoperative kidney injury is taken into account and overdosing does not occur. Similarly to preoperative considerations, postoperative bridging therapy is not necessary in patients on DOACs due to a fast onset of action.

CONCLUSION

- AF is a common arrhythmia characterized by irregular and rapid atrial discharges.
- Risk factors for AF development are multiple and include advanced age, history of obesity, OSA, DM, hypertension, CAD, CHF, valvular heart disease, smoking, and excessive alcohol use.
- Diagnosis is primarily through ECG, which will show irregularly irregular QRS complexes without the presence of P waves.
- Stroke and TIA are the most common sequalae of untreated AF, but their risk may be decreased with the use of chronic anticoagulation.
- Vitamin K antagonists and DOACs are the most commonly used oral anticoagulants.
- Factors determining when patients on the vitamin K antagonist warfarin will need to stop their anticoagulation prior to surgery include the patient's INR, risk of bleeding, and risk of thrombosis, as well as the surgical risk of bleeding.
- Patients at high risk of thrombosis may need bridging therapy to minimize time off systemic anticoagulation.
- Management of DOACs before invasive procedures will depend mainly on renal function.
- Due to the drugs' short half-lives, patients on DOACs have the advantage of continuing their home regimen until shortly before surgery, obviating the need for bridging therapy.
- Regional anesthesia procedures can be safely performed on patients taking DOACs as long as the anticoagulant has been held for a short period of time.

- Reinitiating anticoagulation postoperatively should be decided only after close communication between the surgical and anesthesia teams.

REVIEW QUESTIONS

1. An 80-year-old man with a history of metabolic syndrome including OSA, hypertension, DM, and CHF presents to your preadmission clinic for preoperative evaluation before cholecystectomy. Which one of his comorbidities has the strongest association with the development of AF?

   a. OSA.
   b. Hypertension.
   c. DM.
   d. CHF.

   The correct answer is d.

   Multiple factors are associated with the development of AF. Although both OSA and hypertension have high prevalence in patients with AF, CHF confers the highest relative risk.

2. In the patient presented in Question 1, what is his CHA_2D_2-VASc score?

   a. 2.
   b. 3.
   c. 4.
   d. 5.

   The correct answer is d.

   According to the CHA_2D_2-VASc score, history of CHF, hypertension, DM, vascular disease, age 65–74, and female sex are each 1 point, while age ≥75 and older and prior stroke/TIA are each 2 points. In this patient who is 80 years old, has hypertension, DM, and CHF, his CHA_2D_2-VASc score will be 5.

3. Which DOAC is least dependent on the kidneys for excretion and therefore best used in patients with renal impairment?

   a. Dabigatran.
   b. Rivaroxaban.
   c. Apixaban.
   d. Edoxaban.

   The correct answer is c.

   Dabigatran is excreted 80% unchanged through the kidneys, making it the DOAC most dependent on renal function. Rivaroxaban is 66% kidney-excreted but only 36% unchanged, and edoxaban is excreted 50% unchanged. Apixaban is excreted 27% unchanged through the kidneys, making it least dependent on renal function.

4. Which of the following patients will benefit most from bridging therapy?

   a. A 55-year-old man on warfarin for mechanical mitral valve.
   b. A 70-year-old woman on warfarin for stroke prevention in the setting of AF with a CHA_2DS_2-VASc score of 6.
   c. A 25-year-old woman on dabigatran for recent diagnosis of DVT after a prolonged flight.
   d. A 45-year-old man with history of stage IV colon cancer on apixaban for PE diagnosed 1 month ago.

   The correct answer is a.

   Those patients on warfarin and at high risk of thrombosis, including those with mechanical mitral valve replacements, $CHADS_2$ scores of 5–6, CHA_2DS_2-VASc scores of 7–9, VTE within the past 3 months, and severe thrombophilia will benefit most from bridging therapy. Those at high risk of thrombosis but who have also suffered major bleeding events or ICH within the past 3 months may not tolerate bridging therapy due to high bleeding risk. Patients on DOACs or who are at moderate risk of thrombosis do not require bridging therapy.

5. A 45-year-old woman on rivaroxaban for recent history of DVT after back surgery presents for urgent open reduction and internal fixation of a distal femur fracture. She denies use of other antithrombotic or anticoagulant drugs. She has a normal coagulation profile and a CrCl of 90 mL/min. Her last dose of rivaroxaban was 24 hours ago. Which of the following regional anesthetic procedures is she a candidate for?

   a. Epidural catheter.
   b. Femoral nerve catheter.
   c. Single-shot femoral nerve block.
   d. She is not a candidate for regional anesthesia.

   The correct answer is c.

   The 2018 ASRA guidelines suggest that high-risk regional anesthesia procedures such as an epidural require 2–3 days of DOAC interruption. Reginal procedures at intermediate risk of bleeding, such as single-shot femoral nerve blocks, may be performed with less drug interruption time given the site's ease of compressibility. ASRA does not mention anticoagulation management prior to peripheral nerve catheter placement.

6. In the patient presented in Question 5, what is the best laboratory test to measure plasma rivaroxaban level?

   a. Anti-Xa level.
   b. aPTT.
   c. PT.
   d. INR.

   The correct answer is a.

   In patients taking rivaroxaban or any other factor Xa inhibitors, the most accurate test for drug plasma level is anti-Xa calibrated for that specific anticoagulant or for heparin. If obtaining an anti-Xa level is not possible or requires a significant amount of time, PT can be obtained. PT has a linear relationship with rivaroxaban and edoxaban in the therapeutic and supratherapeutic range. aPTT and INR are not reliable tests for factor Xa inhibitors.

7. A 79-year-old woman with history of hypertension, type 2 diabetes, and smoking presents to the emergency room with productive cough and fever. Vital signs reveal a heart rate of 126 and blood pressure 150/70. ECG shows irregularly irregular QRS complex with no P waves. The patient denies being

diagnosed with AF or a history of palpitations. What is the most appropriate next course of action?

   a. Cardioversion.
   b. Administer beta blocker.
   c. Administer digoxin.
   d. Start heparin drip.

The correct answer is b.

Acute treatment of AF depends on two factors: timing of AF onset and hemodynamic stability. In patients who presents with AF with RVR, cardioversion is desired if there is hemodynamic instability and/or timing of onset is within the past 48 hours. Because AF can lead to blood stasis and atrial clot formation, routine cardioversion is not recommended in chronic AF unless the patient has been adequately anticoagulated and TEE has been performed to rule out atrial thrombosis. This is to minimize the risk of stroke from clot dislodgement once the atrium begins to contract normally again after cardioversion. Instead, desired therapy in these patients will be rate control with a beta blocker or calcium channel blocker and possible oral anticoagulation. Patients who present with asymptomatic AF but are at high risk for AF development should be suspected of having chronic AF and be treated with rate control and further workup.

REFERENCES

1. January CT, Wann LS, Alpert JS, et al. 2014 AHA/ACC/HRS Guideline for the Management of Patients with Atrial Fibrillation: A Report of the American College of Cardiology/American Heart Association Task Force on Practice Guidelines and the Heart Rhythm Society. *J Am Coll Cardiol*. 2014 Dec;64(21):e1–e76.
2. Benjamin EJ, Levy D, Vaziri SM, D'Agostino RB, Belanger AJ, Wolf PA. Independent risk factors for atrial fibrillation in a population-based cohort: The Framingham Heart Study. *JAMA*. 1994 Mar;271(11):840–844.
3. Lau DH, Nattel S, Kalman JM, Sanders P. Modifiable risk factors and atrial fibrillation. *Circulation*. 2017 Aug;136(6):583–596.
4. Gami AS, Hodge DO, Herges RM, et al. Obstructive sleep apnea, obesity, and the risk of incident atrial fibrillation. *J Am Coll Cardiol*. 2007 Feb;49(5):565–571.
5. Huxley RR, Lopez FL, Folsom AR, et al. Absolute and attributable risks of atrial fibrillation in relation to optimal and borderline risk factors: The Atherosclerosis Risk in Communities (ARIC) study. *Circulation*. 2011 Apr;123(14):1501–1508.
6. Stevenson IH, Teichtahl H, Cunnington D, Ciavarella S, Gordon I, Kalman JM. Prevalence of sleep disordered breathing in paroxysmal and persistent atrial fibrillation patients with normal left ventricular function. *Eur Heart J*. 2008 Jul;29(13):1662–1669.
7. Qureshi WT, Alirhayim Z, Blaha MJ, et al. Cardiorespiratory fitness and risk of incident atrial fibrillation: Results from the Henry Ford Exercise Testing (FIT) Project. *Circulation*. 2015 May;131(21):1827–1834.
8. Kim EJ, Yin X, Fontes JD, et al. Atrial fibrillation without comorbidities: Prevalence, incidence and prognosis (from the Framingham Heart Study). *Am Heart J*. 2016 Jul;177:138–144.
9. Dewar RI, Lip GY; Guidelines Development Group for the NICE clinical guideline for the management of atrial fibrillation. Identification, diagnosis and assessment of atrial fibrillation. *Heart*. 2007 Jan;93(1):25–28. doi:10.1136/hrt.2006.099861. Epub 2006 Sep 4. PMID: 16952973; PMCID: PMC1861326.
10. Wyse DG, Waldo AL, DiMarco JP, et al. A comparison of rate control and rhythm control in patients with atrial fibrillation. *N Engl J Med*. 2002 Dec;347(23):1825–1833.
11. Kirchhof P, Camm AJ, Goette A, et al. Early rhythm-control therapy in patients with atrial fibrillation. *N Engl J Med*. 2020 Oct 01;383(14):1305–1316.
12. Staerk L, Sherer JA, Ko D, Benjamin EJ, Helm RH. Atrial fibrillation: Epidemiology, pathophysiology, and clinical outcomes. *Circ Res*. 2017 Apr;120(9):1501–1517.
13. Lip GY, Tse HF, Lane DA. Atrial fibrillation. *Lancet*. 2012 Feb;379(9816):648–661.
14. Olesen JB, Torp-Pedersen C, Hansen ML, Lip GY. The value of the CHA2DS2-VASc score for refining stroke risk stratification in patients with atrial fibrillation with a CHADS2 score 0-1: A nationwide cohort study. *Thromb Haemost*. 2012 Jun;107(6):1172–1179.
15. Jørgensen HS, Nakayama H, Reith J, Raaschou HO, Olsen TS. Acute stroke with atrial fibrillation: The Copenhagen Stroke Study. *Stroke*. 1996 Oct;27(10):1765–1769.
16. Bessissow A, Khan J, Devereaux PJ, Alvarez-Garcia J, Alonso-Coello P. Postoperative atrial fibrillation in non-cardiac and cardiac surgery: An overview. *J Thromb Haemost*. 2015 Jun;13(Suppl 1):S304–12.
17. Harter K, Levine M, Henderson SO. Anticoagulation drug therapy: A review. *West J Emerg Med*. 2015 Jan;16(1):11–17.
18. Jacobs LG. Warfarin pharmacology, clinical management, and evaluation of hemorrhagic risk for the elderly. *Cardiol Clin*. 2008 May;26(2):157–67, v.
19. Ageno W, Gallus AS, Wittkowsky A, Crowther M, Hylek EM, Palareti G. Oral anticoagulant therapy: Antithrombotic Therapy and Prevention of Thrombosis, 9th ed: American College of Chest Physicians Evidence-Based Clinical Practice Guidelines. *Chest*. 2012 Feb;141(2 Suppl):e44S–e88S.
20. Hurlen M, Abdelnoor M, Smith P, Erikssen J, Arnesen H. Warfarin, aspirin, or both after myocardial infarction. *N Engl J Med*. 2002 Sep;347(13):969–974.
21. Otto CM, Nishimura RA, Bonow RO, et al. 2020 ACC/AHA Guideline for the Management of Patients with Valvular Heart Disease: A Report of the American College of Cardiology/American Heart Association Joint Committee on Clinical Practice Guidelines. *Circulation*. 2021 Feb 02;143(5):e72–e227.
22. Gulati G, Hevelow M, George M, Behling E, Siegel J. International normalized ratio versus plasma levels of coagulation factors in patients on vitamin K antagonist therapy. *Arch Pathol Lab Med*. 2011 Apr;135(4):490–494.
23. Sarah S. The pharmacology and therapeutic use of dabigatran etexilate. *J Clin Pharmacol*. 2013 Jan;53(1):1–13.
24. Knauf F, Chaknos CM, Berns JS, Perazella MA. Dabigatran and kidney disease: A bad combination. *Clin J Am Soc Nephrol*. 2013 Sep;8(9):1591–1597.
25. Ganetsky M, Babu KM, Salhanick SD, Brown RS, Boyer EW. Dabigatran: Review of pharmacology and management of bleeding complications of this novel oral anticoagulant. *J Med Toxicol*. 2011 Dec;7(4):281–287.
26. Connolly SJ, Ezekowitz MD, Yusuf S, et al. Dabigatran versus warfarin in patients with atrial fibrillation. *N Engl J Med*. 2009 Sep;361(12):1139–1151.
27. Kubitza D, Berkowitz SD, Misselwitz F. Evidence-based development and rationale for once-daily rivaroxaban dosing regimens across multiple indications. *Clin Appl Thromb Hemost*. 2016 Jul;22(5):412–422.
28. Stacy ZA, Call WB, Hartmann AP, Peters GL, Richter SK. Edoxaban: A comprehensive review of the pharmacology and clinical data for the management of atrial fibrillation and venous thromboembolism. *Cardiol Ther*. 2016 Jun;5(1):1–18.
29. Nafee T, Gibson CM, Yee MK, et al. Betrixaban for first-line venous thromboembolism prevention in acute medically ill patients with risk factors for venous thromboembolism. *Expert Rev Cardiovasc Ther*. 2018 Nov;16(11):845–855.
30. Rupprecht HJ, Blank R. Clinical pharmacology of direct and indirect factor Xa inhibitors. *Drugs*. 2010 Nov;70(16):2153–2170.

31. Samama MM, Meddahi S, Samama CM. Pharmacology and laboratory testing of the oral Xa inhibitors. *Clin Lab Med*. 2014 Sep;34(3):503–517.
32. Patel MR, Mahaffey KW, Garg J, et al. Rivaroxaban versus warfarin in nonvalvular atrial fibrillation. *N Engl J Med*. 2011 Sep;365(10):883–891.
33. Granger CB, Alexander JH, McMurray JJ, et al. Apixaban versus warfarin in patients with atrial fibrillation. *N Engl J Med*. 2011 Sep;365(11):981–992.
34. Douketis JD, Spyropoulos AC, Spencer FA, et al. Perioperative management of antithrombotic therapy: Antithrombotic Therapy and Prevention of Thrombosis, 9th ed: American College of Chest Physicians Evidence-Based Clinical Practice Guidelines. *Chest*. 2012 Feb;141(2 Suppl):e326S–50S.
35. Douketis JD, Spyropoulos AC, Murad MH, et al. Perioperative management of antithrombotic therapy: An American College of Chest Physicians clinical practice guideline. *Chest*. 2022 Nov;162(5):e207–e43.
36. Doherty JU, Gluckman TJ, Hucker WJ, et al. 2017 ACC expert consensus decision pathway for periprocedural management of anticoagulation in patients with nonvalvular atrial fibrillation: A report of the American College of Cardiology Clinical Expert Consensus Document Task Force. *J Am Coll Cardiol*. 2017 Feb;69(7):871–898.
37. Pisters R, Lane DA, Nieuwlaat R, de Vos CB, Crijns HJ, Lip GY. A novel user-friendly score (HAS-BLED) to assess 1-year risk of major bleeding in patients with atrial fibrillation: The Euro Heart Survey. *Chest*. 2010 Nov;138(5):1093–1100.
38. Spyropoulos AC, Douketis JD. How I treat anticoagulated patients undergoing an elective procedure or surgery. *Blood*. 2012 Oct;120(15):2954–2962.
39. Bell BR, Spyropoulos AC, Douketis JD. Perioperative management of the direct oral anticoagulants: A case-based review. *Hematol Oncol Clin North Am*. 2016;30(5):1073–1084.
40. Baron TH, Kamath PS, McBane RD. Management of antithrombotic therapy in patients undergoing invasive procedures. *N Engl J Med*. 2013 May;368(22):2113–2124.
41. Spyropoulos AC, Brohi K, Caprini J, et al. Scientific and Standardization Committee Communication: Guidance document on the periprocedural management of patients on chronic oral anticoagulant therapy: Recommendations for standardized reporting of procedural/surgical bleed risk and patient-specific thromboembolic risk. *J Thromb Haemost*. 2019 Nov;17(11):1966–1972.
42. Horlocker TT, Vandermeuelen E, Kopp SL, Gogarten W, Leffert LR, Benzon HT. Regional anesthesia in the patient receiving antithrombotic or thrombolytic therapy: American Society of Regional Anesthesia and Pain Medicine evidence-based guidelines (4th edition). *Reg Anesth Pain Med*. 2018;43(3):263–309.
43. Douketis JD. Perioperative management of patients who are receiving warfarin therapy: An evidence-based and practical approach. *Blood*. 2011 May;117(19):5044–5049.
44. Syed S, Adams BB, Liao W, Pipitone M, Gloster H. A prospective assessment of bleeding and international normalized ratio in warfarin-anticoagulated patients having cutaneous surgery. *J Am Acad Dermatol*. 2004 Dec;51(6):955–957.
45. Jamula E, Anderson J, Douketis JD. Safety of continuing warfarin therapy during cataract surgery: A systematic review and meta-analysis. *Thromb Res*. 2009 Jul;124(3):292–299.
46. Douketis JD, Spyropoulos AC, Kaatz S, et al. Perioperative bridging anticoagulation in patients with atrial fibrillation. *N Engl J Med*. 2015 Aug;373(9):823–833.
47. Oprea AD, Noto CJ, Halaszynski TM. Risk stratification, perioperative and periprocedural management of the patient receiving anticoagulant therapy. *J Clin Anesth*. 2016 Nov;34:586–599.
48. Siegal D, Yudin J, Kaatz S, Douketis JD, Lim W, Spyropoulos AC. Periprocedural heparin bridging in patients receiving vitamin K antagonists: Systematic review and meta-analysis of bleeding and thromboembolic rates. *Circulation*. 2012 Sep;126(13):1630–1639.
49. Smythe MA, Priziola J, Dobesh PP, Wirth D, Cuker A, Wittkowsky AK. Guidance for the practical management of the heparin anticoagulants in the treatment of venous thromboembolism. *J Thromb Thrombolysis*. 2016 Jan;41(1):165–186.
50. Spyropoulos AC, Turpie AG, Dunn AS, et al. Clinical outcomes with unfractionated heparin or low-molecular-weight heparin as bridging therapy in patients on long-term oral anticoagulants: The REGIMEN registry. *J Thromb Haemost*. 2006 Jun;4(6):1246–1252.
51. Garcia DA, Baglin TP, Weitz JI, Samama MM. Parenteral anticoagulants: Antithrombotic Therapy and Prevention of Thrombosis, 9th ed: American College of Chest Physicians Evidence-Based Clinical Practice Guidelines. *Chest*. 2012 Feb;141(2 Suppl):e24S–e43S.
52. Goudable C, Saivin S, Houin G, et al. Pharmacokinetics of a low molecular weight heparin (Fraxiparine) in various stages of chronic renal failure. *Nephron*. 1991;59(4):543–545.
53. Lim W, Dentali F, Eikelboom JW, Crowther MA. Meta-analysis: Low-molecular-weight heparin and bleeding in patients with severe renal insufficiency. *Ann Intern Med*. 2006 May;144(9):673–684.
54. Fihn SD, Gardin JM, Abrams J, et al. 2012 ACCF/AHA/ACP/AATS/PCNA/SCAI/STS Guideline for the diagnosis and management of patients with stable ischemic heart disease: A report of the American College of Cardiology Foundation/American Heart Association Task Force on Practice Guidelines, and the American College of Physicians, American Association for Thoracic Surgery, Preventive Cardiovascular Nurses Association, Society for Cardiovascular Angiography and Interventions, and Society of Thoracic Surgeons. *J Am Coll Cardiol*. 2012 Dec;60(24):e44–e164.
55. Nutescu EA, Spinler SA, Wittkowsky A, Dager WE. Low-molecular-weight heparins in renal impairment and obesity: Available evidence and clinical practice recommendations across medical and surgical settings. *Ann Pharmacother*. 2009 Jun;43(6):1064–1083.
56. Spyropoulos AC, Al-Badri A, Sherwood MW, Douketis JD. Periprocedural management of patients receiving a vitamin K antagonist or a direct oral anticoagulant requiring an elective procedure or surgery. *J Thromb Haemost*. 2016 05;14(5):875–885.
57. Stevens PE, Levin A. Evaluation and management of chronic kidney disease: Synopsis of the kidney disease: Improving global outcomes 2012 clinical practice guideline. *Ann Intern Med*. 2013 Jun;158(11):825–830.
58. Douketis JD, Healey JS, Brueckmann M, et al. Perioperative bridging anticoagulation during dabigatran or warfarin interruption among patients who had an elective surgery or procedure: Substudy of the RE-LY trial. *Thromb Haemost*. 2015 Mar;113(3):625–632.
59. Beyer-Westendorf J, Gelbricht V, Förster K, et al. Peri-interventional management of novel oral anticoagulants in daily care: Results from the prospective Dresden NOAC registry. *Eur Heart J*. 2014 Jul;35(28):1888–1896.
60. Douketis JD, Spyropoulos AC, Duncan J, et al. Perioperative management of patients with atrial fibrillation receiving a direct oral anticoagulant. *JAMA Intern Med*. 2019 Nov 1;179(11):1469–1478.
61. Halvorsen S, Mehilli J, Cassese S, et al. 2022 ESC Guidelines on cardiovascular assessment and management of patients undergoing noncardiac surgery. *Eur Heart J*. 2022 Oct 14;43(39):3826–3924.
62. Narouze S, Benzon HT, Provenzano D, et al. Interventional spine and pain procedures in patients on antiplatelet and anticoagulant medications (2nd edition): Guidelines from the American Society of Regional Anesthesia and Pain Medicine, the European Society of Regional Anaesthesia and Pain Therapy, the American Academy of Pain Medicine, the International Neuromodulation Society, the North American Neuromodulation Society, and the World Institute of Pain. *Reg Anesth Pain Med*. 2018 Apr;43(3):225–262.
63. Kietaibl S, Ferrandis R, Godier A, et al. Regional anaesthesia in patients on antithrombotic drugs: Joint ESAIC/ESRA guidelines. *Eur J Anaesthesiol*. 2022 Feb 01;39(2):100–132.
64. Li J, Oprea AD. Periprocedural management of patients on oral anticoagulation: Focus on regional anesthesia. *Pol Arch Intern Med*. 2020 Dec 22;130(12):1081–1092.
65. Spyropoulos AC, Al-Badri A, Sherwood MW, Douketis JD. To measure or not to measure direct oral anticoagulants before surgery or invasive procedures: Comment. *J Thromb Haemost*. 2016 12;14(12):2556–2559.

66. Cuker A, Siegal DM, Crowther MA, Garcia DA. Laboratory measurement of the anticoagulant activity of the non-vitamin K oral anticoagulants. *J Am Coll Cardiol*. 2014 Sep;64(11):1128–1139.
67. Dubé C, Douketis JD, Moffat KA, Schulman S, Blais N. Basic coagulation tests as surrogates of dabigatran levels in a pre-operative setting: Analysis of five activated partial thromboplastin time reagents and thrombin time. *Thromb Res*. 2018 Sep;171:62–67.
68. Cuker A, Husseinzadeh H. Laboratory measurement of the anticoagulant activity of edoxaban: A systematic review. *J Thromb Thrombolysis*. 2015 Apr;39(3):288–294.
69. Brinkman HJ. Global assays and the management of oral anticoagulation. *Thromb J*. 2015;13:9.

14.

SEVERE AORTIC STENOSIS

CANDIDATE FOR A SURGICENTER?

Elvera L. Baron and Menachem M. Weiner

STEM CASE AND KEY QUESTIONS

An 87-year-old woman presents for preoperative evaluation prior to extracorporeal shock wave lithotripsy (ESWL), which is only done in our freestanding ambulatory center. She reports that she has severe aortic stenosis (AS).

What additional history should you obtain from a patient presenting for preoperative evaluation with a history of significant cardiac valvular disease?

The patient also reports a history of hypertension for which she takes metoprolol, type II diabetes for which she takes metformin, and urinary stones in her mid-50s that spontaneously passed. She has noticed over the past year that it has become increasingly difficult to walk two city blocks or go up the two flight of stairs to her apartment due to shortness of breath.

Last week she presented to the emergency room with intermittent, sharp, severe left-sided flank pain associated with nausea and vomiting and was diagnosed with bilateral renal calculi.

What are the physical exam findings in a patient with AS?

On physical exam, the patient was noted to be an obese woman with a BMI of 33, unremarkable airway, 3/6 holosystolic murmur at the upper right sternal border, and mild left-sided costovertebral angle tenderness.

What are the available treatments for renal calculi? What is ESWL?

She was discharged home from the emergency room on NSAIDs, with a plan for outpatient urology follow up and possible ESWL.

What preoperative testing is needed for this patient?

A recent ECG revealed normal sinus rhythm. Subsequent echocardiography demonstrated normal left ventricular function (ejection fraction of 55%), moderately hypertrophied left ventricle (LV), severely calcified tricuspid aortic valve, severe AS (aortic valve area [AVA] = 0.85 cm^2, peak pressure gradient [ΔP] = 90 mm Hg), minimal aortic regurgitation, normal right ventricular function, and no other valvular abnormalities.

How is the cardiovascular risk determined for a patient with severe AS presenting for surgery?

The patient's progressively worsening symptoms of exertional dyspnea, coupled with echocardiographic findings, are consistent with diagnosis of severe symptomatic AS. The patient is determined to be at an elevated risk for the procedure due to severe valvular disease, poor functional status, obesity, and a history of diabetes.

What are your anesthetic concerns for a patient with severe AS? What are the hemodynamic goals for patients with AS? How will you monitor blood pressure intraoperatively? What are the potential causes of instability in this patient intraoperatively?

Upon further questioning, the patient remembered that several months ago she underwent screening colonoscopy. She was told by her anesthesiologist at that time that her blood pressure went down and was low during the procedure. The review of the anesthetic record confirmed a prolonged episode of hypotension following induction, which responded to boluses of phenylephrine. Postoperative recovery was unremarkable.

What additional concerns should be considered during preoperative planning?

Additional laboratory data revealed microhematuria with urine specific gravity 1.027 and pH 6.8. Noncontrast computed tomography (CT) scan demonstrated a left-sided 5 mm stone in the upper calyx with mild hydronephrosis and a 4 mm right ureteral nonobstructing stone. The urologist started the patient on tamsulosin and recommended scheduling an outpatient ESWL for treatment of the left-sided stone.

Should a patient with severe AS undergo treatment for the aortic valve prior to undergoing elective surgery?

Based on the patient's severe AS with elevated transaortic gradient, symptoms of exertional dyspnea, and decreased exercise tolerance, aortic valve replacement (AVR) is indicated. Therefore, a discussion is held between the urologists, cardiac surgeons, interventional cardiologists, anesthesiologists, and the patient to determine the risks and benefits of AVR or balloon angioplasty prior to undergoing treatment for her urolithiasis. This shared decision-making process also included discussion about surgical versus transcatheter approaches to AVR. It was determined that the treatment for the urolithiasis was urgent and necessary prior to any aortic valve intervention.

Should a patient with significant valvular disease undergo a procedure in an ambulatory center? Is an open procedure in the main operating room a better option?

Due to the patient's severe AS, the need for a greater level of perioperative monitoring, and risk of complications, the treatment plan for the patient is changed. She is scheduled for flexible ureteroscopy (URS) under general anesthesia with an arterial line for blood pressure monitoring in the hospital. Postoperatively, she recovers in a step-down unit overnight for monitoring.

DISCUSSION

AORTIC STENOSIS OVERVIEW

AS is a progressive disease where patients experience symptoms once the aortic valve orifice is significantly reduced. It is estimated that more than 2% of elderly Americans have AS, with prevalence increasing over the past several decades as the elderly population continues to grow. Common symptoms include chest pain, tachycardia, exertional dyspnea, decreased exercise tolerance, orthopnea, syncope or presyncope, and fatigue.[1,2] On physical exam, a systolic murmur at the right of the sternal border maybe appreciated, and some patients may have evidence of lower extremity peripheral edema. Notably, in adult patients, the physical exam may not be accurate for diagnosis or assessment of the severity of AS.[1,2]

Physiologically, long-standing AS leads to changes in the left ventricle (LV; concentric left ventricular hypertrophy, reduced compliance, increased end-diastolic pressures), which, in turn, predispose the patient to the development of endocardial ischemia and systolic and/or diastolic dysfunction. In these patients, cardiac output can only be increased through an increase in heart rate (HR) because stroke volume (SV) is fixed. Later in the disease, SV cannot be maintained with increased HR, resulting in symptoms with activity or stress. Diastolic dysfunction occurs earlier in the disease; as the LV becomes less compliant, ventricular filling is impaired due to poor diastolic relaxation and progressively relies on the left atrium to fill. Left atrial enlargement and pulmonary hypertension may result.

Etiologies of AS include congenital abnormalities (unicuspid, bicuspid, or quadricuspid valves), age-related calcific degenerative disease, endocarditis, or rheumatic disease. Risk factors for development of AS include older age, congenital valvular disease, history of infections (such as rheumatic fever), cardiovascular risk factors (such as diabetes or hypertension), chronic kidney disease, or history of radiation to the chest.

American Heart Association guidelines classify AS via its stages, ranging from patients at risk for AS (those with bicuspid valves) to those with progressive AS (patients with mild to moderate leaflet calcifications or rheumatic valve changes) to severe asymptomatic and then to severe symptomatic AS.[2] Patient symptoms, valve anatomy and hemodynamics, and resultant LV changes define each stage. Additionally, hemodynamic severity of AS, from mild to severe, is based on the AVA and mean and peak transaortic pressure gradients (in normal flow states). Specifically, an AVA of 1 cm² or less (normal 2.6–3.5 cm²), a V_{max} of 4 m/s or greater, or a mean ΔP of 40 mm Hg or greater are defined as severe AS.[2]

Timely diagnosis of AS is prudent since untreated AS can cause complications such as heart failure, stroke, thromboembolic events, arrhythmias, or endocarditis. Echocardiography is indicated for identifying etiology of AS, assessment of hemodynamic severity, measurement of the LV size and function, prognosis for timing of valve intervention, and examination of other concurrent valvular abnormalities.[2] The key measurements for clinical decision-making are the peak aortic valve velocity, mean pressure gradient, and valve area calculated with the continuity equation.[2] Repeat echocardiography is warranted whenever new signs and symptoms are reported, prior symptoms are worsening, or in situations where a patient with AS is exposed to increased hemodynamic events (such as pregnancy or systemic infection).[2] In some patients, cardiac catheterization maybe helpful in determination of AS severity. In that case, AVA is calculated with the Gorlin formula by using Fick or thermodilution cardiac output measurements.[2] Coronary angiography is also indicated for a select set of patients with AS to rule out concurrent significant coronary artery disease. Finally, exercise/stress testing, which can provide diagnostic and prognostic information, can be used in asymptomatic patients with severe AS but is contraindicated in symptomatic patients with severe AS.[2]

Timing of intervention depends on the severity of patient symptoms and hemodynamic severity found on diagnostic testing. An AS risk score has been developed to estimate risk of cardiovascular events in patients with AS. This risk score incorporates the patient's age, sex, peak aortic jet velocity, troponin measurements, and echocardiographic evidence of LV hypertrophy.[2] A modified score, which additionally incorporates a B-type natriuretic peptide value, has been published in 2009 to select those patients with asymptomatic AS who may benefit from early surgery.[3]

Deciding whether a patient with AS can safely undergo a noncardiac surgical procedure depends on several factors. Severe symptomatic AS is considered an active cardiac condition, and elective surgery is contraindicated because the patient at increased risk for cardiac complications.[4] In the original study, severe AS was associated with a perioperative mortality rate of 13%, compared with 1.6% in patients without AS, likely due an unfavorable anesthetic state caused by anesthetic agents and surgical stress.[1] As such, in cases of symptomatic severe AS, elective surgery should usually be postponed. With the recent advances in anesthetic and surgical approaches, the cardiac risk in patients with significant AS undergoing noncardiac surgery has declined.

Patients with asymptomatic severe AS can undergo mild- to moderate-risk noncardiac surgeries when appropriately monitored.[2] The American College of Surgeons NSQIP Surgical Risk Calculator (www.riskcalculator.facs.org), which uses specific the procedural terminology code of the procedure being performed to enable procedure-specific risk assessment for a wide array of outcomes, can be used to assess cardiac risk.[5] In addition, functional status is a reliable predictor of perioperative and long-term major cardiac events. Patients with reduced functional status preoperatively are at increased risk of perioperative complications.[1]

In a patient where, based on testing and symptoms, an AVR is indicated, a discussion among the surgeons, cardiac surgeons, cardiologists, cardiac interventionalists, and the patient is warranted to determine the risks and benefits of AVR prior to undergoing the noncardiac procedure such as ESWL.[2] For patients who meet indications but are considered high risk or ineligible for surgical AVR, options include proceeding with noncardiac surgery with invasive hemodynamic monitoring and optimization of loading conditions, percutaneous aortic balloon valvuloplasty as a bridging strategy, and transcatheter AVR.[1] A shared decision-making process should drive this decision.

Percutaneous aortic valve balloon dilation is generally recommended for children or young adults, with a limited role described in older patients.[2] Though immediate hemodynamic effect after balloon angioplasty reportedly results in improved transaortic pressure gradients and early symptomatic relief, the AVA is rarely reported to be greater than 1cm^2. The rate of restenosis is very high, occurring within 6–12 months.[2]

HEMODYNAMIC GOALS, INVASIVE MONITORING, AND ANESTHETIC CONSIDERATIONS IN AORTIC STENOSIS

Preoperative assessment of a patient with AS is focused on determining the severity of AS. Patients with AS depend on adequate preload to maintain cardiac output and sufficient diastolic aortic root pressure to maintain coronary perfusion to the hypertrophied LV. Intraoperative management is then directed toward maintaining hemodynamic stability and cardiac output. Since patients with AS have increased myocardial oxygen demand, reduced LV filling, and, over time, decreased contractility, the intraoperative hemodynamic goals include low-normal heart rate, adequate preload and afterload, maintenance of normal contractility, and normal sinus rhythm.

Patients with AS can become acutely hypotensive with administration of anesthesia on induction. The occurrence of hypotension can result in decreased coronary perfusion pressure, development of arrhythmias or ischemia, myocardial injury, cardiac failure, and death. Phenylephrine, an alpha-adrenergic agonist, is a vasopressor of choice for treatment of hypotension in patients with AS to maintain coronary perfusion. Tachycardia should be avoided because it can result in ischemia (due to decreased time spent in diastole for coronary perfusion) and does not allow adequate systolic time for blood to flow across a severely stenotic aortic valve. On the other hand, excessive bradycardia can compromise cardiac output, given the relatively fixed stroke volume. Maintenance of sinus rhythm is crucial to maintain atrial contribution to ventricular filling; atrial fibrillation and supraventricular tachycardias may require immediate synchronized cardioversion to avoid continuous hemodynamic instability, while amiodarone can be used for both supraventricular and ventricular arrhythmias in hemodynamically stable patients. Ventricular ectopy is similarly poorly tolerated and may be treated with lidocaine or amiodarone. Finally, fluid status must be optimized so that the poorly compliant (or noncompliant) LV can maintain stroke volume.[6,7]

Placement of invasive hemodynamic monitors in patients with AS is common. Specifically, arterial catheters are commonly used for beat-to-beat blood pressure monitoring. External defibrillator pads are often placed prior to induction for ease of cardioversion administration as needed, since chest compressions have limited effect on pushing blood through a stenotic aortic valve. Finally, placements of the standard ASA monitors, including five-lead ECG for ischemia and arrhythmia detection, are recommended.[8]

There is conflicting literature supporting one specific anesthetic technique over another in patients with AS.[9] Whichever technique is chosen, the intraoperative hemodynamic goals remain the same until the lesion is fixed. AS is considered a relative contraindication for neuraxial anesthesia due to the resultant sympathectomy, which leads to decrease in preload and systemic vascular resistance, rapid hypotension, and, consequently, compromised coronary perfusion. Among the choices for neuraxial anesthetic administration, epidural, unlike spinal, offers a more gradual decline in hypotension and allows for incremental titration of medications. Alternatively, a spinal with isobaric (rather than hyperbaric) local anesthetic may offer a lower sympathectomy response. If general anesthesia is chosen, the symptomatic response to direct laryngoscopy must be attenuated to prevent development of ischemia. Opioid-based induction is relatively cardiac stable, while any medication that causes myocardial depression, hypotension, tachycardia, or histamine release must be used cautiously. Volatile anesthetics can be used in low concentration to minimize myocardial depression as well. For ESWL in patients with AS, sparse case reports describe use of intrathecal sufentanil,[9] with the majority of literature favoring monitored anesthesia care or general anesthesia.[10]

ANESTHESIA TECHNIQUES FOR ESWL PROCEDURES

ESWL may be performed under neuraxial anesthesia, monitored light sedation, or general anesthesia. Recently the use of ultrasound-guided quadratus lumborum blocks (QLB) for analgesia showed efficacy in abdominal surgery. This block provides anesthesia and analgesia on the anterior and lateral abdominal walls. Yayik et al. studied the use of QLB for analgesia in patients undergoing ESWL and reported that its use reduced extra opioid consumption significantly compared to the control group.[11,12] Similarly, paravertebral blocks have been suggested as anesthetic alternatives for outpatient lithotripsy in selected patients.[13]

Patients with significant cardiovascular disease who need to undergo ESWL, including those with AS, are at higher risk of adverse effects from anesthetic administration. Several case reports have reported successful use of intrathecal sufentanil for analgesia during ESWL, with minimal cardiovascular effects.[9] Severe respiratory depression is a feared complication, and such intrathecal use requires continuous postoperative monitoring for several hours.[9]

CONSIDERATIONS FOR PERFORMING PROCEDURES AT A FREE-STANDING SURGICAL CENTER

Increasing numbers of surgical procedures have migrated from the hospital settings to ambulatory surgical centers (ASCs) over the past few decades. More than 80% of procedures were reportedly performed on an ambulatory basis in 2005, with numbers increasing every year.[14] ESWL is often performed on an outpatient basis at an ASC or a urologist's office. Guidelines have been developed to help clinicians determine which procedures, and on which patients, are safe to perform outside of the hospital. For those procedures requiring increasing depth of sedation, considerations for availability of emergency equipment, adequate monitoring space and equipment, and trained personnel are mandatory. Finally, adherence to state and local laws for office-based surgery is also required.

Administration of safe anesthetics at free-standing ASCs has been made possible by development of shorter-acting medications with fewer hemodynamic side effects and an increase in minimally invasive surgical techniques.[15,16] Metzner et al. examined anesthetic safety concerns for those procedures performed in the hospital versus ASCs. Notably, they reported that more than 50% of lawsuits involved non-operating room locations whenever monitored anesthetic care was provided, and there was a higher incidence of adverse outcomes based on respiratory events in these locations compared to the traditional hospital ORs. Arguably, more than 30% of the respiratory adverse events could have been prevented by additional monitoring techniques.[17]

Components of surgical site safety include physical considerations of the office, surgeon qualifications, and appropriate patient and procedure selection. Specifically, patients with significant comorbidities who are at increased risk of procedural or anesthetic adverse outcomes may not be well suited for ASC.[18,19] It should be noted that some ambulatory centers implemented a policy where procedures only for ASA physical status 1 and 2 patients are performed at their center, while others occasionally accept ASA 3 patient. Other ambulatory centers do not have such policies, and a decision about which patient procedures are performed in an ambulatory versus main hospital settings is individualized for each patient.

The ASA has published guidelines for office-based anesthesia that discusses patient and procedure selection for the office-based practitioner.[20] Although there are few data to support the exclusion of specific procedures or specific patient populations from an office-based surgical setting, certain basic physiologic principles can be applied to these venues. For example, the patient with an anticipated difficult airway is not an ideal candidate for ASC. Since the first step in the ASA-endorsed difficult airway algorithm is to call for help, another experienced provider may not be readily available in the ASC setting. Additionally, certain procedures, such as those that create significant physiologic derangements, may not be well suited for ASC. Finally, patients who may require invasive monitoring during intraoperative management or the postoperative recovery period are better suited for traditional hospital settings. In the case of ESWL, where other treatments for urolithiasis may be more invasive, it is necessary to perform a robust risk-benefit analysis to determine if the risk of treating a patient with significant valvular disease in an ambulatory center may be outweighed by the benefit of the less invasive surgical treatment.

CONCLUSION

- Preoperative evaluation of a patient with symptomatic severe AS must include full history and physical examination, ECG, recent echocardiography, and medical optimization of comorbidities.

- A multidisciplinary discussion is warranted to determine the need for AVR or balloon angioplasty prior to an elective surgical procedure. Most patients with asymptomatic severe AS can safely undergo low- to moderate-risk elective procedures.

- Patients with AS depend on adequate preload to maintain cardiac output and sufficient diastolic aortic root pressure to maintain coronary perfusion to the hypertrophied LV.

- Patients with AS have fixed stroke volume and are highly dependent on normal sinus rhythm for atrial kick, which contributes more than 20% to their (already fixed) stroke volume.

- ESWL may be performed under neuraxial anesthesia, monitored light sedation, or general anesthesia. Severe AS is a relative contraindication to neuraxial anesthesia.

- It is imperative for anesthesiology clinicians to select appropriate patients for an ASC, and they must be vigilant regarding the presence of a patient's high-risk medical comorbidities.

REVIEW QUESTIONS

1. A 73-year-old man with a history of hypertension presents to his cardiologist with progressive worsening of dyspnea on exertion. A loud systolic ejection murmur is heard at the upper right sternal border. Which of the following is the next best step in work up of his symptoms?

   a. Cardiac catheterization.
   b. Transthoracic echocardiography.
   c. Transesophageal echocardiography.
   d. Exercise stress echocardiography.

   The correct answer is b.
   Transthoracic echocardiography is the standard diagnostic test in the initial evaluation of patients with known or

suspected valvular heart disease. It allows for accurate assessment of valve anatomy and etiology, concurrent valve disease, associated abnormalities such as aortic dilation, and ventricular anatomy and function. Transesophageal echocardiography is more invasive and should only be used if transthoracic is inconclusive. If noninvasive testing yields inconclusive results, particularly in the symptomatic patient, or if there is a discrepancy between the noninvasive tests and clinical findings, a hemodynamic cardiac catheterization with direct intracardiac measurements of transvalvular pressure gradients and cardiac output measurements provides valuable clinical information. In asymptomatic patients with severe AS, exercise testing is reasonable to assess physiological changes with exercise and to confirm the absence of symptoms.

2. A 69-year-old man with severe AS presents for endoscopy. Which of the following is the ideal heart rate to maintain during the procedure?

   a. 40 bpm.
   b. 60 bpm.
   c. 80 bpm.
   d. 100 bpm.

The correct answer is b.

One of the main hemodynamic goals for the management in patients with AS is to maintain a relatively slow heart rate. Tachycardia should be avoided because it decreases diastolic filling time, shortens systolic ejection time, and thus decreases cardiac output. On the other hand, blood flow across the stenotic aortic valve is relatively fixed, and severe bradycardia (HR <40 bpm) will result in low cardiac output. The ideal heart rate is usually between 60 and 70 bpm.

3. A 79-year-old man with severe AS presents for ESWL. Which of the following anesthetic techniques is relatively contraindicated?

   a. General anesthesia with inhalational anesthetics.
   b. IV conscious sedation.
   c. General anesthesia with total IV anesthetics.
   d. Spinal anesthesia.

The correct answer is d.

Neuraxial anesthesia, with the risk of sympatholysis and decrease in preload and systemic vascular resistance, is relatively contraindicated in patients with significant AS. It can result in a decrease in cardiac output, arterial blood pressure, and coronary perfusion pressure. It should only be administered if there is an arterial line or very frequent blood pressure monitoring and vasoconstrictor therapy readily available. If a neuraxial technique is chosen, an epidural technique is preferred as it allows for incremental dosing, and thus a sudden drop in systemic vascular resistance can usually be avoided.

4. A 79-year-old man with moderate asymptomatic AS presents for an elective cholecystectomy. Which of the following represents the next best step in his management?

   a. Proceed with surgery.
   b. Balloon valvuloplasty prior to surgery.
   c. Transcatheter aortic valve replacement prior to surgery.
   d. Surgical aortic valve replacement prior to surgery.

The correct answer is a.

Elevated-risk elective noncardiac surgery with appropriate intraoperative and postoperative hemodynamic monitoring is reasonable to perform in patients with asymptomatic moderate or severe AS and normal LV systolic function. AVR prior to elective elevated-risk noncardiac surgery in symptomatic patients with severe AS will prevent hemodynamic instability during as well as after noncardiac surgery. Transcatheter replacement is a reasonable option to avoid delay of semi-urgent noncardiac surgery. In hemodynamically unstable patients at high to prohibitive surgical risk for AVR, balloon aortic valvuloplasty as a bridging strategy may be an option.

5. A 54-year-old woman with a history of supraventricular tachycardia presents for ESWL. Synchronization of the shock waves with which of the following ECG waves will decrease the incidence of arrhythmias?

   a. P.
   b. Q.
   c. R.
   d. T.

The correct answer is c.

Patients with a history of cardiac arrhythmias and those with a pacemaker may be at risk for developing arrhythmias induced by shock waves during ESWL. Synchronization of the shock waves with the R wave on the ECG decreases the incidence of arrhythmias. The shock waves are usually timed to occur 20 ms after the R wave to correspond with the ventricular refractory period. Asynchronous delivery of shock waves is likely safe in patients without heart disease.

6. A 74-year-old man with moderate AS presents for an elective cholecystectomy. The ability to perform which of the following corresponds with moderate functional status?

   a. Climb a flight of stairs.
   b. Golfing with a cart.
   c. Slow ballroom dancing.
   d. Walking at 2–3 mph.

The correct answer is a.

If a patient has not had a recent exercise stress test before noncardiac surgery, functional status can usually be estimated from activities of daily living. Functional capacity is often expressed in terms of metabolic equivalents (METs) and can be classified as excellent (>10 METs), good (7–10 METs), moderate (4–6 METs), poor (<4 METs), or unknown. Examples of activities associated with more than 4 METs are climbing a flight of stairs or walking up a hill, walking on level ground at 4 mph, and performing heavy work around the house. Examples of activities associated with less than 4 METs are slow ballroom dancing, golfing with a cart, playing a musical instrument, and walking at approximately 2–3 mph. Perioperative cardiac and long-term risks are increased in patients unable to perform 4 METs of work during daily activities.

REFERENCES

1. Fleisher LA, Fleischmann KE, Auerbach AD, et al. 2014 ACC/AHA guideline on perioperative cardiovascular evaluation and management of patients undergoing noncardiac surgery: A report of the American College of Cardiology/American Heart Association Task Force on practice guidelines. *J Am Coll Cardiol.* 2014;64: e77–137.
2. Otto CM, Nishimura RA, Bonow RO, et al. 2020 ACC/AHA Guideline for the Management of Patients with Valvular Heart Disease: Executive Summary: A report of the American College of Cardiology/American Heart Association Joint Committee on Clinical Practice Guidelines. *J Am Coll Cardiol.* 2020; S0735-1097.
3. Monin JL, Lancellotti P, Monchi M, et al. Risk score for predicting outcome in patients with asymptomatic aortic stenosis. *Circulation.* 2009;120:69–75.
4. Mittnacht AJ, Fanshawe M, Konstadt S. Anesthetic considerations in the patient with valvular heart disease undergoing noncardiac surgery. *Semin Cardiothorac Vasc Anesth.* 2008;12:33–59.
5. Cohen ME, Ko CY, Bilimoria KY, et al. Optimizing ACS NSQIP modeling for evaluation of surgical quality and risk: Patient risk adjustment, procedure mix adjustment, shrinkage adjustment, and surgical focus. *J Am Coll Surg.* 2013;217:336–46.e1.
6. Frogel J, Galusca D. Anesthetic considerations for patients with advanced valvular heart disease undergoing noncardiac surgery. *Anesthesiol Clin.* 2010;28:67–85.
7. Kennon S, Archbold A. Expert opinion: Guidelines for the management of patients with aortic stenosis undergoing non-cardiac surgery: Out of date and overly prescriptive. *Interv Cardiol.* 2017;12: 133–136.
8. Sowerby RJ, Lantz Powers AG, Ghiculete D, et al. Routine preoperative electrocardiograms in patients at low risk for cardiac complications during shockwave lithotripsy: Are they useful? *J Endourol.* 2019;33:314–318.
9. Eaton MP. Intrathecal sufentanil analgesia for extracorporeal shock wave lithotripsy in three patients with aortic stenosis. *Anesth Analg.* 1998;86:943–944.
10. Thakore P, Liang, TH. Urolithiasis. *StatPearls.* 2020.
11. Yayik AM, Ahiskalioglu A, Alici HA, et al. Less painful ESWL with ultrasound-guided quadratus lumborum block: A prospective randomized controlled study. *Scand J Urol.* 2019;53:411–416.
12. Yayık AM, Ahıskalıoğlu A, Ergüney ÖD, et al. Analgesic efficacy of ultrasound-guided quadratus lumborum block during extracorporeal shock wave lithotripsy. *Agri.* 2020;32:44–47.
13. Hanoura S, Elsayed M, Eldegwy M, et al. Paravertebral block is a proper alternative anesthesia for outpatient lithotripsy. *Anesth Essays Res.* 2013;7:365–370.
14. Shapiro FE, Punwani N, Rosenberg NM, et al. Office-based anesthesia: Safety and outcomes. 2014;119(2):276–285.
15. Tang J, White PF, Wender RH, et al. Fast-track office-based anesthesia: A comparison of propofol versus desflurane with antiemetic prophylaxis in spontaneously breathing patients. *Anesth Analg.* 2001;92:95–99.
16. Sardo ADS, Bettocchi S, Spinelli M, et al. Review of new office-based hysteroscopic procedures 2003–2009. *J Minim Invasive Gynecol.* 2010;17:436–448.
17. Metzner J, Posner KL, Domino KB. The risk and safety of anesthesia at remote locations: The US closed claims analysis. *Curr Opin Anesthesiol.* 2009;22:502–508.
18. Haeck PC, Swanson JA, Iverson RE, et al. Evidence-based safety advisory: Patient assessment and prevention of pulmonary side effects in surgery. Part 2: Patient and procedural risk factors. *Plast Reconstr Surg.* 2009;124:57S–67S.
19. Haeck PC, Swanson JA, Iverson RE, et al. Evidence-based patient safety advisory: Patient selection and procedures in ambulatory surgery. *Plast Reconstr Surg.* 2009;124:6S–23S.
20. American Society of Anesthesiologists. Guidelines for office-based anesthesia: Approved by the ASA House of Delegates on October 13, 1999, and last amended on October 23, 2019. https://www.asahq.org/standards-and-guidelines/guidelines-for-office-based-anesthesia

15.

DOES YOUR CATARACT SURGEON KNOW YOU WERE ADMITTED FOR HEART FAILURE LAST WEEK?

Michael Curtis, Nathaen Weitzel, and Miklos D. Kertai

STEM CASE AND KEY QUESTIONS

A 65-year-old man presents to your preoperative clinic for evaluation prior to cataract surgery scheduled for a week from now. On review of his medical history, he discloses that he had been diagnosed with heart failure several years ago. This has necessitated multiple hospitalizations, including most recently only 1 week ago. He notes that he was very glad to be discharged home because he was worried that this would cause him to miss this cataract surgery that he has been looking forward to for months.

What is heart failure?

Are there any particular review of systems questions or physical exam findings you would want to use to evaluate this patient's status?

Do patients with heart failure commonly present with any other comorbidities?

The patient tells you that he also remembers being told at some point that he has high blood pressure and high cholesterol levels. He mentions that he feels great when he is at home reading the newspaper, but that he gets short of breath relatively quickly while walking around his single-story house. He denies ever having chest pain, but does blame his heavy legs for contributing to the problem.

How would you grade the severity of this patient's heart failure?

Are there any tests you would like to order to further evaluate his cardiac function?

The patient tells you that he has seen a cardiologist regularly since his diagnosis and faithfully takes his medications, though has a hard time remembering what they all are. Based on the list that he brought with him, he appears to take aspirin, rosuvastatin, lisinopril, carvedilol, and furosemide. He is also curious about how he should take these in the coming days before his surgery as he remembers getting instructions for these before a previous surgery.

What medical management exists for heart failure?

Are there any surgical options for treatment of heart failure?

What instructions would give the patient for taking their medications in the days leading up to surgery?

The patient remarks that he has heard about people having heart attacks and strokes while under anesthesia. While he is looking forward to having improved vision, he is appropriately concerned about the potentially negative effects of anesthetics. He is hopeful that you can further explain them to him and bluntly asks if you can quote him specific numbers.

Are there any intraoperative or postoperative risks that are of particular concern for patients with heart failure?

Do all procedures pose the same level of risk to heart failure patients? Or can they be categorized into higher and lower risk procedures?

What scoring systems exist to help one quantify these risks?

Should the patient's cataract surgery be delayed for further patient workup? For medical optimization if needed? Do definitions exist for how time-sensitive a procedure is?

During this discussion of risk and obtaining consent for anesthesia, he nods and remarks that he heard similar things when he got his previously unmentioned implantable cardioverter-defibrillator (ICD) placed to "keep his heart in synchrony." He also heard something similar during discussions about potentially getting a left ventricular assist device (LVAD) or a heart transplant in the future.

Why would an automated ICD—especially one with biventricular pacing—be indicated for heart failure?

If this patient were to already have an LVAD, would you have any other perioperative concerns? What if this patient had previously received an orthotopic heart transplant?

Given the extensive discussion of risk, the patient wants to know what to expect on the day of his cataract surgery. Specifically, if any additional precautions are going to be taken during the surgery to keep him safe.

What monitors would you tell this patient to anticipate on the day of surgery? What if he were undergoing an intra-abdominal procedure necessitating general anesthesia?

DISCUSSION

In the United States, 6.2 million people were estimated by the American Heart Association (AHA) to suffer from heart failure between 2013 and 2016.[1] Given the aging population, anesthesiologists are frequently called upon to care for patients with heart failure. Moreover, novel therapies are emerging, and it is paramount to keep up to date with medications and devices encountered in these patients. Heart failure, with its complicated pathology, varying physiologic underpinnings, degrees of severity, and diverse treatment options, poses many challenges to the anesthesiologist and should be taken seriously in all situations. However, one must also weigh the complexity of the case being performed as well when making choices for an anesthetic plan or monitoring.

While it is still important to know patients' history and their basic pathology for a procedure requiring light sedation and minor fluid shifts (e.g., cataract surgery), the minimal changes to their physiology in such a situation means that the procedure can be performed safely without any of the extensive screening and testing about to be discussed.[2] This is true even in cases of those patients with durable mechanical circulatory support (MCS) devices like LVADs or even those who have previously received a heart transplant. However, in more involved, non-urgent cases—such as a colectomy—these considerations for perioperative testing, medical optimization, and surgical timing should play a more important role.

ETIOLOGY AND PATHOPHYSIOLOGY

Heart failure is a complex clinical syndrome manifesting as the inability of the heart to provide adequate blood flow to meet systemic requirements or accommodate the associated venous return. The diagnosis relies on patient history, physical exam, and confirmation by echocardiography. Coronary (ischemic) heart disease, various cardiomyopathies, hypertension, pericardial disease, and underlying valvular disease are commonly implicated as underlying causes of heart failure. Of these, ischemic heart disease is by far the most common cause, accounting for 62% of cases in one study.[3]

Patients with heart failure may be completely asymptomatic or, depending on the severity, present with a decrease in functional capacity, dyspnea of exertion, or fatigue. Decompensated heart failure manifests as volume overload with weight gain, worsening dyspnea of exertion, orthopnea, paroxysmal nocturnal dyspnea, or nocturia. Accompanying physical examination findings of decompensated heart failure encompass jugular venous distension, presence of pulmonary rales, pleural effusions, peripheral edema, and/or ascites. In terminal phases, a low cardiac output state can lead to inadequate perfusion pressures with cool extremities and hypotension.

Table 15.1 NEW YORK HEART ASSOCIATION (NYHA) FUNCTIONAL CLASSIFICATION FOR HEART FAILURE, WITH SYMPTOMS SHOWN FOR EACH OF THE FOUR CLASSES

NYHA CLASS	SYMPTOMS
I	No limitation of physical activity. Ordinary physical activity does not cause undue fatigue, palpitation, dyspnea (shortness of breath).
II	Slight limitation of physical activity. Comfortable at rest. Ordinary physical activity results in fatigue, palpitation, dyspnea (shortness of breath).
III	Marked limitation of physical activity. Comfortable at rest. Less than ordinary activity causes fatigue, palpitation, or dyspnea.
IV	Unable to carry on any physical activity without discomfort. Symptoms of heart failure at rest. If any physical activity is undertaken, discomfort increases.

A simple and widely used scoring system for the functional severity of heart failure is the New York Heart Association (NYHA) Functional Classification for Heart Failure. In use since 1902, it places patients into one of four categories (Table 15.1) based on subjective symptoms and physical limitations during both rest and activity.[4]

Systolic Versus Diastolic Dysfunction

Another way to further subdivide heart failure is to look at the specific part of the heart that is dysfunctional. Most people think of heart failure as being left ventricular (LV) systolic dysfunction, where the ventricle becomes less efficient at pumping during systole. In the 2022 American Heart Association (AHA)/American College of Cardiology (ACC)/Heart Failure Society of America (HFSA) guidelines, this has been further subdivided into heart failure with reduced ejection fraction (HFrEF), heart failure with mildly reduced ejection fraction (HFmrEF), and heart failure with improved ejection fraction (HFimpEF) (Table 15.2).[5] However, there is also isolated diastolic dysfunction, meaning there are elevated filling pressures for the LV with relatively normal systolic function; this is called heart failure with preserved ejection fraction (HFpEF). Isolated right ventricular (RV) failure is less frequently encountered.

Additional objective criteria exist for grading the severity of both LV systolic and diastolic dysfunction from the American Society of Echocardiography (ASE). LV ejection fraction is used to classify systolic function from hyperdynamic (EF 70%), normal (EF 50–69%) to severely reduced (EF <30%),[6] while a combination of measurements are used to grade diastolic dysfunction from normal to severe/grade III.[7]

Associated Conditions

Given the critical nature of cardiac function to adequate systemic perfusion and the multitude of causes of heart failure,

Table 15.2 **CLASSIFICATION OF HEART FAILURE**

TYPE OF HEART FAILURE	CRITERIA
HFrEF	Current LV ejection fraction ≤40%
HFimpEF	Previous LV ejection fraction ≤40%, but improved to >40% on follow-up measurement
HFmrEF	Current LV ejection fraction 41-49% Evidence of spontaneous or provokable increased LV filling pressures
HFpEF	Current LV ejection fraction ≥50% Evidence of spontaneous or provokable increased LV filling pressures

Derived from Heidenreich PA, et al.[5]

it is not surprising that many conditions frequently are found in these patients. For example, there may be underlying coronary artery disease, severe valvular dysfunction, or a chronic cardiac rhythm disturbance that may be a primary cause or at least a contributing factor to a patient's heart failure. Then, there are the related metabolic and cardiovascular comorbidities. In patients with ischemic heart disease, especially, there is a high incidence of diabetes mellitus—with its micro- and macrovascular complications—as well as obesity, hypertension, and hyperlipidemia.[8,9] Both anemia of chronic disease with decreased erythropoietin production and functional iron deficiency are also prevalent.[10] Chronic hypoxemia can also be present due to other associated conditions such severe chronic obstructive pulmonary disease (COPD) or sleep apnea. In fact, up to 50% of patients with heart failure may have some degree of sleep apnea or hypopnea.[11] This itself can lead to poor sleep quality, which only exacerbates functional impairment and neurohumoral derangement.[12]

On the other hand, heart failure will also lead to dysfunction in multiple other organ systems.[9] It is not uncommon to encounter chronic kidney disease and electrolyte imbalances (e.g., hyponatremia), as well as hepatic congestion and its multiple downstream effects (e.g., hypoalbuminemia, coagulopathy). Respiratory function may also be impaired due to pulmonary edema or pleural effusions related to volume overload seen in heart failure patients.

INTRAOPERATIVE AND POSTOPERATIVE ANESTHETIC RISKS IN HEART FAILURE

Heart failure patients have a significantly increased risk of perioperative mortality—two to four times higher than patients with just isolated coronary disease.[13] When comparing HFpEF and HFrEF directly, it appears that isolated HFpEF patients still have a higher rate of cardiopulmonary complications and mortality than non-heart failure patients, while patients with HFrEF generally have worse overall outcomes than either group.[14–17] Anesthetics can put significant stress on the cardiovascular system in several ways: untreated pain may increase myocardial oxygen demand through tachycardia, while anesthetic-induced vasodilation may decrease perfusion pressure. Both of these can predispose patients to an ischemic event (i.e., myocardial infarction [MI]), and, given that heart failure patients already have marginal cardiac function, this is of particular concern for them.

The fluid and compartmental shifts that can be seen during surgical procedures, as well as with IV fluid administration, also place these patients at particular risk of volume overload. First, this volume may push heart failure patients off the edge of the Frank-Starling curve into decreased cardiac function (i.e., an acute heart failure exacerbation). This also can have many other systemic effects, such as decreased respiratory function from pulmonary edema, renal and/or hepatic congestion, and worsening of underlying electrolyte abnormalities.

Both ischemia and volume overload can also place patients at high risk of developing arrythmias. In particular, atrial stretch can lead to atrial fibrillation and flutter, increasing the risk of both thrombotic events and hemodynamic instability.[18] Lethal arrythmias, such as ventricular tachycardia, can also be seen at higher rates in these patients when placed under the physiologic stress of anesthesia and surgery.[19]

PREOPERATIVE EVALUATION

Preoperative Examination

The preoperative evaluation of patient with heart failure should focus on assessing symptom stability. A change from baseline as far as functional capacity; worsening dyspnea, accompanied by orthopnea; paroxysmal nocturnal dyspnea; and lower extremity edema in addition to weight gain suggest heart failure decompensation. These signs should prompt cancellation of an elective procedure and medical optimization, as well as investigations of the etiology of the decompensating episode (e.g., new ischemia, dietary indiscretions, medication noncompliance). Arrythmias may manifest as palpitations or an irregular heartbeat. Chest pain or dyspneic events may be concerning for ischemic events.

In addition, a review of a patient's medical history, combined with their medication list and previous surgical procedures, may be the first clues into the severity of a patient's condition. For example, a patient who is regularly seen in the medical system with few comorbidities and prescriptions for only low doses of a beta blocker and angiotensin-converting enzyme (ACE) inhibitor is likely to be in better shape than the patient with an automated ICD, diabetes requiring use of long-acting insulin, and taking high doses of daily diuretics.

Assessment of Functional Capacity

Functional status has been traditionally assessed via metabolic equivalents (METs), with 1 MET being defined as the 3.5 mL of oxygen utilization per kilogram per minute it takes to rest in a chair in the sitting position. Various activity scales can help one assess the number of METs a patient can achieve, with ability to reach at least 4 METs—equivalent to walking up a flight of steps without stopping or walking on level ground at

3–4 miles per hour—traditionally being accepted as a good perioperative prognostic indicator.[20,21]

The recent METS study found that a structured questionnaire for functional status—the Duke Activity Status Index (DASI)—was significantly better at classifying a patient's risk of cardiac complications with noncardiac surgery than traditional, subjective provider estimates of functional capacity.[22] The DASI consists of 12 "Yes/No" questions asking if the patient is able to perform a certain activity. Each activity is assigned a point value to be summed, with the METS study showing a DASI score of 34 or greater having a significantly increased risk of 30-day death, MI, or moderate-to-severe complications.

An even more recent study showed that simplified versions of the DASI using only four (M-DASI-4Q) or five (M-DASI-5Q) of the original questions held similar predictive power for 1-year mortality.[23] A "Yes" answer to each question was assigned one point, with the summed number of points being used to predict if a patient could reach a peak utilization of oxygen of 16 mL/kg per minute (approximately 4.5 METs). However, this study lacked the data to show predictive power for cardiac complications, and thus the authors suggested that, for now, it may be used to guide which patients should be referred to cardiopulmonary exercise testing (CPET) for more objective assessment.

Imaging

Generally, an ECG should be ordered for any heart failure patient before an intermediate- or high-risk procedure. Its value is limited prior to low-risk surgeries (such as cataract) and not recommended by the 2014 American College of Cardiology/American Heart Association (ACC/AHA) perioperative guidelines.[20] Nevertheless, if available for review from a patient's medical records, it could point toward concomitant, preexisting ischemic disease (Q waves, left bundle branch block [LBBB]), atrial arrhythmias, or even the presence of a cardiac implantable electronic device.

A chest x-ray could provide additional information when the diagnosis or stability is questionable. However, the majority of times, a thorough history and physical examination provide the answer and chest x-rays are rarely indicated in a patient with known heart failure. If a recent x-ray is available, it could ascertain the presence of cardiomegaly, Kerley B lines (representing interstitial fluid), or pleural effusions.

Echocardiography is the imaging modality recommended for these patients in terms of both diagnosis and follow-up. Knowing a patient's baseline ventricular and valvular function can be invaluable when choosing the appropriate intraoperative management and guiding the need for more invasive monitors. The 2014 ACC/AHA perioperative guidelines deem a preoperative transthoracic echo (TTE) reasonable in patients with dyspnea of unknown etiology, heart failure patients with worsening dyspnea, or stable patients with heart failure who have not had a TTE within the past year.[20] However, some studies have shown only a modest predictive value of echocardiography characteristics like the severity of LV dysfunction and wall motion abnormalities for postoperative cardiovascular complications.[24–26]

This lack of definitive predictive power of traditional preoperative echocardiography may be because it is a window into cardiac function at only one point in time, and the patient may be at a very different state at the actual time of procedure. It is possible that a cardiac-focused point-of-care ultrasound (POCUS) performed immediately preoperatively by anesthesiologists could prove useful, though this depends on having sufficient operator skill to perform the exam and comfortably interpret the results. For example, one should feel comfortable looking for depressed ventricular function, dilatation of the atria and ventricles, overt valvular regurgitation or restricted movement, and evidence of pulmonary edema (e.g., B-lines).

Preoperative stress testing is not necessarily indicated unless there is a strong suspicion for an ischemic etiology with an intervenable lesion.[20] An assessment of a patient's functional status, as discussed above, often provides sufficient information in combination with other recommended perioperative testing.

Laboratory Testing

As discussed above, abnormalities in other organ systems frequently are associated with heart failure, and thus testing is frequently indicated to assess their functionality. A basic metabolic panel (BMP) should be sent to assess renal function and to screen for electrolyte abnormalities, especially with diuretic use. A hemoglobin A1c (HgA1c) can evaluate the control of known diabetes mellitus. A complete blood count (CBC) may also be helpful given the high incidence of anemia in heart failure.[10] Although these additional labs may not directly impact cardiovascular outcomes, they can alter intraoperative anesthetic choices.

Brain Natriuretic Peptide (BNP) and N-Terminal (NT) ProBNP

Brain natriuretic peptide (BNP) and N-terminal (NT)-proBNP (an inert byproduct of the production of the biologically active BNP) are often elevated in volume overloaded states and thus can be used to help assess how well a patient's heart failure is currently controlled.[20] Both have shown an association with perioperative and in-hospital cardiac complications.[27,28]

Based on these studies, the Canadian Cardiovascular Society recommends that a preoperative BNP or NT-proBNP level be drawn any patient who scores 1 or higher on the Revised Cardiac Risk Index (see below), or are age 65 and older, or are age 45 and older with significant cardiovascular disease (including heart failure).[29] They then recommend increased postoperative monitoring (i.e., daily troponin levels for 48–72 hours, a formal ECG in the recovery unit) for cardiovascular events in patients with preop levels of BNP at 92 pg/mL or higher or NT-proBNP at 300 pg/mL or higher. The European Society of Cardiology (ESC) also mentions that ordering preoperative BNP or NT-proBNP levels should be considered in high-risk patients for prognostic purposes, but their guidelines do not mention specific cutoffs or actions to take.[30]

It is important to note that levels may be falsely elevated in chronic kidney disease and falsely low in obesity, which may complicate their interpretation. Patients being treated with sacubitril-valsartan (or other neprilysin inhibitors) will also have inappropriately elevated BNP levels, while NT-pro-BNP should still be reliable.

Troponin

Many recent studies have also evaluated the use of preoperative cardiac troponin levels, with most showing that an elevation—and the degree of elevation—are associated with postoperative major adverse cardiac events (MACE).[31,32] However, its utility is limited in patients with a diagnosis of heart failure with an underlying etiology other than ischemia, and what to do with such information is still subject to debate.[20,33]

PREOPERATIVE RISK CALCULATORS

Revised Cardiac Risk Index

Originally published in 1999, the Revised Cardiac Risk Index (RCRI) is an update to the original Cardiac Risk Index (also known as the Goldman Index) from 1977. It identified six independent risk factors for MACE in noncardiac surgery, which can be used to estimate a percentage risk for patients (Box 15.1).[34]

There are a few limitations to the RCRI, notably that it does not include all-cause mortality given that it specifically focused on MACE. It also included only inpatient events, thus potentially not following patients for a full 30 days after surgery given that many would be discharged before that point.

Box 15.1 RISK FOR PERIOPERATIVE CARDIAC DEATH, NONFATAL MYOCARDIAL INFARCTION, OR NONFATAL CARDIAC ARREST

Revised Cardiac Risk Index (RCRI)

1. History of ischemic heart disease
2. History of congestive heart failure
3. History of cerebrovascular disease (stroke or transient ischemia attack)
4. History of diabetes requiring preoperative insulin use
5. Chronic kidney disease (creatinine >2 mg/dL)
6. Undergoing suprainguinal vascular, intraperitoneal, or intrathoracic surgery

0 predictors = 0.4%, 1 predictor = 0.9%, 2 predictors = 6.6%, ≥3 predictors = >11%.
Adapted from Lee TH, et al.[34]

National Surgical Quality Improvement Program Myocardial Infarction and Cardiac Arrest (NSQIP MICA)

The records of more than 200,000 patients included in the National Surgical Quality Improvement Program (NSQIP) database who underwent surgery in 2007 were evaluated, of which 0.65% experienced a perioperative MI or cardiac arrest.[35] Using a multivariate logistic regression analysis, five predictive factors for perioperative MI and cardiac arrest were identified (Box 15.2).

Box 15.2 FIVE FACTORS FOUND TO BE PREDICTIVE OF PERIOPERATIVE MYOCARDIAL INFARCTION OR CARDIAC ARREST

NSQIP MICA predictive factors

1. Patient age
2. American Society of Anesthesiologists (ASA) class
3. Preoperative creatinine
4. Functional status
5. Procedure being performed

Adapted from Gupta PK, et al.[35]

These five factors are not binary, unlike the RCRI, and rely on a more complicated algorithm (widely available online) to compute a percentage risk. While this cannot be calculated as easily as the RCRI, it was found to outperform that calculator in predictive power and was subsequently revalidated using newer (2008) NSQIP data.

American College of Surgeons National Surgical Quality Improvement Program

The ACS NSQIP Risk Calculator is a free, online tool currently derived from data related to more than 4.3 million operations uploaded into the ACS NSQIP database by participating hospitals.[36] By entering in the type of procedure and 20 patient factors (e.g., age, presence of diabetes, hypertension, etc.), one can get risk predictions for 15 separate outcomes within the first 30 days after surgery, including all-cause mortality and cardiac complications. Although not specifically focused on cardiovascular outcomes, a statistical analysis published using an earlier version of the model from 2013 showed good predictive power in that area.[37]

Surgical Urgency

The ACC/AHA have published consensus definitions for classifying urgency (Table 15.3).[20] These are inherently subjective but may help provide some guidance when determining if it is reasonable to delay a procedure. Of note, the urgency

Table 15.3 CONSENSUS DEFINITIONS FOR THE URGENCY OF A PROCEDURE

URGENCY	DEFINED TIME FRAME	EXAMPLE
Emergent	Surgery within 6 hours	Life or limb threatened, only time for very limited evaluation
Urgent	Surgery in 6–24 hours	Although life or limb threatened, time for limited evaluation
Time-Sensitive	Surgery within 1 week	Oncologic surgery where >1 week delay will negatively impact outcome
Elective	Surgery at any time	Joint replacement where delay will not negatively impact outcome

Adapted from Fleisher LA, et al.[20]

of a procedure is also helpful to consider as a component of perioperative risk itself because some data have shown that emergency procedures have cardiac complications 2–5 times as frequently as those which are elective in nature.[38]

Intrinsic Surgical Risk

Although patient factors often play an important part in determining the risk of MACE, there is greater intrinsic risk involved in some procedures. The 2022 ESC guidelines divide procedures into three general categories based on the 30-day risk of cardiovascular death and/or MI: high-risk (>5%), intermediate-risk (1–5%), and low-risk (<1%).[39,40] As shown in Table 15.4, adapted from these guidelines, open vascular surgery is felt to be higher risk than reconstructive plastic surgery. This is in-line with the RCRI scoring, where intraperitoneal, intrathoracic, and suprainguinal vascular surgeries are assessed as higher risk.

TREATMENT AND MONITORING

Medical Management

Pharmacologic therapy plays a crucial role in the initial management of patients with both HFrEF and HFpEF, with published studies showing symptomatic and mortality benefits for many medications. The 2022 AHA/ACC/HFSA and 2021 ESC guidelines now recommend guideline-directed medical therapy (GDMT) of HFrEF to be comprised of medications from four classes: a beta blocker, a renin-angiotensin system inhibitor (angiotensin converting enzyme [ACE] inhibitor, angiotensin II receptor blocker [ARB], or angiotensin receptor-neprilysin inhibitor [ARNI]), a sodium-glucose cotransporter 2 (SGLT2) inhibitor, and a mineralocorticoid receptor antagonist (MRA).[5,41] Loop diuretics may be used as needed to address volume overload, while additional agents, such as digoxin, statins, soluble guanylate cyclase receptor stimulators, and cardiac myosin activators may be added for select patients.

Current therapy for isolated HFpEF can be markedly different owing to its unique physiology. However, updates in the 2022 AHA/ACC/HFSA guidelines now more closely resemble those for patients with HFrEF, with recommendations including SGLT2 inhibitors, MRAs, and renin-angiotensin system inhibitors.[5] It must be noted, though, that these recommendations generally carry a lower level of evidence.

Beta Blockers

Beta blockers (e.g., carvedilol and metoprolol) have well-established evidence for reduced mortality and morbidity in patients with NYHA functional class II or III heart failure.[42,43] By antagonizing beta-1 receptors, these medications prevent sympathetic cardiac stimulation and reduce renin release from the kidneys. Although a reduction in cardiac output and worsening of functional symptoms may be seen upon initiation, by

Table 15.4 PROCEDURES CATEGORIZED BY RISK OF 30-DAY CARDIOVASCULAR MORTALITY AND/OR MYOCARDIAL INFARCTION

LOW-RISK (<1%)	INTERMEDIATE-RISK (1–5%)	HIGH-RISK (>5%)
Breast	Intraperitoneal (cholecystectomy, hiatal hernia, splenectomy)	Adrenal resection
Dental	Endovascular aneurysm repair	Aortic and major vascular surgery
Eye	Kidney transplant	Duodeno-pancreatic surgery
Endocrine (thyroid)	Gynecologic (major)	Esophagectomy
Gynecologic (minor)	Orthopedic (major, e.g., hip and spine)	Liver resection or transplant
Orthopedic (minor, e.g., meniscectomy)	Peripheral arterial angioplasty	Open lower limb revascularization or amputation
Reconstructive	Urologic (major)	Pneumonectomy
Superficial surgery		Pulmonary transplant
Urologic (minor, e.g., TURP)		Repair of bowel perforation
		Total cystectomy

Adapted from Halvorsen S, et al.[39]

reducing oxygen demand and promoting cardiac remodeling, they can lead to improved cardiac function over the longer term. Several large trials have shown evidence of reduced inpatient mortality when continuing these medications perioperatively for noncardiac surgery if there is a chronic indication for them.[44,45] However, they also concluded that there may be a higher incidence of postoperative hypotension as well.

There are additional caveats to beta blocker use. First, with regards to starting a beta blocker immediately preoperatively, multiple studies have shown that doing so may lead to increased mortality, and thus this practice is not recommended in the 2014 ACC/AHA perioperative guidelines.[20,46–48] Second, the benefits of beta blockers largely only extend to patients with HFrEF—those with isolated HFpEF have not been shown to experience a decrease in all-cause mortality or cardiac death.[49] However, patients with HFrEF should benefit from chronic beta blockade, and a careful perioperative approach while titrating the dose slowly and starting therapy more than a week prior to a planned procedure may be appropriate.[50,51]

Angiotensin Converting Enzyme Inhibitors and Angiotensin II Receptor Blockers

ACE inhibitors (e.g., lisinopril, enalapril) and ARBs (e.g., losartan, valsartan) interrupt the renin-angiotensin-aldosterone system (RAAS) pathway. This has downstream effects such as decreased blood volume—and subsequently pressure—by natriuresis, as well as prevention and possible reversal of ventricular remodeling. They have good evidence for significant mortality and morbidity benefits in patients with HFrEF and thus are standard medical therapy.[52,53] However, multiple studies have failed to demonstrate the same improved outcomes for patients with isolated HFpEF, meaning that ACE inhibitors and ARBs do not currently play an important role in its specific treatment.[54–56]

The majority of current guidelines recommend ACE inhibitors and ARBs use be interrupted 24 hours prior to surgery given concern for an association with refractory hypotension after induction of general anesthesia.[57] However, the impact on clinical outcome of this hypotension is debatable, with some studies showing no significant difference.[58,59] The recent Society for Perioperative Assessment and Quality Improvement (SPAQI) consensus statement recommends a 24-hour discontinuation period when a general anesthetic is anticipated while continuing the ACE/ARB on the day of surgery for patients undergoing procedures under local or monitored anesthesia care.[60]

Angiotensin Receptor-Neprilysin Inhibitors

ARNIs (e.g., sacubitril-valsartan) combine the RAAS pathway interruption of an ARB with the anti-hypertensive action of a neprilysin inhibitor. Neprilysin is the enzyme responsible for the degradation of both atrial and brain natriuretic peptide—both of which exhibit diuretic action—as well as the vasodilatory bradykinin. Recent studies have shown that use of ARNIs reduces the risk of disease progression and sudden cardiac death in HFrEF compared to enalapril (an ACE inhibitor) alone.[61] However, the benefits are less clear for patients with isolated HFpEF as the few studies that exist so far show no improvement in rates of hospitalization or all-cause mortality.[62] As discussed above with ACE inhibitors and ARBs, the decision to discontinue ARNIs the night before surgery over concern for post-induction refractory hypotension is controversial but is generally the accepted approach.[60]

Sodium-Glucose Cotransporter 2 Inhibitors

SGLT2 inhibitors (e.g., dapagliflozin, empagliflozin) are a relatively new pharmacologic therapy in heart failure. The primary mechanism of action is preventing renal reabsorption of glucose from the glomerular filtrate, resulting in lower blood glucose levels and a degree of osmotic diuresis. While their ability to reduce blood glucose levels clearly may be of benefit to patients with type 2 diabetes mellitus (DM2), studies have demonstrated a mortality benefit in HFrEF patients both with and without diabetes.[63,64] Although thorough studies on HFpEF patients are currently lacking, early studies suggest that they may improve diastolic heart function in both diabetic and nondiabetic patients.[65]

Proposed mechanisms for this benefit in nondiabetic patients include inhibition of cardiac fibrosis, reduced endothelial dysfunction, and provision of ketones as an alternative energy supply. SGLT2 inhibitors should be temporarily discontinued 3 days prior to surgery as the stress of the perioperative period may place patients at risk of developing euglycemic diabetic ketoacidosis (DKA).[60,66]

Loop Diuretics

Loop diuretics (e.g., furosemide, bumetanide) are frequently prescribed to help prevent volume overload in heart failure. They block the Cl$^-$ binding site on the renal Na$^+$-K$^+$-2Cl$^-$ symporter, found in the ascending loop of Henle. This results in inhibition of sodium, chloride, and potassium reabsorption, thus leading to diuresis. While they clearly have symptomatic benefits for patients with either HFrEF or HFpEF by reducing volume overload,[67,68] evidence-based survival benefit is thus far limited to small trials.[67,69] Patients are generally instructed to hold loop diuretics on the morning of surgery to prevent hypovolemia-related hypotension on induction of anesthesia, but this is not a strongly established guideline in literature.

Mineralocorticoid Receptor Antagonists

MRAs (e.g., spironolactone, eplerenone) are an alternative class of diuretics that may be given to patients who remain symptomatic despite initiation of all primary therapies. By blocking action of mineralocorticoids like aldosterone, they prevent the reabsorption of sodium and subsequent increase in extracellular volume. However, this mechanism of action increases the risk of hyperkalemia, which necessitates periodic monitoring. There is good evidence that MRAs provide a mortality benefit in HFrEF patients with NYHA II–IV heart failure or those with a recent MI.[70–72] Similar results have been seen for patients with isolated HFpEF, especially those with elevated BNP levels.[73] Like other diuretics, patients are often instructed to hold them on the day of surgery to reduce the likelihood of hypovolemia related hypotension.

Digoxin

Digoxin, once a mainstay of heart failure treatment, is now primarily relegated to providing relief to symptomatic patients who are already on all other primary medical therapies. It provides a combination of increased inotropy and decreased chronotropy by inhibiting Na^+/K^+-ATPase in the myocardium, subsequently leading to increased intracellular calcium. These effects are both helpful in chronic heart failure but can actually exacerbate an acute decompensation.

Digoxin has fallen out of favor as studies demonstrate only a decrease in HFrEF hospitalizations but no change in all-cause mortality.[74] There is similarly no change for mortality for HFpEF with even less evidence that it helps reduce cardiac-related hospitalizations.[75] Its pharmacokinetics and narrow therapeutic window also make it notoriously difficult to manage, with both supratherapeutic levels and withdrawal posing significant risks. For this reason, digoxin should be continued perioperatively in most circumstances.

Statins

Statins (e.g., atorvastatin and rosuvastatin) are widely used for primary prevention of atherosclerotic disease, which itself could worsen cardiovascular function by leading to ischemic injuries. By competitively inhibiting HMG-CoA reductase, statins block the hepatic pathway necessary for cholesterol production. They also have a multitude of lipid-independent (dubbed pleiotropic) effects that theoretically may improve outcomes for heart failure patients, such as inhibition of cytokine activity, improved endothelial function, and maintenance of plaque stability.[76]

Studies have demonstrated mixed results for statins providing significant benefit to patients with HFrEF.[77,78] However, a common practice is to place patients with an LV ejection fraction (EF) of less than 35% on statins, regardless of ischemic versus nonischemic etiology. Studies have shown some observational benefit to all-cause mortality for patients with HFpEF, though mechanisms for this improvement are unclear.[79,80] Regardless, statins should be continued throughout the perioperative period, if possible, with some studies showing postoperative mortality and morbidity benefit with statin use.[81]

Soluble Guanylate Cyclase Stimulators

The endothelial dysfunction and elevated levels of reactive oxygen species seen in heart failure lead to a reduction in nitric oxide (NO) bioavailability, thus inhibiting the cyclic guanylate monophosphate (GMP) pathway.[82] As their name suggests, soluble guanylate cyclase stimulators (e.g., vericiguat) promote the cyclic GMP pathway through both a binding site independent of nitric oxide, as well as sensitizing guanylate cyclase to endogenous NO. This in turn leads to direct myocardial and pulmonary vasodilatory effects.

Recent evidence—most notably from the VICTORIA trial, published in 2020—has shown that vericiguat may decrease the need for hospitalization from heart failure-related causes.[83] However, it did not clearly demonstrate reduction in all-cause or cardiovascular-related death, so the 2021 ESC guidelines currently only say that it should be considered for use at this time.[41]

Cardiac Myosin Activators

Direct cardiac myosin activators (e.g., omecamtiv mecarbil) specifically bind to cardiac myosin, helping to augment the speed of adenosine triphosphate (ATP) hydrolysis and increasing the overall number of myosin heads bound to actin filaments.[84] This effectively results in increased systolic ejection time and stroke volume, as well as improved ventricular remodeling. These drugs have no significant on skeletal or smooth muscle.

This is a relatively new class of medication with a relatively limited number of studies so far. The GALACTIC-HF study did show that omecamtiv mecarbil may delay the time to first heart failure event or cardiovascular death in patients with heart failure, though it did not result in a significant reduction in cardiovascular mortality.[85] Thus, the 2021 ESC guidelines state that at the moment they may be considered as an adjunct to other standard therapies for HFrEF.[41]

Intraoperative Monitoring

The significant anesthetic risks in heart failure raise several questions. For example: Can the procedure be done without undergoing general anesthesia, thus avoiding the cardiopulmonary risks that necessitates? If performing a procedure with just sedation and regional anesthetic is feasible (e.g., for cataract surgery), that may be the safest option for the heart failure patient.

However, if not possible, one may need to take extra precautions for monitoring, depending on the severity of the patient's disease. In patients with advanced heart failure, there should be a low threshold to place an arterial line for pressure monitoring if hemodynamic swings are expected, given their risk of cardiovascular compromise. Similarly, if a complex procedure with large volume shifts is expected, it would not be unreasonable to place a central venous catheter to provide central access for vasopressors or inotropes.

Last, evaluating a patient preoperatively for the risks of transesophageal echo (TEE) probe placement (e.g., difficulty swallowing, known esophageal varices, previous esophageal surgery, etc.) may be prudent. Although usually not necessary outside cardiac surgery, rescue TEE can provide extremely helpful information if a patient becomes hemodynamically unstable and is not responding to provided therapies.

Cardiac Implantable Electronic Devices

Implanted Cardioverter Defibrillators

Patients with systolic heart failure are prone to life-threatening arrythmias (e.g., ventricular tachycardia and ventricular fibrillation), which can lead to sudden cardiac death. Thus, ICDs are indicated for primary prevention of cardiac arrythmias in patients with NYHA class II or worse heart failure and a persistent LVEF of 35% or less after adherence to at least 3 months of optimal medical therapy.[86]

Biventricular pacing, also known as cardiac resynchronization therapy (CRT, also written CRT-D when such therapy is combined with an ICD), is a pacing modality that benefits patients experiencing loss of ventricular synchrony as demonstrated by a wide QRS complex and/or bundle branch block on ECG. In addition to the typical right atrial and RV leads, a third lead is placed in the coronary sinus dedicated to LV pacing. For a heart failure patient who is already a candidate for an ICD to qualify for CRT, they must have a QRS complex of greater than 130 ms combined with an LBBB, or a QRS complex greater than 150 ms regardless of the presence of a bundle branch block.[86]

Pacemakers and ICDs are primarily covered in Chapter 42. However, at minimum, a perioperative evaluation should include an interrogation of the device within the last 6 months. Similarly, one should understand how the device may respond to electrocautery (e.g., disabling pacing or defibrillating the patient) as well as how to turn off these responses if necessary.

Left Ventricular Assist Devices

A wide variety of mechanical circulatory support devices are available for patients with end-stage heart failure, such as the intra-aortic balloon pump (IABP) and Impella micro-axial flow device. However, many of these are by nature limited to the inpatient, intensive-care setting and are thus unlikely to be encountered in the preoperative setting. LVADs are an exception to this, given that they are durable in nature and are increasingly being used as long-term therapy for outpatients.

LVADs are being used in patients with end-stage heart failure as either a bridge to transplant therapy (i.e., until a donor organ is available or myocardial function recovers spontaneously) or as destination therapy (i.e., a permanent solution for patients who are deemed ineligible for transplantation). These devices are reserved for patients with worsening NHYA class IV heart failure not responding to optimal medical management, nor to the use of inotropes and other temporary circulatory support devices. However, 1-year survival for patients with a durable device like an LVAD approaches nearly 80% and 4-year survival is close to 50%.[87]

Currently Available Devices.

In the United States, three primary devices are being used: the HeartMate II (a second-generation device), as well as the HeartMate III and the HeartWare HVAD (both third-generation devices). While the now obsolete first-generation devices (e.g., HeartMate I) provided pulsatile flow, second- and third-generation devices transitioned to continuous flow pumps. The advantage of continuous flow pumps is improved long-term durability due to fewer parts and a smaller device footprint because no blood reservoir is required. The transition from second- to third-generation devices then involved the switch from axial flow to centrifugal flow designs, which shrunk the pump further as well as reduced the risk of both intra-device thrombosis and hemolysis.

Due to the larger pump footprint of the axial-flow HeartMate II, the actual pump has to be implanted into the preperitoneal space of the superior abdomen, with the inflow cannula coming from the apex of the LV and the outflow going to the ascending aorta. The continuous-flow HeartMate III and HVAD are pumps both small enough to be contained fully in the pericardial space. The axial-flow pump of the HeartMate II typically requires a higher speed (up to 15,000 rpm) to maintain output compared to the Heartmate III (up to 9,000 rpm) and the HVAD (up to 4,000 rpm). The third-generation centrifugal-flow devices also have magnetically levitated rotors to reduce points of contact to improve device durability. Both third-generation devices also have washing-cycle functions that can intermittently quickly decrease then increase the pump speed to prevent stasis.

Studies have shown similar 2-year mortality rates between the second- and third-generation devices; however, the third-generation devices both had lower rates of reoperation due to device failure or malfunction.[88,89] However, the HVAD did have a higher rate of stroke within the first 60 days after implantation, which on post-hoc analysis was found to be associated with mean arterial pressures (MAPs) greater than 90 mm Hg. Given these improvements, second-generation devices may become increasingly rare, as they accounted for only 1.8% of LVADs implanted in 2019.[90]

Performance Parameters and Settings.

Several device parameters can be monitored by attaching the device to a console or by accessing the patient controller. These can all provide useful information regarding how the LVAD is functioning in conjunction with the native cardiac output.[91] Of these, only pump speed (i.e., rpm) can be directly changed; all others are indirectly dependent on either the pump speed or other patient factors, such as fluid status, systemic vascular resistance (SVR), and native cardiac activity.

- *Pump speed*: Measured in rpm, this is the only characteristic that can be directly changed. Usually, any large changes are done under guidance by echocardiography to monitor for excessive LV underfilling (that can lead to suction events), as well as volume overload of the RV.

- *Pump power*: Measured in watts (W), this is the power consumption of the pump needed to reach a desired pump speed. Generally, it changes in a linear fashion with pump rpms, but many other factors play a role as well. For example, increased pump power may be indicative of increased SVR (as it takes more power to push blood systemically) or a much more worrisome intra-pump thrombosis.

- *Pump flow*: Measured in liters per minute (L/min), pump flow is calculated from the pump speed and power. It is important to note that this number is calculated, as all modern devices lack a flow sensor for more direct measurements. Also, while analogous to cardiac output, it may not be an accurate assessment of output because it ignores any contribution from the native heart.

- *Pulsatility index (PI)*: This is a dimensionless index that provides insight into the extent of native LVr pulsatility. This single number is only available in HeartMate LVAD models; the HeartWare HVAD only displays a continuous waveform of flow over, from which pulsatility can be inferred. Typically, a low PI is indicative of either low intravascular volume or the lack of significant native cardiac output. However, it could be also the sign of more serious concerns, such as pericardial tamponade.

Given the complexity of these devices, it may be appropriate to have a dedicated mechanical circulatory support technician available during the procedure. This ensures that someone is familiar with the monitoring functionality of the device as well as how to adjust its performance intraoperatively (i.e., pump rpms) if needed. One should also have a low threshold to consult experts familiar with these devices before making settings changes.

Anticoagulation.
Given the inherent risk of thrombosis posed by these devices, patients must be on long-term anticoagulation. Based on the protocols used during the manufacturer studies, all patients should be on warfarin with a goal INR of 2.0 to 3.0, as well as aspirin 81–325 mg/day (the HeartMate trials varied between aspirin doses, while the HeartWare HVAD recommended 325 mg/day in its later studies).[88,89] This strategy is in line with the 2013 International Society for Heart and Lung Transplantation (ISHLT) recommendations that are based on observational studies and expert opinion; however, some individual centers may have adopted their own variations with the addition of either clopidogrel or dipyridamole.[92,93]

Perioperative anticoagulation management is an important topic because in-VAD thrombosis could be a devastating event that results in significant hemodynamic instability or debilitating stroke. However, clear guidelines for management do not exist, meaning that there should be a frank discussion between the surgeon, anesthesiologist, and team managing the patient's VAD on how to balance the risk of surgical bleeding with that of thrombosis. Some institutions have established protocols for discontinuing warfarin anywhere from 3 to 5 days preoperatively and bridging with either a heparin infusion (with a goal PTT of 60–80s) or subcutaneous enoxaparin injections of 1 mg/kg BID.[93–97] Complete reversal of anticoagulation with fresh frozen plasma (FFP), vitamin K, or prothrombin complex concentrates (PCCs) should be avoided unless absolutely needed (e.g., necessary neurologic or ophthalmologic surgery). Anticoagulation should then be restarted as soon possible postoperatively, again balancing this against the risk of bleeding.

Hemodynamic Considerations.
Unfortunately, patients with an LVAD are still subject to hemodynamic instability in some circumstances. They are very dependent on preload conditions because LVAD output cannot exceed the volume that is delivered to it. In severe cases, one may also experience suction events, where the LVAD inflow cannula may get positioned against the LV wall and transiently precludes functional flow. Thus, maintaining euvolemia is critical to adequate LVAD performance.

Similarly, RV function plays a crucial role in maintaining flow because it is responsible for delivering volume to the left side of the heart. This means that anything that impedes its function—including increased pulmonary vascular resistance (PVR) from increased intrathoracic pressure, hypoxemia, or hypercarbia—can have serious consequences for systemic flow. RV failure is also one of the most common complications after LVAD implantation because the LVAD output, when the pump speed is set too high, can potentially overwhelm the capacity of the right heart that is not accustomed to such vigorous left-sided function. If concerned, starting inotropic agents, such milrinone and dobutamine, to augment RV function is a reasonable therapeutic option.

LVADs may provide a limited degree of support when unstable arrhythmias occur, but these rhythm disturbances still prevent optimal LVAD performance and limit systemic outflows. Thankfully, arrhythmias are managed in a similar fashion to all other patients under general anesthesia and do not have special considerations.

LVADs are sensitive to afterload; there is an inverse relationship between pump flow and systemic pressure. In other words, if a patient's pressure increases significantly due to pain or other stimuli, pump flow will drop—unless the pump speed is subsequently increased. The primary concern is that a drop in pump flows can promote stasis, thus increasing the risk for thrombus formation. However, if pressures drop too much, then there is the obvious concern for end-organ perfusion. Thus, one should target a MAP for a patient with an LVAD in the range of 70–80 mm Hg, using vasopressors, vasodilators, or analgesics to achieve this goal.

Intraoperative Monitoring with an LVAD.
Intraoperatively, patients with an LVAD can present a monitoring challenge as their continuous flow devices limit the pulsatility needed by noninvasive blood pressure (NIBP) cuffs and pulse oximetry to reliably provide data. Published reviews suggest that NIBP cuffs are often sufficient for minor procedures, such as endoscopies.[98,99] However, if pulsatility is limited, blood pressure measurement by Doppler is another established noninvasive alternative for monitoring in LVAD patients.[100] One could also consider cerebral oximetry for continuous, noninvasive monitoring of oxygenation in those situations because it does not depend on pulsations like traditional pulse oximetry does.

Invasive monitors (e.g., intra-arterial or central venous catheters) should remain accurate and thus should be strongly considered in cases where pulsatility may diminish (e.g., anticipated large volume shifts or blood loss). TEE may also help direct care in situations with significant hemodynamic instability by providing valuable information about volume status and cardiac function.

Additional Perioperative Considerations.
Several other preoperative considerations should be made for these patients. First is their cardiac status; for example: the original indication for their VAD, the presence of a pacemaker or ICD, and underlying arrhythmias.[101] While thoughtful perioperative management of such additional cardiac implantable electronic devices (CIEDs) is important to maintain sinus rhythm, the value of which was already established in the hemodynamics section above, there are no special considerations for the patient who also has an LVAD. Knowing the therapeutic strategy for the VAD (bridge to transplant or destination therapy) may also inform transfusion decisions: one should minimize blood product administration in transplantation candidates to decrease the risk of alloimmunization, which may increase the difficulty of finding a suitable donor organ match in the future.[102]

Patients may also have signs of end-organ dysfunction (e.g., acute and/or chronic kidney disease, hepatopathy) from either a low cardiac output state or venous congestion from RV functional impairment. Chronic infection is also a significant concern, given that the driveline for the LVAD is tunneled through the chest and is in continuity with the outside world. Apart from the anticoagulation issue discussed above, excessive bleeding may be encountered due to the high rate of acquired von Willebrand's disease from the shear stress-induced proteolysis from the pump.[103]

Power management is yet another issue that has to be considered: while battery systems are available to provide patients a degree of independence and mobility, a full charge typically lasts only on the order of several hours. Thus, the device should be connected to a dedicated, external power source (i.e., wall electrical outlet) whenever possible in the operating room to better protect against any interruption in power.

Finally, in the case of a cardiac arrest, there are a few changes to the typical resuscitation algorithm.[104] First, one needs to check for the characteristic LVAD hum over the precordium to check that the device is working if it is not already hooked up to a monitoring console. If the hum is absent and the power source is disconnected, reconnect the power cable if the LVAD stopped working less than 30 minutes ago. If restarted after 30 minutes of being stopped, the concern is for a significant clot burden in the device, and it could throw an embolus. In the case of VAD failure due to embolism, extracorporeal membrane oxygenation (ECMO) may be needed to bridge the patient to an attempted device exchange.

If there is a hum, then gentle chest compressions can be started just to drive blood through the lungs. Vigorous chest compression may only risk dislodging the implanted inflow or outflow cannulas, which would be fatal, and a functional LVAD should already be providing a degree of systemic circulation anyway.[104,105] The goal of compressions should be to keep the end tidal CO_2 ($P_{ET}CO_2$) above 20 mm Hg. If the ECG shows a shockable rhythm, cardioversion or defibrillation should be performed as long as the defibrillator pads are not positioned directly over the device or its driveline.

Wireless Hemodynamic Monitoring

Wireless hemodynamic monitoring devices (e.g., CardioMEMS) are implantable monitors approved by the US Food and Drug Administration (FDA) for tracking pulmonary artery pressures and heart rates in patients with NYHA class III heart failure—from either HFrEF or HFpEF—who have been hospitalized in the past year. With access to this sort of information, it is hoped that one may be able to intervene early (e.g., adjusting diuretic dose) for patients with an acute exacerbation in their heart failure and ideally avoid the need for hospitalization. A few trials (e.g., the CHAMPION trial) have found that these devices are successful in reducing hospitalizations within 6 and 18 months after implantation.[106] However, the recommendation for implantation from the 2016 ESC heart failure guidelines remains weak, with some concern for bias introduced into these studies by the trial sponsors.[107]

Surgical Management

Outside of mechanical circulatory support and orthotopic heart transplantation, surgical interventions are typically not indicated in heart failure, and the mainstay of medical management is pharmacologic with lifestyle changes. However, in certain instances, there may be an underlying physiologic defect responsible for acute heart failure; for example, severe stenosis and/or regurgitation of the aortic valve. In these cases, addressing the underlying abnormality via surgical intervention is indicated if only to prevent further progression of disease.

Orthotopic Heart Transplantation

Orthotopic heart transplantation is the eventual treatment for symptomatic patients with end-stage heart failure. For listing, typically heart failure patients need to be NYHA functional class IV, refractory to optimal medical therapy, and usually with a peak oxygen consumption (VO_2) of 12 mL/kg/min or less if on beta blocker therapy or 14 mL/kg/min or less if intolerant of beta blockers.[108] Of course, there are other conditions outside of heart failure that may qualify for transplantation listing as well (e.g., intractable life-threatening arrythmias unresponsive to therapies, cardiomyopathies, congenital malformations, etc.). Similarly, there are many contraindications to transplant, such as systemic illness with a life expectancy of less than 2 years despite transplantation, irreversible pulmonary hypertension, and active illicit substance abuse.

Physiologic Changes with a Transplanted Heart.
Heart transplantation is associated with many physiologic changes. First, the process necessitates that the donor heart be denervated in the process: there is a loss of direct sensory, sympathetic, and parasympathetic input. This often leads to a resting heart rate of 90–110 bpm, with reduced variability in response to autonomic reflexes.[109] For example, there may be a

lack of tachycardia in response to orthostatic hypotension or anesthetic-induced vasodilation or bradycardia from baroreceptor reflexes with tracheal intubation.

This has notable implications for the anesthesiologist, such as patients being preload-dependent because a relatively "fixed" heart rate will play less of a role in cardiac output. Similarly, indirect agents (i.e., glycopyrrolate, atropine, ephedrine) and maneuvers (e.g., carotid massage) may have minimal effect in the treatment of bradyarrhythmias or tachyarrhythmias, respectively. Adenosine also has significantly increased potency in the denervated heart, so it may precipitate prolonged asystole.[110]

Agents with direct beta-1 adrenergic activity (i.e., dobutamine, isoproterenol, epinephrine, and norepinephrine) or pacing may be required in the case of bradycardia. As for tachyarrhythmias, amiodarone and verapamil may be reasonable treatment options.[110,111]

Depending on the surgical technique, patients may have two P waves on ECG. This is related to the patient potentially having two sinoatrial nodes: one from the remnants of the native atrium—which is left in place with a biatrial technique—and the other from the donor heart. This should not be confused with a complete heart block. Right bundle branch blocks are also a common finding, occurring in up to 75% of cardiac transplant patients and possibly related to the repeated endomyocardial biopsies used to monitor for graft rejection.[112] Similarly, there is an increased incidence of atrial arrythmias (i.e., atrial fibrillation, atrial flutter) given the surgical disruption of the atria.

Immunosuppression.
The necessary immunosuppression regimens to prevent graft rejection also may present several perioperative challenges. This obviously places the patient at higher risk of infection, and thus both prophylactic antibiotics and sterility during procedures must be taken seriously. This is especially of concern in the early post-transplant phase (i.e., within 6–12 months) or immediately after episodes of acute rejection, when the overall level of immunosuppression is at its highest. Multiple drug-drug interactions encountered with immunosuppressive drugs can also make antibiotic and other medication dosing challenging.

Current agents frequently impact other organ systems. A degree of hepatic and renal dysfunction is common with medications like tacrolimus and mycophenolate, thus routine monitoring with labs is recommended.[111] Calcineurin inhibitors (e.g., tacrolimus, cyclosporine) may also lower the seizure threshold. Long-term corticosteroid use also can lead to adrenal insufficiency or diabetes, meaning that both glucose monitoring and stress-dose steroids may need to be considered. The use of mTOR inhibitors (e.g., sirolimus) may also limit wound healing and increase related complications.[113]

Additional Perioperative Considerations.
Additional considerations include timing of a surgery. In the early post-transplant phase (i.e., the first 6–12 months), patients are at their highest risk of acute graft rejection and are likely on high doses of immunosuppressive medications (which brings along complications, as mentioned above). Thus, it is recommended that all elective surgery be deferred beyond this timeframe when possible.[111]

For all cases, the anesthesiologist should focus on gathering information about the patient's comorbidities and cardiac function (i.e., any signs of rejection on recent biopsy, most recent TTE or ECG results, functional status at home), as well as what immunosuppressive medications they are taking and the doses (i.e., assess for risk of other organ system dysfunction or possible drug-drug interactions). Patients in the late post-transplant phase (i.e., >12 months out) likely will have angiography every several years to evaluate for cardiac allograph vasculopathy, which can lead to perioperative ischemic events and is the most common cause of repeat transplantation.[114]

The choice of anesthetic strategy is important given that these patients can be more sensitive to vasodilatation and the associated drop in preload. General anesthesia without invasive monitors can be safe in straightforward cases with minimal fluid shifts, though regional techniques with sedation may avoid the risk of hypotension when appropriate. However, spinal anesthesia should be used carefully given the sudden drop in vascular tone and preload that its sympathectomy can precipitate. When central access is being considered in higher risk cases, one should be aware that these patients frequently receive their routine cardiac biopsies via the right internal jugular vein, and thus it may have significant scar tissue.

CONSIDERATIONS FOR MINOR, LOW-RISK PROCEDURES

This extensive workup, perioperative medication management, and placement of monitors should be weighed against the risk of the procedure being performed. For simple procedures with minimal cardiovascular impact from either a surgical or anesthetic perspective, such as the cataract surgery posed at the start of this chapter, it would be reasonable to proceed without any preoperative testing. As mentioned, the 2014 ACC/AHA perioperative guidelines state that even foregoing a simple ECG may be reasonable for known heart failure patients undergoing a low-risk procedure.[20] Furthermore, a study analyzing nearly 20,000 cataract surgeries showed no difference in outcomes if routine preoperative testing was performed.[2] Similarly, as discussed above, standard noninvasive monitoring is even sufficient for patients with LVADs undergoing straightforward procedures like endoscopies.[99] And frequently anticoagulation can be continued through those procedures with minimal bleeding risk. So, while truly elective procedures should be delayed for further optimization if a patient is in decompensated heart failure, one should not need to drastically alter their perioperative plans for an otherwise stable patient undergoing a minor procedure.

CONCLUSION

- Heart failure is a serious medical condition with significant morbidity and mortality, and its associated physiologic changes must be considered to provide safe care during the perioperative period.

- Classification of severity is typically done using the NYHA functional classification, though more objective measures of ventricular function via echocardiography do exist.

- A thorough preoperative exam includes looking for signs and symptoms of impaired cardiac function, such as lower extremity edema, dyspnea and/or chest pain on exertion, inability to lie flat, elevated jugular venous pressure, and audible murmurs.

- Preoperative testing should include both recent imaging (e.g., ECG, chest x-ray, and TTE) and laboratory testing (e.g., BNP and/or NT-pro-BNP, electrolytes) to assess cardiac function, current volume status, and presence of other frequently associated comorbidities.

- Scoring systems exists to estimate the rate of major cardiovascular complications in the perioperative setting, such as the RCRI, NSQIP MICA, and ACS NSQIP.

- Beta blockers, ACE inhibitors, ARBs, ARNIs, and other pharmacologic treatments with good evidence exist for treatment of systolic heart failure (HFrEF), though some require careful perioperative management to avoid complications (e.g., euglycemic DKA with SGLT2 inhibitors.) and their use does not necessarily extend to diastolic heart failure (HFpEF) as well.

- Durable implantable devices (e.g., LVADs) for treating heart failure are becoming more frequent and pose their own management problems intraoperatively given their relative lack of pulsatility, unique hemodynamics, and need for anticoagulation.

- Patients who have had an orthotopic heart transplant come with their own perioperative challenges, including loss of autonomic innervation, need for immunosuppression, and ongoing concern for graft rejection.

REVIEW QUESTIONS

1. A 56-year-old male patient with a history of heart failure presents to your preoperative clinic before his scheduled hernia repair. He reports being comfortable while sitting in his favorite chair watching television; however, he reports that he feels out of breath by the time he gets across the house to go to the bathroom. And at this point he will do whatever he can to avoid stairs as they take a significant amount of time to scale and leave him feeling exhausted. What NYHA functional class would you place this patient into?

   a. NYHA functional class I.
   b. NYHA functional class II.
   c. NYHA functional class III.
   d. NYHA functional class IV.

The correct answer is c.

This patient appears to have well-controlled symptoms at rest (e.g., sitting in a chair) but has clear functional limitations with even minimal physical activity (e.g., walking a short distance on a flat surface). This best fits the description of NYHA functional class III heart failure.

2. You are the anesthesiologist for a traumatic femur fracture open reduction and internal fixation (ORIF) in a 65-year-old patient who had an orthotopic heart transplant 6 months ago for her idiopathic cardiomyopathy. Given the complexity of the procedure, the surgeon requests general anesthesia. After induction and securing the airway, the patient becomes progressively more bradycardic and subsequently hypotensive while waiting for the surgical team to prep and drape her. How might you address this hemodynamic instability?

   a. Give a bolus of atropine.
   b. Give a bolus of ephedrine.
   c. Give a bolus of glycopyrrolate.
   d. Give a small bolus of epinephrine.

The correct answer is d.

Patients with an orthotopic heart transplant have a denervated myocardium, meaning that it is going to be relatively unresponsive to external signals from the nervous system. This means that neither painful stimulation nor indirect acting agents (e.g., atropine, glycopyrrolate, ephedrine) will reliably cause a change in heart rate. Agents with direct beta-1 activity (e.g., epinephrine, norepinephrine, dobutamine, isoproterenol) would be needed in this situation.

3. A 73-year-old patient is preparing to have a colectomy for recently diagnosed colon cancer and is discussing his medical history during the preoperative check-in. While he does carry a diagnosis of heart failure, he blames this on his insulin-dependent diabetes and high blood pressure instead of coronary disease, as his recent left heart cath was "clean." He knows that these are high-risk conditions for both strokes and kidney problems and thus feels lucky to have neither of these issues so far. How many predictors would this patient have if one were to calculate his risk via the RCRI?

   a. 1 predictor.
   b. 2 predictors.
   c. 3 predictors.
   d. 4 predictors.

The correct answer is c.

An intraperitoneal surgery, diagnosis of heart failure, and insulin-dependent diabetes are all predictors of increased risk for perioperative MACE. Hypertension itself is not an independent predictor. Even if he were to have an additional predictor in this scenario, the RCRI maxes out 3 or more predictors for a greater than 11% risk of MACE.

4. You are in the preoperative clinic meeting with a patient who recently had a destination-therapy LVAD implanted for end-stage heart failure and who remains on medical therapy. The patient is now scheduled for a laparoscopic cholecystectomy due to recurrent cholecystitis, which is now a more limiting factor in their functional status.

a. Stop their beta blocker—it might cause post-induction bradycardia.
b. Stop their SGLT2 inhibitor—otherwise there is a risk of developing euglycemic DKA.
c. Stop their warfarin without a heparin bridge—the risk of bleeding during the surgery is too high.
d. Stop their statin—the patient may develop a lactic acidosis.

The correct answer is b.

While the timing for SGLT2 inhibitor may be different, often the recommendation is to hold them 72 hours before surgery to prevent developing euglycemic DKA, which is a life-threatening condition if unrecognized. Multiple studies have shown a benefit to continuing chronic beta blocker therapy perioperatively because stopping them may lead to acute rebound tachycardia or hypertension. Statins are typically safe to continue perioperatively, though the traditional teaching is that metformin may lead to a perioperative lactic acidosis if not stopped beforehand. Finally, stopping all anticoagulation in a patient with an LVAD is extremely dangerous due to the risk for thrombus formation—this should only be done in dire situations where the risk of bleeding to the patient outweighs that of device failure or stroke from thrombosis.

5. A patient with long-standing heart failure comes to your clinic to follow-up on TTE results. He had reported irregular bouts of fatigue with physical exertion despite being on an optimal medical regimen that includes a beta blocker and an ACE inhibitor. The echo report documents a LV ejection fraction of 30–35 %, which is actually stable from prior 18 months prior. What would be the most reasonable action to recommend for this patient?

a. Initiate digoxin therapy to reduce his mortality risk.
b. Refer the patient for automated ICD placement for primary prevention of sudden cardiac death.
c. Schedule the patient for regular TTEs every 3 months to monitor his cardiac function.
d. Switch him from lisinopril to losartan as it has better evidence for cardiac remodeling.

The correct answer is b.

ICDs are indicated for primary prevention of sudden cardiac death in patients with an LVEF of 35% or less and NYHA functional class II heart failure despite optimal medical therapy for at least 3 months. While digoxin may provide symptomatic relief for some patients, it has not been shown to provide mortality benefit. A regular TTE on an annual basis may be within the 2014 ACC)/AHA perioperative guidelines for stable heart failure patient with no major recent clinical events, but doing so multiple times a year for such a patient is unnecessary. Finally, the current understanding is that ACE inhibitors (e.g., lisinopril) and ARBs (e.g., losartan) are equally efficacious in outcomes, and there is no need to switch classes if the current medication is well tolerated.

6. A 68-year-old woman with known heart failure with reduced ejection fraction (HFrEF) comes to preoperative clinic before a partial nephrectomy for localized tumor removal in a few weeks. She reports that she feels relatively well; although she has to stop while climbing the hills in her neighborhood to catch her breath, she feels she is able to get around at home and while running errands without issue. She feels like her energy levels improved after she started stable doses of her heart medications (bisoprolol, lisinopril, furosemide) years ago and thankfully have not declined since then. What further preoperative testing would be most helpful to make sure this patient is treated safely?

a. Order a basic metabolic panel (BMP).
b. Send the patient for a dobutamine stress test.
c. Draw a preoperative high-sensitivity troponin.
d. Refer the patient to cardiology for a left heart catheterization.

The correct answer is a.

A BMP may prove helpful both to assess for other comorbidities associated with heart failure (e.g., renal insufficiency, diabetes) as well as for electrolyte abnormalities that may be seen with lisinopril (hyperkalemia) or furosemide (hypokalemia). Neither stress tests nor left heart catheterization are recommended unless there is strong suspicion for an ischemic etiology and an intervenable lesion. While preoperative troponin levels do appear to be associated with perioperative adverse cardiac events, how this information should influence the timing of surgery is still controversial. Thus, preoperative troponins are not recommended in the 2014 ACC/AHA perioperative guidelines.

7. You are taking care of a 77-year-old patient getting a radial ORIF after a recent fall caused a distal radial fracture. The patient has known heart failure with reduced ejection fraction (HFrEF) and chronic renal insufficiency. The patient has slowly become more hypotensive as the case has progressed despite minimal blood loss with tourniquet use. While her MAP in preop was close to 100, now repeated measurements on the blood pressure cuff are in the high 50s and low 60s. Her heart rate is still in the high 80s with no changes on the ECG. What is the most appropriate course of action to address this?

a. Just continue to monitor—there is no need to treat a number if everything else appears stable.
b. Give a bolus of glycopyrrolate—speeding up her heart rate further will increase her cardiac output.
c. Give a fluid bolus by letting the 1 L IV bag quickly run in—she is likely intravascularly depleted given that she has been NPO for hours.
d. Give a bolus of phenylephrine—increasing her SVR will increase her MAP.

The correct answer is d.

Although the etiology of this patient's heart failure is unknown in this scenario, it is reasonable to be concerned that there may be a degree of underlying ischemic disease. Thus, using phenylephrine to increase coronary perfusion pressure to closer to the patient's baseline would be appropriate, while increasing the myocardial oxygen demand further with glycopyrrolate-induced tachycardia may be risky. While it may be true that the patient is hypovolemic, a large fluid bolus over a short period of time may be harmful for a patient with heart failure. Their heart may not be able to accommodate this large increase in preload, potentially leading to even worse cardiac output and/or other adverse effects like pulmonary edema.

8. A 73-year-old patient is getting a lower-extremity skin graft under general anesthesia. They have a HeartWare HVAD LVAD that was placed 1 year ago for nonischemic cardiomyopathy, which has been functioning well, despite residual mild RV dysfunction. They have been adherent to all their medications, including their anticoagulation. Comorbidities include chronic renal insufficiency. Soon after incision, they become hypertensive with MAPs hovering around 100 mm Hg on noninvasive blood pressure cuff and sinus tachycardia on the ECG in the low 100s. An appropriate next action would be

   a. Do nothing—higher pressures mean better systemic perfusion anyway.
   b. Give a bolus of fentanyl and deepen the anesthetic with a goal of getting the MAP down in the 70–80 mm Hg range.
   c. Start milrinone with a bolus followed by infusion—it may lower the blood pressure and help the RV, which is already known to be dysfunctional/
   d. Turn down the pump speed (rpms)—if the MAP is that high, then the patient must not need as much support from their LVAD.

The correct answer is b.

The concern in this question is that the MAP is higher than the typical goal of 70–80 mm Hg for a patient with an LVAD. A high amount of afterload (i.e., MAP) lowers the pump flows (unless the pump speed is increased), which increases the risk of intra-device thrombosis. This could lead to device failure or a devastating embolic event. Turning the pump speed down in response to the pressure may only decrease the flow further and thus is a risky course of action. Typically, adjustments to LVAD device parameters should only be done under expert guidance. While it is true that a bolus of milrinone would likely drop the systemic pressure, it is not clear that this patient needs any RV support. Milrinone is also renally cleared, and thus should only be started cautiously in a patient with renal insufficiency. A more short-acting choice that directly addressed why the patient is hypertensive, such as fentanyl or deeper anesthetic, is a more appropriate choice in this scenario.

REFERENCES

1. Virani SS, Alonso A, Benjamin EJ, et al. Heart disease and stroke statistics-2020 update: A report from the American Heart Association. *Circulation.* 2020;141(9):e139–e596. Epub 2020/01/30. doi:10.1161/CIR.0000000000000757. PubMed PMID: 31992061
2. Schein OD, Katz J, Bass EB, Tielsch JM, et al. The value of routine preoperative medical testing before cataract surgery: Study of medical testing for cataract surgery. *N Engl J Med.* 2000;342(3):168–175. Epub 2000/01/20. doi:10.1056/NEJM200001203420304. PubMed PMID: 10639542
3. He J, Ogden LG, Bazzano LA, Vupputuri S, Loria C, Whelton PK. Risk factors for congestive heart failure in US men and women: NHANES I epidemiologic follow-up study. *Arch Intern Med.* 2001;161(7):996–1002. Epub 2001/04/11. doi:10.1001/archinte.161.7.996. PubMed PMID: 11295963
4. New York Heart Association. *Diseases of the heart and blood vessels: Nomenclature and criteria for diagnosis.* 6th ed. Little; 1964: xxiii.
5. Heidenreich PA, Bozkurt B, Aguilar D, et al. 2022 AHA/ACC/HFSA Guideline for the Management of Heart Failure: A report of the American College of Cardiology/American Heart Association Joint Committee on Clinical Practice Guidelines. *J Am Coll Cardiol.* 2022;79(17):e263–e421. Epub 20220401. doi:10.1016/j.jacc.2021.12.012. PubMed PMID: 35379503
6. American College of Cardiology: American College of Cardiology. Left ventricular ejection fraction LVEF assessment (outpatient setting). 2021. https://www.acc.org/tools-and-practice-support/clinical-toolkits/heart-failure-practice-solutions/left-ventricular-ejection-fraction-lvef-assessment-outpatient-setting
7. Nagueh SF, Smiseth OA, Appleton CP, et al. Recommendations for the evaluation of left ventricular diastolic function by echocardiography: An update from the American Society of Echocardiography and the European Association of Cardiovascular Imaging. *J Am Soc Echocardiogr.* 2016;29(4):277–314. Epub 2016/04/03. doi:10.1016/j.echo.2016.01.011. PubMed PMID: 27037982
8. From AM, Leibson CL, Bursi F, et al. Diabetes in heart failure: Prevalence and impact on outcome in the population. *Am J Med.* 2006;119(7):591–599. Epub 2006/07/11. doi:10.1016/j.amjmed.2006.05.024. PubMed PMID: 16828631
9. Streng KW, Nauta JF, Hillege HL, et al. Non-cardiac comorbidities in heart failure with reduced, mid-range and preserved ejection fraction. *Int J Cardiol.* 2018;271:132–139. Epub 2018/11/30. doi:10.1016/j.ijcard.2018.04.001. PubMed PMID: 30482453
10. Anand IS, Gupta P. Anemia and iron deficiency in heart failure: Current concepts and emerging therapies. *Circulation.* 2018;138(1):80–98. Epub 2018/07/04. doi:10.1161/CIRCULATIONAHA.118.030099. PubMed PMID: 29967232
11. Arzt M, Woehrle H, Oldenburg O, et al. Prevalence and predictors of sleep-disordered breathing in patients with stable chronic heart failure: The SchlaHF Registry. *JACC Heart Fail.* 2016;4(2):116–125. Epub 2015/12/20. doi:10.1016/j.jchf.2015.09.014. PubMed PMID: 26682790
12. Parati G, Lombardi C, Castagna F, et al. Heart failure and sleep disorders. *Nat Rev Cardiol.* 2016;13(7):389–403. Epub 2016/05/14. doi:10.1038/nrcardio.2016.71. PubMed PMID: 27173772
13. van Diepen S, Bakal JA, McAlister FA, Ezekowitz JA. Mortality and readmission of patients with heart failure, atrial fibrillation, or coronary artery disease undergoing noncardiac surgery: An analysis of 38 047 patients. *Circulation.* 2011;124(3):289–296. Epub 2011/06/29. doi:10.1161/CIRCULATIONAHA.110.011130. PubMed PMID: 21709059
14. Fayad A, Ansari MT, Yang H, Ruddy T, Wells GA. Perioperative diastolic dysfunction in patients undergoing noncardiac surgery is an independent risk factor for cardiovascular events: A systematic review and meta-analysis. *Anesthesiology.* 2016;125(1):72–91. Epub 2016/04/15. doi:10.1097/ALN.0000000000001132. PubMed PMID: 27077638
15. Pagel PS, Tawil JN, Boettcher BT, et al. Heart failure with preserved ejection fraction: A comprehensive review and update of diagnosis, pathophysiology, treatment, and perioperative implications. *J Cardiothorac Vasc Anesth.* 2020. Epub 2020/08/05. doi:10.1053/j.jvca.2020.07.016. PubMed PMID: 32747202
16. Huang YY, Chen L, Wright JD. Comparison of perioperative outcomes in heart failure patients with reduced versus preserved ejection fraction after noncardiac surgery. *Ann Surg.* 2020. Epub 2020/06/17. doi:10.1097/SLA.0000000000004044. PubMed PMID: 32541225
17. Lerman BJ, Popat RA, Assimes TL, Heidenreich PA, Wren SM. Association of left ventricular ejection fraction and symptoms with mortality after elective noncardiac surgery among patients with heart failure. *JAMA.* 2019;321(6):572–579. Epub 2019/02/13.

doi:10.1001/jama.2019.0156. PubMed PMID: 30747965; PubMed Central PMCID: PMC6439591
18. Vaporciyan AA, Correa AM, Rice DC, et al. Risk factors associated with atrial fibrillation after noncardiac thoracic surgery: Analysis of 2588 patients. *J Thorac Cardiovasc Surg*. 2004;127(3):779–786. Epub 2004/03/06. doi:10.1016/j.jtcvs.2003.07.011. PubMed PMID: 15001907
19. Cleland JG, Chattopadhyay S, Khand A, Houghton T, Kaye GC. Prevalence and incidence of arrhythmias and sudden death in heart failure. *Heart Fail Rev*. 2002;7(3):229–242. Epub 2002/09/07. doi:10.1023/a:1020024122726. PubMed PMID: 12215728
20. Fleisher LA, Fleischmann KE, Auerbach AD, et al. 2014 ACC/AHA guideline on perioperative cardiovascular evaluation and management of patients undergoing noncardiac surgery: A report of the American College of Cardiology/American Heart Association Task Force on practice guidelines. *J Am Coll Cardiol*. 2014;64(22):e77–137. Epub 2014/08/06. doi:10.1016/j.jacc.2014.07.944. PubMed PMID: 25091544
21. Eagle KA, Berger PB, Calkins H, et al. ACC/AHA guideline update for perioperative cardiovascular evaluation for noncardiac surgery: Executive summary: A report of the American College of Cardiology/American Heart Association Task Force on Practice Guidelines (Committee to Update the 1996 Guidelines on Perioperative Cardiovascular Evaluation for Noncardiac Surgery). *J Am Coll Cardiol*. 2002;39(3):542–553. Epub 2002/02/02. doi:10.1016/s0735-1097(01)01788-0. PubMed PMID: 11823097
22. Wijeysundera DN, Beattie WS, Hillis GS, et al. Integration of the Duke Activity Status Index into preoperative risk evaluation: A multicentre prospective cohort study. *Br J Anaesth*. 2020;124(3):261–270. Epub 2019/12/23. doi:10.1016/j.bja.2019.11.025. PubMed PMID: 31864719
23. Riedel B, Li MH, Lee CHA, et al. A simplified (modified) Duke Activity Status Index (M-DASI) to characterise functional capacity: A secondary analysis of the Measurement of Exercise Tolerance before Surgery (METS) study. *Br J Anaesth*. 2021;126(1):181–90. Epub 2020/07/22. doi:10.1016/j.bja.2020.06.016. PubMed PMID: 32690247
24. Rohde LE, Polanczyk CA, Goldman L, Cook EF, Lee RT, Lee TH. Usefulness of transthoracic echocardiography as a tool for risk stratification of patients undergoing major noncardiac surgery. *Am J Cardiol*. 2001;87(5):505–509. Epub 2001/03/07. doi:10.1016/s0002-9149(00)01421-1. PubMed PMID: 11230829
25. Halm EA, Browner WS, Tubau JF, Tateo IM, Mangano DT. Echocardiography for assessing cardiac risk in patients having noncardiac surgery: Study of Perioperative Ischemia Research Group. *Ann Intern Med*. 1996;125(6):433–441. Epub 1996/09/15. doi:10.7326/0003-4819-125-6-199609150-00001. PubMed PMID: 8779454
26. Park SJ, Choi JH, Cho SJ, et al. Comparison of transthoracic echocardiography with N-terminal pro-brain natriuretic peptide as a tool for risk stratification of patients undergoing major noncardiac surgery. *Korean Circ J*. 2011;41(9):505–511. Epub 2011/10/25. doi:10.4070/kcj.2011.41.9.505. PubMed PMID: 22022325; PubMed Central PMCID: PMC3193041
27. Rodseth RN, Biccard BM, Le Manach Y, et al. The prognostic value of pre-operative and post-operative B-type natriuretic peptides in patients undergoing noncardiac surgery: B-type natriuretic peptide and N-terminal fragment of pro-B-type natriuretic peptide: A systematic review and individual patient data meta-analysis. *J Am Coll Cardiol*. 2014;63(2):170–180. Epub 2013/10/01. doi:10.1016/j.jacc.2013.08.1630. PubMed PMID: 24076282
28. Farzi S, Stojakovic T, Marko T, et al. Role of N-terminal pro B-type natriuretic peptide in identifying patients at high risk for adverse outcome after emergent non-cardiac surgery. *Br J Anaesth*. 2013;110(4):554–560. Epub 2012/12/19. doi:10.1093/bja/aes454. PubMed PMID: 23248094
29. Duceppe E, Parlow J, MacDonald P, et al. Canadian Cardiovascular Society Guidelines on perioperative cardiac risk assessment and management for patients who undergo noncardiac surgery. *Can J Cardiol*. 2017;33(1):17–32. Epub 2016/11/21. doi:10.1016/j.cjca.2016.09.008. PubMed PMID: 27865641
30. Task Force for Preoperative Cardiac Risk A, Perioperative Cardiac Management in Non-cardiac S, European Society of C, Poldermans D, Bax JJ, Boersma E, et al. Guidelines for pre-operative cardiac risk assessment and perioperative cardiac management in non-cardiac surgery. *Eur Heart J*. 2009;30(22):2769–2812. Epub 2009/08/29. doi:10.1093/eurheartj/ehp337. PubMed PMID: 19713421
31. Writing Committee for the VSI, Devereaux PJ, Biccard BM, Sigamani A, et al. Association of postoperative high-sensitivity troponin levels with myocardial injury and 30-day mortality among patients undergoing noncardiac surgery. *JAMA*. 2017;317(16):1642–1651. Epub 2017/04/27. doi:10.1001/jama.2017.4360. PubMed PMID: 28444280
32. Humble CAS, Huang S, Jammer I, Bjork J, Chew MS. Prognostic performance of preoperative cardiac troponin and perioperative changes in cardiac troponin for the prediction of major adverse cardiac events and mortality in noncardiac surgery: A systematic review and meta-analysis. *PLoS One*. 2019;14(4):e0215094. Epub 2019/04/23. doi:10.1371/journal.pone.0215094. PubMed PMID: 31009463; PubMed Central PMCID: PMC6476502
33. De Hert S, Staender S, Fritsch G, et al. Pre-operative evaluation of adults undergoing elective noncardiac surgery: Updated guideline from the European Society of Anaesthesiology. *Eur J Anaesthesiol*. 2018;35(6):407–465. Epub 2018/05/01. doi:10.1097/EJA.0000000000000817. PubMed PMID: 29708905
34. Lee TH, Marcantonio ER, Mangione CM, et al. Derivation and prospective validation of a simple index for prediction of cardiac risk of major noncardiac surgery. *Circulation*. 1999;100(10):1043–1049. Epub 1999/09/08. doi:10.1161/01.cir.100.10.1043. PubMed PMID: 10477528
35. Gupta PK, Gupta H, Sundaram A, et al. Development and validation of a risk calculator for prediction of cardiac risk after surgery. *Circulation*. 2011;124(4):381–387. Epub 2011/07/07. doi:10.1161/CIRCULATIONAHA.110.015701. PubMed PMID: 21730309
36. American College of Surgeons National Surgical Quality Improvement Program. Surgeons ACo. FAQ - ACS Risk Calculator. https://riskcalculator.facs.org/RiskCalculator/faq.html
37. Bilimoria KY, Liu Y, Paruch JL, et al. Development and evaluation of the universal ACS NSQIP surgical risk calculator: A decision aid and informed consent tool for patients and surgeons. *J Am Coll Surg*. 2013;217(5):833–842 e1–3. Epub 2013/09/24. doi:10.1016/j.jamcollsurg.2013.07.385. PubMed PMID: 24055383; PubMed Central PMCID: PMC3805776
38. Mangano DT. Perioperative cardiac morbidity. *Anesthesiology*. 1990;72(1):153–184. Epub 1990/01/01. doi:10.1097/00000542-199001000-00025. PubMed PMID: 2404426
39. Halvorsen S, Mehilli J, Cassese S, et al. 2022 ESC Guidelines on cardiovascular assessment and management of patients undergoing noncardiac surgery. *Eur Heart J*. 2022 Oct 14;43(39):3826–3924.
40. Glance LG, Lustik SJ, Hannan EL, et al. The Surgical Mortality Probability Model: Derivation and validation of a simple risk prediction rule for noncardiac surgery. *Ann Surg*. 2012;255(4):696–702. Epub 2012/03/16. doi:10.1097/SLA.0b013e31824b45af. PubMed PMID: 22418007
41. McDonagh TA, Metra M, Adamo M, et al. 2021 ESC Guidelines for the diagnosis and treatment of acute and chronic heart failure: Developed by the Task Force for the diagnosis and treatment of acute and chronic heart failure of the European Society of Cardiology (ESC). With the special contribution of the Heart Failure Association (HFA) of the ESC. *Eur J Heart Fail*. 2022;24(1):4–131. doi:10.1002/ejhf.2333. PubMed PMID: 35083827
42. Packer M, Bristow MR, Cohn JN, et al. The effect of carvedilol on morbidity and mortality in patients with chronic heart failure: U.S. Carvedilol Heart Failure Study Group. *N Engl J Med*. 1996;334(21):1349–1355. Epub 1996/05/23. doi:10.1056/NEJM199605233342101. PubMed PMID: 8614419

43. Hjalmarson A, Goldstein S, Fagerberg B, et al. Effects of controlled-release metoprolol on total mortality, hospitalizations, and well-being in patients with heart failure: The Metoprolol CR/XL Randomized Intervention Trial in congestive heart failure (MERIT-HF). MERIT-HF Study Group. *JAMA*. 2000;283(10):1295–1302. Epub 2000/03/14. doi:10.1001/jama.283.10.1295. PubMed PMID: 10714728

44. Kertai MD, Cooter M, Pollard RJ, et al. Is compliance with Surgical Care Improvement Project Cardiac (SCIP-Card-2) measures for perioperative beta-blockers associated with reduced incidence of mortality and cardiovascular-related critical quality indicators after noncardiac surgery? *Anesth Analg*. 2018;126(6):1829–1838. Epub 2017/12/05. doi:10.1213/ANE.0000000000002577. PubMed PMID: 29200062

45. Bemenderfer TB, Rozario NL, Moore CG, Karunakar MA. Morbidity and mortality in elective total hip arthroplasty following Surgical Care Improvement Project guidelines. *J Arthroplasty*. 2017;32(8):2359–2562. Epub 2017/04/04. doi:10.1016/j.arth.2017.02.080. PubMed PMID: 28366317

46. Wijeysundera DN, Beattie WS, Wijeysundera HC, Yun L, Austin PC, Ko DT. Duration of preoperative beta-blockade and outcomes after major elective noncardiac surgery. *Can J Cardiol*. 2014;30(2):217–223. Epub 2014/01/01. doi:10.1016/j.cjca.2013.10.011. PubMed PMID: 24373755

47. Bouri S, Shun-Shin MJ, Cole GD, Mayet J, Francis DP. Meta-analysis of secure randomised controlled trials of beta-blockade to prevent perioperative death in non-cardiac surgery. *Heart*. 2014;100(6):456–464. Epub 2013/08/02. doi:10.1136/heartjnl-2013-304262. PubMed PMID: 23904357; PubMed Central PMCID: PMC3932762

48. Chen RJ, Chu H, Tsai LW. Impact of beta-blocker initiation timing on mortality risk in patients with diabetes mellitus undergoing noncardiac surgery: A nationwide population-based cohort study. *J Am Heart Assoc*. 2017;6(1). Epub 2017/01/12. doi:10.1161/JAHA.116.004392. PubMed PMID: 28073770; PubMed Central PMCID: PMC5523631

49. Cleland JGF, Bunting KV, Flather MD, et al. Beta-blockers for heart failure with reduced, mid-range, and preserved ejection fraction: An individual patient-level analysis of double-blind randomized trials. *Eur Heart J*. 2018;39(1):26–35. Epub 2017/10/19. doi:10.1093/eurheartj/ehx564. PubMed PMID: 29040525; PubMed Central PMCID: PMC5837435

50. Oprea AD, Lombard FW, Kertai MD. Perioperative β-adrenergic blockade in noncardiac and cardiac surgery: A clinical update. *J Cardiothorac Vasc Anesth*. 2019 Mar;33(3):817–832.

51. Oprea AD, Wang X, Sickeler R, Kertai MD. Contemporary personalized β-blocker management in the perioperative setting. *J Anesth*. 2020 Feb;34(1):115–133.

52. Flather MD, Yusuf S, Kober L, et al. Long-term ACE-inhibitor therapy in patients with heart failure or left-ventricular dysfunction: A systematic overview of data from individual patients. ACE-Inhibitor Myocardial Infarction Collaborative Group. *Lancet*. 2000;355(9215):1575–1581. Epub 2000/05/23. doi:10.1016/s0140-6736(00)02212-1. PubMed PMID: 10821360

53. Heran BS, Musini VM, Bassett K, Taylor RS, Wright JM. Angiotensin receptor blockers for heart failure. *Cochrane Database Syst Rev*. 2012(4):CD003040. Epub 2012/04/20. doi:10.1002/14651858.CD003040.pub2. PubMed PMID: 22513909; PubMed Central PMCID: PMC6823214

54. Yusuf S, Pfeffer MA, Swedberg K, et al. Effects of candesartan in patients with chronic heart failure and preserved left-ventricular ejection fraction: The CHARM-Preserved Trial. *Lancet*. 2003;362(9386):777–781. Epub 2003/09/19. doi:10.1016/S0140-6736(03)14285-7. PubMed PMID: 13678871

55. Massie BM, Carson PE, McMurray JJ, et al. Irbesartan in patients with heart failure and preserved ejection fraction. *N Engl J Med*. 2008;359(23):2456–2467. Epub 2008/11/13. doi:10.1056/NEJMoa0805450. PubMed PMID: 19001508

56. Cleland JG, Tendera M, Adamus J, et al. The perindopril in elderly people with chronic heart failure (PEP-CHF) study. *Eur Heart J*. 2006;27(19):2338–2345. Epub 2006/09/12. doi:10.1093/eurheartj/ehl250. PubMed PMID: 16963472

57. Brabant SM, Bertrand M, Eyraud D, Darmon PL, Coriat P. The hemodynamic effects of anesthetic induction in vascular surgical patients chronically treated with angiotensin II receptor antagonists. *Anesth Analg*. 1999;89(6):1388–1392. Epub 1999/12/10. doi:10.1097/00000539-199912000-00011. PubMed PMID: 10589613

58. Turan A, You J, Shiba A, Kurz A, Saager L, Sessler DI. Angiotensin converting enzyme inhibitors are not associated with respiratory complications or mortality after noncardiac surgery. *Anesth Analg*. 2012;114(3):552–560. Epub 2012/01/19. doi:10.1213/ANE.0b013e318241f6af. PubMed PMID: 22253266

59. Hollmann C, Fernandes NL, Biccard BM. A systematic review of outcomes associated with withholding or continuing angiotensin-converting enzyme inhibitors and angiotensin receptor blockers before noncardiac surgery. *Anesth Analg*. 2018;127(3):678–687. Epub 2018/01/31. doi:10.1213/ANE.0000000000002837. PubMed PMID: 29381513

60. Sahai SK, Balonov K, Bentov N, et al. Preoperative management of cardiovascular medications: A Society for Perioperative Assessment and Quality Improvement (SPAQI) consensus statement. *Mayo Clin Proc*. 2022 Sep;97(9):1734–1751.

61. McMurray JJ, Packer M, Desai AS, et al. Angiotensin-neprilysin inhibition versus enalapril in heart failure. *N Engl J Med*. 2014;371(11):993–1004. Epub 2014/09/02. doi:10.1056/NEJMoa1409077. PubMed PMID: 25176015

62. Solomon SD, McMurray JJV, Anand IS, et al. Angiotensin-neprilysin inhibition in heart failure with preserved ejection fraction. *N Engl J Med*. 2019;381(17):1609–1620. Epub 2019/09/03. doi:10.1056/NEJMoa1908655. PubMed PMID: 31475794

63. McMurray JJV, Solomon SD, Inzucchi SE, et al. Dapagliflozin in patients with heart failure and reduced ejection fraction. *N Engl J Med*. 2019;381(21):1995–2008. Epub 2019/09/20. doi:10.1056/NEJMoa1911303. PubMed PMID: 31535829

64. Packer M, Anker SD, Butler J, et al. Cardiovascular and renal outcomes with empagliflozin in heart failure. *N Engl J Med*. 2020;383(15):1413–1424. Epub 2020/09/01. doi:10.1056/NEJMoa2022190. PubMed PMID: 32865377

65. Solomon SD, McMurray JJV, Claggett B, et al. Dapagliflozin in heart failure with mildly reduced or preserved ejection fraction. *N Engl J Med*. 2022 Sep 22;387(12):1089–1098.

66. Milder DA, Milder TY, Kam PCA. Sodium-glucose co-transporter type-2 inhibitors: Pharmacology and peri-operative considerations. *Anaesthesia*. 2018;73(8):1008–1018. Epub 2018/03/13. doi:10.1111/anae.14251. PubMed PMID: 29529345

67. Komajda M, Follath F, Swedberg K, et al. The EuroHeart Failure Survey programme: A survey on the quality of care among patients with heart failure in Europe. Part 2: Treatment. *Eur Heart J*. 2003;24(5):464–474. Epub 2003/03/14. doi:10.1016/s0195-668x(02)00700-5. PubMed PMID: 12633547

68. Adamson PB, Abraham WT, Bourge RC, et al. Wireless pulmonary artery pressure monitoring guides management to reduce decompensation in heart failure with preserved ejection fraction. *Circ Heart Fail*. 2014;7(6):935–944. Epub 2014/10/08. doi:10.1161/CIRCHEARTFAILURE.113.001229. PubMed PMID: 25286913

69. Faris RF, Flather M, Purcell H, Poole-Wilson PA, Coats AJ. Diuretics for heart failure. *Cochrane Database Syst Rev*. 2012(2):CD003838. Epub 2012/02/18. doi:10.1002/14651858.CD003838.pub3. PubMed PMID: 22336795

70. RALES Investigators. Effectiveness of spironolactone added to an angiotensin-converting enzyme inhibitor and a loop diuretic for severe chronic congestive heart failure (the Randomized Aldactone Evaluation Study [RALES]). *Am J Cardiol*. 1996;78(8):902–907. Epub 1996/10/15. doi:10.1016/s0002-9149(96)00465-1. PubMed PMID: 8888663

71. Zannad F, McMurray JJ, Krum H, et al. Eplerenone in patients with systolic heart failure and mild symptoms. *N Engl J Med*. 2011;364(1):11–21. Epub 2010/11/16. doi:10.1056/NEJMoa1009492. PubMed PMID: 21073363

72. Pitt B, Remme W, Zannad F, et al. Eplerenone, a selective aldosterone blocker, in patients with left ventricular dysfunction after myocardial infarction. *N Engl J Med*. 2003;348(14):1309–1321. Epub 2003/04/02. doi:10.1056/NEJMoa030207. PubMed PMID: 12668699
73. Pitt B, Pfeffer MA, Assmann SF, et al. Spironolactone for heart failure with preserved ejection fraction. *N Engl J Med*. 2014;370(15):1383–1392. Epub 2014/04/11. doi:10.1056/NEJMoa1313731. PubMed PMID: 24716680
74. Digitalis Investigation Group. The effect of digoxin on mortality and morbidity in patients with heart failure. *N Engl J Med*. 1997;336(8):525–533. Epub 1997/02/20. doi:10.1056/NEJM199702203360801. PubMed PMID: 9036306
75. Ahmed A, Rich MW, Fleg JL, et al. Effects of digoxin on morbidity and mortality in diastolic heart failure: The ancillary digitalis investigation group trial. *Circulation*. 2006;114(5):397–403. Epub 2006/07/26. doi:10.1161/CIRCULATIONAHA.106.628347. PubMed PMID: 16864724; PubMed Central PMCID: PMC2628473
76. Ramasubbu K, Estep J, White DL, Deswal A, Mann DL. Experimental and clinical basis for the use of statins in patients with ischemic and nonischemic cardiomyopathy. *J Am Coll Cardiol*. 2008;51(4):415–426. Epub 2008/01/29. doi:10.1016/j.jacc.2007.10.009. PubMed PMID: 18222351
77. Tavazzi L, Maggioni AP, Marchioli R, et al. Effect of rosuvastatin in patients with chronic heart failure (the GISSI-HF trial): A randomised, double-blind, placebo-controlled trial. *Lancet*. 2008;372(9645):1231–1239. Epub 2008/09/02. doi:10.1016/S0140-6736(08)61240-4. PubMed PMID: 18757089
78. Cleland JG, McMurray JJ, Kjekshus J, et al. Plasma concentration of amino-terminal pro-brain natriuretic peptide in chronic heart failure: Prediction of cardiovascular events and interaction with the effects of rosuvastatin: A report from CORONA (Controlled Rosuvastatin Multinational Trial in Heart Failure). *J Am Coll Cardiol*. 2009;54(20):1850–1859. Epub 2009/11/07. doi:10.1016/j.jacc.2009.06.041. PubMed PMID: 19892235
79. Fukuta H, Sane DC, Brucks S, Little WC. Statin therapy may be associated with lower mortality in patients with diastolic heart failure: A preliminary report. *Circulation*. 2005;112(3):357–363. Epub 2005/07/13. doi:10.1161/CIRCULATIONAHA.104.519876. PubMed PMID: 16009792
80. Alehagen U, Benson L, Edner M, Dahlstrom U, Lund LH. Association between use of statins and mortality in patients with heart failure and ejection fraction of >/=50. *Circ Heart Fail*. 2015;8(5):862–870. Epub 2015/08/06. doi:10.1161/CIRCHEARTFAILURE.115.002143. PubMed PMID: 26243795
81. Berwanger O, Le Manach Y, Suzumura EA, et al. Association between pre-operative statin use and major cardiovascular complications among patients undergoing non-cardiac surgery: The VISION study. *Eur Heart J*. 2016;37(2):177–185. Epub 2015/09/04. doi:10.1093/eurheartj/ehv456. PubMed PMID: 26330424; PubMed Central PMCID: PMC4703907
82. Stasch JP, Pacher P, Evgenov OV. Soluble guanylate cyclase as an emerging therapeutic target in cardiopulmonary disease. *Circulation*. 2011;123(20):2263–73. doi:10.1161/CIRCULATIONAHA.110.981738. PubMed PMID: 21606405; PubMed Central PMCID: PMC3103045
83. Armstrong PW, Pieske B, Anstrom KJ, et al. Vericiguat in patients with heart failure and reduced ejection fraction. *N Engl J Med*. 2020;382(20):1883–1893. Epub 20200328. doi:10.1056/NEJMoa1915928. PubMed PMID: 32222134
84. Kaplinsky E, Mallarkey G. Cardiac myosin activators for heart failure therapy: Focus on omecamtiv mecarbil. *Drugs Context*. 2018;7:212518. Epub 20180423. doi:10.7573/dic.212518. PubMed PMID: 29707029; PubMed Central PMCID: PMC5916097
85. Felker GM, Solomon SD, Claggett B, et al. Assessment of omecamtiv mecarbil for the treatment of patients with severe heart failure: A post hoc analysis of data from the GALACTIC-HF randomized clinical trial. *JAMA Cardiol*. 2022;7(1):26–34. doi:10.1001/jamacardio.2021.4027. PubMed PMID: 34643642; PubMed Central PMCID: PMC8515258
86. Yancy CW, Jessup M, Bozkurt B, et al. 2013 ACCF/AHA guideline for the management of heart failure: A report of the American College of Cardiology Foundation/American Heart Association Task Force on practice guidelines. *Circulation*. 2013;128(16):e240–e327. Epub 2013/06/07. doi:10.1161/CIR.0b013e31829e8776. PubMed PMID: 23741058
87. Kirklin JK, Naftel DC, Pagani FD, et al. Sixth INTERMACS annual report: A 10,000-patient database. *J Heart Lung Transplant*. 2014;33(6):555–564. Epub 2014/05/27. doi:10.1016/j.healun.2014.04.010. PubMed PMID: 24856259
88. Mehra MR, Uriel N, Naka Y, et al. A fully magnetically levitated left ventricular assist device: Final report. *N Engl J Med*. 2019;380(17):1618–1627. Epub 2019/03/19. doi:10.1056/NEJMoa1900486. PubMed PMID: 30883052
89. Rogers JG, Pagani FD, Tatooles AJ, et al. Intrapericardial left ventricular assist device for advanced heart failure. *N Engl J Med*. 2017;376(5):451–460. Epub 2017/02/02. doi:10.1056/NEJMoa1602954. PubMed PMID: 28146651
90. Molina EJ, Shah P, Kiernan MS, et al. The Society of Thoracic Surgeons Intermacs 2020 annual report. *Ann Thorac Surg*. 2021;111(3):778–792. Epub 2021/01/20. doi:10.1016/j.athoracsur.2020.12.038. PubMed PMID: 33465365
91. Lim HS, Howell N, Ranasinghe A. The physiology of continuous-flow left ventricular assist devices. *J Card Fail*. 2017;23(2):169–180. Epub 2016/12/19. doi:10.1016/j.cardfail.2016.10.015. PubMed PMID: 27989869
92. Feldman D, Pamboukian SV, Teuteberg JJ, birks e, lietz k, moore sa, et al. The 2013 International Society for Heart and Lung Transplantation Guidelines for mechanical circulatory support: Executive summary. *J Heart Lung Transplant*. 2013;32(2):157–187. Epub 2013/01/29. doi:10.1016/j.healun.2012.09.013. PubMed PMID: 23352391
93. Rossi M, Serraino GF, Jiritano F, Renzulli A. What is the optimal anticoagulation in patients with a left ventricular assist device? *Interact Cardiovasc Thorac Surg*. 2012;15(4):733–740. Epub 2012/07/05. doi:10.1093/icvts/ivs297. PubMed PMID: 22761118; PubMed Central PMCID: PMC3445379
94. Toeg H, Ruel M, Haddad H. Anticoagulation strategies for left ventricular assist devices. *Curr Opin Cardiol*. 2015;30(2):192–196. Epub 2015/01/13. doi:10.1097/HCO.0000000000000143. PubMed PMID: 25574893
95. Vigneswaran Y, Wang V, Krezalek M, et al. Laparoscopic procedures in patients with cardiac ventricular assist devices. *Surg Endosc*. 2019;33(7):2181–2186. Epub 2018/10/28. doi:10.1007/s00464-018-6497-1. PubMed PMID: 30367296
96. Barbara DW, Wetzel DR, Pulido JN, et al. The perioperative management of patients with left ventricular assist devices undergoing noncardiac surgery. *Mayo Clin Proc*. 2013;88(7):674–682. Epub 2013/07/03. doi:10.1016/j.mayocp.2013.03.019. PubMed PMID: 23809318
97. Degnan M, Brodt J, Rodriguez-Blanco Y. Perioperative management of patients with left ventricular assist devices undergoing noncardiac surgery. *Ann Card Anaesth*. 2016;19(4):676–686. Epub 2016/10/08. doi:10.4103/0971-9784.191545. PubMed PMID: 27716699; PubMed Central PMCID: PMC5070328
98. Stone M, Hinchey J, Sattler C, Evans A. Trends in the management of patients with left ventricular assist devices presenting for noncardiac surgery: A 10-year institutional experience. *Semin Cardiothorac Vasc Anesth*. 2016;20(3):197–204. Epub 2015/12/20. doi:10.1177/1089253215619759. PubMed PMID: 26685184
99. Goudra BG, Singh PM. Anesthesia for gastrointestinal endoscopy in patients with left ventricular assist devices: Initial experience with 68 procedures. *Ann Card Anaesth*. 2013;16(4):250–256. Epub 2013/10/11. doi:10.4103/0971-9784.119167. PubMed PMID: 24107691
100. Bennett MK, Roberts CA, Dordunoo D, Shah A, Russell SD. Ideal methodology to assess systemic blood pressure in patients with continuous-flow left ventricular assist devices. *J Heart Lung Transplant*. 2010;29(5):593–594. Epub 2010/01/12. doi:10.1016/j.healun.2009.11.604. PubMed PMID: 20060321

101. Slaughter MS, Pagani FD, Rogers JG, et al. Clinical management of continuous-flow left ventricular assist devices in advanced heart failure. *J Heart Lung Transplant*. 2010;29(4 Suppl):S1–39. Epub 2010/02/26. doi:10.1016/j.healun.2010.01.011. PubMed PMID: 20181499

102. Chung M. Perioperative management of the patient with a left ventricular assist device for noncardiac surgery. *Anesth Analg*. 2018;126(6):1839–1850. Epub 2017/12/05. doi:10.1213/ANE.0000000000002669. PubMed PMID: 29200070

103. Klovaite J, Gustafsson F, Mortensen SA, Sander K, Nielsen LB. Severely impaired von Willebrand factor-dependent platelet aggregation in patients with a continuous-flow left ventricular assist device (HeartMate II). *J Am Coll Cardiol*. 2009;53(23):2162–2167. Epub 2009/06/06. doi:10.1016/j.jacc.2009.02.048. PubMed PMID: 19497443

104. Peberdy MA, Gluck JA, Ornato JP, et al. Cardiopulmonary resuscitation in adults and children with mechanical circulatory support: A scientific statement from the American Heart Association. *Circulation*. 2017;135(24):e1115–e34. Epub 2017/05/24. doi:10.1161/CIR.0000000000000504. PubMed PMID: 28533303

105. Mabvuure NT, Rodrigues JN. External cardiac compression during cardiopulmonary resuscitation of patients with left ventricular assist devices. *Interact Cardiovasc Thorac Surg*. 2014;19(2):286–289. Epub 2014/05/16. doi:10.1093/icvts/ivu117. PubMed PMID: 24824496

106. Abraham WT, Adamson PB, Bourge RC, et al. Wireless pulmonary artery haemodynamic monitoring in chronic heart failure: A randomised controlled trial. *Lancet*. 2011;377(9766):658–666. Epub 2011/02/15. doi:10.1016/S0140-6736(11)60101-3. PubMed PMID: 21315441

107. Ponikowski P, Voors AA, Anker SD, et al. 2016 ESC Guidelines for the diagnosis and treatment of acute and chronic heart failure: The Task Force for the diagnosis and treatment of acute and chronic heart failure of the European Society of Cardiology (ESC)Developed with the special contribution of the Heart Failure Association (HFA) of the ESC. *Eur Heart J*. 2016;37(27):2129–2100. Epub 2016/05/22. doi:10.1093/eurheartj/ehw128. PubMed PMID: 27206819

108. Mehra MR, Canter CE, Hannan MM, et al. The 2016 International Society for Heart Lung Transplantation listing criteria for heart transplantation: A 10-year update. *J Heart Lung Transplant*. 2016;35(1):1–23. Epub 2016/01/19. doi:10.1016/j.healun.2015.10.023. PubMed PMID: 26776864

109. Ramakrishna H, Jaroszewski DE, Arabia FA. Adult cardiac transplantation: A review of perioperative management Part-I. *Ann Card Anaesth*. 2009;12(1):71–78. Epub 2009/01/13. doi:10.4103/0971-9784.45018. PubMed PMID: 19136760

110. Costanzo MR, Dipchand A, Starling R, et al. The International Society of Heart and Lung Transplantation Guidelines for the care of heart transplant recipients. *J Heart Lung Transplant*. 2010;29(8):914–956. Epub 2010/07/21. doi:10.1016/j.healun.2010.05.034. PubMed PMID: 20643330

111. Jurgens PT, Aquilante CL, Page RL, 2nd, Ambardekar AV. Perioperative management of cardiac transplant recipients undergoing noncardiac surgery: Unique challenges created by advancements in care. *Semin Cardiothorac Vasc Anesth*. 2017;21(3):235–244. Epub 2017/05/04. doi:10.1177/1089253217706164. PubMed PMID: 28466755

112. Pickham D, Hickey K, Doering L, Chen B, Castillo C, Drew BJ. Electrocardiographic abnormalities in the first year after heart transplantation. *J Electrocardiol*. 2014;47(2):135–139. Epub 2013/10/15. doi:10.1016/j.jelectrocard.2013.09.006. PubMed PMID: 24119878; PubMed Central PMCID: PMC3951586

113. Cooper M, Wiseman AC, Zibari G, et al. Wound events in kidney transplant patients receiving de novo everolimus: A pooled analysis of three randomized controlled trials. *Clin Transplant*. 2013;27(6):E625–E635. Epub 2013/09/17. doi:10.1111/ctr.12223. PubMed PMID: 24033455

114. Tjang YS, Tenderich G, Hornik L, Korfer R. Cardiac retransplantation in adults: An evidence-based systematic review. *Thorac Cardiovasc Surg*. 2008;56(6):323–327. Epub 2008/08/16. doi:10.1055/s-2008-1038662. PubMed PMID: 18704853

16.

ECHO SHOWS ELEVATED PULMONARY ARTERY PRESSURE

Debra D. Pulley and Anand Lakshminarasimhachar

STEM CASES AND KEY QUESTIONS

Our first patient is a 50-year-old man with end-stage renal disease (ESRD) on hemodialysis (HD). He now needs revision of his arteriovenous (AV) fistula scheduled in 3 days. During preoperative assessment, he states he is doing well on HD for a year. He states he is not very active but denies any changes in his functional status over the past year. Pulmonary hypertension (PH) is listed on his electronic medical record, and an echocardiogram (echo) from 1 year ago showed elevated systolic pulmonary artery pressure (PAP) of 70 mm Hg.

What type of PH does this patient have, and what needs to be done before surgery?

After a deeper review of his medical records, it is discovered that the echo was performed while the patient was in the hospital with acute volume overload. At that time, his blood pressure was elevated, with ranges above 200/100 mm Hg. He was started on HD and discharged. He states he remembers having a hard time breathing. He also reports that during the hospitalization he lost a lot of fluid in his body and denies any problems now. He has seen his primary care physician (PCP) and nephrologist within the past year with no further workup ordered. Today, his blood pressure is 140/80. You perform a focused history and physical examination to find symptoms/signs of PH, and there are none.

Do you recommend a repeat echo prior to the surgery?

Although the patient may have PH, there was a reason why his PAP was elevated at the time of the echo. He currently has no concerning symptoms/signs of PH, and, reassuringly, you found he had a chest x-ray 6 months ago that did not show any enlargement of the right ventricle (RV) or PA. You decide not to get a repeat echo prior to this surgery.

Our second patient is a 70-year-old woman with a past medical history of coronary artery disease (CAD) who had coronary artery bypass graft (CABG) surgery 3 years ago with ischemic cardiomyopathy (CM). She is anemic and has lost some weight. She is being seen in the preoperative clinic for an esophagogastroduodenoscopy (EGD)/colonoscopy to be scheduled at a freestanding endoscopy facility in 1 week. Her last echo was 1 year ago and showed dilated left ventricle (LV) with ejection fraction (EF) of 40%, systolic PAP of 55 mm Hg, and normal RV function.

What type of pulmonary hypertension does this patient have?

It is most likely this patient has PH and due to LV dysfunction (group 2), but a RHC has never been done to confirm. She recently saw her cardiologist and PCP who both told the patient she needs the EGD/colonoscopy procedure done to evaluate the cause of her anemia, and you agree. During the assessment, she states she is not active because she has no energy. She denies any orthopnea or postural nocturnal dyspnea (PND). On physical examination, there are no rales or peripheral edema. Since she has no signs or symptoms of heart failure and is on guideline-directed medical therapy (GDMT), you decide not to get another echo as it would not likely be different and it would not change her medical management at this time.

Is a free-standing endoscopy facility the appropriate place for her to have her EGD/colonoscopy?

Although not at high risk for developing complications, she is at elevated risk. You talk with her and the gastroenterologist about her risk and recommend that she would be better suited to have the procedure performed at a hospital-centered endoscopy facility where rescue measures can be mobilized rapidly, if needed.

Our third patient is a 59-year-old man with a BMI of 55 presenting for preoperative assessment of a very large hernia. The surgeon has been putting off repair, but the hernia is getting bigger. The surgeon wants your input in optimizing the patient for eventual repair. The patient used to see a pulmonologist, but he refuses to wear the prescribed BiPAP and the pulmonologist "fired him." The patient does see a PCP who has prescribed oxygen 2 L/min at night, which the patient is using.

What is this patient's risk for hernia repair?

Although you are concerned about the much greater risk of emergent surgery for incarcerated bowel than elective repair of the hernia, there are some concerning signs and symptoms. You discuss with the surgeon your concerns and that further workup is needed to have a better risk assessment and potential optimization.

Would you order a preop echo?

Knowing that inadequately treated obstructive sleep apnea (OSA) (and possible obesity hypoventilation syndrome) can lead to pulmonary hypertension and RV dysfunction, you order an echo.

What other tests and optimization would you recommend?

Since laboratory tests have not been done in more than a year, you order a CBC and comprehensive metabolic panel looking for secondary polycythemia, elevated total CO_2, decreased kidney function, and elevated liver enzymes. In addition, you obtain an ECG to identify any concerning signs. While you have the patient in the clinic, you have a conversation to better understand the barriers to compliance with the prescribed BiPAP. Further tests and optimization would depend on these initial tests.

The fourth patient is a 45-year-old woman diagnosed with idiopathic pulmonary arterial hypertension (PAH). She is on three pulmonary vasodilator agents including a subcutaneous pump of treprostinil. She is being seen in the preoperative clinic for a mastectomy to treat breast cancer. She has a PH specialist. Her echo 1 year ago showed systolic PAP 80 with dilated RV and moderate decrease in RV function.

What type of PH does this patient have, and what needs to be done before surgery?

Idiopathic PAH is in group 1. This patient is at high risk for decompensation perioperatively, so before proceeding to surgery you ensure thorough multidisciplinary planning. You repeat an echo to get an accurate picture of her status and if any optimization can be done to decrease her perioperative risk. In addition, you ensure that the surgery be done at a hospital experienced in taking care of patients with PAH.

What should the anesthesiologist be prepared for perioperatively?

As an anesthesiologist, you know that perioperative management should include attention to potential causes of acutely increasing pulmonary pressure and early recognition of PH crisis that can lead to RV failure and death. You use echocardiography to identify the underlying pathophysiology and guide treatment. You also know that, postoperatively, the risk of PH crisis still exists, and you recommend the patient be monitored closely for the next 48–72 hours.

The patient undergoes the surgery. All of her PAH drugs have been continued, including a continuous infusion of treprostinil. She is doing well, but there are no ICU beds available at this time. About an hour later, the PACU RN calls you to tell you that the patient's blood pressure is decreasing.

What do you do when a patient is decompensating in the PACU?

You immediately go to the PACU with your point-of-care ultrasound. Upon examination, you see that there is inadequate filling of both the LV and RV. You rule out any worsening of RV function and give her a small bolus of fluid; her blood pressure stabilizes. Knowing that treprostinil has some antiplatelet effects, you ask the RN the amount of wound drainage. She says there was a lot when the patient first arrived and she emptied the drains several times, but when the surgeon came by to assess, the drainage had really slowed down. The rest of the patient's postoperative course was uneventful.

DISCUSSION

DEFINITION OF PULMONARY HYPERTENSION

Based on recommendations from the 6th World Symposium on Pulmonary Hypertension (WSPH), the definition of PH is an mPAP of 20 mm Hg measured by right heart catheterization (RHC) in the supine position at rest.[1] This was lowered from the previous definition of an mPAP of 25 mm Hg or higher based on evidence showing the upper limit of normal is 20 mm Hg and that patients with pulmonary vascular disease (PVD) below the former threshold of PH are at increased risk of disease progression. Since other processes such as increased cardiac output, increased pulmonary arterial wedge pressure, left-to-right cardiac shunts, and hyperviscosity can elevate mPAP, the task force emphasized the importance of RHC. RHC can identify pre-capillary PH (which can be a sign of pulmonary vascular disease). They proposed pulmonary vascular resistance (PVR) greater than or equal to 3 Woods units (WU) be included in all precapillary PH (see Table 16.1).[2] Box 16.1 shows key concepts in determining pulmonary vascular resistance.[3,4]

Table 16.1 HEMODYNAMIC DEFINITION OF PULMONARY HYPERTENSION (PH)

Precapillary PH	mPAP >20 mm Hg, PAWP	Class 1, 3, 4, 5
Isolated postcapillary PH	mPAP >20 mm Hg	Class 2, 5
Combined post- and precapillary PH	mPAP >20 mm Hg	Class 2, 5
Exercise PH	mPAP/CO slope >3 mm Hg/L/min between rest and exercise	Class 1, 2, 3, 4, 5

Adapted from Humbert M, et al.[2]

> **Box 16.1 KEY CONCEPTS IN DETERMINING PULMONARY VASCULAR RESISTANCE**
>
> The calculation of mean pulmonary artery pressure is analogous to the hydraulic version of Ohm's Law
> I = V/R, where I = Current (flow), V = Voltage (pressure difference), R = Resistance
> CO = mPAP − PCWP/PVR
> mPAP − PCWP (or LAP) = CO × PVR
> Increase in CO or PVR will increase the mPAP
>
> mPAP − PCWP is called the *transpulmonary gradient* (TPG)
> Increased TPG causes increases in PVR.
> A TPG >12 mmHg is a risk factor for right heart failure and usually indicates pulmonary vasoconstriction and possible pulmonary hyperplasia causing increase RV afterload.
> A decrease in TPG and PVR with use of pulmonary vasodilators during RHC is an indicator of possible good response to pulmonary vasodilators intraoperatively.
>
> PAP in diastole − PCWP is called the *diastolic pulmonary gradient* (DPG)
> It is less dependent on preload and cardiac output.
>
> PVR = mPAP − PCWP / CO
> Normal PVR is less than 2 Woods unit or 50–150 dyne-sec-cm^{-5}
> 1 Woods units = 80 dyne-sec-cm^{-5}
> Increased PVR is >3 Woods units or 240 dyne-sec-cm^{-5}
>
> Resistance = Pressure/ Flow
> Pressure = Force/Area = dyne/cm^2
> Flow = Volume/Second = cm^3/Sec
> Hence, Resistance = dyne-sec-cm^{-5}
>
> CO, cardiac output; mPAP, mean pulmonary artery pressure; PCWP, pulmonary capillary wedge pressure; LAP, left atrial pressure; PVR, pulmonary vascular resistance; RHC, right heart catheterization.
> Adapted from Newman JH and Naeije R, et al.[3,4]

CLASSIFICATION OF PULMONARY HYPERTENSION

PH is classified into five different groups based on similar clinical and pathophysiologic mechanisms (see Figure 16.1).[2] It is important to note that, even within each group, there is a heterogeneity of associated diseases. Further complicating classification, a patient's PH may have contributions from several groups.[3,5]

Group 1 is PAH. It includes drug-induced PAH, PAH associated with HIV, PAH associated with portal hypertension, PAH associated with congenital hypertension, and PAH associated with schistosomiasis. Group 2 is PH associated with left-sided heart disease and is the most common form of PH. Left-sided heart disease can include isolated postcapillary hypertension (old term "passive") and combined pre- and postcapillary hypertension (old term "reactive" or "out of proportion").[6] Group 3 is PH associated with lung diseases or hypoxia and is the second most common class of PH. Group 4 is PH associated with chronic PA obstruction. The obstruction can be from thromboemboli or from tumors (such as renal cell cancer). Group 5 is PH associated with unclear or multifactorial mechanisms. This group includes diseases such as sarcoidosis, chronic myeloproliferative disorders, and chronic kidney disease.

SYMPTOMS AND SIGNS OF PULMONARY HYPERTENSION

Symptoms of PH vary depending on the underlying disease and progression of the disease and can include dyspnea on exertion, chest pain, and wheezing. The World Health Organization functional class is used to assess PAH, ranging from class I to class IV according to the amount of physical activity the patient can do.[7] On the physical exam, it is important to look for signs of RV failure. Signs of PH can be seen on the ECG, such as p pulmonale, right axis deviation, RV hypertrophy (RVH), right bundle branch block (RBBB), and RV strain. Similarly, enlargement of the RV and pulmonary artery on radiographic images are signs of PH. Echocardiogram abnormalities include enlarged RA and RV, a basal RV/LV ratio of greater than 1, decreased RV function, and increased estimation of systolic PAP (TR pressure gradient and estimated RAP).[2]

TREATMENT OF PULMONARY HYPERTENSION

The treatment of PH varies depending on the pathophysiology (see Figure 16.1).[2] Patients with PAH group 1 may be treated with calcium channel blockers (if reactive during RHC) and PAH drugs. PAH drugs affect pulmonary vascular disease by various pathways including nitric oxide pathway mediators (e.g., tadalafil, sildenafil, riociguat), endothelin receptor antagonists (e.g., bosentan, ambrisentan), and prostacyclin pathway antagonists (e.g., treprostinil, iloprost).[5] In addition, these drugs may have antiplatelet properties.[8] Patients with PH associated with left heart disease (group 2), lung disease/hypoxia (group 3), unclear/multifactorial (group 5) have treatments focused on the underlying disease. Patients with PH associated with PA obstructions are treated with interventions to remove the obstruction, but also may include medical therapy.

PERIOPERATIVE CARE GUIDELINES

PH is a risk factor for perioperative morbidity/mortality especially in patients with PAH and chronic thromboembolic pulmonary hypertension (CTEPH).[9] Several organizations have recently published recommendations on perioperative management. These include an expert consensus statement published in the *British Journal of Anaesthesia* in 2021,[9] the 2022 ISHLT Consensus statement on management of patients with PH and right heart failure undergoing surgery,[10] and the 2023 AHA Scientific Statement on evaluation and management of PH in noncardiac surgery.[5] Patients at high risk for decompensation perioperatively need to have thorough multidisciplinary

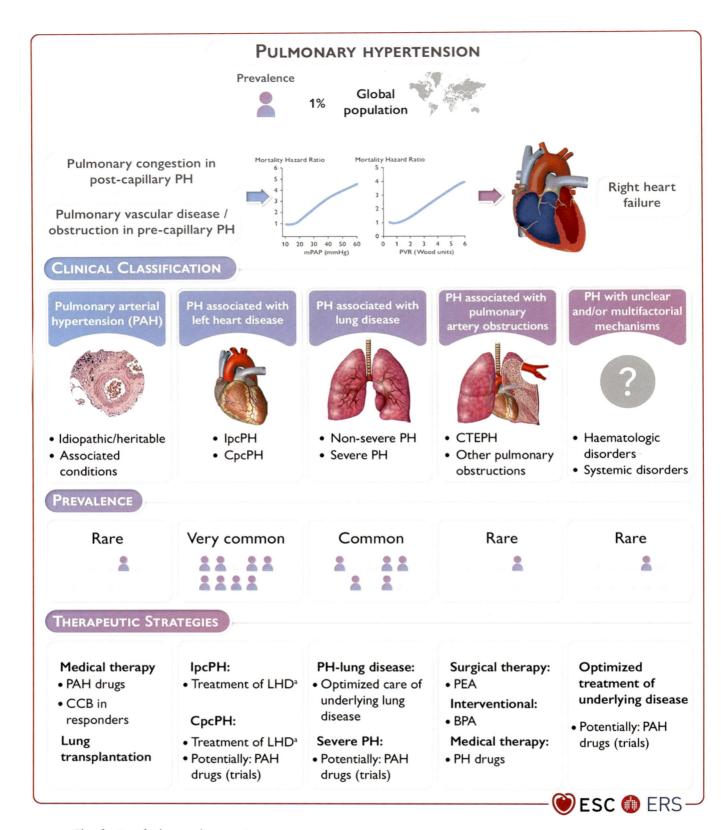

Figure 16.1 Classification of pulmonary hypertension.
Reproduced with permission of the © European Society of Cardiology & European Respiratory Society 2023: European Respiratory Journal 61 (1) 2200879; doi:10.1183/13993003.00879-2022. Published 6 January 2023.

Table 16.2 **RISK OF MORTALITY IN PATIENTS WITH PULMONARY ARTERIAL HYPERTENSION (PAH)**

	LOW RISK	INTERMEDIATE RISK	HIGH RISK
Clinical symptoms/signs of RHF	None	None	Present
Arrhythmia	None	Occasional	Recurrent
WHO functional class	I/II	III	IV
ECHO	Preserved RV function RA area <18 cm^2 No pericardial fluid	Impaired RV function RA area 18–26 cm^2 None or minimal pericardial fluid	Impaired RV function RA area >26 cm^2 Pericardial fluid present
MRI	High RVEF (>54%)	Reduced RVEF (37–54%)	Markedly reduced RVEF (<37%)
RHC	RAP <8 mm Hg	RAP 8–14 mm Hg	RAP >14 mm Hg
	CI >2.5 L/min/m^2	CI 2.0–2.4 L/min/m^2	CI <2.0 L/min/m^2
	SvO$_2$ >65%	SvO$_2$ 60–65%	SvO$_2$ <60%
6MWD	>440 m	165–440 m	<165 m
NT-proBNP	<300 ng/L	300–1,400 ng/L	>1,400 ng/L

PAH, pulmonary artery hypertension; RHF, right heart failure; WHO, World Health Organization; ECHO, echocardiogram; RV, right ventricle; RA right atrium; MRI, magnetic resonance imaging; RVEF, right ventricular ejection fraction; RHC, right heart catheterization; RAP, right atrial pressure; CI, cardiac index; SvO$_2$, mixed venous saturation; 6MWD, 6-minute walk distance; NT-proBNP, N-terminal pro-B-type natriuretic peptide.

Adapted from Price LC, et al.[9]

planning and surgery performed at a facility with expertise in managing these patients. Unfortunately, these consensus statements emphasize that more research with robust data is needed to refine risk factors specific to each PH group in order to develop an individualized approach based the type of PH, its progression, and the complexity of the surgical procedure.

PERIOPERATIVE RISK ASSESSMENT

Highest perioperative risk has been associated with patients with group 1 PAH and CTEPH (group 4) patients.[9] Table 16.2 identifies variables that predict mortality in patients with PAH; however, these variables have not been validated for perioperative risk.[9] Table 16.3 lists helpful tools to assess risk for each PH group, but there are limitations with all tools.[5,9,10] Risk will also vary with the type of surgery. High-risk surgeries include emergent major surgery, cardiovascular surgery, liver transplantation, and any operation with anticipated large fluid shifts and/or blood loss.[10]

MANAGEMENT OF PULMONARY HYPERTENSIVE CRISIS AND ACUTE RIGHT VENTRICULAR FAILURE

Essential to management of patients with PH is knowledge of situations that can lead to worsening of RV preload and afterload leading to pulmonary hypertensive crisis (PHC) and acute RV failure (RVF) and the spiral that can lead to death (see Figure 16.2).[5] Management of this event needs to be immediate and can be intensive. The primary goal is to reduce PAP and improve RV function to maintain adequate systemic perfusion. Some key management strategies are

Table 16.3 **TOOLS TO ASSESS PERIOPERATIVE RISK IN PULMONARY HYPERTENSION**

PAH (GROUP 1)	REVEAL 2.0 ESC RISK GUIDELINES
PH associated with LHD (Group 2)	2014 ACC/AHA on cardiac evaluation for noncardiac surgery
PH associated with lung disease and/or hypoxia (Group 3)	ARISCAT
CTEPH (Group 4)	REVEAL 2.0
PH with unclear/multifactorial (Group 5)	None

PAH, pulmonary artery hypertension; ESC, European Society of Cardiology; PH, pulmonary hypertension; LHD, left heart disease; ACC, American College of Cardiology; AHA, American Heart Association; CTEPH; chronic thromboembolic pulmonary hypertension.

Adapted from Rajagopal S, et al.; Price LC, et al.; McGlothlin DP, et al.[5,9,10]

1. *Oxygen therapy*: Administer supplemental oxygen to improve oxygenation and alleviate hypoxemia. Maintaining adequate oxygen levels helps reduce pulmonary vasoconstriction and decreases the workload on the RV. Avoid hypercarbia, acidosis, and increased airway pressure, which may worsen PH.

2. *Hemodynamic support*: Use invasive monitoring techniques such as arterial lines, central venous catheters, and pulmonary artery catheters (in high-risk cases) to closely monitor hemodynamic parameters. This allows for real-time assessment of cardiac function and fluid status. Transesophageal and transthoracic echocardiography are

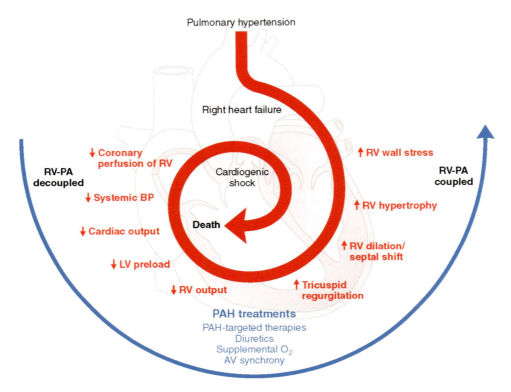

Figure 16.2 Worsening of right-sided heart failure in pulmonary hypertension.
Reprinted with permission from Circulation. 2023;147:1317–1343. ©2023 American Heart Association, Inc.

also very useful tools to assess and manage volume status and right heart failure.

3. *Fluid management*: Optimize fluid status carefully. PHC can be exacerbated by fluid overload, which increases RV afterload. Diuretics may be necessary to achieve euvolemia and reduce RV preload.

4. *Vasodilator therapy*: Administer pulmonary vasodilators to reduce PAP and decrease RV afterload. Inhaled nitric oxide (iNO) is the preferred vasodilator, but other options such as inhaled or IV prostacyclin analogs (e.g., epoprostenol) or phosphodiesterase inhibitors (e.g., sildenafil) can be considered. These medications should be administered under expert supervision.

5. *Inotropic support*: Consider the use of inotropic agents, such as dobutamine or milrinone, to enhance contractility and improve RV function. These agents can help maintain systemic perfusion while reducing RV filling pressures. Epinephrine infusion may be needed to support RV function in case of significant RV dysfunction. Norepinephrine and/or vasopressin may be needed for vasopressor support, with vasopressin having less vasoconstrictor effects on the pulmonary circulation.

6. *Mechanical circulatory support*: In severe cases of RVF when pharmacological interventions are ineffective, mechanical circulatory support devices like extracorporeal membrane oxygenation (ECMO) or RV assist devices (RVADs) may be necessary to provide temporary or long-term support. A specialized team should manage these interventions.

7. *Treatment of underlying cause*: Identify and address the underlying cause of the pulmonary hypertensive crisis. This may involve treating infections, resolving thromboembolic events, or managing acute exacerbations of preexisting PH.

8. *Expert consultation*: Involvement of a multidisciplinary team, including cardiologists, cardiac anesthesiologists, critical care specialists, and pulmonary hypertension experts, is crucial for the optimal management of RVF during a pulmonary hypertensive crisis. Their expertise can guide treatment decisions and provide appropriate support.

It is important to note that the management of RVF during a pulmonary hypertensive crisis should be tailored to the individual patient's condition. The strategies mentioned above provide a general framework, but each case may require specific adjustments based on the clinical scenario. As mentioned earlier, use of the echocardiogram can be invaluable in helping identify the pathophysiology and guide treatment.[2,5,9,10] Last, it is recommended that patients should be closely monitored postoperatively for 48–72 hours due to risk of decompensation.[9]

CONCLUSION

- PH is caused by a diverse group of disease processes.
- Identifying the type of PH is essential for appropriate treatment.
- PH is a risk factor for perioperative mortality especially in patients with PAH and CTEPH.
- Perioperative strategies to reduce the risk of acute RV failure include attention to causes of acute PH and use of echocardiography to guide treatment.
- Be alert for future updates in perioperative risk stratification in patients with PH; meanwhile, use a pragmatic approach.

REVIEW QUESTIONS

1. Which group of PH is drug-induced PAH?

    a. Group 1.
    b. Group 2.
    c. Group 3.
    d. Group 4.

    The correct answer is a.
    Drug-induced PAH is group 1.[1]

2. Which group of PH is PH is associated with infection with schistosomiasis?

    a. Group 1.
    b. Group 3.
    c. Group 4.
    d. Group 5.

    The correct answer is a.
    PH associated with infection with schistosomiasis is group 1 PAH.[1]

3. What group of PH has the highest prevalence?

    a. Group 1.
    b. Group 2.
    c. Group 3.
    d. Group 5.

    The correct answer is b.
    PH associated with left heart disease (group 2) is the most common.[2]

4. What group of PH has the second highest prevalence?

    a. Group 1.
    b. Group 3.
    c. Group 4.
    d. Group 5.

    The correct answer is b.
    PH associated with lung disease or hypoxia (group 3).[2]

5. Which of the following has not been found to cause development of PAH?

    a. Fenfluramine.
    b. Phentermine.
    c. Methamphetamines.
    d. Dasatinib.

    The correct answer is b.
    The combination of fenfluramine and phentermine produced in the 1990s caused some patients to develop PAH. Fenfluramine was the primary cause, not phentermine.[1]

6. Which of the following statements is not true about the WSPH hemodynamic classification of PH?

    a. Precapillary PH: mPAP of greater than 20 mg Hg, PAWP 15 mm Hg or less, PVR greater than 2 WU.
    b. Isolated postcapillary PH: mPAP of greater than 20 mm Hg, PAWP greater than 15 mm Hg, PVR less 2 WU or less.
    c. Combined pre- and postcapillary PH: mPAP of greater than 20 mm Hg, PAWP greater than 15 mm Hg, PVR greater than 2 mm Hg.
    d. Did not include a definition for exercise PH.

    The correct answer is d.
    A definition for exercise PH was included.[5]

7. Symptoms and signs suggestive of PH include all *except*

    a. Dyspnea on exertion.
    b. PA enlargement of chest x-ray.
    c. Enlarged RA.
    d. Basal RV/LV ratio of less than 1 on echo.

    The correct answer is d.
    A basal RV/LV ratio 1 or greater is suggestive of PH.[2]

8. Which of the following pulmonary vasodilator/pathway affected is not correct?

    a. Sildenafil/nitric oxide pathway.
    b. Bosentan/endothelin receptor antagonist.
    c. Riociguat/endothelin receptor antagonist.
    d. Treprostinil/prostacyclin pathway.

    The correct answer is c.
    Riociguat affects the nitric oxide pathway.[5]

9. Potentially deleterious effects of CO_2 insufflation during laparoscopic surgery on patients with PH leading to RV failure include all but the following:

    a. Vagal reaction.
    b. Systemic hypercarbia.
    c. Large fluid shifts leading to RV dilation.
    d. Increase in inspiratory airway pressure altering RV preload and afterload.

    The correct answer is c.

Large fluid shifts can lead to RV dilation, but laparoscopic surgeries typically have less fluid shifts or blood loss than open surgeries.[10]

10. Which is not correct about the progression of worsening right-sided heart failure in patients with PH that can lead to a vicious spiral and death?

   a. Increased RV wall stress → RV hypertrophy → RV dilation/septal shift → increased tricuspid regurgitation (TR).
   b. Increased TR → RV dilation/septal shift → RV hypertrophy → increased RV wall stress.
   c. Increased TR → decreased RV output → decreased LV preload → decreased cardiac output.
   d. Decreased systemic BP → decreased coronary perfusion of RV → cardiogenic shock → death.

The correct answer is b.

PH leads to increased RV wall stress → RV hypertrophy → RV dilation/septal shift → increased TR → decreased RV output → decreased LV preload → decreased cardiac output → decreased systemic BP → decreased coronary perfusion of RV → cardiogenic shock → death.[5]

REFERENCES

1. Simonneau G, Montani D, Celermajer DS, et al. Haemodynamic definitions and updated clinical classification of pulmonary hypertension. *Eur Respir J.* 2019 Jan;53:1801913. doi:10.1183/13993003.01913-2018
2. Humbert M, Kovacs G, Hoeper MM, et al. 2022 ESC/ERS Guidelines for the diagnosis and treatment of pulmonary hypertension. *Eur Respir J.* 2023 Jan;61(1):2200879. doi:10.1183/13993003.00879-2022
3. Newman JH. Pulmonary hypertension by the method of Paul Wood. *Chest.* 2020 Sep;158(3):1164–1171. doi:10.1016/j.chest.2020.02.035
4. Naeije R, Vachiery JL, Yerly P, Vanderpool R. The transpulmonary pressure gradient for the diagnosis of pulmonary vascular disease. *Eur Respir J.* 2013 Jan;41(1):217–223. doi:10.1183/09031936.00074312
5. Rajagopal S, Ruetzler K, Ghadimi K, et al. Evaluation and management of pulmonary hypertension in noncardiac surgery: A scientific statement from the American Heart Association. *Circulation.* 2023 Apr 25;147(17):1317–1343. doi:10.1161/CIR.0000000000001136
6. Vachiéry JL, Adir Y, Barberà JA, et al. Pulmonary hypertension due to left heart diseases. *J Am Coll Cardiol.* 2013 Dec 24;62(25 Suppl):D100–D108. doi:10.1016/j.jacc.2013.10.033
7. Highland KB, Crawford R, Classi P, et al. Development of the Pulmonary Hypertension Functional Classification Self-Report: A patient version adapted from the World Health Organization Functional Classification measure. *Health Qual Life Outcomes.* 2021 Aug 24;19(1):202. doi:10.1186/s12955-021-01782-0
8. Rogula SP, Mutwil HM, Gąsecka A, Kurzyna M, Filipiak KJ. Antiplatelet effects of prostacyclin analogues: Which one to choose in case of thrombosis or bleeding? *Cardiol J.* 2021;28(6):954–961. doi:10.5603/CJ.a2020.0164
9. Price LC, Martinez G, Brame A, et al. Perioperative management of patients with pulmonary hypertension undergoing non-cardiothoracic, non-obstetric surgery: A systematic review and expert consensus statement. *Br J Anaesth.* 2021 Apr;126(4):774–790. doi:10.1016/j.bja.2021.01.005
10. McGlothlin DP, Granton J, Klepetko W, et al. ISHLT consensus statement: Perioperative management of patients with pulmonary hypertension and right heart failure undergoing surgery. *J Heart Lung Transplant.* 2022 Sep;41(9):1135–1194. doi:10.1016/j.healun.2022.06.013

17.

SHOULDER REPLACEMENT IN PATIENT WHO HAD A HEART AND LUNG TRANSPLANT

Caroline R. Gross and Zdravka Zafirova

STEM CASE AND KEY QUESTIONS

A 48-year-old woman presented to the orthopedic surgeon with complaints of progressive deep and pulsating pain radiating from the right shoulder to the elbow, significantly restricted active movement, and preserved passive movement. The symptoms have become debilitating and have limited her daily activities. Her past medical history was significant for idiopathic pulmonary hypertension and cardiomyopathy, leading to heart and single left lung transplantation 3 years prior. She denied allergies to medications. She was diagnosed with osteonecrosis of the humeral head and was scheduled for a shoulder arthroplasty.

What preoperative evaluation should be performed? What history and clinical status information needs to be elicited?

The preoperative evaluation should document vital signs, including baseline heart rate, blood pressure, and oxygen saturation; orthostatic vital signs may be indicated based on symptoms. Along with a comprehensive multisystem history and physical examination, a detailed cardiopulmonary physical examination should be performed. Evidence of cardiopulmonary dysfunction should be elicited, including chest pain, ischemia, dyspnea, orthopnea, exercise intolerance, and arrhythmia.[1–3] Signs and symptoms of respiratory insufficiency can present diagnostic challenges as they may result from cardiac or pulmonary dysfunction, including graft dysfunction and airway complications following lung transplantation.[3,4]

The clinician should investigate any history of infection and current symptoms of infection, being aware that typical inflammatory symptoms, including fever and leukocytosis, may be attenuated by immunosuppression therapy.[5] A review of preexisting microbiological studies may reveal resistant pathogens and guide antibiotic prophylaxis. Symptoms and results of surveillance studies such as biopsy, MRI, and molecular studies guide the diagnosis and treatment of graft rejection and should be reviewed at the preoperative visit. The presence of active infection or rejection is likely to warrant postponement of surgery to allow for treatment of these conditions, except in the case of emergencies.

The patient underwent myocardial biopsy 4 months ago, without reported evidence of rejection. She denied chest pain, dyspnea, or cough. Her physical examination demonstrated height 164 cm, weight 56 kg, blood pressure 131/78, heart rate 102, pulse oximetry on room air 95%; normal S1 and S2, no jugular venous distention (JVD), no peripheral edema or cyanosis, no heart murmurs, and clear lungs with slightly reduced bibasilar breath sounds.

What testing should be done, and what is the optimal timing of the preoperative visit?

The preoperative assessment should allow time for gathering of multidisciplinary medical information, performance of any indicated testing, and adjustment of medication regimens. The timing of elective and semi-elective surgery can be affected by the discovery of infection or rejection. A preoperative CBC is indicated preoperatively, as anemia and cytopenia are common in the transplant population and can be addressed prior to surgery. Leukocytosis may point to possible infection. Blood type, screen, and cross-match prior to surgeries with potential for blood loss and transfusion are critical and should be done in advance to assure the availability of cross-matched blood. Renal and hepatic function assessment with blood urea nitrogen (BUN), creatinine (Cr), electrolytes, and liver function tests should be obtained. The increased incidence of arrhythmia and conduction abnormalities warrants baseline ECG in these patients, which can also demonstrate signs of ischemia or heart failure.[1] The presence of a pacemaker necessitates a recent interrogation of its programming and potential adjustment in the immediate preoperative period. The chest x-ray may display signs of infection, rejection, and other complications, including decompensation of cardiovascular disease.[6] Computed tomography (CT) aids in further evaluation of cardiopulmonary abnormalities.[6] Pulmonary function tests should be considered in patients with underlying abnormalities and in the setting of new or worsening respiratory symptoms.

Her preoperative laboratory testing revealed white blood cell (WBC) 9 K/μL, hemoglobin (Hgb) 9.8 g/dL, platelets 178 K/μL, Cr 1.2 mg/dL, and normal electrolytes, transaminases, and bilirubin. The patient's ECG demonstrated first-degree atrioventricular (AV) block, occasional VPCs, and normal ST segments. Chest x-ray revealed a prominent right hilar region.

Is infection screening recommended? What infectious precautions should be considered in these patients?

Signs and symptoms suggestive of infection should be investigated. The immunosuppressed state of organ transplant recipients predisposes them to increased incidence and severity of opportunistic infections, while the inflammatory response and thus the clinical presentation may be attenuated. In addition to continuation of chronic antimicrobial prophylaxis, these patients may necessitate broader prophylaxis in the perioperative period as well as a low threshold for initiation of targeted antimicrobial therapy even with subtle signs of infection. SARS-CoV-2 screening before surgery is guided by the current standards and regional infection prevalence.[7-9] These patients warrant enhanced exposure precautions in regard to SARS-CoV-2, including mask utilization and respiratory precautions by all staff.[7-9]

Is an echocardiogram necessary? Is a stress test or coronary perfusion study indicated? Why?

The presence of symptoms should guide the decision to perform further testing. While echocardiography and advanced studies are not indicated for asymptomatic patients without major risk factors for cardiac disease in the general population, patients with heart and lung transplant warrant specific considerations.[10,11] Frequently, the etiology of symptoms such as dyspnea or exercise intolerance may be difficult to ascertain on clinical basis alone and cardiopulmonary testing is needed to guide diagnosis and therapy. Furthermore, cardiac allograft vasculopathy can be challenging to identify due to reduced symptomatology and underestimation of its severity on imaging.[12,13] Therefore, consideration should be given to cardiac testing even in asymptomatic patients. The assessment of biventricular function and possible valvular abnormalities with echocardiography is recommended.[10,11]

On further questioning, she stated that she had mild chronic exertional dyspnea, unchanged for some time; her metabolic equivalents (METs) score was estimated to be 4. The decision was made to perform a transthoracic echocardiogram (TTE), which demonstrated mildly reduced biventricular function with an ejection fraction (EF) of 47%, mild pulmonary hypertension, and mild mitral and tricuspid insufficiency. A myocardial single-photon emission CT (SPECT) was performed by her cardiologist after the preoperative clinic visit and revealed no significant abnormalities.

How should her medications be managed in the perioperative period?

Immunosuppression and antimicrobial prophylaxis should be continued in the perioperative period. Current therapeutic drug levels should be documented for medications requiring monitoring. Adjustments of doses should be made based on monitoring results and changes in clinical status.[5]

The patient's medication regimen included prednisone, mycophenolate, tacrolimus, valacyclovir, and hydrocodone/acetaminophen. The tacrolimus level had been checked by her cardiologist and was in the therapeutic range. She received instructions to continue her medications up to the time of surgery. For her anemia, she was prescribed iron supplementation.

On the day of surgery, she arrived in the preoperative area after fasting for 8 hours. She had taken all her medications with sips of water 3 hours prior.

What are the anesthetic options for shoulder replacement? What are the advantages of each?

Total shoulder replacement can be performed using general anesthesia (GA), regional anesthesia, or combination of both modalities. Advantages of GA include patient comfort and cooperation. Shoulder surgery frequently is performed in the beach chair position, which can be uncomfortable for extended periods of time.[14]

Interscalene block (ISB) is the regional anesthetic of choice for total shoulder replacement. The benefits of ISB include intra- and postoperative pain control, decreased opioid utilization, and isolated upper extremity muscle relaxation to facilitate surgery. The combination of GA and ISB can be used for the benefits of both.

What are the risks of an ISB? Are there specific concerns in a patient with a history of heart-lung transplantation?

There is a nearly 100 % rate of ipsilateral phrenic nerve paralysis after an ISB. In a patient with residual pulmonary disease following heart-lung transplantation, this can precipitate shortness of breath or respiratory insufficiency. Although the risk of pneumothorax is lower with an ISB than with other types of brachial plexus blocks (such as a supraclavicular block), this complication may be tolerated poorly in a patient with underlying pulmonary disease.[14]

The surgery will be performed on the right shoulder, and the patient has previously had a left single lung transplant. How does this affect your decision to perform regional anesthesia?

This laterality improves the safety profile of an ISB. This patient's two lungs have distinctly different anatomy and physiology. The transplanted left lung is relatively normal in terms of its compliance and ability to perform gas exchange. The native right lung, however, is diseased with impaired function. The risks of an ISB (specifically, phrenic nerve paralysis) are lessened if performed on the side of the diseased lung as it contributes less to overall respiratory function.[14]

The patient was brought into the operating room and was positioned supine on the operating room table.

What monitors are required for this case?

Standard American Society of Anesthesiologists (ASA) monitors are required. These include continuous monitoring of oxygenation (by pulse oximetry), end-tidal carbon dioxide (by side-stream capnography), blood pressure, ECG, and temperature. An arterial catheter should be placed in this patient for serial arterial blood gas (ABG) monitoring given her residual lung disease. Since she has relatively normal cardiac function and no recent changes in functional status, central venous catheter and pulmonary artery catheters are not required.[15-18]

After the placement of monitors, an uncomplicated ISB is performed under ultrasound guidance using 25 mL of bupivacaine 0.5%. In the operating room, the block effect is tested and appears adequate. Immediately after incision, however, the patient complains of sharp shoulder pain. The decision was made to convert to GA.

How should anesthesia be induced?

Induction of anesthesia requires careful titration of medications to avoid hypotension. The transplanted heart lacks sympathetic innervation and thus, will not compensate for hypotension with reflex tachycardia. Therefore, it is important to maintain adequate preload and systemic vascular resistance. If time permits, a crystalloid bolus should be considered prior to induction of anesthesia. Appropriate medications include etomidate 0.2–0.4 mg/kg or propofol 1–2 mg/kg along with bolus doses of phenylephrine to maintain a mean arterial pressure within 20% of the patient's baseline.

The rate of gastroesophageal reflux disease (GERD) is high in lung transplant recipients. In the absence of other risk factors for aspiration, such as a full stomach or traumatic injury, however, a rapid-sequence induction is not required.[19,20]

The induction and intubation are uneventful. What ventilator settings should be used?

The goals are to optimize oxygenation and ventilation while minimizing peak airway pressures. The initial ventilator settings are assist-control volume control with tidal volumes 6–8 cc/kg and FiO_2 0.6–0.8. After a baseline ABG, respiratory rate can be adjusted based on $PaCO_2$ and FiO_2 can be titrated based on PaO_2.

A baseline ABG showed pH 7.38, $PaCO_2$ 56, PaO_2 130, and bicarbonate 29.6 on FiO_2 0.80.

How do you interpret these results?

This patient has compensated respiratory acidosis and reduced oxygenation. The elevated bicarbonate in a patient with elevated $PaCO_2$ and normal pH suggests a chronic process.

After the patient was positioned in the beach chair position, the blood pressure decreased from 120/75 to 80/55.

How should hypotension be managed?

A crystalloid bolus is reasonable in the setting of hypotension associated with induction of anesthesia or change in patient positioning, as the transplanted heart is denervated and preload dependent. Direct-acting adrenergic agents such as phenylephrine and epinephrine can be administered. Vasopressin is also an option as its action is independent of the adrenergic system, and it has negligible impact on the heart rate.

As the incision is closed, the blood loss for the case is estimated to be 300 mL.

Should the patient receive a blood transfusion?

Without hemodynamic changes or evidence of end-organ hypoperfusion, a blood transfusion is not indicated. The equation for maximum allowable blood loss is:

$$\text{Maximum allowable blood loss} = \text{Estimated blood volume} \frac{(\text{Starting Hct} - \text{Target Hct})}{\text{Starting Hct}}$$

(Estimated blood volume in milliliters.)

A target hemoglobin greater than 8.0 g/dL is reasonable for this patient. To achieve this, the maximum allowable blood loss is approximately 680 mL (greater than the estimated blood loss).[21–25]

Upon the completion of surgery, an ABG showed pH 7.39, $PaCO_2$ 51, PaO_2 145, and bicarbonate 28 while the patient was breathing spontaneously on FiO_2 0.70.

Should this patient be extubated? Would you reverse the muscle relaxation? With which agent?

Yes, this patient is a candidate for extubation. Hypercapnia is present, but her $PaCO_2$ is only slightly elevated from baseline, and most importantly, her pH is normal. Her oxygenation on FiO_2 0.70 is lower than expected; therefore, a recruitment maneuver should be performed. She should be extubated to supplemental oxygen.

Cholinesterase inhibitors are used for muscle relaxation reversal. While not expected to cause bradycardia in transplant patients, reports of bradyarrhythmia have been published.[26] Anticholinergic drugs will not increase heart rate due to denervation of the transplanted heart. Sugammadex may be a safe alternative for reversal.[27–29]

In the PACU, the patient complains of significant right shoulder pain.

Is it appropriate to reattempt an ISB?

No, it is unsafe to repeat an ISB. The maximum safe dose of bupivacaine for brachial plexus blocks is 2.5 mg/kg, which is 140 mg in this patient. She received 25 mL of bupivacaine 0.5% during the initial block, which is equal to 125 mg. To administer additional bupivacaine at this point would put the patient at risk for local anesthetic toxicity. Pain must be managed with a combination of opioids and adjuvant medications.

One hour following the surgery, the patient develops respiratory distress in the PACU. Her respiratory rate is 30 breaths per minute, she is using accessory muscles during inspiration, and her SpO_2 is 86% on 5 L supplemental oxygen via nasal cannula.

What is the next step?

The patient needs additional oxygen and her nasal cannula should be exchanged for bilevel positive airway pressure (BiPAP) or high-flow nasal cannula. Given her increased work of breathing, evidenced by accessory muscle use and tachypnea, she likely will benefit from BiPAP, which will improve ventilation in addition to oxygenation. While respiratory support is increased, it is important to consider the cause of the patient's deterioration. The differential diagnosis is broad and includes common postoperative problems, such as pain, atelectasis, or bronchospasm, as well as more serious complications, such as pulmonary embolism, aspiration, or pneumothorax. An ABG and chest x-ray are indicated.

The patient's symptoms improve and SpO_2 increases to 96% on BiPAP with inspiratory pressure 10 cm H_2O, end-expiratory pressure 5 cm H_2O, and FiO_2 0.70. Chest x-ray shows bibasilar atelectasis.

Does this patient require ICU admission?

Yes, this patient should be transferred to the ICU. Given her medical comorbidities and requirement for noninvasive positive-pressure ventilation, she should be monitored closely with serial exams and ABGs to ensure her respiratory status continues to improve.

DISCUSSION

The number of heart, lung, and combined heart-lung transplantations performed in the United States is increasing and post-transplantation survival is improving.[30-32] According to the Organ Procurement and Transplantation Network, 89,342 heart, 50,034 lung, and 1,486 heart-lung transplants were performed in the United States between 1988 and 2023. In 2022 alone, 4,111 heart, 2,692 lung, and 51 heart-lung transplants were performed.[30] Current 1- and 5-year survival after heart, lung, and combined heart-lung transplantation is 90–91% and 77–78%, 86–89% and 52–58%, and 76–83% and 35–62%, respectively.[30-32] A considerable number of these patients will present for noncardiothoracic surgeries.

The unique anatomy and physiology of patients following transplantation must be considered by the anesthesiologist.[1,2] The transplanted heart lacks sensory, sympathetic, and parasympathetic innervation; although after a period of time some reinnervation may occur, it is generally incomplete and unreliable. The heart retains alpha- and beta-adrenergic receptors, thus it remains responsive to circulating catecholamines as well as the normal Frank-Starling mechanism. Despite resting tachycardia (typically 90–110 beats per minute), the ability to increase heart rate in response to increased cardiac output (CO) demand is impaired. While intrinsic impulse formation and conductivity are preserved, various rhythm alterations may be noted including atrial flutter and fibrillation, brady-arrhythmias, and conduction abnormalities. A permanent pacemaker, or rarely, an implantable cardioverter-defibrillator (ICD) may be required following cardiac transplantation. During the preoperative evaluation, the programming of these devices should be documented and adjusted according to the perioperative needs. Respiratory variations and the responses to carotid massage and Valsalva maneuvers are impaired. Cardiac output is maintained via stroke volume and is preload-dependent. The compensatory responses to vasodilation, vasoconstriction, and hypovolemia are compromised, thus predisposing patients to exaggerated hypotension, orthostasis, and significant hypertension.[1,2]

For transplant recipients, the impact of infection and immunosuppressive therapy must be considered. Infections are a significant risk for morbidity and mortality. The clinician should exercise vigilance as the attenuation of typical inflammatory signs and symptoms by the immunosuppression regimen leads to diagnostic difficulty. Immune defenses are impaired, resulting in increased frequency and severity of infectious complications. Infections can include opportunistic and nosocomial respiratory, mediastinal, blood, and genitourinary bacterial, fungal, viral, and parasitic syndromes. Pathogens affecting this population include *Pneumocystis*, *Legionella*, *Toxoplasma*, cytomegalovirus (CMV), herpes, candida, and aspergillus. For lung transplant recipients, infection with common respiratory viruses and SARS-CoV-2 are a significant concern. Early therapy with anti-spike monoclonal antibodies in patients with SARS-CoV-2 may improve outcomes.

Lung transplantation is a therapeutic option for patients with severe acute respiratory distress syndrome resulting from SARS-CoV-2 infection. Intra- and postoperative outcome differences have been identified in lung transplant recipients with SARS-CoV-2 infection compared to transplant recipients with chronic end-stage lung disease without SARS-CoV-2 infection. These include higher incidence of intraoperative venoarterial extracorporeal membrane oxygenation use, longer median allograft ischemic time, more days on mechanical ventilation, longer ICU and hospital lengths of stay, and increased incidence of primary graft dysfunction.[7,8,9] The rate of performance status improvement in SARS-CoV-2 patients is higher, while antibody-mediated rejection incidence is lower. The differences in long-term outcomes such as survival are yet to be defined.

The incidence of airway complications after lung transplantation is 2–18%. These complications may develop in the acute postoperative period or occur later, due to the impact of the disrupted bronchial blood circulation, prolonged donor lung ischemic time, surgical techniques, infection, and exposure to prolonged postoperative mechanical ventilation. Anastomotic complications such as infection, bleeding, dehiscence, and necrosis present in the acute postoperative period, while tracheo- and bronchomalacia, airway stenosis, excess granulation tissue, and fistulas are a delayed concern.[4]

Allograft rejection remains a significant cause of acute graft dysfunction, chronic organ failure, morbidity, and mortality. Acute rejection in heart transplants occurs within the first 6 months and can be symptomatic (signs of heart failure and arrythmia) or asymptomatic, thus surveillance biopsies at regular intervals are warranted. Cardiac allograft vasculopathy (CAV) is a manifestation of chronic rejection and occurs in 8% and 32% of patients during the first 1 and 5 years after transplantation, respectively.[13] CAV may be asymptomatic or underestimated on standard imaging, posing a diagnostic challenge. Stress echocardiography and myocardial perfusion imaging as well as coronary angiography remain the standard diagnostic modalities; intravascular ultrasonography is the most sensitive.[10,11,13] CAV has been associated with significantly increased risk of sudden cardiac death.

Following lung transplantation, acute rejection results in perivascular, interstitial, and airspace infiltrates and bronchiolitis; it can present with dyspnea, cough, sputum production, hypoxemia, fever, or leukocytosis. Chronic rejection is characterized by inflammation and fibrotic changes with resulting bronchiolitis obliterans. Asymptomatic rejection is diagnosed by invasive biopsy.

The incidence of neurologic complications in heart and lung transplant recipients is 10–30% and includes stroke, posterior reversible encephalopathy syndrome (PRES), and neuropathies. Hypertension, renal, hepatic, and pancreatic dysfunction, hyperglycemia, and hyperlipidemia can be a result of immunosuppression or associated patient comorbidities.

Commonly used immunosuppressive medications have several important adverse effects and drug interactions.[5] Steroids may cause hyperglycemia, hypertension, hyperlipidemia, osteoporosis and necrosis, and adrenal suppression; the risk of the latter should warrant consideration of perioperative stress-dose steroids. Cyclosporine and tacrolimus are associated with nephrotoxicity, hepatotoxicity, neuropathy, hyperglycemia, hyperkalemia, hypomagnesemia, and reduction of the seizure threshold; cyclosporine has multiple drug-drug interactions. Mycophenolate, azathioprine, and sirolimus are associated with cytopenia and gastrointestinal toxicity.

An important goal of the preoperative assessment for a transplant recipient is determination of cardiopulmonary functional status. For heart transplant recipients, this includes an evaluation for signs and symptoms of coronary disease and heart failure such as chest pain, dyspnea on exertion, or orthopnea. For lung transplant recipients, this includes symptoms of residual pulmonary disease, such as wheezing or shortness of breath. Other key organ dysfunctions should be identified through history, physical examination, and targeted preoperative studies. Lower extremity edema, elevated JVD, and pulmonary crackles could represent new or worsening heart failure with volume overload. Wheezing or decreased air sounds could indicate residual reactive airway disease. A baseline neurologic examination should be documented, particularly when regional anesthesia is considered. For any organ recipient, is important to inquire about any procedures (catheterizations, biopsies, stents, pacemaker insertions) performed since the transplantation.

Any patient with prior heart or lung transplantation undergoing noncardiothoracic surgery should have a CBC, basic metabolic panel, and coagulation studies prior to surgery. A type and screen should be collected for any patient undergoing a surgery with significant anticipated blood loss (>500 mL). Transplant patients frequently have anemia and are at increased risk of intraoperative transfusion. Preoperative interventions to treat anemia may include nutrition adjustment and medications, such as iron or erythropoietin-stimulating drugs. Finding appropriate cross-matched blood may be more challenging due to antibodies related to prior transfusions and transplant. The risk of sensitization to HLA antigens and predisposition to antibody-mediated rejection of the transplanted organ associated with blood product transfusion has been raised; however, studies have also suggested a reduction in graft rejection linked to pre-transplant transfusions. Leukocyte reduction of packed red blood cells to be transfused may reduce the risk of HLA sensitization and CMV transmission; however, the benefit of leukoreduction in reducing HLA sensitization has been questioned in recent studies. CMV-negative transplant recipients require CMV-safe blood units—the choice to use CMV-seronegative donors versus leukoreduction to control the exposure to CMV remains debated.

Heart or lung transplant recipients should receive an ECG prior to any noncardiothoracic surgery. It should be compared to the most recent available studies to identify any interval developments. ECG changes associated with heart transplant include two P waves, AV and bundle branch blocks, and dysrhythmia. A new arrhythmia or ST segment elevations or T-wave inversions could indicate rejection or ischemia and should prompt further investigation.

Chest x-ray, CT scan, MRI, and other imaging modalities can help to identify a wide range of abnormalities and complications, including infection, acute rejection, heart failure, bronchiolitis obliterans, post-transplantation lymphoproliferative disorder, and disease recurrence in the transplanted lung, as well as airway complications such as bronchial dehiscence, stricture formation, and bronchomalacia.[6] The use of these studies is guided by clinical presentation. However, even in asymptomatic lung transplant patients, a chest x-ray before any intermediate- or high-risk procedure is advisable. Additional preoperative tests should be considered for patients with recent changes in functional status. In a lung transplant recipient, new symptoms of cough or shortness of breath should prompt pulmonary function tests. In a heart transplant recipient, new symptoms of chest pain or dyspnea should prompt a preoperative echocardiogram and possibly stress test or myocardial perfusion study and angiography. Heart transplant recipients should be regarded as a unique patient population in terms of the use of cardiac testing, indications for interventions, and their impact on outcomes.

A review of medications is an important part of the preoperative evaluation, and a comprehensive plan for drug management should be instituted with multidisciplinary team involvement. In addition to appropriate continuation, interruption, and appropriate adjustment of cardiovascular, pulmonary, and endocrine medications, particular attention must be given to the immunosuppressant and antimicrobial prophylactic and therapeutic regimens. These therapies should be continued without interruption in the perioperative period, using IV medications in lieu of oral drugs as necessary. Furthermore, typical perioperative surgical infection prophylaxis may require broadening based on the presence of preexisting pathogens and their drug sensitivities. Nutrition optimization and other preventative measures may be instituted at this time.

General, regional, and neuraxial anesthesia all have been performed safely in patients following heart and lung transplantation.[15–18] The choice of anesthetic depends on the surgery to be performed, the patient's current cardiac and pulmonary function, the presence of additional comorbidities, provider experience, and patient preferences. Benefits of general anesthesia (GA) include control of the airway and breathing as well as patient comfort, especially during prolonged cases that require specific positioning. Disadvantages of GA include often challenging intra- and postoperative ventilation strategies in patients with poor lung compliance. Prolonged intubation following GA places patients at risk for pneumonia and other pulmonary complications. Nasotracheal intubations should be avoided in these patients due to infectious concerns. Benefits of regional anesthesia include improved postoperative pain control, decreased opioid utilization, and isolated extremity muscle relaxation to facilitate surgery. Risks of regional anesthesia are rare and include nerve damage and hematoma. In lung transplant patients, the risks of phrenic nerve paralysis and pneumothorax are of particular concern as they increase the risk of pulmonary complications, morbidity, and mortality. Upper extremity nerve blocks performed ipsilateral to the transplanted "healthy" lung should be avoided. In heart transplant recipients, neuraxial anesthesia should be used with caution. The transplanted heart may not compensate for vasodilatation; thus special attention should be directed toward preload optimization and vasopressor support.

The choice of intraoperative monitors depends on the patient's comorbidities, functional status, and the surgery to be performed. Standard ASA monitors—including pulse oximetry, end-tidal carbon dioxide, noninvasive blood pressure, continuous ECG, and temperature—should be used on all patients. An arterial catheter should be used in all patients with post-transplant disease including heart failure, valvulopathy, coronary artery disease, or significant respiratory dysfunction. It is reasonable to place the arterial line prior to induction of anesthesia to allow for careful titration of medications for hemodynamic stability. For patients with post-transplant lung disease, an arterial line is indicated for serial ABG analyses. It may be useful to collect a baseline ABG in patients without recent laboratory studies. In patients with normal post-transplant heart and lung function, an arterial line is indicated for cases with significant expected blood loss or fluid shifts. Most noncardiothoracic surgeries on transplant recipients are performed without intraoperative transesophageal echocardiography (TEE). However, TEE can be considered if intraoperative hemodynamic instability is expected or the patient has evidence of cardiopulmonary decompensation.

Choice of anesthetic medications, including muscle relaxants, should be informed by the presence of cardiovascular, renal, and liver dysfunction. In cases where contractility of the transplanted heart is preserved, the cardiodepressant effects of inhaled and IV anesthetics are well-tolerated; however, the stabilizing effect of ketamine on hemodynamics is attenuated. Anesthesiologists should account for interactions between immunosuppressant and anesthetic drugs. Cyclosporine and tacrolimus can lower the seizure threshold, and acid-base disturbances can compound the risk of seizures. Cyclosporine augments the action of neuromuscular relaxants (NMR), and prolonged paralysis may be seen.

The cardiopulmonary pathology of transplant recipients guides perioperative hemodynamic management. Fluid boluses should be used to augment cardiac output in the preload dependent transplanted heart. Direct vasoactive medications are used for blood pressure support, and chronotropic and inotropic agents may be required to maintain higher heart rate and cardiac output. Epinephrine, dobutamine, isoproterenol, and phosphodiesterase-3 inhibitors such as milrinone are utilized. Ephedrine and dopamine, while helpful, may be less predictable in their hemodynamic effects as their action is partially indirect; phenylephrine is effective for blood pressure support without accompanying reflex bradycardia. Beta blockers should be avoided, and potent direct vasodilators should be titrated slowly. Amiodarone can be used for arrhythmia control, but cautiously due to potential bradycardia. The anticholinergic agents atropine and glycopyrrolate are ineffective for heart rate support, and paradoxical bradycardia has been described.[26,27] Cholinesterase inhibitors are not expected to produce customary bradycardia when used for reversal of NMR in heart transplant recipients and their safety has been demonstrated; however, reports of severe bradycardia and asystole have been reported and may be linked to reinnervation.[26,27] An anticholinergic agent added to a reversal agent is beneficial in attenuating some peripheral muscarinic effects. Sugammadex has been safely used for reversal in these patients.[28,29]

In the postoperative period, these patients may require close observation in a monitored setting such as an ICU or stepdown unit.

CONCLUSION

- Heart and lung transplant recipients present increasingly for noncardiothoracic surgery and pose unique clinical challenges requiring focused preoperative evaluation.

- The preoperative evaluation should focus on the evaluation of cardiopulmonary status and may prompt more extensive testing beyond the standard recommendations for non-transplant patients.

- Unique post-transplant cardiovascular physiology includes disruptions in the conduction system and autonomic innervation. While the responses to circulating catecholamines and the Frank-Starling mechanism are preserved, the compensatory responses to hypo- and hypertension and stress are blunted.

- Preexisting lung disease as well as post-transplant complications including acute and chronic rejection and infection predispose lung transplant recipients to perioperative pulmonary complications.

- The preoperative evaluation should address management of immunosuppression regimens and assess for evidence of infection and graft rejection.

- General and regional anesthesia may be utilized safely according to surgical needs, with consideration of pathophysiological changes related to the transplant.

- Intraoperative monitoring should be tailored to each patient. Invasive monitors to consider include arterial, central venous, and pulmonary artery catheters as well as perioperative echocardiography.

- The plan for airway management should consider possible post-transplant airway issues and aspiration risk.

- Postoperative recovery may require more extensive monitoring in a higher acuity unit such as an ICU or step-down unit.

REVIEW QUESTIONS

1. Which of the following regarding the preoperative evaluation of heart and lung transplant patients is correct?

    a. The cardiopulmonary examination is the only relevant focus of the evaluation.
    b. The pathology and clinical presentation of cardiovascular disease in heart transplant patients is the same as in non-transplant patients.
    c. Obtaining a preoperative ECG is advisable to identify conduction abnormalities and arrhythmias.
    d. Immunosuppression therapy should be held preoperatively due to concern for infection.

    The correct answer is c.

    While the cardiopulmonary assessment is an essential component of the preoperative evaluation, other organ systems in post-transplant patients may be affected, and any abnormalities should be identified and addressed. In addition to the typical risk factors and pathology of cardiovascular disease, transplant patients are at risk for CAV and other cardiovascular complications related to the disruption of normal physiology as well as rejection and infection. These disorders may be asymptomatic and may be underestimated by basic testing. Recent ECG, compared with previous ones, can identify preexisting and new-onset arrhythmias and conduction abnormalities frequently encountered in these patients. While concern for infectious complications in immunosuppressed patients is ever-present, immunosuppression therapy should not be interrupted.[1,12,13]

2. Pathophysiologic alterations after heart and lung transplantation may include all of the following, *except*

    a. Conduction abnormalities and arrhythmias.
    b. Disruption of the autonomic innervation of the heart.
    c. Preservation of responses to circulating catecholamines.
    d. Impairment of the Frank-Starling mechanisms.

    The correct answer is d.

    The transplanted heart is denervated and thus lacks normal sensory, sympathetic, and parasympathetic responses; delayed reinnervation is incomplete and unreliable. However, the heart retains alpha- and beta-adrenergic receptor sensitivity and responsiveness to circulating catecholamines as well as the normal Frank-Starling mechanisms. The intrinsic impulse formation and conductivity may be preserved; however, arrhythmias and conduction abnormalities are not uncommon.[1,2]

3. All of the following regarding post-transplant complications are correct, *except*

    a. Heart transplant rejection can be asymptomatic or present with signs of heart failure, CAV, and arrhythmia.
    b. Patients with heart transplant are at increased risk of coronary artery disease, which may be asymptomatic and underestimated on testing.
    c. The demonstration of inflammatory infiltrates in transplanted lungs should be treated immediately with antimicrobial agents.
    d. Evidence of neurologic complications should be evaluated and documented in the preoperative evaluation of transplant recipients.

    The correct answer is c.

    Acute and chronic heart transplant rejection may present with heart failure, arrhythmia, or accelerated coronary artery disease but is frequently asymptomatic, and regular surveillance with testing and biopsy is indicated. Patients with CAV may also lack symptoms, and the standard clinical testing may underestimate the degree of the disease.

    Interstitial and airspace inflammation in the transplanted lung may indicate rejection rather than infection and may require enhancement of the immunosuppression regimen; therefore, while surveillance for infections should be undertaken, antimicrobial agents should not be the first line of therapy in the absence of high suspicion or evidence of infection. The incidence of neurologic complications, including neuropathies, stroke, and PRES is estimated at 10–30%.[1,2,13,31,32]

4. Regarding lung transplantation and SARS-CoV-2 infection, all of the following statements are correct, *except*

    a. Enhanced respiratory exposure prophylaxis should be practiced in the hospital care of these patients.
    b. The incidence of graft rejection is consistently higher in lung transplant recipients with end-stage lung disease due to SARS-CoV-2.
    c. Prolonged mechanical ventilation and ICU and hospital lengths of stay are likely in lung transplant recipients with end-stage lung disease due to SARS-CoV-2.
    d. Early therapy of SARS-CoV-2 infection in lung transplant patients improves outcomes.

    The correct answer is b.

    Immunosuppression of transplant recipients increases the risk of severe SARS-CoV-2 infection, and respiratory protection by the clinical staff is advised in the care of these patients. Lung transplant recipients with end-stage lung disease due to SARS-CoV-2 are more likely to experience longer time on mechanical ventilation and longer ICU and hospital stays. The incidence of graft rejection, particularly antibody-mediated, appears to be lower in these patients.[8–10]

5. Which of the following statements regarding perioperative considerations for patients after heart and lung transplantation is correct?

    a. Transfusion of blood products always reduces the risk of organ rejection.

b. The risk of sensitization to HLA antigens may be ameliorated by leukoreduction of packed red blood cells.
c. CMV-negative blood transfusion is not necessary as most of the population is CMV-positive.
d. CMV is not linked to CAV.

The correct answer is b.

Blood product transfusion predisposes transplant patients to sensitization to HLA antigens and potential antibody-mediated donor organ rejection; however, the immune interactions are complex and there is evidence that pre-transplant transfusion may be associated with reduced incidence of graft rejection. The units of packed red blood cells to be transfused should be leukoreduced. While a substantial portion of the population is CMV-positive, including many transplant recipients, CMV-negative transplant recipients require CMV-safe blood. CMV can lead to overt clinical infection and may contribute to CAV.[21–25]

6. Which of the following is correct regarding anesthetic techniques for patients after heart and lung transplantation?

a. These patients are at risk for aspiration and rapid-sequence induction should always be performed.
b. The performance of regional anesthesia for upper extremity surgery should never be done on the side of the transplanted lung.
c. Neuraxial anesthesia should not be done in heart transplant patients.
d. Both general and regional anesthesia may contribute to the risk of perioperative pulmonary complications in lung transplant patients.

The correct answer is d.

General and regional anesthesia can be performed safely. However, airway complications, challenges with ventilation, and the potential for prolonged ventilation of lung transplant patients may contribute to postoperative pulmonary complications. Such risk is augmented by preoperative cardiopulmonary dysfunction. The potential for aspiration exists; however, it is related more to typical aspiration risk factors and less to the transplant itself. Therefore, the indications for rapid-sequence induction should be based on the standard assessment of risk and NPO status. The site of nerve blocks for upper extremity surgery should be carefully considered. A brachial plexus block with significant risk of phrenic nerve paralysis or pneumothorax should be avoided, particularly on the side of the "healthy" transplanted lung. Blocks performed more distally, in the absence of risk of local anesthetic translocation higher into the nerve sheaths, should not present an issue. Neuraxial anesthesia is not contraindicated but should be performed with caution due to the physiology of the denervated heart; special attention should be directed toward preload optimization and hemodynamic support with vasopressors.[17–19]

7. Correct statements regarding the perioperative management of heart and lung transplant patients include all of the following, *except*

a. In heart transplant patients, the hemodynamic effects of ketamine are attenuated.
b. The reversal of NMR never results in bradycardia.
c. Anticholinergic agents do not prevent bradycardia reliably with administration of NMR reversal.
d. Prolonged NMR effect may be seen as a result of immunosuppressive therapy.

The correct answer is b.

In the denervated transplanted heart, the stabilizing effect of ketamine on hemodynamics is attenuated and thus unreliable. The cholinesterase inhibitors used for reversal of NMR in heart transplant recipients generally do not produce bradycardia, and their safety as well as that of sugammadex has been demonstrated. However, reports of severe bradycardia and asystole have been reported with cholinesterase inhibitors. Caution should be exercised with reversal agents, especially because anticholinergics are ineffective at increasing heart rate. Certain immunosuppressants such as cyclosporine augment the action of NMR and prolonged paralysis may be seen.[17,18,26–29]

REFERENCES

1. Birati EY, Rame JE. Post-heart transplant complications. *Crit Care Clin*. 2014;30:629–637.
2. McCartney SL, Patel C, Del Rio JM. Long-term outcomes and management of the heart transplant recipient. *Best Pract Res Clin Anaesthesiol*. 2017;31(2):237–248.
3. Costa J, Benvenuto LJ, Sonett JR. Long-term outcomes and management of lung transplant recipients. *Best Pract Res Clin Anaesthesiol*. 2017;31(2):285–297.
4. Kim HH, Jo KW, Shim TS, et al. Incidence, risk factors, and clinical characteristics of airway complications after lung transplantation. *Sci Rep*. 2023;13:667.
5. Ivulich S, Westall G, Dooley M, et al. The evolution of lung transplant immunosuppression. *Drugs*. 2018;78:965–982.
6. Li Ng Y, Paul N, Patsios D, et al. Imaging of lung transplantation: Review. *Am J Roentgenol*. 2009;192:S1–S13.
7. Kurihara C, Manerikar A, Querrey M, et al. Clinical characteristics and outcomes of patients with COVID-19-associated acute respiratory distress syndrome who underwent lung transplant. *JAMA*. 2022;327:652–661.
8. Bermudez C, Bermudez F, Courtwright A, et al. Lung transplantation for COVID-2019 respiratory failure in the United States: Outcomes 1-year posttransplant and the impact of preoperative extracorporeal membrane oxygenation support. *J Thorac Cardiovasc Surg*. 2023:S0022-5223(23)00340–00349.
9. Casutt A, Papadimitriou-Olivgeris M, Ioakeim F, et al. Outcomes of SARS-CoV-2 infection among lung transplant recipients: A single center retrospective study. *Transpl Infect Dis*. 2023;25:e14007.
10. Sade LE, Eroğlu S, Yüce D, et al. Follow-up of heart transplant recipients with serial echocardiographic coronary flow reserve and dobutamine stress echocardiography to detect cardiac allograft vasculopathy. *J Am Soc Echocardiogr*. 2014;27:531–539.
11. Badano LP, Miglioranza MH, Edvardsen T, et al. European Association of Cardiovascular Imaging/Cardiovascular Imaging Department of the Brazilian Society of Cardiology recommendations for the use of cardiac imaging to assess and follow patients after heart transplantation. *Eur Heart J Cardiovasc Imaging*. 2015;16(9):919–948.
12. Alba AC, Foroutan F, Ng Fat Hing NKV, et al. Incidence and predictors of sudden cardiac death after heart transplantation: A systematic review and meta-analysis. *Clin Transplant*. 2018;32(3):e13206.

13. Agarwal S, Parashar A, Kapadia SR, et al. Long-term mortality after cardiac allograft vasculopathy: Implications of percutaneous intervention. *JACC Heart Fail*. 2014;2(3):281–288.
14. Schoch BS, Barlow JD, Schleck C, et al. Shoulder arthroplasty for atraumatic osteonecrosis of the humeral head. *J Shoulder Elbow Surg*. 2016;25:238–245.
15. Herborn J, Parulkar S. Anesthetic considerations in transplant recipients for nontransplant surgery. *Anesthesiol Clin*. 2017;35(3):539–553.
16. Jurgens PT, Aquilante CL, Page RL, et al. Perioperative management of cardiac transplant recipients undergoing noncardiac surgery: Unique challenges created by advancements in care. *Semin Cardiothorac Vasc Anesth*. 2017;21(3):235–244.
17. Shaw IH, Kirk IJB, Conacher ID. Anaesthesia for patients with transplanted hearts and lungs undergoing non-cardiac surgery. *Br J Anaesth*. 1991; 67: 772–778.
18. Blasco LM, Parameshwar J, Vuylsteke A. Anesthesia for noncardiac surgery in the heart transplant recipient. *Curr Opin Anaesthesiol*. 2009; 22: 109–113.
19. Wood RK. Esophageal dysmotility, gastro-esophageal reflux disease, and lung transplantation: What is the evidence? *Curr Gastroenterol Rep*. 2015;17(12):48.
20. Jamie Dy F, Freiberger D, Liu E, et al. Impact of gastroesophageal reflux and delayed gastric emptying on pediatric lung transplant outcomes. *J Heart Lung Transplant*. 2017;36(8):854–861.
21. Kotter JR, Drakos SG, Horne BD, et al. Effect of blood product transfusion-induced tolerance on incidence of cardiac allograft rejection. *Transplant Proc*. 2010;42:2687–92.
22. Mason D, Little S, Nowicki E, et al. Temporal pattern of transfusion and its relation to rejection after lung transplantation. *J Heart Lung Transplant*. 2009; 28:558–563.
23. Fernández FG, Jaramillo A, Ewald G, et al. Blood transfusions decrease the incidence of acute rejection in cardiac allograft recipient. *J Heart Lung Transplant*. 2005;24:S255–261.
24. Sarkar RS, Philip J, Yadav P, et al. Transfusion medicine and solid organ transplant—Update and review of some current issues. *Med J Armed Forces India*. 2013;69:162–167.
25. Scornik JC, Meier-Kriesche HU. Blood transfusions in organ transplant patients: Mechanisms of sensitization and implications for prevention. *Am J Transplant*. 2011;11:1785–1791.
26. Bertolizio G, Yuki K, Odegard K, Collard V, Dinardo J. Cardiac arrest and neuromuscular blockade reversal agents in the transplanted heart. *J Cardiothorac Vasc Anesth*. 2013;27:1374–1378.
27. Barbara DW, Christensen JM, Mauermann WJ, et al. The safety of neuromuscular blockade reversal in patients with cardiac transplantation. *Transplantation*. 2016;100(12):2723–2728.
28. Tezcan B, Şaylan A, Bölükbaşı D, et al. Use of sugammadex in a heart transplant recipient: Review of the unique physiology of the transplanted heart. *J Cardiothorac Vasc Anesth*. 2016;30(2):462–465.
29. Varela N, Golvano M, Pérez-Pevida B. Safety of sugammadex for neuromuscular reversal in cardiac transplant patients. *J Cardiothorac Vasc Anesth*. 2016;30:e37.
30. Organ Procurement and Transplantation Network National Database. https://optn.transplant.hrsa.gov/data/view-data-reports/national-data/
31. Chambers DC, Cherikh WS, Goldfarb SB, et al. The international thoracic organ transplant registry of the International Society for Heart and Lung Transplantation: Thirty-fifth adult lung and heart-lung transplant report—2018; Focus theme: Multiorgan transplantation. *J Heart Lung Transplant*. 2018;37(10):1169–1183.
32. Khush KK, Cherikh WS, Chambers DC, et al. The international thoracic organ transplant registry of the International Society for Heart and Lung Transplantation: Thirty-fifth adult heart transplantation report—2018; Focus theme: Multiorgan transplantation. *J Heart Lung Transplant*. 2018;37(10):1155–1168.

PULMONARY

18.

COPD

STILL SMOKING, STILL WHEEZING

Wesley Rajaleelan and Jean Wong

STEM CASE AND KEY QUESTIONS

A 55-year-old man with a history of chronic obstructive pulmonary disease (COPD) and is still smoking has had worsening back pain with radiation to his left leg for the past 2 months. A recent MRI reveals spondylolisthesis of L3–L5 and spinal stenosis. The spine surgeon suggests a lumbar laminectomy, and the patient has been referred to the preoperative clinic for a preoperative assessment prior to surgery.

What are salient history, physical examination and investigations you'd like to obtain when seeing this patient during the preoperative period?

He started smoking at the age of 16 and has been smoking 30 cigarettes a day ever since. He gives a history of chronic cough for the past 10 years with recurrent chest infections and has occasionally used bronchodilators along with antibiotics during his chest infections in the past. He also reports dyspnea with exertion upon climbing a flight of stairs but is currently not using any bronchodilators. There are no other changes in his symptoms or exacerbation of symptoms or hospitalizations.

A physical examination reveals the patient has a barrel-shaped chest, pursed-lip breathing with increased expiratory time, and clubbing. Upon auscultation, the patient has coarse breath sounds and expiratory wheezing.

In addition to your history and physical examination, what additional testing would you request? Is there any indication to order preoperative pulmonary function tests (PFTs)? What do you expect to see on the PFTs? Is there an indication to order a chest x-ray?

The patient's previous PFT shows a decline of forced expiratory volume in 1 second (FEV_1), inadequate lung emptying on expiration, and subsequent static and dynamic hyperinflation.[1] This indicates airflow obstruction. The patient's room air oxygen saturation is 95%. An ECG shows right-heart hypertrophy but no changes suggestive of ischemic heart disease. There is no indication for a chest radiograph.

Are there any implications of smoking in a patient complaining of back pain?

He has been complaining of chronic sharp shooting pain across his lower back radiating to his left lower limb, which is preventing him from working. In a cross-sectional study by Green et al. of 34,535 patients in the United States, they found the prevalence of back pain to be 28%. They also found a significant association between back pain and smoking.[2]

Is there any cardiac testing indicated in a patient with COPD? If so, which test would you order? ECG? Echocardiogram?

An ECG shows right-heart hypertrophy but no changes suggestive of ischemic heart disease. The prevalence of pulmonary hypertension (PH) has a linear relationship with the severity of COPD, and moreover severe PH is almost always related with cor pulmonale. In these conditions, an echocardiogram proves useful in detecting early cardiac complications of COPD.[3,4]

What medications would you expect a patient to be on for COPD, depending on its severity? What are pharmacologic options for preoperative optimization?

The patient, who was on bronchodilators prior to surgery, is referred to a pulmonologist prior to surgery for preoperative optimization of his COPD. The pulmonologist prescribes an inhaled corticosteroid and antimuscarinics as well as a short antibiotic course.

What are the benefits of quitting smoking before surgery?

The patient is advised that it is critical that he quit smoking prior to surgery to improve his chances for an optimal surgical outcome of his spine surgery. The perioperative period provides an excellent window of opportunity to address the risks posed by smoking. At least 4 weeks of abstinence reduces the risk of postoperative respiratory complications. Notably, for bone healing, smoking cessation started as late as at the time of surgery improves outcomes.[5] Studies have shown that patients are receptive to smoking cessation therapies.

What nonpharmacological and behavioral modifications may help this patient quit smoking before surgery?

He is given brief counseling by the anesthesiologist and referred to a telephone quit line for further counseling and follow-up to support his quit attempt. He should also be referred to an addiction specialist or a nicotine dependence clinic for follow-up of care to aid in smoking cessation.[6,7]

What is this patient's risk of postoperative pulmonary complications? Should elective surgery be postponed?

The risk of this patient developing postoperative pulmonary complications is quite high given his symptomatology. His elective surgery should be postponed for preoperative optimization of his respiratory status.

DISCUSSION

COPD is characterized by an abnormal airway inflammatory response and irreversible airflow obstruction occurring in response to long-term exposure to inhaled particles from noxious compounds, and gases from cigarette smoke and air pollution.[8,9] Remodeling of the small airway compartment and loss of the elastic recoil by the airway, hypersecretion of mucus (chronic bronchitis), tissue destruction (emphysema), and disruption of normal defense mechanisms leads to airway inflammation and fibrosis.[8,9] Patients with COPD may present with associated comorbidities and symptom exacerbations which can affect the overall quality of life. As the disease progresses, hypertrophy of the vascular smooth muscle ensues, with collagen deposition and destruction of the ciliary bed leading to PH and cor pulmonale.[10,11]

Smoking is the main cause of COPD, which can present as two different phenotypes, the "pink puffers" and the "blue bloaters." The "pink puffers" present with breathlessness, hyperinflation, hypoxemia, and hypocarbia, in contrast to "blue bloaters" who present with hypoxemia, secondary polycythemia, PH, cor pulmonale, and carbon dioxide retention.[10,11]

HISTORY

A complete history and physical examination at the preoperative anesthesia clinic is of paramount importance when assessing patients with COPD.

A detailed history of medications used to control disease, number of exacerbations, and previous hospitalizations should be obtained. In addition, a detailed smoking history including onset of smoking and the number of cigarettes smoked in pack-years is useful. Symptom control (cough, sputum production, dyspnea, wheezing) or any recent changes in these symptoms should be elicited as well as comorbidities such as coronary artery disease or cerebrovascular disease since these are the top two causes of death in individuals with COPD.[12–14] The need for home oxygen indicates severe COPD and increases the risk for postoperative complications.

In patients with COPD, physical examination can reveal a range of findings from a clear chest examination to end-expiratory wheezing, dyspnea at rest, and pursed-lip breathing. Wheezing is usually a sign of uncontrolled COPD or a COPD exacerbation. Use of accessory muscles of respiration is a concerning finding in patients with COPD pointing to the severity or lack of symptom control. An elevated jugular venous pressure may indicate right-heart failure.[15–18]

INVESTIGATIONS

The 2020 American College of Physicians (ACP) guidelines recommended that routine preoperative chest radiographs should not be routinely performed in patients to predict risk of postoperative pulmonary complications. However, PFTs may be useful for patients with a worsening in symptoms to discern the cause of dyspnea.[8] A systematic review also concluded that routine chest radiographs were not associated with a decrease in morbidity or mortality.[19]

Preoperative PFTs may aid in diagnostic evaluation, assess disease severity, monitor the progression of the disease, and evaluate response to bronchodilators.[18–20] Preoperative cardiac evaluation in a patient with COPD may aid in evaluating worsening symptoms, assessing cardiovascular risks, determining baseline cardiac status, and helping prepare the patient for pulmonary rehabilitation.[18,20,21]

Preoperative evaluation of a patient's exercise capacity is reflective of their cardiopulmonary status. If a patient is able to climb two flights of stairs or walk more than 0.4 miles or 3.5 miles/hour without stress-induced dyspnea, these are equivalent to the 4 metabolic equivalents (METs) that are minimally recommended before elective surgery.[15,16] A complete blood profile may show polycythemia and increased white blood cell counts.[22]

SEVERITY OF COPD

Assessing the severity of COPD includes assessment of symptomatology, diagnostic PFTs, and the impact of the disease on quality of life and activities of daily living. The key components that aid in diagnosing the severity of COPD are

1. Evaluation of symptomatology based on the presenting symptoms such as coughing, wheezing, sputum production, and shortness of breath.

2. Pulmonary function tests (FEV_1, forced vital capacity [FVC] and diffusing capacity for carbon monoxide [DLCO]) play a vital role in assessing the severity of COPD.

3. Frequency of acute exacerbation of COPD often provides us with valuable insight into the severity and control of COPD. More frequent hospital visits during exacerbations are associated with more severe disease.[23–25]

TREATMENT OF COPD

Prevention and Maintenance

Smoking cessation is the single most important key factor in preventing the progression of COPD.[24,25] Smoking cessation can reverse some of the smoking-induced pathologic changes that lead to an increased risk of perioperative complications.[24,25]

Vaccinations such as the influenza vaccination and pneumococcal PCV13 and PPSV23 are recommended for those older than 65. PPSV23 has been shown to reduce the incidence of community-acquired pneumonia in patients with COPD.[24,25]

Preoperative Management of Stable COPD

There are no medications that improve lung function decline in patients with COPD, albeit pharmacotherapy is used to decrease exacerbations and prevent complications. The agents used include[26–28]

- Muscarinic antagonists
- Beta-2 agonists
- Combination therapy

Muscarinic Antagonists

Anticholinergics have an important role to play in the management of COPD as a bronchodilator. These synthetic quaternary congeners of atropine like ipratropium bromide, oxitropium bromide, and tiotropium bromide are commonly used.[26–28] These drugs have a relatively shorter duration of action and are commonly used in conjunction with beta adrenergic agents such as formoterol and albuterol.[26–28] These drugs work by binding to the muscarinic receptors, blocking the action of acetylcholine and thereby reducing the bronchomotor tone, effectively leading to bronchodilation.[26–28]

Beta-2 Agonists

Beta-2 agonists are drugs that act specifically at the beta-2 receptors found in the smooth muscle by stimulating receptors, which in turn increases cyclic adenosine monophosphate (cAMP) and produce antagonism to bronchoconstriction.[26–28] These agents can be classified as short-acting and long-acting beta-2 agonists, as seen in Box 18.1. In an acute exacerbation, these bronchodilators have significant effects for improving FEV_1, lung volumes, dyspnea, exacerbation rate, and the number of hospitalizations in patients with COPD. Beta-2 agonists also produce increased heart rate and have the ability to precipitate cardiac rhythm disturbances in patients with existing heart conditions.[26–28]

Long-acting beta-2 agonists (LABA) and long-acting muscarinic antagonists (LAMA) remain the cornerstone of management of COPD treatment. Recently, several combination inhalers containing LABA have been introduced, such as indacaterol/glycopyrronium and vilanterol/umeclidinium.[26,28] Ultra-LABAs, such as indacaterol and olodaterol, have been recently developed, providing prolonged bronchodilation compared to standard LABA. The Global Initiative for Chronic Obstructive Lung Disease (GOLD) was launched in 1997, in collaboration with the National Heart, Lung, and Blood Institute, National Institutes of Health (US) and the World Health Organization. The 2021 GOLD guidelines suggest the usage of LABA and LAMA for treating stable COPD.[27] GOLD has also been promoting the ABCD assessment of patients with COPD based on their severity at presentation and the risk of acute severe exacerbations. GOLD classified patients into groups based on symptom severity and risk for exacerbations.[27] Group A included patients with mild symptoms and low risk of exacerbations. Group B included patients with severe disease with low exacerbation risk, group C included patients with low symptom severity with high risk of exacerbation, and group D included patients presenting with severe symptoms with a high risk of symptom exacerbation[27] (Table 18.1).

GOLD also suggested the use of LABA and LAMA in combination for patients in group B presenting with persistent symptoms and patients in group C with further symptom exacerbation and the addition of inhaled corticosteroids for patients in group D.[26–28]

Box 18.1 SMOKING CESSATION COUNSELING

Ask, Advise, Assess, Assist, and Arrange

- Ask to identify all tobacco users at all visits.
- Advise tobacco users in a clear and personalized manner to quit at every visit.
- Assess willingness to make a quit attempt.
- Assist by offering medications and counseling.
- Arrange for follow-up meetings beginning the first week after the quit date.

Ask, Advise, and Refer

- Ask to identify all tobacco users at all visits.
- Advise tobacco users briefly to quit and offer cessation assistance via the quitline.
- Refer tobacco users to quitline-delivered counseling and the quitline numbers.

Ask, Advise, and Connect

- Ask to identify all tobacco users at all visits.
- Advise them briefly to quit and offer cessation assistance to quit.
- Connect tobacco users directly with quitline-delivered counseling through an automated connection system.

Table 18.1 GOLD CLASSIFICATION OF PATIENT GROUPS

Group A	Mild symptoms and low risk of exacerbations
Group B	Severe disease with low exacerbation risk
Group C	Low symptom severity with high risk of exacerbation
Group D	Severe symptoms with a high risk of symptom exacerbation

MANAGEMENT OF ACUTE EXACERBATIONS

Seventy to eighty percent of COPD exacerbations are triggered by bacterial and viral infections, and the remaining

20–30% are due to prolonged exposure to environmental pollutants.[26–28] COPD exacerbations may be mimicked by other medical conditions, and the presence of congestive heart failure and pneumonia may be difficult to distinguish from an acute exacerbation.[26–28]

Based on severity, an exacerbation may be managed with bronchodilators, corticosteroids, and antibiotics.[26–28] Short-acting inhaled beta-2 agonists and short-acting muscarinic antagonists remain mainstays in the treatment of symptoms and airflow obstruction during exacerbations in the perioperative period. There is no evidence of a difference between classes of short-acting bronchodilators in improvement in lung function.[26–28]

Based on the current recommendations of using antibiotics for acute exacerbations in COPD that shows reduced short-term mortality and treatment failure, the GOLD guidelines recommend the use of antibiotics in those patients whose exacerbation symptoms indicate a probable bacterial infection such as increased sputum volume and purulence.[26–28]

Systemic corticosteroids have clearly been shown to reduce the length of hospitalizations, improve lung function and symptoms, and reduce the risk of treatment failure and relapse.[29,30] A large cohort study in the United States showed that patients receiving low-dose methylprednisolone of less than 240 mg/day versus high-dose methylprednisolone of greater than 240 mg/day had better outcomes.[29] Higher doses were associated with longer ICU stays, longer hospital admissions, and higher costs as well as more steroid-related adverse events.[29] A recent meta-analysis suggested that a 5-day course of oral corticosteroids was sufficient to treat hospitalized patients with an exacerbation, and outcomes were not inferior to one method of administration.[30] The role of systemic corticosteroids is highly debated. There is no strong evidence for route of administration or duration of treatment.[29,30] The GOLD guidelines recommend a dose of 30–40 mg prednisolone equivalent per day, preferably oral route, for 10–14 days.[27] It is important to note that systemic corticosteroids are not recommended for long-term use as per the American Thoracic Society (ATS) statement.[8]

OPTIMIZATION OF A COPD PATIENT IN PREPARATION FOR SURGERY

Preoperative preparation of patients with COPD should include continuation of LABA and LAMA until the day of surgery in all symptomatic patients and patients with bronchial hyper-reactivity. Short-term treatment with systemic or inhaled corticosteroids has been shown to improve the lung function and decrease the incidence of wheezing following endotracheal intubation without the risk of infection or wound dehiscence.[26–28] Antibiotics are given when the character of sputum or bronchoalveolar lavage changes, suggesting an infection, and the surgical procedure should be postponed for at least 2 weeks.[26–28]

SMOKING AND NICOTINE: PATHOPHYSIOLOGIC EFFECTS

Respiratory System

The noxious toxins found in cigarette smoke causes increased mucus secretion, reduced ciliary clearance, and impaired tracheobronchial tree clearance, thus disrupting the epithelial lining of the lung and increasing epithelial permeability.[31] Nicotine promotes loss of elastin in the lung tissues causing increased closing volumes leading to emphysema and thereby increasing the alveolar volume.[31] It also stimulates the vagal response and parasympathetic ganglia, causing bronchoconstriction and increased airway resistance.[31] The increased closing volume predisposes patients to atelectasis when the smaller airways begin to close.[31,32] Pulmonary surfactant is markedly reduced, with an increase in proteolytic enzymes. The lung loses its elastic properties, resulting in emphysema and increased risk for infections.[31,32]

Cardiovascular System

Nicotine is a sympathetic stimulant, thereby increasing the heart rate and systolic and diastolic blood pressures. Smoking also increases peripheral vascular resistance, increasing myocardial contractility, in turn increasing the oxygen consumption of the myocardial muscle.[31–33] An increase in the coronary vascular resistance leads to a decrease in the coronary blood flow, resulting in decreased oxygen supply of the myocardium and subendocardial ischemia of the myocardium.[31–33]

Carbon monoxide (CO) plays a major role in cigarette smoke-induced cardiovascular diseases. The main mechanism by which CO causes heart disease is by the production of hypoxia.[33] The effects of CO are more profound in the myocardium than in the peripheral tissues. The extraction of oxygen is up to four times more in the myocardium than in the peripheral tissues. CO may also have direct effects on the myocardium. It causes increased heart rate and pulse pressure compared to the same degree of anoxia produced by inhalation of nitrogen.[33] CO is also implicated in the process of atherosclerosis and known to potentiate platelet aggregation and thrombosis.[33]

Hematopoietic System

Cigarette smoke contains active molecules like nitrosamines, low-molecular-weight phenols, aldehydes, hydrogen cyanides, and polycyclic hydrocarbons which causes oxidative stress by production of free radicals.[22] The effects of pro-oxidants on red blood cell membranes causes hemolysis, and, to compensate for this effect,[22] smoking increases synthesis of hemoglobin, red blood cells, white blood cells, and platelet reactivity, increasing the production of fibrinogen.[22,32] Hematocrit increases, which, in turn, increases blood viscosity, causing a pro-coagulable state and increasing the chances of thrombosis.[22]

In addition, nicotine increases "platelet stickiness," producing a hypercoagulable state thereby increasing the risk of thrombotic events.[22] Chronic exposure to CO causes hemoglobin (Hb) to bind to CO to form carboxyhemoglobin, which causes a shift of the Hb disassociation curve to the left, resulting in less oxygen availability for tissue metabolism. To compensate for this reduced availability of oxygen, smokers compensate by increasing erythrocyte synthesis, resulting in higher Hb values and increased hematocrit.[33]

Gastrointestinal System

Nicotine increases gastric acid and pepsinogen secretion and is strongly associated with increased risk of developing gastroesophageal reflux and peptic ulcer disease. Nicotine is known to decrease gastric motility, and it decreases the lower esophageal tone.[31]

Renal System

Nicotine is known to cause glomerular inflammation, glomerulonephritis, and urethral obstruction.[31] Nicotine has also been found to increase albumin excretion, decrease glomerular filtration rate, and promote renal artery stenosis. There is an impaired response of the kidneys to the increased systemic blood pressure in smokers.[31]

Smoking and Back Pain

Back pain has been found to be significantly more common in current smokers compared to reformed ex-smokers or never smokers (36.9%, 33.1%, and 23.5%, respectively; P < 0.01 in a study on 34,525 adults).[34] Another meta-analysis observed that smokers had a higher prevalence of back pain than non-smokers (odds ratio [OR] 1.30)[35] with the association between smoking and low back pain being strongest for chronic and disabling low back pain. Former smokers had a higher prevalence of low back pain when compared with never smokers, but a lower prevalence of low back pain than current smokers. In the cohort studies, both former and current smokers had an increased incidence of low back pain (OR 1.32 and OR 1.31, respectively) compared with never smokers.[35] They also found that the association between current smoking and the incidence of low back pain was stronger in adolescents (OR 1.82) than in adults (OR 1.16).[35]

Importantly, all of the studies show a dose-response relation between the number of cigarettes smoked and chronic low back pain.[34,35]

SMOKING AND SURGICAL OUTCOMES

Smoking is a risk factor for increased mortality and perioperative complications.[14] Moller et al. in a retrospective study of 811 patients demonstrated that smoking was the single most important risk factor for the development of postoperative complications and the need for postoperative ICU admission.[14] A systematic review of 18 large cohort studies showed that current smoking increases hospital mortality by about 20% and major postoperative complications by 40%.[36]

Smoking and Osteogenesis and Wound Healing

In a cohort study, it was found that the bone mineral content was lower at the femoral neck, tibia, calcaneus, and, to a lesser extent, at the lumbar spine and carpal bones in smokers versus nonsmokers.[37] A 5-year longitudinal study showed that men who started smoking at a younger age had considerably smaller increases in total body and lumbar spine bone mineral content and substantially greater decrease of the total hip and femoral neck bone mineral content than did men who were nonsmokers at both baseline and the follow-up visit.[37]

Epidemiological surveys found that smoking in postmenopausal women led to significantly more cortical bone loss than in nonsmoking postmenopausal women.[38] Nicotine has an anti-estrogenic affect. Smoking may nullify the protective skeletal effects of usual doses of estrogen replacement, and higher doses must be used to achieve clinical effects comparable to those observed in nonsmokers.[37,38]

The pathogenesis of bone mass loss related to smoking occurs directly due to toxic activity of smoke on bone cells and indirectly by involvement of sexual, calcitrophic, and adrenocortical hormones. Smoking causes decreased osteogenesis, angiogenesis, and collagen synthesis, which impairs osteoclast and osteoblast activity balance. This causes decreased bone mineral complex.[37–39]

Smoking causes delayed wound healing in fractures. In a study on 146 closed grade 1 open tibia shaft fractures treated with cast immobilization and operative management, the median time for healing for current smokers was significantly higher than nonsmokers (269 days vs. 136 days P < 0.05).[40]

Nicotine, being a potent vasoconstrictor, reduces blood flow, which is of paramount importance to healing bone tissue; it inhibits the proliferation of fibroblasts essential for healing and increases platelet adhesiveness, favoring microvascular occlusion.[40,41]

Gronkjaer et al. in a meta-analysis of 107 studies found that patients who had smoked preoperatively had more than twice the risk of developing postoperative wound complications compared to those who had never smoked. The risk of general infections was increased by 54% among patients who smoked preoperatively compared to patients who never smoked.[42]

Quitting smoking 3–4 weeks prior to surgery reduced the risks of wound complications.[5] Nasell et al., in a randomized controlled trial (RCT) found that postoperative deep wound infections were more common among smokers as compared to nonsmokers, and smokers had six times higher odds in developing postoperative complications in ankle fracture fixations.[43]

Postoperative Respiratory Complications in Smokers

Smokers have 2.5 times the risk of developing postoperative pulmonary complications as compared to nonsmokers.[16] In a large study of 600,000 patients undergoing major surgery using the American College of Surgeons National Surgical Quality Improvement Program Database, the adjusted odds for respiratory events was higher in current versus past smokers (odds ratio [OR] 1.45, 95% confidence interval [CI] 1.40, 1.51 vs. OR 1.13, 95% CI 1.08, 1.18).[16]

Postoperative Cardiovascular Complications in Smokers

Musallam et al. also examined 30-day postoperative mortality, arterial events such as myocardial infarction or cerebrovascular accidents, and venous events. They found that after adjusting for potential confounders, only current smokers had increased odds of mortality after surgery (OR 1.17, 95% CI 1.10, 1.24), and the 30-day postoperative mortality for cardiovascular and arterial events was significantly higher among current versus past smokers (OR 1.65, 95% CI 1.51, 1.81 vs. OR 1.2, 95% CI 1.09, 1.31).[16]

REVERSIBILITY OF SMOKING-INDUCED PATHOLOGIC CHANGES

Although current smokers with more than a 20-pack year exposure are more likely to have postoperative morbidity and mortality, former smokers, may not be at greater risk of postoperative mortality even if they have an extensive past history of smoking.[16,42] Smoking cessation is of prime importance before surgery and long-term to stop the progression of COPD.[42]

Abstinence and complete cessation of smoking leads to remarkable improvement in FEV_1 on PFTs. However, reduction in the number of cigarettes smoked each day or intermittent quitting did not achieve the same result of improvement in FEV_1 achieved with complete and sustained cessation, unless the percentage of reduction was more than 85%. This reaffirms the need for complete smoking cessation.[44]

Benefits of Quitting Smoking Before Surgery

The perioperative period represents a high-impact opportunity as a "teachable moment" for smoking cessation.[7,45] Mills et al. in a meta-analysis reported a 41% risk reduction of postoperative complications in patients who had quit smoking preoperatively.[15] Wong et al., in another meta-analysis, reported that at least 4 weeks of abstinence were needed to show a reduction in complications, and the longer the abstinence, the greater the risk reduction compared to shorter periods of abstinence from smoking.[6]

For patients who cannot quit completely before surgery, Glassman et al. observed favorable outcomes in patients who quit smoking postoperatively.[46] The rates of non-union were significantly higher in smokers when compared to nonsmokers, and patients who had stopped smoking after surgery resumed full active work and reported higher patient satisfaction scores compared to patients who had continued to smoke (P < 0.005).[46]

PREOPERATIVE SMOKING CESSATION INTERVENTIONS

Similar to studies conducted in the community, intensive behavioral support and pharmacotherapy are effective for increasing abstinence in the surgical population. A systematic review of 13 trials concluded that a combination of intensive behavioral support and pharmacotherapy initiated as late as 4 weeks before surgery reduced postoperative complications and increased the likelihood of long-term abstinence.[47] A smoking cessation program started 6–8 weeks before surgery reduced postoperative pulmonary complications and morbidity.[48] Lifestyle changes including smoking cessation and respiratory exercise training have been shown to decrease the incidence of postoperative pulmonary complications among smokers and helped patients quit smoking.[47,48]

Brief interventions provided less than 4 weeks before surgery are likely to increase abstinence but have not demonstrated a significant effect on postoperative complications.[48] The exceptions were the studies led by Glassman et al., where postoperative abstinence after spine surgery reduced risks for non-union,[46] and Nasell et al. where abstinence after acute upper and lower limb fracture surgery reduced the odds of postoperative complications by 2.5 times.[5]

Patients with COPD who still smoke may have a high degree of nicotine dependence and find it difficult to quit smoking. The difficulty in quitting smoking is primarily attributed to nicotine, the addictive substance in tobacco.[49,50]

In a Cochrane review including 53 studies with more than 25,000 participants, behavioral support (brief advice and counseling) and nicotine replacement therapy (NRT), varenicline, and bupropion were effective in helping people to stop smoking.[49] These interventions included brief advice or counseling, individual and group behavioral therapy, telephone counseling, self-help groups, and self-help materials.[7,48]

Behavioral Therapy

Several strategies have been suggested to facilitate the delivery of smoking cessation treatment in hospital and healthcare settings.[50–55] The most notable are the 5A approach (Ask, Advise, Assess, Assist, and Arrange) which was recommended for primary care.[56] It is a brief goal-directed approach to effectively address tobacco use with patients with the goal of meeting the tobacco user's readiness to quit. This model involves Asking every patient at every visit about their tobacco usage, Advising the smoking patient to quit, Assessing their willingness to quit, Assisting the patients to quit, and Arranging for follow-up.[56]

The 5A approach was modified by the American Society of Anesthesiologists (ASA) to Ask, Advice, and Refer (AAR) as seen in Box 18.1. Using this approach, the smokers are identified, briefly advised, and referred to resources such as telephone quit line counseling and follow-up. An Ask, Advise, and Connect approach has shown that directly connecting smokers using an electronic connection system within the patient's health record (electronic referrals) to resources such as quit lines significantly increased the treatment enrollment compared with the AAR approach (see Box 18.1).[56] More recently, opt-out approaches have been suggested to increase abstinence.

Advice given by physicians to their smoking patients has been shown to promote smoking cessation. Even brief advice increases the odds of quitting, but increased intensity (frequency or duration) of such advice is associated with an additional benefit. A brief advice intervention is likely to increase the quit rate by 1–3%.[53–56] The quit rates can be quite variable, ranging from 1% to 14% across trials studied. However, the relative effect of the intervention is less variable because trials with low quit rates generally have low rates of intervention.[53–56] During the preoperative visit, anesthesiologists should briefly counsel their patients about the benefits of smoking cessation and support smoker's self-efficacy by focusing on their strengths and previous successes.[56] Patient involvement in the decision-making process through the use of simple practical tools such as decision aids not only facilitates clinician–patient conversations about smoking but also reduces patient uncertainty in the decision-making.[56]

Referral to telephone quit lines have been shown to be effective in various populations and is free and widely available. The magnitude of quit line impact has been measured in a variety of context and research studies.[56,57] Phone counseling interventions have been associated with better smoking cessation rates in both the short and long term.[56,57] Text messaging and online chat support is also provided by some quit lines.

Online or e-learning may be an alternative to providing intensive in-person counseling and education for surgical patients. These online modules enable the patients to interact, receive personalized feedback, and simulate counseling sessions. In a prospective multicenter study, Wong et al. assessed 459 smokers undergoing elective noncardiac surgery in a preoperative smoking cessation intervention which included a patient e-learning program, brief advice, smoking cessation educational pamphlets, quit lines, and pharmacotherapy.[7] The 6 months point prevalence of abstinence was 22% which is much higher than unassisted quit rates.[7]

PHARMACOTHERAPY

First-line medications recommended to assist with smoking cessation are nicotine replacement, bupropion, and varenicline.

Nicotine Replacement Therapies

NRT is the most common form of smoking cessation pharmacotherapy. Albeit there were concerns with the use of NRT in patients with cardiovascular risks, a subsequent large trial has shown a lack of association between nicotine patches and acute cardiovascular risk in patients who continued to smoke when using NRT.[58]

Nicotine is the principal neuromodulator of the psychopharmacological effects associated with addiction.[52–55] NRTs reduce the motivation to consume tobacco and the psychophysiological withdrawal symptoms through the delivery of nicotine.[52–55] The evidence that NRT helps individuals to quit smoking is now well established, and many clinical guidelines recommend NRT as the first line of pharmacological treatment to quit smoking. NRT was the first proven effective pharmacotherapy for smoking cessation, increasing quit rates by 50–70% when combined with behavioral therapy.[52–55] NRTs are available in various formulations including long-acting nicotine patches, short-acting gum, lozenges, inhalers, and as nasal spray.[52–55] Various forms of NRT are shown in Table 18.2.

Nicotine stimulates neural nicotinic acetylcholine receptors in the ventral tegmental area of the brain, causing release of dopamine in the nucleus accumbens. This leads to a reduction in nicotine withdrawal symptoms in smokers who abstain from smoking. It does not completely eliminate the symptoms of withdrawal because none of the available nicotine delivery systems reproduces the rapid and high levels of arterial nicotine achieved when cigarette smoke is inhaled.[52–55]

A meta-analysis of 150 studies has shown that the effectiveness of NRT is largely independent of the intensity of additional support and the medical setting in which it is offered.[59]

Bupropion

Bupropion, an antidepressant, is both a norepinephrine and dopamine reuptake inhibitor, which potentiates the monoaminergic neurotransmission by a different mechanism compared to other antidepressants. The primary metabolite, hydroxy bupropion, decreases the reuptake of dopamine and norepinephrine into presynaptic neuronal membranes that mimic presynaptic neuronal activity.[48,54] In addition, the acute administration of bupropion reduces the firing of dopamine and norepinephrine neurons in a dose-dependent manner. One placebo-controlled trial tested the efficacy of bupropion in the perioperative setting and showed that those patients receiving 7 weeks of bupropion before surgery were more likely to stop smoking or reduce their cigarette consumption at the time of surgery and 3 weeks after surgery.[60]

Varenicline

Varenicline is a nicotinic acetylcholine receptor partial agonist that acts by reducing withdrawal symptoms and blunting of pleasurable effects of smoking.[51,54,61] In a multicenter RCT, 286 surgical patients were randomized to receive varenicline or placebo for 12 weeks and monthly counseling. Varenicline increased the likelihood of abstinence by 45% compared with placebo at 12 months after surgery. There were also a significantly lower number of cigarettes smoked by the individuals who continued to smoke.[61]

In another prospective, multicenter RCT, 296 patients were randomized to participate in a smoking cessation program which included 10–15 minutes of counseling, pharmacotherapy with varenicline, an educational pamphlet, and a fax referral to a telephone quit line or brief advice and self-referral to a telephone quit line.[62] The perioperative smoking cessation program with counseling and varenicline increased

Table 18.2 PHARMACOTHERAPIES FOR SMOKING CESSATION

MEDICATIONS	BENEFITS	PRECAUTIONS	HOW TO USE
Nicotine gum	Prevents overeating and provide additional help to reduce cravings	Difficult to use correctly (the rate of chewing affects nicotine delivery), no eating or drinking 20 minutes before or during use	1 piece every 1–2 hours for 6 weeks, then gradual reduction over 6 weeks
Nicotine Lozenges	Prevents overeating and provides additional help to reduce cravings	May be difficult to use correctly, no eating or drinking 20 minutes before or during use	Weeks 1–6: Every 1–2 hours Weeks 7–9: Every 2–4 hours Weeks 10–12:1 Every 4–8 hours
Nicotine patch	Automatically gives the right dose in a 24-hour period and reduces cravings	Nocturnal nicotine may disturb sleep, not recommended if psoriasis and eczema	If >10 cigs/day: 1 patch/day 21 mg for 4 weeks 14 mg 4 weeks 7 mg 4 weeks (12 weeks total) If <10 cigs/d: 14 mg 4 weeks 7 mg 4 weeks
Nicotine inhaler	Helps smokers with strongly conditioned smoking associated behavior	Looks and feels like a cigarette, but may induce bronchospasm	6–16 cartridges/day for 6 weeks, followed by gradual reduction over 6 weeks
Nicotine nasal spray	Faster relief, very useful for heavy Smokers	May cause nasal irritation, risk of nicotine overdose and long-term addiction	1–2 sprays/hour for 12 weeks
Bupropion	Easy to use Reduces withdrawal symptoms and rewarding effects	Possible insomnia and dry mouth; contraindicated in patients predisposed to seizures or with eating disorders	Start 1–2 weeks before quitting, 150 mg OD for 3 days followed by 150 mg BID for 12 weeks
Varenicline	Easy to use Reduces withdrawal symptoms and rewarding effects	Possible insomnia and Nausea; caution in patients predisposed to seizures, suicidality, operating heavy machinery	Start 1–2 weeks before quitting, 0.5 mg OD for 3 days followed by 0.5 mg BID for 4 days, then 1 mg BID for 12 weeks

OD, once a day; BID, twice a day.

abstinence from smoking 1, 3, 6, and 12 months after surgery compared to the brief intervention.[62]

Electronic (E-) Cigarettes

E-cigarettes were found to lead to a similar rate of smoking cessation on the day of surgery and up to 6 months after surgery compared to patients randomized to NRT in a small pilot study of 30 patients.[63] More research needs to be conducted on the use of e-cigarettes as a smoking cessation aid for surgical patients.

CONCLUSION

- Patients with COPD who continue to smoke are challenging to manage perioperatively.
- Medical treatment of exacerbations of COPD should be undertaken prior to surgery to reduce risks and ensure an optimal outcome.
- Avoiding postoperative pulmonary complications is the goal in the perioperative management of smokers with preexisting COPD.
- The perioperative period provides an appropriate window of opportunity to address the risks posed by smoking. This period represents a high-impact opportunity as a "teachable moment" for smoking cessation for surgical patients.
- At least 4 weeks of smoking cessation has been shown to be effective in reducing respiratory and other complications; however, even quitting at the time of surgery and after surgery reduces risks of non-union after spine surgery.
- A holistic approach involving pharmacological and behavioral therapies has been shown to be effective for helping patients quit smoking prior to and after surgery. However, providing these interventions in routine practice can be difficult. Future studies should investigate how these interventions can be practically implemented.

REVIEW QUESTIONS

1. Which is not part of the COPD spectrum?

    a. Emphysema.
    b. Chronic bronchitis.
    c. Idiopathic pulmonary disease.
    d. Chronic cough.

The correct answer is c.

Idiopathic pulmonary disease is a restrictive lung disease and does not fall under the obstructive disease spectrum. All the other options are diseases that are part of the COPD spectrum.

2. Which of the following is inconsistent with long-term sequelae of COPD?

    a. Erythrocytosis.
    b. Hypercapnia.
    c. Hypoxemia.
    d. Leucopenia.

The correct answer is d.

Chronic exposure to CO causes hemoglobin to bind to CO to form carboxyhemoglobin, which causes the shift of the Hb disassociation curve to the left, resulting in less oxygen availability for tissue metabolism. To compensate for this reduced availability of oxygen, smokers compensate by increasing erythrocyte synthesis, resulting in higher Hb values and increased hematocrit. Hypercapnia occurs as a result of chronic carbon dioxide retention, and hypoxia ensues because of less oxygen available for tissue metabolism. Leukocytosis is common, whereas leucopenia does not occur.

3. Treatment options of COPD include

    a. Muscarinic antagonists.
    b. Beta-2 agonists.
    c. Inhaled corticosteroids.
    d. All of the above.

The correct answer is d.

Treatment options for COPD include muscarinic antagonists, beta-2 agonists, and inhaled corticosteroids. All of these agents can be used for prevention, maintenance, and treatment of COPD.

4. Which option is true with regards to behavioral therapy for smoking cessation?

    a. Ask, advise, and refer.
    b. Ask, advise, and connect.
    c. Ask, advise, assess, assist, and arrange.
    d. All of the above.

The correct answer is d.

Ask, advise, and refer (AAR), Ask, advise, and connect (AAC), Ask, advise, assess, assist, and arrange (5A's) are all behavioral strategies that have been suggested to facilitate the delivery of smoking cessation treatment in hospital and healthcare settings. The AAR and AAC approaches are more practical in the perioperative setting than the 5A's approach which is suggested for primary practice.

5. Which of the statements is false?

    a. Cigarette smoking cessation improves postoperative outcomes.
    b. COPD is an obstructive lung disease.
    c. The airflow obstruction in COPD is completely reversible.
    d. Muscarinic antagonists, antibiotics, inhaled corticosteroids, and supplemental oxygen are part of the treatment regimen of patients with COPD.

The correct answer is c.

The airflow obstruction in COPD is not completely reversible. However, stopping smoking will prevent further deterioration, and stopping at least 4 weeks before surgery will decrease the risks for perioperative complications.

6. First-line pharmacological agents to help smokers quit include all of the following *except*

    a. Nicotine replacement therapy.
    b. E-cigarettes.
    c. Bupropion.
    d. Varenicline.

The correct answer is b.

NRT, bupropion, and varenicline are all considered first-line pharmacological agents that have been shown in clinical trials to increase abstinence. Currently, e-cigarettes are not considered first-line agents to help smokers quit. There is only a pilot study in surgical patients investigating whether e-cigarettes are effective in increasing abstinence.

7. Which statement with regards to carbon monoxide is true?

    a. Weakly binds to hemoglobin.
    b. Shifts the oxygen disassociation curve to the left.
    c. Causes leucopenia.
    d. Exhibits a strong ionotropic effect.

The correct answer is b.

CO generated from smoking strongly binds to hemoglobin to form carboxyhemoglobin, which shifts the Hb disassociation curve to the left. This causes decreased oxygen to the tissues, increased hematocrit, and is a weak inotrope.

REFERENCES

1. Rabe KF, Watz H. Chronic obstructive pulmonary disease. *Lancet*. 2017;389(10082):1931–1940. doi:10.1016/S0140-6736(17)31222-9.
2. Green BN, Johnson CD, Snodgrass J, Smith M, Dunn AS. Association between smoking and back pain in a cross-section of adult Americans. *Cureus*. 2016;8(9):e806. https://doi.org/10.7759%2Fcureus.806.
3. Dias-Fuentes G, Hashmi HRT, Venkatram S. Perioperative evaluation of patients with pulmonary conditions undergoing non cardiothoracic surgery. *Health Serv Insights*. 2016;9(Suppl 1):9–23. https://doi.org/10.4137%2FHSI.S40541.

4. MacNee W. ABC of Chronic obstructive pulmonary disease Pathology, pathogenesis, and pathophysiology. *BMJ*. 2006;332(7551):1202–1204. PMCID: PMC1463976
5. Nåsell H, Adami J, Samnegård E, Tønnesen H, Ponzer S. Effect of smoking cessation intervention on results of acute fracture surgery: A randomized controlled trial. *J Bone Joint Surg Am*. 2010;92(6):1335–1342. doi:10.2106/JBJS.I.00627.
6. Wong J, Lam DP, Abrishami A, et al. Short term preoperative smoking cessation and post-operative complications: A systematic review and meta analysis. *Can J Anesth*. 2012;59(3):268–279. doi:10.1007/s12630-011-9652-x.
7. Wong J, Raveendran R, Chuang J, et al. Utilizing patient e-learning in an intervention study on preoperative smoking cessation. *Anesth Analg*. 2018;126(5):1646–1653. doi:10.1213/ANE.0000000000002885.
8. Nici L, Mammen MJ, Charbek E, et al. Pharmacologic management of chronic obstructive pulmonary disease: An official American Thoracic Society Clinical Practice Guideline [published correction appears in *Am J Respir Crit Care Med*. 2020 Sep 15;202(6):910]. *Am J Respir Crit Care Med*. 2020;201(9):e56–e69. doi:10.1164/rccm.202003-0625ST.
9. IARC Working Group on the Evaluation of Carcinogenic Risks to Humans. Tobacco smoke and involuntary smoking. *IARC Monogr Eval Carcinog Risks Hum*. 2004;83:1–1438. PMID: 15285078. PMCID: PMC4781536.
10. Gupta NK, Agrawal RK, Srivastav AB, Ved ML. Echocardiographic evaluation of heart in chronic obstructive pulmonary disease patient and its co-relation with the severity of disease. *Lung India*. 2011;28(2):105–109. doi:10.4103/0970-2113.80321.
11. Mathews AM, Wysham NG, Xie J, et al. Hypercapnia in advanced chronic obstructive pulmonary disease: A secondary analysis of the National Emphysema Treatment Trial. *Chronic Obstr Pulm Dis*. 2020;7(4):336–345. doi:10.15326/jcopdf.7.4.2020.0176.
12. Lumb A, Biercamp C. Chronic obstructive pulmonary disease and anaesthesia. *Cont Educ Anaesth Crit Care Pain*. 2014;14(1):1–5. https://doi.org/10.1093/bjaceaccp/mkt023.
13. Turan A, Mascha EJ, Roberman D. Smoking and perioperative outcomes. *Anesthesiology*. 2011;114(4):837–846. doi:10.1097/ALN.0b013e318210f560.
14. Moller AM, Villebro N, Pedersen T. Effect of preoperative smoking intervention on post operative complications: A randomized control trial. *Lancet*. 2002;359(9301):114–117. doi:10.1016/S0140-6736(02)07369-5.
15. Mills E, Eyawo O, Lockhart I. Smoking cessation reduces post-operative complications: A systematic review and meta-analysis. *Am J Med*. 2011 Feb;124(2):144–154. doi:10.1016/j.amjmed.2010.09.013.
16. Musallam KM, Rosendaal FR, Zaatari G, et al. Smoking and the risk of mortality in vascular and respiratory events in patients undergoing major surgery. *JAMA Surg*. 2013;148(8):755–762. doi:10.1001/jamasurg.2013.2360.
17. Gupta D, Agarwal R, Aggarwal AN. Guidelines for diagnosis and management of COPD. *Lung India*. 2013;30(3):228–267. doi:10.4103/0970-2113.116248.
18. Labaki WW, Rosenberg SR. Chronic obstructive pulmonary disease. *Ann Intern Med*. 2020;173(3):ITC17–ITC32. doi:10.7326/AITC202008040.
19. Joo HS, Wong J, Naik VN, et al. The value of screening of preoperative chest X-rays: Systematic review. *Can J Anesth*. 2005;52(6):568–574. doi:10.1007/BF03015764.
20. Vagvolgyi A, Rozgonyi Z, Kerti M, et al. Effectiveness of perioperative pulmonary rehabilitation in thoracic surgery. *J Thoracic Disease*. 2017;9(6):1584–1591. doi:10.21037/jtd.2017.05.49.
21. Bobbio A, Chetta A, Ampollini L, et al. Preoperative pulmonary rehabilitation in patients undergoing lung resection in non small cell lung cancer. *Eur J Cardio-Thorac Surg*. 2008;33(1):95–98. doi:10.1016/j.ejcts.2007.10.003.
22. Malenica M, Prnjavorac B, Bego T, et al. Effect of cigarette smoking on hematological parameters in a healthy population. *Med Arch*. 2017;71(2):132–136. doi:10.5455/medarh.2017.71.132-136.
23. Ko FW, Chan KP, Hui DS, et al. Acute exacerbation of COPD. *Respirology*. 2016;21(7):1152–1165. doi:10.1111/resp.12780.
24. Wedzicha JA, Miravitlles M, Hurst JR, et al. Management of COPD exacerbations. *Eur Respir J*. 2017 Mar 15;49(3):1–6. doi:10.1183/13993003.00791-2016.
25. Myles PS, Iacono GA, Hunt JO, et al. Risk of respiratory complications and wound infections in patients undergoing ambulatory surgery: Smokers versus nonsmokers. *Anaesthesia*. 2002;97(4):842. doi:10.1097/00000542-200210000-00015.
26. Pierre S, Rivera C, La Maitere B, et al. Guidelines on smoking management during the perioperative period. *Anaesth Crit Care Pain Med*. 2017;36(3):195–200. doi:10.1016/j.accpm.2017.02.002.
27. Global initiative for chronic obstructive lung disease (GOLD). Global strategy for the diagnosis, management, and prevention of chronic obstructive pulmonary disease. 2021. https://staging.goldcopd.org/wp-content/uploads/2020/11/GOLD-REPORT-2021-v1.1-25Nov20_WMV.pdf
28. Malerba M, Foci V, Patrucco F, et al. Single inhaler LABA/LAMA for COPD. *Front Pharmacol*. 2019;10:390. doi:10.3389/fphar.2019.00390.
29. Walters JA, Gibson PG, Wood-Baker R. Systemic corticosteroids for acute exacerbations of COPD. *Cochrane Database Syst Rev*. 2009;(1):CD001288. doi:10.1002/14651858.CD001288.pub3.
30. Kiser TH, Allen RR, Valuck RJ, et al. Outcomes associated with corticosteroid dosage in critically ill patients with acute exacerbations of chronic obstructive pulmonary disease. *Am J Respir Crit Care Med*. 2014;189(9):1052–1064. doi:10.1164/rccm.201401-0058OC.
31. Beck ER, Taylor RF, Lee LY, Frazier DT. Bronchoconstriction and apnea induced by cigarette smoke: Nicotine dose dependence. *Lung*. 1986;164(5):293–301. doi:10.1007/BF02713653.
32. Azhar N. Pre-operative optimisation of lung function. *Indian J Anaesth*. 2015;59(9) 550–556. doi:10.4103/0019-5049.165858.
33. Zevin S, Saunders S, Gourlay SG, Jacob P, Benowitz NL. Cardiovascular effects of carbon monoxide and smoking. *J Am Coll Cardiol* 2001;38(6):1633–1638. doi:10.1016/s0735-1097(01)01616-3.
34. Abate M, Vanni D, Pantalone A, Salini V. Cigarette smoking and musculoskeletal disorders. *Muscles Ligaments Tendons J*. 2013;9:3(2):63–69. doi:10.11138/mltj/2013.3.2.063.
35. Shiri R, Karppinen J, Leino-Arjas P, Solovieva S, Viikari-Juntura E. The association between smoking and low back pain: a meta analysis. *Am J Med*. 2010;123(1):87.e7–35. doi:10.1016/j.amjmed.2009.05.028.
36. Theadom A, Cropley M. Effects of preoperative smoking cessation on the incidence and risk of intraoperative and postoperative complications in adult smokers: A systematic review. *Tob Control*. 2006;15(5):352–358. doi:10.1136/tc.2005.015263.
37. Rudäng R, Darelid A, Nilsson M, et al. Smoking is associated with impaired bone mass development in young adult men: A 5 year longitudinal study. *J Bone Miner Res*. 2012;27(10):2189–2197. doi:10.1002/jbmr.1674.
38. Noale M, Maggi S, Crepaldi G. Osteoporosis among Italian women at risk: The Osteolab Study. *J Nutr Health Aging*. 2012;16(6):529–533. doi:10.1007/s12603-011-0359-z.
39. Gerdhem P, Obrant KJ. Effects of cigarette-smoking on bone mass as assessed by dual-energy X-ray absorptiometry and ultrasound. *Osteoporos Int*. 2002;13(12):932–936. doi:10.1007/s001980200130.
40. Sanjay N, Shanthappa AH. Effect of smoking on the healing of tibial shaft fractures in a rural Indian population. *Cureus*. 2022;14(3):e23018. doi:10.7759/cureus.23018
41. Ziran BH, Hendi P, Smith WR, Westerheide K, Agudelo JF. Osseous healing with a composite of allograft and demineralized bone matrix: Adverse effects of smoking. *Am J Orthop*. 2007;36:207–209. PMID:17515188
42. Grønkjær M, Eliasen M, Skov-Ettrup LS, et al. Preoperative smoking status and post-operative complications: A systematic review and meta-analysis. *Ann Surg*. 2014;259(1):52–71. doi:10.1097/SLA.0b013e3182911913.
43. Nåsell H, Ottosson C, Törnqvist H, Lindé J, Ponzer S. The impact of smoking on complications after operatively treated ankle fractures—A follow-up study of 906 patients. *J Orthop Trauma*. 2011;25(12):748–755. doi:10.1097/BOT.0b013e318213f217.

44. Sørensen LT, Hørby J, Pilsgaard B, Jorgensen T. Smoking as a risk factor in wound healing and infection in breast cancer surgery. *Eur J Surg Oncol*. 2002;28(8):815–820. doi:10.1053/ejso.2002.1308.
45. McBride CM, Emmons KM, Lipkus IM. Understanding the potential of teachable moments: The cause of smoking cessation. *Health Educ Res*. 2003;18(2):156–170. doi:10.1093/her/18.2.156.
46. Glassman SD, Anagnost SC, Parker A, et al. The effect of cigarette smoking and smoking cessation on spinal fusion. *Spine*. 2000;25(20):2608–2615. doi:10.1097/00007632-200010150-00011.
47. Thomsen T, Villebro N, Møller AM. Interventions for preoperative smoking cessation. *Cochrane Database Syst Rev*. 2014;2014(3):CD002294. doi:10.1002/14651858.CD002294.pub4.
48. Yousefzadeh A, Chung F, Wong DT, Warner DO, Wong J. Smoking cessation: The role of the Anesthesiologist. *Anesth Analg*. 2016;122(5):1311–1320. doi:10.1213/ANE.0000000000001170.
49. Stead LF, Perera R, Bullen C, et al. Nicotine replacement therapy for smoking cessation. *Cochrane Database Syst Rev*. 2012:11–17:CD000146. doi:10.1002/14651858.CD000146.pub4.
50. Roberts E, Eden Evins A, McNeill A, Robson D. Efficacy and tolerability of pharmacotherapy for smoking cessation in adults with serious mental illness: a systematic review and network meta-analysis. *Addiction*. 2016;111(4):599–612. doi:10.1111/add.13236.
51. Rennard S, Hughes J, Cinciripini PM, et al. A randomized placebo-controlled trial of varenicline for smoking cessation allowing flexible quit dates. *Nicotine Tob Res*. 2012;14(3): 343–350. doi:10.1093/ntr/ntr220.
52. Silagy C, Lancaster T, Stead L, Mant D, Fowler G. Nicotine replacement therapies for smoking cessation. *Cochrane Database Syst Rev*. 2004;3:CD000146. doi:10.1002/14651858.CD000146.pub2.
53. Molyneux A. Nicotine replacement therapies. *BMJ*. 2004;328(7437):454–456. doi:10.1136/bmj.328.7437.454.
54. Ebbert JO, Hatsukami DK, Croghan IT, et al. Combination of varenicline and bupropion SR for tobacco-dependence treatment in cigarette smokers: A randomized trial. *JAMA*. 2014;311(2):155–163. doi:10.1001/jama.2013.283185.
55. Clinical practice guideline treating tobacco use and dependence 2008 Update Panel, Liaisons, and Staff. A clinical practice guideline for treating tobacco use and dependence: 2008 update. A U.S. Public Health Service report. *Am J Prev Med*. 2008 Aug;35(2):158–176. doi:10.1016/j.amepre.2008.04.009.
56. Vidrine JI, Shete S, Cao Y, et al. Ask-Advice-Connect: A new approach to smoking treatment delivery in healthcare setting. *JAMA Intern Med*. 2013;173(6):458–464. doi:10.1001/jamainternmed.2013.3751.
57. Moyers TB, Miller WR, Hendrickson SML. How does motivational interviewing work? Therapist interpersonal skill predicts client involvement within motivational interviewing sessions. *J Consult Clin Psychol*. 2005;73(4):590–598. doi:10.1037/0022-006X.73.4.590.
58. Benowitz NL, Pipe A, West R, et al. Cardiovascular safety of varenicline, bupropion, and nicotine patch in smokers a randomized clinical trial. *JAMA Intern Med*. 2018;178(5):622–631. doi:10.1001/jamainternmed.2018.0397.
59. Wu P, Wilson K, Dimoulas P, Mills EJ. Effectiveness of smoking therapies: A systematic review and meta-analysis. *BMC Public Health*. 2006;6:300–306. doi:10.1186/1471-2458-6-300.
60. Myles PS, Leslie K, Angliss M, Mezzavia P, Lee L. Effectiveness of bupropion as an aid to stopping smoking before elective surgery: A randomised controlled trial. *Anaesthesia*. 2004;59(11):1053–1058. doi:10.1111/j.1365-2044.2004.03943.x.
61. Wong J, Abrishami A, Yang Y, et al. A perioperative smoking cessation intervention with varenicline: A double-blind, randomized, placebo-controlled trial. *Anesthesiology*. 2012;117(4):755–764. doi:10.1097/ALN.0b013e3182698b42.
62. Wong J, Abrishami A, Riazi S, et al. A perioperative smoking cessation intervention with varenicline, counselling, and fax referral to a telephone quitline vs a brief intervention: A randomized control trial. *Anesth Analg*. 2017;125(2):571–579. doi:10.1213/ANE.0000000000001894.
63. Lee SM, Tenney R, Wallace AW, Arjomandi M. E-cigarettes versus nicotine patches for perioperative smoking cessation: A pilot randomized trial. *PeerJ*. 2018;6:e5609. doi:10.7717/peerj.5609.

19.

SEVERE OSA IN THE AMBULATORY SETTING

Sean Love, Chelsey Santino, and Tina Tran

STEM CASE AND KEY QUESTIONS

A 54-year-old man with past medical history significant for hypertension and obesity (BMI 39 kg/m^2) is diagnosed with a rotator cuff tear. His orthopedic surgeon recommends arthroscopy and surgical repair at a nearby ambulatory surgery center (ASC). The patient has never had surgery. Due to pain from his rotator cuff, he is unable to reach for objects with his arm and is eager to undergo surgery to treat the problem. The orthopedic surgeon refers the patient to a perioperative optimization clinic associated with his practice for evaluation prior to scheduling surgery.

What are the risk factors for obstructive sleep apnea (OSA)? What screening tools can be used to determine a patient's risk for having OSA?

The patient is evaluated by a provider (usually an anesthesiologist or a nurse practitioner) in the perioperative optimization clinic. A STOP-Bang questionnaire is used to determine the patient's risk for having OSA. The patient reports that he frequently experiences fatigue during the day, awakens frequently at night, and sometimes wakes up gasping for air. He has been told that he snores loudly at night. Based on this information, his STOP-Bang score is 7 out of 8 possible points, placing him at high risk for having OSA. The provider informs the patient that, based on current guidelines, it is not mandatory that he undergo formal testing to diagnose OSA prior to surgery, but obtaining a formal diagnosis and beginning treatment may decrease his risk of experiencing complications.

What are some concerns for performing anesthesia on a patient with OSA? How is OSA diagnosed? What therapies are employed to treat OSA? How long should a patient wait to undergo elective surgery after beginning treatment for OSA?

Patients with OSA are at increased risk for perioperative complications including cardiac arrhythmias, hypoxemia, hypercarbia, and difficult airway management. After a discussion of these risks, the patient is referred for a sleep study, or polysomnogram, which is the gold standard for diagnosing OSA. Based on this exam, the patient is diagnosed with moderate to severe OSA. The patient subsequently discusses treatment options with this primary care physician and decides to begin a nutrition and exercise program aimed at losing weight. He also agrees to begin using a continuous positive airway pressure (CPAP) device while sleeping to help with his breathing.

Even a modest amount of weight loss on the order of 10–15% can result in significant reduction in the severity of OSA, leading to important physiologic benefits. While the ability to lose weight and the rate of weight loss will be different for everyone, usually a modest reduction in weight can be achieved in as little as 4–8 weeks. Meanwhile, the benefits of using a CPAP device usually start to be seen over a similar timeframe. Often patients report that it takes a couple weeks to adjust to using and being able to sleep with the CPAP machine running at night. For those who remain compliant with the regimen, improvements in fatigue, alertness and energy levels, and memory are typically experienced within the first few weeks of usage. Improvements in physiology, including reduction in blood pressure or severity of pulmonary hypertension for patients diagnosed with these conditions, are often observed around the same timeframe. For these reasons, a patient who has just begun therapy for OSA may benefit by waiting at least 4–8 weeks before scheduling elective surgery.

What are important intraoperative and postoperative considerations in patients with OSA? What techniques can anesthesiologists employ to mitigate risk associated with performing anesthesia on patients with OSA?

Several anesthetic options exist for a patient undergoing rotator cuff repair. The type of anesthesia a patient receives should be chosen after carefully weighing the risks and benefits of different techniques in the context of the patient's comorbidities and the nature of the surgery. A regional anesthetic technique, or nerve block, could be performed under some degree of sedation. With a nerve block, the patient would be able to breathe spontaneously, usually without need for respiratory support. If a general anesthetic (GA) is preferred instead, usually an endotracheal tube or a laryngeal mask airway (LMA) would be placed. A combined approach in which both a GA and nerve block are utilized can minimize perioperative opioid requirements. High or repetitive doses of opioids can depress respiratory function in a patient already at risk of respiratory compromise due to OSA. Each of these approaches offers certain advantages and disadvantages which need to be carefully and collaboratively reviewed by the anesthesiologist, surgeon, and patient.

A regional technique with light to moderate sedation would allow the patient to breathe spontaneously with supplemental oxygen, potentially avoiding the need for airway manipulation or device insertion. Local analgesia provides improved postoperative pain control and decreased need for opioid administration. Risks of a regional anesthetic with a nerve block include bleeding, nerve damage, and the need to convert to GA in the middle of the case in the event of airway compromise and/or block failure. Some patients may wish to be fully asleep for the case, which would be a contraindication to a regional anesthetic technique utilizing light to moderate sedation.

GA would most likely necessitate the placement of a breathing device in the airway to facilitate ventilation (endotracheal tube or LMA), which could be difficult if the patient has challenging anatomy or is prone to desaturation due to obesity and decreased functional residual capacity. Anesthesia providers employing a GA should limit the amount of opioid-based medications they administer to the patients because it can compromise respiratory function. A multimodal approach to pain management should be utilized and include non-opioid analgesics.

The patient understands the risks and benefits of each approach and wishes to proceed with surgery. He is instructed to bring his CPAP machine with him on the day of surgery for use in the postoperative care unit, if needed.

What is a suitable surgical setting for high-risk patients with severe OSA? What steps should be taken by the anesthesiologist to prepare for the potential challenges posed by a patient with OSA?

A collaborative decision should be made by all clinical providers involved in the patient's care regarding the optimal location for a patient with severe OSA to undergo surgery. This decision should be based on several factors including: OSA severity, response to treatment, the presence of comorbidities, the nature of the surgery, the type of anesthesia needed, anticipated opioid requirements, and the resources available in the PACU, including nursing skillset, staffing ratios, and monitoring equipment. If the patient has medical comorbidities that are not optimized, will likely require high or repetitive doses of opioids, or is not able to use the CPAP machine after surgery, it may be best to perform the surgery in a hospital setting to allow for increased monitoring capabilities, resources, and the ability to admit the patient for observation or intervention if complications were to arise secondary to his OSA.

Because the patient has been compliant with his CPAP therapy, has agreed to bring the device on the day of surgery, and is medically optimized, the anesthesiologist in the perioperative optimization clinic determines that it would be safe for the surgery to proceed in an ASC.

The anesthesia provider on the morning of surgery examines the patient by performing an airway exam, which is notable for a large neck circumference, large tongue, normal thyromental distance, and a Mallampati score of II. The anesthesiologist identifies several risk factors for difficult mask ventilation including male gender, obesity, and a history of OSA requiring CPAP therapy. The anesthesiologist confirms that the ASC has video laryngoscopes and fiberoptic scopes available in their difficult airway cart should the need for advanced equipment arise. After reviewing the risks and benefits of general versus a regional anesthetic, the patient elects to undergo regional anesthesia with light to moderate sedation.

What regional anesthesia techniques could be offered? What risk factors are associated with regional anesthesia for shoulder surgery? Are there regional techniques that should be avoided in patients with OSA?

In the preoperative preparation area, an interscalene block is administered under ultrasound guidance. The anesthesiologist tells the patient that he may experience some shortness of breath. Interscalene blocks are associated with phrenic nerve paralysis, leading to a reduction in diaphragmatic excursion and pulmonary function which lead to symptomatic dyspnea, especially in patients with abnormal pulmonary function. The patient receives midazolam for sedation during block placement. He confirms that his shoulder, arm, and fingers feel weak and numb and denies any shortness of breath or difficulty breathing. The anesthesiologist transports the patient to the OR and surgery proceeds. The patient receives mild sedation for the case.

What medications could be used to provide sedation while minimizing the risks of airway obstruction? What are potential problems that can be encountered while employing sedation and a regional anesthetic technique?

The anesthesiologist utilizes a dexmedetomidine infusion to provide anxiolysis, analgesia, and sedation without suppressing respiratory drive. The patient occasionally snores during the surgery but is arousable to voice, indicating a light plane of sedation. The patient receives supplemental oxygen via a nasal cannula, and his vital signs are stable.

Approximately 30 minutes into the surgery, the patient complains of sharp pain at the surgical site not relieved with local analgesia injection and increased sedation. The team decides to convert to a GA with insertion of an LMA. The patient is given propofol for induction, and the anesthesiologist has difficulty ventilating the patient with a face mask.

What interventions can be utilized to assist with difficult ventilation and intubation?

Difficulty with mask ventilation may necessitate the use of an oropharyngeal or nasopharyngeal airway device in addition to maneuvers such a chin lift or a jaw thrust. Once adequate mask ventilation is confirmed, the anesthesiologist decides to proceed using the difficult airway algorithm. An LMA is inserted and proper positioning is confirmed via tidal volumes and capnography. Surgery concludes uneventfully and the patient is ready to emerge from anesthesia.

What additional preparations are needed prior to removal of an LMA? What are the risks and benefits of removing the LMA deep (spontaneous ventilation without gag reflex to oropharyngeal suctioning) versus awakening the patient (patient cooperates with hand squeezing and mouth opening) prior to removal of the LMA?

Given the challenges encountered with mask ventilation after induction, the anesthesiologist decides that the patient should be awake and responding appropriately to commands prior to removing the LMA. Potential adverse clinical outcomes after removal of the LMA prior to the patient being awake are airway obstruction and/or laryngospasm and higher risk of abrupt desaturation with brief periods of apnea, particularly in patients with OSA.

After the patient is awake and following commands, the LMA is removed. The patient is brought to the recovery room, where he tells his nurse that he is experiencing moderate pain in his shoulder. Non-opioid analgesics including acetaminophen and ibuprofen are administered, and nursing alternates the application of heat and ice packs to the surgical site to further aid in pain control. The surgeons prescribe the patient a short course of oxycodone for the patient to take as needed for pain management upon returning home.

What discharge criteria are used to safely discharge a patient with severe OSA who receives GA? How does this differ for someone who does not have sleep apnea?

The patient maintains stable oxygen saturation levels on room air without intervention. He is alert, his pain is well controlled, and he denies having nausea. The anesthesiologist instructs the patient to wear his CPAP as prescribed, use the opioids prescribed to him as needed and in combination with non-opioid analgesics, to sleep in an inclined position, and to have someone stay with him to monitor him for respiratory compromise during sleep. The patient expresses that he understands these instructions and meets criteria for discharge.

DISCUSSION

OSA is a chronic condition characterized by episodes of partial or complete collapse of the airway with an associated decrease in oxygenation saturation or arousal from sleep.[1] It is estimated that almost 1 billion people are affected by OSA, with a prevalence exceeding 50% in some countries.[2] Risk factors include male gender, advanced age, and elevated BMI.[3] OSA is associated with a three- to four-fold increased risk of being difficult to mask ventilate and difficult to intubate.[4] Unfortunately, OSA is undiagnosed in many patients presenting for surgery. Predictive clinical features include loud snoring, gasping, temporary cessation of respiration during sleep, obesity, and enlarged neck circumference. Validated tools, such as the STOP-Bang questionnaire, can be used in the perioperative setting to determine a patient's risk of having OSA. Definitive diagnosis is established via polysomnography. CPAP is the gold standard treatment, the use of which may decrease perioperative complications.[5]

ETIOLOGY, PATHOGENESIS, AND SYMPTOMS

OSA is characterized by repeated obstruction of the pharyngeal airway during sleep, resulting in hypoxia and/or hypercapnia. The pathogenesis is postulated to be due to the interaction between upper airway anatomy and sleep-related changes such as reduced upper airway muscle activity and tone.

During sleep, the lumen of the upper airway becomes deformable, rendering it susceptible to closing in the presence of decreased transmural pressure. This narrowing leads to increased airway resistance, increased turbulence, and decreased inspiratory flow, causing fluttering of the soft palate and pharyngeal soft tissue. Collectively, these changes can lead to snoring, which is an almost universal finding in patients with OSA.[6] Severe narrowing of the airway leading to complete closure results in apneic episodes observed in those with OSA.

Factors that increase the collapsibility of the upper airway structures often lead to a higher risk of OSA. These factors include large tongue size, increased size of the lateral pharyngeal walls, increased soft tissue volume, and enlarged tonsils.[7] Tonsillar enlargement is particularly relevant in pediatric patients in whom a linear relationship between tonsillar size and severity of OSA has been observed.[8] Increased soft tissue mass is commonly seen in obese patients who have increased adiposity of the upper airway, neck, or tongue, which leads to increased collapsing tissue pressure in the pharynx.[7] However, increased soft tissue aggregation in the upper airway independent of BMI and neck circumference can be seen in families and is thought to be a heritable trait.[9] Patients with this phenotype may not raise suspicion for having OSA but upon evaluation may be at similar risk for adverse outcomes.

Common presenting symptoms of OSA include daytime sleepiness, nonrestorative sleep, loud snoring, witnessed apnea by a sleep partner, awakening with choking or gasping, nocturnal restlessness, insomnia with frequent awakenings, lack of concentration, and headaches.

COEXISTING SYNDROME: OBESITY HYPOVENTILATION SYNDROME

Obesity hypoventilation syndrome (OHS) is a diagnosis distinct from but often coexisting with OSA. It is estimated that 10–20% of obese patients with OSA also have OHS, while approximately 90% of patients with OHS concurrently have OSA.[10] OHS is defined by the triad of obesity (BMI ≥30 kg/m^2), daytime hypoventilation with associated hypercarbia ($PaCO_2$ ≥45 mm Hg), and hypoxemia (PaO_2 ≤70 mm Hg) in the presence of sleep-disordered breathing without other known causes of hypoventilation. An elevated bicarbonate due to metabolic compensation for chronic respiratory acidosis should lead the clinician to suspect the presence of OHS. A threshold bicarbonate of 27mEq/L has been identified as being 92% sensitive in identifying hypercapnia on arterial blood gas.[11] In severe cases, patients with OHS may have facial plethora secondary to polycythemia and/or pulmonary hypertension from chronic hypoxia and hypercarbia, which can lead to dyspnea on exertion, elevated jugular venous pressure, hepatomegaly, and right heart failure. Although pulmonary function tests can be useful in ruling out underlying causes of hypoventilation, normal results do not exclude the diagnosis of OHS. Patients suspected of having right heart dysfunction should undergo echocardiography. CPAP or in some cases bilevel positive airway pressure (BiPAP) is the treatment of choice for patients with OHS.[11] These forms of positive pressure ventilation should be used in the postoperative period in patients who are prescribed them or as a means of rescue in patients with OHS who have not been prescribed such therapies.

> *Box 19.1* **STOP-BANG QUESTIONNAIRE**
>
> **S**noring (Do you Snore loudly?)
> **T**iredness (Do you feel Tired during the day?)
> **O**bserved Apnea (Has someone Observed you stop breathing/coughing/choking during your sleep?)
> High Blood **P**ressure (Are you have or are being treated for high blood Pressure?)
> **B**MI (Is your Body Mass Index greater than 35 kg/m2?)
> **A**ge (Is your Age older than 50 years old?)
> **N**eck circumference (Is your Neck circumference greater than 16 inches/40 cm?)
> **G**ender (Are you male Gender?)
>
> Score 1 point for each positive answer.
> Scoring interpretation: 0–2 = low risk, 3–4 = moderate risk, ≥5 = high risk

Table 19.1 APNEA-HYPOPNEA INDEX (AHI) FOR DIAGNOSIS OF OBSTRUCTIVE SLEEP APNEA SEVERITY

APNEA SEVERITY	APNEA-HYPOPNEA INDEX (AHI) (EVENTS PER HOUR OF SLEEP)
Normal (No OSA)	<5
Mild	5 ≤ AHI < 15
Moderate	15 ≤ AHI < 30
Severe	≥30

SCREENING

Several validated screening tools exist for OSA. The STOP-Bang Questionnaire was developed and validated for use in the perioperative setting and is recommended for use by several professional anesthesia organizations.[2,13–16] The sensitivity of this screening questionnaire has been shown to be greater than 85% with a specificity ranging from 25% to 85% depending on the population in whom the questionnaire is administered. The tool appears to have the highest specificity among obese men.[12–14] The tool itself is an eight-question, yes/no questionnaire (see Box 19.1). Each "yes" answer earns a point. The sum of the points is used to risk-stratify the patient for OSA. Scores of 0–2 indicate a minimal risk for OSA, scores of 3–4 indicate intermediate risk, and a score of 5 or greater indicates an elevated risk for OSA.

DIAGNOSIS

Nocturnal polysomnography is used to definitively diagnose OSA via quantification of the Apnea-Hypopnea Index (AHI). *Apnea* refers to complete obstruction of airflow, whereas *hypopnea* is partial obstruction of airflow. Both must last a minimum of 10 seconds to qualify as an apneic or hypopneic event. Hypopnea is considered significant if it leads to either a decrease in oxygen saturation of 3% or greater or causes arousal from sleep. The AHI is derived from the total number of episodes of apnea and hypopnea divided by the total sleep time. Severity of OSA is indicated by an increasing AHI, with the minimum for diagnosis of OSA being five episodes per hour with symptoms of OSA or 15 episodes per hour without symptoms.[17] Severe OSA is characterized by 30 or more apneic or hypopneic episodes per hour.[18] See Table 19.1 for AHI event per hour diagnosis criteria.

Polysomnography is performed at an overnight sleep center where comprehensive information about sleep patterns are recorded, including brain activity via electroencephalography (EEG), eye movement via electrooculography (EOG), muscle movement via electromyography (EMG), and cardiac rhythm via ECG. Additional patient sleep pattern evaluations include breathing function, respiratory airflow, respiratory efforts, and oxygen saturation to determine an AHI.

Home sleep apnea testing for diagnosis of OSA can also be performed in the appropriate patient population. Generally, home testing is considered appropriate for patients with a high pretest probability of moderate to severe uncomplicated OSA on the basis of clinical symptoms. It is within this population that the sensitivity and specificity of OSA is highest, making home sleep apnea testing a viable alternative to in-laboratory polysomnography.[19]

TREATMENT

A variety of treatment modalities exist for OSA. CPAP is the first-line treatment and is considered the gold standard. CPAP works as a pneumatic splint to keep the soft tissue of the upper airway from collapsing. It has been shown to improve the sleep indices and overall quality of life in patients with OSA. In addition, CPAP use in patients with OSA has been shown to lower blood pressure, improve left ventricular ejection fraction in patients with comorbid heart failure, reduce the incidence of stroke and arrhythmias, and reduce the risk of fatal and nonfatal cardiovascular events.[20–24] Varying rates of patient compliance with CPAP therapy are observed, which can be a potential barrier to successful treatment.

Other modalities of treatment exist but are less effective. Oral appliances can be used with varying success. Weight loss is recommended as a long-term treatment often used in tandem with CPAP.[25,26] While weight loss may not be practical in the setting of perioperative optimization, it can provide long-term benefits to the patient, especially in patients with severe OSA.[26] In rare instances, surgery can also be employed to reduce the amount of soft tissue in the airway (uvulopalatopharyngoplasty), although this is typically performed as a last resort given the morbid and irreversible nature of the procedure.

PREOPERATIVE EVALUATION

Ideally, patients with diagnosed or suspected OSA should be identified prior to the day of surgery to allow for evaluation, workup, preparation, and management. This can be initiated by direct consultation from the operating surgeon to the anesthesiologist or via an appointment with a preanesthesia or perioperative optimization clinic (if available). The preoperative evaluation should include a medical record review, patient and/or family member interview, physical examination, and review of pertinent radiological and laboratory studies.

Medical record review should include a review of the patient's past medical and surgical history, medications, allergies, and appropriate review of systems. Additional information might be needed if the patient has a history of a difficult airway, cardiovascular or pulmonary problems, elevated BMI, congenital conditions such as Down syndrome or acromegaly, and disease states such as cerebral palsy or neuromuscular disease. If sleep studies have been completed, they should be reviewed to assess the severity of OSA.

The patient and/or family interview should include questions targeted at determining the extent of snoring, apneic episodes, arousals from sleep, headaches, and daytime somnolence or fatigue. The patient's partner may be able to assist in determining certain risk factors that the patient may not be aware of, such as snoring intensity and frequency of apneic episodes. If collateral input is not available, a STOP-Bang Questionnaire can be performed to assist with risk stratification.

The physical exam should include evaluation of the external airway, oropharyngeal and nasopharyngeal structures, neck circumference, tonsillar size, tongue size, and neck range of motion. Several observational studies have identified the following as being associated with OSA: neck circumference greater than 17 inches in men and greater than 16 inches in women, anatomical nasal obstruction, craniofacial abnormalities affecting the airway, and enlarged tonsils touching or nearly touching in the midline.[27]

If features of the preoperative evaluation are suggestive of OSA, the surgeon and anesthesiologist should discuss the benefits of obtaining a sleep study and initiating therapy if the patient is diagnosed with OSA.

PERIOPERATIVE RISKS

Patients with OSA are at risk for multiple perioperative complications including a three- to four-fold higher risk of difficult mask ventilation and intubation.[14] Additionally, OSA is associated with multiple comorbidities which may increase the need for respiratory interventions, prolong length of stay, and increase perioperative mortality.[28,29]

INPATIENT VERSUS OUTPATIENT MANAGEMENT

The decision of whether a surgery is safe to schedule in an ambulatory setting is an important one and must be carefully considered by both the patient's surgeon and anesthesia provider. In making this determination, several factors should be considered including the nature of the surgery (including its urgency, complexity, and duration), the type of anesthesia administered (general, regional, and/or sedation), the status of the patient (including the presence and severity of comorbidities including OSA), need for postoperative pain control, adequacy of postdischarge observation, and resources available at the outpatient facility.[30]

At the time of publication, only one professional anesthesia organization specifically addresses and provides guidance on performing anesthesia in the outpatient setting for patients with OSA. The Society for Ambulatory Anesthesia (SAMBA) has published a consensus statement on preoperative selection of adult patients with OSA which specifically addresses the candidacy of patients with OSA for ambulatory surgery. They determined that patients with a diagnosis of OSA with medically optimized comorbid conditions can be considered for ambulatory surgery if they are able to use CPAP in the postoperative period. SAMBA specifically recommends the use of the STOP-Bang questionnaire for preoperative screening during the patient selection process. Patients suspected of having OSA through screening can be considered for ambulatory surgery if postoperative pain can be managed with predominantly non-opioid techniques.[31]

Other professional organizations have developed task forces and guidelines which address perioperative management of OSA but, to date, do not provide specific guidance on outpatient versus inpatient management. The American Society of Anesthesiologists (ASA) Task Force on Perioperative Management of Obstructive Sleep Apnea concluded that there is a lack of compelling evidence with regards to patient selection for appropriateness of inpatient versus ambulatory settings.[30]

REGIONAL ANESTHESIA

Regional anesthesia involves the injection of a local anesthetic, typically performed under ultrasound guidance, into the vicinity of nerves that provide sensation to the surgical site. While the benefit of regional anesthetic techniques is to provide targeted analgesia, regional anesthesia is not without risks. These include damage to nerves and surrounding structures, bleeding, infection, and reactions to local anesthetics, including allergic reactions and local anesthetic toxicity syndrome (LAST). Other risks exist specific to the type of regional anesthetic technique being employed. Several different regional anesthetic blocks can provide patients with analgesia while undergoing shoulder surgery.

One of the most common regional nerve blocks performed for shoulder surgery is the interscalene block, which is performed at the level of the interscalene groove. The principal advantage of this block for shoulder surgery is that it targets the brachial plexus at the level of the C5–C7 nerve roots and early trunks. By successfully blocking the brachial plexus at this level, distal branches are anesthetized, and excellent anesthesia and analgesia of the shoulder can be achieved.

One challenge of the interscalene block is its proximity to the phrenic nerve, which arises from the C3, C4, and C5 nerve roots and crosses under the prevertebral fascia from the upper lateral border of the anterior scalene muscle before descending medially along the anterior scalene muscle toward its target at the diaphragm. Performance of an interscalene block leads invariably to an ipsilateral phrenic nerve palsy, which causes a transient hemidiaphragm palsy. Hemidiaphragm palsy can lead to a decrease in a patient's forced expiratory volume, forced vital capacity, and peak expiratory flow rate. M-mode ultrasound studies of lung function show a corresponding reduction or obliteration of caudal motion of the diaphragm. Hemidiaphragm paralysis is usually well-tolerated in patients able to compensate by using accessory muscles to maintain relatively normal respiratory physiology.

For a patient with OSA, transient hemidiaphragm paralysis could exacerbate the risk for desaturation and insufficient ventilation in the postoperative setting, especially in the presence of sedatives. For this reason, the anesthesiologist and patient may wish to select a different regional technique. The risk of hemidiaphragm paralysis could be reduced by performing the regional nerve block more distally, farther away from the level of the roots. Specifically, a suprascapular nerve block could be performed. This type of block would mitigate risk for phrenic nerve palsy and transient hemidiaphragm paralysis. However, as the block is performed more distally, analgesia at the level of the shoulder can be less effective.

RECOMMENDATIONS FOR THE PERIOPERATIVE PRACTITIONER

OSA increases the risks of perioperative complications and should be recognized and managed in the perioperative period to minimize postoperative morbidity and mortality.[32] It is well established that anesthetic medications can impact upper airway physiology, arousal responses, muscle activation, and ventilatory drive, all of which place the patient with OSA at increased risk. Several professional anesthesia organizations have produced statements or guidelines for the perioperative management of OSA based on current evidence and expert opinion.

The Society of Anesthesia and Sleep Medicine (SASM) Guideline on Intraoperative Management of Adult Patients with Obstructive Sleep Apnea provides several recommendations for anesthesia providers caring for patients with known or suspected OSA. First, routine screening for OSA is recommended for adult patients, acknowledging that patients with OSA are at increased risk for being difficult to mask and/or intubate. The guideline addresses several medications commonly administered in the perioperative setting in terms of their risk when used in patients with OSA. Specifically, the guideline states that when propofol is used for procedural sedation, it may increase the risk for respiratory compromise and hypoxemic events, requiring increased vigilance on behalf of the anesthesia provider who chooses to use this medication. The guideline states that opioids should be used with caution given their propensity to depress respiratory efforts. In addition, neuromuscular blocking agents may confer increased risk of respiratory complications if not adequately reversed. The guidelines mention that ketamine and alpha-2 agonists such as dexmedetomidine have favorable respiratory profiles, but current understanding of their effects on patients with OSA is limited, and there are no official recommendation regarding the use of these medications. The guideline also states that regional anesthesia may be advantageous compared to GA but does not recommend its use over GA given the lack of evidence on the use of regional anesthesia specifically in patients with OSA.[28]

The American Society of Anesthesiologists (ASA) Task Force on Perioperative Management of Obstructive Sleep Apnea acknowledges that OSA confers increased perioperative risk and confirms that patient selection is important for reducing this risk in patients with OSA.[30] According to this task force, anesthesiologists and surgeons should collaborate to identify, optimize, and create an appropriate perioperative plan for patients with known or suspected OSA. The task force recommends that the anesthesiologist be prepared to enact the difficult airway algorithm given the increased risk for difficult ventilation and intubation in this patient population. The group also acknowledges that the potential for postoperative respiratory compromise is high in patients with OSA and states that the selection of intraoperative medications should be carefully considered. If moderate sedation is employed, the task group recommends that continuous capnography be utilized. The task force recommends that GA with a secure airway be used in favor of deep sedation given the propensity of patients with OSA to obstruct in response to doses of medication used in deep sedation. If GA is employed, the task force recommends that the patient be fully awake, responding to commands, and able to demonstrate that they can protect their airway prior to proceeding with extubation, at which time patients should be fully reversed from neuromuscular blockade, and extubation should be performed in the lateral or semi-upright position if possible. The task force recommends that a multimodal approach to analgesia be utilized to reduce or eliminate the need for opioids. The group recommends that regional anesthesia be employed to reduce the need for GA and to further decrease or eliminate the need for systemic opioids. In addition, the task force recommends that patients should bring their CPAP machine for use in the postoperative period. Last, the task force cautions providers that patients with OSA may require extended monitoring in the postoperative period due to higher risk of airway obstruction and central respiratory depression, and patients with severe OSA may need to be admitted for monitoring overnight if they do not meet discharge criteria from the PACU in a reasonable timeframe, especially if they are being discharged to an unmonitored setting.[30]

CONCLUSION

- OSA is caused by repeated obstruction of the pharyngeal airway during sleep, which can result in hypoxia and hypercapnia.
- An overnight polysomnogram is the gold standard for diagnosing OSA.
- CPAP is the first-line therapy for patients diagnosed with OSA. Weight loss is also commonly recommended if the patient has a high BMI.
- OSA is associated with increased risk for difficult mask ventilation, difficult intubation, and overall increased perioperative clinical challenges.

- The perioperative practitioner should risk-stratify patients with known or suspected OSA.
- The STOP-Bang questionnaire was developed and validated for use in the surgical patient population and is a reliable method of risk stratification in patients with suspected OSA.
- Current guidelines state that patients with OSA can have surgery in the outpatient setting if they have been medically optimized prior to proceeding with surgery.
- A multidisciplinary plan should be developed for the patient with OSA regarding the location of surgery, with consideration of the resources available and the plan for anesthesia.
- Regional anesthesia should be considered in patients with OSA given increased risk for difficult mask ventilation and intubation.
- Opioid-sparing anesthetic techniques are advised for patients with OSA due to the respiratory depressant effect of opioids.
- Patients who use CPAP therapy at home should bring their CPAP for use after surgery.

REVIEW QUESTIONS

1. OSA has a higher prevalence in patients with which of the following characteristic?

   a. Female sex.
   b. Patients who smoke.
   c. Patients with high BMI.
   d. Young patients.

   The correct answer is c.

   The prevalence of undiagnosed OSA is high in the general population. It has a higher prevalence in male patients, older patients, and patients with high BMIs.[33,34]

2. What is the definitive objective diagnosis for OSA?

   a. STOP-Bang questionnaire.
   b. Witness account of apnea and obstruction.
   c. Berlin questionnaire.
   d. Polysomnography.

   The correct answer is d.

   No clinical model can accurately predict the severity of OSA. Objective testing is required to make the definitive diagnosis. The two accepted methods of testing are polysomnography and home testing with portable monitors. Patients with significant medical comorbidities are recommended to obtain the sleep study in a controlled, monitored setting.[35,36]

3. What is a common universal clinical finding in patients with OSA?

   a. Loud snoring.
   b. Obesity.
   c. Large tonsils.
   d. Daytime somnolence.

   The correct answer is a.

   During sleep, the lumen of the upper airway becomes more deformable, rendering it susceptible to closing in the presence of decreased transmural pressure. This narrowing leads to increased airway resistance, increased turbulence, and decreased inspiratory flow, causing fluttering of the soft palate and pharyngeal soft tissue. Collectively, these changes can lead to snoring, which is an almost universal finding in patients with OSA.[6]

4. What is the gold standard for treatment of OSA?

   a. Oral/dental appliances.
   b. CPAP.
   c. Rapid weight loss.
   d. Uvulopalatopharyngoplasty (UPPP) surgery.

   The correct answer is b.

   Other modalities of treatment exist but are not as effective as CPAP. Oral appliances can be used with some success. Weight loss is also recommended as a long-term treatment often used in tandem with CPAP. While weight loss may not be practical in the setting of perioperative optimization, it can provide long-term benefits to the patient, especially in patients with severe OSA.[26]

5. What factors increase the risks for perioperative complications in patients with OSA?

   a. Female gender.
   b. CPAP use.
   c. Orthopedic surgery.
   d. Use of perioperative opioids.

   The correct answer is d.

   The respiratory depressant effect of opioids may lead to increased respiratory complications and should be used with caution. The role of regional anesthetic techniques may be advantageous compared to GA, allowing for avoidance of upper airway instrumentation and neuromuscular blocking medications, effective pain management, reduced opioid consumption, and significant suppression of the systemic stress response.[28]

6. SAMBA recommends that patients with known OSA are appropriate for ambulatory surgery if

   a. They receive medical clearance from their primary care doctor or pulmonologist.
   b. They have lost weight and feel their OSA symptoms have improved.
   c. They are compliant with CPAP use and are able to do so in the postoperative period.
   d. They live with someone who could observe their respiratory patterns.

   The correct answer is c.

   SAMBA has published a consensus statement on preoperative selection of adult patients with OSA which specifically addresses the candidacy of OSA patients for ambulatory surgery. They determined that patients with a known diagnosis of OSA with medically optimized comorbid conditions can be considered for ambulatory surgery if they are able to use CPAP in the postoperative period.[31]

7. Potential benefits of regional anesthesia over GA in patients with OSA include

   a. Avoiding instrumentation of the airway, such as intubation.
   b. Eliminating the need for opioids for pain management.
   c. Negating the need for difficult airway equipment and supplies.
   d. Ability to perform the surgery at an ASC rather than in a hospital setting.

   The correct answer is a.

   If GA is employed, the patient should be fully awake, responding to commands, and able to demonstrate full protection of their airway prior to extubation. Patients should be fully reversed from neuromuscular blockade. Extubation should be performed in the lateral or semi-upright position if possible. Regional anesthesia should be employed when possible to reduce reliance on GA and decrease or eliminate the need for systemic opioids.[30]

8. The ASA Task Force on Perioperative Management of Obstructive Sleep Apnea recommends the following consideration to decrease the risk of perioperative complications in patients who have OSA:

   a. Administer deep sedation rather than GA.
   b. The preferred airway device is an LMA rather than an ETT.
   c. Discharge patients when they demonstrate appropriate use of their CPAP machine.
   d. Admit patients for overnight monitoring if they do not meet PACU discharge criteria.

   The correct answer is d.

   Patients should be advised to bring their CPAP machine for use in the postoperative period. Patients with OSA may require extended monitoring in the postoperative period due to higher risk of airway obstruction and central respiratory depression. Patients with severe sleep apnea may need to be admitted for overnight monitoring if they do not meet PACU discharge criteria, especially if they are being discharged to an unmonitored setting.[30]

REFERENCES

1. Balk EM, Moorthy D, Obadan NO, et al. Diagnosis and treatment of obstructive sleep apnea in adults: Comparative effectiveness review no. 32. AHRQ publication no. 11-EHC052-EF. Agency for Health Care Research and Quality; July 2011.
2. Benjafield A, Ayas N, Eastwood P, et al. Estimation of the global prevalence and burden of obstructive sleep apnoea: A literature-based analysis. *Lancet Respir Med*. 2019;7. doi:10.1016/S2213-2600(19)30198-5.
3. Franklin KA, Lindberg E. Obstructive sleep apnea is a common disorder in the population a review on the epidemiology of sleep apnea. *J Thorac Dis*. 2015;7:1311–1322.
4. Nagappa M, Wong DT, Cozowicz C, Ramachandran SK, Memtsoudis SG, Chung F. Is obstructive sleep apnea associated with difficult airway? Evidence from a systematic review and meta-analysis of prospective and retrospective cohort studies. *PLoS One*. 2018 Oct 4;13(10):e0204904. doi:10.1371/journal.pone.0204904. PMID: 30286122; PMCID: PMC6171874
5. Gupta RM, Parvizi J, Hanssen AD, Gay PC. Postoperative complications in patients with obstructive sleep apnea syndrome undergoing hip or knee replacement: A case-control study. *Mayo Clin Proc*. 2001;76:897–905.
6. Dempsey JA, Veasey SC, Morgan BJ, O'Donnell CP. Pathophysiology of sleep apnea [published correction appears in *Physiol Rev*. 2010 Apr;90(2):797–798]. *Physiol Rev*. 2010;90(1):47–112. doi:10.1152/physrev.00043.2008
7. Schwab RJ, Pasirstein M, Pierson R, et al. Identification of upper airway anatomic risk factors for obstructive sleep apnea with volumetric magnetic resonance imaging. *Am J Respir Crit Care Med*. 2003 Sep 1;168(5):522–530. doi:10.1164/rccm.200208-866OC. Epub 2003 May 13. PMID: 12746251.
8. Soultan Z, Wadowski S, Rao M, Kravath RE. Effect of treating obstructive sleep apnea by tonsillectomy and/or adenoidectomy on obesity in children. *Arch Pediatr Adolesc Med*. 1999;153(1):33–37. doi:10.1001/archpedi.153.1.33
9. Redline S, Tishler PV, Tosteson TD, et al. The familial aggregation of obstructive sleep apnea. *Am J Respir Crit Care Med*. 1995 Mar;151(3 Pt 1):682–687. doi:10.1164/ajrccm/151.3_Pt_1.682. PMID: 7881656
10. Kessler R, Chaouat A, Schinkewitch P, Faller M, Casel S, Krieger J, Weitzenblum E. The obesity-hypoventilation syndrome revisited: A prospective study of 34 consecutive cases. *Chest*. 2001;120:369–376.
11. Edmond H, Chau L, Lam D, et al. Obesity hypoventilation syndrome: A review of epidemiology, pathophysiology, and perioperative considerations. *Anesthesiology*. 2012;117:188–205. doi:https://doi.org/10.1097/ALN.0b013e31825add60
12. Chung F, Yegneswaran B, Liao P, et al. STOP questionnaire: A tool to screen patients for obstructive sleep apnea. *Anesthesiology*. 2008 May;108(5):812–821. doi:10.1097/ALN.0b013e31816d83e4. PMID: 18431116
13. Chung F, Subramanyam R, Liao P, Sasaki E, Shapiro C, Sun Y. High STOP-Bang score indicates a high probability of obstructive sleep apnoea. *Br J Anaesth*. 2012;108(5):768–775. doi:10.1093/bja/aes022
14. Nagappa M, Liao P, Wong J, et al. Validation of the STOP-Bang questionnaire as a screening tool for obstructive sleep apnea among different populations: A systematic review and meta-analysis. *PLoS One*. 2015 Dec 14;10(12):e0143697. doi:10.1371/journal.pone.0143697. PMID: 26658438; PMCID: PMC4678295
15. Boynton G, Vahabzadeh A, Hammoud S, Ruzicka DL, Chervin RD. Validation of the STOP-BANG questionnaire among patients referred for suspected obstructive sleep apnea. *J Sleep Disord Treat Care*. 2013 Sep 23;2(4):10.4172/2325-9639.1000121. doi:10.4172/2325-9639.1000121. PMID: 24800262; PMCID: PMC4008971
16. Urman RD, Chung F, Gan TJ. Obstructive sleep apnea and ambulatory surgery: Who is truly at risk? *Anesth Analg*. 2019 Aug;129(2):327–329. doi:10.1213/ANE.0000000000004217
17. Epstein LJ, Kristo D, Strollo PJ Jr, et al. Adult Obstructive Sleep Apnea Task Force of the American Academy of Sleep Medicine: Clinical guideline for the evaluation, management and long-term care of obstructive sleep apnea in adults. *J Clin Sleep Med*. 2009;5:263–276. PMID: 19960649
18. Iber C, Ancoli-Israel S, Chesson AL, Quan SF. *The AASM Manual for the Scoring of Sleep and Associated Events*. American Academy of Sleep Medicine; 2007.
19. Kapur VK, Auckley DH, Chowdhuri S, Kuhlmann DC, Mehra R, Ramar K, Harrod CG. Clinical practice guideline for diagnostic testing for adult obstructive sleep apnea: An American Academy of Sleep Medicine clinical practice guideline. *J Clin Sleep Med*. 2017;13(3):479. Epub 2017 Mar 15.

20. Kasai T, Floras JS, Bradley TD. Sleep apnea and cardiovascular disease: A bidirectional relationship. *Circulation*. 2012;126(12):1495–1510.
21. Marin JM, Carrizo SJ, Vicente E, Agusti AG. Long-term cardiovascular outcomes in men with obstructive sleep apnoea-hypopnoea with or without treatment with continuous positive airway pressure: An observational study. *Lancet*. 2005;365(9464):1046–1053.
22. Phillips CL, Grunstein RR, Darendeliler MA, et al. Health outcomes of continuous positive airway pressure versus oral appliance treatment for obstructive sleep apnea: A randomized controlled trial. *Am J Respir Crit Care Med*. 2013;187(8):879–887.
23. Iftikhar IH, Valentine CW, Bittencourt LR, et al. Effects of continuous positive airway pressure on blood pressure in patients with resistant hypertension and obstructive sleep apnea: A meta-analysis. *J Hypertens*. 2014;32(12):2341–2350.
24. Kaneko Y, Floras JS, Usui K, et al. Cardiovascular effects of continuous positive airway pressure in patients with heart failure and obstructive sleep apnea. *N Engl J Med*. 2003;348(13):1233–1241.
25. Joosten SA, Hamilton GS, Naughton MT. Impact of weight loss management in OSA. *Chest*. 2017 Jul;152(1):194–203. doi:10.1016/j.chest.2017.01.027. Epub 2017 Feb 6. PMID: 28185772
26. Hudgel DW, Patel SR, Ahasic AM, et al.; American Thoracic Society Assembly on Sleep and Respiratory Neurobiology. The role of weight management in the treatment of adult obstructive sleep apnea: An official American Thoracic Society Clinical practice guideline. *Am J Respir Crit Care Med*. 2018 Sep 15;198(6):e70–e87. doi:10.1164/rccm.201807-1326ST. PMID: 30215551
27. Dahlqvist J, Dahlqvist A, Marklund M, Berggren D, Stenlund H, Franklin KA. Physical findings in the upper airways related to obstructive sleep apnea in men and women. *Acta Otolaryngol*. 2007;127:623–630.
28. Memtsoudis SG, Stundner O, Rasul R. The impact of sleep apnea on postoperative utilization of resources and adverse outcomes. *Anesth Analg*. 2014;118:407–418.
29. Mokhlesi B, Hovda MD, Vekhter B, et al. Sleep-disordered breathing and postoperative outcomes after elective surgery: Analysis of the nationwide inpatient sample. *Chest*. 2013;144:903–914.
30. American Society of Anesthesiologists Task Force. Practice guidelines for the perioperative management of patients with obstructive sleep apnea: An updated report by the American Society of Anesthesiologists Task Force on Perioperative Management of Patients with Obstructive Sleep Apnea. *Anesthesiology* 2014;120:268–286. doi:https://doi.org/10.1097/ALN.0000000000000053
31. Joshi GP, Ankichetty SP, Gan TJ, Chung F. Society for Ambulatory Anesthesia consensus statement on preoperative selection of adult patients with obstructive sleep apnea scheduled for ambulatory surgery. *Anesth Analg*. 2012 Nov;115(5):1060–1068. doi:10.1213/ANE.0b013e318269cfd7. Epub 2012 Aug 10. PMID: 22886843
32. Abdelsattar ZM, Hendren S, Wong SL, Campbell DA Jr, Ramachandran SK. The impact of untreated obstructive sleep apnea on cardiopulmonary complications in general and vascular surgery: A cohort study. *Sleep*. 2015;38(8):1205–1210. Published 2015 Aug 1. doi:10.5665/sleep.4892
33. Fassbender P, Herbstreit F, Eikermann M, Teschler H, Peters J. Obstructive sleep apnea: A perioperative risk factor. *Dtsch Arztebl Int*. 2016 Aug;113(31–32):524.
34. Young T, Skatrud J, Peppard PE. Risk factors for obstructive sleep apnea in adults. *JAMA*. 2004;291:2013–2016.
35. Amra B, Rahmati B, Soltaninejad F, Feizi A. Screening questionnaires for obstructive sleep apnea: An updated systematic review. *Oman Med J*. 2018 May;33(3):184–192.
36. Epstein LJ, Kristo D, Strollo PJ Jr, et al. Clinical guideline for the evaluation, management, and long-term care of obstructive sleep apnea in adults. *J Clin Sleep Med*. 2010 Jun 15;5(3):263–276.

20.

COVID-19

Robert Fong

STEM CASE AND KEY QUESTIONS

The 2020 SARS-CoV-2 (COVID-19) global pandemic[1] produced dramatic upheavals in healthcare delivery systems, forcing many areas of medical care provision including surgery to be put on hold in the early stages as limited resources were devoted to the care of those infected. While hospitals have largely adapted their processes to safely resume operations and surgical volumes in many healthcare systems have returned to pre-pandemic levels, increasing numbers of surgical candidates who are either newly infected with or have had a history of COVID-19 infection present a new challenge to the field of perioperative medicine. SARS-CoV-2 has the potential to affect virtually every organ system in the acute phase, engendering a spectrum of illness ranging from completely asymptomatic to critically ill and even fatal. It has been well documented that undergoing surgery in the context of active infection with SARS-CoV-2 is a risky proposition,[2] with significantly increased perioperative morbidity and mortality, as well as engendering risk of exposure to perioperative providers and staff. Additionally, many in the recovery phase of COVID-19 illness have been shown to have lasting effects and disability months after initial infection,[3] with potential implications for long-term perioperative risk.

A 66-year-old African American woman presents for a remote telemedicine visit to the anesthesia preoperative clinic, referred by colorectal surgery. At the start of the interview, the patient says "I am having cancer surgery next week and I just tested positive for COVID." Review of the electronic medical record prior to the visit reveals that the patient was just diagnosed with T3N1M0 colon cancer, discovered during colonoscopy for anemia and unexplained 15-pound weight loss over the past 6 months. Her history is significant for well-controlled hypertension treated with hydrochlorothiazide and lisinopril. She has a BMI of 39 kg/m^2, and vital signs at her last in person hospital encounter 1 week ago were unremarkable. Bloods drawn during that encounter are only significant for a hemoglobin of 9.6 mg/dL, decreased from 12.1 mg/dL 6 months prior, and a serum creatinine of 1.3 mg/dL The patient has thus far elected not to receive vaccination for COVID.

What tests are available for detection of COVID-19 infection, and what are their performance characteristics?

Several testing modalities exist for the detection of SARS-CoV-2 infection. Reverse transcriptase polymerase chain reaction (RT-PCR) methods aimed at detecting viral nucleic acid in respiratory samples, such as nasal swabs or bronchial aspirates are considered the diagnostic gold standard.[4] Saliva-based nucleic amplification tests (NAAT) have also become available and have been shown to have similar diagnostic accuracy to nasopharyngeal swab NAAT testing.[5] Based on systematic reviews, 70% sensitivity and 95% specificity are reasonable lower-limit estimates of the performance of nucleic acid-based detection methods.[6] The ability to detect active infection with these techniques depends on the source and quality of specimen collection and the stage of disease and degree of viral replication and clearance. For example, samples obtained by broncho-alveolar lavage have the highest diagnostic yield followed in order by sputum samples, nasal swabs, and throat swabs.[7,8]

Antigen-based tests are immunological assays designed to detect specific viral antigens and thus identify active infection. They are approved for analysis of samples obtained by nasopharyngeal or nasal swabbing, which are placed directly into an extraction reagent and are capable of returning results within 15–30 minutes. These tests are relatively inexpensive and are often performed in a point-of-care format. While their specificity approaches that of NAAT's when performed correctly, their sensitivity tends to be lower[9] in part due inability to detect low antigen levels before symptom onset or later in the course of infection when viral copy number decreases.

Serological antibody testing has also been developed aimed at identifying prior infection. As these tests are not useful for diagnosing active infection, they will not be discussed further. The performance characteristics by manufacturer of the myriad NAAT, antigen, and antibody tests can be found on the US Food and Drug Administration (FDA)'s list of in vitro diagnostics Emergency Use Authorizations.[10]

The patient states that she went to a drive-up testing center 2 days prior after she learned that her son, who had visited 5 days ago, had since tested positive for COVID-19 after developing flu-like symptoms. She describes having her nose swabbed and getting her positive result within an hour while she waited. She does not recall the specific name of the test she was administered and has misplaced the hard copy of her test result she was given. She currently endorses no new symptomatology and states she feels at her baseline level of health.

Should this patient receive a repeat confirmatory PCR test administered at your medical center?

The patient's test result was very likely obtained from an antigen-based immunoassay. Based on the performance characteristics described above, the high specificity of these tests renders a positive result extremely compelling. False-positive tests are nevertheless possible and more likely in areas where disease prevalence is lower. Bayesian decision heuristics commonly employed in medical decision-making require consideration of pretest probability and testing characteristics to compute a post-test probability of disease to inform further action. To this end, a group at the Cleveland clinic has developed a quantitative risk prediction model using a development cohort of more than 11,000 patients of whom approximately 7% tested positive for COVID and tested it on a validation group of more than 2,200 patients of whom close to 300 tested positive.[11] This calculator, which includes cancer as a known risk factor, is freely available at https://riskcalc.org/COVID19. The Centers for Disease Control and Prevention (CDC) provides a useful qualitative framework for aiding decision-making regarding ordering confirmatory NAAT testing after antigen testing.[12] They group patients into low-, intermediate-, and high-risk groups (see Figure 20.1) based on symptomatology and known exposure to COVID-19.

As this patient is currently asymptomatic but had a known exposure to her son, she is in the intermediate-risk category, for which the CDC recommends confirmatory testing with NAAT. Additionally, you enter your patient's data into the online COVID-19 risk calculator, which returns a pre-test probability of 20%. The test positivity rate reported for your local area has been holding steady at about 8%. As you do not know the manufacturer of the test she received, you use an estimate of sensitivity (56%) and specificity (99%) reported by the Infectious Disease Society of America (IDSA) and the CDC as an average over many antigen tests studied[13] and compute a post-test probability of 93%. Because critical management decisions regarding your patient's cancer care hinge on her COVID infection status, you order a confirmatory PCR test at your medical center, which she comes in to take later that afternoon.

What are the most common symptoms of COVID infection? Are they different among cancer patients?

Fever, dry cough, and fatigue have been identified as the most common symptoms of COVID-19 infection in cancer patients. Other common symptoms include dyspnea, rigors, myalgias, headaches, and loss of taste or smell. This is very similar to symptomatology of those who do not have cancer, although dyspnea can be more severe, particularly in those with lung malignancies.[14]

The next morning you are informed that your patient's confirmatory COVID test returned a positive result. You contact the patient to inform her, and she reports developing a cough as well as feeling feverish and fatigued overnight. You inform her that in light of her active COVID-19 infection, you will need to discuss the timing of her planned operation with her surgical team.

Your patient, alarmed at the prospect of postponing her cancer surgery, asks why delaying the operation would even be under consideration. How do you reply?

Accumulated evidence makes it quite clear that undergoing surgery in the context of active COVID infection places an individual at significantly elevated risk for morbidity and mortality, particularly among those who are unvaccinated. The *Lancet* reported the first large, international multicenter cohort study of more than 1,100 surgical patients who tested positive for SARS-CoV-2 within 7 days of or 30 days after surgery.[15] Approximately one-quarter of the surgeries were elective in this study, which reported a 23.8% 30-day mortality and pulmonary complications in 51.2%. Of those who developed pulmonary complications, 38% died within 30 days.

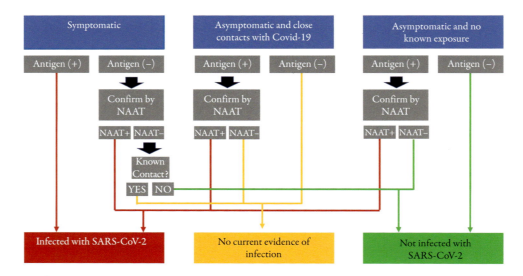

Figure 20.1 Antigen testing algorithm.
Adapted from Interim Guidance for Antigen Testing for SARS-CoV-2. Centers for Disease Control and Prevention (CDC). https://www.cdc.gov/coronavirus/2019-ncov/lab/resources/antigen-tests-guidelines.html

Thirty-day mortality was found to be associated with male gender, age older than 70, American Society of Anesthesiologists (ASA) grades 3–5, malignant versus benign or obstetric diagnosis, emergency versus elective surgery, and major versus minor surgery. A subsequent meta-analysis encompassing more than 2,900 patients confirmed a 30-day high mortality among COVID positive surgical patients of 20% and also reported a postoperative ICU admission rate of 15%.[16]

You explain to the patient that having surgery while actively ill with COVID engenders significantly elevated perioperative risk. You reassure her that you will have a thoughtful interdisciplinary discussion with her surgeons and cancer care team to carefully weigh the risks and benefits of delaying her operation and agree on the duration of that delay.

Do patients with cancer have increased morbidity and mortality from COVID-19 infection?

Patients with cancer have been found to be more significantly likely to contract SARS-CoV-2, possibly as a consequence of immune dysregulation.[17] Conflicting studies regarding the severity of COVID infection in cancer patients abound in the literature. Some report increased mortality and likelihood of ICU admission in those with cancer[18,19] while a more limited number report similar outcomes of COVID-19 infection between those with cancer and those without.[20] Hematologic[21] and lung malignancies[22] have been identified specifically as portending worse outcomes and severe illness in COVID infection, likely the consequence of immune dysregulation in the former case and decreased underlying pulmonary function secondary to associated comorbidities like chronic obstructive pulmonary disease (COPD) and smoking history as well as immunosuppressive cancer treatment regimens in the latter. A recent study conducted in Louisiana compared more than 300 COVID-positive patients diagnosed with cancer over 2 months to more than 4,800 without cancer.[23] After controlling for age, race, sex, and comorbidities, those with cancer were still more likely to die than those without (odds ratio [OR] 2.10; 95% confidence interval [CI] 1.44, 2.87). Multivariate analysis revealed higher mortality with age older than 65 years, male gender, chronic kidney disease, obesity, active or progressive cancer, and recent anticancer therapy.

Concerned about your patient's prognosis in light of her active cancer, older age, hypertension, obesity, and renal dysfunction you conclude the call by advising her regarding warning signs and symptoms that should prompt her to seek emergency medical care including worsening dyspnea, chest pain, mental status changes, or neurological symptoms.

Do guidelines exist regarding timing of surgery after COVID-19 infection?

The ASA and the Anesthesia Patient Safety Foundation (APSF) have issued guidelines regarding the timing of nonurgent surgery after confirmed COVID-19 infection.[24] Recommended waiting periods were created to serve the dual goals of ensuring that the patient is no longer a viral transmission risk as well as minimizing postoperative complications. With respect to the former goal, providers are advised to follow a time- and symptom-based approach in which patients are deemed no longer infectious when symptoms have improved, 24 hours have passed since the last fever without the use of antipyretics, and a defined interval has passed since the first appearance of symptoms or since the recording of a positive test result in those who are asymptomatic. The duration of this interval is 10 days for those who are asymptomatic or experienced mild illness, defined as those who do not develop pneumonia or an oxygen requirement, and 10–20 days for those who suffered severe or critical illness. These intervals reflect the time after symptom onset beyond which replication-competent virus can no longer be detected in these groups.

With regard to suggested waiting periods to minimize perioperative risk, recommendations were drawn from data showing increased perioperative pulmonary complications within the first 4 weeks of infection,[25] prolonged pulmonary dysfunction out to 3 months after recovering from acute respiratory distress syndrome (ARDS),[26] and diabetes as a significant risk factor for severe illness and hospitalization.[27] Recommended waiting periods are

- 4 weeks for a patient who did not experience respiratory symptoms.
- 6 weeks for a patient who had respiratory symptoms but did not require hospitalization.
- 8–10 weeks for a symptomatic patient who is diabetic, immunocompromised, or hospitalized.
- 12 weeks for a patient who was in the ICU due to COVID-19 infection

Subsequent to these initial recommendations, a multicenter, international prospective cohort study of more than 140,000 surgical patients, of whom more than 3,100 tested positive for SARS-CoV-2, was reported.[28] Using logistic regression models to calculate adjusted 30-day mortality stratified by time intervals after COVID-19 diagnosis, the study found that mortality returns to the COVID-negative baseline after 7 weeks for those who have recovered from a symptomatic perspective but remains elevated for those with persistent symptomatology. The ASA/APSF timing guidelines were updated in February 2022 to recommend that "elective surgery should be delayed for 7 weeks after a SARS-CoV-2 infection in *unvaccinated* patients that are asymptomatic at the time of surgery."[29]

The June 2023 update advises against elective surgery within 2 weeks of diagnosis. Between 2 and 7 weeks, risk-benefit considerations should include risks of delaying, comorbidities, complexity of surgery, and severity and status of infection.[29]

A nationwide analysis of 938 COVID-positive patients identified in a Veteran's Affairs registry reported 90-day mortality compared to procedure-matched COVID-negative controls and found an increased mortality in successive 2-week post-COVID positive intervals out to 9 weeks.[30] A retrospective cohort study of more than 220,000 patients that grouped them into different time windows after COVID diagnosis found that fully vaccinated patients did not manifest significantly elevated risk for postoperative complications.[31] A recent prospective study in 41 French centers of 4,928 patients with a better than 90% vaccination rate, of whom 705 had preoperative Omicron-dominant COVID infection, demonstrated no increase in the incidence of postoperative respiratory complications if the patients were asymptomatic on the day of surgery.[32] Taken together, these studies suggest that the decision regarding surgical timing after COVID positivity should consider vaccination status and symptomatic severity and weigh the potential risks of postoperative complications against morbidity engendered by delaying surgery rather than dogmatically adhering to fixed time intervals.

Given that the patient is unvaccinated and currently symptomatic, you recommend a 7- to 8-week waiting period from the point of view of perioperative risk when you confer with the surgical team, acknowledging that she is still in the early stages of her COVID infection so that, if her illness were to become more severe or require hospitalization, that recommended wait time would increase. Taking this under advisement, the surgical team plans to discuss the surgical and oncologic treatment plan at their remote tumor board meeting the next day and asks that you join on the conference call if you are available.

Are there decision tools to help assess the risks inherent in delaying cancer surgery?

Cancer treatment has been an area of particular concern throughout the pandemic as delays in care have raised the specter of disease progression and worsened outcomes.[33] Many oncological subspecialties have reevaluated their treatment paradigms to manage the challenges of surgical timing as well as the risks inherent in immunosuppressed patients receiving chemotherapy requiring repeat in-person treatment visits with the potential for viral exposure. Fortunately, as many healthcare systems resume near-normal operations and surgical capacity is restored, the need to delay cancer surgeries due to resource availability has diminished significantly. Nevertheless, the problem of surgical timing for cancer patients who contract COVID-19 will persist for some time.[34] Throughout the pandemic, studies have appeared in the literature that have attempted to quantify the risks and downstream consequences of delaying cancer care.[35,36] While an exhaustive review of this area is falls well beyond the scope of the present discussion, one particular analysis by Turaga et al.[37] that seeks to quantify the impact of delaying cancer surgery will be highlighted here as an example of a useful tool to guide decision-making. Based on computing hazard ratios for mortality and tumor progression beyond current median wait times for cancer surgery, this modeling study draws data from the National Cancer Database to describe a "safe postponement period" (SPP) for individual cancer types, both in the context of a surgery-first approach as well as in the context of neoadjuvant chemotherapy preceding surgery. For example, with respect to colon cancer, the SPP for colon cancer is 5 weeks from diagnosis for a surgery first approach, and 24 weeks from diagnosis for surgery after chemotherapy.

At the multidisciplinary tumor board remote meeting, you voice your concerns regarding increased perioperative risk to this patient in the context of her active and symptomatic COVID infection and voice your recommendation of a 7-week waiting period. The possibility of changing the treatment approach to a chemotherapy-first strategy was considered,[38] as they had taken this approach for several patients early in the pandemic when the medical center had a moratorium on all but urgent and emergent surgeries. The oncology team points out that the safety of receiving chemotherapy in the context of active COVID-19 infection has not been definitively established. Some studies reported an increase in mortality for COVID-positive patients receiving chemotherapy,[39–41] while others have not, suggesting instead that the death rates for those with cancer and COVID-19 are driven by advanced age, male gender, and noncancer comorbidities.[42–44] However, given the particularly myelosuppressive effects of the FOLFOX regimen they would consider for this patient, starting chemotherapy in the context of active COVID infection is deemed too high risk. After continued deliberation, you and those in attendance agree to schedule her operation in 4 weeks, at which time the patient will be no longer infectious and at the limit of the SPP for her cancer. You request that the patient return to preoperative clinic in 3 weeks to evaluate her recovery and for thorough preoperative evaluation and risk assessment.

Should this patient undergo repeat PCR testing prior to her scheduled surgery in 4 weeks?

Persistent positive tests have been reported out to 90 days after initial infection,[45] and the CDC currently does not recommend repeat testing within that window for those who are asymptomatic or have recovered to avoid subjecting patients to unnecessary quarantine restrictions. These repeat positive tests are thought to be due in the vast majority of cases to residual but not replication-competent viral particles.[46,47] For those who develop new symptoms, however, repeat testing may be considered.

A joint statement put forth by the ASA and APSF in December 2022 recommended against routine preoperative COVID testing of asymptomatic patients,[48] and, as such, the policy at your medical center, which required a SARS-CoV-2 test result within 72 hours of all scheduled nonurgent or emergent operating room cases without exception, was recently amended. As long as the patient remains asymptomatic up to the time of her rescheduled surgery she will not require retesting.

How do you plan to approach preoperative assessment when the patient presents to clinic? What tests will you order?

Many individuals will experience persistent effects of COVID-19 long after initial infection. Among those with potential implications for perioperative risk include diminished lung function, new arrhythmias or heart failure, decreased renal function, and persistent inflammation.[3] Thus the goal of preoperative assessment is to evaluate the completeness of recovery from infection and return to pre-COVID baseline health and function. Given the recency of the pandemic, evidence-based recommendations derived from large prospective studies for the preoperative evaluation and testing of surgical candidates who are recovering or have recovered from COVID-19 illness are not yet available. Thus, a reasonable initial approach is to screen for those long-term effects that have been commonly observed in observational studies of those who have recovered from COVID-19 infection, particularly those that are likely to impact perioperative risk.

When the patient presents to clinic, you plan to conduct a thorough history and physical examination aimed at identifying any new or persistent symptomatology in the aftermath of this patient's COVID-19 infection. You plan to assess her activity tolerance using a 6-minute walk test, screen for potential arrhythmias with a preoperative ECG, and send laboratory testing to screen for renal dysfunction, coagulopathy, persistent inflammation, and cardiac dysfunction. These will include basic metabolic panel (BMP), CBC, coagulation studies, fibrinogen, d-dimer, NT-pro-BNP, troponin (cTn), ferritin, and LDH. The decision to order additional testing such as chest x-ray or transthoracic echocardiogram (TTE) will be driven by abnormalities revealed by history, physical exam, or biomarker values.

Three days later, you learn that your patient has been admitted to the ICU with worsening dyspnea and fatigue, as well as acute-onset the day prior of abdominal pain and bloating, vomiting, and inability to tolerate oral intake. On admission, she was found to be febrile to 38.4°C, tachycardic with a heart rate of 115, mildly hypotensive compared to her baseline with a blood pressure of 102/64, and mildly tachypneic. She is currently maintaining oxygen saturations in the low 90s with the help of supplemental oxygen by facemask. Admission labs are remarkable for a hemoglobin of 8.4 mg/dL, mild leukopenia, and a serum creatinine of 1.5 mg/dL. Chest computed tomography (CT) scan reveals bilateral ground-glass opacities concentrated in the lower lobes of the lungs in a peripheral distribution intermixed with some areas of focal consolidation, solidifying a diagnosis of COVID-19 pneumonia.[49] Abdominal CT obtained by the consulting surgical service is consistent with her clinical presentation of complete large bowel obstruction with stricturing observed at the site of her tumor, and the surgical team recommends urgent surgery within the next 12 hours.

What are the most important perioperative considerations given the current state of the patient?

This patient is at extremely high risk, as outlined above, for perioperative morbidity and mortality due to her active, symptomatic SARS-CoV-2 infection, and evolving COVID pneumonia requiring supplemental oxygen support. Additionally, emergency surgery for cancer-related bowel obstruction carries an elevated risk of surgical morbidity and mortality on its own.[50] The patient is anemic, likely due to ongoing blood loss from her colon cancer, and is developing acute kidney injury likely secondary to dehydration but also possibly as a result of her COVID-19 infection. The patient will require general endotracheal anesthesia with a rapid-sequence induction for any operative procedure given her risk of aspiration secondary to her obstructive pathology. Patients hospitalized with active COVID infection tend to have reduced pulmonary reserve, and she will likely experience an accelerated decline in oxygen saturation upon induction. Additionally, these patients can be particularly prone to hypotension during induction,[51] and close hemodynamic monitoring will be indicated. This patient is actively infectious, and protection of perioperative providers and staff from exposure will be of paramount importance, particularly during aerosolizing procedures such as airway instrumentation. Specific recommendations for mitigating exposure risk will be reviewed below but broadly involve appropriate procedural site selection to ensure the availability of negative-pressure containment, judicious use of proper personal protective equipment (PPE), procedural modifications during airway management, and fastidious hand hygiene and equipment decontamination.

An interdisciplinary meeting is held with representatives of the surgical, anesthesia, and critical care teams in attendance to discuss the optimal management of the patient in this high-risk clinical context. After consideration of the significant risks inherent in performing urgent surgery given her current state of health, the decision is made to opt for endoscopic placement of a self-expandable metal stent (SEMS) to relieve the obstruction, a procedure sometimes used as a bridge until definitive surgical resection,[52] particularly for patients who are at high risk for perioperative mortality. The surgical team explains that successful stent deployment would be a temporizing measure that would allow time for the patient's condition and perioperative risk profile to improve as well increase the likelihood of a successful laparoscopic resection. Recent analysis has shown that while surgery within 7 days of stenting results in the highest disease-free and overall survival, the decrement in these primary outcomes becomes much more significant after a 14-day interval, particularly for stage III cancers.[53] Therefore, balancing the significant perioperative risk to the patient in her current state of critical illness against worsened downstream oncologic outcome of waiting too long to operate, a plan is made to perform laparoscopic resection in 2 weeks assuming successful stent placement. Acknowledging the possibility that the patient's clinical trajectory with respect to COVID infection could worsen rather than improve in that interval, all are nevertheless in agreement to proceed with this plan. The patient is scheduled as an urgent add-on case in the endoscopy suite for later in the day.

In the next few hours, what steps should be taken to optimize the patient for endoscopic stent placement? What tests or lab would you perform?

A nasogastric tube is placed in the ICU for decompressive purposes, IV access is obtained, and the patient is started on fluid resuscitation with crystalloid solution. An arterial line is placed for hemodynamic and blood gas monitoring. The first arterial blood gas drawn demonstrates a mild respiratory alkalosis with a pH of 7.48 and pCO_2 of 32, as well as a paO_2 of 70 on 15 L O_2 by non-rebreather facemask. A 12-lead ECG is obtained, significant only for sinus tachycardia. The intensive care team performs a bedside TTE and notes grossly normal biventricular function and no regional wall motion abnormalities. Coagulation labs including d-dimer and fibrinogen are sent and found to be within normal limits. A blood sample is sent for ABO verification and type and screen in anticipation of the possibility of transfusion during this admission. Procalcitonin is an inflammatory biomarker that has been shown to be associated with bacterial infection when its levels are elevated.[54] A procalcitonin level is ordered and is found to be less than 0.1 mcg/L. In light of this result and the observation of mild leukopenia, the likelihood of bacterial superinfection in this patient is deemed low, and antibiotic therapy is not initiated. After weighing the patient's risk of bleeding against the hypercoagulability risk engendered by COVID infection,[55] the decision is made to initiate prophylactic-dose heparin. Finally, driven by the results of the RECOVERY trial that showed a mortality benefit to patients hospitalized with COVID-19 who required supplemental oxygen or were mechanically ventilated of a dexamethasone course as compared to standard of care,[56] the ICU fellow suggested starting the patient on a course of dexamethasone. This suggestion was vetoed by the ICU attending who cited the results of the more recent COVIDICUS multicenter randomized control trial of 546 ICU patients with COVID hypoxic respiratory failure that demonstrated no difference in 60-day mortality for patients who received dexamethasone courses.[57]

After 8 hours, the endoscopy suite is ready to receive the patient, and she is transported directly into a procedural room that has been retrofitted early in the pandemic to have negative-pressure capability. All members of the care team and periprocedural staff are outfitted with PPE appropriate for airborne precautions. Immediately prior to induction, all present exit the procedural room with the exception of the two anesthesia providers managing the airway. After an extended period of spontaneously breathing pre-oxygenation by mask, rapid sequence induction with propofol and succinylcholine is followed by facile endotracheal tube placement using a video laryngoscope. Ten minutes later, the procedural team re-enters the room to begin the procedure. After induction and throughout the procedure, occasional IV boluses of phenylephrine are needed to support the patient's hemodynamics. Oxygen saturations of 89–92% are observed throughout the procedure on volume-controlled ventilation with 100% FiO_2, tidal volume of 6 cc/kg, and PEEP of 5 cm H_2O. After approximately 45 minutes, the stent is successfully deployed. At the conclusion of the procedure, the decision is made to keep the patient intubated for transport back to the ICU given the marginal oxygenation throughout the procedure.

After 4 days, the patient's oxygenation and general condition improve, and she is able to be extubated to high-flow nasal cannula. Her supplemental oxygen requirement gradually decreases over the next several days, and her renal function improves to near baseline with adequate urine output. With the colonic stent in place, she is able to tolerate a soft diet. After continued observation and clinical improvement, she undergoes successful laparoscopic hemicolectomy with anastomosis as planned 14 days after stent placement followed by uneventful recovery.

DISCUSSION

PANDEMIC COURSE

Since the first reports of the novel coronavirus, SARS-CoV-2, in December 2019 in Wuhan China,[58] more than 680 million people have been infected worldwide, of which more than 6.8 million have succumbed. As of the current writing, the United States accounts for a sixth of all reported cases with a death toll of greater than 1.1 million. In addition to the physical toll exacted on those who have contracted the virus, the global pandemic has had profound effects on mental health,[59] the economy,[60] and healthcare delivery systems.[61] As the rapid spread of the virus has strained hospital resources in many areas and increased the risk to patients and providers of in-person care, physicians have had to make difficult choices regarding prioritizing or delaying medical services. Surgical procedures are invasive, resource intensive, and potentially aerosolizing and as such have been particularly vulnerable to postponement or deferment. During the early months of the pandemic, many states issued moratoria on elective surgery in the face of limiting supplies of PPE and diversion of resources to treat critically ill COVID patients. A survey of 25 hospital systems across the United States revealed a 35% average decrease in surgical volume from March through July of 2020, during the height of the first pandemic wave as compared to the same time period in 2019.[62] In many locales, surgical volumes have since returned to pre-pandemic levels as testing and PPE have become more widely available and hospital systems have adapted new strategies and protocols to mitigate exposure risk and safely resume operations. In December 2020, Pfizer-BioNTech and Moderna released COVID-19 vaccines to the public, the accelerated development, production, and distribution of which were fueled in large part by Operation Warp Speed, a multibillion-dollar federal program.[63]

Multiple strains and variants with varying infectivity and severity profiles have emerged and proliferated differentially worldwide since the beginning of the pandemic. In the United States, Alpha was the first variant to emerge by the end of 2020 and caused more serious illness. The original vaccines released were effective against this variant, and, by spring of 2021, it was supplanted by the Delta variant, which caused more deadly disease in the unvaccinated and more effectively evaded vaccine-induced immunity. This prompted recommendations for the vaccinated to receive booster shots. By November of 2021, the Omicron variant quickly surpassed Delta in new cases due to its enhanced transmissibility, and its subvariants remain dominant in the United States as of this writing. Fortunately, these Omicron variants have been shown to cause milder disease.[64] By the end of 2021, estimates of infection and vaccination-induced immunity in the United States exceeded 95%, driving a significant decline in hospitalization and death rates. In May 2023, the CDC declared the termination of the COVID Public Health Emergency.[65]

Despite these promising developments, the new operational equilibria established by healthcare delivery systems have been metastable and fragile. New and more virulent strains have recently emerged against which the extant vaccines have questionable efficacy,[66] while growing reports of COVID-19 reinfection[67] call into question the durability of acquired immunity. Meanwhile, the resolve within many segments of the population to continue the preventative practices of masking, social distancing, and isolation has continued to erode.[68] Taken together these imminent threats maintain the ever-present specter of rapid disease resurgence with the potential to overwhelm the capacity of local healthcare delivery systems and force a renewed curtailing of elective procedures. Therefore, decisional algorithms that were developed early in the pandemic[69] to thoughtfully triage surgical candidates will continue to be necessary. In any event, as viral penetrance within the population continues to increase, there will be an increasing number of surgical candidates who present with either active or previous COVID-19 infection. In the former case, the question of appropriate timing of surgery relative to infection will require consideration of the patient's disease burden and perioperative risk, consequences of delaying surgery, exposure risk to healthcare providers, resource availability, disease trajectory in the local community, and any applicable municipal mandates. In cases of previous COVID-19 infection, an accurate assessment of perioperative risk that takes into account any long-term sequelae of viral infection as well as consequent efforts to optimize these patients with regard to their acquired comorbidities will be of paramount importance.

VIRAL BIOLOGY

Like the severe acute respiratory syndrome (SARS) and Middle East respiratory syndrome (MERS) outbreaks of 2002 and 2012, respectively, the pathogen responsible for the 2020 pandemic is a beta-coronavirus with a likely zoonotic origin.[70] Among the several structural proteins encoded by its single-stranded, positive-sense RNA genome, the heterotrimeric Spike (S) glycoprotein mediates host cell entry by binding to angiotensin converting enzyme 2 (ACE 2). After receptor binding, serine protease TMPRSS2 cleaves S protein to facilitate membrane fusion. Both ACE 2 and TMPRSS2 are expressed on respiratory epithelial cells, explaining the infectivity, pathogenesis, and tissue tropism of the virus. After virus internalization and uncoating, two long open reading frames of the viral RNA are immediately translated, producing polyproteins that are processed into individual nonstructural proteins that form the viral transcription and replication complex. After replication of the viral genome and expression of structural and capsid proteins, virions are assembled and extruded from the host cell by exocytosis. SARS-CoV-2 manifests numerous adaptations throughout its replicative cycle that facilitate evasion of host innate immune response. These include extensive glycosylation of S protein, genome RNA modification, creation of protected viral replication organelles within host cells, suppression of host interferon production, and expression of accessory proteins that interfere with innate immune processes.[71]

CLINICAL COURSE

The clinical course of COVID infection is critically dependent on the vaccination status of the patient as well as the particular viral strain or variant infecting the patient. Those who are vaccinated experience mostly asymptomatic to mild infection not requiring hospitalization, and the currently dominant Omicron variants produce milder disease with reduced long-term sequelae than the initial and previous variants. The available clinical data summarized below skew toward earlier viral variants infecting unvaccinated patients and should thus be interpreted as representing a "worst-case" baseline of COVID infection. That said, the continued prevalence of COVID infection in the population coupled with the continued rapid mutation of the virus leaves open the possibility of future strains that could cause more severe disease, manifest greater virulence and transmissibility, or evade current population immunity.

The incubation period of the virus has been reported to be within 14 days, although most of those infected who develop symptoms will do so within 4–5 days,[72] when viral replication is particularly active. Approximately one-third of individuals who are infected remain asymptomatic,[73] although cross-sectional surveys that have informed this estimate show wide variation and differing ranges of symptoms assessed. These asymptomatic individuals who may not be aware that they are infected have been a significant public health concern with respect to their potential role in disease spread. Among those who do manifest signs of infection, the most commonly reported symptoms include cough, myalgia, and headaches. Other symptoms reported include dyspnea, anosmia, sore throat, diarrhea, nausea, and vomiting.[74] Less commonly, some infected individuals have manifested conjunctivitis[75] or a number of varied dermatological findings including reddish-purple nodules on the digits that have been called "COVID toes."[76]

Symptomatic infection exhibits a wide range of severity. In a report of more than 44,000 infected patients from the Chinese Center for Disease Control and Prevention,[77] 81% exhibited mild symptoms, 14% experienced severe symptoms (defined as dyspnea, hypoxia, or greater than 50% lung involvement on imaging in the first 48 hours), and 5% became critically ill with respiratory failure, shock, or multiorgan dysfunction. The overall case fatality rate is estimated to be in the 0.5–1% range,[78] although the existence of undiagnosed fatal infections[79] as well as undiagnosed cases among the asymptomatic engender significant uncertainty in establishing the numerator and denominator used to arrive at this estimate. Mortality is significantly higher among hospitalized COVID patients and even higher among those requiring mechanical ventilation—as high as 25% and 60%, respectively, according to data from a New York City health system in the early stages of the pandemic.[27] Fortunately, increased resource availability and advances in care have dramatically increased survival among these critically ill patients,[80] although the improvement may be partially explained by the increase in numbers of younger, healthier individual contracting the virus.

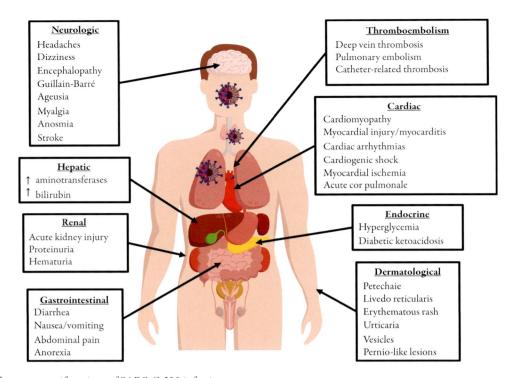

Figure 20.2 Extrapulmonary manifestations of SARS-CoV-2 infection.
Adapted from Gupta A, Madhavan MV, Sehgal K, et al. Extrapulmonary manifestations of COVID-19. *Nat Med*. Jul 2020;26(7):1017–1032.

Those who are admitted for COVID pneumonia develop dyspnea at a median of 5 days and are hospitalized at a median of 7 days after initial appearance of symptoms. This coincides with a period of immune activation and cytokine release after viral replication has subsided. In as many as 20% of those hospitalized, this can progress to ARDS. Up to 25% of hospitalized individuals will require mechanical ventilation.[81]

The most common extrapulmonary effects of SARS-CoV-2 infection have been observed in the cardiovascular system and include myocardial injury manifest as cardiac enzyme leak (seen in 20–30% of those hospitalized with COVID-19 and up to 55% of those with preexisting cardiovascular disease), cardiomyopathy, acute coronary syndrome, cardiogenic shock, acute cor pulmonale, and arrhythmias.[82] The etiology of these cardiac effects is likely multifactorial, a combination of inflammation, hypercoagulability, elevated catecholamines, and direct viral invasion of cardiac myocytes. Myocardial injury has been significantly associated with mortality in the acute phase of infection, even in those without prior cardiovascular disease. Data out of Wuhan, China reported arrhythmia in 17% of those hospitalized and 44% of those requiring ICU care.[83] New-onset atrial fibrillation has been the most commonly observed arrhythmia after sinus tachycardia, although heart block and ventricular arrhythmias have also been seen.[84]

SARS-CoV-2 has been shown to be neurotropic, and infection has been associated with a myriad of nervous system manifestations caused by a combination of direct viral effects, inflammation, and coagulopathy.[85] Encephalopathy has been the most common among these, reported in up to 7% of hospitalized patients and 69% of those requiring intensive care. Cerebrovascular disease has emerged as a serious complication, occurring in 2–6% of those hospitalized. Particularly alarming have been the reports of large-vessel stroke as a presenting symptom of COVID infection in some younger individuals.[86] Encephalitis and Guillain-Barré have been identified as inflammatory complications of viral infection in a small number of individuals. Notably, the presence and extent of these neurologic sequelae are often independent of the severity of respiratory symptoms. For an excellent and comprehensive review of these and other extrapulmonary complications of SARS-CoV-2 infection, the reader is referred to Gupta et al.[87] and Figure 20.2 adapted therefrom.

RISK FACTORS FOR SEVERE INFECTION

Older age and comorbidity burden have been overwhelmingly associated with increased severity of and mortality due to COVID-19. In multiple cohorts internationally, older patients have accounted for a disproportionate percentage of those hospitalized and critically ill.[77,81,88,89] Numerous studies confirm significantly increased mortality in older individuals, as high as 10–27% in those older than 85 years.[90–92] For example, in a 1-month period early in the pandemic, individuals older than 65 years accounted for more than 80% of COVID-related deaths in the United States.[93] Despite this heavy toll exacted by SARS-CoV-2 on the elderly, it is important to note that a significant number of younger individuals have succumbed to COVID-19 illness as well.

Individuals with comorbidities are much more likely to die from COVID-19 illness than those who have none—by a factor of 12, for example, reported in a study of 300,000 COVID-infected patients in the United States.[74] Among 355

Table 20.1 **ESTABLISHED RISK FACTORS FOR AND LABORATORY VALUES ASSOCIATED WITH SEVERE COVID-19 INFECTION**

ESTABLISHED RISK FACTORS	LABORATORY FEATURES	
Cancer	Abnormality	Possible threshold
Chronic kidney disease (CKD)	Elevations in:	
Chronic obstructive pulmonary disease (COPD)	D-dimer	>1,000 ng/mL (normal range: <500 ng/mL)
Down syndrome	CRP	>100 mg/L (normal range: <8.0 mg/L)
Immunocompromised state from solid organ transplant	LDH	>245 units/L (normal range: 110–210 units/L)
Obesity (BMI ≥30 kg/m^2)	Troponin	>2× the upper limit of normal (normal range for troponin T high sensitivity: females 0–9 ng/L; males 0–14 ng/L)
Pregnancy	Ferritin	>500 mcg/L (normal range: females 10–200 mcg/L; males 30–300 mcg/L)
Serious cardiovascular disease • Heart failure • Coronary artery disease (CAD) • Cardiomyopathies	CPK	>2× the upper limit of normal (normal range: 40–150 units/L)
Sickle cell disease	Decrease in:	
Smoking	Absolute lymphocyte count	<800/microl (normal range for age ≥21 years: 1,800–7,700/microl)
Type 2 diabetes mellitus		

Adapted from CDC. Coronavirus Disease 2019 (COVID-19): Who is at increased risk for severe illness? People of any age with underlying medical conditions. http://www.cdc.gov/coronavirus/2019-ncov/need-extra-precautions/people-with-medical-conditions.html; and Gandhi RT, et al. COVID-19: Clinical Features. https://www.uptodate.com/contents/covid-19-clinical-features

patients who died of COVID-19 in Italy, the mean number of their comorbidities was 2.7.[90] Table 20.1 reproduces a list of comorbidities associated with severe disease compiled by the CDC. Those who are elderly with multiple comorbidities are particularly vulnerable to severe and fatal disease, an unfortunate reality underlying the tragedy of the many who have died from viral outbreaks in nursing homes and long-term care facilities.[93]

Male gender[94,95] and depressed socioeconomic status have also been associated with severe illness and mortality. The healthcare disparities engendered by the latter are largely responsible for the poorer outcomes of COVID infection documented for Black, Hispanic, and South Asian individuals.[96–100] A number of laboratory abnormalities have been shown to correlate with severe illness and are summarized in Table 20.1.

LONG-TERM EFFECTS OF COVID

As the pandemic progresses, it has become increasingly apparent that many who have contracted SARS-CoV-2 and recovered from its acute effects suffer from lingering symptoms and long-term sequelae. As many as 80% of those who have had symptomatic infection experience the persistence for weeks to months of at least one of those symptoms. These individuals are often dubbed "COVID long haulers" and their lasting symptoms termed "long COVID syndrome."[101] Recognizing the scope of this problem, many healthcare systems have established post-COVID care clinics to manage these long-term effects.

A recent study by Huang and colleagues reported the follow-up out to 6 months of more than 1,700 patients who were hospitalized with SARS-CoV-2 in Wuhan China.[3] To date it represents the largest cohort study of post-COVID patients encompassing the longest duration of follow-up. Of those included in the analysis, 76% continued to endorse at least one symptom 6 months after initial infection, with fatigue and muscle weakness representing the most common persistent symptom, present in 63% of respondents. Sleeping difficulties were reported in 26% and anxiety and depression in 23%. Follow-up in this study also included 6-minute walk testing and blood draws for laboratory assays, as well as pulmonary function testing and chest CT for random samples of patients stratified by disease severity. Subject to the caveat that pre-COVID baselines were not available for most of the patients, 22–29% across severity scales performed less than the lower limit of normal in the 6-minute walk test and 22–56% manifested diffusion impairments during pulmonary function testing. Notably, 38% of those who were infected with SARS continue to have decreased diffusion capacity 15 years later, portending possibly permanent damage for many infected with COVID-19. The most common CT finding in

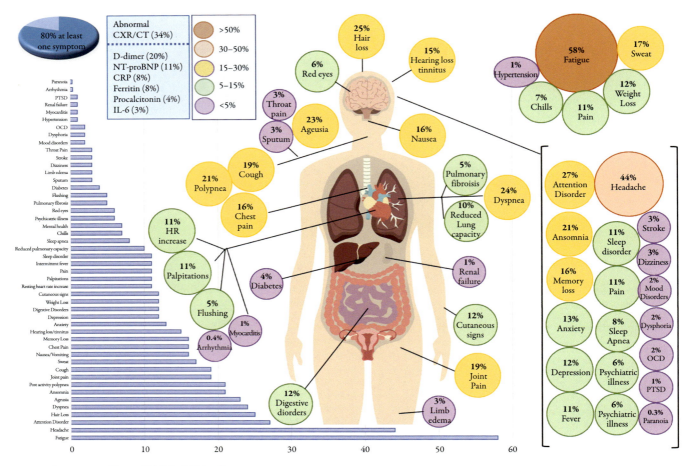

Figure 20.3 Long-term effects of SARS-CoV-2 infection.
Adapted from Lopez-Leon S, Wegman-Ostrosky T, Perelman C, et al. More than 50 long-term effects of COVID-19: A systematic review and meta-analysis. *medRxiv*. 2021 Jan 30.

the Huang study, corroborated by other radiological follow-up studies of post-COVID patients,[102] was pulmonary interstitial change, consistent with fibroblast proliferation in the convalescent phase of the disease. While only 4% of the patients in the study were critically ill in the ICU during their initial infection, data in the critical care literature document significant long-term disability in many who have survived ARDS or prolonged mechanical ventilation.[103]

A recent meta-analysis encompassing more than 47,000 patients and 15 studies largely corroborated this characterization of the lasting effects of SARS-CoV-2 infection and additionally identified a total of 50 long-term symptoms experienced by COVID-19 survivors.[104] Notable among these with regard to potential implications for future preoperative assessment include dyspnea (24%), chest pain (16%), palpitations (11%), new-onset diabetes (4%), sleep apnea (8%), and limb edema (3%). See Figure 20.3 for a complete list. The myriad long-term effects documented in this analysis highlight the capability of the virus to affect multiple organ systems as well as engender end organ effects that were not apparent during the initial phase of the illness. As a poignant illustration of this, Huang and colleagues noted a decline in estimated glomerular filtration rate in 13% of patients who did not develop acute kidney injury during their initial illness.[3]

A cohort study reported in the *Journal of the American Medical Association* (JAMA) of 100 patients recently recovered from COVID-19 has drawn attention to persistent cardiac effects, reporting 78% with cardiac involvement demonstrable by MRI and 60% with evidence of ongoing myocardial inflammation.[105] Significantly, these effects were found to be independent of preexisting conditions, illness severity in the acute phase acute, and the time from the original diagnosis. Arrhythmias have been shown to persist in a significant number of those who develop them in the acute phase of COVID-19 infection, but also to onset during the recovery phase in others.[84]

Lasting neurological effects have been a particularly debilitating feature for some COVID long haulers, likely the result of persistent neuroinflammation and direct neuronal damage. Headaches, abnormalities in taste and smell, tremors, and insomnia as well as memory, concentration, and cognitive impairments that have been characterized as "COVID fog" are among the numerous chronic manifestations that have been described.[106] Further characterization of these lasting health effects with respect to preexisting comorbidities and patient demographics, as well as continued follow-up over a longer time horizon will be necessary and informative in guiding long-term care of survivors. Nevertheless, it is already clear that, like its predecessors that have caused more limited disease outbreaks in years past, this coronavirus will leave many that it has infected with some degree of permanent disability.

PREOPERATIVE ASSESSMENT

During the early months of the pandemic, many healthcare systems halted elective surgeries due to limited supplies of PPE, diversion of resources to care for rapidly growing numbers of the critically ill, and mitigation of infectious risk to patients and perioperative care providers. As hospitals have adapted their operations to the COVID landscape and surgical volumes have recovered to pre-pandemic levels despite the continued spread of the virus, an increasing number of surgical candidates will present who are either newly infected with COVID or have recovered from previous COVID infection. Given the wide spectrum of severity of initial infection, the increased perioperative risk to patients and providers of having surgery in the acute phase of viral infection, and the incidence of long-term multiorgan effects that can linger after recovery, surgical timing, preoperative assessment, and optimization of these patients require a thoughtful and multidisciplinary approach. With regard to those surgical candidates who test positive for COVID-19 infection, the current recommendations with regard to surgical timing and the principles that underlie them have been discussed above.

When the decision is ultimately reached regarding timing of surgery for a patient who has had COVID, what are the important preoperative considerations that need to be taken into account to optimize the patient's outcome? Evidence to inform a systematic approach to preoperative assessment of surgical candidates who have had COVID has thus far been limited. Within this background of uncertainty, a report from the Oregon Health and Science University offers the first and most systematic published guidance in this regard.[107] The product of multidisciplinary collaboration among perioperative stakeholders within the organization including surgery, anesthesiology, and hospital administration, their protocol adopts a holistic framework that incorporates current understanding of the effects, both short- and long-term, of viral infection as well as perioperative risk and outcomes of those infected. A comprehensive evaluation in the anesthesia preoperative clinic serves as the cornerstone of the approach.

The authors draw analogies to recovery from other medical events including upper respiratory infections, myocardial infarction, and stroke to guide surgical timing in those who have tested positive. Those who have asymptomatic infection are advised to wait a minimum of 4 weeks before having surgery, while those who are symptomatic at least 6–8 weeks. No specific recommendations are provided regarding those who were critically ill, although the implication is that thorough history and examination will be conducted to assess whether patients who have experienced any level of illness severity have returned to their pre-COVID baseline health and functioning. These intervals are consistent with those recommended by the ASA and APSF outlined above. Recommendations are targeted toward cardiopulmonary assessment, evaluation of coagulation and nutrition, and testing for markers of inflammation and are stratified by the severity of initial illness and the nature of the intended surgery. The specific protocol for testing is summarized in Table 20.2.

Table 20.2 **PROTOCOL FOR THE PREOPERATIVE ASSESSMENT OF COVID-19 SURVIVORS, STRATIFIED BY SEVERITY OF ILLNESS AND NATURE OF PLANNED PROCEDURE**

STEP/TEST	MINOR PROCEDURES/ WITHOUT GENERAL ANESTHESIA ASYMPTOMATIC	SYMPTOMATIC	MAJOR PROCEDURES ASYMPTOMATIC	SYMPTOMATIC
CXR	No, if pulmonary exam and O₂ saturation normal	No, if pulmonary exam and O₂ sat normal	Yes	Yes
ECG	Yes	Yes	Yes	Yes
Echo	No, if cardiac exam and vitals normal	No, if cardiac exam, NT-pro-BNP and vitals normal	No, if cardiac exam, NT-pro-BNP and vitals normal	Determined by H&P
CMP	Yes	Yes	Yes	Yes
CBC	Yes	Yes	Yes	Yes
PTT	No	Consider based on severity of illness	Yes	Yes
D-dimer	No	Yes	Yes	Yes
Fibrinogen	No	Consider based on severity of illness	Yes	Yes
NT-pro-BNP	No	Yes	Yes	Yes
LDH, ferritin, prealbumin	No	Consider based on severity of illness	No	Consider based on severity of illness

Adapted from Bui N, et al.[107]

The approach to ordering testing is largely driven by findings from history and physical exam and additionally informed by patient- and procedure-specific risk, consistent with current principles of preoperative assessment in other contexts. For example, imaging by chest x-ray is indicated by persistence of pulmonary symptoms, abnormalities found on pulmonary exam. or oxygen saturation measurement, or in the case of major surgical procedures or those requiring general anesthesia. While many post-COVID patients are likely to manifest long-term decrements in diffusing capacity for carbon monoxide (DLCO),[108] the authors do not recommend pulmonary function testing since it is known to be of limited utility in preoperative assessment outside of lung reduction surgery. Six-minute walk testing may be a more useful functional study to assess cardiopulmonary capacity as it has been shown in some studies to be predictive of postoperative pulmonary complications.[109] Echocardiogram is indicated by symptomatology, elevated NT-pro-BNP levels, or abnormal cardiac exam findings. Abnormal results obtained from these studies would prompt consultation of appropriate specialists to assist in optimizing the candidate for surgery.

Other preoperative tests proposed by the authors are conducted for screening purposes, performed on all surgical candidates regardless of type of surgery or severity of initial COVID-19 illness. These are geared toward identifying markers of persistent subclinical COVID complications, persistent inflammation, or identifying abnormalities that have been observed in some studies to develop in the convalescent phase of infection, such as arrhythmia or renal dysfunction. To this end, BMP, CBC, and ECG are recommended for all post-COVID patients. Additional markers of inflammation, coagulation, or nutritional status such as d-dimer, fibrinogen, PTT, LDH, ferritin, and pre-albumin are recommended for all except those who experienced an asymptomatic illness course and are candidates for undergoing minor procedures. While observational studies have chronicled abnormalities of numerous biomarker levels including these and others during the acute phase of infection and attempted to use them to predict illness severity, little is currently known regarding the relationship of these biomarker levels to predicting perioperative risk during the recovery phase of viral illness. Nevertheless, until these risks can be precisely quantified by future studies, it is reasonable to suspect that those with persistent inflammation, coagulopathy, or metabolic disturbances would be at elevated risk of perioperative and postoperative complications.

Finally, the authors advocate applying the Edmonton Frail Scale (EFS) to evaluate those post-COVID surgical candidates older than 65 years or those who experienced severe initial illness. The concept of frailty, defined as "a biologic syndrome of a decreased physiological reserve, resulting from the cumulative declines of multiple organ systems, which predisposes one to adverse outcomes when exposed to stressors such as surgery" has emerged recently as a useful predictive tool in the preoperative evaluation of elderly patients.[110] The EFS has been validated for use by nongeriatricians for particular categories of surgery and consists of 11 questions over multiple domains of health and function. Given the multiorgan system impact of COVID-19 illness, the disproportionate toll of infection on the elderly, and the persistence of some degree of long-term debility in many, such an assessment of frailty is well conceived and likely to yield useful insight to aid in preoperative risk assessment. The ability of frailty assessment to predict postoperative morbidity in the context of COVID infection is a promising area of future investigation.

PERIOPERATIVE MANAGEMENT

As discussed above, the general approach to surgical candidates who have tested positive for COVID is to delay surgery until they have recovered from acute infection, are no longer infectious, and have returned as much as possible to their pre-COVID baseline health and functioning. This acknowledges the significantly greater risk of postoperative complications that accompany undergoing surgery while in the acute phase of viral infection and protects healthcare providers from exposure. In the case of urgent or time-sensitive surgery, however, the risks of delaying the procedure must be weighed against these risks, and, in some circumstances, it may be determined to be in the best interest of the patient to proceed with surgery even though they are recently COVID-positive, acutely symptomatic, and/or still infectious. In these situations, guidelines for prevention of viral transmission to care providers in the operating theater has been put forth by a number of organizations including the Anesthesia Patient Safety Foundation (APSF)[111] and the ASA[112] with input from the CDC.

Proper use of PPE and meticulous hand hygiene are the mainstays of preventing viral transmission in the perioperative setting. SARS-CoV-2 is transmitted primarily through contact with respiratory droplets over a short range (<6 feet) in most circumstances. As such, droplet precautions in most contexts are sufficient to prevent viral spread. In the perioperative setting, however, numerous procedures, including airway management in the course of providing anesthesia, generate aerosol,[113] thus increasing the risk of airborne transmission. As such, all personnel in the operating room should observe airborne precautions, the most important element of which is wearing either an N-95 mask or a powered air purifying respirator (PAPR). While both will afford protection against aerosol transmission, the latter has the advantage of not requiring fit testing and being able to be repeatedly disinfected and reused. Additional protective equipment is aimed at preventing skin contamination by droplets and includes eye protection in the form of goggles and/or face shields (eyeglasses alone are insufficient to protect against airborne droplets), water-resistant gowns, gloves, and disposable hair and beard covers. All perioperative providers and staff should be proficient in proper PPE donning and doffing procedures so as not to risk exposure when removing potentially contaminated elements.[114] During transport, COVID-positive patients should have a facemask applied if spontaneously breathing and a filtering heat moisture exchanger (HME) should be interposed between the Ambu-bag and endotracheal tube for intubated patients. Data are inconsistent with regard to quantifying the actual risk to providers and staff of infection during aerosolizing procedures, but the impression thus far is that in environments where proper PPE is freely available and used appropriately, the incidence of infection is low.[115] In fact, at least one study found that anesthesia providers and intensive care staff (who most routinely encounter COVID-positive patients and perform aerosolizing procedures) actually had lower rates of infection than other groups of healthcare providers,[116] suggesting that constant vigilance and fastidious adherence to PPE usage guidelines are effective at preventing infection.

Operating room or procedural suite equipment and surfaces as well as the anesthesia machine have significant potential for contamination by respiratory droplets or aerosol. As such, rigorous protocols for decontamination are necessary to prevent viral transmission to healthcare staff and other patients. Terminal cleaning procedures often include the use of UV light or vaporized hydrogen peroxide, as well as allowing sufficient time for air exchanges to reduce the aerosol burden in the operating room. With respect to the anesthesia machine, the use of filters rated for viral particles is an important precaution for preventing contamination of the internal components. Two filters should be employed, one at the airway Y-piece and the other guarding the connection of the expiratory limb of the airway circuit to the machine. It is important to note that while HME devices are commonly used in airway circuits, only models that specifically contain filters are effective for blocking viral particles. All disposable components of the airway circuit including the gas sample line should be disposed of after use with a COVID-positive patient. The absorbent canister and the gas analyzer water trap do not need to be replaced if the filters were positioned appropriately during use of the anesthesia machine.

Little data exist regarding peri- and postoperative outcomes of those who have recovered from SARS-CoV-2 infection. In the absence of specific evidence to inform anesthetic choice and conduct in this population, providers should apply current evidence-based principles governing perioperative management of any abnormalities discovered during preoperative assessment and testing. With respect to COVID-positive patients still in the active phase of infection for whom the decision is made to proceed with urgent or time-sensitive surgery, perioperative considerations center around managing elevated perioperative risk and mitigating healthcare worker exposure. As outlined above, pulmonary and thromboembolic complications constitute the most common sources of postoperative morbidity in these patients and likely contribute to increased perioperative mortality. Regional and neuraxial anesthesia are not contraindicated in the context of active COVID infection and may be favored in circumstances that permit their application in order to avoid general anesthesia, endotracheal intubation, and accompanying aerosolization of airway secretions. Of note in this regard, many patients with COVID-19 are prophylactically anticoagulated, impacting the feasibility or timing of neuraxial anesthesia. When providing sedation, a surgical mask should be placed over the nasal cannula, and the oxygen flow rate kept to the minimum necessary to maintain oxygenation to minimize airway aerosol. If a regional technique with sedation is the chosen approach, care should be taken to avoid the need for conversion to general anesthesia requiring airway instrumentation during the procedure.

When providing general anesthesia to COVID-positive patients, rapid-sequence induction and intubation are preferred to minimize the need for mask ventilation and the duration of provider exposure to airway secretions. A review of more than 200 patients critically ill with COVID infection revealed that they are particularly prone to hypoxemia and hypotension during intubation after induction with propofol.[46] In these particularly high-risk patients, use of alternative induction agents that engender less hypotension such as ketamine or etomidate may be beneficial, and fluid and vasopressor support may be additionally necessary to maintain hemodynamics. With respect to the specifics of airway management, recommendations derived largely from expert opinion are available.[117–119] Before attempting intubation, the patient should be thoroughly preoxygenated to hedge against potential reduced physiological pulmonary reserve and avoid the need for rescue ventilation. Video laryngoscopy is recommended to facilitate rapid and facile placement of the endotracheal tube while increasing the distance between the anesthesia provider's face and the patient's mouth.[120] In the event that mask ventilation is necessary or unavoidable, maintain a tight mask seal, employing two providers if necessary, and ventilate at low pressures with low volumes. Consider the use of a supraglottic airway device (SGA) in preference to masking if rescue ventilation is needed. Awake fiberoptic intubation should be avoided if at all possible, as patient coughing will create significant aerosol burden. If there is no other option, thorough oropharyngeal topicalization with liquid lidocaine or lidocaine jelly should be ensured prior to scope insertion. After placement of the endotracheal tube, inflate the cuff prior to connection of the breathing circuit and ensure that a filter is present and remains attached to the endotracheal tube during any circuit disconnections. The intubating provider should wear double gloves during the procedure and dispose of the outer gloves immediately after tube placement. More aerosol is generated during extubation than during intubation, to a degree quantitatively similar to that created during a volitional cough.[121] As such, the patient's mouth should be covered by a towel or sheet when removing the endotracheal tube. Lidocaine, opioid, or dexmedetomidine administered during emergence can be considered to minimize coughing during extubation.[122] Finally, limiting the number of people in the room to only those necessary during airway management procedures will help ensure the safety of the care team and staff.

CONCLUSION

- SARS-CoV-2 infection can have effects on virtually every organ system and cause a spectrum of illness ranging from asymptomatic to critically ill or even fatal.

- Cardiopulmonary manifestations of viral infection are common and underlie the increased perioperative morbidity and mortality experienced by those who undergo surgery in the active phase of viral infection.

- With the exception of emergent, urgent, or time-sensitive procedures, surgery should be delayed for those infected with COVID-19 until they are no longer infectious and have returned to their pre-COVID baseline level of health and functioning.
- Vaccination confers a significant protective effect against severe illness as well as the risk of postoperative complications after COVID infection.
- In the case of time-sensitive procedures, such as cancer surgery, multidisciplinary planning is recommended to weigh the increased perioperative risk of those still in the active phase of infection against the risk of morbidity engendered by surgical delay.
- For those who undergo surgery while actively infected with COVID-19, intraoperative considerations center around mitigating exposure risk to perioperative providers and staff; recognizing systemic effects of viral infection such as decreased cardiopulmonary reserve, coagulopathy, and inflammation; and managing the correspondingly increased perioperative risk to the patient.
- Many who recover from COVID-19 will experience long-term effects and disability including but not limited to decreased pulmonary function, arrhythmias, renal dysfunction, neurological symptoms, and persistent inflammation.
- Preoperative assessment for surgical candidates who have recovered from COVID-19 centers around identifying these persistent effects and engaging specialty consultation as needed to optimize their status with respect to any acquired comorbidities.

REVIEW QUESTIONS

1. According to the CDC Antigen Test Algorithm, for which of the following individuals who have received a COVID-19 antigen test result would confirmatory NAAT be most indicated?

   a. Asymptomatic with no known exposures and a negative antigen test result.
   b. Asymptomatic with close contact to COVID-19 and a negative antigen test result.
   c. Asymptomatic with close contact to COVID-19 and a positive antigen test result.
   d. Symptomatic with a positive antigen test result.

   The correct answer is c.

   The CDC antigen Test algorithm[12] sorts individuals into low, medium, and high pretest probability with respect to its recommendations regarding confirmatory NAAT testing. The individual described in choice a has a low pretest probability of having COVID-19, so a negative antigen test alone is sufficient to rule out infection. The individual described in D has a high pretest probability of having COVID-19, so a positive antigen test is sufficient to consider the patient infected. Individuals described in B and D are in the intermediate category of pretest probability, having had exposure but not symptomatic. In this group, a negative antigen test is taken as sufficient to consider the individual as not having evidence of infection currently, acknowledging that should the individual develop symptoms they should be retested. A positive antigen test in this group should be confirmed with a NAAT test, thus C is correct.

2. Which of the following statements is most accurate concerning the infectious risk of a SARS-CoV-2 positive individual?

   a. If the individual is asymptomatic, he or she is not infectious.
   b. If the individual is symptomatic, he or she is considered infectious for no longer than 7 days after his or her symptoms began.
   c. If the individual is hospitalized with severe illness or immunocompromised, he or she may be considered infectious for up to 20 days after his or her symptoms began.
   d. If the individual tests positive again after 45 days after the initial appearance of symptoms, he or she is likely infectious even if his or her symptoms have continuously improved or resolved.

   The correct answer is c.

   Asymptomatic spread has been partially responsible for the rapid propagation of the SARS-CoV-2 virus throughout the pandemic. Individuals will have a period of infectiousness before symptoms develop or even if they are ultimately asymptomatic in their own course. CDC guidelines regarding the period during which COVID-positive individuals are considered infectious are based on the ability to detect replication-competent virus.[24] For asymptomatic individuals, the upper limit of this interval is 10, not 7 days after first appearance of symptoms. In some instances, NAAT tests have yielded positive results out to 90 days after initial infection. In most cases, this has been shown to be the result of residual viral particles that are no longer replication-competent.[43] Thus, the CDC does not recommend retesting within 90 days of confirmed infection unless symptoms are not improving or new symptoms develop. Those who have severe illness or immunocompromise are considered infectious for a longer duration, 20 days per CDC guidelines.

3. Which of the following is most accurate regarding the extrapulmonary manifestations of SARS-CoV-2 infection?

   a. Cardiac manifestations of COVID-19 illness occur almost exclusively in those with preexisting cardiac disease.
   b. The occurrence and severity neurologic manifestations of COVID-19 illness correlates with the severity of pulmonary involvement.
   c. Heart block is the most common arrythmia associated with SARS-CoV-2 infection.
   d. New-onset arrythmias have been observed to occur in the convalescent phase of COVID-19 illness.

   The correct answer is d.

SARS-CoV-2 can have effects on virtually every organ system.[87] Outside of the respiratory effects of viral infection, the cardiovascular system is the most commonly affected. More than half of the cardiac manifestations, which include cardiomyopathy, acute coronary syndrome, cardiogenic shock, acute cor pulmonale, and arrhythmias, occur in those with no previous history of cardiac disease.[82] While heart block has been seen with COVID-19 infection, sinus tachycardia and atrial fibrillation have been the most commonly observed arrythmias. New-onset arrhythmias have been observed not infrequently to occur in the recovery phase of infection.[84] Neurologic manifestations of COVID-19 illness can be particularly debilitating, and their occurrence and severity are not correlated with the severity of respiratory symptoms.[85]

4. Which of the following is most accurate regarding patients with cancer who are also infected with COVID-19?

   a. Receiving chemotherapy in the context of active COVID-19 infection has been definitively shown to be safe.
   b. COVID-19 infection in the context of breast cancer is associated with worse outcomes than in the context of hematologic malignancies.
   c. Although individuals with cancer are not more likely than those without to contract COVID-19, the illness they experience if they do is often more severe.
   d. For some cancers for which surgery is the preferred initial treatment option, the recommended surgical delay periods based on concurrent COVID-19 illness status engender an increased risk of worsened oncologic outcomes, such as cancer recurrence or spread.

The correct answer is d.

Patients with cancer are both more likely to be infected with SARS-CoV-2 than patients without[17] and experience more severe disease. Lung and hematologic, not breast cancers are associated with the worst outcomes in the context of COVID-19 infection.[21,22] While the evidence is not unanimous, many studies demonstrate worse outcomes for patients receiving chemotherapy when they are infected with COVID-19, attributed largely to the immunosuppression.[39-41] Choice d is correct, supporting the wisdom of thoughtful multidisciplinary discussion and planning to carefully weigh the risks of undergoing surgery before full recovery from COVID-19 infection against the risks of worsened oncologic outcomes engendered by delaying surgery.

5. Which of the following is most accurate regarding perioperative risk in the context of COVID-19 infection?

   a. Current evidence indicates that 30-day postoperative mortality for patients who have recovered symptomatically from COVID-19 infection returns to the baseline level of those not infected with COVID-19 about 4 weeks after appearance of symptoms.
   b. Postoperative cardiac complications represent the most common source of perioperative morbidity and mortality in patients with active COVID-19 infection.
   c. Current estimates of 30-day postoperative mortality for patients who have active COVID-19 infection in the perioperative period fall in the range of 20–25%.
   d. Female gender is associated with greater 30-day postoperative mortality for patients who have active COVID-19 infection in the perioperative period.

The correct answer is c.

Having surgery when actively infected with COVID-19, particularly when symptomatic, severely, or critically ill, incurs significant risk. Currently available cohort data place the 30-day postoperative mortality in the range of 20–25%.[15,16] Pulmonary complications are the most common form of postoperative morbidity and account for a significant portion of the mortality. Postoperative mortality has been shown to be associated with male gender, age older than 70, ASA grades 3–5, malignant versus benign or obstetric diagnosis, emergency versus elective surgery, and major versus minor surgery. A recent study showed that the postoperative mortality rate for those infected with COVID-19 in the perioperative period returns to the COVID-negative baseline 7 weeks after the appearance of symptoms if the symptoms have resolved by then.[28]

6. A 71-year-old man presents to anesthesia preoperative clinic scheduled for robotic assisted laparoscopic prostatectomy (RALP) for prostate cancer in 2 weeks. He has recovered from confirmed COVID-19 illness that started 10 weeks ago and required several days in the hospital and supplemental oxygen but not ICU care. While he endorses feeling much better now, he still complains of lingering fatigue as well as getting winded and feeling his heart pounding with exertion to a degree that he did not before contracting COVID. His past medical history is otherwise significant only for well-controlled hypertension. Which of the following tests or labs would be least useful in the preoperative assessment of this patient?

   a. Pulmonary function testing (PFT).
   b. ECG.
   c. BMP.
   d. Six-minute walk testing.

The correct answer is a.

It is becoming increasingly evident that many who have been infected with SARS-CoV-2 will have lasting effects months after initial infection.[104] Persistent fatigue is among the most common of these long-term effects. Many manifest persistent deficits in pulmonary function or DLCO.[3] This patient has been left with dyspnea on exertion, suggesting that this may be the case. Six-minute walk testing to assess functional capacity has been shown to be predictive of postoperative complications[109] and thus would have value in this case. While PFTs might reveal abnormalities in respiratory mechanics or diffusion, this modality has been shown to have limited value in preoperative assessment for most nonthoracic surgery. New-onset arrhythmias have been observed in the recovery period of COVID-19 infection.[92] Given this fact and the patient's symptomatology on exertion, ECG would be a useful study. BMP to assess electrolytes and renal function is useful, as renal dysfunction is not uncommon among those infected with COVID-19. New-onset renal dysfunction has been observed in those without previous dysfunction, as well as in the convalescent phase of illness.[3]

7. Which of the following intraoperative airway management techniques is consistent with expert recommendations regarding minimizing viral transmission risk when the patient is COVID positive?

  a. Favor awake fiberoptic intubation to decrease the need for mask ventilation and increase the distance between the patient's mouth and the airway manager.
  b. When attaching the airway circuit to the endotracheal tube, ensure that there are two viral filtering HME devices, the first interposed between the endotracheal tube and the Y-piece of the circuit, and the second interposed between the anesthesia machine and the inspiratory limb of the airway circuit.
  c. When mask ventilation is necessary, do so using large-volume breaths to decrease the frequency with which breaths need to be delivered.
  d. Prior to induction, allow the spontaneously breathing patient an extended period of time for preoxygenation.

The correct answer is d.

Airway management procedures are aerosol-generating and engender risk of viral transmission to healthcare providers and perioperative staff. Expert recommendations to minimize this risk have been articulated in the literature.[117–119] Answer d maximizes the time to desaturation available to the operator to successfully intubate the patient, thus decreasing the chance of mask or rescue ventilation which can disperse viral aerosol. If mask ventilation is necessary, a tight mask seal should be ensured and the patient ventilated at low volumes and pressures to minimize aerosol dispersal. When attaching the airway circuit to the endotracheal tube, the second viral filtering HME filter should be interposed between the anesthesia machine and the expiratory limb of the airway circuit to prevent contamination of the anesthesia machine. Awake fiberoptic intubation should be avoided if at all possible, as coughing during the procedure would produce significant aerosol burden.

REFERENCES

1. Cucinotta D, Vanelli M. WHO declares COVID-19 a pandemic. *Acta Biomed*. Mar 19 2020;91(1):157–160. doi:10.23750/abm.v91i1.9397
2. Huang G. High mortality is expected in patients who have COVID-19 during the postoperative period. *CMAJ*. 2020 Jul 20;192(29):E847. doi:10.1503/cmaj.75781
3. Huang C, Huang L, Wang Y, et al. 6-month consequences of COVID-19 in patients discharged from hospital: A cohort study. *Lancet*. 2021 Jan 16;397(10270):220–232. doi:10.1016/S0140-6736(20)32656-8
4. Boger B, Fachi MM, Vilhena RO, Cobre AF, Tonin FS, Pontarolo R. Systematic review with meta-analysis of the accuracy of diagnostic tests for COVID-19. *Am J Infect Control*. 2021 Jan;49(1):21–29. doi:10.1016/j.ajic.2020.07.011
5. Butler-Laporte G, Lawandi A, Schiller I, et al. Comparison of saliva and nasopharyngeal swab nucleic acid amplification testing for detection of SARS-CoV-2: A systematic review and meta-analysis. *JAMA Intern Med*. 2021 Mar 1;181(3):353–360. doi:10.1001/jamainternmed.2020.8876
6. Watson J, Whiting PF, Brush JE. Interpreting a COVID-19 test result. *BMJ*. 2020 May 12;369:m1808. doi:10.1136/bmj.m1808
7. Bwire GM, Majigo MV, Njiro BJ, Mawazo A. Detection profile of SARS-CoV-2 using RT-PCR in different types of clinical specimens: A systematic review and meta-analysis. *J Med Virol*. 2021 Feb;93(2):719–725. doi:10.1002/jmv.26349
8. Wang W, Xu Y, Gao R, et al. Detection of SARS-CoV-2 in different types of clinical specimens. *JAMA*. 2020 May 12;323(18):1843–1844. doi:10.1001/jama.2020.3786
9. Lisboa Bastos M, Tavaziva G, Abidi SK, et al. Diagnostic accuracy of serological tests for COVID-19: Systematic review and meta-analysis. *BMJ*. 2020 Jul 1;370:m2516. doi:10.1136/bmj.m2516
10. Food and Drug Administration (FDA). In vitro diagnostics EUA. https://www.fda.gov/medical-devices/coronavirus-disease-2019-covid-19-emergency-use-authorizations-medical-devices/in-vitro-diagnostics-euas
11. Jehi L, Ji X, Milinovich A, et al. Individualizing risk prediction for positive coronavirus disease 2019 testing: Results from 11,672 patients. *Chest*. 2020 Oct;158(4):1364–1375. doi:10.1016/j.chest.2020.05.580
12. CDC. Interim guidance for antigen testing for SARS-CoV-2. https://www.cdc.gov/coronavirus/2019-ncov/lab/resources/antigen-tests-guidelines.html.
13. Dinnes J, Deeks JJ, Adriano A, et al. Rapid, point-of-care antigen and molecular-based tests for diagnosis of SARS-CoV-2 infection. *Cochrane Database Syst Rev*. 2020 Aug 26;8:CD013705. doi:10.1002/14651858.CD013705
14. Liu C, Zhao Y, Okwan-Duodu D, Basho R, Cui X. COVID-19 in cancer patients: Risk, clinical features, and management. *Cancer Biol Med*. 2020 Aug 15;17(3):519–527. doi:10.20892/j.issn.2095-3941.2020.0289
15. Gómez Rosado JC, Toro López MDD, Capitan-Morales LC. Mortality and pulmonary complications in patients undergoing surgery with perioperative SARS-CoV-2 infection: An international cohort study. *Lancet*. 2020 Jul 4;396(10243):27–38. doi:10.1016/s0140-6736(20)31182-x
16. Abate SM, Mantefardo B, Basu B. Postoperative mortality among surgical patients with COVID-19: A systematic review and meta-analysis. *Patient Saf Surg*. 2020;14:37. doi:10.1186/s13037-020-00262-6
17. Wang Q, Berger NA, Xu R. Analyses of risk, racial disparity, and outcomes among US patients with cancer and COVID-19 infection. *JAMA Oncol*. 2021 Feb 1;7(2):220–227. doi:10.1001/jamaoncol.2020.6178
18. Giannakoulis VG, Papoutsi E, Siempos, II. Effect of cancer on clinical outcomes of patients with COVID-19: A meta-analysis of patient data. *JCO Glob Oncol*. 2020 Jun;6:799–808. doi:10.1200/GO.20.00225
19. Williamson EJ, Walker AJ, Bhaskaran K, et al. Factors associated with COVID-19-related death using OpenSAFELY. *Nature*. 2020 Aug;584(7821):430–436. doi:10.1038/s41586-020-2521-4
20. Brar G, Pinheiro LC, Shusterman M, et al. COVID-19 Severity and outcomes in patients with cancer: A matched cohort study. *J Clin Oncol*. 2020 Nov 20;38(33):3914–3924. doi:10.1200/JCO.20.01580
21. Vijenthira A, Gong IY, Fox TA, et al. Outcomes of patients with hematologic malignancies and COVID-19: A systematic review and meta-analysis of 3377 patients. *Blood*. 2020 Dec 17;136(25):2881–2892. doi:10.1182/blood.2020008824
22. Luo J, Rizvi H, Preeshagul IR, et al. COVID-19 in patients with lung cancer. *Ann Oncol*. 2020 Oct;31(10):1386–1396. doi:10.1016/j.annonc.2020.06.007
23. Lunski MJ, Burton J, Tawagi K, et al. Multivariate mortality analyses in COVID-19: Comparing patients with cancer and patients without cancer in Louisiana. *Cancer*. 2021 Jan 15;127(2):266–274. doi:10.1002/cncr.33243

24. American Society of Anesthesiologists. APSF and ASA joint statement on elective surgery and anesthesia for patients after COVID-19 infection. https://www.asahq.org/in-the-spotlight/coronavirus-covid-19-information

25. Glasbey JC, Nepogodiev D, Omar O, et al. Delaying surgery for patients with a previous SARS-CoV-2 infection. *Br J Surg*. 2020 Nov;107(12):e601–e602. doi:10.1002/bjs.12050

26. Hsieh MJ, Lee WC, Cho HY, et al. Recovery of pulmonary functions, exercise capacity, and quality of life after pulmonary rehabilitation in survivors of ARDS due to severe influenza A (H1N1) pneumonitis. *Influenza Other Respir Viruses*. 2018 Sep;12(5):643–648. doi:10.1111/irv.12566

27. Petrilli CM, Jones SA, Yang J, et al. Factors associated with hospital admission and critical illness among 5279 people with coronavirus disease 2019 in New York City: Prospective cohort study. *BMJ*. 2020 May 22;369:m1966. doi:10.1136/bmj.m1966

28. Nepogodiev D, Simoes JFF, Li E, et al. Timing of surgery following SARS-CoV-2 infection: An international prospective cohort study. *Anaesthesia*. 2021 Mar 9. doi:10.1111/anae.15458

29. American Society of Anesthesiologists. ASA and APSF joint statement on elective surgery / procedures and anesthesia for patients after COVID-19 infection. https://www.asahq.org/about-asa/newsroom/news-releases/2022/02/asa-and-apsf-joint-statement-on-elective-surgery-procedures-and-anesthesia-for-patients-after-covid-19-infection

30. Kougias P, Sharath SE, Zamani N, Brunicardi FC, Berger DH, Wilson MA. Timing of a major operative intervention after a positive COVID-19 test affects postoperative mortality: Results from a nationwide, procedure-matched analysis. *Ann Surg*. 2022;276(3):554–561.

31. Le ST, Kipnis P, Cohn B, Liu VX. COVID-19 vaccination and the timing of surgery following COVID-19 infection. *Ann Surg*. 2022;276(5):265–272.

32. Garnier M, Constantin JM, Cinotti R, et al.; DROMIS-22 Study Group and the SFAR Research Network. Association of preoperative COVID-19 and postoperative respiratory morbidity during the Omicron epidemic wave: The DROMIS-22 multicentre prospective observational cohort study. *EClinicalMedicine*. 2023;58:101881.

33. Bakouny Z, Hawley JE, Choueiri TK, et al. COVID-19 and cancer: Current challenges and perspectives. *Cancer Cell*. 2020 Nov 9;38(5):629–646. doi:10.1016/j.ccell.2020.09.018

34. Bartlett DL, Howe JR, Chang G, et al. Management of cancer surgery cases during the COVID-19 pandemic: Considerations. *Ann Surg Oncol*. 2020 Jun;27(6):1717–1720. doi:10.1245/s10434-020-08461-2

35. Hartman HE, Sun Y, Devasia TP, et al. Integrated survival estimates for cancer treatment delay among adults with cancer during the COVID-19 pandemic. *JAMA Oncol*. 2020 Dec 1;6(12):1881–1889. doi:10.1001/jamaoncol.2020.5403

36. Sud A, Jones ME, Broggio J, et al. Collateral damage: The impact on outcomes from cancer surgery of the COVID-19 pandemic. *Ann Oncol*. 2020 Aug;31(8):1065–1074. doi:10.1016/j.annonc.2020.05.009

37. Turaga KK, Girotra S. Are we harming cancer patients by delaying their cancer surgery during the COVID-19 pandemic? *Ann Surg*. 2020 Jun 2. doi:10.1097/sla.0000000000003967

38. Lou E, Subramanian S. Changing oncology treatment paradigms in the COVID-19 pandemic. *Clin Colorectal Cancer*. 2020 Sep;19(3):153–155. doi:10.1016/j.clcc.2020.05.002

39. Crolley VE, Hanna D, Joharatnam-Hogan N, et al. COVID-19 in cancer patients on systemic anti-cancer therapies: Outcomes from the CAPITOL (COVID-19 Cancer PatIenT Outcomes in North London) cohort study. *Ther Adv Med Oncol*. 2020;12:1758835920971147. doi:10.1177/1758835920971147

40. Tang LV, Hu Y. Poor clinical outcomes for patients with cancer during the COVID-19 pandemic. *Lancet Oncol*. 2020 Jul;21(7):862–864. doi:10.1016/S1470-2045(20)30311-9

41. Park R, Lee SA, Kim SY, de Melo AC, Kasi A. Association of active oncologic treatment and risk of death in cancer patients with COVID-19: A systematic review and meta-analysis of patient data. *Acta Oncol*. 2021 Jan;60(1):13–19. doi:10.1080/0284186x.2020.1837946

42. Chin IS, Galavotti S, Yip KP, et al. Influence of clinical characteristics and anti-cancer therapy on outcomes from SARS-CoV-2 infection: A systematic review and meta-analysis of 5,678 cancer patients. *medRxiv*. https://www.medrxiv.org/content/10.1101/2020.12.15.20248195v1.full

43. Lee LY, Cazier JB, Angelis V, et al. COVID-19 mortality in patients with cancer on chemotherapy or other anticancer treatments: A prospective cohort study. *Lancet*. 2020 Jun 20;395(10241):1919–1926. doi:10.1016/s0140-6736(20)31173-9

44. Kuderer NM, Choueiri TK, Shah DP, et al. Clinical impact of COVID-19 on patients with cancer (CCC19): A cohort study. *Lancet*. 2020 Jun 20;395(10241):1907–1918. doi:10.1016/s0140-6736(20)31187-9

45. Yahav D, Yelin D, Eckerle I, et al. Definitions for coronavirus disease 2019 reinfection, relapse and PCR re-positivity. *Clin Microbiol Infect*. 2021 Mar;27(3):315–318. doi:10.1016/j.cmi.2020.11.028

46. Liotti FM, Menchinelli G, Marchetti S, et al. Assessment of SARS-CoV-2 RNA test results among patients who recovered from COVID-19 with prior negative results. *JAMA Intern Med*. 2020 Nov 12. doi:10.1001/jamainternmed.2020.7570

47. Song KH, Kim DM, Lee H, et al. Dynamics of viral load and anti-SARS-CoV-2 antibodies in patients with positive RT-PCR results after recovery from COVID-19. *Korean J Intern Med*. 2021 Jan;36(1):11–14. doi:10.3904/kjim.2020.325

48. Anesthesia Patient Safety Foundation. ASA and APSF updated statement on perioperative testing for SARS-CoV-2 in the asymptomatic patient. https://www.apsf.org/news-updates/asa-and-apsf-updated-statement-on-perioperative-testing-for-sars-cov-2-in-the-asymptomatic-patient/

49. Kaufman AE, Naidu S, Ramachandran S, Kaufman DS, Fayad ZA, Mani V. Review of radiographic findings in COVID-19. *World J Radiol*. 2020 Aug 28;12(8):142–155. doi:10.4329/wjr.v12.i8.142

50. Bakker IS, Snijders HS, Grossmann I, Karsten TM, Havenga K, Wiggers T. High mortality rates after nonelective colon cancer resection: Results of a national audit. *Colorectal Dis*. 2016 Jun;18(6):612–21. doi:10.1111/codi.13262

51. Yao W, Wang T, Jiang B, et al. Emergency tracheal intubation in 202 patients with COVID-19 in Wuhan, China: Lessons learnt and international expert recommendations. *Br J Anaesth*. 2020 Jul;125(1):e28–e37. doi:10.1016/j.bja.2020.03.026

52. van Hooft JE, van Halsema EE, Vanbiervliet G, et al. Self-expandable metal stents for obstructing colonic and extracolonic cancer: European Society of Gastrointestinal Endoscopy (ESGE) Clinical Guideline. *Endoscopy*. 2014 Nov;46(11):990–1053. doi:10.1055/s-0034-1390700

53. Kye BH, Kim JH, Kim HJ, et al. The optimal time interval between the placement of self-expandable metallic stent and elective surgery in patients with obstructive colon cancer. *Sci Rep*. 2020 Jun 11;10(1):9502. doi:10.1038/s41598-020-66508-6

54. Han J, Gatheral T, Williams C. Procalcitonin for patient stratification and identification of bacterial co-infection in COVID-19. *Clin Med (Lond)*. 2020 May;20(3):e47. doi:10.7861/clinmed.Let.20.3.3

55. Ortega-Paz L, Capodanno D, Montalescot G, Angiolillo DJ. Coronavirus disease 2019-associated thrombosis and coagulopathy: Review of the pathophysiological characteristics and implications for antithrombotic management. *J Am Heart Assoc*. 2021 Feb 2;10(3):e019650. doi:10.1161/jaha.120.019650

56. Horby P, Lim WS, Emberson JR, et al. Dexamethasone in hospitalized patients with COVID-19. *N Engl J Med*. 2021 Feb 25;384(8):693–704. doi:10.1056/NEJMoa2021436

57. Bouadma L, Mekontso-Dessap A, Burdet C, et al. High-dose dexamethasone and oxygen support strategies in intensive care unit patients with severe COVID-19 acute hypoxemic respiratory failure: The COVIDICUS Randomized Clinical Trial. *JAMA Intern Med*. 2022;182(9):906–916

58. Lu H, Stratton CW, Tang YW. Outbreak of pneumonia of unknown etiology in Wuhan, China: The mystery and the miracle. *J Med Virol*. 2020 Apr;92(4):401–402. doi:10.1002/jmv.25678
59. Xiong J, Lipsitz O, Nasri F, et al. Impact of COVID-19 pandemic on mental health in the general population: A systematic review. *J Affect Disord*. 2020 Dec 1;277:55–64. doi:10.1016/j.jad.2020.08.001
60. Nicola M, Alsafi Z, Sohrabi C, et al. The socio-economic implications of the coronavirus pandemic (COVID-19): A review. *Int J Surg*. 2020 Jun;78:185–193. doi:10.1016/j.ijsu.2020.04.018
61. Blumenthal D, Fowler EJ, Abrams M, Collins SR. COVID-19: Implications for the health care system. *N Engl J Med*. 2020 Oct 8;383(15):1483–1488. doi:10.1056/NEJMsb2021088
62. Berlin G BD, Gibler K, Schulz J. Cutting through the COVID-19 surgical backlog. McKinsey & Company. 2020. https://www.mckinsey.com/industries/healthcare-systems-and-services/our-insights/cutting-through-the-covid-19-surgical-backlog
63. Uttarilli A, Amalakanti S, Kommoju PR, et al. Super-rapid race for saving lives by developing COVID-19 vaccines. *J Integr Bioinform*. 2021 Mar 24. doi:10.1515/jib-2021-0002
64. CDC COVID-19 Response Team. SARS-CoV-2 B.1.1.529 (Omicron) variant—United States, December 1–8, 2021. *MMWR Morb Mortal Wkly Rep*. 2021;70(50):1731–1734.
65. Silk BJ, Scobie HM, Duck WM, et al. COVID-19 surveillance after expiration of the public health emergency declaration – United States, May 11, 2023. *MMWR Morb Mortal Wkly Rep*. 2023;72:523–528.
66. Rubin R. COVID-19 vaccines vs variants: Determining how much immunity is enough. *JAMA*. 2021;325(13):1241–1243. doi:10.1001/jama.2021.3370
67. SeyedAlinaghi S, Oliaei S, Kianzad S, et al. Reinfection risk of novel coronavirus (COVID-19): A systematic review of current evidence. *World J Virol*. 2020 Dec 15;9(5):79–90. doi:10.5501/wjv.v9.i5.79
68. Crane MA, Shermock KM, Omer SB, Romley JA. Change in reported adherence to nonpharmaceutical interventions during the COVID-19 pandemic, April–November 2020. *JAMA*. 2021 Mar 2;325(9):883–885. doi:10.1001/jama.2021.0286
69. Prachand VN, Milner R, Angelos P, et al. Medically necessary, time-sensitive procedures: Scoring system to ethically and efficiently manage resource scarcity and provider risk during the COVID-19 pandemic. *J Am Coll Surg*. 2020 Aug;231(2):281–288. doi:10.1016/j.jamcollsurg.2020.04.011
70. Tizaoui K, Zidi I, Lee KH, et al. Update of the current knowledge on genetics, evolution, immunopathogenesis, and transmission for coronavirus disease 19 (COVID-19). *Int J Biol Sci*. 2020;16(15):2906–2923. doi:10.7150/ijbs.48812
71. Hu B, Guo H, Zhou P, Shi ZL. Characteristics of SARS-CoV-2 and COVID-19. *Nat Rev Microbiol*. 2021 Mar;19(3):141–154. doi:10.1038/s41579-020-00459-7
72. Lauer SA, Grantz KH, Bi Q, et al. The incubation period of coronavirus disease 2019 (COVID-19) from publicly reported confirmed cases: Estimation and application. *Ann Intern Med*. 2020 May 5;172(9):577–582. doi:10.7326/m20-0504
73. Oran DP, Topol EJ. The proportion of SARS-CoV-2 infections that are asymptomatic: A systematic review. *Ann Intern Med*. 2021 Jan 22. doi:10.7326/M20-6976
74. Stokes EK, Zambrano LD, Anderson KN, et al. Coronavirus disease 2019 case surveillance – United States, January 22–May 30, 2020. *MMWR Morb Mortal Wkly Rep*. 2020 Jun 19;69(24):759–765. doi:10.15585/mmwr.mm6924e2
75. Nasiri N, Sharifi H, Bazrafshan A, Noori A, Karamouzian M, Sharifi A. Ocular manifestations of COVID-19: A systematic review and meta-analysis. *J Ophthalmic Vis Res*. 2021;16(1):103–112. doi:10.18502/jovr.v16i1.8256
76. Genovese G, Moltrasio C, Berti E, Marzano AV. Skin manifestations associated with COVID-19: Current knowledge and future perspectives. *Dermatology*. 2021;237(1):1–12. doi:10.1159/000512932
77. Wu Z, McGoogan JM. Characteristics of and important lessons from the coronavirus disease 2019 (COVID-19) outbreak in China: Summary of a report of 72 314 cases from the Chinese Center for Disease Control and Prevention. *JAMA*. 2020 Apr 7;323(13):1239–1242. doi:10.1001/jama.2020.2648
78. Meyerowitz-Katz G, Merone L. A systematic review and meta-analysis of published research data on COVID-19 infection fatality rates. *Int J Infect Dis*. 2020 Dec;101:138–148. doi:10.1016/j.ijid.2020.09.1464
79. Weinberger DM, Chen J, Cohen T, et al. Estimation of excess deaths associated with the COVID-19 pandemic in the United States, March to May 2020. *JAMA Intern Med*. 2020 Oct 1;180(10):1336–1344. doi:10.1001/jamainternmed.2020.3391
80. Dennis JM, McGovern AP, Vollmer SJ, Mateen BA. Improving survival of critical care patients with coronavirus disease 2019 in England: A national cohort study, March to June 2020. *Crit Care Med*. 2021 Feb 1;49(2):209–214. doi:10.1097/CCM.0000000000004747
81. Wang D, Hu B, Hu C, et al. Clinical characteristics of 138 hospitalized patients with 2019 novel coronavirus-infected pneumonia in Wuhan, China. *JAMA*. 2020 Mar 17;323(11):1061–1069. doi:10.1001/jama.2020.1585
82. Kang Y, Chen T, Mui D, et al. Cardiovascular manifestations and treatment considerations in COVID-19. *Heart*. 2020 Aug;106(15):1132–1141. doi:10.1136/heartjnl-2020-317056
83. Guo T, Fan Y, Chen M, et al. Cardiovascular implications of fatal outcomes of patients with coronavirus disease 2019 (COVID-19). *JAMA Cardiol*. 2020 Jul 1;5(7):811–818. doi:10.1001/jamacardio.2020.1017
84. Babapoor-Farrokhran S, Rasekhi RT, Gill D, Babapoor S, Amanullah A. Arrhythmia in COVID-19. *SN Compr Clin Med*. 2020 Aug 14:1–6. doi:10.1007/s42399-020-00454-2
85. Ellul MA, Benjamin L, Singh B, et al. Neurological associations of COVID-19. *Lancet Neurol*. 2020 Sep;19(9):767–783. doi:10.1016/S1474-4422(20)30221-0
86. Oxley TJ, Mocco J, Majidi S, et al. Large-vessel stroke as a presenting feature of COVID-19 in the young. *N Engl J Med*. 2020 May 14;382(20):e60. doi:10.1056/NEJMc2009787
87. Gupta A, Madhavan MV, Sehgal K, et al. Extrapulmonary manifestations of COVID-19. *Nat Med*. 2020 Jul;26(7):1017–1032. doi:10.1038/s41591-020-0968-3
88. Chen N, Zhou M, Dong X, et al. Epidemiological and clinical characteristics of 99 cases of 2019 novel coronavirus pneumonia in Wuhan, China: A descriptive study. *Lancet*. 2020 Feb 15;395(10223):507–513. doi:10.1016/S0140-6736(20)30211-7
89. Verity R, Okell LC, Dorigatti I, et al. Estimates of the severity of coronavirus disease 2019: A model-based analysis. *Lancet Infect Dis*. 2020 Jun;20(6):669–677. doi:10.1016/S1473-3099(20)30243-7
90. Onder G, Rezza G, Brusaferro S. Case-fatality rate and characteristics of patients dying in relation to COVID-19 in Italy. *JAMA*. 2020 May 12;323(18):1775–1776. doi:10.1001/jama.2020.4683
91. Richardson S, Hirsch JS, Narasimhan M, et al. Presenting characteristics, comorbidities, and outcomes among 5700 patients hospitalized with COVID-19 in the New York City area. *JAMA*. 2020 May 26;323(20):2052–2059. doi:10.1001/jama.2020.6775
92. Severe outcomes among patients with coronavirus disease 2019 (COVID-19) – United States, February 12–March 16, 2020. *MMWR Morb Mortal Wkly Rep*. 2020 Ma4 27;69(12):343–346. doi:10.15585/mmwr.mm6912e2
93. McMichael TM, Currie DW, Clark S, et al. Epidemiology of COVID-19 in a long-term care facility in King County, Washington. *N Engl J Med*. 2020 May 21;382(21):2005–2011. doi:10.1056/NEJMoa2005412
94. Peckham H, de Gruijter NM, Raine C, et al. Male sex identified by global COVID-19 meta-analysis as a risk factor for death and ITU admission. *Nat Commun*. 2020 Dec 9;11(1):6317. doi:10.1038/s41467-020-19741-6
95. Kragholm K, Andersen MP, Gerds TA, et al. Association between male sex and outcomes of Coronavirus Disease 2019 (COVID-19): A Danish nationwide, register-based study. *Clin Infect Dis*. 2020 Jul 8. doi:10.1093/cid/ciaa924
96. Moore JT, Ricaldi JN, Rose CE, et al. Disparities in incidence of COVID-19 among underrepresented racial/ethnic groups in

96. counties identified as hotspots during June 5–18, 2020–22 States, February–June 2020. *MMWR Morb Mortal Wkly Rep.* 2020 Aug 21;69(33):1122–1126. doi:10.15585/mmwr.mm6933e1
97. Price-Haywood EG, Burton J, Fort D, Seoane L. Hospitalization and mortality among Black patients and White patients with COVID-19. *N Engl J Med.* 2020 Jun 25;382(26):2534–2543. doi:10.1056/NEJMsa2011686
98. Escobar GJ, Adams AS, Liu VX, et al. Racial disparities in COVID-19 testing and outcomes: Retrospective cohort study in an integrated health system. *Ann Intern Med.* 2021 Feb 9. doi:10.7326/M20-6979
99. Kabarriti R, Brodin NP, Maron MI, et al. Association of race and ethnicity with comorbidities and survival among patients with COVID-19 at an urban medical center in New York. *JAMA Netw Open.* 2020 Sep 1;3(9):e2019795. doi:10.1001/jamanetworkopen.2020.19795
100. Gold JAW, Rossen LM, Ahmad FB, et al. Race, ethnicity, and age trends in persons who died from COVID-19–United States, May-August 2020. *MMWR Morb Mortal Wkly Rep.* 2020 Oct 23;69(42):1517–1521. doi:10.15585/mmwr.mm6942e1
101. Marshall M. The lasting misery of coronavirus long-haulers. *Nature.* 2020 Sep;585(7825):339–341. doi:10.1038/d41586-020-02598-6
102. Han X, Fan Y, Alwalid O, et al. Six-month follow-up chest CT findings after severe COVID-19 pneumonia. *Radiology.* 2021 Apr;299(1):E177–E186. doi:10.1148/radiol.2021203153
103. Herridge MS, Cheung AM, Tansey CM, et al. One-year outcomes in survivors of the acute respiratory distress syndrome. *N Engl J Med.* 2003 Feb 20;348(8):683–693. doi:10.1056/NEJMoa022450
104. Lopez-Leon S, Wegman-Ostrosky T, Perelman C, et al. More than 50 long-term effects of COVID-19: A systematic review and meta-analysis. *medRxiv.* 2021 Jan 30. doi:10.1101/2021.01.27.21250617
105. Puntmann VO, Carerj ML, Wieters I, et al. Outcomes of cardiovascular magnetic resonance imaging in patients recently recovered from coronavirus disease 2019 (COVID-19). *JAMA Cardiol.* 2020 Nov 1;5(11):1265–1273. doi:10.1001/jamacardio.2020.3557
106. Baig AM. Deleterious outcomes in long-hauler COVID-19: The effects of SARS-CoV-2 on the CNS in chronic COVID syndrome. *ACS Chem Neurosci.* 2020 Dec 16;11(24):4017–4020. doi:10.1021/acschemneuro.0c00725
107. Bui N, Coetzer M, Schenning KJ, O'Glasser AY. Preparing previously COVID-19-positive patients for elective surgery: A framework for preoperative evaluation. *Perioper Med (Lond).* 2021 Jan 7;10(1):1. doi:10.1186/s13741-020-00172-2
108. Guler SA, Ebner L, Beigelman C, et al. Pulmonary function and radiological features four months after COVID-19: First results from the national prospective observational Swiss COVID-19 lung study. *Eur Respir J.* 2021 Jan 8. doi:10.1183/13993003.03690-2020
109. Ramos RJ, Ladha KS, Cuthbertson BH, et al. Association of six-minute walk test distance with postoperative complications in non-cardiac surgery: A secondary analysis of a multicentre prospective cohort study. [Association entre la distance parcourue pendant le test de marche de six minutes et les complications postoperatoires en chirurgie non cardiaque: Une analyse secondaire d'une etude de cohorte prospective multicentrique.] *Can J Anaesth.* 2021 Apr;68(4):514–529. doi:10.1007/s12630-020-01909-9
110. He Y, Li LW, Hao Y, et al. Assessment of predictive validity and feasibility of Edmonton Frail Scale in identifying postoperative complications among elderly patients: A prospective observational study. *Sci Rep.* 2020 Sep 7;10(1):14682. doi:10.1038/s41598-020-71140-5
111. Zucco L LN, Ketchandji D, Aziz M, Ramachandran SK. An update on the perioperative considerations for COVID-19 severe acute respiratory syndrome coronavirus-2 (SARS-CoV-2). *APSF Newsletter.* 2020;35(2):33–68.
112. American Society of Anesthesiologists. COVID-19 information for health care professionals. https://www.asahq.org/about-asa/governance-and-committees/asa-committees/committee-on-occupational-health/coronavirus?&ct=ab9ea2535282bd626450c-60f6a5b17460fbc9fa6fe3e5b12d615e21b48bf895914ce9d-05c8e5b2793b65895e2f6b30f5873aaad789319543706056fa5767c289
113. Tran K, Cimon K, Severn M, Pessoa-Silva CL, Conly J. Aerosol generating procedures and risk of transmission of acute respiratory infections to healthcare workers: A systematic review. *PLoS One.* 2012;7(4):e35797. doi:10.1371/journal.pone.0035797
114. Tomas ME, Kundrapu S, Thota P, et al. Contamination of health care personnel during removal of personal protective equipment. *JAMA Intern Med.* 2015 Dec;175(12):1904–10. doi:10.1001/jamainternmed.2015.4535
115. Liu M, Cheng SZ, Xu KW, et al. Use of personal protective equipment against coronavirus disease 2019 by healthcare professionals in Wuhan, China: Cross sectional study. *BMJ.* 2020 Jun 10;369:m2195. doi:10.1136/bmj.m2195
116. Cook TM, Lennane S. Occupational COVID-19 risk for anaesthesia and intensive care staff—Low-risk specialties in a high-risk setting. *Anaesthesia.* 2021 Mar;76(3):295–300. doi:10.1111/anae.15358
117. Cook TM, El-Boghdadly K, McGuire B, McNarry AF, Patel A, Higgs A. Consensus guidelines for managing the airway in patients with COVID-19: Guidelines from the Difficult Airway Society, the Association of Anaesthetists the Intensive Care Society, the Faculty of Intensive Care Medicine and the Royal College of Anaesthetists. *Anaesthesia.* 2020 Jun;75(6):785–799. doi:10.1111/anae.15054
118. Cook TM, McGuire B, Mushambi M, et al. Airway management guidance for the endemic phase of COVID-19. *Anaesthesia.* 2021 Feb;76(2):251–260. doi:10.1111/anae.15253
119. Orser BA. Recommendations for endotracheal intubation of COVID-19 patients. *Anesth Analg.* 2020 May;130(5):1109–1110 doi:10.1213/ane.0000000000004803
120. Hall D, Steel A, Heij R, Eley A, Young P. Videolaryngoscopy increases "mouth-to-mouth" distance compared with direct laryngoscopy. *Anaesthesia.* 2020 Jun;75(6):822–823. doi:10.1111/anae.15047
121. Brown J, Gregson FKA, Shrimpton A, et al. A quantitative evaluation of aerosol generation during tracheal intubation and extubation. *Anaesthesia.* 2021 Feb;76(2):174–181. doi:10.1111/anae.15292
122. Peng PWH, Ho PL, Hota SS. Outbreak of a new coronavirus: What anaesthetists should know. *Br J Anaesth.* 2020 May;124(5):497–501. doi:10.1016/j.bja.2020.02.008

GASTROINTESTINAL

21.

CIRRHOSIS AND TRULY ELECTIVE MAJOR SURGERY

Sofia S. Jakab and Adriana D. Oprea

STEM CASE AND KEY QUESTIONS

A 55-year-old woman noticed a lump in her right breast when showering. She went for further evaluation at a local women's clinic. She was found to have a 5 cm breast lesion, with biopsy showing invasive ductal carcinoma. She saw a breast surgeon who recommended mastectomy and immediate transverse rectus abdominus myocutaneous (TRAM) flap reconstruction. She presents for preoperative evaluation. She mentions a liver "illness," but she does not know details. Her primary care doctor retired a few years ago. She has not had any medical follow-up since, and she does not recall other medical problems. She had no prior surgery or hospitalizations. She does not take any medications. She works as a court clerk. She is sedentary; she gained 20 lbs over the past month, and noticed shortness of breath when walking upstairs, but otherwise no symptoms. She rarely drinks any alcohol. She never smoked or used any drugs. Her blood pressure is 160/95, heart rate 98, respiratory rate 16, SpO$_2$ 95% on room air, weight 220 lbs, BMI 38. Her exam is remarkable for palmar erythema, a few spider angiomas on the chest; her cardiopulmonary exam is normal; her abdomen is soft but distended, making it difficult to assess the liver span or splenomegaly; there is 2+ pedal edema. Recent laboratory values are remarkable for a platelet count of 80,000/microL, INR 1.7, bilirubin 1.5 mg/dL, AST 90 U/L, ALT 40 U/L, albumin 3.1 g/dL, creatinine 0.6 mg/dL, sodium 136 mEq/L. Chest x-ray is normal, except for prominent pulmonary arteries.

What makes you suspect she may have cirrhosis?

Any patient with chronic liver disease can develop cirrhosis. Diagnosis of cirrhosis can be suggested by clinical findings (firm and/or enlarged left liver lobe, splenomegaly, spider angioma, or palmar erythema), laboratory data (thrombocytopenia, liver synthetic dysfunction with abnormal albumin, INR, bilirubin), or liver fibrosis scores such as FIB-4 (gihep.com/calculators/hepatology/fibrosis-4-score/), and can be confirmed by imaging showing high liver stiffness (by elastography techniques), nodular surface of the liver, or features of portal hypertension (splenomegaly, recanalized umbilical vein, portosystemic collaterals).

What else do you want to know about this patient?

You receive records from the office of her former primary care doctor. Three years ago, she had an abdominal ultrasound done for abnormal liver tests, which showed a fatty liver with a nodular surface and enlarged spleen. There was no ascites. She also had an upper endoscopy, which showed small esophageal varices. Her hepatitis C testing was negative. Other labs at that time were remarkable for triglycerides 330 mg/dL, HDL cholesterol 30 mg/dL, LDL cholesterol 190 mg/dL, Hb A1c 6.2%.

What are the stages of cirrhosis and their prognostic significance?

What scoring systems can help predict postoperative outcomes in patients with cirrhosis?

What is the significance of esophageal varices found 3 years prior? Any other testing or treatment necessary?

What laboratory values are important for this patient's preoperative evaluation?

It is just a mastectomy with TRAM flap reconstruction, do you need to get an echocardiogram?

What are the cardiopulmonary complications of cirrhosis that may impact her intra- and postoperative course?

You discuss with the patient your concerns that she has cirrhosis and that she needs further evaluation, including, at the minimum, a hepatology consult and echocardiogram. She tells you that she just saw a cardiologist the day before. You obtain her echocardiogram, which showed normal left ventricle with an ejection fraction of 70%, a slightly dilated right ventricle with an estimated right ventricular systolic pressure of 80 mm Hg, no valvular disease, and no other cardiac abnormalities but likely ascites. In addition, the laboratories she had in the morning are back, remarkable for platelets 35,000/microL, INR 2.7, albumin 2.4 g/dL, bilirubin 3.2 mg/dL, creatinine 2.1, and sodium 128 mEq/L.

How does this information change your preoperative evaluation and recommendations?

Is the presence of ascites of importance for the planned surgery?

What worries you most about her latest laboratories, and what do you need to do next?

You send her to the emergency room for further evaluation and likely hospital admission. At the end of the day, you check to see what happened. A diagnostic paracentesis showed spontaneous bacterial peritonitis (SBP); hepatology service was consulted, and the patient was admitted.

What are your recommendations to the medical team regarding specific medical problems that need to be optimized before she can undergo mastectomy?

What are your options to control her coagulopathy perioperatively? Given the complexity of this patient's situation, a multidisciplinary discussion involving the hepatologist, transplant surgeon, oncologist, breast surgeon, and anesthesiologist addressed the following questions: (1) What is her prognosis related to her liver disease, if no transplant is done? (2) What is the cancer-free period she needs to achieve before being accepted as a liver transplant candidate? (3) What is her prognosis related to her breast cancer, if no treatment is received? (4) What are the potential risks/complications from mastectomy given her decompensated liver disease? The presence of ascites makes TRAM flap reconstruction a difficult choice as it will further increase the risk of abdominal wall hernias. In addition, if the patient's ascites proves to be recurrent or refractory (requiring large-volume paracentesis despite maximum dose or diuretics, or because titration of diuretics cannot be attained given the development of diuretic-induced complications), the only therapeutic option is a transjugular intrahepatic portosystemic shunt (TIPS), which lowers portal pressure by shunting the blood from a branch of the portal vein into a branch of hepatic vein. The echocardiographic findings of dilated right ventricle and elevated right ventricular systolic pressure could be secondary to portopulmonary hypertension, which is a major contraindication to TIPS as TIPS would increase cardiac preload and risk of right-sided heart failure. If she does not have portopulmonary hypertension, TIPS could be considered, but only after her active infection resolves and if her liver function improves to a Model for End-Stage Live Disease (MELD) score of less than 18.

You tell the rest of the team that if the final recommendation is to proceed with mastectomy (and probably no breast reconstruction) as soon as she is optimized, she would need at the minimum the following: evidence of successful treatment of SBP based on repeat ascites fluid analysis; right-heart catheterization to evaluate for portopulmonary hypertension (alternatively, careful diuresis with repeat echocardiogram to see if improvement occurs in her right ventricular size and pressure with diuresis); stabilization of renal function; and assessment of nutritional status. Once her infection and renal function are improved, you would like to get a thromboelastogram and fibrinogen level to assess her coagulopathy and decide if and what blood products she would require perioperatively.

DISCUSSION

Chronic liver diseases (CLD) pose a major public health problem, with a worldwide prevalence of 844 million people and mortality rate of 2 million deaths per year, comparable with diabetes, pulmonary, and cardiovascular diseases.[1] The prevalence of CLD and cirrhosis is underestimated because many patients are asymptomatic and not aware of their liver problems. In a recent study, about 633,000 people in the United States were found to have abnormal liver tests and high fibrosis scores with a high likelihood of having cirrhosis, but 69% of those did not know of having liver disease.[2] Despite significant improvements in therapies for chronic hepatitis B and C, many patients are diagnosed and treated when they have cirrhosis and remain at risk for further complications such as liver cancer and end-stage liver disease. Furthermore, the risk of cirrhosis in patients with nonalcoholic fatty liver disease, the most common CLD in the United States, will continue to increase given the lack of active policies to engage the public and healthcare clinicians in strategies targeting early diagnosis and treatment.[3]

Any patient with CLD or chronic abnormalities in liver enzymes and/or risk factors for liver disease (chronic alcohol use, transfusion of blood products, substance use, tattoos, or family history of liver disease) should be suspected of cirrhosis, and part of their evaluation should focus on excluding or confirming cirrhosis.

ETIOLOGY

The most common causes of cirrhosis are nonalcoholic fatty liver disease, alcoholic liver disease, and chronic hepatitis C. Nonalcoholic fatty liver disease, frequently seen in patients with metabolic syndrome, has become a leading cause of liver-related morbidity and need for liver transplantation.[4] Less common causes are autoimmune hepatitis, primary biliary cholangitis, primary sclerosing cholangitis, or genetic conditions such as hemochromatosis or alpha-1 antitrypsin deficiency.

CLINICAL STAGES

Clinical presentation and complications of cirrhosis are secondary to portal hypertension and liver insufficiency. Patients with cirrhosis develop increased intrahepatic resistance to portal blood flow secondary to fibrosis and architecture distortion (mechanical component) and increased hepatic vascular tone (functional component), ultimately resulting in portal hypertension. Portal pressure is estimated by measuring the hepatic venous pressure gradient (HVPG) through transjugular hepatic vein balloon catheterization. HVPG is the difference between the wedged (occluded) hepatic vein pressure and the free hepatic vein pressure and normally is less than 5 mm Hg.[5,6] Worsening portal hypertension correlates closely with development of complications such as ascites/hepatic hydrothorax, variceal bleeding (VB), or portosystemic encephalopathy (when the blood shunted through portosystemic collaterals is not detoxified by the liver) and causes splenomegaly and hypersplenism with thrombocytopenia/pancytopenia, or it can affect other organs leading to portopulmonary hypertension or HRS. Liver insufficiency is manifested as hypoalbuminemia, muscle wasting, jaundice, coagulopathy, and hepatic encephalopathy (HE; from failure of the detoxification function of the liver).

Cirrhosis has two clinical stages: compensated and decompensated, each with distinct presentation and prognosis.[7] The *compensated stage* is asymptomatic, with a median survival of more than 12 years, and it is at this stage when the diagnosis of cirrhosis is difficult to make and requires a high index of suspicion. This compensated stage is divided into mild portal hypertension (HVPG of 5–9 mm Hg), and clinically significant portal hypertension (CSPH) when HVPG is 10 mm Hg or more, associated with a higher risk of decompensation or liver cancer.[8] Some patients can remain compensated, others can develop complications that define their progression to decompensated cirrhosis, such as VB, ascites and/or HE, or further decompensations with refractory ascites, recurrent VB, and refractory HE. Overall, *decompensated cirrhosis* is associated with a median survival of less than 2 years.[6,7] Of note, patients who require ongoing treatment to control their cirrhosis complications (diuretics for ascites, laxatives for encephalopathy, endoscopic or interventional radiology procedures for bleeding varices) are still staged as decompensated cirrhosis even if they no longer have clinical ascites, encephalopathy, or VB.

Only with significant improvement in liver function (albumin, INR, bilirubin) after removal, suppression, or cure of the primary etiology of cirrhosis (as seen with sustained alcohol abstinence, sustained viral suppression for hepatitis B, or viral elimination for hepatitis C) can patients who achieve resolution of ascites (off diuretics), encephalopathy (off laxatives/rifaximin), and absence of recurrent variceal hemorrhage (for at least 12 months) be considered *recompensated*.[5]

DIAGNOSIS

In patients with compensated cirrhosis, the diagnosis is suspected from physical exam findings (spider angiomas, palmar erythema, palpable left lobe of the liver, small liver span, splenomegaly) or laboratory abnormalities. A low platelet count of less than 150,000/microL is often the first sign[9] or a low/low-normal albumin level (<3.8 g/dL). Another red flag for cirrhosis is an AST greater than ALT in patients with no alcohol use, especially if in the past ALT was higher than AST; this is related to increased leakage of mitochondrial AST in cirrhosis.[10] Elevated bilirubin and elevated INR occur usually later. Imaging studies could also incidentally detect cirrhosis by findings such as nodular liver, splenomegaly, and/or portosystemic collaterals. Recently, significant advances in noninvasive methods to detect severe fibrosis and cirrhosis have led to changes in clinical practice, using elastography techniques (transient elastography [Fibroscan] or MR elastography) to assess liver stiffness rather than liver biopsy.[11] If a patient has elastography findings concordant with the clinical, laboratory, and radiologic features suggestive of cirrhosis, the diagnosis of cirrhosis can be established without a liver biopsy. If there is discordance, a liver biopsy may be necessary to make the correct diagnosis. Of note, a patient with compensated cirrhosis may lack any abnormalities on exam, laboratory testing, or imaging, and the diagnosis is based on liver stiffness measurement and/or liver biopsy.

In patients with decompensated cirrhosis, liver biopsy is rarely needed as the history and physical exam are very suggestive. These patients have a history of VB, current or past ascites or jaundice, or HE. Of note, the presence of varices on endoscopy or imaging indicates clinically significant portal hypertension, but it does not define decompensated cirrhosis in the absence of prior VB. On exam, most patients have sarcopenia (temporal wasting, decreased upper and lower extremity muscle mass) in addition to the classical findings of cirrhosis (spider angiomas, palmar erythema, ascites, caput medusae, jaundice, asterixis). Their laboratory results are markedly abnormal with thrombocytopenia, liver synthetic dysfunction (low albumin, elevated bilirubin, INR), electrolytes abnormalities (especially hyponatremia), and renal dysfunction. Imaging will show nodular liver, ascites, splenomegaly, and portosystemic collaterals very consistent with the diagnosis of cirrhosis.

MANAGEMENT

Management of patients with cirrhosis is complex given their several and severe complications.

Screening and Surveillance for High-Risk Gastroesophageal Varices

The risk of first VB is 5–15% per year, highest in patients with large varices, or with varices having endoscopic red wale marks (areas of thinning of the variceal wall). All patients with cirrhosis need upper endoscopy to screen for these high-risk varices which require primary prophylaxis with a nonselective beta blocker (propranolol, nadolol, carvedilol) or endoscopic variceal ligation (EVL) to prevent VB, in accordance with the most recent American Association for the Study of Liver Diseases guidance.[6] Patients with no varices or small varices need repeat endoscopy every 1–3 years, depending on their cirrhosis stage, findings on the last endoscopy, and if their liver disease is active (ongoing alcohol use, untreated viral hepatitis) or inactive. This paradigm has recently changed, using nonselective beta blockers for treatment of CSPH rather than just high-risk varices,[5] with the goal of preventing any complications that define decompensations (VB, ascites, or HE).

Variceal Bleeding

VB is associated with high mortality, especially if other decompensating events are present: 80% 5-year mortality versus 20% 5-year mortality if VB is the only complication of cirrhosis.[12] Specific treatments aim to decrease portal pressure or locally treat the bleeding varices. They include octreotide infusion (decreases portal hypertension by inducing splanchnic vasoconstriction), antibiotics (decrease risk of rebleeding and mortality by decreasing infections, especially SBP which can increase splanchnic vasodilatation and portal pressure), endoscopic treatment (mainly EVL, less commonly sclerotherapy), temporizing measures (Blakemore balloon tamponade or covered self-expanding esophageal metal stents), and interventional radiology therapies (TIPS, coil-embolization of varices, balloon-occluded retrograde transvenous obliteration [BRTO]). Unless TIPS was placed with optimal decrease of the portosystemic gradient to less than 12 mm Hg, all patients with prior VB need secondary prophylaxis of VB with both a nonselective beta blocker and EVL.[6,13]

Ascites and Hepatic Hydrothorax

Ascites and hepatic hydrothorax are characterized by low levels of fluid protein (<2.5 g/dL) and fluid albumin (a difference between serum and fluid albumin of >1.1). Ascites is the most common decompensation of cirrhosis and is associated with 50% mortality at 2 years. Optimal control of ascites can be achieved using a combination of a low-salt diet, diuretics (spironolactone, which acts on the renin-angiotensin-aldosterone system, one of the first compensatory mechanisms activated in cirrhosis, and furosemide, a loop diuretic), large-volume paracentesis with albumin infusion, and TIPS placement if there is refractory ascites requiring frequent large-volume paracentesis. Percutaneous catheters can be used for palliative management of ascites in patients with poor prognosis. Patients with ascites are at risk of developing complicated abdominal wall hernias and, most importantly, spontaneous bacterial peritonitis and HRS, which are associated with a significant increase in mortality. NSAIDs should be avoided because they reduce natriuresis, decrease glomerular filtration pressure by causing vasodilatation of the efferent renal arterioles, and could precipitate renal failure. The management of hepatic hydrothorax is similar with ascites, including a low-salt diet, diuretics, and TIPS placement. Drainage using a chest tube should be avoided given complications such as leakage and renal/electrolyte abnormalities, although select patients may need pigtail catheter placement.[14]

Spontaneous Bacterial Peritonitis

The most life-threatening complication of ascites is SBP, an infection of the ascites fluid that occurs "spontaneously," in the absence of a recognizable cause such as perforated viscus. It is considered that gut bacterial translocation causes transient bacteremia which infects the ascites fluid (hematogenous seeding). The diagnosis of SBP cannot be made just on clinical symptoms as many patients lack the classical symptoms of fever, abdominal pain, leukocytosis, and instead present with HE or just worsening creatinine and/or bilirubin. It requires ascites fluid analysis showing a neutrophil count greater than 250/mm^3. When ascites cultures are positive (only in up to 50% of patients), it is a monobacterial infection, usually with enteric organisms. Anaerobic, fungal, or polymicrobial infections should be further investigated for secondary peritonitis. The initial treatment of SBP includes antibiotics and albumin infusion, especially in the setting of renal dysfunction because SBP can precipitate HRS. After completing the treatment for SBP, secondary prophylaxis with long-term antibiotics (usually ciprofloxacin) is recommended.[14]

Hepatorenal Syndrome

HRS is the most dreaded complication of cirrhosis, with a median survival of 1 month. It occurs when sodium and water retention do not compensate enough to overcome the renal hypoperfusion induced by splanchnic and systemic vasodilation in patients with decompensated cirrhosis, and the only mechanism left to increase glomerular filtration pressure is intrarenal vasoconstriction.[15] Vasoconstrictor therapy with terlipressin (now available in the United States) or norepinephrine in combination with albumin, or renal replacement therapy are used, but the only treatment to significantly impact survival is liver transplantation.[15,16]

Hepatic Encephalopathy

Patients with cirrhosis can develop HE before they have significant liver insufficiency if they have large or multiple spontaneous portosystemic collaterals which divert the portal flow away from the liver and the blood is not detoxified in the liver. It is important to identify these patients who could benefit from embolization of those shunts to prevent multiple hospitalizations and when typical encephalopathy therapies such as lactulose or rifaximin are not enough.[17] For patients with severe synthetic dysfunction, embolization of portosystemic shunts will not lead to substantial improvement in their symptoms and the only definitive treatment is liver transplantation. The most critical part in the management of HE, regardless of the underlying pathophysiologic mechanism (shunting vs. liver insufficiency), is to identify, treat, and avoid precipitants such as infection, bleeding, electrolyte and renal abnormalities, dehydration, narcotics, sedatives, and constipation.[18] Of note, there is no utility to "trending" ammonia levels because treatment optimization relies on clinical symptoms (inversion of sleep/wake pattern, changes in mood/personality, forgetfulness, slowness, confusion, disorientation).

Screening for Liver Cancer

All patients with cirrhosis require imaging of their liver every 6 months to screen for liver cancer, which significantly increases mortality risk especially in patients with compensated cirrhosis.[19]

Liver Transplantation

Liver transplantation should be considered in any patient with decompensated cirrhosis and no psychosocial or medical contraindications, but it requires a thorough evaluation.[20] Organ allocation is based on the MELD score (using creatinine, INR, bilirubin, Na), but, given the shortage of available organs, only about 6,000 patients are transplanted each year from a wait list of approximately 14,000–16,000 (optn.transplant.hrsa.gov/data/).

Acute-on-Chronic Liver Failure

In patients with cirrhosis, an acute insult such as ischemia (from infection, VB, surgery), alcoholic hepatitis, acute viral hepatitis, or drug-induced injury could precipitate worsening liver failure (with worsening jaundice, ascites, coagulopathy) associated with one or more extrahepatic organ failures (kidney, brain, cardiovascular, respiratory) and poor prognosis. This entity was defined as acute-on-chronic liver failure (ACLF) and is clinically useful to assess patient's prognosis, urgency of liver transplantation, or futility of further treatment.[21]

SCORING SYSTEMS TO PREDICT POSTOPERATIVE MORTALITY IN CIRRHOSIS

Initial models to stratify the surgical risk in patients with cirrhosis used the Child-Turcotte-Pugh (CTP) score and the MELD score (Figure 21.1). The original CTP score was developed in 1964, by Child and Turcotte,[22] with the goal of assessing preoperative morbidity and mortality in patients with cirrhosis undergoing surgery, although it does not consider any surgery-specific variables and it was never validated. The CTP score includes five categories: bilirubin, albumin, INR, ascites, and encephalopathy. Most patients with compensated cirrhosis have a CTP score of 5–6 (class A), and most patients with decompensated cirrhosis and high risk for morbidity/mortality with surgical procedures have a CTP score of 10–15 (class C). Overall, patients with CTP class A cirrhosis have no contraindication for surgery, while patients with CTP class C cirrhosis should not undergo elective surgery; only selected patients with CTP class B cirrhosis should be considered for elective surgery. Mansour et al.[23] showed postoperative mortality rates of 10%, 30%, and 82% in patients with CTP classes A, B, and C, respectively.

The MELD score (Figure 21.1) was developed to predict mortality post TIPS, defining a cutoff MELD of 18 to identify patients at risk for liver failure due to their decreased hepatic reserve.[24] Later, the MELD score was validated as a predictor of 3-month mortality for patients listed for liver transplantation.[25] It is used for organ allocation in liver transplant candidates because it is based only on objective parameters (bilirubin, INR, creatinine; Na was added in 2016). Northup et al.[26] found a 1% increase in postoperative mortality for each MELD point until 20 and a 2% increase in mortality with each MELD point after 20.

The first dedicated surgical risk prediction model validated in patients with cirrhosis was the Mayo Postoperative Surgical Risk score (MRS), which combines the MELD score, American Society of Anesthesiologist (ASA) class, and age (Figure 21.1) and predicts the postoperative mortality risk at 7 days, 30 days, 90 days, 1 year, and 5 years.[27]

These prediction models (CTP, MELD, MRS) were potentially suboptimally calibrated, leading to overestimation of surgical risk[28] and did not consider surgery type, which constitutes a major predictor of surgical risk in patients with cirrhosis.[29] Mahmud et al.[30] used population-level data to derive and internally validate a novel cirrhosis surgical risk model the VOCAL-Penn score (VPS, Figure 21.1), which includes age, preoperative albumin, platelet count, bilirubin, surgery category, emergency indication, fatty liver disease, ASA classification, and obesity (www.vocalpennscore.com). The VPS demonstrated superior discrimination to MELD, MELD-Na, CTP, and MRS when estimating mortality at 30, 90, and 180 postoperative days in a Veterans Health Administration internal validation and was subsequently externally validated in two non-Veterans Health Administration independent health systems.[31] In contrast to other risk stratification models, the VPS has been expanded to predict 90-day postoperative hepatic decompensation.[32]

PREOPERATIVE EVALUATION IN CIRRHOSIS

The risk of perioperative morbidity and mortality in patients with cirrhosis is related to the complexity of their pathophysiologic derangements driven by the liver synthetic dysfunction and portal hypertension, which could lead to significant intra- and postoperative consequences. Baseline factors contributing to an increased surgical risk in patients with cirrhosis are risk of intraoperative bleeding given portosystemic collaterals, coagulopathy, thrombocytopenia, and fibrinolytic abnormalities; renal dysfunction; increased susceptibility to infection; potential for a thrombophilic state and predisposition to venous thromboembolism; impaired hepatic drug metabolism and elimination; and malnutrition.[33] Possible postoperative complications in patients with cirrhosis include hepatic

Parameter	VOCAL-Penn	Mayo Risk Score	MELD-Na	Child-Turcotte-Pugh score
Age	Years	Years	>12 years	
BMI	<30 (Y/N)			
Etiology of cirrhosis	NAFLD (Y/N)	Alcohol/cholestatic Viral/others		
Decompensation of cirrhosis	ASA class 3: compensated 4: decompensated	ASA class 3: compensated 4: decompensated		Ascites (0/slight/moderate) Hepatic encephalopathy (0/grade 1–2/grade 3–4)
Laboratory	Albumin Total bilirubin Platelet count	Total bilirubin, INR Creatinine	Total bilirubin, INR Creatinine Na	Albumin Total bilirubin, INR
Surgery type	Abd (lap vs open) Abd wall Vascular Major ortho Chest/cardiac	All major surgeries (no specific choice)		
Emergency	Y/N			

Figure 21.1 Clinical parameters used for predictive scores in patients with cirrhosis undergoing surgery.

decompensation with ACLF and multisystem organ failure; acute worsening of portal hypertension, including development/worsening of ascites; HE and/or VB (in addition, liberal use of blood products, volume overload, and infections can also increase the risk of VB); renal dysfunction; heart failure, especially if cirrhotic cardiomyopathy or portopulmonary hypertension is present; medication-related complications, particularly from opiates, with worsening HE; decreased wound healing in the setting of malnutrition; and decreased postoperative recovery secondary to sarcopenia.[33]

Therefore, in addition to achieving optimal control of ascites, VB risk, and HE prior to surgery, patients with cirrhosis require evaluation of the effect of cirrhosis on their cardiopulmonary status, hemostasis, and nutrition.

CARDIOPULMONARY COMPLICATIONS OF CIRRHOSIS

Patients with cirrhosis may have cardiopulmonary complications that need to be considered in the setting of surgical procedures, such as cirrhotic cardiomyopathy, hepatopulmonary syndrome, and portopulmonary hypertension.

Cirrhotic cardiomyopathy may be present in up to 50% of patients with cirrhosis and is characterized by a combination of systolic dysfunction, impaired diastolic relaxation, and electrophysiological disturbances such as prolonged QT_C interval. This predisposes patients to poorly tolerate volume overload, and it may contribute to the development of HRS and ACLF.[34] Also, because of a blunted response to pharmacologic or physiologic stress, it can result in overt heart failure. In addition, patients with metabolic syndrome (especially if cirrhosis is secondary to nonalcoholic steatohepatitis) have additional risk factors for coronary artery disease and cardiac morbidity/mortality.

The major pulmonary complications of cirrhosis are hepatopulmonary syndrome (HPS), portopulmonary hypertension (POPH), and hepatic hydrothorax.[35] HPS occurs in 5–30% of patients with cirrhosis, and it manifests as hypoxia due to the development of intrapulmonary vascular dilatations. It leads to increased mortality and impaired quality of life, and it may require increased intraoperative oxygen concentration. POPH is defined as development of pulmonary arterial hypertension in the setting of portal hypertension, and it is present in 5–10% of patients with cirrhosis, causing increased mortality independent of their liver disease. POPH is probably the most important condition to recognize preoperatively because it can cause intra- and postoperative complications. It is suspected if there are radiologic findings of a prominent main pulmonary artery, but this is a late sign. Echocardiogram with measurement of right ventricular systolic pressure (RVSP) is recommended as a screening test for patients undergoing evaluation for liver transplantation because moderate to severe POPH not responsive to treatment is an absolute contraindication for liver transplant. In most patients with cirrhosis, an elevated RVSP will reflect hyperdynamic circulation (elevated cardiac output and pulmonary pressure but normal pulmonary vascular resistance) or volume overload (with elevated pulmonary artery wedge pressure), rather than true POPH, when pulmonary vascular resistance is significantly elevated.[35]

HEMOSTASIS IN CIRRHOSIS

Hemostasis in patients with cirrhosis requires special consideration perioperatively as they usually have deficits of both procoagulant and anticoagulant factors. Despite elevated PT/INR and thrombocytopenia, most patients are actually "rebalanced," and some can have a higher chance of thrombosis than of bleeding.[36] In fact, INR is not predictive of bleeding complications in patients with cirrhosis, and preoperative fresh frozen plasma transfusions are not beneficial. Similarly, platelet transfusion targeting a platelet count higher than 50,000/microL are not associated with less bleeding complications.[37] Thrombopoietin analogues and receptor agonists could be used to increase platelet count in patients with cirrhosis prior to invasive procedures, but there is no clear guidance if/when to use these agents instead of platelet transfusion.[38] Cryoprecipitate is transfused to increase the fibrinogen level to 100 mg/dL perioperatively, although there are no controlled trials in patients with cirrhosis.[37] Thromboelastography and rotational thromboelastometry are emerging as more specific tests to evaluate hemostasis in patients with cirrhosis and guide use of blood products.[39]

NUTRITIONAL STATUS IN CIRRHOSIS

Malnutrition is present in more than 80% of patients with cirrhosis,[40] but an accurate assessment of their nutritional status is challenging: their weight is affected by fluid retention, and serum albumin will be decreased by the liver synthetic dysfunction and infections, so other measurements such as triceps skin fold, mid-arm muscle circumference, or muscle function (frailty scores) are more important. Even if low serum albumin is associated with higher postoperative mortality, using albumin infusion does not have any impact, but perioperative nutritional support does improve the complication rates following surgery.[41,42]

In summary, a complete preoperative evaluation in patients with cirrhosis includes

- Etiology of liver disease
- Stage of cirrhosis: compensated or decompensated
- History of clinical decompensation (VB, ascites, encephalopathy, jaundice), and their current treatment (diuretics, beta blockers, TIPS, endoscopic banding)
- Documentation of specific exam findings suggestive of cirrhosis, in particular assessment of ascites, HE, nutritional status
- Last upper endoscopy and liver imaging findings
- Evaluation of cardiopulmonary complications of cirrhosis
- Laboratory data including albumin, bilirubin, PT/INR, creatinine, Na

- MELD score, CTP score, VOCAL-Penn score
- Assessment of whether the procedure should be delayed to allow for patient optimization or until after liver transplantation
- Assessment of futility especially if a high-risk patient is not a transplant candidate

Ideally, the following should be implemented and/or optimized for patients with cirrhosis undergoing elective or semielective surgery:

- Control ascites (in some patients TIPS is placed preoperatively)
- Assess and reduce the risk of VB (upper endoscopy and proper primary/secondary prophylaxis of VB)
- Control HE
- Assess and correct hemostatic parameters
- Assess and optimize nutritional status, including use of enteral nutrition
- If possible, postpone surgery until hepatitis C treatment is completed, to avoid interruptions
- Achieve stable treatment of autoimmune hepatitis and chronic hepatitis B
- Insist on alcohol abstinence

CONCLUSION

- Assess for cirrhosis in patients with chronic liver disease or risk factors.
- Recognize clinical, laboratory, and imaging findings suggestive of cirrhosis.
- Use VOCAL-Penn score to assess the perioperative risk in patients with cirrhosis. CTP score and MELD score help appreciate the severity of liver disease; MELD is objective and validated to assess 3-month mortality in patients with cirrhosis; organ allocation for liver transplantation is based on MELD.
- Beware of cardiopulmonary complications of cirrhosis: cirrhotic cardiomyopathy, hepatopulmonary syndrome, portopulmonary hypertension.
- Involve hepatology team to optimize patient's status regarding control of ascites, encephalopathy, risk of VB, nutritional status, and hemostasis.

REVIEW QUESTIONS

1. Which of the following makes you suspect cirrhosis?

   a. Heterogeneous liver on ultrasound.
   b. Serum albumin of 4 g/dL.
   c. Platelet count of 145,000/microL.
   d. AST 100 U/L, ALT 150 U/L.

   The correct answer is c.

   A decreasing platelet count over the years, especially when it gets to less than 150,000/microL is most often the first sign of cirrhosis.[9] Portal hypertension in cirrhosis causes splenomegaly and hypersplenism, with thrombocytopenia, followed by leukopenia and anemia. Many patients get a bone marrow biopsy before they get diagnosed with cirrhosis. Other laboratory abnormalities suggestive of cirrhosis is albumin less than 3.8 g/dL, AST>ALT in the absence of alcohol. Also, imaging with nodular liver or features of portal hypertension (portosystemic collaterals, splenomegaly, ascites) indicate cirrhosis in the right clinical situation.

2. What are the cirrhosis complications that define decompensated cirrhosis?

   a. Large varices on endoscopy.
   b. Prior VB.
   c. 4+ edema.
   d. Sarcopenia.

   The correct answer is b.

   Cirrhosis has two clinical stages: compensated and decompensated, each with distinct presentation and prognosis.[7] The compensated stage is asymptomatic, with a median survival of more than 12 years. The decompensated stage includes patients who have obvious clinical complications of cirrhosis such as VB, ascites, and/or HE, with a median survival of less than 2 years.[6,7] The presence of varices on endoscopy or portosystemic collaterals on imaging indicates clinically significant portal hypertension and higher risk for decompensation and mortality, but it does not define decompensated cirrhosis in the absence of prior VB.

3. What score best predicts postoperative risk in patients with cirrhosis?

   a. FIB-4.
   b. MELD score.
   c. VOCAL-Penn score.
   d. CTP score.

   The correct answer is c.

   For patients with cirrhosis undergoing surgical procedures, scoring systems helpful to predict their perioperative morbidity and mortality include the MELD score, CTP score, Mayo Postoperative Surgical Risk Score, and the VPS. The VPS demonstrated superior mortality prediction to MELD, MELD-Na, CTP, and MRS at 30, 90, and 180 postoperative days.[30]

4. What are the parameters we use to calculate the CTP score?

   a. INR, bilirubin, creatinine, albumin, sodium.
   b. INR, bilirubin, albumin, sodium, nutritional status.
   c. INR, bilirubin, albumin, ascites, size of varices.
   d. INR, bilirubin, albumin, ascites, HE.

   The correct answer is d.

The original CTP score was developed in 1964, by Child and Turcotte,[22] with the goal of assessing preoperative morbidity and mortality in patients with cirrhosis undergoing surgery. The initial score included five categories: bilirubin, albumin, ascites, encephalopathy, and nutritional status. In 1973, Pugh replaced nutritional status with PT/INR to eliminate the least objective part of the score, but even this version still includes subjective categories (ascites, encephalopathy) and uses arbitrary cutoffs for albumin, bilirubin, and PT/INR. The CTP score was never validated, although it is widely used in clinical practice and has stood the test of time.

5. What echocardiographic findings could suggest cardiopulmonary complications from cirrhosis?

   a. Wall motion abnormality.
   b. Tricuspid regurgitation.
   c. Dilated left atrium.
   d. Elevated RVSP.

The correct answer is d.

Elevated RVSP on echocardiogram needs further investigation for POPH. In most patients with cirrhosis, an elevated RVSP will reflect hyperdynamic circulation (elevated cardiac output and pulmonary pressure but normal pulmonary vascular resistance) or volume overload (with elevated pulmonary artery wedge pressure) rather than true POPH, when pulmonary vascular resistance is significantly elevated.[35]

6. Which of the following blood products are most beneficial for a patient with cirrhosis and INR 2, platelet count of 55,000/L, hemoglobin 8 g/dL, and fibrinogen 90 mg/dL, about to undergo urgent hernia repair?

   a. Cryoprecipitate.
   b. Fresh frozen plasma.
   c. Platelet transfusion.
   d. PRBC.

The correct answer is a.

Liberal use of blood products, especially PRBC, may precipitate VB by increasing portal hypertension. Cryoprecipitate is transfused to increase the fibrinogen level to 100 mg/dL perioperatively, although there are no controlled trials in patients with cirrhosis. INR is not predictive of bleeding complications in patients with cirrhosis, and preoperative fresh frozen plasma transfusions are not beneficial. Similarly, platelet transfusion targeting a platelet count higher than 50,000/microL are not associated with less bleeding complications.[37] Thromboelastography and rotational thromboelastometry are emerging as more specific tests to evaluate hemostasis in patients with cirrhosis and guide use of blood products.[39]

7. When reviewing medical records from the last admission of a patient with cirrhosis scheduled for cholecystectomy, you note the following: your patient presented with hematemesis and was found to have bleeding esophageal varices which were banded; his ascites analysis showed WBC 400/microL, 25% PMN; his ammonia level was 200 umol/L; he was not confused or disoriented. What medications should this patient be taking?

   a. Ciprofloxacin.
   b. Nadolol.
   c. Lactulose.
   d. Metoprolol.

The correct answer is b.

All patients with prior VB need secondary prophylaxis of variceal bleeding with both nonselective beta blocker (such as nadolol) and endoscopic band ligation.[6] SBP is diagnosed if the PMN count is higher than 250/microL. The decision to treat HE is based on clinical symptoms, not on ammonia level.

REFERENCES

1. Byass P. The global burden of liver disease: A challenge for methods and for public health. *BMC Med.* 2014;12:159. doi:10.1186/s12916-014-0159-5
2. Scaglione S, Kliethermes S, Cao G, et al. The epidemiology of cirrhosis in the United States: A population-based study. *J Clin Gastroenterol.* 2015;49:690–696. doi:10.1097/MCG.0000000000000208
3. Marcellin P, Kutala BK. Liver diseases: A major, neglected global public health problem requiring urgent actions and large-scale screening. *Liver Int.* 2018;38 Suppl 1:2–6. doi:10.1111/liv.13682
4. Younossi ZM, Wong G, Anstee QM, et al. The global burden of liver disease. *Clin Gastroenterol Hepatol.* 2023;21(8):1978–1991. doi:10.1016/j.cgh.2023.04.015
5. de Franchis R, Bosch J, Garcia-Tsao G, et al. Baveno VII Faculty. Baveno VII renewing consensus in portal hypertension. *J Hepatol.* 2022;76:959–974. doi:10.1016/j.jhep.2021.12.022
6. Garcia-Tsao G, Abraldes JG, Berzigotti A, et al. Portal hypertensive bleeding in cirrhosis: Risk stratification, diagnosis, and management: 2016 Practice guidance by the American Association for the Study of Liver Diseases. *Hepatology.* 2017;65(1):310–335. doi:10.1002/hep.28906
7. D'Amico G, Garcia-Tsao G, Pagliaro L. Natural history and prognostic indicators of survival in cirrhosis: A systematic review of 118 studies. *J Hepatol.* 2006;44(1):217–231. doi:10.1016/j.jhep.2005.10.013
8. Ripoll C, Groszmann R, Garcia-Tsao G, et al. Hepatic venous pressure gradient predicts clinical decompensation in patients with compensated cirrhosis. *Gastroenterology.* 2007;133(2):481–488. doi:10.1053/j.gastro.2007.05.024
9. Berzigotti A, Seijo S, Arena U, et al. Elastography, spleen size, and platelet count identify portal hypertension in patients with compensated cirrhosis. *Gastroenterology.* 2013;144(1):102–111.e1. doi:10.1053/j.gastro.2012.10.001
10. Sheth SG, Flamm SL, Gordon FD, et al. AST/ALT ratio predicts cirrhosis in patients with chronic hepatitis C virus infection. *Am J Gastroenterol* 1998;93:44–48. doi:10.1111/j.1572-0241.1998.044_c.x
11. European Association for Study of Liver; Asociacion Latinoamericana para el Estudio del Higado. EASL-ALEH clinical practice guidelines: Non-invasive tests for evaluation of liver disease severity and prognosis. *J Hepatol.* 2015;63(1):237–264. doi:10.1016/j.jhep.2015.04.006
12. D'Amico G, Bernardi M, Angeli P. Towards a new definition of decompensated cirrhosis. *J Hepatol.* 2022;76(1):202–207. doi:10.1016/j.jhep.2021.06.018
13. Jakab SS, Garcia-Tsao G. Evaluation and management of esophageal and gastric varices in patients with cirrhosis. *Clin Liver Dis.* 2020;24(3):335–350. doi:10.1016/j.cld.2020.04.011
14. Biggins SW, Angeli P, Garcia-Tsao G, et al. Diagnosis, evaluation, and management of ascites, spontaneous bacterial peritonitis and hepatorenal syndrome: 2021 Practice guidance by the American Association for the Study of Liver Diseases. *Hepatology.* 2021;74(2):1014–1048. doi:10.1002/hep.31884
15. Patidar KR, Piano S, Cullaro G, et al.; HRS-Harmony Consortia. Recent advances in the management of hepatorenal syndrome: A

US perspective. *Clin Gastroenterol Hepatol*. 2023;21(4):897–901.e1. doi:10.1016/j.cgh.2022.12.034
16. Glass L, Sharma P. Evidence-based therapeutic options for hepatorenal syndrome. *Gastroenterology*. 2016 Apr;150(4):1031–1033.
17. Laleman W, Simon-Talero M, Maleux G, et al. Embolization of large spontaneous portosystemic shunts for refractory hepatic encephalopathy: A multicenter survey on safety and efficacy. *Hepatology*. 2013;57(6):2448–2457. doi:10.1002/hep.26314
18. European Association for the Study of the Liver. EASL clinical practice guidelines on the management of hepatic encephalopathy. *J Hepatol*. 2022;77(3):807–824. doi:10.1016/j.jhep.2022.06.001
19. Marrero JA, Kulik LM, Sirlin CB, et al. Diagnosis, staging, and management of hepatocellular carcinoma: 2018 Practice guidance by the American Association for the Study of Liver Diseases. *Hepatology*. 2018;68(2):723–750. doi:10.1002/hep.29913.
20. Martin P, DiMartini A, Feng S, et al. Evaluation for liver transplantation in adults: 2013 Practice guideline by the American Association for the Study of Liver Diseases and the American Society of Transplantation. *Hepatology*. 2014;59(3):1144–1165. doi:10.1002/hep.26972
21. Bajaj JS, O'Leary JG, Lai JC, et al. Acute-on-chronic liver failure clinical guidelines. *Am J Gastroenterol*. 2022;117(2):225–252. doi:10.14309/ajg.0000000000001595
22. Child CG, Turcotte JG. Surgery and portal hypertension. *Major Probl Clin Surg*. 1964;1:1–85.
23. Mansour A, Watson W, Shayani V, et al. Abdominal operations in patients with cirrhosis: Still a major surgical challenge. *Surgery*. 1997;122:730–736. doi:10.1016/s0039-6060(97)90080-5
24. Kamath PS, Wiesner RH, Malinchoc M, et al. A model to predict survival in patients with end-stage liver disease. *Hepatology*. 2001 Feb;33(2):464–470. doi:10.1053/jhep.2001.22172
25. Wiesner R, Edwards E, Freeman R, et al. United Network for Organ Sharing Liver Disease Severity Score Committee. Model for end-stage liver disease (MELD) and allocation of donor livers. *Gastroenterology*. 2003 Jan;124(1):91–96. doi:10.1053/gast.2003.50016
26. Northup PG, Wanamaker RC, Lee VD, et al. Model for End-Stage Liver Disease (MELD) predicts nontransplant surgical mortality in patients with cirrhosis. *Ann Surg*. 2005;242(2):244–251. doi:10.1097/01.sla.0000171327.29262.e0
27. Teh SH, Nagorney DM, Stevens SR, et al. Risk factors for mortality after surgery in patients with cirrhosis. *Gastroenterology*. 2007;132(4):1261–1269. doi:10.1053/j.gastro.2007.01.040
28. Kim SY, Yim HJ, Park SM, et al. Validation of a Mayo post-operative mortality risk prediction model in Korean cirrhotic patients. *Liver Int*. 2011;31(2):222–228. doi:10.1111/j.1478-3231.2010.02419.x
29. Mahmud N, Fricker Z, Serper M, et al. In-hospital mortality varies by procedure type among cirrhosis surgery admissions. *Liver Int*. 2019;39(8):1394–1399. doi:10.1111/liv.14156
30. Mahmud N, Fricker Z, Hubbard RA, et al. Risk prediction models for post-operative mortality in patients with cirrhosis. *Hepatology*. 2021;73:204–218. doi:10.1002/hep.31558
31. Mahmud N, Fricker Z, Panchal S, et al. External validation of the VOCAL-Penn cirrhosis surgical risk score in 2 large, independent health systems. *Liver Transpl*. 2021;27:961–970. doi:10.1002/lt.26060
32. Mahmud N, Fricker Z, Lewis JD, et al. Risk prediction models for postoperative decompensation and infection in patients with cirrhosis: A Veterans Affairs cohort study. *Clin Gastroenterol Hepatol* 2022;20(5):e1121–e1134. doi:10.1016/j.cgh.2021.06.050
33. Northup PG, Friedman LS, Kamath PS. AGA clinical practice update on surgical risk assessment and perioperative management in cirrhosis: *Expert Review. Clin Gastroenterol Hepatol*. 2019;17(4):595–606. doi:10.1016/j.cgh.2018.09.043
34. Izzy M, VanWagner LB, Lin G, et al. Redefining cirrhotic cardiomyopathy for the modern era. *Hepatology*. 2020;71(1):334–345. doi:10.1002/hep.30875
35. Machicao VI, Balakrishnan M, Fallon MB. Pulmonary complications in chronic liver disease. *Hepatology*. 2014;59(4):1627–1637. doi:10.1002/hep.26745
36. Drolz A, Horvatits T, Roedl K, et al. Coagulation parameters and major bleeding in critically ill patients with cirrhosis. *Hepatology*. 2016;64(2):556–568. doi:10.1002/hep.28628
37. Northup PG, Garcia-Pagan JC, Garcia-Tsao G, et al. Vascular liver disorders, portal vein thrombosis, and procedural bleeding in patients with liver disease: 2020 Practice guidance by the American Association for the Study of Liver Diseases. *Hepatology*. 2021;73(1):366–413. doi:10.1002/hep.31646
38. Terrault N, Chen YC, Izumi N, et al. Avatrombopag before procedures reduces need for platelet transfusion in patients with chronic liver disease and thrombocytopenia. *Gastroenterology*. 2018;155(3):705–718. doi:10.1053/j.gastro.2018.05.025
39. De Pietri L, Bianchini M, Montalti R, et al. Thrombelastography-guided blood product use before invasive procedures in cirrhosis with severe coagulopathy: A randomized, controlled trial. *Hepatology*. 2016;63(2):566–573. doi:10.1002/hep.28148
40. Maharshi S, Sharma BC, Srivastava S. Malnutrition in cirrhosis increases morbidity and mortality. *J Gastroenterol Hepatol*. 2015;30:1507–1513. doi:10.1111/jgh.12999
41. Jie B, Jiang ZM, Nolan MT, Zhu SN, Yu K, Kondrup J. Impact of preoperative nutritional support on clinical outcome in abdominal surgical patients at nutritional risk. *Nutrition*. 2012;28:1022–1027. doi:10.1016/j.nut.2012.01.017
42. Lai J, Tandon P, Bernal, W, et al. Malnutrition, frailty, and sarcopenia in patients with cirrhosis: 2021 Practice guidance by the American Association for the Study of Liver Diseases. *Hepatology*. 2021;74(3):1611–1644. doi:10.1002/hep.32049

NEUROLOGICAL

22.

PATIENT HAS SEIZURES AND NEEDS "CLEARANCE"

Ramanjot S. Kang, Ashley Mathew, and Shirley Avraham

STEM CASE AND KEY QUESTIONS

A 7-year-old 25 kg nonverbal female with a past medical history of epilepsy and global developmental delay presents for preoperative clearance for an upcoming laparoscopic umbilical hernia repair. Her seizures, which typically present as grand mal/tonic-clonic, have been well controlled on her current regimen of levetiracetam and carbamazepine. Her seizure medications are taken BID with yogurt. Her mother reports that the last seizure was 1 week ago, and seizures occur on average once every 2 weeks.

What defines a seizure? What is the definition of epilepsy?

A seizure is defined as abnormal electrical activity in the brain resulting from excessive and hypersynchronous discharge of neurons.[1] Epilepsy is a disease associated with spontaneously recurring seizures. Traditionally epilepsy was characterized by two or more unprovoked seizures occurring more than 24 hours apart in the absence of a precipitating factor.[2]

What are the underlying causes/pathophysiology of seizures?

Potential underlying mechanisms of seizure disorder include (1) loss of inhibitory activity, (2) enhanced release of excitatory amino acids, and (3) enhanced neuronal firing. Specific precipitating factors include febrile seizures in children until age 6, alcohol withdrawal, metabolic derangements, toxicity, brain trauma, infection, or stroke. A seizure provoked by a reversible insult is not classified as epilepsy because it is not a chronic state.[1]

What is the incidence of epilepsy in the general population? What is the incidence in the pediatric population?

Approximately 1.2% of the US population had an active epilepsy diagnosis in 2015.[3,4] Epilepsy is one of the most common chronic neurologic conditions in children. It affects 0.5 to 1% of children. Patients at the extremes of age, pediatric and elderly, have the highest incidence. Approximately 1 out of 150 children is diagnosed with epilepsy during the first 10 years of life, with the highest rate observed during infancy.[3] Up to one-third of epilepsy patients can continue to have seizures despite medical therapy, known as *refractory epilepsy*.[1]

What are the different classifications of seizures? How do they differ in their presentations?

Seizures may be localized to a specific area in the brain (partial/focal seizures) or may be generalized. Focal seizures have the potential to become generalized. Depending on the cortical area affected, focal seizures manifest different motor, sensory, or psychiatric symptoms. Generalized seizures produce bilaterally symmetric electrical activity, resulting in loss of consciousness and/or abnormal motor activity. Generalized seizures are further classified by the type of motor activity, such as tonic, clonic, or myoclonic[5] (Box 22.1).

What are the treatment options for epilepsy? Antiepileptic drugs (AEDs) versus surgical? Other therapies?

Treatment options for epilepsy include AEDs; surgical procedures, including resection of structural lesions; deep brain stimulation (DBS); and implantation of devices such as a vagal nerve stimulator (VNS). Various diets, such as the ketogenic diet, have also been shown to be effective in seizure control.[3]

You are seeing this patient in the preoperative clinic. Knowing that epilepsy is associated with increased risk of perioperative complications, what are your perioperative considerations for this patient?

Box 22.1 **SEIZURE CLASSIFICATION ACCORDING TO THE INTERNATIONAL LEAGUE AGAINST EPILEPSY (ILAE)**

Focal seizures
    With aura
    With motor features
    With autonomic features
    With dyscognitive features
    Without dyscognitive features
Generalized seizures
    Tonic-clonic
    Absence
    Clonic
    Tonic
    Atonic
    Myoclonic
    Unknown

Adapted from Fisher et al.[6]

The patient should bring documentation and/or consult notes from their neurologist or primary care physician with details regarding current seizure status. It is important that the patient stays up to date with follow-up as regular dose adjustments are needed based on normal pediatric growth weight gain. Anesthetic evaluation should focus on the underlying cause of seizure (if applicable), type of seizure, and medications used for treatment (Tables 22.1 and 22.2). A number of medications used in the perioperative period can interact with AEDs or affect seizure threshold.[7,8]

It is also important to know if the patient is using alternative therapies such as VNS or is on a ketogenic diet. An implanted VNS would affect the intraoperative use of electrocautery. A patient on a ketogenic diet requires glucose level and intraoperative acid-base monitoring as the diet may precipitate metabolic acidosis.[11]

In the case of elective surgery, seizures should be well controlled and the patient's exposure to potential triggers should be limited prior to the scheduled case. Perioperative seizures may result in aspiration, and the postictal state may be confused with delayed awakening from anesthesia.[10]

What instructions will you give her mother regarding medication administration on the day of surgery?

It is imperative that antiseizure medication be continued throughout the perioperative period to maintain therapeutic levels (Box 22.2). The surgical time should be scheduled to accommodate medication administration. The mother should be advised to administer the antiseizure medication as prescribed the day of surgery.[10] NPO guidelines should be strictly followed—yogurt is considered a solid food.[12] Her mother should try give the dose with water, clear apple juice, or, if needed a small amount of clear gelatin (contains protein so not true "clear" liquid.) However, if the surgery requires electroencephalography (EEG) monitoring and localization, AEDs may be held in order to invoke intraoperative seizures.[13]

Any laboratory studies needed? Any imaging studies needed?

Due to possible metabolic and hematologic derangements caused by antiseizure medications, it is reasonable to request a recent blood count and metabolic panel.[15] New imaging studies are not needed (unless there is a known structural abnormality and unexplained change in pattern of the seizures).

Table 22.1 PREANESTHETIC EVALUATION

Etiology	Known cause: structural abnormality, disease state, or idiopathic
Signs and symptoms of the seizures	Generalized "full body" seizures or focal seizures
Structural lesions in the brain where the seizures originate.	May not be fully appreciated prior to surgery, as some procedures involve detailed mapping (electrocorticography) of the suspected brain areas.
Is it part of a syndrome?	What other manifestations may be included in the syndrome?
Triggering events	If applicable, in general it would be prudent to avoid triggering agents/activities

Adapted from Ruskin, et al.[9]

Table 22.2 COMMONLY USED ANTIEPILEPTIC DRUGS, MECHANISMS OF ACTION, AND COMMON SIDE EFFECTS

DRUG	MECHANISM OF ACTION	MAJOR SIDE EFFECTS	COMMENTS
Phenytoin	Blocks voltage sensitive Na$^+$ channels	Dizziness, drowsiness, blurry vision, ataxia, fatigue, nausea, constipation	Low therapeutic index, enzyme inducer, megaloblastic anemia
Phenobarbital	Potentiates GABAergic inhibition	Sedation, dizziness, confusion	
Carbamazepine	Blocks voltage-sensitive Na channels	Aplastic anemia, leukopenia, hepatotoxicity, ataxia, sedation	SIADH/hyponatremia
Oxcarbazepine		Visual disturbance	Enzyme inducer
Valproic acid	Increases synthesis and release of GABA, inhibits NMDA receptors	Sedation, tremor thrombocytopenia, hepatotoxicity	
Lamotrigine	Blocks voltage sensitive Na$^+$ channels	Stevens-Johnson syndrome, ataxia, sedation	Levels increased by valproic acid
Ethosuximide	Reduces low-threshold T-type Ca$^+$ currents	Drowsiness, nausea	
Vigabatrin	GABA analogue	Visual field deficits	
Topiramate	Potentiates GABAergic inhibition	Paresthesia, speech difficulty, renal stones	Pulmonary embolism

Adapted from Butterworth, et al.[10]

Box 22.2 PERIOPERATIVE MEDICATION MANAGEMENT FOR PATIENTS WITH EPILEPSY

Preoperative management
    Consult with primary care doctor or neurologist
    Clarify usual seizure types, frequency, and triggers
    Review medication regimen, review rescue medication regimen
    Check AED level
Management for minor surgery
    Schedule surgery to allow for usual morning and evening dose of medication
    Avoid prolonged fasting
Management for major surgery
    Ensure regular medications up to fasting
    Use intravenous preparations of drugs when necessary
    If IV dose of regular drugs not possible, administer:
    Phenytoin: IV load 15–20 mg/kg at rate of 50 mg/minute, then twice daily maintenance dose of 2.5–5.0 mg/kg
    Benzodiazepine: Give IV as rescue

Adapted from Cote, et al.[14]

AED levels may not be required unless there has been an adjustment in dose or change in renal or hepatic function that may contribute to change in drug metabolism or excretion.[15]

You are now the anesthesiologist on the day of surgery. What questions will you ask the mother?

A comprehensive preoperative exam should be performed on this medically complex child, including surgical history and details from prior anesthetics. Details should be obtained regarding the patient's seizure history, such as type of seizure, frequency, and last witnessed seizure. A thorough review of all medications and dose schedules should be obtained. Baseline mental status should be well documented. Any preoperative anxiety should be alleviated by use of premedication or parental presence because stress can induce seizures.

During your preoperative evaluation, her mother states that the morning AED dose was delayed. It was administered mixed in yogurt at 8 a.m. Surgery is scheduled for 1 p.m. What is your plan?

Yogurt is considered a solid and requires a complete 6- to 8-hour NPO time.[12] Since this is an elective nonurgent surgery, it is advised to wait at least 6 hours to minimize the risk of aspiration. The mother and the surgery team should be involved in this discussion to postpone.

It is now 3 p.m. and the patient is appropriately NPO. What is your anesthetic plan? How will you induce anesthesia in this patient, IV versus mask induction? What are the considerations for each?

General anesthesia with standard American Society of Anesthesiologists (ASA) monitors is preferred in this patient for laparoscopic umbilical hernia repair. Induction in this patient can be achieved via IV, IM, or mask, depending on provider preference and patient behavior.

IV induction requires patient cooperation. IV placement can be accomplished by prepping with a eutectic mixture of local anesthetics (EMLA) cream or lidocaine patch, followed by standard IV induction with propofol, fentanyl, and muscle relaxant if needed. Mask induction can be achieved using sevoflurane with or without nitrous, followed by IV placement. Anesthesia can be maintained with inhalational agents, propofol, fentanyl, with or without dexmedetomidine. The airway should be secured with an endotracheal tube. Postoperative pain control may be supplemented by bilateral transversus abdominis plane (TAP) regional block, rectus sheath block, or local anesthetic injection by the surgeon. Any use of local anesthetic requires the calculation of maximal recommended dose to avoid systemic toxicity. Local anesthetics can readily cross the blood–brain barrier resulting in seizure and coma.[13]

Any concern with interactions of anesthetic agents and AEDs? Which anesthetic agents will you avoid, if any?

Drugs with epileptogenic potential should be avoided, which theoretically include enflurane, ketamine, and methohexital.[5] Large doses of atracurium, cisatracurium, and meperidine should be avoided due to the epileptogenic potential of metabolites.[5] Laudanosine, a metabolite of atracurium and cisatracurium, and normeperidine, a metabolite of meperidine, have both been shown to decrease seizure threshold.[9] It is also important to be aware of hepatic microsomal enzyme induction which can occur due to chronic AED use. Enzyme induction may increase dosing requirement and frequency of administration of a number of IV anesthetics and nondepolarizing muscle relaxants.[15,16]

The surgical time is longer than expected. The patient's next levetiracetam dose is due in 1 hour. What is your plan when the dose is due?

The plan is to administer the next dose parenterally in 1 hour. AEDs should be administered parenterally where possible. IV forms of phenytoin, sodium valproate, and levetiracetam are available (where IV doses are equivalent to oral doses), and carbamazepine is available as a suppository. If the patient's regular AED is not available in parenteral formulation, advice should be sought from a neurologist regarding alternatives that may be used to cover the perioperative period.[10]

Shortly after bringing your patient to PACU, she has a grand mal seizure. You're immediately called to the bedside. What is your management?

First priorities in seizures are airway protection, oxygenation, assessment of cardiorespiratory function, and establishment of IV access. Initial therapy for seizures is a benzodiazepine. If the seizure does not terminate consider an IV bolus of an AED such as phenytoin or phenobarbital.[13] Refractory seizures, known as *status epilepticus* (SE), may require use of general anesthesia, including propofol, benzodiazepine, and barbiturates.[13]

The patient is ready to be discharged home. What are your instructions to her mother?

Her mother should be advised to continue AED as prescribed. If the patient is on a ketogenic diet, the diet should be resumed. The patient should be observed closely after surgery as anesthetics and/or their interaction with AEDs or surgical stress itself may precipitate seizures.

DISCUSSION

Seizures are sudden, uncontrolled, electrical disturbances in the brain that can result from pathology within the central nervous system (CNS), systemic disease, or may be idiopathic. Whereas seizures are acute, *epilepsy* constitutes a more chronic neurologic condition in which an individual has two or more unprovoked seizures occurring more than 24 hours apart. The overall prevalence of epilepsy in the general population is 1–2%, with children and elderly being most affected.[3,4] The diagnosis of seizure disorder is mainly clinical and may include imaging and laboratory studies(lab/s) to identify any structural or metabolic cause.

ETIOLOGY AND PATHOPHYSIOLOGY

A seizure is defined as a transient occurrence of signs and/or symptoms that result from abnormal excessive or synchronous neuronal activity in the brain.[1,6] The International League Against Epilepsy (ILAE) has classified seizures into two main categories: focal and generalized (Box 22.1). Focal seizures arise from one brain hemisphere, while generalized seizures arise from both hemispheres.[6]

Furthermore, seizures may be provoked or unprovoked. Seizures may be provoked by a variety of causes, including electrolyte abnormalities, infections, tumors, and certain medications. Unprovoked seizures are often the result of a predisposition, either due to a genetic cause or another insult to the brain, that recur without warning.

Ultimately, seizures occur when there is an abnormal synchronous firing of a large group of neurons. This occurs as a result of excitation of susceptible neurons and can either be provoked by a triggering event or unprovoked and the result of an underlying process.

PRESENTATION

Given that seizures result from abnormal neuronal activity, they can present in various ways. Signs and symptoms of seizures may include confusion, uncontrollable jerking motions, and loss of consciousness. The presentation of seizures may also vary depending on the type of seizure an individual has.

ASSOCIATED DISORDERS

Patients with epilepsy are at an increased risk for a wide range of medical conditions (Table 22.3). These include other neurologic conditions such as stroke, metabolic derangements resulting from diabetes or hypertension, and cancer.

Table 22.3 CONDITIONS MORE PREVALENT IN PEOPLE WITH EPILEPSY THAN IN THE GENERAL POPULATION

Diabetes	Bronchitis/emphysema
Stroke	Heart disease
Asthma	High blood pressure
Cancer	Thyroid conditions
Arthritis	Back problems
Allergies	Glaucoma
Cataracts	Fibromyalgia

Adapted from Prasad, et al.[17]

Accordingly, patients with seizure disorders must be evaluated for concomitant conditions upon diagnosis.

DIAGNOSIS

Based on a patient's symptoms and medical history, several tests may be performed to help establish the diagnosis of a seizure disorder. First, a neurologic exam is often completed to establish a patient's baseline motor and functional status. This would also help in determining if there are other intracranial processes contributing to a patient's seizure activity. Lab work would include chemistry looking for electrolyte abnormalities or metabolic derangements contributing to the seizure activity. A lumbar puncture may be performed to rule out an infectious cause of seizures in the presence of other suggestive features such as fever. Continuous EEG monitoring may be employed to localize the foci of seizures—this may be done in an outpatient setting, at home, or the patient may be admitted to the hospital for observation. Last, imaging, such as MRI, computed tomography (CT), and positron emission tomography (PET) may also be utilized to detect lesions in the brain, bleeding, or cysts. Ultimately, the diagnosis of seizure disorders is based on a patient's clinical presentation. The tests and procedures above may help in establishing a diagnosis and determining if there are treatable causes for seizures.

CURRENT TREATMENT

There are several treatment options available for patients with seizures.

Medical Management

The choice of AED depends on the type of seizure, the efficacy of a drug for a patient, and the adverse drug profile (Table 22.1). Although monotherapy is preferable, polytherapy may be utilized for patients in whom seizures remain uncontrolled. AEDs are classified according to their mechanism of action. The three main mechanisms through which AEDs exert their effect include: (1) gamma aminobutyric acid (GABA) receptors, (2) glutamate receptors, and (3) sodium channels.[18]

In most patients, seizures may be controlled with medical therapy alone. In fact, studies show that AED therapy is effective in about 70% of patients.[19] However, it is important to note that medical management controls seizure activity but does not treat the underlying condition or halt the progression of disease. For patients whose seizures are well controlled, certain factors may still precipitate seizures. Last, even for patients in whom medical therapy is effective, side effects of AEDs may necessitate that they trial other treatment modalities.

Surgical Resection

Surgical resection is often reserved for patients who fail medical management or those who have adverse side effects to AEDs. Several types of surgeries may be employed to treat seizures that are refractory to medical therapy. These include focal resection, temporal lobe resection, frontal lobe resection, parietal and occipital lobe resection, or lesionectomies. Together, all of these surgeries seek to locate and excise seizure foci that has been identified on electroencephalography.[20]

Deep Brain Stimulation

DBS involves the implantation of a device that targets epileptic foci in the brain. Electrodes are placed after mapping to stimulate target regions. The electrodes are then connected to a stimulator which is placed in the chest well. The underlying mechanism of DBS involves cellular inhibition or excitation (neuromodulation) within the target structure. The stimulation will then either help to disrupt seizure propagation or raise the overall seizure threshold.[21]

Vagal Nerve Stimulation

VNS is used to treat medically refractory epilepsy and medically refractory severe depression. The mechanism of action is unclear but may involve stimulation of the limbic system, locus coeruleus, and amygdala. The stimulator is implanted subcutaneously, with electrodes around the left vagus nerve because placement around the right vagal nerve has greater stimulation of the sinoatrial node which may result in bradycardia. These devices work to inhibit seizure activity at the brainstem and cortical levels. Side effects may include bradycardia, hoarseness, superior laryngeal nerve injury, cough, dyspnea, hematoma, and seizures.[22]

Diets

The ketogenic diet is a special high-fat, low-carbohydrate, and low-protein diet that has been shown to be a potential treatment for epilepsy.[19] The goal of this diet is to mimic fasting states and, as a result, cause the body to use fats as a primary fuel source. Although the exact mechanism is unclear, it is thought that the diet works through multiple pathways to cause biochemical alterations which impact neuronal hyperexcitability.

PREOPERATIVE EVALUATION

Metabolic/Electrolyte Derangements

Metabolic disturbances including hypoglycemia and hyponatremia can present with seizures. Most of the patients without underlying epilepsy who experienced perioperative seizures have a metabolic disorder. Patients should be screened for electrolyte abnormalities such as hyponatremia following transurethral surgery and hypercalcemia following thyroid or parathyroid surgery.[23] Sepsis can also cause seizures and should be evaluated in any patient with an obvious source of infection. Patients with seizures in the setting of metabolic derangements generally do not require AED treatment, and correction of causative metabolic abnormality mostly suffices.[23]

Continuation of AED Therapy

Patients with epilepsy undergoing surgery should be maintained on their antiepileptic medications as close to baseline as possible. They should be instructed to take their morning dose of antiepileptic medications with a sip of water before surgery. Antiepileptic medications should be reinstated as soon as possible after the surgery. If enteral options are not possible, IV equivalents of these agents should be started in the postoperative period. A number of IV formulations are available: phenytoin, valproic acid, levetiracetam, phenobarbital, and lacosamide.[20]

INTRAOPERATIVE CONSIDERATIONS

AED Enzyme Induction

Various AEDs are known enzyme inducers, specifically cytochrome P450 and glucuronyl transferase (GT) enzymes. This can reduce the serum concentration of drugs that are substrates of the enzyme, causing reduced pharmacological effects.[24] Known enzyme-inducing AEDs include phenytoin, carbamazepine, and phenobarbital.[25] Newer-generation AEDs do not demonstrate enzyme induction.

Inhalational Agents

General anesthesia inhalational agents have been shown to have both pro- and anticonvulsant properties. When administered in low doses, inhalational agents have been shown to induce EEG-identified epileptiform activity. This is most likely due to inhibition of inhibitory CNS neurotransmission leading to unchecked excitatory neurotransmission in cortical and subcortical brain regions. However, with increasing doses of inhalational agent there is eventual burst suppression and isoelectricity on EEG[15] (Table 22.4).

Opiates

Seizures occur when there is a decrease in seizure threshold. Opiates may cause a decrease in seizure threshold and accordingly potentiate seizure activity in individuals who have a propensity for seizures as a result of some other process. Chronic

Table 22.4 INHALATIONAL AGENTS AND SEIZURE THRESHOLD

PROCONVULSANT	ANTICONVULSANT	NO EFFECT
Enflurane	Halothane	Nitrous oxide
Sevoflurane (low dose)	Enflurane	
	Isoflurane	
	Sevoflurane (high dose)	
	Desflurane	

anticonvulsant therapy has been linked to increased intraoperative fentanyl requirements.[26] In general, patients undergoing neurologic surgery have been shown to have lower analgesic requirements than those undergoing non-neurologic surgery.[27] However, studies have shown a dose-effect relationship between the number of anticonvulsants received and fentanyl requirements.[26]

IV Anesthetic Agents

Patients on enzyme-inducing AEDs have been shown to have resistance to dexmedetomidine due to increased plasma clearance.[28] Types of anesthesia may influence the threshold for seizures. Anesthetics such as etomidate are proconvulsive at a lower dose and anticonvulsant at a higher dose.[23] The barbiturates (thiopental, methohexital, and pentobarbital) and propofol are well established for the treatment of refractory SE.[29] All agents have been reported to produce excitatory activity, such as myoclonus, opisthotonos, and, rarely, generalized seizures on induction of anesthesia. The highest incidence appears to be with etomidate, followed by thiopental, methohexital, and propofol.[30] At higher doses, all agents act as anticonvulsants.[31]

Ketamine is a noncompetitive glutamate antagonist acting at N-methyl-D-aspartate (NMDA) receptors. Low doses may facilitate seizures, but at doses that produce sedative or anesthetic effects, ketamine shows anticonvulsant properties.[29]

Benzodiazepines

All benzodiazepines in clinical practice possess potent anticonvulsant properties.[29] Diazepam, midazolam, and lorazepam are widely used to terminate episodes of SE.

Local Anesthetics

Local anesthetics cause an inhibition of membrane depolarization and, as a result, cause increased neuronal excitability which leads to seizures. Accordingly, careful attention must be paid to local anesthetic dosing for patients—especially those with seizure disorders. Local anesthetic systemic toxicity (LAST) may precipitate seizures in individuals without a history of seizures as well and must be ruled out as a cause of new seizures.

Neuromuscular Blocking Agents

Long-term AED therapy specifically with phenytoin and carbamazepine has been associated with resistance to non-depolarizing neuromuscular blockers (NDNMB).[32] Possible mechanisms include upregulation of acetylcholine (Ach) receptors, decreased sensitivity of Ach receptors, competition of binding sites, and hepatic enzyme induction leading to increased NDNMB metabolism.[32]

ACUTE MANAGEMENT OF SEIZURE IN PERIOPERATIVE PERIOD

Breakthrough Seizure

The occurrence of perioperative seizures in patients with a pre-existing seizure disorder is unclear. Several factors may increase a patient's risk of perioperative seizures, including medications administered, timing of medication administration, missed doses of antiepileptic medications, and sleep deprivation.

Presentation

Perioperative seizures can cause brain damage due to hypoxia, apnea, prolonged postoperative mechanical ventilation, and delayed awakening from anesthesia. Physiological cardiac and respiratory regulation may be impaired. There may be tachycardia and tachypnea, apnea, and bradycardia or sudden death due to autonomic instability, which causes cardiac arrhythmias or neurogenic pulmonary edema.[33]

Under general anesthesia, due to the routine use of dense neuromuscular blockade, it is difficult to detect intraoperative seizures. Therefore, intraoperative seizures are mostly of the nonconvulsive type. Though EEG is considered the gold standard in the detection of nonconvulsive seizures, the routine use of the same in the intraoperative period is far from conventional and is technically challenging.[34] Perioperative use of bispectral index (BIS), patient state index (PSI), and burst suppression ratio (BSR) may be used as a substitute for EEG, but further studies are required to determine their ability in the timely detection of intraoperative seizures.[34]

Management

According to the American Association of Neurology (AAN) Practice Guidelines, elevated serum prolactin, twice the baseline value, 10–20 minutes after a suspected seizure, is considered to be a useful adjunct to diagnose a generalized tonic-clonic seizure.[35]

Management includes maintaining a patent airway with adequate ventilation and protecting the patient from injuries resulting from seizures.

Should convulsions persist for more than 5 minutes, IV benzodiazepine should be used. The drug of choice is lorazepam. Alternatively, diazepam (5–20 mg) may be used. If convulsions persist, a second dose of benzodiazepine with phenytoin (20 mg/kg over 30 minutes) may be used. For refractory seizures, phenobarbital (1.5 mg/kg/min or 100 mg/70 kg/min can be used with a maximum dose of 20 mg/kg or 1,000 mg/70 kg), midazolam (0.1–0.3 mg/kg in 2–5 minutes, followed by infusion of 0.05–0.4 mg/kg/hour), propofol (1–2 mg/kg followed infusion of 2–10 mg/kg/h), thiopental (5–10 mg/kg in 10 minutes, followed by infusion of 100–400 mg/h), lidocaine (1.5–2 mg/kg in 2–5 minutes, followed by infusion of 2–3 mg/kg/h for 12 hours), isoflurane (0.5–1.5%) and ketamine (50–100 mg followed by infusion of 50–100 mg/h).[33]

STATUS EPILEPTICUS

SE is considered the most extreme form of seizure and is a medical emergency. Seizures, as stated above, are defined by the ILAE as transient occurrences of signs and/or symptoms due to abnormal excessive or synchronous neuronal activity in the brain.[6] In contrast, SE involves seizures that are prolonged or occur repeatedly at brief intervals. However, due to the limited knowledge of the pathophysiology of SE and the need to treat patients quickly, the definition of SE has changed over time. As of 2015, the ILAE Task Force on Classification of Status Epilepticus has proposed SE to be a condition that results from "the failure of the mechanisms responsible termination or from the initiation of mechanisms which lead to abnormally prolonged seizures (after time point t_1) ... long-term consequences (after time point t_2), including neuronal death, neuronal injury, and alterations of neuronal networks, depending on the type and duration of seizures."

Presentation

Based on the definition of SE in Table 22.5, the classification of a seizure as SE is based on two different time points (t_1 and t_2). The first, t_1, indicates a point in time where the seizure can be considered prolonged and the second, t_2, the point in time where a seizure may cause long-term consequences.

Management

The prognosis of SE is correlated with the duration of the seizures. The longer the seizures, the greater the probability for neuronal injury.[6] Accordingly, management of SE revolves around decreasing the duration of seizures. After a diagnosis of SE is made, treatment should be initiated immediately. Treatment involves supportive therapy including oxygen and hemodynamic support with IV fluids. Obtaining IV access is an important next step in order to obtain laboratory tests to ascertain a complete blood count, electrolyte levels, a glucose level, and antiepileptic drug levels, as well as a toxic drug screen. If seizures persist following supportive measures, IV antiepileptic agents should be started (Table 22.2).

CONCLUSION

- Anesthesiologists encounter seizure disorders commonly in the perioperative setting.
- Due to several reasons, patients with seizure disorders undergoing surgical procedures under anesthesia can have an increased frequency of seizures.
- In the preoperative assessment of patients with seizure disorders, it is important to understand how well-controlled a patient's seizure activity is and to identify the type of seizures, the frequency, severity, and the factors triggering the seizures; the use of anticonvulsant drugs and possible interactions with drugs used in anesthesia; and the presence of ketogenic diet and any neurostimulation and its implications in anesthetic techniques.
- It is essential to understand the pro- and anticonvulsant properties of drugs used in anesthesia, thus minimizing the risk of seizure activity in the intra- and postoperative phases.

REVIEW QUESTIONS

1. A 52-year-old man with a history of seizure disorder is scheduled to undergo spinal anesthesia for left total knee arthroplasty. In the PACU, he suffers refractory SE. Which of the following medications would be the most effective anticonvulsant?

   a. Phenobarbital.
   b. Propofol.
   c. Methohexital.
   d. Lorazepam.

   The correct answer is d.

Table 22.5 THE INTERNATIONAL LEAGUE AGAINST EPILEPSY (ILAE) TASK FORCE ON STATUS EPILEPTICUS (SE) OPERATIONAL DEFINITION OF SE

TYPE OF SE	WHEN A SEIZURE IS LIKELY TO BE PROLONGED LEADING TO CONTINUOUS SEIZURE ACTIVITY (T_1)	WHEN A SEIZURE MAY CAUSE LONG TERM CONSEQUENCES (T_2)
Tonic-clonic SE	5 minutes	30 minutes
Focal SE with impaired consciousness	10 minutes	>60 minutes
Absence status epilepticus	10–15 minutes	Unknown

Adapted from Trinka, et al.[36]

First-line treatment includes benzodiazepines and phenytoin. Refractory seizures can be managed with benzodiazepines, propofol, short-acting barbiturates, or phenobarbital. The benzodiazepines, such as lorazepam, are particularly effective for seizures. Phenytoin is less effective but is not associated with respiratory depression, which can be seen with benzodiazepines and barbiturates.

2. A 42-year-old man with a history of well-controlled epilepsy undergoes an uneventful laparoscopic cholecystectomy. After arrival to PACU, he suffers a tonic-clonic seizure. Which of the following is true regarding benzodiazepine administration?

   a. A benzodiazepine should be administered immediately.
   b. The patient should be treated with a benzodiazepine if he fails treatment with an antiepileptic.
   c. A benzodiazepine should never be given.
   d. A benzodiazepine should be given after expert consultation.

The correct answer is a.
The first-line therapy for SE are benzodiazepines.

3. A 5-year-old child with a history of epilepsy is undergoing resection of seizure foci under general anesthesia. Which of the following medications is most likely to produce seizure on EEG?

   a. Midazolam.
   b. Methohexital.
   c. Sevoflurane.
   d. Nitrous oxide.

The correct answer is b.
Injection of methohexital (0.25–0.5 mg/kg) has been shown to activate EEG seizure discharges in patients with epilepsy.[37] Midazolam and high-dose volatile anesthetics can depress cerebral electrical activity. Nitrous oxide has been shown to have little effect on seizure threshold.[37]

4. A 5-year-old child with a history of epilepsy is undergoing resection of seizure foci under general anesthesia. Which of the following interventions is most likely to produce seizure on EEG?

   a. Hyperventilation.
   b. Hypoventilation.
   c. Trendelenburg position.
   d. Normocapnic ventilation.

The correct answer is a.
Hyperventilation is a technique that may be used to lower seizure threshold and produce seizure activity on EEG. The mechanism is thought to be due to cerebral vasospasm caused by respiratory alkalosis/hypocapnia.[16]

5. An 8-year-old boy with a history of epilepsy treated with valproic acid is scheduled for an appendectomy. Which of the following is most likely a result of treatment with valproic acid?

   a. Hyperkalemia.
   b. Gingival hyperplasia.
   c. Coagulopathy.
   d. Weight gain.

The correct answer is c.
A known side effect of many AEDs is hematologic function abnormalities. Valproic acid, a commonly used anticonvulsant, can induce thrombocytopenia in 5–18% of patients.[8] The exact mechanism through which valproic acid can cause thrombocytopenia is unknown, but potential processes include decreased platelet production due to bone marrow toxicity and increased disruption of platelets.[8]

Questions 6 and 7 are part of a set.

6. A 9-year-old boy with a history of epilepsy on AEDs is being admitted for open reduction and internal fixation (ORIF) of a radius fracture after fall. Perioperative considerations should include

   a. Holding AEDs morning of surgery.
   b. Increased requirement of NDNMB.
   c. Decreased need for opioids postoperatively.
   d. Methohexital is a good choice for induction.

The correct answer is b.
Long-term AED use is associated with resistance to NDNMB. This is thought to be due to induction of hepatic drug metabolism, increased NDNMB protein binding, and/or upregulation of Ach receptors.[16] It is crucial to take AEDs as prescribed, including the day of surgery, to maintain therapeutic levels.[4] Methohexital is associated with increased seizure activity.[37]

7. The patient in Question 6 is given oral midazolam as a premedication. However, after 30 minutes, there is no apparent effect. Which medication is the patient most likely taking for his seizures?

   a. Gabapentin.
   b. Lamotrigine.
   c. Levetiracetam.
   d. Carbamazepine.

The correct answer is d.
Medications that induce CYP-3A4 include carbamazepine, phenytoin, phenobarbital, St. John's wort, dexamethasone, topiramate, and oxcarbazepine. Chronic use of these medications may make premedication with commonly used benzodiazepines such as midazolam and diazepam less effective.

8. Which of the following is considered an excitatory neurotransmitter in the CNS?

   a. Glutamate.
   b. GABA.
   c. Glycine.
   d. Calcium.

The correct answer is a.
Glutamate is the main excitatory neurotransmitter, whereas glycine and GABA are the two primary inhibitory neurotransmitters in the somatosensory system.

9. A 65-year-old woman with seizure disorder treated with carbamazepine is presenting for routine preoperative evaluation prior to elective lumbar discectomy. Which of the following metabolic derangements is most likely to be seen?

　a. Na + 156.
　b. Na + 118.
　c. K + 5.1.
　d. Mg + 1.2.

The correct answer is b.

Carbamazepine causes an increase in antidiuretic hormone (ADH) which leads to abnormal sensitivity of renal tubules to ADH activity. This causes increased expression of aquaporin 2 channels in the renal tubules.[38]

10. What is the mechanism of action of phenytoin?

　a. Calcium channel blocker.
　b. GABA potentiation.
　c. Na$^+$ channel blocker.
　d. NMDA inhibition.

The correct answer is c.

Phenytoin is used in the management of generalized or partial seizures through its effect on sodium conductance in motor neurons by either promoting sodium efflux or inhibiting sodium influx. By acting on sodium channels, phenytoin stabilizes and slows conduction velocity of neuronal membranes for pharmacologic control of seizures. Side effects of phenytoin include gingival hyperplasia, dermatitis, and resistance to nondepolarizing muscle relaxants with chronic use.

11. A patient receives a stellate ganglion block with 0.25% bupivacaine 2 mL with epinephrine 1:200,000. Approximately 30 seconds after the injection, the patient experiences a seizure. What is the most likely cause?

　a. Reaction to epinephrine in the anesthetic solution.
　b. Vertebral artery injection of bupivacaine.
　c. New-onset seizure activity unrelated to stellate ganglion block.
　d. Anaphylactoid reaction to bupivacaine.

The correct answer is b.

The patient is most likely experiencing seizure secondary to CNS toxicity after injection into the vertebral artery during stellate ganglion block. The stellate ganglion is located at the fusion of the inferior cervical and first thoracic ganglions at the level of the C7 transverse process. Complications of stellate ganglion block include local anesthetic systemic toxicity due to IV or intra-arterial injection. The toxic dose for intra-arterial injection (e.g., in the vertebral or carotid arteries) is lower due to a higher concentration of local anesthetic in the neurovascular tree. Subarachnoid injection, intraneural injection, pneumothorax, esophageal perforation, and chylothorax are other possible complications.

12. A 63-year-old patient with metastatic carcinoma and chronic renal failure is started on high-dose meperidine therapy for cancer-related pain. A few days after initiation of treatment, the patient begins to develop tremors, fasciculations, mydriasis, and hyperreflexia. Which of the following is most likely the cause of symptoms?

　a. Progression of metastatic disease causing neurologic symptoms.
　b. Seizures from normeperidine toxicity.

The correct answer is b.

Meperidine has an active metabolite that is excreted by the kidneys. The accumulation of the active metabolite of meperidine, normeperidine, is neurotoxic and can cause seizures.

13. Which of the following is true for the placement of a VNS for the treatment of medically refractory seizures?

　a. Placement is usually performed under MAC.
　b. Postoperative complications include hoarseness and cough.
　c. The electrode array is placed around the right vagus nerve.
　d. It is recommended that patients discontinue their anticonvulsants the day of surgery to minimize interference with the VNS.

The correct answer is b.

VNS can be used for the treatment of medically refractory seizures. The stimulator is implanted subcutaneously with electrodes around the left vagus nerve. One potential complication after placement is hoarseness and cough.[22]

14. Physiologic changes associated with electroconvulsive therapy include all of the following *except*

　a. An initial sympathetic surge causing hypertension and tachycardia.
　b. An increase in cerebral blood flow and metabolism.
　c. Alterations in glucose homeostasis.
　d. ECG changes unaccompanied by enzyme leak.

The correct answer is a.

Electroconvulsive therapy causes a generalized tonic-clonic seizure by electrical stimulation of the brain. Cerebral blood flow and metabolism increase dramatically. From a cardiovascular standpoint, there is an initial parasympathetic surge (primarily during the electrical stimulation) with severe bradycardia or asystole. This is followed by a sympathetic surge causing hypertension and tachycardia, ST-segment depression and T-wave inversion not associated with myocardial enzyme changes, and, rarely, ventricular tachycardia. Glucose homeostasis is affected variably with both improved and worse control.[24]

15. A 28-year-old woman underwent a cesarean delivery at 35 weeks of gestation because of severe preeclampsia. Nearly 48 hours after delivery she experiences a generalized tonic-clonic seizure. Which of the following is *most* likely the anticonvulsant of choice?

　a. Levetiracetam.
　b. Magnesium sulfate.
　c. Phenytoin.
　d. Lorazepam.

The correct answer is b.

The anticonvulsant indicated for the treatment of eclampsia is magnesium sulfate. Eclamptic seizures are tonic-clonic in nature, typically self-limiting and of short duration, and do not usually recur. For the majority of these patients, the initial seizure occurs during labor or within the first 48 hours after delivery.

REFERENCES

1. Basic mechanisms underlying seizures and epilepsy. In: Bromfield EB, Cavazos JE, Sirven JI, eds. *An Introduction to Epilepsy*. American Epilepsy Society; 2006:1–26.
2. Fisher RS, Acevedo C, Arzimanoglou A, et al. ILAE Official Report: A practical clinical definition of epilepsy. *Epilepsia (Copenhagen)*. 2014;55(4):475–482.
3. Modalsli Aaberg K, Gunnes N, Johanne Bakken I, et al. Incidence and prevalence of childhood epilepsy: A nationwide cohort study. *Pediatrics*. 2017;139(5):2016–3908.
4. Cheng MA, Tempelhoff R. Anesthesia and epilepsy. *Curr Opin Anaesthesiol*. 1999;12(5):523–528.
5. Niesen AD, Jacob AK, Aho LE, et al. Perioperative seizures in patients with a history of a seizure disorder. *Anesth Analg*. 2010;111(3):729–735.
6. Fisher RS, Cross JH, French JA, et al. Operational classification of seizure types by the International League Against Epilepsy: Position paper of the ILAE Commission for Classification and Terminology. *Epilepsia*. 2017;58:522–530.
7. Kofke WA. Anesthetic management of the patient with epilepsy or prior seizures, *Curr Opin Anaesthesiol*. 2010;23(3):391–399.
8. Buoli M, Serati M, Botturi A, et al. The risk of thrombocytopenia during valproic acid therapy: A critical summary of available clinical data. *Drugs R D*. 2018;18(1):1–5.
9. Ruskin K, Rosenbaum S, Rampil I, eds. *Fundamentals of Neuroanesthesia: A Physiologic Approach to Clinical Practice*. Oxford University Press; 2013. https://oxfordmedicine.com/view/10.1093/med/9780199755981.001.0001/med-9780199755981
10. Butterworth JF, Mackey DC, Wasnick JD. *Morgan & Mikhail's Clinical Anesthesiology*. 6th ed. McGraw-Hill Education LLC; 2018.
11. Stafstrom CE, Carmant L. Seizures and epilepsy: An overview for neuroscientists. *Cold Spring Harb Perspect Med*. 2015;5(6):a022426.
12. American Society of Anesthesiologists. Practice guidelines for preoperative fasting and the use of pharmacologic agents to reduce the risk of pulmonary aspiration: Application to healthy patients undergoing elective procedures: An updated report by the American Society of Anesthesiologists Task Force on Preoperative Fasting and the Use of Pharmacologic Agents to Reduce the Risk of Pulmonary Aspiration. *Anesthesiology*. 2017;126:376–393.
13. Kelso ARC, Cock HR. Status epilepticus. *Pract Neurol*. 2005;5:322–333.
14. Cote C, Lerman J, Anderson B. *A Practice of Anesthesia for Infants and Children*. Elsevier; 2017.
15. Constant I., Seeman R., Murat I. Sevoflurane and epileptiform EEG changes [review article]. *Pediatr Anesth*. 2005;15:266–274.
16. Koh JL, Egan B, McGraw T. Pediatric epilepsy surgery: Anesthetic considerations. *Anesthesiol Clin*. 2012;30(2):191–206.
17. Prasad VN, Chawla HS, Goyal A, Gauba K, Singhi P. Incidence of phenytoin induced gingival overgrowth in epileptic children: A six month evaluation. *J Indian Soc Pedod Prev Dent*. 2002 Jun;20(2):73–80.
18. Macdonald RL, Kelly KM. Antiepileptic drug mechanisms of action. *Epilepsia*. 1995;36(S2–S12):1528–1157.
19. D'Andrea Meira I, Romão TT, Pires do Prado HJ, Krüger LT, Pires MEP, da Conceição PO. Ketogenic diet and epilepsy: What we know so far. *Front Neurosci*. 2019;13:5.
20. Dhallu MS, Baiomi A, Biyyam M, Chilimuri S. Perioperative management of neurological conditions. *Health Serv Insights*. 2017. doi:10:1178632917711942
21. Zangiabadi N, Ladino LD, Sina F, Orozco-Hernández JP, Carter A, Téllez-Zenteno JF. Deep brain stimulation and drug-resistant epilepsy: A review of the literature. *Front Neurol*. 2019;10:601.
22. Ben-Menachem E. Vagus-nerve stimulation for the treatment of epilepsy. *Lancet Neurol*. 2002;1(8):477–482.
23. Dhallu MS, Baiomi A, Biyyam M, Chilimuri S. Perioperative management of neurological conditions. *Health Serv Insights*. 2017. doi:10:1178632917711942
24. Patsalos PN, Perucca E. Clinically important drug interactions in epilepsy: General features and interactions between antiepileptic drugs. *Lancet Neurol*. 2003;2(6):347–356.
25. Perucca E. Clinically relevant drug interactions with antiepileptic drugs. *Br J Clin Pharmacol*. 2006;61(3):246–255.
26. Tempelhoff R, Modica PA, Spitznagel EL. Anticonvulsant therapy increases fentanyl requirements during anaesthesia for craniotomy. *Can J Anaesth*. 1990;37:327–332.
27. Dunbar PJ, Visco E, Lam AM. Craniotomy procedures are associated with less analgesic requirements than other surgical procedures. *Anesth Analg*. 1999;88(2):335–340.
28. Flexman AM, Wong H, Riggs KW, et al. Enzyme-inducing anticonvulsants increase plasma clearance of dexmedetomidine: A pharmacokinetic and pharmacodynamic study. *Anesthesiology*. 201;120(5):1118–1125.
29. Modica PA, Tempelhoff R, White PF. Pro- and anticonvulsant effects of anesthetics (Part II). *Anesth Analg*. 1990;70(4):433–444.
30. Hymes JA. Seizure activity during isoflurane anesthesia. *Anesth Analg*. 1985;64(3):367–368.
31. Reddy RV, Moorthy SS, Dierdorf SF, Deitch RD Jr, Link L. Excitatory effects and electroencephalographic correlation of etomidate, thiopental, methohexital, and propofol. *Anesth Analg*. 1993;77(5):1008–1011.
32. Alloul K, Whalley DG, Shutway F, Ebrahim Z, Varin F. Pharmacokinetic origin of carbamazepine-induced resistance to vecuronium neuromuscular blockade in anesthetized patients. *Anesthesiology*. 1996;84(2):330–339.
33. Maranhão MV, Gomes EA, de Carvalho PE. Epilepsy and anesthesia. *Rev Bras Anestesiol*. 2011;61(2):232–136.
34. Ajayan N. Multimodal monitoring to aid detection and management of intraoperative seizures: A case report. *J Clin Monit Comput*. 2021;35(1):209–212.
35. Chen DK, So YT, Fisher RS; Therapeutics and Technology Assessment Subcommittee of the American Academy of Neurology. Use of serum prolactin in diagnosing epileptic seizures: Report of the Therapeutics and Technology Assessment Subcommittee of the American Academy of Neurology. *Neurology*. 2005;65(5):668–675.
36. Trinka E, Cock H, Hesdorffer D, et al. A definition and classification of status epilepticus: Report of the ILAE Task Force on Classification of Status Epilepticus. *Epilepsia*. 2015;56:1515–1523. https://doi.org/10.1111/epi.13121
37. Soriano SG, Martyn JA. Antiepileptic-induced resistance to neuromuscular blockers: Mechanisms and clinical significance. *Clin Pharmacokinet*. 2004;43:71–81.
38. de Bragança AC, Moyses ZP, Magaldi AJ. Carbamazepine can induce kidney water absorption by increasing aquaporin 2 expression. *Nephrol Dial Transplant*. 2010;25(12):3840–3845.

23.

CLINICAL APPLICATION OF PERIOPERATIVE BRAIN HEALTH

Samuel N. Blacker

STEM CASE AND KEY QUESTIONS

A prominent 69-year-old neurosurgeon presents for a preoperative anesthesia evaluation a week prior to a scheduled prostatectomy. The patient is accompanied by his adult daughter.

What additional elements of the preoperative evaluation should be conducted for this patient?

The patient is taking simvastatin for hyperlipidemia and lisinopril for hypertension. He is active and still operating. The patient admits that he is more fatigued at the end of the day recently and has had some weight loss recently.

When asked about past surgical history, the patient's daughter related that after a right inguinal hernia repair 1 year ago, under general anesthesia (GA), the patient experienced 3 days of confusion postoperatively and it delayed his hospital discharge.

Define delirium and postoperative cognitive dysfunction (POCD). What risk factors does this patient have for delirium and postoperative cognitive dysfunction?

The patient's daughter and the patient's wife were very distressed by the postoperative events, but the patient has no memory of the first 3 postoperative days. The patient reports he feels fine.

Also, since the surgery a year ago, the daughter relates her father has been a bit more forgetful, has trouble remembering the name of his new granddaughter, and has lost his keys several times. This was not noted prior to the surgery.

What screening should be done preoperatively to assess risks for delirium and POCD?

The patient laughs when administered a Mini-Cog test. The patient is able to recall the three words and draw a clock face without difficulty.

Does this patient meet the criteria for frailty? What are the postoperative risks for a patient meeting frailty criteria?

The patient's weight has decreased since the surgery a year ago and his BMI is now noted as 22 kg/m² and was 24 kg/m² 1 year ago. The patient's daughter relates that he has been noted to eat less and overall is less energetic at home and at work in the hospital. The patient is also not able to conduct rounds as quickly at the hospital and has been arriving late to the operating room.

What can be done perioperatively to prevent delirium and POCD postoperatively?

Different anesthetic options are presented to the patient. The patient does not want GA because he is very concerned about his family's distress regarding his postoperative course with the last surgery.

What are the risks associated with spinal versus GA in relation with the outcomes of delirium and POCD?

The patient and family members agree to proceed with a combined spinal/epidural anesthetic. However, in the operating room the patient is very uncomfortable with positioning and the spinal is technically difficult. The anesthesia team is unable to place a spinal or epidural after multiple attempts. The patient is very uncomfortable and anxious, and the decision is made to convert to GA.

The surgery is successful and the patient is extubated. An hour later, prior to PACU discharge, the anesthesiologist is paged. The patient is not cooperative and pulling at his IV lines.

What is occurring and is there anything available for treatment?

The patient is given IV dexmedetomidine, 4 mcg at a time, for a total of 20 mcg in the PACU. The patient's family is brought to his bedside, but he does not recognize his daughter. The patient is restrained as he continues to be combative and pull at his IV lines.

Later on the ward, the patient is intermittently lucid and confused. This lasts for 2 days, and the patient then remains consistently at baseline mental status and able to be discharged home.

DISCUSSION

Perioperative brain health guidelines have been developed to enable the creation of care pathways and multidisciplinary teams to identify and care for elderly patients.[1,2] Perioperative brain health best practices are targeted to prevent delirium and postoperative cognitive dysfunction (POCD) which can have a lasting impact on health outcomes. The American Society of Anesthesiologists (ASA) and the American Association of Retired Persons (AARP), as well as the Fifth International Perioperative Neurotoxicity workgroup have all published best practice recommendations.[3-5] The American Society for Enhanced Recovery and Perioperative Quality Initiative have also issued a Joint Consensus Statement on Postoperative Delirium Prevention.[6] Recommendations also exist for nonagenarians and centenarians.[7]

Delirium is a fluctuating and acute clouding of consciousness diagnosed utilizing the *Diagnostic and Statistical Manual of Mental Disorders* (DSM-5) criteria.[8]

1. Disturbance in attention and awareness
2. Disturbance in cognition
3. Develops over a short period of time
4. Disturbances not better explained by other disorder
5. Direct physiological consequence of another medical condition

The anesthetic is the "other medical condition" in the case of delirium after surgery.

There are two types of post anesthetic delirium, emergence delirium and postoperative delirium. *Emergence delirium* is delirium upon anesthesia emergence and in the PACU.[9] Delirium occurring up to 72 hours after an anesthetic is *postoperative delirium*.[10] Despite having defined time intervals, postoperative delirium and emergence delirium are frequently used interchangeably in the literature.[11]

Postoperative/emergence delirium can also present as either hypoactive or hyperactive. The majority of postoperative delirium cases are hypoactive and therefore may be overlooked.[12]

POCD can last months to years and cause significant morbidity. POCD can only be diagnosed utilizing neurocognitive testing and is more useful as a research term rather than a clinical term.[13] There are a variety of neurocognitive tests used in the literature, making study comparisons difficult. Neurocognitive tests that utilize different testing methods measure different cognitive domains with inconsistent accuracy, sensitivity and specificity.

Because POCD is more a research term, rather than a clinical term, the need for consistent clinical terminology was proposed in December 2018, utilizing the DSM-5 diagnosis of *neurocognitive dysfunction* (NCD).[14] NCD is clinically diagnosed when there is a cognitive concern with objective evidence of a cognitive deficit. NCD is either mild or major based on the maintenance or interruption of activities of daily living (ADL). NCD after an anesthetic is diagnosed as three separate entities based on proximity to one of three time intervals.

1. *Surgery to 30 days after surgery*: Delayed neurocognitive recovery.
2. *Thirty days after surgery to 1 year after surgery*: Mild or major postoperative neurocognitive disorder (PNCD)
3. *If PNCD lasts beyond 1 year from surgery*: POCD

PATHOGENESIS

The developed adult brain is not static, and both anatomic and physiologic changes of aging may begin as early as the fourth decade.[15] As the brain ages the nervous system mass and density, receptor density, and neurotransmitters all decrease. Also, as the brain ages, the blood–brain barrier has a reduced integrity along with decreased neurogenesis, atrophy of prefrontal white matter, and impairment of anti-inflammatory feedback. The changes clinically manifest as decreased cognitive reserve, processing speed, reasoning, memory, and spatial cognitive abilities and also increased sensitivity to medications.[16] After surgery and an anesthetic, these changes in addition to altered synaptic activity from activation of the immune system and inflammatory cascade increase the risk for postoperative delirium and POCD/NCD.[17,18]

SCREENING FOR DELIRIUM AND POCD/PNCD

The American College of Surgeons (ACS) published guidelines recommending patients older than 65 and anyone at risk for preoperative cognitive impairment should be screened along with an assessment of cognitive ability and capacity.[19] The screening tests can help guide preoperative counseling and risk assessment.

Preoperative cognitive impairment is common in elderly patients and screening tools can help assess at-risk patients.[20] A variety of cognitive assessment tools are available, but tools that are accurate and brief are needed for surgical assessments. The Mini-Cog and Mini Mental Status Exam (MMSE) are both designed to be brief.[21] The MMSE has high sensitivity and specificity, but it can take 7–10 minutes to administer, which can be onerous in a rushed preoperative setting. The Mini-Cog however, takes 2–4 minutes to conduct and is recommended by the ACS and American Geriatric Society (AGS). The Mini-Cog has good sensitivity, but lower specificity that the MMSE.[22]

The Mini-Cog consists of the patient repeating three unrelated words, drawing a clock with a specific time, and then recalling the three unrelated words.[23] The patient receives 1 point for each correct word and either 2 points for drawing a correct clock or 0 points for an incorrect clock. The test is a screening test, where 0–2 points suggests impairment and 3–5 points suggests no impairment.

The screening tool are relatively quick and powered to detect probable impairment. In a study of 211 elderly patients without known dementia scheduled for an elective hip or knee replacement, the Mini-Cog was used to screen for cognitive impairment.[24] Fifty (24%) of the patients screened demonstrated probable cognitive impairment, with a Mini-Cog score of less than or equal to 2. Also, the patients with probable preoperative cognitive impairment were more likely to develop postoperative delirium, stay in the hospital longer, and be discharged to a care facility rather than home. A 2022 retrospective study demonstrated 21% of elderly surgical patients were cognitively impaired and had higher rates of postoperative delirium.[25] Preoperative cognitive training and may also help in patients without known preexisting cognitive impairment.[26,27]

Other risk factors for delirium and POCD/NCD include multimorbidity, poor cognitive function, anemia, poor nutrition, intraoperative blood loss, preoperative anxiety, untreated pain, and IV opioid use.[28,29,30,31] Most risk factors are difficult to modify in a preoperative setting.

SCREENING FOR FRAILTY

Frailty is an independent risk factor for postoperative delirium, and elderly patients should be assessed for frailty.[32,33,34,35] Frailty is a decrease in physiologic reserve which exceeds expected decline based on age alone; it consists of five elements.[36]

1. Weight loss
2. Weakness
3. Slow walking speed
4. Self-reported exhaustion
5. Low physical activity

A variety of screening assessments are available to assess for frailty.[37,38] The ACS and AGS recommends a frailty score based from the five frailty elements.[39,40] A patient receives 1 point for each of the five elements and then is risk-stratified into not frail, pre-frail, and frail. Pre-frail and frail patients are at increased risk of delirium, longer length of hospital stay, and increased risk of discharge to a care facility.[41]

Mitigation of frailty involves geriatric specialty consultation.[42] Preoperatively, exercise and nutritional prehabilitation may also decrease postoperative complications in a frail patient.[43,44]

PERIOPERATIVE DELIRIUM PREVENTION

Nonpharmacologic Prevention Strategies

Hospital-wide delirium prevention protocols can reduce delirium postoperatively.[45,46] Protocols include cognitive screening, ensuring that family or friends accompany the patient, ensuring medication dosing and timing are correct, availability of hearing aids and glasses if needed, proximity to a window, and availability of familiar objects as well as a clock and calendar to assist the patient with orientation.[47] However, barriers exist to implementation as a survey of 1,737 anesthesiologists showed low compliance with frailty and delirium screening as well as patient and family education.[48]

Pharmacologic Prevention Strategies

Perioperative avoidance of medications with anticholinergic properties, corticosteroids, benzodiazepines, meperidine, and starting more than five new medications can reduce postoperative delirium risk.[49]

Anesthesia Technique

There is no consensus regarding a superior anesthesia technique or medications to prevent delirium and POCD/NCD, in elderly surgical patients. Spinal and epidural anesthesia, compared to GA, has been studied for both delirium and POCD with mixed results.[50,51,52,53,54] A meta-analysis of 49 controlled trials and observational studies of elderly patients noted increased occurrence of delirium with the use of GA compared to local, spinal, or regional anesthesia (28% vs. 20%).[55] Prospective, randomized studies assessing spinal versus GA regarding POCD/NCD alone have not elicited a difference.[56,57,58] Combining thoracic epidural analgesia with a GA was shown to reduce postoperative delirium for the first 7 postoperative days compared to GA alone in 1,802 elderly patients receiving either thoracic or abdominal surgery.[59] The combined epidural and GA group did have more hypotension than the GA alone group.

Comparisons of GA techniques comparing the use of propofol-based total intravenous anesthesia (TIVA) and volatile agent have been conducted. No difference was found in postoperative delirium in a Cochrane meta-analysis of 321 patients from five trials.[60] However, the Cochrane meta-analysis conducted for POCD, reviewing seven studies with 869 participants, showed a reduction of POCD with use of TIVA.

Examining delayed neurocognitive recovery specifically, a propofol-based anesthetic versus a sevoflurane-based anesthetic was examined for 554 elderly patients undergoing laparoscopic abdominal surgery. Both group's anesthetics were titrated to a bispectral index score of 40–60. No statistical difference in delayed neurocognitive recovery at 5–7 days was seen between the two groups.[61]

Medication Strategies

Beyond anesthetic techniques, adjuncts such as ketamine and dexmedetomidine have been studied relative to postoperative delirium and POCD.

Ketamine was evaluated in a 2018 meta-analysis for both delirium and POCD.[62] Four randomized studies involving both high- and low-dose ketamine demonstrated no postoperative delirium reduction with ketamine. The largest study in the analysis cautioned against using ketamine for elderly patients due to negative experiences with ketamine use.[63] Examining POCD in three trials, the evidence was deemed low quality; however, a single bolus of ketamine at anesthesia induction reduced POCD.[64]

The literature regarding dexmedetomidine and postoperative delirium is more extensive compared to other medications. Examining both elderly and non-elderly patients, two meta-analyses revealed a reduction of postoperative delirium with dexmedetomidine use compared to placebo and other sedatives.[65,66] This held for use preoperatively, intraoperatively, and postoperatively. Another meta-analysis of 15 studies pooling 2,183 patients also showed intraoperative infusions of dexmedetomidine of 0.1–0.7 mcg/kg/hr reduced the delirium incidence in adults undergoing noncardiac surgery.[67]

The literature examining only elderly patients is more heterogeneous regarding intraoperative and postoperative use of dexmedetomidine for cardiac and noncardiac surgery populations.[68,69,70,71,72,73,74] Dexmedetomidine, when compared to propofol sedation, was associated with less postoperative delirium in a retrospective study of elderly patients receiving lower extremity surgery under spinal anesthesia.[75]

Other potential delirium prevention strategies have been studied as well. Administration of the cholinergic medication physostigmine at induction and for 24 hours afterward was studied prospectively in 261 double-blinded adult liver surgery patients.[76] The incidence of delirium was not statistically significant between the placebo and physostigmine groups (15% and 20%), and the POCD incidence was not different at discharge, 3 months, or 1 year postoperatively.

Benzodiazepine use has also been examined regarding risks of complication in general. Examining total knee arthroplasty patients, Hernandez et al. noted that patients taking preoperative outpatient benzodiazepines had higher rates of postoperative delirium, surgical revision, and femur fracture fixation.[77] However, recent evidence has questioned withholding benzodiazepines because anxiety is a delirium risk factor. In a retrospective review of 1,266 patients, Wang et al. found that even for the elderly (mean age 72.2 ± 5.6 years) who received midazolam immediately preoperatively, postoperative delirium incidence was similar to those patients who did not received midazolam (23.3% in the midazolam group and 24.93% in the non-midazolam group). More recent literature has shown that only postoperative benzodiazepine use was associated with delirium.[78] Another retrospective review examined perioperative benzodiazepine use and noted that postoperative delirium incidence was higher in patients who discontinued benzodiazepines prior to surgery compared to those who continued benzodiazepine use or initiated use preoperatively.[79] A small prospective observational study of 40 elderly endoscopy patients receiving propofol found no incidence of delirium with additional preprocedural midazolam use.[80] Also, continuation of long-term anticholinergic mediations was not associated with development of delirium in postoperative elderly patients.[81]

Other Modalities

Blood Pressure Management

Blood pressure targets for anesthetic management have been evaluated. Perioperative hypotension (mean arterial pressure [MAP] <65 mm Hg) has been associated with delirium in surgical patients. In a randomized controlled trial, Hu et al. evaluated 322 elderly patients undergoing noncardiac surgery and compared patients with MAPs between 60–70 mm Hg and 90–100 mm Hg.[82] The group with the higher MAP had a lower postoperative delirium incidence and also shorter duration when it did occur. However, overall postoperative adverse events were not reduced. Also, a retrospective cohort analysis of 1,083 patients demonstrated an increased risk of postoperative delirium with increased duration of an intraoperative MAP of less than 65 mm Hg.[83] Another retrospective multicenter cohort study also demonstrated a relationship between a duration-dependent MAP of less than 55 mm Hg and postoperative delirium.[84] Other factors such as variability of MAP, along with higher sevoflurane concentrations and greater anesthetic depth, were found to be associated with increased postoperative delirium in a prospective, cross-sectional trial of 80 adult surgery patients.[85] Interestingly, the time of MAP at less than 60 mm Hg or less than 70% of baseline were not different, only the variance of the MAP.

Processed Electroencephalogram

The use of a processed electroencephalogram (EEG) monitoring has been evaluated for its role in postoperative cognitive outcomes of elderly patients. A Cochrane meta-analysis of three studies totaling 2,197 elderly patients revealed a lower rate of postoperative delirium (15.2% vs. 21.3%) with use of bispectral index monitor-guided GA versus clinical signs-guided anesthesia.[86] POCD was also included in the meta-analysis and bispectral index-guided anesthesia was associated with a lower rate of POCD at 12 weeks only. POCD at 1 weeks and 52 weeks after surgery was not effected.

Several other studies examining processed EEG monitoring and postoperative delirium have been less favorable.[87,88] A 2020 meta-analysis of five studies concluded EEG-guided anesthetics did not reduce postoperative delirium.[89] However, a 2021 meta-analysis of eight studies concluded that bispectral index monitoring can reduce the incidence of postoperative delirium in elderly surgical patients in a mixed surgical cohort.[90] However, examining cardiac, orthopedic, and colon surgery there was no difference in the incidence of postoperative delirium.

A 2020 Joint Consensus statement by the American Society for Enhanced Recovery and Perioperative Quality Initiative recommends EEG monitoring for overall anesthetic management, including preventing unintended burst suppression.[91] However, processed EEG monitoring had insufficient evidence to recommend its use to reduce the risk of postoperative delirium and postoperative neurocognitive disorder.

The heterogeneity may be explained by some patients having increased susceptibility for delirium as studies demonstrating that patients with EEG suppression at lower volatile anesthetic concentrations have an increased incidence of postoperative delirium.[92,93] EEG burst suppression and the connection to delirium was evaluated in a 2022 study. Patients who demonstrated lower brain anesthetic resistance were anesthetized with less anesthesia and were at higher risk for delirium.[94] The processed EEG may give insight into delirium risk rather than preventing it. Also, burst-suppression may not confer any perioperative neuroprotection and may be unnecessary.[95]

Cerebral Oximetry

Cerebral oxygenation is a modality that has been considered to improve brain health outcomes. The Best Practice Guidelines for Postoperative Brain Health discuss cerebral perfusion optimization, however no definitive measurement has been established.[96] Cerebral oximetry is not correlated with any outcome, and there are mixed results in the literature regarding delirium and POCD outcomes.[97,98,99,100,101,102] A Cochrane review of perioperative active cerebral near-infrared spectroscopy monitoring of brain oxygenation found low-quality evidence and uncertain effects on postoperative delirium and POCD.[103]

Ventilation

Lung-protective ventilation and its effects on delirium have been evaluated in the elderly surgical population. Tidal volumes of 6 mL/kg at 15 times a minute with 5 cm H_2O positive end-expiratory pressure (PEEP) and lung recruitment every 30 minutes versus 8 mL/kg at 12 breaths a minute was found to lower serum inflammatory markers, improve cerebral oxygenation, and reduce postoperative delirium in elderly spine surgery patients.[104]

SURGERY

The surgical experience can influence declines in cognitive function, as seen in two long-term cohort studies.[105,106] The Whitehall II cohort study found cognitive changes correlated with surgery. The authors also noted large medical events, such as stroke, were associated with worse cognitive declines than with surgery. The Oxford Project to Investigate Memory and Ageing (OPTIMA) cohort found cognitive decline associated with surgery in patients with preexisting cognitive impairment. However, patients with no preexisting cognitive impairment did not have associated cognitive declines after surgery.

Postoperative Screening and Diagnosis

After surgery, validated tools such as the Confusion Assessment Method (CAM) and the Confusion Assessment Method for the Intensive Care Unit (CAM-ICU) may be utilized to diagnose clinical delirium.[107] The tools can be utilized for hypoactive delirium as well, which is not overt and more difficult to diagnose.[108] Delirium is a fluctuating disease, and timing of the assessment is paramount. In a postoperative cardiothoracic ICU setting, assessments for delirium occurring twice daily (in the morning and evening) for 4 days detected 97% (confidence interval [CI] 91-99%) of delirium.[109] Ninety percent of cases were detected in the first 3 days.

TREATMENT OPTIONS

When a patient is diagnosed with delirium, mitigating risk factors and ensuring the proper utilization of preventive strategies, such as early ambulation and reorienting the patient, are paramount.[110,111] Medications, such as haloperidol or other antipsychotic medications, can be utilized for a short treatment course if the patient is a danger to themselves or healthcare personnel.[112,113] Medications, however, are not associated with changes in outcomes for ICU patients with delirium.[114,115] However, use of dexmedetomidine was studied in a 2019 Cochrane review. Dexmedetomidine use may shorten delirium duration, but it is not associated with reduced delirium incidence, days with coma, physical restraint use, length of stay, long-term cognitive outcomes, or mortality for any studied medication compared to placebo.[116]

POCD treatment is limited, and the workup includes ruling out other diseases and organic causes. If no primary cause is found, treatment of POCD includes supportive therapy for the patient and family, adequate analgesia, management of symptoms, and ensuring family members have access to resources to help care for a family member with POCD.[117] POCD treatment is also limited by the difficulty of diagnosis, as it is a research term and not a clinical diagnosis. The change to use of the clinical term "neurocognitive dysfunction" may improve disease recognition.[118]

CONCLUSION

- Perioperative brain health best practices are targeted to prevent delirium and POCD.
- The terminology for POCD is changing based on DSM criteria of NCD.
- Preoperative screening of patients older than 65 and with cognitive risk factors should be conducted preoperatively to assess perioperative risk of delirium and cognitive dysfunction.
- No single anesthetic technique has been shown to be superior in preventing delirium and POCD/NCD.
- Medication adjuncts such as dexmedetomidine may help prevent delirium in at-risk patients.
- Other modalities, such as intraoperative EEG monitoring, may prevent delirium by reducing time under burst suppression.
- Nonpharmacologic strategies and ruling out organic causes should be utilized to treat delirium prior to pharmacologic modalities.

REVIEW QUESTIONS

1. A previously functional 89-year-old man had surgery 5 months ago and is noted to no longer be able to perform personal hygiene and is forgetting the names of his grandchildren. What type of cognitive dysfunction is occurring?

    a. Delayed neurocognitive recovery.
    b. Mild postoperative neurocognitive disorder.
    c. Major postoperative neurocognitive disorder.
    d. Postoperative cognitive dysfunction.

The correct answer is c.

NCD is clinically diagnosed when there is a cognitive concern with objective evidence of a cognitive deficit. NCD with maintenance of activities of daily living (ADL) is considered mild NCD; if ADLs are interrupted, then it is major NCD. NCD after an anesthetic is diagnosed as three separate entities based on proximity to one of three time intervals[119]:

1. *Surgery to 30 days after surgery*: Delayed neurocognitive recovery
2. *30 days after surgery to 1 year after surgery*: Mild or major PNCD
3. *If PNCD lasts beyond 1 year from surgery*: Postoperative cognitive dysfunction

This patient is 5 months past surgery and cannot maintain ADLs and has a noted cognitive concern. This patient meets criteria for major postoperative neurocognitive disorder.

2. A 65-year-old woman is recovering after surgery for a femur fracture 2 weeks ago. Her daughter notes the patient is leaving the stove on and forgetting names and where she left items, such as her keys. What type of cognitive dysfunction is occurring?

   a. Delayed neurocognitive recovery.
   b. Mild postoperative neurocognitive disorder.
   c. Major postoperative neurocognitive disorder.
   d. Postoperative cognitive dysfunction.

The correct answer is a.

NCD is clinically diagnosed when there is a cognitive concern with objective evidence of a cognitive deficit. NCD with maintenance of ADLs is considered mild NCD; if ADLs are interrupted, then it is major NCD. NCD after an anesthetic is diagnosed as three separate entities based on proximity to one of three-time intervals (see Answer in Question 1).[120]

This patient is 2 weeks out from surgery and maintaining ADLs; however, there is a noted cognitive concern. This patient meets criteria for delayed neurocognitive recovery.

3. A patient is diagnosed with delirium in the recovery room after a surgery. The patient is not violent, but is in distress and does not know where they are or the date. What is the best initial step for treatment?

   a. Haloperidol.
   b. Dexmedetomidine.
   c. Reorient the patient.
   d. Restrain the patient.

The correct answer is c.

When a patient is diagnosed with delirium, mitigating risk factors and ensuring the proper utilization of preventive strategies, such as early ambulation and reorienting the patient, are paramount.[121,122] If the patient is violent or a risk to themselves or staff, medications can be utilized.[123,124] Medications, however, are not associated with changes in outcomes for ICU patients with delirium.[125,126,127]

4. Which of the following is not part of the Mini-Cog screening assessment?

   a. Spelling "world" backward.
   b. Drawing a clock.
   c. Repeating three words immediately.
   d. Repeating three words after a period of time.

The correct answer is a.

The Mini-Cog consists of the patient repeating three unrelated words, drawing a clock at a specific time, and then recalling the three words.[128] The patient receives 1 point for each correct word and either 2 points for drawing a correct clock or 0 points for an incorrect clock. The test is a screen, where 0–2 points suggests impairment and 3–5 points suggests no impairment. Spelling "world" backward is not part of the Mini-Cog screening.

5. Which of the following can help reduce burst suppression incidence with GA?

   a. Volatile agents.
   b. Propofol.
   c. Processed EEG.
   d. Cerebral oximetry.

The correct answer is c.

No definitive evidence exists for a best anesthetic to reduce postoperative delirium. Processed EEG monitoring has been studied to reduce postoperative delirium. A 2020 Joint Consensus statement by the American Society for Enhanced Recovery and Perioperative Quality Initiative recommends EEG monitoring for overall anesthetic management, including preventing unintended burst suppression.[129] However, processed EEG monitoring had insufficient evidence to recommend its use to reduce the risk of postoperative delirium and postoperative neurocognitive disorder.

6. Which of the following medications can reduce the duration of delirium?

   a. Haloperidol.
   b. Dexmedetomidine.
   c. Quetiapine.
   d. Midazolam.

The correct answer is b.

Medications such as haloperidol or other antipsychotic medications can be utilized for a short treatment course if the patient is a danger to themselves or healthcare personnel.[130,131] Medications, however, are not associated with changes in outcomes for ICU patients with delirium.[132,133] However, use of dexmedetomidine was studied in a 2019 Cochrane review. Dexmedetomidine use may shorten delirium duration, but it is not associated with reduced delirium incidence, days with coma, physical restraint use, length of stay, long-term cognitive outcomes, or mortality for any studied medication compared to placebo.[134]

7. Which of the following is not a component of a frailty assessment?

   a. Weight loss.
   b. Slow walking speed.
   c. Reduced sleep.
   d. Weakness.

The correct answer is c.

Frailty is a decrease in physiologic reserve, which exceeds expected decline based on age alone and consists of five elements[135]:

1. Weight loss
2. Weakness
3. Slow walking speed
4. Self-reported exhaustion
5. Low physical activity

Reduced sleep can be a component of normal aging, but is not a component of frailty.

REFERENCES

1. Decker J, Kaloostian CL, Gurvich T, et al. Beyond cognitive screening: Establishing an Interprofessional Perioperative Brain Health Initiative. *J Am Geriatr Soc.* 2020;68(10):2359–2364. doi:10.1111/jgs.16720
2. Vacas S, Canales C, Deiner SG, Cole D. Perioperative brain health in the older adult: A patient safety imperative. *Anesth Analg.* 2022 Aug;135(2):316–328. doi:10.1213/ANE.0000000000006090
3. https://www.asahq.org/brainhealthinitiative/news/calltoaction
4. Berger M, Schenning KJ, Brown CH 4th, et al. Best practices for postoperative brain health: Recommendations from the Fifth International Perioperative Neurotoxicity Working Group. *Anesth Analg.* 2018;127(6):1406–1413. doi:10.1213/ANE.0000000000003841
5. Peden CJ, Miller TR, Deiner SG, Eckenhoff RG, Fleisher LA; Members of the Perioperative Brain Health Expert Panel. Improving perioperative brain health: An expert consensus review of key actions for the perioperative care team. *Br J Anaesth.* 2021;126(2):423–432. doi:10.1016/j.bja.2020.10.037
6. Hughes CG, Boncyk CS, Culley DJ, et al. American Society for Enhanced Recovery and Perioperative Quality Initiative Joint Consensus Statement on Postoperative Delirium Prevention. *Anesth Analg.* 2020;130(6):1572–1590. doi:10.1213/ANE.0000000000004641
7. Irwin MG, Ip KY, Hui YM. Anaesthetic considerations in nonagenarians and centenarians. *Curr Opin Anaesthesiol.* 2019;32(6):776–782. doi:10.1097/ACO.0000000000000793
8. American Psychiatric Association. Delirium. In *Diagnostic and statistical manual of mental disorders.* 5th ed. American Psychiatric Association; 2013.
9. Shim JJ, Leung JM. An update on delirium in the postoperative setting: prevention, diagnosis and management. *Best Pract Res Clin Anaesthesiol.* 2012;26(3):327–343. doi:10.1016/j.bpa.2012.08.003
10. Silverstein JH, Timberger M, Reich DL, Uysal S. Central nervous system dysfunction after noncardiac surgery and anesthesia in the elderly. *Anesthesiology.* 2007;106(3):622–628. doi:10.1097/00000542-200703000-00026
11. Berian JR, Zhou L, Russell MM, et al. Postoperative delirium as a target for surgical quality improvement. *Ann Surg.* 2018;268(1):93–99. doi:10.1097/SLA.0000000000002436
12. Girard TD, Exline MC, Carson SS, et al. Haloperidol and ziprasidone for treatment of delirium in critical illness. *N Engl J Med.* 2018;379(26):2506–2516. doi:10.1056/NEJMoa1808217
13. Needham MJ, Webb CE, Bryden DC. Postoperative cognitive dysfunction and dementia: What we need to know and do. *Br J Anaesth.* 2017;119(suppl_1):i115–i125. doi:10.1093/bja/aex354
14. Evered L, Silbert B, Knopman DS, et al. Recommendations for the Nomenclature of Cognitive Change Associated with Anaesthesia and Surgery-2018. *Anesthesiology.* 2018;129(5):872–879. doi:10.1097/ALN.0000000000002334
15. Maguire SL, Slater BMJ. Physiology of ageing. *Anaesth Intensive Care Med.* 2010;11(7):290–292. doi:10.1016/j.mpaic.2010.04.004
16. Benavides-Caro CA. Anaesthesia and the elderly patient, seeking better neurological outcomes. *Colombian J Anesthesiol.* 2016;44(2):128–133.
17. Saxena S, Maze M. Impact on the brain of the inflammatory response to surgery. *Presse Med.* 2018;47(4 Pt 2):e73–e81. doi:10.1016/j.lpm.2018.03.011
18. Strøm C, Rasmussen LS, Sieber FE. Should general anaesthesia be avoided in the elderly?. *Anaesthesia.* 2014;69(Suppl 1):35–44. doi:10.1111/anae.12493
19. Mohanty S, Rosenthal RA, Russell MM, Neuman MD, Ko CY, Esnaola NF. Optimal perioperative management of the geriatric patient: A best practices guideline from the American College of Surgeons NSQIP and the American Geriatrics Society. *J Am Coll Surg.* 2016;222(5):930–947. doi:10.1016/j.jamcollsurg.2015.12.026
20. Weiss Y, Zac L, Refaeli E, et al. Preoperative cognitive impairment and postoperative delirium in elderly surgical patients: A retrospective large cohort study. *Ann Surg.* doi:10.1097/SLA.0000000000005657
21. Berger M, Schenning KJ, Brown CH 4th, et al. Best practices for postoperative brain health: Recommendations from the Fifth International Perioperative Neurotoxicity Working Group. *Anesth Analg.* 2018;127(6):1406–1413. doi:10.1213/ANE.0000000000003841
22. Berger M, Schenning KJ, Brown CH 4th, et al. Best Practices for postoperative brain health: Recommendations from the Fifth International Perioperative Neurotoxicity Working Group. *Anesth Analg.* 2018;127(6):1406–1413. doi:10.1213/ANE.0000000000003841
23. Mohanty S, Rosenthal RA, Russell MM, Neuman MD, Ko CY, Esnaola NF. Optimal perioperative management of the geriatric patient: A best practices guideline from the American College of Surgeons NSQIP and the American Geriatrics Society. *J Am Coll Surg.* 2016;222(5):930–947. doi:10.1016/j.jamcollsurg.2015.12.026
24. Culley DJ, Flaherty D, Fahey MC, et al. Poor performance on a preoperative cognitive screening test predicts postoperative complications in older orthopedic surgical patients. *Anesthesiology.* 2017;127(5):765–774. doi:10.1097/ALN.0000000000001859
25. Weiss Y, Zac L, Refaeli E, et al. Preoperative cognitive impairment and postoperative delirium in elderly surgical patients: A retrospective large cohort study. *Ann Surg.* doi:10.1097/SLA.0000000000005657
26. O'Gara BP, Mueller A, Gasangwa DVI, et al. Prevention of early postoperative decline: A randomized, controlled feasibility trial of perioperative cognitive training. *Anesth Analg.* 2020;130(3):586–595. doi:10.1213/ANE.0000000000004469
27. Humeidan ML, Reyes JC, Mavarez-Martinez A, et al. Effect of cognitive prehabilitation on the incidence of postoperative delirium among older adults undergoing major noncardiac surgery: The Neurobics randomized clinical trial. *JAMA Surg.* 2021;156(2):148–156. doi:10.1001/jamasurg.2020.4371
28. Scholz AF, Oldroyd C, McCarthy K, Quinn TJ, Hewitt J. Systematic review and meta-analysis of risk factors for postoperative delirium among older patients undergoing gastrointestinal surgery. *Br J Surg.* 2016;103(2):e21–e28. doi:10.1002/bjs.10062
29. Raats JW, Steunenberg SL, de Lange DC, van der Laan L. Risk factors of post-operative delirium after elective vascular surgery in the elderly: A systematic review. *Int J Surg.* 2016;35:1–6. doi:10.1016/j.ijsu.2016.09.001
30. Assefa MT, Chekol WB, Melesse DY, Nigatu YA. Incidence and risk factors of emergence delirium after anesthesia in elderly patients at a postanesthesia care unit in Ethiopia: Prospective observational study. *Patient Relat Outcome Meas.* 2021;12:23–32. Published 2021 Feb 9. doi:10.2147/PROM.S297871
31. Ansaloni L, Catena F, Chattat R, et al. Risk factors and incidence of postoperative delirium in elderly patients after elective and emergency surgery. *Br J Surg.* 2010;97(2):273–280. doi:10.1002/bjs.6843
32. Makary MA, Segev DL, Pronovost PJ, et al. Frailty as a predictor of surgical outcomes in older patients. *J Am Coll Surg.* 2010;210(6):901–908. doi:10.1016/j.jamcollsurg.2010.01.028

33. Susano MJ, Grasfield RH, Friese M, et al. Brief preoperative screening for frailty and cognitive impairment predicts delirium after spine surgery. *Anesthesiology*. 2020;133(6):1184–1191. doi:10.1097/ALN.0000000000003523
34. Mauri V, Reuter K, Körber MI, et al. Incidence, risk factors and impact on long-term outcome of postoperative delirium after transcatheter aortic valve replacement. *Front Cardiovasc Med*. 2021;8:645724. doi:10.3389/fcvm.2021.645724
35. Mazzola P, Tassistro E, Di Santo S, et al. The relationship between frailty and delirium: Insights from the 2017 Delirium Day study [published online ahead of print, 2021 Mar 31]. *Age Ageing*. 2021;afab042. doi:10.1093/ageing/afab042
36. Rockwood K, Stadnyk K, MacKnight C, McDowell I, Hébert R, Hogan DB. A brief clinical instrument to classify frailty in elderly people. *Lancet*. 1999;353(9148):205–206. doi:10.1016/S0140-6736(98)04402-X
37. Shem Tov L, Matot I. Frailty and anesthesia. *Curr Opin Anaesthesiol*. 2017;30(3):409–417. doi:10.1097/ACO.0000000000000456
38. Nidadavolu LS, Ehrlich AL, Sieber FE, Oh ES. Preoperative evaluation of the frail patient. *Anesth Analg*. 2020;130(6):1493–1503. doi:10.1213/ANE.0000000000004735
39. Fried LP, Tangen CM, Walston J, et al. Frailty in older adults: Evidence for a phenotype. *J Gerontol A Biol Sci Med Sci*. 2001;56(3):M146–M156. doi:10.1093/gerona/56.3.m146
40. Makary MA, Segev DL, Pronovost PJ, et al. Frailty as a predictor of surgical outcomes in older patients. *J Am Coll Surg*. 2010;210(6):901–908. doi:10.1016/j.jamcollsurg.2010.01.028
41. Qiu C, Chan PH, Zohman GL, et al. Impact of anesthesia on hospital mortality and morbidities in geriatric patients following emergency hip fracture surgery. *J Orthop Trauma*. 2018;32(3):116–123. doi:10.1097/BOT.0000000000001035
42. Braude P, Goodman A, Elias T, et al. Evaluation and establishment of a ward-based geriatric liaison service for older urological surgical patients: Proactive care of Older People undergoing Surgery (POPS)-Urology. *BJU Int*. 2017;120(1):123–129. doi:10.1111/bju.13526
43. McIsaac DI, MacDonald DB, Aucoin SD. Frailty for perioperative clinicians: A narrative review. *Anesth Analg*. 2020;130(6):1450–1460. doi:10.1213/ANE.0000000000004602
44. Norris CM, Close JCT. Prehabilitation for the frailty syndrome: Improving outcomes for our most vulnerable patients. *Anesth Analg*. 2020;130(6):1524–1533. doi:10.1213/ANE.0000000000004785
45. Siddiqi N, Harrison JK, Clegg A, et al. Interventions for preventing delirium in hospitalised non-ICU patients. *Cochrane Database Syst Rev*. 2016;3:CD005563. doi:10.1002/14651858.CD005563.pub3
46. Deeken F, Sánchez A, Rapp MA, et al.; PAWEL Study Group. Outcomes of a delirium prevention program in older persons after elective surgery: A stepped-wedge cluster randomized clinical trial. *JAMA Surg*. 2022 Feb 1;157(2):e216370. doi:10.1001/jamasurg.2021.6370. Epub 2022 Feb 9. PMID: 34910080; PMCID: PMC8674802.
47. https://www.asahq.org/brainhealthinitiative/toolsforpatients/sixtips
48. Deiner S, Fleisher LA, Leung JM, et al. Adherence to recommended practices for perioperative anesthesia care for older adults among US anesthesiologists: results from the ASA Committee on Geriatric Anesthesia-Perioperative Brain Health Initiative ASA member survey. *Perioper Med (Lond)*. 2020;9:6. doi:10.1186/s13741-020-0136-9
49. American Geriatrics Society Expert Panel on Postoperative Delirium in Older Adults. Postoperative delirium in older adults: best practice statement from the American Geriatrics Society. *J Am Coll Surg*. 2015;220(2):136–48.e1. doi:10.1016/j.jamcollsurg.2014.10.019
50. Weinstein SM, Poultsides L, Baaklini LR, et al. Postoperative delirium in total knee and hip arthroplasty patients: A study of perioperative modifiable risk factors. *Br J Anaesth*. 2018;120(5):999–1008. doi:10.1016/j.bja.2017.12.046
51. Sieber FE, Zakriya KJ, Gottschalk A, et al. Sedation depth during spinal anesthesia and the development of postoperative delirium in elderly patients undergoing hip fracture repair [published correction appears in Mayo Clin Proc. 2010 Apr;85(4):400. Dosage error in article text]. *Mayo Clin Proc*. 2010;85(1):18–26. doi:10.4065/mcp.2009.0469
52. Ehsani R, Djalali Motlagh S, Zaman B, Sehat Kashani S, Ghodraty MR. Effect of general versus spinal anesthesia on postoperative delirium and early cognitive dysfunction in elderly patients. *Anesth Pain Med*. 2020;10(4):e101815. doi:10.5812/aapm.101815
53. Kamitani K, Higuchi A, Asahi T, Yoshida H. Postoperative delirium after general anesthesia vs. spinal anesthesia in geriatric patients. *Masui*. 2003;52(9):972–975.
54. Li T, Li J, Yuan L, et al. Effect of regional vs general anesthesia on incidence of postoperative delirium in older patients undergoing hip fracture surgery: The RAGA randomized trial. *JAMA*. 2022;327(1):50–58. doi:10.1001/jama.2021.22647
55. Silva AR, Regueira P, Albuquerque E, et al. Estimates of geriatric delirium frequency in noncardiac surgeries and its evaluation across the years: A systematic review and meta-analysis. *J Am Med Dir Assoc*. 2021;22(3):613–620.e9. doi:10.1016/j.jamda.2020.08.017
56. Williams-Russo P, Sharrock NE, Mattis S, Szatrowski TP, Charlson ME. Cognitive effects after epidural vs general anesthesia in older adults: A randomized trial. *JAMA*. 1995;274(1):44–50.
57. Tzimas P, Samara E, Petrou A, Korompilias A, Chalkias A, Papadopoulos G. The influence of anesthetic techniques on postoperative cognitive function in elderly patients undergoing hip fracture surgery: General vs spinal anesthesia. *Injury*. 2018;49(12):2221–2226. doi:10.1016/j.injury.2018.09.023
58. Silbert BS, Evered LA, Scott DA. Incidence of postoperative cognitive dysfunction after general or spinal anaesthesia for extracorporeal shock wave lithotripsy. *Br J Anaesth*. 2014;113(5):784–791. doi:10.1093/bja/aeu163
59. Li YW, Li HJ, Li HJ, et al. Delirium in older patients after combined epidural-general anesthesia or general anesthesia for major surgery: A randomized trial. *Anesthesiology*. 2021;135(2):218–232. doi:10.1097/ALN.0000000000003834
60. Miller D, Lewis SR, Pritchard MW, et al. Intravenous versus inhalational maintenance of anaesthesia for postoperative cognitive outcomes in elderly people undergoing non-cardiac surgery. *Cochrane Database Syst Rev*. 2018;8(8):CD012317. Published 2018 Aug 21. doi:10.1002/14651858.CD012317.pub2
61. Li Y, Chen D, Wang H, et al. Intravenous versus volatile anesthetic effects on postoperative cognition in elderly patients undergoing laparoscopic abdominal surgery. *Anesthesiology*. 2021;134(3):381–394. doi:10.1097/ALN.0000000000003680
62. Hovaguimian F, Tschopp C, Beck-Schimmer B, Puhan M. Intraoperative ketamine administration to prevent delirium or postoperative cognitive dysfunction: A systematic review and meta-analysis. *Acta Anaesthesiol Scand*. 2018;62(9):1182–1193. doi:10.1111/aas.13168
63. Avidan MS, Maybrier HR, Abdallah AB, et al. Intraoperative ketamine for prevention of postoperative delirium or pain after major surgery in older adults: An international, multicentre, double-blind, randomised clinical trial [published correction appears in Lancet. 2017 Jul 15;390(10091):230]. *Lancet*. 2017;390(10091):267–275. doi:10.1016/S0140-6736(17)31467-8
64. Hovaguimian F, Tschopp C, Beck-Schimmer B, Puhan M. Intraoperative ketamine administration to prevent delirium or postoperative cognitive dysfunction: A systematic review and meta-analysis. *Acta Anaesthesiol Scand*. 2018;62(9):1182–1193. doi:10.1111/aas.13168
65. Flükiger J, Hollinger A, Speich B, et al. Dexmedetomidine in prevention and treatment of postoperative and intensive care unit delirium: A systematic review and meta-analysis. *Ann Intensive Care*. 2018;8(1):92. doi:10.1186/s13613-018-0437-z
66. Zhang J, Yu Y, Miao S, et al. Effects of peri-operative intravenous administration of dexmedetomidine on emergence agitation after general anesthesia in adults: A meta-analysis of randomized controlled trials. *Drug Des Devel Ther*. 2019;13:2853–2864. doi:10.2147/DDDT.S207016
67. Govêia CS, Miranda DB, Oliveira LVB, Praxedes FB, Moreira LG, Guimarães GMN. Dexmedetomidine reduces postoperative

cognitive and behavioral dysfunction in adults submitted to general anesthesia for non-cardiac surgery: Meta-analysis of randomized clinical trials [published online ahead of print, 2021 Feb 19]. *Braz J Anesthesiol*. 2021;S0104-0014(21)00062-2. doi:10.1016/j.bjane.2021.02.020

68. Lee C, Lee CH, Lee G, Lee M, Hwang J. The effect of the timing and dose of dexmedetomidine on postoperative delirium in elderly patients after laparoscopic major non-cardiac surgery: A double blind randomized controlled study. *J Clin Anesth*. 2018;47:27-32. doi:10.1016/j.jclinane.2018.03.007

69. Deiner S, Luo X, Lin HM, et al. Intraoperative infusion of dexmedetomidine for prevention of postoperative delirium and cognitive dysfunction in elderly patients undergoing major elective noncardiac surgery: A randomized clinical trial. *JAMA Surg*. 2017;152(8):e171505. doi:10.1001/jamasurg.2017.1505

70. Subramaniam B, Shankar P, Shaefi S, et al. Effect of intravenous acetaminophen vs placebo combined with propofol or dexmedetomidine on postoperative delirium among older patients following cardiac surgery: The DEXACET randomized clinical trial [published correction appears in *JAMA*. 2019 Jul 16;322(3):276]. *JAMA*. 2019;321(7):686-696. doi:10.1001/jama.2019.0234

71. Su X, Meng ZT, Wu XH, et al. Dexmedetomidine for prevention of delirium in elderly patients after non-cardiac surgery: A randomised, double-blind, placebo-controlled trial. *Lancet*. 2016;388(10054):1893-1902. doi:10.1016/S0140-6736(16)30580-3

72. Djaiani G, Silverton N, Fedorko L, et al. Dexmedetomidine versus propofol sedation reduces delirium after cardiac surgery: a randomized controlled trial. *Anesthesiology*. 2016;124(2):362-368. doi:10.1097/ALN.0000000000000951

73. Li CJ, Wang BJ, Mu DL, et al. Randomized clinical trial of intraoperative dexmedetomidine to prevent delirium in the elderly undergoing major non-cardiac surgery. *Br J Surg*. 2020;107(2):e123-e132. doi:10.1002/bjs.11354

74. Hu J, Zhu M, Gao Z, et al. Dexmedetomidine for prevention of postoperative delirium in older adults undergoing oesophagectomy with total intravenous anaesthesia: A double-blind, randomised clinical trial. *Eur J Anaesthesiol*. 2021;38(Suppl 1):S9-S17. doi:10.1097/EJA.0000000000001382

75. Park JW, Kim EK, Lee HT, Park S, Do SH. The effects of propofol or dexmedetomidine sedation on postoperative recovery in elderly patients receiving lower limb surgery under spinal anesthesia: A retrospective propensity score-matched analysis. *J Clin Med*. 2021;10(1):135. doi:10.3390/jcm10010135

76. Spies CD, Knaak C, Mertens M, et al. Physostigmine for prevention of postoperative delirium and long-term cognitive dysfunction in liver surgery: A double-blinded randomised controlled trial [published online ahead of print, 2021 Jan 28]. *Eur J Anaesthesiol*. 2021. doi:10.1097/EJA.0000000000001456

77. Hernandez NM, Cunningham DJ, Hinton ZW, Wu CJ, Seyler TM. Are patients taking benzodiazepines at increased risk for complications following primary total knee arthroplasty? *J Arthroplasty*. 2021;36(5):1611-1616. doi:10.1016/j.arth.2020.12.004

78. Duprey MS, Devlin JW, Griffith JL, et al. Association between perioperative medication use and postoperative delirium and cognition in older adults undergoing elective noncardiac surgery. Anesth Analg. 2022 Jun;134(6):1154-1163. doi:10.1213/ANE.0000000000005959

79. Omichi C, Ayani N, Oya N, et al. Association between discontinuation of benzodiazepine receptor agonists and post-operative delirium among inpatients with liaison intervention: A retrospective cohort study. *Compr Psychiatry*. 2021;104:152216. doi:10.1016/j.comppsych.2020.152216

80. Lee D, Petersen F, Wu M, et al. A prospective observational cohort pilot study of the association between midazolam use and delirium in elderly endoscopy patients. *BMC Anesthesiol*. 2021;21(1):53. doi:10.1186/s12871-021-01275-z

81. Heinrich M, Müller A, Cvijan A, et al. Preoperative comparison of three anticholinergic drug scales in older adult patients and development of postoperative delirium: A prospective observational study. *Drugs Aging*. 2021;38(4):347-354. doi:10.1007/s40266-021-00839-5

82. Hu AM, Qiu Y, Zhang P, et al. Higher versus lower mean arterial pressure target management in older patients having non-cardiothoracic surgery: A prospective randomized controlled trial. *J Clin Anesth*. 2021;69:110150. doi:10.1016/j.jclinane.2020.110150

83. Maheshwari K, Ahuja S, Khanna AK, et al. Association between perioperative hypotension and delirium in postoperative critically ill patients: A retrospective cohort analysis. *Anesth Analg* 2020;130(3):636-643. doi:10.1213/ANE.0000000000004517

84. Wachtendorf LJ, Azimaraghi O, Santer P, et al. Association between intraoperative arterial hypotension and postoperative delirium after noncardiac surgery: A retrospective multicenter cohort study. *Anesth Analg*. 2022 Apr;134(4):822-833. doi:10.1213/ANE.0000000000005739

85. Jung C, Hinken L, Fischer-Kumbruch M, et al. Intraoperative monitoring parameters and postoperative delirium: Results of a prospective cross-sectional trial. *Medicine (Baltimore)*. 2021;100(1):e24160. doi:10.1097/MD.0000000000024160

86. Punjasawadwong Y, Chau-In W, Laopaiboon M, Punjasawadwong S, Pin-On P. Processed electroencephalogram and evoked potential techniques for amelioration of postoperative delirium and cognitive dysfunction following non-cardiac and non-neurosurgical procedures in adults. *Cochrane Database Syst Rev*. 2018;5(5):CD011283. Published 2018 May 15. doi:10.1002/14651858.CD011283.pub2

87. Wildes TS, Mickle AM, Ben Abdallah A, et al. Effect of electroencephalography-guided anesthetic administration on postoperative delirium among older adults undergoing major surgery: The ENGAGES randomized clinical trial. *JAMA*. 2019;321(5):473-483. doi:10.1001/jama.2018.22005

88. Yang Y, Song Y, Song C, Li C. Comparison of bispectral index-guided individualized anesthesia with standard general anesthesia on inadequate emergence and postoperative delirium in elderly patients undergoing esophagectomy: A retrospective study at a single center. *Med Sci Monit*. 2020;26:e925314. doi:10.12659/MSM.925314

89. Sun Y, Ye F, Wang J, et al. Electroencephalography-guided anesthetic delivery for preventing postoperative delirium in adults: An updated meta-analysis. *Anesth Analg*. 2020;131(3):712-719. doi:10.1213/ANE.0000000000004746

90. Shan W, Chen B, Huang L, Zhou Y. The effects of bispectral index-guided anesthesia on postoperative delirium in elderly patients: A systematic review and meta-analysis. *World Neurosurg*. 2021;147:e57-e62. doi:10.1016/j.wneu.2020.11.110

91. Chan MTV, Hedrick TL, Egan TD, et al. American Society for Enhanced Recovery and Perioperative Quality Initiative Joint Consensus Statement on the role of neuromonitoring in perioperative outcomes: Electroencephalography. *Anesth Analg*. 2020;130(5):1278-1291. doi:10.1213/ANE.0000000000004502

92. Soehle M, Dittmann A, Ellerkmann RK, Baumgarten G, Putensen C, Guenther U. Intraoperative burst suppression is associated with postoperative delirium following cardiac surgery: A prospective, observational study. *BMC Anesthesiol*. 2015;15:61. doi:10.1186/s12871-015-0051-7

93. Fritz BA, Maybrier HR, Avidan MS. Intraoperative electroencephalogram suppression at lower volatile anaesthetic concentrations predicts postoperative delirium occurring in the intensive care unit. *Br J Anaesth*. 2018;121(1):241-248. doi:10.1016/j.bja.2017.10.024

94. Cooter Wright M, Bunning T, Eleswarpu S, et al. A processed electroencephalogram–based brain anesthetic resistance index is associated with postoperative delirium in older adults: A dual center study. *Anesth Analg*. 2022 Jan;134(1):149-158. doi:10.1213/ANE.0000000000005660

95. Ma K, Bebawy JF. Electroencephalographic burst-suppression, perioperative neuroprotection, postoperative cognitive function, and mortality: A focused narrative review of the literature. *Anesth Analg*. 2022 Jul;135(1):79-90. doi:10.1213/ANE.0000000000005806

96. Berger M, Schenning KJ, Brown CH 4th, et al. Best practices for postoperative brain health: Recommendations from

97. Soh S, Shim JK, Song JW, Kim KN, Noh HY, Kwak YL. Postoperative delirium in elderly patients undergoing major spinal surgery: Role of cerebral oximetry. *J Neurosurg Anesthesiol.* 2017;29(4):426–432. doi:10.1097/ANA.0000000000000363
98. Schoen J, Meyerrose J, Paarmann H, Heringlake M, Hueppe M, Berger KU. Preoperative regional cerebral oxygen saturation is a predictor of postoperative delirium in on-pump cardiac surgery patients: A prospective observational trial. *Crit Care.* 2011;15(5):R218. doi:10.1186/cc10454
99. Kim J, Shim JK, Song JW, Kim EK, Kwak YL. Postoperative cognitive dysfunction and the change of regional cerebral oxygen saturation in elderly patients undergoing spinal surgery. *Anesth Analg.* 2016;123(2):436–444. doi:10.1213/ANE.0000000000001352
100. Zheng F, Sheinberg R, Yee MS, Ono M, Zheng Y, Hogue CW. Cerebral near-infrared spectroscopy monitoring and neurologic outcomes in adult cardiac surgery patients: A systematic review. *Anesth Analg.* 2013;116(3):663–676. doi:10.1213/ANE.0b013e318277a255
101. Shaefi S, Marcantonio ER, Mueller A, et al. Intraoperative oxygen concentration and neurocognition after cardiac surgery: Study protocol for a randomized controlled trial. *Trials.* 2017;18(1):600. doi:10.1186/s13063-017-2337-1
102. Fontes MT, McDonagh DL, Phillips-Bute B, et al. Arterial hyperoxia during cardiopulmonary bypass and postoperative cognitive dysfunction. *J Cardiothorac Vasc Anesth.* 2014;28(3):462–466. doi:10.1053/j.jvca.2013.03.034
103. Yu Y, Zhang K, Zhang L, Zong H, Meng L, Han R. Cerebral near-infrared spectroscopy (NIRS) for perioperative monitoring of brain oxygenation in children and adults. *Cochrane Database Syst Rev.* 2018;1(1):CD010947. doi:10.1002/14651858.CD010947.pub2
104. Wang J, Zhu L, Li Y, Yin C, Hou Z, Wang Q. The potential role of lung-protective ventilation in preventing postoperative delirium in elderly patients undergoing prone spinal surgery: A preliminary study. *Med Sci Monit.* 2020;26:e926526. doi:10.12659/MSM.926526
105. Patel D, Lunn AD, Smith AD, Lehmann DJ, Dorrington KL. Cognitive decline in the elderly after surgery and anaesthesia: Results from the Oxford Project to Investigate Memory and Ageing (OPTIMA) cohort. *Anaesthesia.* 2016;71(10):1144–1152. doi:10.1111/anae.13571
106. Krause BM, Sabia S, Manning HJ, Singh-Manoux A, Sanders RD. Association between major surgical admissions and the cognitive trajectory: 19 year follow-up of Whitehall II cohort study. *BMJ.* 2019;366:l4466. doi:10.1136/bmj.l4466
107. Inouye SK, van Dyck CH, Alessi CA, Balkin S, Siegal AP, Horwitz RI. Clarifying confusion: The confusion assessment method. A new method for detection of delirium. *Ann Intern Med.* 1990;113(12):941–948. doi:10.7326/0003-4819-113-12-941
108. Hosker C, Ward D. Hypoactive delirium. *BMJ.* 2017;357:j2047. doi:10.1136/bmj.j2047
109. Hamadnalla H, Sessler DI, Troianos CA, et al. Optimal interval and duration of CAM-ICU assessments for delirium detection after cardiac surgery. *J Clin Anesth.* 2021;71:110233. doi:10.1016/j.jclinane.2021.110233
110. Robinson TN, Eiseman B. Postoperative delirium in the elderly: diagnosis and management. *Clin Interv Aging.* 2008;3(2):351–355. doi:10.2147/cia.s2759
111. Takahashi N, Hiraki A, Kawahara K, et al. Postoperative delirium in patients undergoing tumor resection with reconstructive surgery for oral cancer. *Mol Clin Oncol.* 2021;14(3):60. doi:10.3892/mco.2021.2222
112. Vochteloo AJ, Moerman S, van der Burg BL, et al. Delirium risk screening and haloperidol prophylaxis program in hip fracture patients is a helpful tool in identifying high-risk patients, but does not reduce the incidence of delirium. *BMC Geriatr.* 2011;11:39. doi:10.1186/1471-2318-11-39
113. Duning T, Ilting-Reuke K, Beckhuis M, Oswald D. Postoperative delirium: Treatment and prevention. *Curr Opin Anaesthesiol.* 2021;34(1):27–32. doi:10.1097/ACO.0000000000000939
114. Rood PJT, Zegers M, Slooter AJC, et al. Prophylactic haloperidol effects on long-term quality of life in critically ill patients at high risk for delirium: Results of the REDUCE study. *Anesthesiology.* 2019;131(2):328–335. doi:10.1097/ALN.0000000000002812
115. Girard TD, Exline MC, Carson SS, et al. Haloperidol and ziprasidone for treatment of delirium in critical illness. *N Engl J Med.* 2018;379(26):2506–2516. doi:10.1056/NEJMoa1808217
116. Burry L, Hutton B, Williamson DR, et al. Pharmacological interventions for the treatment of delirium in critically ill adults. *Cochrane Database Syst Rev.* 2019;9(9):CD011749. doi:10.1002/14651858.CD011749.pub2
117. Pappa M, Theodosiadis N, Tsounis A, Sarafis P. Pathogenesis and treatment of post-operative cognitive dysfunction. *Electron Physician.* 2017;9(2):3768–3775. doi:10.19082/3768
118. Evered L, Silbert B, Knopman DS, et al. Recommendations for the nomenclature of cognitive change associated with anaesthesia and surgery-2018. *Br J Anaesth.* 2018;121(5):1005–1012. doi:10.1016/j.bja.2017.11.087
119. Evered L, Silbert B, Knopman DS, et al. Recommendations for the nomenclature of cognitive change associated with anaesthesia and surgery-2018. *Br J Anaesth.* 2018;121(5):1005–1012. doi:10.1016/j.bja.2017.11.087
120. Evered L, Silbert B, Knopman DS, et al. Recommendations for the nomenclature of cognitive change associated with anaesthesia and surgery-2018. *Br J Anaesth.* 2018;121(5):1005–1012. doi:10.1016/j.bja.2017.11.0874
121. Robinson TN, Eiseman B. Postoperative delirium in the elderly: diagnosis and management. *Clin Interv Aging.* 2008;3(2):351–355. doi:10.2147/cia.s2759
122. Takahashi N, Hiraki A, Kawahara K, et al. Postoperative delirium in patients undergoing tumor resection with reconstructive surgery for oral cancer. *Mol Clin Oncol.* 2021;14(3):60. doi:10.3892/mco.2021.2222
123. Vochteloo AJ, Moerman S, van der Burg BL, et al. Delirium risk screening and haloperidol prophylaxis program in hip fracture patients is a helpful tool in identifying high-risk patients, but does not reduce the incidence of delirium. *BMC Geriatr.* 2011;11:39. doi:10.1186/1471-2318-11-39
124. Duning T, Ilting-Reuke K, Beckhuis M, Oswald D. Postoperative delirium: Treatment and prevention. *Curr Opin Anaesthesiol.* 2021;34(1):27–32. doi:10.1097/ACO.0000000000000939
125. Rood PJT, Zegers M, Slooter AJC, et al. Prophylactic haloperidol effects on long-term quality of life in critically ill patients at high risk for delirium: Results of the REDUCE study. *Anesthesiology.* 2019;131(2):328–335. doi:10.1097/ALN.0000000000002812
126. Girard TD, Exline MC, Carson SS, et al. Haloperidol and ziprasidone for treatment of delirium in critical illness. *N Engl J Med.* 2018;379(26):2506–2516. doi:10.1056/NEJMoa1808217
127. Burry L, Hutton B, Williamson DR, et al. Pharmacological interventions for the treatment of delirium in critically ill adults. *Cochrane Database Syst Rev.* 2019;9(9):CD011749. doi:10.1002/14651858.CD011749.pub2
128. Mohanty S, Rosenthal RA, Russell MM, Neuman MD, Ko CY, Esnaola NF. Optimal perioperative management of the geriatric patient: A best practices guideline from the American College of Surgeons NSQIP and the American Geriatrics Society. *J Am Coll Surg.* 2016;222(5):930–947. doi:10.1016/j.jamcollsurg.2015.12.026
129. Chan MTV, Hedrick TL, Egan TD, et al. American Society for Enhanced Recovery and Perioperative Quality Initiative Joint

Consensus Statement on the role of neuromonitoring in perioperative outcomes: Electroencephalography. *Anesth Analg.* 2020;130(5):1278–1291. doi:10.1213/ANE.0000000000004502

130. Vochteloo AJ, Moerman S, van der Burg BL, et al. Delirium risk screening and haloperidol prophylaxis program in hip fracture patients is a helpful tool in identifying high-risk patients, but does not reduce the incidence of delirium. *BMC Geriatr.* 2011;11:39. doi:10.1186/1471-2318-11-39

131. Duning T, Ilting-Reuke K, Beckhuis M, Oswald D. Postoperative delirium: Treatment and prevention. *Curr Opin Anaesthesiol.* 2021;34(1):27–32. doi:10.1097/ACO.0000000000000939

132. Rood PJT, Zegers M, Slooter AJC, et al. Prophylactic haloperidol effects on long-term quality of life in critically ill patients at high risk for delirium: Results of the REDUCE study. *Anesthesiology.* 2019;131(2):328–335. doi:10.1097/ALN.0000000000002812

133. Girard TD, Exline MC, Carson SS, et al. Haloperidol and ziprasidone for treatment of delirium in critical illness. *N Engl J Med.* 2018;379(26):2506–2516. doi:10.1056/NEJMoa1808217

134. Burry L, Hutton B, Williamson DR, et al. Pharmacological interventions for the treatment of delirium in critically ill adults. *Cochrane Database Syst Rev.* 2019;9(9):CD011749. doi:10.1002/14651858.CD011749.pub2

135. Rockwood K, Stadnyk K, MacKnight C, McDowell I, Hébert R, Hogan DB. A brief clinical instrument to classify frailty in elderly people. *Lancet.* 1999;353(9148):205–206. doi:10.1016/S0140-6736(98)04402-X

24.

RESTRICTIVE LUNG DISEASE FROM PARKINSON'S DISEASE RIGIDITY

IS IT REAL?

Shilpa Rao

STEM CASE AND KEY QUESTIONS

A 75-year-old male patient with Parkinson's disease (PD) presents for elective placement of a deep brain stimulator (DBS) depth electrode connector and generator placement. He underwent implantation of depth electrodes 14 days prior. Significant past medical history includes PD, hypertension, and long-standing interstitial lung disease. Medications include carbidopa-levodopa 25 mg/100 mg three times a day. On examination, he is rigid, with a slightly hoarse voice, as well as having a shuffling gait. His previous anesthetic history is unremarkable.

What is PD? What is the underlying pathology, and what are current treatment options?

PD is a neurodegenerative disorder of the central nervous system caused by loss of dopaminergic neurons in the substantia nigra. Multiple treatment modalities are available, including medical management and surgical placement of a DBS.

Would you like to obtain a more detailed preoperative history and preoperative laboratory tests? Why are they relevant?

A detailed history and examination are important to identify perioperative risk factors such as aspiration risk or the potential for a difficult airway. Routine preoperative testing is not indicated in patients with PD and is usually dictated by other underlying comorbidities.

When is additional cardiopulmonary testing indicated?

Depending on the presence of individual risk factors and the patient's reported functional capacity, additional cardiac testing (ECG, echocardiogram) may be required. Pulmonary function tests (PFTs) aid in diagnosis of underlying restrictive lung disease, sometimes seen in patients with PD.

What instructions would you give the patient regarding preoperative antiparkinsonian medications?

To minimize time gaps between dosage intervals which can potentially lead to disease exacerbations, all antiparkinsonian medications should be taken on the morning of surgery.

You notice that this patient is on levodopa. What medications would you avoid in the perioperative period?

Monoamine oxide inhibitors are avoided in these patients as they can cause an acute hypertensive episode. Phenothiazines, butyrophenones, droperidol, and metoclopramide can exacerbate symptoms of PD.

What monitors would you like to use on this patient? Any additional preparation for airway management?

Standard American Society of Anesthesiologists monitors are required. An arterial catheter may be considered for invasive blood pressure monitoring.

What are the risks associated with general anesthesia (GA), and how will you prepare for them?

Important risks include the possibility of a difficult airway, risk of aspiration, and autonomic dysfunction.

You place an IV line in the preoperative holding area after adequate assessment of the patient. The patient appears calm, although his wife mentions he gets very agitated in unfamiliar surroundings. During a rapid-sequence induction of GA, the patient begins to flail and pulls out his IV line. You notice about half the dose of propofol is already administered before the line is out. What do you do next?

The immediate concerns are patient safety and maintaining the airway while preventing aspiration. Falls and secondary injury must be prevented and additional help should be called into the operating room. A second IV line should be quickly established by an experienced anesthesia clinician while a second clinician is managing the airway. If the patient is apneic, gentle manual ventilation should be performed to prevent gastric insufflation. Once a new and patent IV line is established, the rest of anesthesia induction may proceed as originally planned.

You successfully perform rapid-sequence induction using propofol and rocuronium and intubate the patient using a video laryngoscope. After visually confirming the endotracheal tube pass through the vocal cords, you attach the tube to the anesthesia *circuit and notice that there is no end tidal CO_2. What is the next step?*

The first step is confirming correct endotracheal tube placement by video laryngoscope and/or fiberoptic scope. In addition, the circuit and end tidal connections must be quickly inspected to ensure there are no disconnections. Mucus plugs blocking the endotracheal tube can be suctioned with a soft suction catheter. Bronchospasm should be considered in the differential diagnosis, as long at the endotracheal tube's position is confirmed visually.

You resolve the issue, and the surgery commences. What are your choices for perioperative pain management and why?

Multimodal analgesia must be considered. These involve short-acting opiates such as small doses of fentanyl, IV acetaminophen, NSAIDs, and local anesthesia around the surgical site.

You notice that the peak airway pressures have increased since you intubated the patient. What is your next step?

Auscultation of bilateral lung fields can help diagnose causes of increased peak airway pressure such as endobronchial intubation/bronchospasm and these must be treated accordingly. Mechanical obstructions in the circuit, patient biting on the endotracheal tube, and a stuck inspiratory valve can also contribute to increased peak airway pressures.

The surgery is completed and you extubate the patient after he meets extubation criteria. Half an hour later, you get a stat call from a PACU nurse who mentions the patient has labored breathing. What is your next step?

A quick and focused assessment is important. Any additional narcotics or sedatives administered in the PACU must be noted, and one must follow-up with the PACU team to note the timing of the last levodopa dose as skipped doses may lead to PD exacerbation. If indeed this is due to missed doses and patient is not cooperative to take oral medications, a nasogastric tube must be passed to administer levodopa. Ventilation must be assisted with bag mask if respirations are inadequate.

DISCUSSION

DEFINITION AND PATHOPHYSIOLOGY

PD is a slowly progressive neurodegenerative disorder involving the central nervous system, caused by the deficiency of dopaminergic fibers in substantia nigra. It was originally described in 1817, by James Parkinson. The peak age of onset is in the sixties and the course of illness ranges from 10 to 25 years. Approximately 0.3% of the general population and 3% of the population older than 65 years have PD.[1]

Etiology is multifactorial, with genetic and environmental factors. Age is the biggest risk factor, with the median age of onset being 60 years.[2] There is an inverse correlation between cigarette smoking and PD. A large meta-analysis including 44 case-control studies and 8 cohort studies from 20 countries showed an inverse correlation between smoking and PD, with a pooled relative risk of 0.39 for current smokers although the underlying mechanism is not completely understood.[3] There are further inconclusive associations between caffeine intake, use of pesticides, heavy metals exposure and the development of PD.

Genetic causes have been identified with several distinct mutations. Recently, nine mutations involving a novel gene leucine-rich repeat kinase 2 *(LRRK2)*, have been identified as the cause of autosomal-dominant PD in kindreds, while other cases had been previously linked to the *PARK8* locus on chromosome 12.[4]

DIAGNOSIS

There is no "gold standard" for the diagnosis of PD. Rather, it is based on the clinical features as mentioned below, with some laboratory tests to corroborate. Fluorodopa positron emission tomography (PET) measures levodopa uptake into dopamine nerve terminals, showing a decline of about 5% per year of striatal uptake. This diagnostic test reveals decreased dopaminergic nerve terminals in the striatum in both PD and the Parkinson-plus syndromes (PS) that include cognitive deficits, dementia, or cranial nerve involvement in addition to PD but does not distinguish between them. A marked response to levodopa is helpful in the differential diagnosis, indicating presynaptic dopamine deficiency with intact postsynaptic dopamine receptors, features typical of PD.[5]

A biopsy of substantia nigra may demonstrate depletion of dopaminergic cells, but this is rarely needed for confirmation of diagnosis.

Neurologic Manifestations

Main clinical features include the presence of motor symptoms such as resting tremor, bradykinesia, postural instability, and shuffling gait. The tremor associated with PD is often described as "pill rolling," consisting of back-and-forth repeated movements of the fingers. Rigidity is associated with constant tension and contraction of the muscle "cogwheel"-like. One of the most disabling symptoms is bradykinesia, where there is associated loss of spontaneous movement and severe slowing down of activities of daily living (ADLs). Commonly seen non-motor symptoms include emotional instability, depression, unpredictable mood and cognitive changes, difficulty swallowing, and dysarthria. Many of the non-motor symptoms precede the onset of motor symptoms by many years. There is now a great deal of evidence supporting the fact that the disease may begin in the peripheral autonomic nervous system and/or the olfactory bulb, with the pathology then spreading through the central nervous system and affecting the lower brainstem structures before involving the substantia nigra.[6] As the disease progresses, symptoms worsen over time and difficult to manage non-motor symptoms such as autonomic dysfunction, orthostatic hypotension, and urinary incontinence can lead to a poor overall quality of life.

Cognitive Manifestations

There may be varying degrees of cognitive impairment during the course of PD. Mild impairment is often noticed in early stages of the disease and does not interfere in ADLs. As the disease progresses, there may be worsening cognitive decline, manifested as difficulty focusing or carrying out complex tasks, impaired executive function, slowing of thinking and processing information, memory problems, and visual-spatial difficulties. There may or may not be associated dementia in advanced PD. Cognitive impairment can be diagnosed by obtaining a detailed history from the patient and family members, as well as performing a Mini-Mental Status Examination (MMSE) or Montreal Cognitive Assessment.

Cardiovascular Manifestations

PD is associated with autonomic dysfunction and impaired regulation of myocardial function. Clinical manifestations include heart rate variability, which may be one of the early clinical features. Cardiac involvement in PD/PS includes cardiac autonomic dysfunction, cardiomyopathy, coronary heart disease, arrhythmias, conduction defects, sudden cardiac death (SCD), and sudden unexpected death in PD.[7]

Multisystem atrophy (formerly called Shy Drager syndrome) shares many clinical features of PD including autonomic dysfunction and sensory-motor symptoms, and it has an overall worse prognosis, with poor response to levodopa treatment.

Pulmonary Manifestations

A variety of pulmonary complications are seen in PD, and they pose significant challenges in the perioperative period. Lee et al. evaluated symptom burden experienced by patients with PD with 35.8% reporting shortness of breath on exertion and 17.9% cough and 13% sputum production.[8] Both obstructive and restrictive lung disease patterns can be seen and can coexist in a single patient. Patient symptomatology such as difficulty coughing, hoarseness, and difficulty clearing secretions should alert the anesthesiologist to an increased risk of perioperative pulmonary complications such aspiration or bronchospasm.

Weakness of inspiratory muscles can lead to dyspnea, tachypnea, and impaired functional capacity. Weakness of expiratory muscles can lead to weak cough and inability to clear secretions. These can predispose patients to aspiration during the perioperative period.

Seccombe et al. measured spirometry, lung volumes, respiratory muscle strength, response to hypoxic gas inhalation, and hypercapnic ventilatory response in 19 patients with PD. Normal lung function was observed in 16 patients, mild airflow limitation was observed in 1 patient, and 2 patients demonstrated restrictive dysfunction based on total lung capacity.

The authors demonstrated impaired respiratory drive/response to hypercapnia, and the abnormal occlusion pressure response indicated central drive impairment.[9]

Ultimately, there is the presence of abnormal pulmonary function associated with PD, but debate continues as to the predominant pattern.

MEDICAL MANAGEMENT OF PARKINSON'S DISEASE

Medical management is usually the first line of treatment for PD. Levodopa is one of the commonly used medications in PD. Levodopa (metabolic precursor of dopamine) is taken orally and is rapidly absorbed from the small intestine. Onset of action is usually within 30 minutes, and it has a short half-life of up to 3 hours. After absorption, it crosses the blood–brain barrier and is converted to dopamine, thereby increasing dopamine concentrations in the brain and causing symptomatic relief. It is usually combined with carbidopa, which inhibits the decarboxylase enzyme in the periphery thus preventing its conversion to dopamine in the blood and thereby allowing more levodopa to cross the blood–brain barrier.

The levodopa-carbidopa combination is very effective in ameliorating symptoms in the initial stages of PD. In early PD, the duration of the beneficial effects of levodopa may exceed the plasma lifetime of the drug, suggesting that the nigrostriatal dopamine system retains some capacity to store and release dopamine. A principal limitation of long-term levodopa therapy is that this apparent buffering capacity is lost over time and the patient's motor state may fluctuate dramatically with each dose of levodopa.[10] Over time, there is wearing off of the effectiveness of levodopa, leading to fluctuations in clinical course (on-off phenomenon), in addition to triggering of dyskinesia/dystonia with rising and falling levels of levodopa. Increasing dopamine concentrations in the blood leads to undesirable side effects such as nausea, confusion, and hallucinations. All of the above factors lead to limitations of levodopa use, although it is still considered the most effective first line of treatment for symptom control.

It is important to minimize prolonged interruptions between levodopa (half-life is 1–3 hours) dosing to avoid exacerbations in disease control.

Catechol-O-methyltransferase (COMT) inhibitors extend the availability of levodopa in the plasma and brain by decreasing its peripheral degradation and slowing its elimination rate.[11] For patients with the "wearing off" phenomenon who are receiving optimal doses of levodopa, the addition of a COMT inhibitor can increase the "on" time (period of time experiencing symptom relief) and reduce "off" time (duration of time experiencing little to no therapeutic benefit).[12] Currently, there are three medications in this category: tolcapone, entacapone, and opicapone. Tolcapone is associated with significant side effects including hepatotoxicity and is discontinued from clinical use. Entacapone is generally well tolerated.

A combination of levodopa/carbidopa/entacapone was developed to minimize the on-off phenomenon.

Directly acting dopamine receptor agonists (bromocriptine, ropinirole, pramipexole) have the advantage of potentially fewer toxic metabolites and not requiring enzymatic conversion to active metabolite. These are often used in conjunction with levodopa/carbidopa combinations. A recent study described increased perioperative complications associated with use of rotigotine.[13]

Bromocriptine is an ergot derivative and a partial antagonist of dopamine D_1 receptor. Ropinirole and pramipexole have selective dopamine D_2 receptor activity and are well absorbed orally. The above medications are also effective in treating the on-off phenomenon. Some of the side effects and disadvantages include confusion/hallucinations, orthostatic hypotension, and the requirement of several weeks to achieve clinically significant doses.[11]

Apomorphine is an injectable medication (0.02–0.06 mL, 3–6 mg three times per day), given subcutaneously. Advantages include rapid onset of action and use as rescue therapy to offset the on-off phenomenon. It can also be used in patients who are unable to take oral medications due to severe rigidity. A transdermal patch of rotigotine has also been developed, designed to provide continuous drug delivery 24 hours per day.[12]

Selective monoamine oxidase (MAO-I) B inhibitors (rasagiline or selegiline, at doses <10 mg/day) have been used with modest effect on the clinical course of PD. Mechanisms of action include ability to slow the metabolism of dopamine in striatum. Use of MAO-I in combination with selective serotonin reuptake inhibitors or other serotoninergic agents (such as meperidine) can potentially cause serotonin syndrome and has significant intraoperative implications to the treating anesthesiologist.

Other classes of antiparkinsonian drugs include anticholinergics (trihexyphenidyl), N-methyl-D-aspartic acid (NMDA) antagonists (amantadine), and adenosine 2a receptor antagonist (istradefylline).[14]

SURGICAL MANAGEMENT OF PARKINSON'S DISEASE

Surgical management mainly consists of implantation of DBS with connector and generator placement. During the last 15 years, DBS has been established as a highly effective therapy for advanced, medically refractory PD. DBS targets placement of depth electrodes in the subthalamic nucleus, and the principal benefit is the overall reduction of undesirable side effects associated with medication therapy and improved quality of life. Appropriate patient selection is important prior to undergoing DBS implantation.

Inclusion criteria for DBS implantation are idiopathic PD, improvement in response to dopaminergic medication, and refractory symptoms.

Relative exclusion criteria include advanced age (>75years), coexisting severe comorbidity, malignancy or chronic immunosuppression, brain atrophy, and severe psychiatric disorder with cognitive deficits.[15] The implantation procedure requires a highly specialized center with stereotactic navigation facilities, specialized equipment and personnel, and experienced neurosurgeons. The surgery can be done in two stages, the first involving placement of targeted depth electrodes and the second stage involving lead connectors and generator placement. Subsequently patients may return for replacement of the generator battery every 5–6 years.

The first stage of implantation can be performed under local/regional anesthesia with sedation (asleep-awake-asleep technique) if the patient is found suitable and cooperative. Another option is GA under continuous MRI and navigation system software (e.g., ClearPoint) guidance if the patient is deemed unsuitable for awake technique. The second stage of the procedure involving lead connectors and generator placement is usually performed under GA.

Other surgical treatment options include pallidotomy (surgical destruction of globus pallidus) and thalamotomy, but with the advent and success of DBS implantation, these techniques are less frequently performed.

Anesthetic Implications and Management

Given the complexity of PD, a multidisciplinary approach to perioperative care of these patients while following enhanced recovery after surgery (ERAS) principles could minimize complications while improving patient outcomes (Table 24.1).[16]

Preoperative Considerations

A preoperative anesthesia visit can aid in obtaining adequate history and physical examination, as well as assessment of underlying risk factors for a safe anesthetic.

These patients are also typically older than 65 years and may have associated comorbidities. A detailed history regarding the natural course of the disease; exacerbations; and medications taken including type, dose, and frequency must be obtained, along with other medical history. Instructions regarding medication intake prior to surgery must be given to the patient/caregiver. Prior anesthetic records, if available, must be reviewed in detail.

Physical examination must include cardiovascular, respiratory, and neurologic examination and a complete 10-system review. A detailed airway examination is important to note any cervical spine rigidity or limited range of motion that may warrant a difficult airway.

Cardiovascular workup is dictated by comorbidities. It may be difficult to obtain an exercise stress test in these patients due to symptoms, hence a pharmacologic stress test and echocardiogram may be needed in selected patient population. PFTs may be required if the etiology of dyspnea remains in question.

Obtaining consent for anesthesia and surgical procedure may be challenging if the patient has underlying cognitive dysfunction. This can be identified by performing a quick mini-cognitive test (comprising of a three-item recall test and a scored drawing test) and a Mini Mental Status Examination. In such a scenario, a healthcare power of attorney should be identified ahead of time for discussion.

All antiparkinsonian medications should be continued, including on the day of surgery, to avoid exacerbation of the

Table 24.1 KEY ELEMENTS OF ENHANCED RECOVERY SURGICAL PROGRAM FOR PATIENTS WITH PARKINSON'S DISEASE

Preoperative	Early neurology referral to optimize Parkinson's disease symptoms and antiparkinsonian medications
	Minimize fasting times and continue antiparkinsonian medication if possible
	Swallowing therapy to decrease aspiration risk
	Preventive opioid-sparing multimodal analgesia
	Avoidance of sedative drugs
	Prehabilitation in patients with advanced disease
Intraoperative	Regional anesthesia or local analgesia where possible
	Processed electroencephalography-guided general anesthesia
	Avoidance of triggers of postoperative delirium
	Prevention of hypothermia
	Prevention of postoperative nausea and vomiting but avoiding dopamine antagonists
	Multimodal opioid-sparing analgesia
	Early tracheal extubation for neuromonitoring
Postoperative	Noise- and stress-reduced environment in recovery
	Screening for delirium in recovery (delirium may be hypoactive)
	Early resumption of enteral feeding and antiparkinsonian medication
	Personal case management by nurses trained in Parkinson's disease care
	Prevention and treatment of infections (e.g., chest physiotherapy, incentive spirometry, urinary catheter care)
	Referral to physiotherapy for early mobilization and fall prevention
	Early discharge and referral to occupational therapy and social workers to aid transition from hospital to home
	Rehabilitation in centers trained in Parkinson's disease management

With permission from Yim RLH.[16]

disease. The only exception is DBS placement under a monitored anesthesia care technique, where these medications may be held on the day of surgery.[17]

Intraoperative Considerations

Anesthetic Techniques

Depending on the surgical site, patients with PD may be amenable to local-regional anesthesia or general endotracheal anesthesia. Regardless of the anesthetic or surgical technique, standard monitors as designated by the American Society of Anesthesiologists (ASA) are required in all patients. Invasive hemodynamic monitoring may be considered depending on the comorbidities and type of surgery.

Advantages of local-regional anesthesia include avoiding hemodynamic variability as well as the aspiration risk associated with GA and endotracheal intubation. An adequately placed regional block minimizes the need for extra narcotics, thereby minimizing unwanted side effects such as nausea or excessive sedation. However, the main disadvantage of this technique is patient cooperation as well as need for sedation due to incomplete regional technique.

Advantages of GA include securing of airway and the ability to provide appropriately relaxed muscles most of the commonly performed procedures. Risks associated with GA in a patient with PD include aspiration, more hemodynamic variability, and possibility of a difficult airway.

When indicated, a rapid-sequence induction and intubation may be necessary to safely secure the airway and minimize the risk of aspiration. If a difficult airway is suspected due to limited neck range of movement or rigidity, using a video laryngoscope may be a safer option to visualize and secure the airway. Propofol can be used as an induction agent, but its facilitatory effects on gamma aminobutyric acid (GABA)ergic transmission and inhibitory effects on glutamate transmission may be responsible for involuntary movements or dyskinesias seen in patients with PD.[18] Inhalational agents such as sevoflurane can be safely used in patients with PD with results similar to propofol.[19] Processed EEG monitoring is encouraged to avoid undesirable depth of anesthesia. Ketamine is generally avoided due to its sympathomimetic effects, which may be undesirable in an elderly patient with PD and underlying cardiac comorbidities. Non-depolarizing neuromuscular blocking agents have been safely used in patients with PD. Directly acting vasopressors such as phenylephrine may be required to treat intraoperative hypotension.

Pain Management Options

Potent opioids such as fentanyl can cause skeletal muscle rigidity when given rapidly in higher doses. Possible explanations include inhibition of striatal release of GABA and increased dopamine production; however, this responds to administration of neuromuscular blockade. In addition, patients with PD may be sensitive to the respiratory depressant effects of narcotics during both the intraoperative and postoperative periods. It is recommended to minimize doses of narcotics in these patients and encourage use of non-narcotic multimodal analgesia such as acetaminophen, NSAIDS, or local anesthesia (when amenable).

Perioperative Complications

Intraoperative exacerbations of PD are difficult to recognize under GA with muscle relaxation. Under local-regional anesthesia, it usually manifests as skeletal muscle tremors, rigidity, and increasing feelings of discomfort. Care must be taken to appropriately redose levodopa intraoperatively, via nasogastric tube under GA, as these manifestations may not be recognized in an asleep patient. Patients with PD are predisposed to increased risk of postoperative delirium, confusion, and hallucinations.[20]

Medications that can worsen PD symptoms (phenothiazines, butyrophenones, haloperidol, metoclopramide) must be avoided in the perioperative period. The anesthesiologist must expect and be prepared to treat intraoperative autonomic instability manifesting as excessive blood pressure and

Table 24.2 SUMMARY OF COMMONLY OBSERVED NON-MOTOR SYMPTOMS IN PARKINSON'S DISEASE, PERIOPERATIVE RISK FACTORS, AND PREVENTION

NON-MOTOR DOMAINS	COMMON NON-MOTOR SYMPTOMS	PERIOPERATIVE RISK FACTORS	PREVENTION
Cardiovascular	Orthostatic intolerance, syncope	Change in fluid status, low salt intake, effect of anesthetics and new medications (i.e., sleep aids).	Careful management of fluid status, high salt diet if needed, limit drugs that cause orthostatic hypotension, leg stockings.
Sleep/fatigue	Excessive daytime sleepiness, insomnia, restless legs, and fatigue, RBD	Frequent nursing assessments, pain associated with surgery, change in sleep pattern, medications with sedative effect (i.e., antipsychotic)	Identify the cause of sleep disturbance, limit sleep interruption, avoid sedative drugs during the day. Cognitive-behavioral therapy for insomnia, pharmacological treatment (dopamine agonists, melatonin, eszopiclone).
Perceptual problems	Hallucinations, delusions, and double vision	Postoperative delirium or exacerbation of preexisting psychosis due to infection, fluid-electrolyte imbalance, adverse drug reactions (i.e., anticholinergic).	Careful assessment of treatment regimen and drug-drug interaction, identify and treat infection and fluid-electrolyte imbalance promptly.
Gastrointestinal	Dysphagia, constipation	Immobility, change in diet, adverse drug reactions (i.e., opioids), sub-optimal oral care, oral secretion.	Early mobility with physical therapy, raise the head of the bed, adapt diet consistency, use bowel regimen, good oral hygiene.
Secretion	Sialorrhea, increased respiratory secretions	Immobility and supine position.	Importance of early mobility and incentive spirometry to prevent aspiration.
Urinary	Urgency, frequency, retention, nocturia	Urinary tract infections, adverse drug reactions (i.e., anticholinergic).	Early mobility with physical therapy, maintain good hydration, careful assessment of drug side effects, early identification and treatment of infection.
Mood/cognition	Poor attention, memory impairment, apathy, anxiety, and depression	Maybe worsened in the perioperative state, social isolation, and hypoactive delirium.	Maintain circadian rhythm, frequent reorientation, early mobility, minimize deliriogenic drugs, consider antidepressant drugs if comorbid depression.
Miscellaneous	Pain	Immobility, change in treatment for Parkinson's disease (off symptom).	Pain associated with Parkinson's disease should be differentiated from the pain related to surgery and treated appropriately.

With permission from Lenka et al.[21]

---

heart rate changes in response to stimuli, medications, or position changes.

Parkinsonism-hyperpyrexia syndrome is another feared complication manifested by rigidity, bradykinesia or akinesia, hyperpyrexia, rhabdomyolysis, autonomic dysfunction, and altered mental status. It is similarly precipitated by a decreased intake of dopamine agonists or increased intake of dopamine antagonists (e.g., haloperidol).[16]

Other perioperative potential complications are summarized in Table 24.2.[21]

SPECIFIC CONSIDERATIONS FOR DBS PLACEMENT

As discussed earlier, anesthetic management for DBS implantation has been successfully performed under local-regional anesthesia with appropriate scalp blocks in suitable patients. One of the major requirements for this technique is an awake and cooperative patient. A detailed preoperative discussion is essential to ensure patient cooperation through various stages of the procedure. In addition to adequate IV access and standard ASA monitoring, a stereotactic frame is applied on the patient's forehead and scalp under local anesthesia, followed by a computed tomography (CT) scan to ensure correct placement. Supplemental oxygen is usually provided via a nasal cannula. Sedation is then instituted in the form of propofol infusion (50–100 mcg/kg/min, titrated to effect) and/or dexmedetomidine (0.2–0.7 mcg/kg/hr, titrated to effect) with intermittent narcotic boluses (e.g., fentanyl 25–50 mcg) as required. Caution must be used in this technique to minimize airway obstruction and/or apnea since access to head and neck to rescue the airway is limited once the stereotactic frame is placed and fixed. Surgical drapes must be placed in an appropriate manner to allow visualization of the patient's airway and breathing. An alternate technique is placement of laryngeal mask airway (LMA) for the asleep part and then removing the LMA for the awake part of the procedure. This may sometimes be required if the patient is deemed at risk for airway obstruction with sedation (e.g., obesity, severe sleep apnea, etc.) An arterial line is typically placed to monitor blood pressure intraoperatively. After burr holes and/or mini craniotomy is performed, the patient is then wakened for the DBS placement. It must be noted that the induced/elicited hand tremors as part of DBS placement testing may interfere with the pulse oximeter and arterial waveforms, giving rise to artifacts. After confirmation of appropriate placement and neurologic intactness, sedation is restarted for the remainder of the procedures and closure.

If GA is chosen, the patient is intubated after appropriate induction of anesthesia. The procedure is then performed under continuous MRI/software navigation guidance, and the patient is extubated at the end of the surgery after meeting extubation criteria. Special anesthetic considerations include placement of MRI-compatible monitors, equipment, and anesthesia machine.

A major intraoperative concern is intracranial hemorrhage during the placement of depth electrodes. In an awake patient, it manifests as rapid decline in mental status and/or focal neurological deficits. An emergency airway plan must be discussed ahead of time with the surgical team should this unfortunate intraoperative event occur. Appropriate blood pressure management is critical intraoperatively to reduce the possibility of this event. Selective beta blockers that do not cross the blood–brain barrier, such as labetalol, can be used. Alternatively, hydralazine can also be used. Propranolol should be avoided as it can cross the blood–brain barrier and can decrease/inhibit tremors.

POSTOPERATIVE CONSIDERATIONS

Emergence and awakening from GA may be associated with worsening of confusion and delirium.[22] The cause may be multifactorial, including age, medications, preexisting cognitive deficits, or unfamiliar environment. This event must be anticipated, and care must be taken to prevent patient injury and/or disconnection of lines and protection of the airway until the patient is reoriented. Once the patient has appropriately recovered, it is important to restart prior PD medications to minimize gaps in treatment.

RESTRICTIVE LUNG DISEASE

Etiology

Restrictive lung diseases comprise of a wide range of diseases causing reduced lung volumes. Broadly, they can be classified into

1. Diseases affecting the lung parenchyma, such as interstitial lung disease, idiopathic pulmonary fibrosis, sarcoidosis, systemic lupus erythematosus, and various other autoimmune diseases with pulmonary involvement; pneumonitis resulting from chemical exposure/viruses; or residual postinfectious lung scarring.
2. Diseases affecting the chest wall/thoracic cage, such as severe kyphoscoliosis, obesity, and neuromuscular diseases affecting chest wall muscles (e.g., myasthenia gravis, myopathies, amyotrophic lateral sclerosis, quadriplegia, phrenic nerve neuropathy).

Diagnosis

Signs and symptoms of restrictive lung disease are often nonspecific in the initial stages. Often, the patient may complain of shortness of breath with exertion or "difficulty catching a breath." Eliciting a history of exposure to chemicals/asbestos may be a valuable aid in diagnosis. Symptoms specific to neuromuscular diseases such as double vision with myasthenia gravis may be seen.

Imaging studies greatly aid in the diagnosis. Chest x-ray may reveal reticular/reticulonodular opacities or increased interstitial markings; however, these are not specific to any particular disease process. Bilateral hilar lymphadenopathy may suggest sarcoidosis.

High-resolution CT scan of the chest aids in better delineation of the pathologic process and the extent of pulmonary alveolar involvement. Upper lung zone predominance is observed in sarcoidosis/chronic pneumonitis, and lower lung zone infiltration is observed in patients with idiopathic pulmonary fibrosis.

PFTs can differentiate between obstructive lung disease and restrictive lung disease. In restrictive lung disease, both forced expiratory volume in 1 second during maximal effort (FEV_1) and forced vital capacity (FVC) are reduced, with greater reduction in FVC; thus the ratio of FEV_1/FVC is normal or increased higher than 80%.

A lung biopsy can aid in definitive diagnosis but is an invasive procedure associated with risks, hence may not be always necessary.

To diagnose diseases affecting the chest wall or thoracic cage, chest radiographic imaging is one of the primary techniques. The degree and severity of kyphoscoliosis can be determined by measuring the Cobb angle. Anteroposterior and lateral views are typically performed.

Treatment

Treatment strategies depend on the underlying diagnosis. In certain conditions such as kyphoscoliosis, surgical correction can improve underlying lung function when performed in the early stages. Medical management of myasthenia gravis consists of acetylcholine esterase inhibitors, corticosteroids, immunosuppressants, or plasmapheresis. Thymectomy can be beneficial if an underlying thymoma is present.

Supplemental oxygen is the mainstay of therapy for most of the intrinsic lung disorders causing restrictive lung disease. Additionally, corticosteroids and immunosuppressants can be used in certain autoimmune diseases with pulmonary involvement. Advanced stages of pulmonary involvement in idiopathic pulmonary fibrosis may need a lung transplant.

Anesthetic Implications

Preoperative optimization prior to elective surgery includes smoking cessation and bronchodilators in select patients.

These patients are at increased risk of rapid onset of oxygen desaturation and hypoxia during induction and emergence from anesthesia due to reduced pulmonary reserve. Reduced compliance may increase the risk of barotrauma during positive-pressure ventilation. Smaller tidal volumes and lung-protective ventilation strategies (lower tidal volume and increased respiratory rate) may be required. In addition, avoiding hypoxia/hypercarbia and acidosis can prevent worsening of underlying pulmonary hypertension during the perioperative period.

Patients with underlying restrictive lung disease are at increased risk of perioperative pulmonary complications, especially if VC is less than 15 mL/kg, FVC is less than 50% of predicted, or resting $PaCO_2$ is greater than 45 mm Hg. Perioperative adverse events include bronchospasm, rapid onset of desaturation, and increased ventilator dependence in the postoperative period due to inability to extubate. Patients with underlying restrictive lung disease are sensitive to the respiratory depressant effects of narcotics, and minimizing narcotics and adopting multimodal analgesia during the perioperative period is beneficial.

Hence, a thorough understanding of the underlying disease process, treatment history, and appropriate anesthetic technique will aid in successful management of patients with various degrees of restrictive lung disease.

CONCLUSION

- An increasing number of patients with PD present for DBS and other elective/emergent surgery.
- Important considerations include understanding the disease pathogenesis, natural course, and progression, as well as its various therapeutic modalities.
- Difficult airway must be anticipated and prepared for accordingly.
- Associated risk of aspiration with induction of anesthesia should be anticipated.
- Potential drug interactions must be anticipated in the perioperative period.
- It is important to minimize gaps in treatment (especially levodopa) in the perioperative period.
- Patients with underlying restrictive lung disease have significant anesthetic implications and must be recognized and appropriately treated.

REVIEW QUESTIONS

1. What is the underlying disease pathogenesis in PD?

   a. Depletion of norepinephrine in substantia nigra.
   b. Depletion of dopamine in substantia nigra.
   c. Elevated catecholamine levels in adrenal gland.
   d. Excessive thyroxine hormone secretion.

The correct answer is b.

The main abnormality in patients with PD is the loss of pigmented cells in the substantia nigra with replacement gliosis, the causes of which can be multifactorial. More importantly, the clinical features are due to an imbalance between acetylcholine and dopamine secretion, with cholinergic overgrowth and deficiency of dopaminergic neurons.

2. What is the first line of therapy in patients with PD?

   a. Levodopa.
   b. DBS insertion.
   c. Selegiline.
   d. Pallidotomy.

The correct answer is a.

Levodopa is usually the first line of treatment in PD. Medical therapy is typically begun with levodopa/carbidopa combination, with good clinical effects and resolution of symptoms in the initial phase. However, as the disease progresses, the effectiveness varies and side effects such as confusion and hallucinations begin to occur along with the on-off phenomenon and exacerbations of PD in between doses. Surgical therapy such as DBS and pallidotomy are usually not the first line of therapy. Selegiline can be added during the course of treatment, but it is not usually the first line of therapy.

3. All of the following are side effects of levodopa therapy *except*:

   a. Nausea.
   b. Confusion.
   c. On-off phenomenon.
   d. Isolated arm weakness.

The correct answer is d.

Unfortunately, levodopa therapy is associated with multiple side effects, commonly ranging from nausea and vomiting, loss of appetite, confusion/hallucinations, agitation, abnormal movements, and mood variations. Over a period of time, patients may experience increasing side effects from the therapy which may be worse than the disease process itself. Due to progression of the disease, patients may also experience an "on-off" phenomenon where the therapeutic effects last for a shorter period of time and wear off more quickly, resulting in increasing dosages/frequency of levodopa or addition of a second line of medical treatment.

4. Important anesthetic implications in patients in PD include

   a. Possible difficult intubation.
   b. Risk of aspiration.
   c. Emergence delirium.
   d. All of the above.

The correct answer is d.

Anesthetic management of patients with PD is associated with multiple challenges, including possible difficult intubation due to rigidity, risk of aspiration from full stomach/improper gastric emptying or nausea, and confusion and delirium on awakening from GA. Clinicians should be cognizant of these and other potential issues such as medication interactions and should be adequately prepared to manage accordingly.

5. DBS involves placement of depth electrodes in the
   a. Subthalamic nuclei.
   b. Medullary body.
   c. Cerebellum.
   d. Temporal lobe.

The correct answer is a.

Surgical implantation of depth electrodes (DBS) has gained popularity due to its effectiveness, minimally invasive nature, relative safety, and reduction in the dosages of medications used to treat PD. This procedure involves unilateral or bilateral placement of depth electrodes in the subthalamic nuclei, which are then connected to a generator with a battery implanted in a subcutaneous pocket in the chest wall. Other than PD, DBS therapy is also approved to treat essential tremor, refractory epilepsy, and dystonia.

6. Recommended treatment strategies to control intraoperative blood pressure during DBS implantation include all of the following *except*
   a. Labetalol.
   b. Nitroglycerine.
   c. Propranolol.
   d. Hydralazine.

The correct answer is c.

Propranolol is a nonselective beta blocker which can cross the blood–brain barrier and inhibit tremors thereby interfering with the surgical confirmation of appropriate placement of DBS electrodes. Other medications listed can be used to treat increases in blood pressure readings intraoperatively. Cardiovascular changes in DBS surgery are complex, and a retrospective study which analyzed 79 DBS procedures found that approximately 82% showed hemodynamic events (hypertension, bradycardia, tachycardia). The incidence of an intracranial bleed can vary between 0.5% and 5%, and hypertensive episodes are associated with this event. Hence, perioperative blood pressure control is important.[20,23]

7. Recommended strategies to treat postoperative pain include
   a. Minimize narcotics.
   b. Injection of local anesthesia at the surgical site.
   c. IV acetaminophen.
   d. All of the above.

The correct answer is d.

Patients with PD are sensitive to the respiratory depressant effects of narcotics due to advanced age and preexisting mental status. It is recommended that narcotics be minimized in the perioperative period and pain treated with adjuncts to avoid side effects as well as to facilitate postoperative neurologic examination. Non-narcotic adjuncts are well tolerated.

REFERENCES

1. DeLong MR JJ. Parkinson's disease and other movement disorders. In: Fauci AS, Braunwals E, Kasper DL, Hauser SL, Longo DL, Jameson JL, Loscalzo J, eds. *Harrison's Principles of Internal Medicine*. 17th ed. McGraw Hill; 2008:2406–2417.
2. Lees AJ, Hardy J, Revesz T. Parkinson's disease. *Lancet*. 2009 Jun 13;373(9680):2055–2066.
3. Hernán MA, Takkouche B, Caamaño-Isorna F, Gestal-Otero JJ. A meta-analysis of coffee drinking, cigarette smoking, and the risk of Parkinson's disease. *Ann Neurol*. 2002 Sep;52(3):276–284.
4. Di Fonzo A, Tassorelli C, De Mari M, et al. Comprehensive analysis of the LRRK2 gene in sixty families with Parkinson's disease. *Eur J Hum Genet*. 2006 Mar;14(3):322–331.
5. Fahn S. Parkinson's disease and related disorders. In: Hazzard WR, Halter JB, eds. *Principles of Geriatric Medicine and Gerontology*. New York: McGraw Hill; 2003:1401–1408.
6. Katzenschlager R, Head J, Schrag A, et al. Fourteen-year final report of the randomized PDRG-UK trial comparing three initial treatments in PD. *Neurology*. 2008 Aug 12;71(7):474–480.
7. Scorza FA, Fiorini AC, Scorza CA, Finsterer J. Cardiac abnormalities in Parkinson's disease and Parkinsonism. *J Clin Neurosci*. 2018 Jul;53:1–5.
8. Lee MA, Prentice WM, Hildreth AJ, Walker RW. Measuring symptom load in idiopathic Parkinson's disease. *Parkinsonism Relat Disord*. 2007 Jul;13(5):284–289.
9. Seccombe LM, Giddings HL, Rogers PG, et al. Abnormal ventilatory control in Parkinson's disease: Further evidence for non-motor dysfunction. *Respir Physiol Neurobiol*. 2011 Dec 15;179(2–3):300–304.
10. Goldenberg MM. Medical management of Parkinson's disease. *P T*. 2008 Oct;33(10):590–606.
11. Ruottinen HM, Rinne UK. Entacapone prolongs levodopa response in a one month double blind study in parkinsonian patients with levodopa related fluctuations. *J Neurol Neurosurg Psychiatry*. 1996 Jan;60(1):36–40.
12. Adler CH, Singer C, O'Brien C, et al. Randomized, placebo-controlled study of tolcapone in patients with fluctuating Parkinson disease treated with levodopa-carbidopa. Tolcapone Fluctuator Study Group III. *Arch Neurol*. 1998 Aug;55(8):1089–1095.
13. Nakadate Y, Nakashige D, Omori K, Matsukawa T. Risk factors for postoperative complications in patients with Parkinson disease: A single center retrospective cohort study. *Medicine (Baltimore)*. 2023 Apr 25;102(17):e33619.
14. Anderson SD, Shah NK, Yim J, Epstein BJ. Efficacy and safety of ticagrelor: A reversible P2Y12 receptor antagonist. *Ann Pharmacother. United States*. 2010 Mar;44(3):524–537.
15. Aminoff MJ. Pharmacologic management of parkinsonism and other movement disorders. In: Katzung BG, ed. *Basic and Clinical Pharmacology*. 10th ed. McGraw Hill; 2007:442–451.
16. Yim RLH, Leung KMM, Poon CCM, Irwin MG. Peri-operative management of patients with Parkinson's disease. *Anaesthesia*. 2022 Jan;77(Suppl 1):123–133.
17. Oprea AD, Keshock MC, O'Glasser AY, et al. Preoperative management of medications for neurologic diseases: Society for Perioperative Assessment and Quality Improvement consensus statement. *Mayo Clin Proc*. 2022 Feb;97(2):375–396.
18. Leegwater-Kim J; Waters C. Parkinsonism. In: Rakel RE Bope ET, eds. *Conn's Current Therapy*. WB Saunders; 2008:931–936.
19. Zhou Y, Li Z, Ma Y, et al. The effect of Propofol versus Sevoflurane on postoperative delirium in Parkinson's disease patients undergoing deep brain stimulation surgery: An observational study. *Brain Sci*. 2022 May 25;12(6):1–10.
20. Groiss SJ, Wojtecki L, Südmeyer M, Schnitzler A. Deep brain stimulation in Parkinson's disease. *Ther Adv Neurol Disord*. 2009 Nov;2(6):20–28.
21. Lenka A, Mittal SO, Lamotte G, Pagan FL. A pragmatic approach to the perioperative management of Parkinson's disease. *Can J Neurol Sci*. 2021 May;48(3):299–307.
22. Golden WE, Lavender RC, Metzer WS. Acute postoperative confusion and hallucinations in Parkinson disease. *Ann Intern Med*. 1989 Aug 01;111(3):218–222.
23. Chowdhury T, Wilkinson M, Cappellani RB. Hemodynamic perturbations in deep brain stimulation surgery: First detailed description. *Front Neurosci*. 2017;11:477.

25.

A 56-YEAR-OLD WITH A RECENT CVA FOR ELECTIVE SURGERY

HOW SOON IS TOO SOON?

Debra D. Pulley

STEM CASE AND KEY QUESTIONS

A 56-year-old man presents to the preoperative clinic for assessment prior to total hip replacement in 4 weeks. As you are about to ask him about his medical history, he asks you "Can you get a stroke during an operation?"

What are the mechanisms of perioperative stroke?

You tell him that a stroke can occur during an operation when there is not enough blood and/or oxygen perfusing the cells in the brain. This can happen from a blood clot or low blood pressure. He then asks you what his risk is.

What is the incidence of perioperative stroke?

You tell him that, overall, the risk of stroke is low but it varies with the type of surgery and patient risk factors. His surgery is at a lower risk than other surgeries such as cardiac and vascular surgery. You ask him why he is concerned. He tells you his primary care physician (PCP) has been warning him that if he does not quit smoking and get his blood pressure under control, he will have a stroke.

What factors increase the risk of perioperative stroke?

He has no other significant medical history. His blood pressure is 200/100 mm Hg, heart rate 75, and pulse oximetry is 94%. He denies any symptoms of transient ischemic attacks (TIAs), angina, or arrhythmias. On physical exam, his lungs are clear and heart sounds are normal with regular rate and no murmurs. He is limited by his hip pain, but his functional capacity is greater than 4 METs. You tell him that although he has risk factors that will increase his risk of stroke, he does not have major risk factors that are associated with perioperative stroke. However, his overall risk for surgery will be improved if he can get his blood pressure under control and stop smoking. He agrees to meet with his PCP. Unfortunately, 2 weeks later, the patient is in the emergency department with an acute stroke. He is being transferred to the neuroradiology suite to have an emergent thrombectomy under anesthesia.

Is there a preferred anesthetic for acute stroke? What are your goals for anesthetic management?

You plan on a general anesthesia with an endotracheal tube because the patient is not cooperative and you are concerned he will move during critical portions of the procedure. You maintain cerebral perfusion pressure and normocapnia throughout the procedure. A thrombus is successfully removed from the middle cerebral artery. Post-procedure, the patient's hemiplegia improves, and after a week in the hospital, he is discharged to a rehabilitation facility. One month later, the orthopedic surgeon informs you that the patient's hip pain is severely inhibiting the patient's rehabilitation after the stroke. The patient and his family really want the surgeon to fix the hip.

When should elective surgery proceed after a stroke?
Discussions occur among you, the surgeon, the neurologist, the patient, and his family concerning the optimal timing due to increased risk of proceeding too soon. Three months later, while continuing aspirin, the patient had his hip surgery and is doing well.

DISCUSSION

Stroke can have devastating consequences especially when it occurs perioperatively. The incidence of stroke varies depending on the surgery being performed. The incidence in cardiac surgery is the highest but has great variability from coronary artery bypass graft (CABG) to multiple valve surgery (1–10%).[1] Vascular is the next highest (descending thoracic 7% and carotid endarterectomy 2.3%). The incidence in noncardiac, nonvascular, and non-neurological surgery is between 0.1% and 1.0%.[2] Since many strokes are not clinically recognized (known as *covert stroke*), the actual incidence is higher than reported (7%).[3] In spite of concurrent reductions in perioperative acute myocardial infarction/death, unfortunately, the incidence of perioperative stroke has been increasing.[4]

MECHANISMS FOR PERIOPERATIVE STROKE

Ischemic strokes are much more prevalent than hemorrhagic strokes, with the incidence of hemorrhagic being only 1–4% of all perioperative strokes.[1] The Trial of Org 10172 in Acute

Stroke Treatment (TOAST) classification divides ischemic stroke into large-artery atherosclerosis, cardioembolism, small-artery occlusion (lacunar), stroke of other determined etiology, and stroke of undetermined etiology.[5] Using the TOAST criteria for ischemic stroke, cardioembolism due to atrial fibrillation has been reported to be a dominant mechanism in noncardiac/noncarotid surgery along with thrombotic events causing large-vessel occlusion and less likely small-vessel occlusion.[6,7] Other etiologies include anemic tissue hypoxia and cerebral hypoperfusion. In about 30% of cases, the etiology of the stroke remained undetermined.

RISK FACTORS FOR PERIOPERATIVE STROKE

Patient risk factors for perioperative stroke include age, cerebrovascular disease, valvular heart disease, atrial fibrillation, coronary artery disease, kidney disease, patent foramen ovale (PFO), diabetes mellitus, hypertension, chronic obstructive pulmonary disease, and congestive heart failure.[7] As stated earlier, the type of surgery has a big impact on the overall risk of stroke. Surgeries that include manipulation of the heart and vessels leading to the brain are more likely to have cardioembolism. Emergency surgery is also a risk, along with postoperative hypotension.[8] The risk of perioperative stroke in greatest within 3 days of surgery.[7] Newly started beta blockers increased the risk of perioperative stroke and mortality in the POISE trial.[9] Several risk calculators are available including the American College of Surgeons (ACS) National Surgical Quality Improvement Program (NSQIP) surgical risk calculator[10] and the Gupta Myocardial Infarct or Cardiac Arrest (MICA)[11] that scored well in stroke prediction in patients undergoing noncardiac surgery but not as well for patients undergoing vascular surgery.[12]

PERIOPERATIVE MANAGEMENT TO REDUCE RISK OF PERIOPERATIVE STROKE

The American Heart Association (AHA)/American Society of Anesthesiologists (ASA) published considerations for reducing stroke in patients undergoing cardiac and thoracic aortic surgeries.[13] Also in 2020, the Society for Neuroscience in Anesthesiology and Critical Care published guidelines.[14] In 2021, the AHA/ASA published guidelines for reducing stroke in patients undergoing noncardiac, non-neurological surgery.[2] Preoperatively, recommendations include perioperative stroke risk assessment, appropriate decision-making on when to stop/start anticoagulation, consideration of symptomatic carotid artery stenosis for revascularization, and delaying surgery if the patient had a recent stroke. In addition, it was not recommended that patients be screened for PFO, but if they have already been determined to need PFO closure, this procedure can be done before elective surgery. Intraoperatively, patients at high risk of stroke should have normocapnia maintained. Currently, there is not sufficient evidence to recommend specific blood pressure thresholds, but hypotension can lead to hypoperfusion. Postoperatively, if a patient has a stroke,

Box 25.1 **FAAST TEST**

FACE	Uneven smile?
	Facial droop?
ARM	Arm/leg numbness?
	Arm/leg weakness?
	Not due to surgery (limb procedures)?
ANESTHESIA	Residual anesthetic effect?
SPEECH	Slurring speech?
	Difficulty to speak or to understand?
TIME	*Get help immediately—"Time is Brain"*

Adapted from Sun et al[15]

endoluminal thrombectomy should be performed if criteria are met. To help with early detection of stroke, a simple tool is shown in Box 25.1.[15]

ANESTHETIC MANAGEMENT FOR ENDOLUMINAL THROMBECTOMY OF ACUTE STROKE

At present, there is no evidence-based algorithm to decide whether the procedure should be done under sedation or under general anesthesia.[16] Clinical decision-making has to be done quickly and is based on individual circumstances.

TIMING OF SURGERY AFTER STROKE

It is well recognized that autoregulation of the cerebral vessels is impaired after acute stroke.[17] For years, it had been reasonable to assume that elective surgery should be delayed until autoregulation is no longer impaired. A retrospective Danish nationwide cohort study was published in 2014 that showed risk of perioperative stroke, major adverse cardiac event, and 30-day mortality was increased after a stroke, and the risk did not level off until about 9 months later.[18] This led to many recommending delay in surgery for 6–12 months. Then, in 2022, a much larger cohort study was published that showed the risk of surgery after stroke was not reduced by delaying surgery more than 90 days.[19] The study also verified that patients who have surgery within 30 days of a stroke had an eight-fold higher risk of stroke than did patients without a previous stroke. If surgery cannot be delayed for 90 days after a stroke, then shared decision-making can be useful.[20] Questions that need to be answered include: What are the benefits of surgery? How risky is it? What are the consequences if surgery is delayed? Are there any alternatives to surgery? And what are the patient's goals and values?

CONCLUSION

- Perioperative stroke leads to increased morbidity and mortality.

- Risk of perioperative stroke varies with the type of procedure (highest in cardiovascular surgeries).
- Patient risk factors for stroke include recent stroke, age, valvular heart disease, coronary artery disease, atrial fibrillation, PFO, and renal disease.
- Early recognition of perioperative stroke and treatment options such as endoluminal thrombectomy can improve patient outcomes.
- Current evidence suggests that the risk of proceeding with elective surgery after an acute stroke levels off after 90 days.

REVIEW QUESTIONS

1. Which one of the following statements about perioperative stroke is incorrect?

    a. Perioperative stroke is decreasing in frequency.
    b. Perioperative stroke incidence varies with patient risk factors and type of surgery.
    c. Many perioperative strokes are not clinically recognized and are known as covert strokes.
    d. Hemorrhagic strokes account for 1–4% of all perioperative strokes.

The correct answer is a.
In spite of reductions in rate of death and MI, perioperative ischemic stroke is increasing in noncardiac surgery.[4]

2. Which of the following elective surgeries has the highest risk of perioperative stroke?

    a. Multiple valve surgery.
    b. Carotid endarterectomy.
    c. CABG.
    d. Orthopedic surgery.

The correct answer is a.
Multiple valve surgery has the highest risk.[1,2]

3. Which of the following is not true concerning risk factors for perioperative stroke?

    a. Chronic kidney disease increases risk.
    b. Valvular heart disease increases risk.
    c. Intraoperative hypotension (mean arterial pressure [MAP] <65 mm Hg) increases risk.
    d. Postoperative hypotension (MAP <65 mm Hg) increases risk.

The correct answer is c.
Intraoperative hypotension, defined as a MAP of lower than 65 mm Hg, did not increase risk of stroke.[8]

4. Which one of these actions is not part of the current recommendations for reducing perioperative stroke risk in noncardiac nonvascular non-neurologic surgery?

    a. Perform a preoperative risk assessment.
    b. Delay urgent surgery for PFO closure if patient has already been determined to need closure.
    c. Delay surgery if a patient had a recent stroke.
    d. Normocapnia should be maintain intraoperatively.

The correct answer is b.
The AHA/ASA guidelines specifically state not to delay urgent surgery for PFO closure.[2]

5. Which of the following complications is increased when proceeding with elective surgery after a recent stroke?

    a. Stroke.
    b. Major adverse cardiac event.
    c. Mortality.
    d. All of the above.

The correct answer is d.
The risk for all of the listed complications is increased.[17]

REFERENCES

1. Vlisides P, Mashour GA. Perioperative stroke. *Can J Anaesth*. 2016 Feb;63(2):193–204. doi:10.1007/s12630-015-0494-9
2. Benesch C, Glance LG, Derdeyn CP, et al. Perioperative neurological evaluation and management to lower the risk of acute stroke in patients undergoing noncardiac, nonneurological surgery: A scientific statement from the American Heart Association/American Stroke Association. *Circulation*. 2021 May 11;143(19):e923–e946. doi:10.1161/cir.0000000000000968
3. Neuro VI. Perioperative covert stroke in patients undergoing non-cardiac surgery (NeuroVISION): A prospective cohort study. *Lancet*. 2019 Sep 21;394(10203):1022–1029. doi:10.1016/S0140-6736(19)31795-7
4. Smilowitz NR, Gupta N, Ramakrishna H, Guo Y, Berger JS, Bangalore S. Perioperative major adverse cardiovascular and cerebrovascular events associated with noncardiac surgery. *JAMA Cardiol*. 2017 Feb 1;2(2):181–187. doi:10.1001/jamacardio.2016.4792
5. Yu S, Li P. Cognitive declines after perioperative covert stroke: Recent advances and perspectives. *Curr Opin Anaesthesiol*. 2020 Oct;33(5):651–654. doi:10.1097/aco.0000000000000903
6. Vlisides PE, Moore LE. Stroke in surgical patients: A narrative review. *Anesthesiology*. 2021;134(3):480–492. doi:10.1097/aln.0000000000003664
7. Grau AJ, Eicke M, Burmeister C, Hardt R, Schmitt E, Dienlin S. Risk of ischemic stroke and transient ischemic attack is increased up to 90 days after non-carotid and non-cardiac surgery. *Cerebrovasc Dis*. 2017;43(5-6):242–249. doi:10.1159/000460827
8. Vasivej T, Sathirapanya P, Kongkamol C. Incidence and risk factors of perioperative stroke in noncardiac, and nonaortic and its major branches surgery. *J Stroke Cerebrovasc Dis*. 2016 May;25(5):1172–1176. doi:10.1016/j.jstrokecerebrovasdis.2016.01.051
9. Group PS, Devereaux PJ, Yang H, et al. Effects of extended-release metoprolol succinate in patients undergoing non-cardiac surgery (POISE trial): A randomised controlled trial. *Lancet*. 2008 May 31;371(9627):1839–1347. doi:10.1016/S0140-6736(08)60601-7
10. Bilimoria KY, Liu Y, Paruch JL, et al. Development and evaluation of the universal ACS NSQIP surgical risk calculator: A decision aid and informed consent tool for patients and surgeons. *J Am Coll Surg*. 2013 Nov;217(5):833–842 e1-3. doi:10.1016/j.jamcollsurg.2013.07.385
11. Gupta PK, Gupta H, Sundaram A, et al. Development and validation of a risk calculator for prediction of cardiac risk after surgery. *Circulation*. 2011 Jul 26;124(4):381–387. doi:10.1161/CIRCULATIONAHA.110.015701
12. Wilcox T, Smilowitz NR, Xia Y, Berger JS. Cardiovascular risk scores to predict perioperative stroke in noncardiac surgery. *Stroke*. 2019 Aug;50(8):2002–2006. doi:10.1161/STROKEAHA.119.024995

13. Gaudino M, Benesch C, Bakaeen F, et al. Considerations for reduction of risk of perioperative stroke in adult patients undergoing cardiac and thoracic aortic operations: A scientific statement from the American Heart Association. *Circulation*. 2020 Oct 6;142(14):e193-e209. doi:10.1161/CIR.0000000000000885
14. Vlisides PE, Moore LE, Whalin MK, et al. Perioperative care of patients at high risk for stroke during or after non-cardiac, non-neurological surgery: 2020 Guidelines from the Society for Neuroscience in Anesthesiology and Critical Care. *J Neurosurg Anesthesiol*. 2020;32(3):210–226. doi:10.1097/ana.0000000000000686
15. Sun Z, Yue Y, Leung CCH, Chan MTV, Gelb AW. Clinical diagnostic tools for screening of perioperative stroke in general surgery: A systematic review. *Br J Anaesth*. 2016;116(3):328–338. doi:https://doi.org/10.1093/bja/aev452
16. Hindman BJ, Dexter F. Anesthetic management of emergency endovascular thrombectomy for acute ischemic stroke, Part 2: Integrating and applying observational reports and randomized clinical trials. *Anesth Analg*. 2019 Apr;128(4):706–717. doi:10.1213/ane.0000000000004045
17. Aries MJ, Elting JW, De Keyser J, Kremer BP, Vroomen PC. Cerebral autoregulation in stroke: A review of transcranial Doppler studies. *Stroke*. 2010 Nov;41(11):2697–2704. doi:10.1161/STROKEAHA.110.594168
18. Jorgensen ME, Torp-Pedersen C, Gislason GH, et al. Time elapsed after ischemic stroke and risk of adverse cardiovascular events and mortality following elective noncardiac surgery. *JAMA*. 2014 Jul 16;312(3):269–277. doi:10.1001/jama.2014.8165
19. Glance LG, Benesch CG, Holloway RG, et al. Association of time elapsed since ischemic stroke with risk of recurrent stroke in older patients undergoing elective nonneurologic, noncardiac surgery. *JAMA Surg*. 2022 Aug 1;157(8):e222236. doi:10.1001/jamasurg.2022.2236
20. Sturgess J, Clapp JT, Fleisher LA. Shared decision-making in peri-operative medicine: A narrative review. *Anaesthesia*. 2019 Jan;74(Suppl 1):13–19. doi:10.1111/anae.14504

RENAL

26.

AVOIDING EXACERBATION OF CHRONIC KIDNEY DISEASE

Emily Y. Xue, David Moore, and Alexander F. Arriaga

STEM CASE AND KEY QUESTIONS

A 69-year-old man was recently diagnosed with a pancreatic mass which was determined to be pancreatic adenocarcinoma. He is scheduled for a Whipple procedure and presents for preoperative evaluation. He has a history of hypertension and type 2 diabetes mellitus, which are managed with hydrochlorothiazide, lisinopril, metformin, and glargine insulin. On preoperative laboratory tests his creatinine is elevated to 1.46 mg/dL (estimated glomerular filtration rate [eGFR] 46 mL/min/1.73m^2).

What other laboratory tests or workup should be performed for the preoperative evaluation of this patient?

Physical examination reveals well-controlled hypertension with blood pressure at 118/71, heart rate 65, and SpO$_2$ 99% on room air. He is 1.73 m tall and weighs 92 kg (BMI 31). Airway examination reveals a Mallampati class of III with full dentures and a large beard. He denies knowing any history of "kidney issues," but review of available records shows a creatinine of 1.3–1.6 mg/dL over the past several years. Other laboratory values reveal sodium of 138 mEq/L, potassium of 3.9 mEq/L, bicarbonate of 24 mEq/L, blood urea nitrogen (BUN) of 20 mg/dL, hematocrit of 32.5, and hemoglobin A1c of 6.9 g/dL.

What comorbidities are commonly associated with chronic kidney injury or diabetes mellitus? What comorbidities are particularly important for the anesthesiologist to evaluate, given the perioperative risk they pose?

How are chronic kidney disease (CKD) and acute kidney injury (AKI) diagnosed and graded?

Records also reveal no other known cardiac or pulmonary issues. An ECG shows normal sinus rhythm without evidence of ischemia. On review of systems, he denies recent illness, peripheral edema, orthopnea, shortness of breath, weight gain or weight loss, or changes in urination. He denies recent antibiotics or chronic use of NSAIDs. He states that he is retired from an office job but has an active social life and drives around town for errands. He has trouble walking long distances or taking stairs due to osteoarthritis in his knees and does not regularly exercise, though he denies chest pain or dyspnea with exertion. Based on risk factors for major adverse cardiac events perioperatively (MACE) and unclear history on his functional status/metabolic equivalents (METS), a pharmacologic myocardial perfusion scan is ordered. The test reveals a normal ejection fraction with mild diastolic dysfunction and no evidence of ischemia. The plan is made to proceed to surgery.

What are the risk factors for perioperative AKI in this patient? What other perioperative risks may be increased by CKD?

On the day of surgery, what considerations are important for minimizing risks for AKI?

The patient is instructed to hold lisinopril and metformin on the day of surgery. His other medications are taken as usual. In the preoperative holding area, fingerstick blood glucose is 124 mg/dL. An epidural and arterial line are placed prior to entering the OR.

What medications can be appropriately used during induction and maintenance of anesthesia for a patient with renal impairment?

After induction of anesthesia with propofol and fentanyl, the anesthesiologist has difficulty mask ventilating the patient despite using two hands and an oral airway, thus the decision is made to give 100 mg of succinylcholine and proceed with intubation. The patient is intubated uneventfully via direct laryngoscopy. The ECG tracing on the monitor is observed carefully and no changes are seen. The anesthesiologist gives rocuronium for maintenance of muscle relaxation; the patient has return of two twitches on train-of-four stimulation within 30 minutes. Maintenance of anesthesia is achieved with inhaled desflurane. The epidural is started with continuous bupivacaine 0.125%.

What are some possible implications of this patient's diabetes mellitus on intraoperative management?

What intraoperative parameters should be observed to reduce the risk of AKI?

What is the evidence supporting the use of "renal protective" agents such as mannitol, fenoldopam, low-dose dopamine, alpha-2 agonists, or diuretics?

Initially urine output is 75–100 mL/hour. However, in hour 4 of the surgery increased bleeding is noted with estimated blood loss reaching 900 mL. For maintenance of a mean arterial pressure (MAP) of higher than 65, increasing boluses of phenylephrine and ephedrine are needed, and 1 L of lactated Ringers and 500 mL of 5% albumin are given. Despite this, urine output decreases to 20 mL/hour. The patient is transfused 1 unit of packed red blood cells (PRBCs). Surgical control of bleeding is achieved, and the case is completed.

Due to hypotension, the epidural infusion rate is decreased, and the epidural is not bolused prior to the end of the case. Additional hydromorphone is given for pain control. IV ketorolac is not given.

What is the workup for intraoperative or postoperative AKI? What are common mechanisms for AKI in the perioperative period?

In the PACU, the patient's creatinine is 1.55 mg/dL. Urine output continues at approximately 20–30 mL/hour. He receives multiple boluses of 500 mL of lactated Ringer's. Urinalysis reveals a few non-dysmorphic red blood cells and hyaline casts, but no muddy brown casts are seen. Over the next few days, urine output gradually increases to 40–50 mL/hour; creatinine trends upward and peaks at 2.3 mg/dL before decreasing.

What is the mechanism for contrast-induced kidney injury? List some proposed methods for prophylaxis and treatment.

On postoperative day 4, the patient develops abdominal pain with concern for intra-abdominal bleeding or infection. The surgical team orders computed tomography (CT) abdomen/pelvis with IV contrast. After discussion with radiology, it is determined that appropriate sensitivity of the study requires IV contrast. The patient is given IV hydration and oral N-acetylcysteine prior to receiving contrast for renal protection. Fortunately, no evidence of significant bleeding or infection is noted. The patient's abdominal pain improves, and he is discharged 7 days later.

DISCUSSION

Definition and Manifestations of Chronic Kidney Disease and Acute Kidney Injury

CKD affects millions of patients and can have important perioperative implications. Data from the National Health and Nutrition Examination Survey (NHANES III) indicate an incidence of chronic kidney impairment of any severity of approximately 10% in US adults, with an additional 0.1% affected by end-stage renal disease (ESRD).[1] Given such a broad population, understanding the severity of CKD is also important to clinical decision-making as the manifestations of this disease can range from generally asymptomatic to life-threatening. A widely used framework for grading CKD comes from the National Kidney Foundation KDOQI and KDIGO guidelines, which define CKD as decreased kidney function (as measured by GFR) or evidence of kidney damage which is present for at least 3 months.[1,2] GFR can be estimated through a calculation based on serum creatinine and demographic factors, and it is generally accepted as a better description of kidney function than serum creatinine levels. The KDIGO guidelines also take into account albuminuria for grading severity. Based on this classification, a GFR of less than 60 mL/min/1.73m^2 for at least 3 months is indicative of "moderate" kidney disease with likely clinical ramifications and correlates to CKD stage III. As the kidney has significant reserve, a GFR of less than 60 mL/min/1.73m^2 actually represents loss of approximately half of normal kidney function.[2,3] Stage IV CKD occurs with severely reduced kidney function (GFR 15–29), and stage V occurs in ESRD requiring dialysis. Stages I and II (GFR of $\geq$90 and 60–89, respectively) occur when there is evidence of kidney damage (e.g., proteinuria, biopsy results, etc.) but GFR is either normal or only mildly decreased. In some populations such as the elderly, elevation in creatinine with a GFR of more than 60 is not considered abnormal (Table 26.1).

Manifestations of CKD can vary based on severity. The most common etiologies of CKD in the US are hypertension, diabetes, and glomerulonephritis, and thus evaluation of a patient's symptoms should also take these conditions into account.[3,4] With increasing loss of kidney function, especially in class IV or V CKD, patients are at risk for volume overload, electrolyte abnormalities (in particular hyperkalemia, hyponatremia, hyperphosphatemia), and hyperchloremic metabolic acidosis. These abnormalities may be mild and manageable by medical therapy in stable patients or dialysis in patients with ESRD, but they may become exacerbated by illness or surgery.[4,5] Patients may have baseline chronic anemia due to impaired renal erythropoietin production, and they may have platelet dysfunction due to uremia. Evaluation and management of these factors will be discussed below.

AKI should also be a serious consideration in the perioperative period. The Acute Kidney Injury Network (AKIN)

Table 26.1 STAGES OF CHRONIC KIDNEY DISEASE (CKD) BASED ON NKF/DOQI GUIDELINES

STAGING OF CHRONIC KIDNEY DISEASE (CKD)

Stage I	GFR $\geq$90 mL/min/1.73m^2	Evidence of kidney damage with normal GFR
Stage II	GFR 60–90 mL/min/1.73m^2	Kidney damage with mild decrease in GFR
Stage III	GFR 30–59 mL/min/1.73m^2	Moderately decreased GFR
Stage IV	GFR 60–90 mL/min/1.73m^2	Severely decreased GFR
Stage V	GFR <15 mL/min/1.73m^2 or renal replacement therapy (RRT)	Kidney failure

Diagnosis of chronic kidney disease requires duration of at least 3 months.

GFR, glomerular filtration rate.

Table 26.2 ACUTE KIDNEY INJURY NETWORK (AKIN) AND RISK, INJURY, FAILURE, LOSS, ESKD (RIFLE) CRITERIA FOR ACUTE KIDNEY INJURY; BOTH CLASSIFICATIONS ARE BASED ON CHANGES IN SERUM CREATININE (OR GFR) AND URINE OUTPUT

COMPARING AKIN AND RIFLE CRITERIA FOR ACUTE KIDNEY INJURY

SERUM CREATININE CRITERIA				URINE OUTPUT (UOP) CRITERIA
AKIN		**RIFLE**		
Stage 1	Cr increases by 1.5–2× or ≥ 0.3 mg/dL	Risk	Cr increases by 1.5× or GFR decreases by >25%	UOP <0.5 mL/kg/hr × 6 hours
Stage 2	Cr increases by 2–3×	Injury	Cr increases by 2× or GFR decreases by >50%	UOP <0.5 mL/kg/hr × 12 hours
Stage 3	Cr increases by 3.0× or renal replacement therapy (RRT)	Failure	Cr increases by 3× or GFR decreases by >75% or Cr ≥4 mg/dL	UOP <0.3 mL/kg/hr × 12 hours or anuria × 24 hours
Receiving RRT is considered stage 3 regardless of stage prior to RRT		Loss	Persistent acute renal failure for >4 weeks	
		ESKD	End-stage kidney disease for >3 months	

staging system and Risk, Injury, Failure, Loss, ESRD (RIFLE) criteria are two frequently used systems for classifying AKI (Table 26.2).[6,7] An increase in serum creatinine of 150% or decreased urine output of less than 0.5 mL/kg/hour for 6 hours is indicative of the first stage of AKI in each of these criteria, with further increases in creatinine and decreased urine output representing increasing severity of AKI. The RIFLE criteria also recognizes that AKI may lead to persistent renal failure. Loss of kidney function is defined as persistent acute renal failure for longer than 4 weeks and CKD as renal failure for longer than 3 months. Etiologies for AKI may generally be divided into three broad categories of prerenal (e.g., decreased perfusion to kidneys), intrinsic renal (e.g., due to acute tubular necrosis, acute interstitial nephritis, glomerulonephritis), or postrenal (e.g., obstructive) causes, which may help with diagnosis and treatment of underlying cause of AKI. Effective management of AKI and measures to prevent progression from mild to severe stages of kidney injury can be critical for preserving kidney function as well as reducing morbidity and mortality. Multiple studies have shown worsened outcomes with development of AKI in inpatients, which occurs fairly frequently (some studies stating up to 5–7% of inpatients).[8,9] In one study examining more than 19,000 patients at a large academic medical center, development of AKI while admitted was associated with increased mortality and length of stay, with progressively worse outcomes with larger creatinine increases.[10]

PREOPERATIVE EVALUATION OF CHRONIC KIDNEY DISEASE

In patients with elevated creatinine or decreased GFR preoperatively, whether due to "known" CKD or an incidental laboratory finding, it is important to evaluate for severity and possible associated conditions of chronic kidney injury, and these findings should be used to help inform perioperative decision-making. In addition, if the etiology of CKD is known, optimization of any underlying causes is also prudent.

Preoperative workup for patients with CKD should be influenced by the type of surgery (i.e., less investigation may be needed for a day surgery case compared to a high-risk surgery). If previous laboratory results are available, correlating recent creatinine and GFR to a patient's trend can be useful in determining if creatinine elevation is chronic or acute. If AKI is diagnosed prior to an elective surgery, some sources advocate delaying surgery until AKI workup is completed.[3] In CKD patients, bare minimum laboratories would include a basic metabolic panel to evaluate for common electrolyte abnormalities like hyperkalemia or acidemia and trend creatinine/GFR and CBC for anemia (though platelets may be dysfunctional in advanced CKD, patients are not usually thrombocytopenic). It has been suggested that bleeding time assay may be the best way to quantify coagulopathy in CKD; however, the clinical utility of this may be questionable.[4] As previously stated, most patients with mild kidney impairment will likely be asymptomatic and likely without significant sequelae of kidney failure on exam, but patients with stage IV or V CKD should be assessed for signs of volume overload like pitting edema, orthopnea, and elevated jugular venous pressure (JVP), or for altered mental status that may be due to uremia.

In addition, common comorbid conditions of CKD should also be appropriately evaluated preoperatively. Management of diabetes and hypertension, two of the most common etiologies of CKD in the United States, is very important. Patients with hypertension and CKD are sometimes on an angiotensin converting enzyme inhibitor (ACEI) or angiotensin II receptor blocker (ARB) given the benefits in slowing progression of proteinuria. It should be noted that especially with new initiation of ACEIs or ARBs patients can have creatinine elevations as well as hyperkalemia, which usually stabilize.[3]

CKD itself has also been associated with increased risk for cardiovascular disease and coronary artery disease (CAD), a risk that is increased further when patients also have diabetes, hypertension, and other comorbid disease.[11] As recognized in the 2014 American College of Cardiology (ACC)/American Heart Association (AHA) Guidelines for perioperative cardiovascular examination, CKD with creatinine of greater than 2 mg/dL is one of the Revised Cardiac Risk Index (RCRI) criteria for increased risk of major adverse cardiac events (MACE) perioperatively. These events include myocardial infarction, pulmonary edema, ventricular fibrillation, cardiac arrest, and complete heart block. The other risk criteria identified are insulin-dependent diabetes mellitus, history of cerebrovascular disease, ischemic heart disease, congestive heart failure (CHF), and high-risk surgery (intrathoracic, intra-abdominal, suprainguinal vascular). Patients with two or more risk factors have a substantially higher risk for MACE than with one or zero, and such patients may warrant further cardiovascular workup if they have impaired functional status.[12] Two other major surgical risk calculators, the American College of Surgeons (ACS) National Surgical Quality Improvement Program (NSQIP) surgical risk calculator and the Myocardial Infarct or Cardiac Arrest (MICA) calculator also take into account kidney function, including creatinine of greater than 1.5 mg/dL or acute renal failure, respectively.[13,14] Though a simple creatinine cutoff is not perfect and can correlate to different GFR in different patients, it is a useful tool to prompt closer scrutiny of cardiovascular disease and function and possibly intervention or medical optimization prior to surgery given the elevated risks.

PERIOPERATIVE RISKS IN CKD PATIENTS

Many studies have shown an increased risk for adverse perioperative outcomes in patients with CKD or AKI. In addition, the risk for developing AKI or renal failure is itself increased in patients with preexisting kidney dysfunction. One large meta-analysis examined 49 studies (mostly on cardiac and vascular surgery) and found that CKD was associated with both short- and long-term effects. Having an eGFR of less than 60 mL/min/1.73m^2 (the cutoff in the study) was associated with approximately 3 times increased risk of 30-day mortality and AKI, as well as about 1.5 times increased risk of long-term all-cause mortality and MACE. The analysis also noted that the relative risk for 30-day mortality increased with progressively lower eGFR.[15] Another study that examined 49,000 patients undergoing "major general surgery" from the NSQIP database found an association between modest creatinine elevation (>1.5 mg/dL) and increased 30-day mortality and morbidity (encompassing multiple cardiac, respiratory, infectious, and hemorrhagic complications).[16] The cause for the association between kidney disease and adverse outcomes is likely multifactorial. Some of the manifestations of kidney disease, like anemia, coagulopathy, and acidosis, can have significant effects perioperatively. In addition, many of the common pathologies for kidney disease (hypertension, diabetes) are also risk factors for cardiovascular disease, which may also increase risk.

It is also important to understand risk factors for AKI or progression to acute renal failure in the perioperative period. A study by Kheterpal et al. examined more than 65,000 cases to identify factors that were associated with the development of acute renal failure and/or need for renal replacement therapy after major noncardiac surgery. They identified seven preoperative factors that had a significant association with eGFR less than 50 in the first seven postoperative days: age, emergent surgery, liver disease, BMI, high-risk surgery, peripheral vascular occlusive disease, and chronic obstructive pulmonary disease (COPD) on chronic bronchodilators. They also identified several intraoperative factors including vasopressor infusion use, total vasopressor dose, and use of intraoperative diuretics. In addition, the study found that patients who developed acute renal failure had increased 30-day and 1-year mortality.[9] Definitions of high-risk surgery vary among sources but usually can include intrathoracic, intraperitoneal or intra-abdominal, suprainguinal vascular surgeries and those involving large blood loss or fluid shifts.[9,12] A general surgery AKI risk index has also been proposed that divides patients into classes I–V based on the number of preoperative risk factors among age 56 or older, male sex, active CHF, ascites, hypertension, emergency surgery, intraperitoneal surgery, mild or moderate CKD, and diabetes mellitus on oral or insulin therapy. In validation studies, patients of class I (0–2 risk factors) have very low risk of developing perioperative AKI (approximately 0.2%), ranging to patients in class V (6+ risk factors) who may have up to 9.5% risk.[17]

PERIOPERATIVE MANAGEMENT FOR PREVENTING ACUTE KIDNEY INJURY

As discussed previously, management of patients undergoing surgery with CKD should start with a thorough preoperative evaluation for manifestations of kidney failure, functional status, and common comorbidities as well as optimization of these factors as much as possible. Patients with increased risk for AKI based on patient and surgical factors should have even closer scrutiny both before and during surgery.

There are no particular guidelines for intraoperative monitoring in patients with CKD, however in addition to standard American Society of Anesthesiologists (ASA) monitors, it is reasonable to consider whether bladder catheterization (to monitor hourly urine output) and/or an arterial line (for close hemodynamic monitoring and drawing serial labs) are suitable for the planned surgery, especially in high-risk patients or if expecting large hemodynamic shifts or blood loss.

Acute Disease Quality Initiative and PeriOperative Quality Initiative groups have published a consensus statement on addressing prevention of perioperative AKI.[18] (Figure 26.1)

Preoperatively, optimizing the CKD is paramount. In addition, the most obvious intervention is to avoid or discontinue known nephrotoxins whenever feasible. Of course, sometimes these agents are necessary for diagnostic or therapeutic management, so consideration of the risks and benefits of each intervention is necessary. Common nephrotoxic

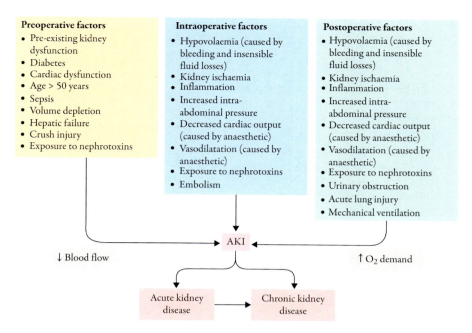

Figure 26.1 Perioperative factors for acute kidney injury. From Prowle JR. *Nat Rev Nephrol.* 2021 Sep;17(9):605–618.

agents include NSAIDs, ACE inhibitors, aminoglycosides, acyclovir, penicillin, cephalosporins, ciprofloxacin, HIV protease inhibitors, cyclosporine, and tacrolimus.[5]

Radiocontrast agents causing contrast-induced nephropathy are also a frequent concern, especially in patients with CKD. If they cannot be avoided, prehydration with IV (not oral) crystalloid has been shown to decrease contrast-induced AKI, and there is some evidence for the role of N-acetylcysteine.[19]

In addition, holding ACE/ARBs prior to surgery has long been a controversial topic. However, the VISION study, a large prospective cohort study published in 2017, found that holding ACEIs/ARBs for 24 hours before surgery was associated with decreased likelihood of death, stroke, myocardial injury, and intraoperative hypotension.[20] Based on these data it would be reasonable to hold ACEIs/ARBs prior to surgery.[21] Other antihypertensives can usually be continued if blood pressure is well-controlled.

No preoperative pharmacologic interventions have helped prevent AKI.[18]

Intraoperatively, in terms of anesthetic management, general and regional anesthesia are both acceptable for patients with CKD, with neither appearing to confer an advantage for preventing AKI. Maintaining adequate perfusion to the renal vasculature is the most important factor in avoiding prerenal AKI, and the kidneys can be very susceptible to compromise during anesthesia given the many changes in vascular resistance and volume status that occur with anesthetic agents and during surgery. To this end, prevention of hypotension and appropriate fluid management are important. In normal kidneys, autoregulation of blood flow (i.e., the ability of the renal vasculature to maintain relatively constant perfusion) can be maintained at MAPs of 80–180 mm Hg[5]; thus, especially when MAP is less than this autoregulation limit, renal blood flow becomes directly dependent on systemic pressure. A large study published in *Anesthesiology* investigated what MAP is adequate for renal and cardiac perfusion (based on AKI and myocardial injury). It found a threshold MAP of less than 55 mm Hg where a statistically significant increase in AKI and myocardial injury occurred and that increased duration of hypotension was associated with greater risk.[22] It has also been suggested that avoiding relative hypotension based on a patient's baseline blood pressure (>30% from baseline) may be effective for maintaining renal perfusion,[23] and, in a similar vein, avoiding hypertension out of the autoregulatory range should also occur. The results of an interventional trial of use of a MAP target of greater than 65 mm Hg as part of a goal-directed strategy have added weight to these observational data, demonstrating fewer postoperative complications (including AKI) and shorter length of hospital stay; this is currently the recommended target to decrease the risk of AKI.[18,24]

Intraoperative fluid management may be more difficult in patients with more severe CKD given a higher risk for volume overload, which must be balanced with supporting perfusion with adequate preload. One meta-analysis of multiple studies on perioperative hemodynamic optimization suggests that goal-directed fluid therapies may reduce the incidence of perioperative AKI.[25] The randomized controlled trials included in the analysis differed in their approaches but largely studied the use of fluids, blood transfusion, +/− inotropes (mainly dobutamine), or vasodilators to achieve hemodynamic optimization based on targets of cardiac index, oxygen delivery, stroke volume variation, and systemic vascular resistance, among others. The authors of the meta-analysis concluded that use of these strategies was associated with a statistically significant decrease in perioperative AKI. In addition, while most of the studies included fluid-loading preoperatively, they also found that implementing these therapies intraoperatively or postoperatively could also decrease incidence of AKI. It has also been suggested that use of balanced physiologic crystalloids, instead of hyperchloremic solutions like 0.9% saline, may confer advantage in avoiding AKI.[23] As such, when possible, use of goal-directed fluid therapies may be one approach to fluid management for avoiding AKI.

Myoglobin/hemoglobin (e.g., in the setting of rhabdomyolysis) can have direct tubular effects. There is theoretical risk for nephrotoxicity from compound A in low-flow sevoflurane anesthesia, however this has not been substantiated in human studies.

Beyond this, there is a burgeoning literature regarding possible pharmacologic interventions for preventing intraoperative AKI, though many interventions remain controversial. A Cochrane review published in 2013 investigated several perioperative medications including dopamine and dopamine analogues, diuretics, calcium channel blockers, ACE inhibitors, N-acetylcysteine, atrial natriuretic peptide, sodium bicarbonate, antioxidants, and erythropoietin; based on the heterogeneity of the available studies, the review did not identify any interventions that appeared to offer benefit in preventing AKI.[26] A 2021 systematic review found that alpha-2 agonists such as dexmedetomidine or clonidine may have some benefit in reducing AKI and need for renal replacement therapy.[27] Dopamine has been shown in some trials to increase urine output without decreasing AKI incidence.[28] There is some evidence for fenoldopam, a dopamine-1 receptor agonist that decreases systemic vascular resistance without decreasing renal perfusion, in decreasing incidence of AKI, though a meta-analysis did not show any change in mortality or need for dialysis.[29] Diuretics like furosemide have also not been shown to prevent AKI.[30]

Postoperative factors that could decrease the risk of postoperative AKI are maintenance of adequate perfusion (as previously discussed), avoidance of nephrotoxins, and postoperative glycemic control.[18] Studies have shown that while hyperglycemia may not be a risk factor for postoperative AKI, glycemic variability does.[31,32] The recent consensus statement recommends postoperative glycemic targets of less than 180 mg/dL.[18]

CONCLUSION

- CKD is defined as decreased kidney function (based on GFR) with a duration of at least 3 months, with a wide range of severity and clinical manifestations.[1,2]

- AKI can be diagnosed based on increases in creatinine or decreased urine output.[6,7] AKI can be broadly divided into prerenal, intrinsic renal, or postrenal etiologies.

- AKI in hospitalized patients, including in the perioperative period, has been associated with adverse outcomes including increased mortality and length of stay. More severe AKI has been associated with increasingly poor outcomes.[8–10]

- Preoperative workup for patients with CKD or elevated creatinine should be tailored to the severity of disease and underlying etiology, if known. Reasonable preoperative labs include basic metabolic panel and CBC. Physical exam should evaluate for volume overload and altered mental status.

- Common comorbid conditions of CKD include diabetes, hypertension, and CAD.[3,11]

- The VISION study found that holding ACEIs or ARBs for 24 hours prior to surgery was associated with decreased risk of death, stroke, myocardial injury, and intraoperative hypotension.[20]

- CKD with elevated creatinine is a risk factor for MACE based on the ACC/AHA guidelines for perioperative risk assessment, as well as on the ACS NSQIP MICA and surgical risk calculators. Patients should be evaluated for cardiovascular risk and possible preoperative optimization or treatment.

- Preexisting CKD is associated with increased risk for developing perioperative AKI.[15] CKD has also been associated with increased risk for perioperative 30-day mortality, 1-year mortality, MACE, and morbidity including cardiac, pulmonary, infectious, and hemorrhagic complications.[16]

- Risk factors for perioperative AKI include age, emergent surgery, liver disease, BMI, high-risk surgery, peripheral vascular occlusive disease, and COPD. Intraoperative risks include vasopressor infusion use, total vasopressor dose, and intraoperative diuretics.[9]

- Intraoperative management for preventing AKI should focus on preventing hemodynamic instability. Renal autoregulation occurs at MAPs of 80–180 mm Hg.[5] A MAP of less than 55 mm Hg is associated with increased risk for AKI and myocardial injury.[22]

- Use of goal-directed fluid management strategies and physiologic crystalloids may be useful for preventing perioperative AKI.[23,25]

- Common nephrotoxic agents include NSAIDs, ACEIs, aminoglycosides, acyclovir, penicillin, cephalosporins, ciprofloxacin, HIV protease inhibitors, cyclosporine, tacrolimus, and radiocontrast agents.[5] These should be avoided if possible if there is concern for AKI.

REVIEW QUESTIONS

1. A 64-year-old man with a history of hypertension, hyperlipidemia, diabetes mellitus type 2 (on insulin), and CKD (baseline creatinine of 2.0) was incidentally diagnosed with localized adenocarcinoma of the ascending colon. He now presents to preoperative clinic preceding his laparoscopic right hemicolectomy. He gardens and says he can climb two flights of stairs without stopping, but rarely engages in more vigorous physical activity. On review of systems, he feels fine. Aside from preoperative labs, what is the next best step in his preoperative workup?

a. Obtain a transthoracic echocardiogram (TTE).
b. Obtain exercise stress test.
c. Proceed with surgery.
d. Cardiology referral for coronary angiogram.

The correct answer is c.

Proceed with surgery. This patient has three RCRI risk factors (insulin-dependent diabetes, Cr of 2.0, and intra-abdominal surgery) and is therefore at elevated risk of adverse cardiac events according to the RCRI criteria.[14] However, this patient has adequate functional status (MET ≥4). Current guidelines advise against further cardiac testing in this scenario (answers a, b, d) because these tests are unlikely to change management.[12] Answer a would be correct if the patient endorsed new symptoms of CHF like dyspnea on exertion, orthopnea, or peripheral edema. Answer b might be appropriate in certain situations when patients are high risk, there is clinical suspicion of CAD, and the patient has poor functional status. Answer d would be most appropriate if the patient had new angina symptoms, concern for acute coronary syndrome, or recent positive stress test, and the surgery was completely elective.

2. A 72-year-old patient with CKD stage IV (eGFR 15–29 mL/min/1.73m^2) complicated by anemia, hypertension, and multiple electrolyte derangements undergoes cystoscopy, lithotripsy, and stent placement for ureteral stones under general anesthesia with endotracheal intubation and exhibits prolonged emergence. Which of these agents will likely have the *least* change in pharmacokinetics in patients with CKD compared to patients with normal kidney function?

a. Meperidine.
b. Vecuronium.
c. Midazolam.
d. Sevoflurane.

The correct answer is d.

Sevoflurane. Volatile anesthetics can be safely used in patients with CKD. Their metabolism and elimination is independent of the kidneys, thus there is little concern for accumulation of metabolites or prolonged effect due to slow elimination as in some other common anesthetic drugs.[5] Choice a is incorrect because meperidine's active metabolite, normeperidine, is cleared by renal excretion and can accumulate in patients with CKD and lead to seizures. Similarly, morphine is metabolized into the active agent morphine-6-glucuronide, which is renally cleared and should also be avoided in patients with CKD.[4] Vecuronium can usually be used in patients with kidney disease, but its active metabolites are partially renally cleared so it may exhibit prolonged duration of action. Midazolam also may have prolonged action due to accumulation of active metabolites; in addition, hypoalbuminemia in patients with severe CKD and volume overload can reduce protein-binding, especially of medications such as midazolam that are highly protein-bound.

3. A 23-year-old man with no known medical history is brought in emergently for exploratory surgery for a gunshot wound to the abdomen. He receives a massive blood transfusion and requires splenectomy and bowel resection. The abdominal aorta is cross-clamped for 25 minutes. In the ICU postoperatively, urine output declines to 5–10 cc/hour for more than 6 hours. No change occurs after multiple fluid boluses. Creatinine is now 3.0 mg/dL. What is the next best step for management of his AKI?

a. Give additional 1L of crystalloid in 250 cc boluses.
b. Obtain urinalysis and urine sediment.
c. Obtain central access and proceed with hemodialysis.
d. Resume maintenance IVF and trend creatinine.

The correct answer is b.

Obtain urinalysis and urine sediment. Though it is most likely that this young, previously healthy patient's oliguric AKI is due to hypoperfusion in the setting of massive blood loss, management of AKI should evaluate for prerenal, intrinsic renal, and postrenal causes. Obtaining a urine sediment in particular can help determine if intrinsic renal etiologies such as acute tubular necrosis (ATN), acute interstitial nephritis (AIN), vasculitides, or other pathology are present, which may have an important influence on management. Though this is not an option in the question, renal ultrasound and examination of urinary catheter would also be warranted to evaluate for postrenal causes of oliguria. We have established that fluid boluses (choice a) are not improving urine output, and continuing to bolus without evaluating for possible progression to acute renal failure can lead to volume overload. Proceeding directly to hemodialysis in a patient without clear indications for dialysis such as acidosis, electrolyte derangements, uremia, or volume overload is unnecessary and poses its own risks. Simply trending creatinine will not help elucidate the underlying cause of oliguria.

4. A 56-year-old woman with a history of hypertension, diastolic heart failure, COPD, and current cigarette smoking is scheduled to undergo video-assisted thoracic surgery (VATS) wedge resection for a right upper lobe lung nodule. Her medications are amlodipine, lisinopril, metoprolol, albuterol, and tiotropium inhalers. What is the *most* appropriate management of her medications on the day of surgery?

a. Hold amlodipine.
b. Hold metoprolol.
c. Hold lisinopril.
d. Hold tiotropium.

The correct answer is c.

Hold lisinopril; continue amlodipine, metoprolol, and tiotropium. The VISION study, a large prospective cohort study, found that holding ACEIs/ARBs for 24 hours prior to surgery was associated with decreased likelihood of death, stroke, myocardial injury, and intraoperative hypotension.[20] Given these findings, holding lisinopril would be appropriate. Other antihypertensives such as amlodipine, a calcium channel blocker, can generally be continued on the day of surgery. Given the patient's COPD and current smoking, continuing inhalers on the day of surgery (choice d) is the correct decision. Continuing beta blockers in patients who have been on them chronically is a class I recommendation from the ACC/

AHA 2014 guideline on perioperative cardiovascular evaluation and management[12]; thus this patient who has been on beta blocker therapy should have metoprolol continued on the day of surgery (choice b).

REFERENCES

1. K/DOQI clinical practice guidelines for chronic kidney disease: Evaluation, classification, and stratification. *Am J Kidney Dis*. 2002 Feb;39(2 Suppl 1):S1–266.
2. Group KDIGOKCW. KDIGO 2012 clinical practice guideline for the evaluation and management of chronic kidney disease. *Kidney International Supplements*. 2013;3(19–62).
3. Kalamas AG, Niemann CU. Patients with chronic kidney disease. *Med Clin North Am*. 2013 Nov;97(6):1109–1122.
4. Palevsky PM. Perioperative management of patients with chronic kidney disease or ESRD. *Best Pract Res Clin Anaesthesiol*. 2004 Mar;18(1):129–144.
5. Anesthesia for patients with kidney disease. In: Butterworth IV JF, Mackey DC, Wasnick JD, eds. *Morgan and Mikhail's Clinical Anesthesiology*. 7th ed. McGraw-Hill; 2022:679–697.
6. Bellomo R, Ronco C, Kellum JA, Mehta RL, Palevsky P. Acute renal failure: Definition, outcome measures, animal models, fluid therapy and information technology needs: The Second International Consensus Conference of the Acute Dialysis Quality Initiative (ADQI) Group. *Crit Care*. 2004 Aug;8(4):R204–R212.
7. Mehta RL, Kellum JA, Shah SV, et al. Acute Kidney Injury Network: Report of an initiative to improve outcomes in acute kidney injury. *Crit Care*. 2007;11(2):R31.
8. Nash K, Hafeez A, Hou S. Hospital-acquired renal insufficiency. *Am J Kidney Dis*. 2002 May;39(5):930–936.
9. Kheterpal S, Tremper KK, Englesbe MJ, et al. Predictors of postoperative acute renal failure after noncardiac surgery in patients with previously normal renal function. *Anesthesiology*. 2007 Dec;107(6):892–902.
10. Chertow GM, Burdick E, Honour M, Bonventre JV, Bates DW. Acute kidney injury, mortality, length of stay, and costs in hospitalized patients. *J Am Soc Nephrol*. 2005 Nov;16(11):3365–3370.
11. Manjunath G, Tighiouart H, Ibrahim H, et al. Level of kidney function as a risk factor for atherosclerotic cardiovascular outcomes in the community. *J Am Coll Cardiol*. 2003 Jan 1;41(1):47–55.
12. Fleisher LA, Fleischmann KE, Auerbach AD, et al. 2014 ACC/AHA guideline on perioperative cardiovascular evaluation and management of patients undergoing noncardiac surgery: A report of the American College of Cardiology/American Heart Association Task Force on practice guidelines. *J Am Coll Cardiol*. 2014 Dec 9;64(22):e77–137.
13. Cohen ME, Ko CY, Bilimoria KY, et al. Optimizing ACS NSQIP modeling for evaluation of surgical quality and risk: Patient risk adjustment, procedure mix adjustment, shrinkage adjustment, and surgical focus. *J Am Coll Surg*. 2013 Aug;217(2):336–346.e1.
14. Gupta PK, Gupta H, Sundaram A, et al. Development and validation of a risk calculator for prediction of cardiac risk after surgery. *Circulation*. 2011 Jul 26;124(4):381–387.
15. Mooney JF, Ranasinghe I, Chow CK, Perkovic V, Barzi F, Zoungas S, et al. Preoperative estimates of glomerular filtration rate as predictors of outcome after surgery: A systematic review and meta-analysis. *Anesthesiology*. 2013 Apr;118(4):809–824.
16. O'Brien MM, Gonzales R, Shroyer AL, et al. Modest serum creatinine elevation affects adverse outcome after general surgery. *Kidney Int*. 2002 Aug;62(2):585–592.
17. Kheterpal S, Tremper KK, Heung M, et al. Development and validation of an acute kidney injury risk index for patients undergoing general surgery: Results from a national data set. *Anesthesiology*. 2009 Mar;110(3):505–515.
18. Prowle JR, Forni LG, Bell M, et al. Postoperative acute kidney injury in adult non-cardiac surgery: Joint consensus report of the Acute Disease Quality Initiative and PeriOperative Quality Initiative. *Nat Rev Nephrol*. 2021 Sep;17(9):605–618.
19. Khwaja A. KDIGO clinical practice guidelines for acute kidney injury. *Nephron Clin Pract*. 2012;120(4):c179–c184.
20. Roshanov PS, Rochwerg B, Patel A, et al. Withholding versus continuing angiotensin-converting enzyme inhibitors or angiotensin II receptor blockers before noncardiac surgery: An analysis of the vascular events in noncardiac surgery patients cohort evaluation prospective cohort. *Anesthesiology*. 2017 Jan;126(1):16–27.
21. Sahai SK, Balonov K, Bentov N, et al. Preoperative management of cardiovascular medications: A Society for Perioperative Assessment and Quality Improvement (SPAQI) consensus statement. *Mayo Clin Proc*. 2022 Sep;97(9):1734–1751.
22. Walsh M, Devereaux PJ, Garg AX, Kurz A, Turan A, Rodseth RN, et al. Relationship between intraoperative mean arterial pressure and clinical outcomes after noncardiac surgery: Toward an empirical definition of hypotension. *Anesthesiology*. 2013 Sep;119(3):507–515.
23. Zarbock A, Milles K. Novel therapy for renal protection. *Curr Opin Anaesthesiol*. 2015 Aug;28(4):431–438.
24. Calvo-Vecino JM, Ripollés-Melchor J, Mythen MG, et al. Effect of goal-directed haemodynamic therapy on postoperative complications in low-moderate risk surgical patients: A multicentre randomised controlled trial (FEDORA trial). *Br J Anaesth*. 2018 Apr;120(4):734–744.
25. Brienza N, Giglio MT, Marucci M, Fiore T. Does perioperative hemodynamic optimization protect renal function in surgical patients? A meta-analytic study. *Crit Care Med*. 2009 Jun;37(6):2079–2090.
26. Zacharias M, Mugawar M, Herbison GP, et al. Interventions for protecting renal function in the perioperative period. *Cochrane Database Syst Rev*. 2013 Sep 11;2013(9):Cd003590.
27. Pathak S, Olivieri G, Mohamed W, et al. Pharmacological interventions for the prevention of renal injury in surgical patients: A systematic literature review and meta-analysis. *Br J Anaesth*. 2021 Jan;126(1):131–138.
28. Friedrich JO, Adhikari N, Herridge MS, Beyene J. Meta-analysis: Low-dose dopamine increases urine output but does not prevent renal dysfunction or death. *Ann Intern Med*. 2005 Apr 5;142(7):510–524.
29. Gillies MA, Kakar V, Parker RJ, Honoré PM, Ostermann M. Fenoldopam to prevent acute kidney injury after major surgery—A systematic review and meta-analysis. *Crit Care*. 2015 Dec 25;19:449.
30. Lassnigg A, Donner E, Grubhofer G, Presterl E, Druml W, Hiesmayr M. Lack of renoprotective effects of dopamine and furosemide during cardiac surgery. *J Am Soc Nephrol*. 2000 Jan;11(1):97–104.
31. Adler CH, Singer C, O'Brien C, et al. Randomized, placebo-controlled study of tolcapone in patients with fluctuating Parkinson disease treated with levodopa-carbidopa. Tolcapone Fluctuator Study Group III. *Arch Neurol*. 1998 Aug;55(8):1089–1095.
32. Song JW, Shim JK, Yoo KJ, Oh SY, Kwak YL. Impact of intraoperative hyperglycaemia on renal dysfunction after off-pump coronary artery bypass. *Interact Cardiovasc Thorac Surg*. 2013 Sep;17(3):473–478.

HEMATOLOGY

27.

PREOPERATIVE ANEMIA MANAGEMENT

EVALUATION AND TREATMENT

Kenneth Cummings

STEM CASE AND KEY QUESTIONS

An otherwise healthy 36-year-old woman presents to your preoperative clinic 3 weeks prior to a scheduled abdominoplasty. She lost a significant amount of weight after a prior gastric bypass surgery, leading to excess abdominal skin. Her preoperative laboratory evaluation is significant for a hemoglobin (Hgb) of 7 g/dL.

What is the definition of anemia? What are possible causes?

The patient underwent her bariatric surgery 2 years ago and is now at a near-normal BMI. She recalls being told that she needed to take "a bunch of vitamins and other stuff" that tended to cause abdominal discomfort and constipation as well as "some kind of vitamin shot every few months" after her surgery. She moved after 1 year and was lost to follow-up with the bariatric surgeon. She felt well and was annoyed by the number of pills and injections so decided to stop taking them.

What signs and symptoms might one expect to find from anemia?

On further questioning, she admits that she feels tired most of the time but has always attributed it to being the mother of two school-age children. She does not report any excessive menstrual blood loss (actually minimal due to the presence of an intrauterine device) or other obvious sources of bleeding. In the exam room, she has a large cup of diet cola and is chewing on the ice in the cup. On physical examination, she is tachycardic with somewhat pale nail beds and conjunctiva. The remainder of the exam is normal.

Are there further laboratory studies needed to better define her anemia?

You order additional laboratory studies including a full blood count with differential and red blood cell indices, reticulocyte count, iron studies, and vitamin B_{12} and folate levels. Her hemoglobin is 7.2 g/dL with a mean corpuscular volume of 70 fL and a reticulocyte percentage of 0.5%. Her platelet count is 650,000 per microL. Her ferritin level is 55 mcg/L with a transferrin saturation of 10%. Her B_{12} and folate studies are normal.

What is the likely cause of her anemia? Is there any other evaluation that should be performed? Does it need treatment? If so, how?

You provide her with a referral to a local gastroenterologist to rule out gastrointestinal blood loss as a contributor to her anemia. Because her surgery is elective and there are several weeks available, you arrange for treatment with IV iron infusions and schedule a vitamin B_{12} injection.

How much iron should she receive? What formulation? How quickly will there be a response?

She is scheduled to receive infusions at your hospital's infusion center. Because of restrictions from her insurance coverage, she receives 5 infusions of iron sucrose over 2 weeks. She complains about the inconvenience but follows through with the process. One week after the infusion series ends, her hemoglobin has improved to 9 g/dL.

Are there any risks to administering IV iron formulations?

She tolerates the infusions well. During her third session, she complains of muscle aches and feeling flushed. The infusion is paused for 20 minutes, and she feels much better. The infusion is restarted at half the rate and continues uneventfully. Her final two infusions continue at the slower rate without any issues.

What about her normal B_{12} and folate levels? Does she need treatment? What will you counsel her about iron and other substrates going forward?

With the patient's permission, you contact her bariatric surgeon who recommends a colleague with whom to follow-up in your area. The patient is agreeable to seeing her after surgery and grudgingly agrees to restart her postoperative dietary supplements and vitamin injections.

DISCUSSION

DEFINITION AND IMPLICATIONS

Anemia (Hgb <12 g/dL in women, <13 g/dL in men) is a syndrome reflecting inadequate total red blood cell (RBC) mass. In the perioperative patient, there is abundant evidence linking anemia with increased morbidity and mortality. For example, the adjusted odds of death or cardiac events (cardiac arrest or myocardial infarction [MI]) was inversely related to the preoperative hematocrit in one study of veterans undergoing noncardiac surgery, with an increased risk seen in even "mild" anemia.[1] Also, a large observational study from Australia found an increased rate of hospital readmission in patients who were anemic at hospital discharge (14.1% vs. 7.4%).[2]

EVIDENCE FOR PREOPERATIVE CORRECTION OF ANEMIA

Despite the evidence showing deleterious effects of perioperative anemia, studies evaluating the benefits of treating anemia have been sparse. The most relevant evidence comes from the PREVENTT trial,[3] a randomized controlled trial (RCT) evaluating the efficacy of iron infusion in anemic patients before open abdominal surgery. Patients with preoperative anemia ($N = 487$) were randomized to 1,000 mg of ferric carboxymaltose or placebo 10–42 days before surgery. There were no significant differences between the groups in transfusion rate, death, or any other safety endpoints.

The major criticism of the PREVENTT trial, however, is that the cause of the patients' anemia was not determined. All anemic patients were included, not just those with iron deficiency. A recent secondary analysis attempted to address this shortcoming. Blood samples collected as part of the trial were analyzed for iron deficiency, and any association of iron status with the trial outcomes was assessed. Unfortunately, there was no beneficial effect of iron infusion detected even in patients identified as iron deficient.[4]

However, it remains logical to assume that correcting a condition associated with significantly increased perioperative complications is a rational thing to do, even if the current literature is insufficient.

IDENTIFICATION OF THE CAUSE OF ANEMIA

Anemia can result from several (sometimes coexisting) etiologies, broadly categorized into decreased production, blood loss, and accelerated RBC destruction. Any approach to the anemic patient should include a search for potential sources of blood loss, evaluation of the adequacy of substrates for RBC production, and an assessment of renal function. Figure 27.1 outlines one conceptual framework for approaching the diagnosis and treatment of preoperative anemia.

TREATMENT OPTIONS

In this case, the patient has iron deficiency anemia, and this discussion will focus on that condition. Oral iron replacement is an option if there are 4–6 weeks available prior to surgery. Oral iron is very poorly absorbed (a few milligrams per day) and is associated with a very high rate of gastrointestinal side effects (nausea, abdominal pain, diarrhea, constipation, black stool). If oral iron is used, once-daily (40–60 mg) or alternate-day (80–100 mg) dosing should be used to prevent increased hepcidin levels. Dietary factors also impact iron absorption, and the concomitant intake of acidic substances (vitamin C supplements, orange juice) may be helpful. A repeat hemoglobin level should be checked at 4 weeks to evaluate response.[5]

A much more time-efficient method of iron administration is by IV infusion. It is preferable for patients undergoing surgery within several weeks, who have severe anemia (Hgb <10 g/dL), or who cannot tolerate oral iron. In this case, a repeat hemoglobin level should be checked at 2–3 weeks after infusion to assess for response. Although variable, hemoglobin increases from 2 to 5 g/dL are typical after a full course of therapy.[6,7]

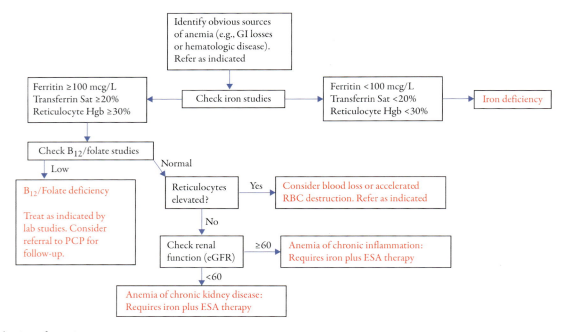

Figure 27.1 Evaluation of anemia.

If preoperative treatment is not feasible, one could certainly arrange for IV iron infusion in the immediate postoperative period, even during the hospital stay. This would provide needed substrate for RBC production given both the anemia and likely recent surgical blood loss. This practice (possibly combined with erythropoiesis-stimulating agent [ESA] use) is recommended in an international consensus statement on managing postsurgical anemia.[8]

AVAILABLE FORMULATIONS AND POTENTIAL RISKS OF IV IRON

The major differences between the available iron formulations come from how tightly the iron is bound to a carbohydrate carrier molecule. Formulations with tightly bound iron (low-molecular-weight [LMW] iron dextran, ferric carboxymaltose, iron isomaltoside, ferumoxytol) allow rapid infusion of large doses. Less tightly bound formulations (iron gluconate, iron sucrose) have much lower single-infusion dose limits, which leads to the need for repeated infusions. These two formulations, however, are much less expensive and thus are commonly favored by insurance companies. Table 27.1 summarizes key features of the commonly available iron formulations.[9]

Although a total body iron deficit can be calculated using the Ganzoni formula,[10] in practice, a 1,000 mg total dose is chosen because that is the maximum allowable dose in the United States. Because of this limit, some iron formulations (e.g., ferric carboxymaltose or LMW iron dextran) can provide a "total dose infusion" in just a single infusion session.

Early safety concerns arose from high-molecular-weight iron dextran formulations that had an unacceptably high incidence of hypersensitivity reactions. The currently available formulations do not have this problem although a test dose is still recommended when administering LMW iron dextran. Fortunately, the rate of serious adverse events with modern iron formulations is less than 1 in 250,000 doses.[11] There are adverse events, however, the most serious (and uncommon) being complement activation-related pseudo allergy (CARPA). The CARPA syndrome is referred to as a "pseudoallergy" in that it is not IgE-mediated but rather involves the direct systemic activation of the complement cascade with serious consequences such as cardiovascular collapse, respiratory distress, and others.[12] Much more common minor reactions include chest tightness, myalgias/arthralgias, or flushing. These minor reactions can be treated by pausing the infusion and resuming after symptoms resolve. Switching to another formulation may also be helpful for subsequent infusions.

Concerns about increased infection risk after iron infusion have not been borne out, and the infectious risks (among many others) associated with allogeneic transfusion are almost certainly higher than with IV iron.[13]

THE ROLE FOR ERYTHROPOIESIS-STIMULATING AGENTS

ESAs are recombinant forms of erythropoietin, typically epoetin alfa or darbepoetin. In nonsurgical settings, they are used to treat anemia of chronic kidney disease and in oncology. Multiple studies in various surgical populations (orthopedic, oncologic, gynecologic) have shown improved hemoglobin concentrations and decreased rates of perioperative transfusion with the preoperative use of iron infusion combined with ESA treatment.[11] It is reasonable to use these agents in patients with anemia of inflammation or with chronic kidney disease (with a higher hemoglobin target than usual).

In long-term ESA use, as in chronic kidney disease, targeting normal hemoglobin levels is associated with thromboembolism. In the acute preoperative setting, however, there is no convincing evidence of increased risk if appropriate venous thromboembolism (VTE) prophylaxis is used. The higher rate of VTE seen in one study of patients undergoing spine surgery was confounded by the fact that none of the patients received pharmacologic VTE prophylaxis.[14] It may therefore be reasonable to avoid ESA use in patients with a history of VTE, but an individualized approach to the risks and benefits should be taken.

PATIENT BLOOD MANAGEMENT

Preoperative treatment of anemia is part of a larger concept described as *patient blood management* (PBM). This is a patient-centered, systematic, evidence-based approach to improve patient outcomes by reducing unnecessary transfusion.[15] It is a global approach that incorporates preoperative, intraoperative, and postoperative strategies.

The preoperative phase consists of screening for anemia in high-risk patients (large expected perioperative blood loss or known risk for anemia), identifying causes, and treating as

Table 27.1 COMMONLY USED INTRAVENOUS IRON FORMULATIONS

	IRON SUCROSE	IRON GLUCONATE	LOW-MOLECULAR-WEIGHT IRON DEXTRAN	FERUMOXYTOL	IRON ISOMALTOSIDE	FERRIC CARBOXYMALTOSE
Maximum single dose (mg)	200	125	20 mg/kg	510	20 mg/kg	15–20 mg/kg
Interval between infusions	1,000 mg per 14 days	8 infusions in 14 days	Daily	3–8 days	1 week	1 week
Total dose infusion?	No	No	Yes	Yes	Yes	Yes

appropriate. Simultaneously, planning for perioperative needs should occur: identifying the patient's values about transfusion, arranging for blood conservation strategies if appropriate, and managing patients' anticoagulation (if applicable).

The intraoperative period includes contributions from both the surgical and anesthesiology teams. Minimization of coagulopathy is accomplished by maintaining normothermia, avoiding dilutional coagulopathy, and using antifibrinolytic agents as appropriate.[16] Use of RBC salvage can be helpful if there is a large expected blood loss. Finally, the surgical contribution at this phase consists of a focus on meticulous hemostasis.

Postoperatively, PBM consists of reducing ongoing blood loss (such as from excessive blood testing) and minimizing factors that can exacerbate bleeding (such as ongoing coagulopathy). Following evidence-based transfusion practices is key. It is also important to note that IV iron infusion or other targeted anemia treatments in the postoperative period are always an option if clinically indicated.

CONCLUSION

- Evaluation of an anemic patient should include a search for potential sources of blood loss, evaluation of substrates for RBC production, and assessment of renal function.
- Iron infusion treatment is an option to treat patients who have iron deficiency anemia.
- PBM incorporates preoperative, intraoperative, and postoperative strategies.
- The PREVENTT trial showed no beneficial effect of iron infusion in anemic patients undergoing major abdominal surgery.
- More research is needed on preoperative treatment of patients with anemia.

REVIEW QUESTIONS

1. What is not the expected laboratory finding in iron deficiency with anemia (IDA)?

    a. Hemoglobin level is decreased.
    b. Ferritin level is decreased.
    c. Total iron-binding capacity (TIBC) is decreased.
    d. Transferrin saturation is decreased.

The correct answer is c.
TIBC is increased in IDA and decreased in anemia due to inflammation.[11]

2. What is not the expected laboratory finding in mixed anemia (anemia due to inflammation and IDA)?

    a. Hemoglobin is decreased.
    b. Ferritin level is normal.
    c. TIBC is variable.
    d. Transferrin saturation is decreased.

The correct answer is d.
Transferrin saturation is normal in mixed anemia.[11]

3. Which of the following is not true on the use of oral iron to treat anemia?

    a. Patients may complain of abdominal pain.
    b. Patient's stool may turn black.
    c. Can exacerbate colitis in patients with inflammatory bowel disease.
    d. Patient adherence is greater than 50%.

The correct answer is d.
Patient adherence is less than 50%.[11]

4. Which of the following IV iron formulations is associated with the greatest risk for hypersensitivity reactions and a test dose is recommended?

    a. Iron gluconate.
    b. Iron sucrose.
    c. LMW iron dextran.
    d. Ferric carboxymaltose.

The correct answer is c.
Hypersensitivity reactions are possible with all iron infusions but most commonly with LMW iron dextran.[11]

5. Which of the following is not true about tranexamic acid?

    a. Tranexamic acid is an antifibrinolytic drug.
    b. Tranexamic acid has been shown to decrease the incidence and severity of bleeding in patients undergoing cesarean delivery.
    c. Tranexamic acid has been shown to decrease the incidence and severity of bleeding in patients undergoing cardiac surgery.
    d. Tranexamic acid has been shown to decrease the incidence of thrombotic events.

The correct answer is d.
A concern for routinely giving tranexamic acid in surgery is the potential risk for increasing thrombotic events not decreasing them, although the POISE-3 study did not show an increase in the incidence of thrombotic events.[16]

REFERENCES

1. Wu WC, Schifftner TL, Henderson WG, et al. Preoperative hematocrit levels and postoperative outcomes in older patients undergoing noncardiac surgery. *JAMA*. 2007;297(22):2481–2488.
2. Collaborative TPS. The management of peri-operative anaemia in patients undergoing major abdominal surgery in Australia and New Zealand: A prospective cohort study. *Med J Aust*. 2022;217(9):487–493.
3. Richards T, Baikady RR, Clevenger B, et al. Preoperative intravenous iron to treat anaemia before major abdominal surgery (PREVENTT): A randomised, double-blind, controlled trial. *Lancet*. 2020;396(10259):1353–1361.
4. Richards T, Miles LF, Clevenger B, et al. The association between iron deficiency and outcomes: A secondary analysis of the intravenous iron therapy to treat iron deficiency anaemia in patients undergoing major abdominal surgery (PREVENTT) trial. *Anaesthesia*. 2023;78(3):320–329.

5. Muñoz M, Acheson AG, Auerbach M, et al. International consensus statement on the peri-operative management of anaemia and iron deficiency. *Anaesthesia*. 2017;72(2):233–247.
6. Amrane S, Skupski B, Prasad N, Tsai T. Intravenous iron infusion as an alternative to blood transfusion in severely anemic gynecologic patients [5Q]. *Obstet Gynecol*. 2016;127:140S.
7. Cançado RD, de Figueiredo PO, Olivato MC, Chiattone CS. Efficacy and safety of intravenous iron sucrose in treating adults with iron deficiency anemia. *Revista brasileira de hematologia e hemoterapia*. 2011;33(6):439–443.
8. Muñoz M, Acheson AG, Bisbe E, et al. An international consensus statement on the management of postoperative anaemia after major surgical procedures. *Anaesthesia*. 2018;73(11):1418–1431.
9. Peters F, Ellermann I, Steinbicker AU. Intravenous iron for treatment of anemia in the 3 perisurgical phases: A review and analysis of the current literature. *Anesth Analg*. 2018;126(4):1268–1282.
10. Ganzoni AM. [Intravenous iron-dextran: Therapeutic and experimental possibilities]. *Schweiz Med Wochenschr*. 1970;100(7):301–303.
11. Warner MA, Shore-Lesserson L, Shander A, Patel SY, Perelman SI, Guinn NR. Perioperative anemia: Prevention, diagnosis, and management throughout the spectrum of perioperative care. *Anesth Analg*. 2020;130(5):1364–1380.
12. Szebeni J. Complement activation-related pseudoallergy: A stress reaction in blood triggered by nanomedicines and biologicals. *Mol Immunol*. 2014;61(2):163–173.
13. Avni T, Bieber A, Grossman A, Green H, Leibovici L, Gafter-Gvili A. The safety of intravenous iron preparations: Systematic review and meta-analysis. *Mayo Clin Proc*. 2015;90(1):12–23.
14. Stowell CP, Jones SC, Enny C, Langholff W, Leitz G. An open-label, randomized, parallel-group study of perioperative epoetin alfa versus standard of care for blood conservation in major elective spinal surgery: Safety analysis. *Spine (Phila Pa 1976)*. 2009;34(23):2479–2485.
15. Shander A, Hardy JF, Ozawa S, et al. A global definition of patient blood management. *Anesth Analg*. 2022;135(3):76–488.
16. Devereaux PJ, Marcucci M, Painter TW, et al. Tranexamic acid in patients undergoing noncardiac surgery. *N Engl J Med*. 2022;386(21):1986–1997.

28.

PROLONGED PTT IN A HEALTHY PATIENT

Nicole Verdecchia and Khoa Nguyen

STEM CASE AND KEY QUESTIONS

A 3-year-old boy with a history of sleep-disordered breathing and obstructive sleep apnea (OSA) is scheduled to undergo a tonsillectomy. You are performing a screening preoperative evaluation over the phone. His parents state that he has no other medical history and is otherwise healthy.

What is OSA syndrome? What are the indications for tonsillectomy?

Smith's *Anesthesia for Infants and Children* defines OSA as a disorder of breathing during sleep characterized by prolonged partial upper airway obstruction or intermittent complete obstruction with or without snoring and associated with moderate to severe oxygen desaturation that disrupts normal sleep time breathing and normal sleep patterns.[1] The most common cause for OSA is adenotonsillar hypertrophy causing narrowing of the upper airway. The peak prevalence of OSA in children is between 2 and 8 years of age. The two most common indications for tonsillectomy include recurrent throat infections and sleep-disordered breathing. Other indications for tonsillectomy include adenotonsillar hyperplasia with OSA, failure to thrive, abnormal dentofacial growth, malignancy, and hemorrhagic tonsillitis.[2,3]

What type of preoperative testing or information is needed prior to surgery? Are routine laboratory tests indicated?

You perform a careful review of the patient's medical history, and there is no personal or family history of bleeding events. You decide no preoperative testing is indicated.

What tests would you order in a child with a positive history of bleeding?

Unknown to you, the surgeon had already ordered a complete blood count and coagulation studies. The platelets are within normal limits, but the partial thromboplastin time (PTT) is noted to be 50.

The child's mother asks about the significance of the abnormal value. What do you tell her?

An isolated abnormal PTT in the absence of a bleeding history could represent a spurious value. When corroborated with a positive history of bleeding events, the most likely diagnoses are von Willebrand disease (vWD) followed by hemophilias or other factor deficiencies or inhibitors.

While you are speaking to the mother, the surgeon calls and tells you that he would like to proceed with the case despite the abnormal laboratory values due to the patient's lack of history of bleeding. How do you respond? What is the risk of proceeding with surgery with a prolonged PTT during tonsillectomy?

Undiagnosed coagulopathy can lead to post-tonsillectomy hemorrhage, which is considered a surgical emergency. Primary tonsillar hemorrhage occurs within the first 24 hours of surgery, and secondary bleeding occurs within 2 weeks.[4]

The risk of post-tonsillectomy hemorrhage increases with increasing age, male gender, recurrent tonsillitis, previous peritonsillar abscess, multiple bleeding episodes, and inherited or acquired coagulopathies (aspirin or anticoagulant therapy).[4]

Primary hemorrhage occurs in 0.2–2.2% and secondary hemorrhage in 0.1–3% of patients, often resulting in readmission and increased healthcare costs.[4]

Are there any other further laboratory tests that you need to order? Is a hematology consult indicated?

With an unexpected abnormal PTT, hematology should be consulted to determine a diagnosis, if any. Due to the complexity of laboratory testing and diagnosis of different coagulation disorders, an expert should be consulted.

What additional tests should be ordered to clarify the diagnosis?

Screening tests for vWD include plasma von Willebrand factor (vWF) antigen levels (vWF:Ag); plasma vWF activity, which is represented by ristocetin cofactor activity (vWF:RCo); and factor VIII activity. Based on the results of the tests, the child is diagnosed with type 1 vWD.

What are types of vWD, and how are they diagnosed? Are treatment modalities different?

Based on the results of the tests the child is diagnosed with type 1 vWD. The hematologist recommends desmopressin prior to tonsillectomy, and the procedure is uneventful.

In PACU, after several hours, the patient develops profuse bleeding from their mouth. What will you do?

Post-tonsillectomy hemorrhage is considered a surgical emergency. The patient should undergo a rapid-sequence induction to minimize the aspiration risk due to possible blood in the stomach. A difficult airway must be anticipated due to edema and blood in the airway. Multiple suction catheters should be available to help with visualization of the airway. Fluid management is also important as patients are often anemic and hypovolemic. Adequate IV access should be obtained, and blood products available.

DISCUSSION

PREOPERATIVE EVALUATION OF THE PEDIATRIC PATIENT

In general, all pediatric patients should undergo a full history and physical examination. Previous anesthesia history should be elicited, including previous airway management techniques and any risk factors for a difficult airway or airway abnormalities. Evaluating the cardiopulmonary system is also very important given the effects of anesthesia on these organ systems. If the patient has a history of congenital heart disease, it may be necessary to view a preoperative echocardiogram, ECG, or review recent heart catheterization reports. If the patient has pulmonary disease, it is necessary to view any sleep studies and pulmonary function tests, and discern what medications they are currently using. Medication lists should be reviewed, with attention to which medications are given on the day of surgery. Recent upper respiratory tract infections are an important thing to ask about, especially in the ear nose and throat (ENT) patient population, due to the increased risk of reactivity associated with the infectious process. Specific attention should be placed to a history of easy bruising, epistaxis, prolonged bleeding after other surgeries or dental extractions, or family history of bleeding diathesis. A significant bleeding history may lead to an increased risk of hemorrhage intraoperatively or postoperatively. Many institutions routinely draw preoperative laboratories including platelet counts and coagulation studies. Other important parts of the history include sleep patterns, snoring, poor school performance, or behavior problems that may elicit the risk of airway obstruction.

Tonsillectomy surgery is one of the most common pediatric surgical procedures performed annually in the United States and accounts for 16% of ambulatory surgeries in patients younger than 15 years of age.[3,5]

One of the most feared complications of tonsillectomy is post-tonsillectomy hemorrhage. This has led many hospital systems to routinely perform coagulation testing on pediatric patients, especially because tonsillectomy might be the first surgery or hemostatic challenge that a child has.[6–10] The rate of post-tonsillectomy hemorrhage ranges from 0% to 7% in different sources as described above.[6–10]

There have been several studies examining this issue, and there have been controversial conclusions. There is a group that recommends no screening at all, while some recommend screening only patients who have a positive history for bleeding or coagulation disorders, and some screen every patient routinely regardless of history.[11]

In the group that recommends no screening at all, the rationale is that bleeding complications are rare, and, even when coagulation screening is performed routinely, bleeding complications cannot be predicted or prevented. Coagulation disorders were not reliably detected by laboratory screening or by history alone.[11–14]

Many studies have been done that showed no differences in coagulation laboratory tests in bleeders versus nonbleeders, indicating that these tests do not predict bleeding outcomes.[15–21] Burk et al. performed a study that showed a large number of false positives, leading to unnecessary further testing.[10] In this study, they concluded that routine testing has a low predictive value due to poor sensitivity of testing and low prevalence of bleeding.[10] Sarny et al. showed that a positive history was significantly predictive of bleeding episodes, but positive laboratory values for coagulopathy were not associated with increased hemorrhage risk.[12] Asaf et al. concluded that coagulation screening tests should not be performed unless there is a positive medical history of bleeding tendency.[22] Eberl et al. showed that the positive predictive value of coagulation screening was 6.8% whereas history alone predicted 9.2% of bleeding episodes.[19]

On the other hand, Kang et al., Tami et al., Smith et al., and Licameli et al. showed elevated PTT in the bleeding populations in their studies. In this group of studies, routine screening for coagulation disorders identified patients who might bleed intraoperatively, leading to prevention.[23–26] They believe that patient history may not always identify bleeding disorders, and patient reliability must be questioned.[26]

The largest study performed, which included 4,374 children, compared bleeding complications in a group of patients who were selectively screened versus routinely screened and found that there were fewer bleeding episodes in the selective screening group compared with the routinely screened group.[7] Furthermore, the patients who did have bleeding disorders were not discovered by routine preoperative testing but were known in advance.[7]

BLEEDING DISORDERS IN PEDIATRIC PATIENTS

There are three phases of hemostasis: the endothelial injury and platelet plug, the coagulation cascade, and termination of clotting by antithrombotic mechanisms.[1,27–29]

The initial response for primary hemostasis is the platelet plug, which is activated by endothelial injury. When platelets encounter an injured endothelium, they undergo physical and biochemical changes leading to adhesion, activation, and aggregation[1,29–32] (Figure 28.1).

Secondary hemostasis via the clotting cascade occurs next and involves a series of pro-enzymes, enzymes, and clotting factors. Multiple cofactors are involved in this process.[29,32,33]

The third phase is the termination of coagulation and fibrinolysis. This involves antithrombin, tissue factor inhibitor, and protein C. Additionally, plasminogen binds to fibrin and to tissue plasminogen activator to form plasmin, which breaks down clot. Protein C works by inhibiting Va and VIIIa, and protein C requires a cofactor called Protein S.[1,29,34,35]

The extrinsic pathway begins when the endothelial vessel wall is damaged and causes the release of tissue factor, which initiates plasma-mediated hemostasis.[36] Tissue factor (TF) is a cofactor that assists in the production of activated

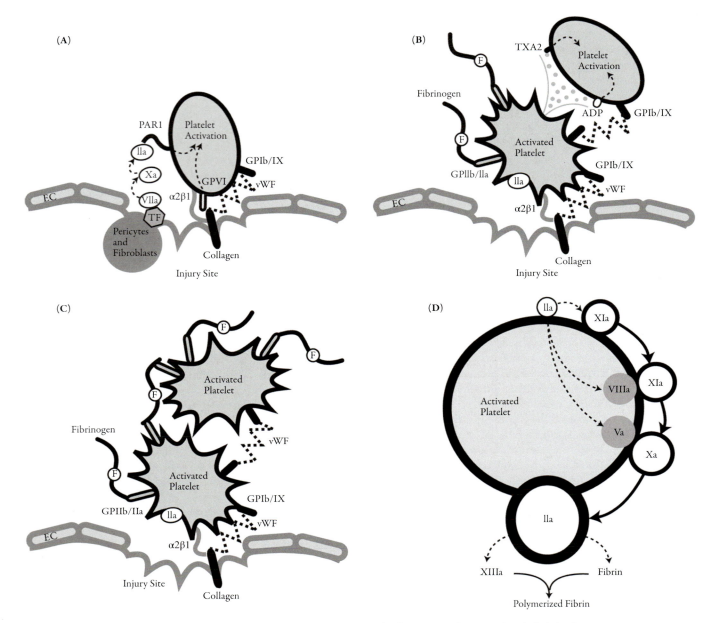

Figure 28.1 Clot formation at injury site. A. At the site of injured endothelial cells (EC), platelets adhere to subendothelial collagen via interactions between von Willebrand factor (vWF) and platelet-surface glycoprotein receptor (GP), GPIb/IX. The platelet integrin receptor (α2β1) reinforces the binding to collagen. Trace amounts of thrombin are generated during the initiation phase of coagulation by FXa via interactions between circulating FVIIa and tissue factor (TF) expressed on subendothelial pericytes and fibroblasts. B. Platelets activated by collagen and thrombin release adenosine-diphosphate (ADP) and thromboxane (TXA2), which activate platelets in the vicinity. C. Activated platelets express GPIIb/IIIa and capture fibrinogen (F). On the activated platelet surface, thrombin-mediated feedback activations of FXI, FVIII, and FV result in the propagation phase of thrombin generation. Sustained activation of prothrombin is feasible via formation of tenase (activated FIX-FVIII) and prothrombinase (activated FX-FV). D. Polymerization of fibrin is achieved by thrombin-activated FXIII during the propagation phase.
With permission from Bolliger D. Anesthesiology. 2010 Nov;113(5):1205–1219.

factor VII. The TF–VII complex then activates factor X in the final common pathway, as well as factor IX from the intrinsic pathway. The extrinsic pathway is responsible for initiating clotting.[29,32–35]

The intrinsic pathway, on the other hand, is activated by contact with a negatively charged surface. This starts with factor XII, which subsequently activates factor XI, which then activates factor IX. Factor IX forms a complex with factor VIII to activate factor X in the common pathway. Factor VIII can be activated by both factor X and thrombin, which is a positive feedback loop. The intrinsic pathway is responsible for the amplification of the clotting cascade.[36,37]

Both the extrinsic and intrinsic pathways converge to form the final common pathway, which includes factor Xa, factor V, prothrombin (II), and fibrinogen (I). More specifically, factor Xa linked to cofactor Va converts prothrombin (II) to thrombin (IIa). Thrombin proceeds to convert fibrinogen to fibrin. Thrombin also assists in activating factors XI, VIII, and V.[29,37] Finally, factor XIII stabilizes and crosslinks the overlapping fibrin strands.[29]

LABORATORY TESTS EVALUATING COAGULATION

Most clotting factors are made in the liver. However, factor VIII and vWF are made in endothelial cells. Some factors depend on vitamin K, including VII, IX, X, protein C, and protein S.[1,29]

Prothrombin time (PT) is a measure of the extrinsic and final common pathway of the coagulation cascade. It represents the number of seconds for a patient's plasma to clot after being exposed to calcium and thromboplastin, which is an activator of the extrinsic pathway.[28]

The activated partial thromboplastin time, or PTT, measures the intrinsic and final common pathway of the coagulation cascade. This represents the number of seconds for a patient's plasma to clot after calcium and phospholipid are added, which activate the intrinsic pathway. No tissue factor is present, unlike in the measurement of PT.[28]

DIFFERENTIAL DIAGNOSIS OF COAGULATION DISORDERS

Disorders of coagulation can involve platelets, the coagulation cascade, or the fibrinolytic system. There are many inherited and/or acquired disorders within each system.

Inherited platelet disorders are very rare and include syndromes such as Wiskott-Aldrich syndrome, Bernard-Soulier syndrome, and X-linked thrombocytopenia, among many others.[38] Acquired platelet disorders are comprised of antiplatelet drugs such as aspirin, clopidogrel, prasugrel, ticlopidine, abciximab, eptifbatide, and tirofiban[39,40]; liver dysfunction; renal disease; disseminated intravascular coagulation (DIC); myeloproliferative disorders; trauma, immune thrombocytopenia (ITP); and many more.[1,28,41–43]

Inherited coagulation disorders can involve the intrinsic or extrinsic pathway. Inherited coagulation disorders involving the intrinsic pathway include vWD, hemophilia A and B, factor XI deficiency, factor XIII deficiency, and acquired factor inhibitors.[28,39]

Acquired coagulation disorders also can be separated by intrinsic or extrinsic pathway mechanisms. Heparin and low-molecular-weight heparin (LMWH) have a greater effect on the intrinsic pathway, while warfarin and other vitamin K-dependent anticoagulant drugs affect the extrinsic pathway.[39,44] Liver failure and DIC can affect coagulation factors from both pathways.[41,43]

Disorders of platelets will result in thrombocytopenia or abnormal platelet morphology and a prolonged bleeding time. Disorders of the extrinsic pathway will result in a prolonged INR, while disorders of the intrinsic pathway result in prolonged PTT. Clinical context and other laboratory tests must be taken into consideration to further pinpoint a diagnosis.[28]

DIFFERENTIAL DIAGNOSIS OF AN ISOLATED ELEVATED PTT

The differential diagnosis includes disorders that prolong PTT but likely have normal platelet count and normal PT/INR. These include vWD, hemophilia A or B, factor VIII, IX, or XI deficiencies, or intrinsic pathway factor inhibitors, heparin, LMWH, direct thrombin inhibitors, liver disease, disseminated intravascular coagulation, vitamin K deficiency or vitamin K dependent factor deficiency, and antiphospholipid antibody syndrome.[1,28]

Liver disease, vitamin K deficiency, vitamin K-dependent factor deficiencies, and DIC present with other laboratory abnormalities such as thrombocytopenia, prolonged INR, and abnormal liver function tests (LFTs), and these should not be present in an otherwise healthy child. Factors involved in the final common pathway also affect the PT/INR.

Another cause of elevated PTT is lupus anticoagulant, which may not correlate to clinical bleeding.[45,46] In fact, in 36% of cases referred for consultation in one study, abnormal PTT indicated no risk of bleeding disorders and may have been artifactually elevated.[46] One example of this is that factor XII defects can cause PTT elevation but have no clinical significance.[7]

COAGULATION DISORDERS IN PEDIATRIC POPULATION

The most common bleeding disorder in this population is vWD, which, despite having low vWF levels, may show normal PTT on screening tests. In fact, stress, underlying disease, and blood type can cause changes in vWF levels, which makes diagnosis difficult to pinpoint, especially on screening laboratory values.[47–50] The laboratory diagnosis of vWD is complicated, requiring four different tests.[51] Therefore, even if PTT is routinely done on patients, vWD diagnosis may be missed. The clinical history would be valuable in diagnosing this disorder prior to tonsillectomy to avoid hemorrhage. Since the disease is usually autosomal dominant, a family history would be likely to reveal the diagnosis. Moreover, another study showed that there was no significant difference in the number of bleeding events between patients with vWD and patients without vWD based on laboratory values alone.[51]

The second most common bleeding disorder in this population is hemophilia.[1] Again, this is a difficult disease to screen for because the predictive value of screening tests is low. PTT is insensitive, hemophilia is rare, and only severe or moderate types can even be detected.[15,29,52]

Von Willebrand Disease

vWD is the most common inherited bleeding disorder and is defined as either a qualitative or quantitative deficiency in vWF). vWF is a multimeric glycoprotein made in endothelial cells and megakaryocytes. vWF plays an important role in platelet adhesion during tissue injury by binding to platelets at the glycoprotein Ib receptor and endothelial cells. It also carries factor VIII in plasma, which contributes to fibrin clot formation. Patients with vWD present with history of easy bruising, recurrent epistaxis, menorrhagia, and mucocutaneous bleeding.[53-59]

There are multiple types of vWD. Type I is characterized by a qualitative deficiency of vWF, is autosomal dominant, and accounts for 75% of patients. Type II is also autosomal dominant and characterized by a qualitative defect in the vWF. Type 2A accounts for 10–15% of cases and has smaller, ineffective vWF multimers. Type IIb makes up 5% of cases and is characterized by abnormal vWF that binds more readily to platelets, which causes sequestration of platelets. This can lead to thrombocytopenia. Type III is the rarest and most severe as the patient has no detectable vWF. Types 2M and 2N are also extremely rare and produce defects in binding to platelets and factor VIII. There are many genetic mutations within the vWF gene that have been identified in vWD.[53-59]

Diagnosis of vWD

The diagnosis of vWD is complicated as there are multiple lab tests that fluctuate, making diagnosis difficult. In addition, the several types of vWD are managed differently. Guidelines and recommendations are provided by a panel of experts that describe when it is appropriate to order specific lab testing after initial screening is complete[59] (Figure 28.2).

The initial workup of any type of bleeding disorder includes platelet count and coagulation studies like PTT. Other tests of interest include closure time with PFA-100, which analyzes platelet function; plasma vWF antigen levels (vWF:Ag); plasma vWF activity, which is represented by ristocetin cofactor activity (vWF:RCo) that measures interaction with platelets and vWF collagen binding; and factor VIII activity. vWF multimer size distribution using gel electrophoresis and ristocetin-induced platelet aggregation (RIPA) can also be completed.[54,59] Finally, vWF:CB, a comparison of vWF collagen binding with vWF multimer distribution, has been shown to be a sensitive screening test for vWD types 2A and 2B.[54,55,60] There are also newer tests that measure the platelet-binding activity of vWF, called vWF:GP1bM and vWF:GPIbR, that are more accurate than the vWF:RCo, and these are now recommended for use.[59]

Laboratory findings for type I vWD include increased bleeding time, normal platelet count, reduced vWF antigen, reduced ristocetin cofactor activity, and reduced factor VIII activity with a normal vWF:RCo/vWF:Ag ratio. There is a decrease in normal vWF multimers.[54-57,59,60]

Type IIa vWD laboratory values show normal platelet counts, increased bleeding time, reduced vWF:RCo/vWF:Ag ratio, and normal to slightly low vWF antigen levels.[54,59]

In type IIb vWD, the bleeding time is elevated, the platelet count is reduced, the vWF:Ag is normal or slightly reduced, and the vWF:RCo/vWF:Ag ratio is markedly reduced.[54-57,60]

If a diagnosis of vWD cannot be made by these laboratory values, then further lab testing must be completed to determine an alternative diagnosis.

Treatment Options in vWD

It is impossible to treat vWD without determining the type of vWD the patient has. Most commonly, patients have type I vWD and can be treated with desmopressin (DDAVP). Normally, a trial of DDAVP would be completed to assess response prior to surgery or actual need. Another option is to treat with vWF-containing concentrates, such as Humate-P and Alphanate. If a patient has type IIb vWD, DDAVP will worsen their clinical symptoms and cause further thrombocytopenia. DDAVP is also not useful in type III vWD. In these cases, patients must be treated with vWF-containing concentrates. Other options include antifibrinolytics, estrogen therapy, or topical therapy with thrombin or fibrin sealant. Of note, cryoprecipitate is not recommended for treatment of vWD.[55-57,61,63]

Hemophilias

Hemophilia A is an X-linked disorder of factor VIII deficiency, occurs in 1/5,000 male births, and is more likely to be severe. Hemophilia B is an X-linked disorder of factor IX deficiency and occurs in 1/30,000 male births. These deficiencies in clotting factors lead to spontaneous bleeding within joints, deep muscles, or other organ systems.[64] Classically, laboratory values include a prolonged PTT with normal PT since factors are involved in the intrinsic pathway. However, mild forms of the disease may have normal PTT values. The diagnosis is confirmed with factor level testing, and mixing studies will show a correction of PTT as long as there are no additional inhibitors present.[1,29,64]

Diagnosis and Management of Hemophilias

Hemophilia is often diagnosed after a patient presents with a bleeding episode, whether it be spontaneous or after a procedure. Other times, patients have laboratory tests drawn and an isolated aPTT is discovered. The confirmation of a hemophilia diagnosis requires several steps.[65] First, heparin contamination must be ruled out in a patient with an elevated aPTT. The next step is to complete a mixing study where the patient's plasma is mixed with normal plasma with normal clotting factors. If the aPTT does not correct to a normal value, an acquired hemophilia with a factor VIII or factor IX inhibitor is likely, and this commonly developed in hemophilia patients. If mixing study results in correction of aPTT, then hereditary hemophilia may be likely. A low factor VIII level must also be demonstrated for hemophilia A, and low factor IX must be demonstrated for hemophilia B. Other factor deficiencies or a lupus anticoagulant must also be ruled out with the appropriate testing.[65,66]

The primary goal in management for hemophilia is to prevent hemorrhage. For hemophilia A treatment options include desmopressin or factor concentrates. For major surgeries the levels of factor VIII should be kept between 80%

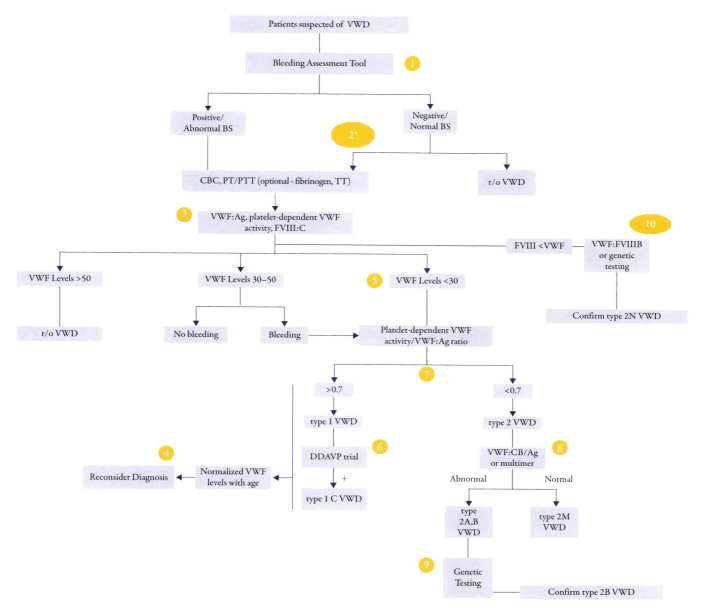

Figure 28.2 An overall algorithm addressing the diagnosis of vWD. The numbers in the yellow circles correspond to guideline questions. vWF levels refer to vWF antigen (vWF:Ag) and/or platelet-dependent vWF activity. The algorithm says vWF level 30–50 for simplicity; this refers to vWF levels of 0.30–0.50 IU/mL, with the caveat that the lower limit of the normal range as determined by the local laboratory should be used if it is <0.50 IU/mL.
*Men and children, referred to a hematologist and/or first-degree relative affected with vWD. BS, bleeding score; CBC, complete blood count; DDAVP, desmopressin; FVIII, factor FVIII; FVIII:C, FVIII coagulant activity; PT, prothrombin time; PTT, partial thromboplastin time; r/o, rule out; TT, thrombin time; vWF:CB/Ag, ratio of vWF collagen binding to antigen; vWF:FVIIIB, vWF FVIII binding.
With permission from James PD. *Blood Adv*. 2021 Jan 12;5(1):280–300.

and 100% whereas for minor procedures levels of more than 40% should suffice. It is important to note that giving factor VIII concentrate is often ineffective if the patient has inhibitors to this factor, so bypassing that part of the coagulation cascade is necessary using activated prothrombin complex concentrate/factor eight inhibitor bypassing activity (FEIBA) or recombinant factor VII.[65,66]

In patients with hemophilia B, desmopressin is not an option, and the coagulopathy is corrected by factor IX concentrates or prothrombin complex concentrates.

CONCLUSION

- The goal of preoperative testing is to predict patients who will bleed postoperatively after tonsillectomy. History alone may not be enough to predict this risk. However, it is not clear that coagulation studies preoperatively will predict this risk either.

- If a normal patient has an abnormal coagulation study incidentally, it is not clear if this would predict bleeding.

- Based on extensive literature, the American Academy of Otolaryngology, Head and Neck Surgery recommends performing coagulation screening tests only in patients with suspicious histories and not routinely.[6,7,67] There are several reasons for this recommendation that involve the insensitive nature of testing rare diseases, the poor cost effectiveness of these tests, and the lack of data showing that abnormal testing predicts bleeding.

- Due to the large number of surgeries performed annually and the low rate of hemorrhage, it is not cost effective to test every patient routinely. In fact, it is estimated to cost more than a half billion dollars to routinely screen for bleeding disorders during tonsillectomy.[48,67] Furthermore, having abnormal coagulation lab values does not necessarily lead to bleeding diathesis, and many coagulopathies are clinically insignificant.

REVIEW QUESTIONS

1. The most common indication for tonsillectomy in pediatric patients is

    a. Failure to thrive.
    b. Malignancy.
    c. Abnormal dentofacial growth.
    d. Sleep disordered breathing.

The correct answer is d.

The most common indication for tonsillectomy in pediatric patients is sleep disordered breathing.

2. Which of the following is the coagulopathy most commonly see in pediatric patients presenting for tonsillectomy?

    a. Hemophilia A.
    b. vWD.
    c. Hereditary thrombocytopenia
    d. Hemophilia B.

The correct answer is b.

The most common cause of coagulopathy in pediatric patients presenting for tonsillectomy is vWD, while the hemophilias are less prevalent.

3. Which of the following must be treated with von Willebrand concentrate instead of DDAVP?

    a. vWD type I.
    b. vWD type IIa.
    c. vWD type IIb.
    d. Hemophilia A.

The correct answer is c.

Desmopressin is contraindicated in treating vWD type IIb, where DDAVP will release hyperfunctional vWD multimers with the potential of increased platelet aggregation and worsening thrombocytopenia.

4. The risk of post-tonsillectomy hemorrhage increase with all of the following *except*:

    a. Increasing age.
    b. Female gender.
    c. Recurrent tonsillitis.
    d. Previous peritonsillar abscess.

The correct answer is b.

Males are at risk of increased posttonsillectomy bleed, as are those with recurrent tonsillitis, previous peritonsillar abscess, and increasing age.

5. The American Academy of Otolaryngology, Head and Neck Surgery do not recommend routine preoperative coagulation screening for tonsillectomy due the following reasons:

    a. Insensitive nature of testing rare diseases.
    b. Poor cost effectiveness.
    c. Lack of data to support that abnormal tests predict postoperative bleeding.
    d. All the above.

The correct answer is d.

There are several reasons for this recommendation which involve the insensitive nature of testing for rare diseases, the poor cost effectiveness of these tests, and the lack of data showing that abnormal testing predicts bleeding.

REFERENCES

1. Vanderhoek SM, Dalesio NM, Schwengel DA. Anesthesia for otorhinolaryngologic surgery. In: Davis PJ, Cladis FP, Motoyama EK, eds. *Smith's Anesthesia for Infants and Children*. 8th ed. Elsevier Health Sciences; 2017:917–944.
2. Darrow DH, Siemens C. Indications for tonsillectomy and adenoidectomy. *Laryngoscope*. 2002;6–10.
3. Patel HH, Straight CE, Lehman EB, Tanner M, Carr MM. Indications for tonsillectomy: A 10 year retrospective review. *Int J Pediatr Otolaryngol*. 2014;78:2151–2155.
4. Myssiorek D, Alvi A. Post-tonsillectomy hemorrhage: An assessment of risk factors. *Int J Pediatr Otorhinolaryngol*. 1996;27:35–43.
5. Baugh RF, Archer SM, Mitchell RB, et al. Clinical practice guidelines: Tonsillectomy in children. *Otolaryngol Head Neck Surg*. 2011;144(IS)SI–S30.
6. Hartnick CJ, Ruben RJ. Preoperative coagulation studies prior to tonsillectomy. *Arch Otolaryngol Head Neck Surg*. 2000;126:684–686.
7. Zwack GC, Derkay CS. The utility of preoperative hemostatic assessment in adenotonsillectomy. *Int J Pediatr Otorhinolaryngol*. 1997;39:67–76.
8. Osborne MS, Clark MPA. The surgical arrest of post-tonsillectomy haemorrhage: Hospital episode statistics 12 years on. *Ann R Coll Surg Engl*. 2018;100(5):406–408.
9. Johnson RF, Chang A, Mitchell RB. Nationwide readmissions after tonsillectomy among pediatric patients – United States. *Int J Pediatr Otolaryngol*. 2018;107:10–13.
10. Burk CD, Miller L, Handler SD, Cohen AR. Preoperative history and coagulation screening in children undergoing tonsillectomy. *Pediatrics*. 1992;89(1):691–695.
11. D Kendrick, K Gibbin. An audit of the complications in pediatric tonsillectomy, adenoidectomy and adenotonsillectomy. *Clin Otolaryngol*. 1993;18:115–117.
12. Sarny S, Ossimitz G, Habermann W, Stammberger H. Preoperative coagulation screening prior to tonsillectomy in adults: Current practice and recommendations. *Eur Arch Otorhinolarngol*. 2013;270(3):1099–1104.
13. Gabriel P, Mazoit X, Ecoffey C. Relationship between clinical history, coagulation tests, and perioperative bleeding during tonsillectomies in pediatrics. *J Clin Anesth*. 2000;12:288–291.

14. Bidlingmaier C, Olivieri M, Stelter K, et al. Postoperative bleeding in paediatric ENT surgery: First results of the German ESPED trial. *Hamostaseologie*. 2010;30:S108–S111.
15. Manning SC, Beste D, McBride T, Goldberg A. An assessment of preoperative coagulation screening for tonsillectomy and adenoidectomy. *Int. J. Pediatr. Otorhinolaryngol*. 1987;13:237–244.
16. Close HL, Kryzer TC, Nowlin JH, Alving BM. Hemostatic assessment of patients before tonsillectomy: A prospective study. *Otolaryngol. Head Neck Surg*. 1994;11(6):733–738.
17. Handler SD, Miller L, Richmond KH, Baranak CC. Post tonsillectomy hemorrhage: Incidence, prevention and management. *Laryngoscope*. 1986;96:1243–1247.
18. Thomas GK, Arbon RA. Preoperative screening for potential T and A bleeding. *Arch Otolaryngol Head Neck Surg*. 1970;91:453–456.
19. Eberl W, Wendt I, Schroeder HG. Preoperative coagulation screening prior to adenoidectomy and tonsillectomy. *Klin Padiatr*. 2005;217:20–24.
20. Eisert S, Hovermann M, Bier H, Gobel U. Preoperative screening for coagulation disorders in children undergoing adenoidectomy (AT) and tonsillectomy (TE): Does it prevent bleeding complications? *Klin Padiatr*. 2006;218:334–339.
21. Schwaab M, Hansen S, Gurr A, Dazert S. Significance of blood tests prior to adenoidectomy. *Laryngorhinootologie*. 2008;87:100–106.
22. Asaf T, Reuveni H, Yermiahu T, et al. The need for routine preoperative coagulation screening tests (Prothrombin time PT/partial thromboplastin time PTT) for healthy children undergoing elective tonsillectomy and/or adenoidectomy. *Int J Pediatri Otorhinolaryngol*. 2001;61:217–222.
23. Licameli GR, Jones DT, Santosuosso J, et al. Use of a preoperative bleeding questionnaire in pediatric patients who undergo adenotonsillectomy. *Otolaryngol Head Neck Surg*. 2008;139:546–550.
24. Smith PS, Orchard PJ, Lekas MD. Predicting bleeding in common ear, nose and throat procedures: A prospective study. *R. I. Med. J*. 1990;73:103–106.
25. Tami TA, Parker GS, Taylor RE. Post-tonsillectomy bleeding: An evaluation of risk factors. *Laryngoscope*. 1987;97:1307–1311.
26. Kang J, Brodsky L, Daniger I, Volk M, Stanievich J. Coagulation profile as a predictor for post-tonsillectomy and adenoidectomy (T+A) hemorrhage. *Int J Pediatr Otorhinolaryngol*. 1994;28:157–165.
27. Bolliger D, Gorlinger K, Tanaka KA. Pathophysiology and treatment of coagulopathy in massive hemorrhage and hemodilution. *Anesthesiology*. 2010;113(5):1205–1219.
28. Kamal AH, Tefferi A, Pruthi RK. How to interpret and pursue an abnormal prothrombin time, activated partial thromboplastin time, and bleeding time in adults. *Mayo Clin Proc*. 2007;82:864–873.
29. Hilgartner MW, Corrigan JJ Jr. Coagulations. In: Miller DR, Baehner RL, Miller LP, eds. *Blood Diseases of Infancy and Childhood*. 7th ed. CV Moseby; 1995:924–986.
30. Broos K, Feys HB, De Meyer SF, et al. Blood platelet biochemistry. *Thromb Res*. 2012;129:245–249.
31. Broos K, Feys HB, De Meyer SF, et al. Platelets at work in primary hemostasis. *Blood Rev*. 2011;25:155–167.
32. Furie B, Furie BC. Mechanisms of thrombus formation. *N Engl J Med*. 2008;359:938–949.
33. Hoffman M. Remodeling the blood coagulation cascade. *J Thromb Thrombolysis*. 2003;16:17–20.
34. Rezaie AR. Regulation of the protein C anticoagulant and antiinflammatory pathways. *Curr Med Chem*. 2010;19:2059–2069.
35. Schenone M, Furie BC, Furie B. The blood coagulation cascade. *Curr Opin Hematol*. 2004;11:272–277.
36. Furie B, Furie BC. In vivo thrombus formation. *J Thromb Haemost*. 2007;5:12–17.
37. Crawley JT, Zanardelli S, Chion CK, et al. The central role of thrombin in hemostasis. *J Thromb Haemost*. 2007;5:95–101.
38. Bolton-Maggs PH, Chalmers EA, Collins PW, et al. A review of inherited platelet disorders with guidelines for their management on behalf of the UKHCDO. *Br J Haematol*. 2006;135:603.
39. Roberts HR, Monroe DM, Escobar MA. Current concepts of hemostasis: Implications for therapy. *Anesthesiology*. 2004;100:722–730.
40. Hall R, Mazer CD. Antiplatelet drugs: A review of their pharmacology and management in the perioperative period. *Anesth Analg*. 2011;112:292–318.
41. Tripodi A, Mannucci PM. The coagulopathy of chronic liver disease. *N Engl J Med*. 2011;365:147–156.
42. Kaw D, Malhotra D. Platelet dysfunction and end-stage renal disease. *Semin Dial*. 2006;19:317–322.
43. Kaneko T, Wada H. Diagnostic criteria and laboratory tests for disseminated intravascular coagulation. *J Clin Exp Hematop*. 2011;51:67–76.
44. Mannucci PM, Franchini M. Old and new anticoagulant drugs: A minireview. *Ann Med*. 2011;43:116–123.
45. Fuller AM. Evauulation and management of coagulation disorders in elective surgical patients. *Laryngoscope*. 1981;91:1484–1500.
46. Lind SE. The bleeding time does not predict surgical bleeding. *Blood* 1991;77(12):2547–2551.
47. Bolger WE, Parsons DS, Potempa L. Preoperative hemostatic assessment of the adenotonsillectomy patient. *Arch Otolaryngol Head Neck Surg*. 1990;103:396–405.
48. Derkay CS. Pediatric otolaryngology procedures in the United States. *Int J Pediatr Otorhinolarynol*. 1977–1987;25:1–12.
49. Perry JJ, Alving BM. Von Willebrand's disease. *Am. Family Pract*. 1990;41:219–224.
50. Cox Gill J. Diagnosis and treatment of von Willebrand disease. *Hematol Oncol Clin North Am*. 2004;18:1277–1299, viii.
51. Krishna P, Lee D. Post-tonsillectomy bleeding: A meta-analysis. *Laryngoscope*. 2001;111:1358–1361.
52. Derkay CS, Werner E, Plotnick E. Management of children with von Willebrand disease undergoing adenotonsillectomy. *Am J Otolaryngol*. 1996;17:172–177.
53. Sadler JE. New concepts in von Willebrand disease. *Annu Rev Med*. 2005;56:173–191.
54. de Faria FC, Henneberg R, do Nascimento AJ, Kubo KS, Frigeri HR, da Silva PH. Von Willebrand disease lab diagnosis. *Indian J Hematol Blood Transfus*. 2016;32(2):135–140.
55. Yawn BP, Nichols WL, Rick ME. Diagnosis and management of Von Willebrand disease: Guidelines for primary care. *American Academy of Family Physicians*. 2009;80(11):1261–1268.
56. Peyvandi F, Garagiola I, Baronciani L. Role of von Willebrand factor in haemostasis. *Blood Transfus*. 2011;9:S3–S8.
57. Nichols WL, Hultin MB, James AH, et al. von Willebrand disease (vWD): Evidence-based diagnosis and management guidelines, the National Heart, Lung, and Blood Institute (NHLBI) Expert Panel report (USA). *Haemophilia*. 2008;14:171.
58. O'Brien SH, Saini, S. von Willebrand disease in pediatrics: Evaluation and management. *Hematol Oncol Clin N Am*. 2019;33(3):425–438.
59. James, PD, Connell NT, Ameer B, et al. ASH ISTH NHF WFH 2021 guidelines on the diagnosis of von Willebrand disease. *Blood Adv*. 2021;5(1):280–300.
60. Greaves M, Watson HG. Approach to the diagnosis and management of mild bleeding disorders. *J Thromb Haemost*. 2007;5:167–174.
61. Leebeek FWG, Eikenboom JCJ. Von Willebrand's disease. *N Engl J Med*. 2016;375:2067–2080.
62. Harper P, Favaloro EJ, Curtin J, Barnes C, Dunkley S. Human plasma-derived FVIII/vWD concentrate (Biostate): A review of experimental and clinical pharmacokinetic, efficacy and safety data. *Drugs Context*. 2016;8(5):212–229.
63. Lusher JM. Clinical guidelines for treating von Willebrand disease patients who are not candidates for DDAVP—A survey of European physicians. *Haemophilia*. 1998;4(Suppl 3):11.
64. Carcao MD. The diagnosis and management of congenital hemophilia. *Semin Thromb Hemost*. 2012;28:727.
65. Charlebois J, Rivard GE, St-Louis J. Management of acquired hemophilia A: Review of current evidence. *Transfus Apheresis Sci*. 2018;57(6):717–720.
66. Franchini M, Mannuucci P. Hemophilia A in the third millennium. *Blood Rev*. 2013;27(4):179–184.
67. The American Academy of Otolaryngology-Head and Neck Surgery. Clinical Indicators Compendium. Alexandria, VA: American Academy of Otolaryngology-Head and Neck Surgery; 1999.

ENDOCRINE

29.

ELEVATED GLUCOSE ON ADMISSION FINGERSTICK

HOW HIGH CAN WE GO?

Lindsay E. Carafone, Colin E. Bauer, Joshua D. Miller, and Steven D. Wittlin

STEM CASE AND KEY QUESTIONS

An obese 47-year-old woman with history of hypertension, hyperlipidemia, and uncontrolled type 2 diabetes (T2DM) presents to her primary care physician (PCP) with worsening, months-long, postprandial, colicky, right upper quadrant abdominal pain and is diagnosed with cholelithiasis. She is referred to a surgeon and advised to undergo elective laparoscopic cholecystectomy.

Which surgical procedures are impacted by presence of T2DM? What key elements in this patient's history must be addressed preoperatively?

Prior to scheduling her surgery and at the surgeon's request, the patient visits the hospital's preoperative evaluation clinic for "medical clearance." Review of her history reveals a maternal family history of T2DM as well as a personal history of hypertension of 6 years' duration, well-controlled on thiazide and angiotensin-converting enzyme (ACE) inhibitor, and hyperlipidemia of 8 years' duration on atorvastatin (recent LDL-C = 87 mg/dL). She was diagnosed with T2DM 11 years ago at an annual physical examination with her PCP.

What is the impact of disease duration on complication risk in patients with DM? Which diabetes-associated complications can specifically impact perioperative risk?

At time of DM diagnosis, she was started on 500 mg extended-release metformin by mouth daily, rapidly titrated to the current dose of 1,000 mg twice daily. Five years ago, the sulfonylurea, glimepiride, was added to her regimen, and, last year, she began taking the noninsulin, injectable glucagon-like-peptide-1 (GLP1) receptor agonist, liraglutide, once daily. At her most recent PCP visit last month, the long-acting basal insulin, glargine, was added to her regimen, 20 units at bedtime.

How does medication regimen impact perioperative planning in patients with T2DM undergoing surgery? What issues specific to insulin use must be addressed in patients with DM undergoing surgery? What laboratory testing is essential to assessing glycemic control and perioperative risk in patients with DM?

The patient reports monitoring her home "fingerstick" glucose 2–3 times daily before meals. Her most recent dilated eye examination was 6 months prior to presentation and normal by report. On physical examination in clinic, the patient has a BMI of 36 kg/m² blood pressure of 132/76 mm Hg, and pulse of 72 beats per minute (bpm). She appears nontoxic and has slight acanthosis at the neck along with mild dorsocervical fullness. She has centripetal obesity with nonviolaceous striae and mild tenderness to deep palpation of the right upper abdominal quadrant. In addition to an unremarkable ECG, point-of-care hemoglobin A1c (HbA1c) testing in clinic was 8.2%.

What is the relationship between HbA1c and risk of perioperative complications?

The patient has strong bilateral dorsalis pedis pulses and no pedal edema. She has decreased sensation to monofilament testing in the lower extremities at the first and second digits. She has decreased vibratory perception to 128 Hz tuning fork in the great toes bilaterally. She does not have any evidence of skin breakdown, ulceration, or Charcot foot. The remainder of the examination was unremarkable.

What perioperative complications may develop in patients with diabetes-related microvascular comorbidities? How might presence of diabetes-related complications specifically impact intraoperative anesthesia care?

The patient is scheduled for elective laparoscopic cholecystectomy the following week.

What diabetes-specific instructions are needed to prepare this patient for surgery? What diabetes-specific information should be conveyed to the surgical team?

In addition to fasting on the night prior to procedure, the patient is advised to hold her metformin 24 hours prior to surgery. She is further advised to take two-thirds the dose of her nighttime basal insulin the night prior to surgery and to hold her glimepiride and liraglutide on the morning of surgery. She is scheduled as one of the first cases on the morning of surgery.

How frequently should a patient with DM assess blood sugar in the days preceding elective surgery? What treatment options can patients consider to address preoperative hyperglycemia leading up to surgery?

The patient follows the clinic's preoperative medication recommendations. She arrives to the ambulatory surgery center on the morning of her scheduled surgery. In the preoperative assessment area, capillary fingerstick glucose is 325 mg/dL. She otherwise appears well, euvolemic with vital signs within normal limits.

Is a single glucose assessment enough data to inform a decision to proceed with surgery in patients with DM? What other data are needed to risk-stratify patients with DM on the morning of surgery?

Following initial glucose assessment, the patient receives 6 units of rapid-acting, SQ insulin lispro. The case is delayed and a recheck 2 hours later shows a fingerstick blood glucose of 163 mg/dL. She then undergoes an uneventful elective laparoscopic cholecystectomy lasting just over an hour. While in recovery, fingerstick glucose was 182 mg/dL. The patient was discharged home 12 hours postoperatively, advised to slowly advance her diet in the coming days and to resume her home diabetes regimen. She follows up with her surgeon 1 week postoperatively and with her PCP shortly thereafter.

DISCUSSION

The diabetes epidemic affects more than 37 million Americans— 11.3% of the US population. Additionally nearly 40% of US adults aged 18 year or older suffer from pre-diabetes.[1] There are approximately 1.4 million new cases of DM diagnosed annually in the United States.[1] Diabetes is classified by the pathogenesis of the disease in the individual. At least 90–95% of people with DM have type 2 with relative insulin deficiency due to a combination of decreased insulin production and insulin resistance. It has been suggested that the pathogenesis of T2DM falls along a spectrum from primary insulin deficiency to major insulin resistance.[2] The remaining 5–10% of patients with DM have type 1 due to pancreatic beta-cell failure or other secondary types. Complications from uncontrolled and long-standing DM are numerous. Diabetes, along with its comorbidities, can greatly impact perioperative risk for all types of surgeries, from elective to emergent. Thorough preoperative assessment of patients with diabetes is imperative in ensuring that patients are optimized for surgery and that safety is addressed throughout the spectrum of perioperative care.

DIAGNOSIS

Diagnostic criteria for DM, as established by the American Diabetes Association, are[3]

1. Symptoms of hyperglycemia (such as polyuria, polydipsia, polyphagia) plus a random plasma glucose 200 mg/dL (11.1 mmol/L) or higher

or

2. Fasting plasma glucose level 126 mg/dL (7.0 mmol/L) or higher performed after no caloric intake for at least 8 hours

or

3. HbA1c 6.5% (48 mmol/mol) or higher

or

4. Two-hour plasma glucose 200 mg/dL (11.1 mmol/L) or higher during an oral glucose tolerance test (OGTT)

LONG-TERM COMPLICATIONS AND ASSOCIATED PERIOPERATIVE RISK

Chronic hyperglycemia results in end-organ pathology including nephropathy, coronary artery disease, cerebrovascular disease, retinopathy, peripheral neuropathy, cardiac autonomic neuropathy, gastroparesis, and peripheral vascular disease, among others. Peripheral vascular disease puts patients at greater risk for surgical site infections and poor wound healing.[4]

Patients with DM may have difficulty with glycemic control with concurrent risk of hypoglycemia. Repeated hypoglycemic episodes may cause hypoglycemia unawareness in that neuroglycopenic symptoms only occur at increasingly lower glucose thresholds. Alternatively, patients may have hyperglycemia, glucose toxicity, and can develop diabetic ketoacidosis (DKA) or hyperglycemic hyperosmolar state (HHS) with alterations in mentation.

Autonomic dysfunction is present in as many as 90% of patients with.[5] The natural history of T2DM is to have progressive deterioration over time.[6] Older patients have significantly increased risk, especially with concomitant hypertension. Dysfunction is suggested by orthostasis, resting tachycardia, decreased heart rate variability, exercise intolerance, coronary artery calcium score, silent ischemia, early satiety, diarrhea, impotence, urinary retention, and/or abnormal sweating, and may predict adverse cardiac events.[7-9] Patients with DM may develop limited joint mobility (also known as *cheiroarthropathy*), which is due to glycosylation of collagen tissues. Common manifestations include short stature and tight waxy skin, which may make venipuncture more difficult. If the joints involved include the temporomandibular joint, the atlantooccipital joint, or the cervical spine, endotracheal intubation may be challenging.

PREOPERATIVE EVALUATION: DIABETES-SPECIFIC ELEMENTS

In addition to standard elements of the preoperative evaluation, such as the history, physical, and routine laboratory evaluation, several items are highly relevant for the evaluation of patients with DM and are listed in Box 29.1.

Preoperative evaluation for diabetic microvascular complications, such as neuropathy and retinopathy, is vital. Prior

> *Box 29.1* ELEMENTS OF PREOPERATIVE DIABETES RISK ASSESSMENT
>
> 1. Diabetes type
> 2. Disease duration/context of initial diagnosis
> 3. If type 1 diabetes: coexisting autoimmune diseases, history of ketosis
> 4. Known complications
> 5. Associated comorbidities
> 6. Home diabetes regimen (oral agents, insulin type/frequency, last medication adjustment)
> 7. Frequency/severity of hypoglycemia and methods of hypoglycemia treatment
> 8. Hemoglobin A1c
> 9. Home glucose monitoring (fingerstick blood glucose versus continuous glucose monitor)
> 10. Renal function
> 11. If insulin pump use, obtain settings from patient or endocrinologist
>
> Adapted from Miller JD.[10]

to scheduling surgery, and in order to adequately prepare the surgical team, the patient should be screened for signs of autonomic neuropathy. Diabetic autonomic neuropathy is a significant contributor to intraoperative cardiovascular morbidity.[11]

A recent determination of the HbA1c is useful for risk stratification, though some data suggest that perioperative blood sugar is at least as, if not more, important than HbA1c in predicting poor outcomes.[12] Preoperative hyperglycemia was associated with myocardial injury after noncardiac surgery and 30-day mortality in a recent study.[13] Evaluation of current electrolytes, as well as blood urea nitrogen and creatinine, are important for patients with known kidney disease and for those at risk. Routine urinalysis may show proteinuria, which precedes declining renal function.

Assessment of diabetes-related risk burden should allow for adequate attention to preoperative glycemic control. Evidence of poor glycemic control and/or the presence of unaddressed complications should prompt delay of elective surgery to better optimize the patient's diabetes care.

Of note, time to developing diabetes-related complications averages 10 years following initial diagnosis/recognition of the disease.[14,15] Thus, particular attention should be paid to screening for complications in individuals with longer diabetes duration.

In addition to routine airway, cardiovascular, and pulmonary examination conducted during the preoperative evaluation, physical examination should evaluate for cheiroarthropathy. Typical findings include the prayer sign (inability to approximate the palms when hands are held together with palms facing and fingertips touching).

As mentioned, long duration of poorly controlled diabetes predisposes to the development of macro- and microvascular complications. It is a well known fact that patients with diabetes can have silent ischemia, therefore vigilance should be paramount when recommending additional preoperative cardiac workup for patients undergoing high-risk noncardiac procedures and who are at elevated cardiac risk (>1% risk of major adverse cardiac events).[16]

Diabetes control is only one of the pillars of the preoperative optimization, the other being optimization of associated comorbidities, which in themselves can lead to poor postoperative outcomes.

On the day of surgery, specific questions for patient history and review of systems include time of last oral intake as well last dose and type of insulin administered. Fingerstick blood glucose should be determined in the preoperative holding area.

RISK STRATIFICATION USING HBA1C: ACCEPTED THRESHOLDS

HbA1c is a measure of the glycosylation of hemoglobin in erythrocytes. It reflects the estimated average blood glucose (eAG) values over the preceding 3-month period prior to lab draw, allowing providers to assess treatment compliance and effectiveness. This relationship is based on the formula $28.7 \times HbA1c - 46.7 = eAG$. Table 29.1 shows the relationship between the HbA1c and the average measure of blood glucose.[17]

In general, a goal HbA1c less than 7.0% is recommended for most patients to avoid long-term complications of DM. Tighter glycemic goals are appropriate for patients who are at lower risk of hypoglycemia. Higher, individualized A1c targets are established when potential harms outweigh benefits of tighter glycemic control, as in patients with significant risk

Table 29.1 RELATIONSHIP BETWEEN HBA1C AND AVERAGE MEASURE OF BLOOD GLUCOSE

HBA1C (%)	EAG (MG/DL)	EAG (MMOL/L)
6.0	126	7.0
6.5	140	7.8
7.0	154	8.6
7.5	169	9.4
8.0	183	10.1
8.5	197	10.9
9.0	212	11.8
9.5	226	12.6
10.0	240	13.4
10.5	254	14.2

of hypoglycemia, limited life expectancy, longer disease duration, or severe comorbidities.[18]

There is no consensus in the surgical community about optimal A1c for risk stratification of elective surgery as most research has focused on the effects of acute hyperglycemia on surgical outcomes. The American Diabetes Association and the Endocrine Society recommend targeting an A1c of less than 8% when possible prior to elective surgeries.[19,20] There is some data to suggest that patients with a preoperative HbA1c greater than 8% have worse outcomes.[21] However, these data are retrospective: prospective studies need to be completed before definitive optimization targets can be determined. At some centers, lower preoperative A1c targets have been established for patients with DM pursuing elective joint replacement. This practice is based on the risk hyperglycemia poses to postoperative healing and joint infections. However, there is not sufficient data to determine the optimal A1c for minimizing risk of postoperative complications such as infection.[22]

It is important to note that because HbA1c reflects a 3-month average of blood glucose values, the HbA1c will lag behind improvements in glucose values made during a shorter time period leading up to surgery. Therefore a patient may have improvement of blood glucose values into the normal range over a period of weeks yet still have an elevated HbA1c. Such a patient should not be delayed for surgery on the basis of a repeat elevated HbA1c at less than 3 months because the level would not have had time to reflect the improved glycemic control.

IMMEDIATE EFFECTS OF HYPERGLYCEMIA ON PERIOPERATIVE RISK

Hyperglycemia in the perioperative period is associated with worse outcomes when compared to patients without diabetes as well as to patients with diabetes who have better glucose control.[23]

Hyperglycemia is an independent marker of in-hospital mortality in patients without a diagnosis of diabetes.[24] Perioperative hyperglycemia is also associated with increased length of stay and hospital complications after noncardiac surgery.[25] Multiple mechanisms are proposed to increase risk and may relate to physiologic changes associated with hyperglycemia, including increases in reactive oxygen species, burden of inflammation, and impaired white blood cell function.

In the preoperative period, multiple etiologies for hyperglycemia may exist: patients routinely omit medications such as metformin; preoperative instructions regularly suggest patients should lower their insulin dosing while they are NPO; due to circadian rhythms, patients undergoing early morning surgery may have a physiologic surge in cortisol; the "dawn phenomenon" which has been associated with nocturnal growth hormone spikes can worsen morning insulin resistance and increase hepatic gluconeogenesis; preoperative anxiety may further increase serum cortisol levels. The impact of cortisol (Figure 29.1) on blood glucose is complex and multifactorial.[26,27] Stress hyperglycemia, in and of itself, has a negative impact on wound healing and increases risk of perioperative complications and mortality.[28]

While hyperglycemia is associated with worse outcomes, tight glycemic control may be inappropriate for some patients owing to risks associated with hypoglycemia. Moderate control of blood glucose is currently advocated, and different societies have varying target serum glucose levels, with most societies targeting a blood glucose of 140–180 mg/dL for the majority of hospitalized patients. The Society for Ambulatory Anesthesia currently recommends blood glucose levels of less than 180 mg/dL (10 mM) during the perioperative period,[29] although more liberal targets (<250 mg/dL) may be appropriate for patients undergoing ambulatory procedures where concerns for delayed wound healing or postoperative infections are not an issue (e.g., cataract surgery). The American Diabetes Association recommends a perioperative target blood glucose range of 100–180 mg/dL within 4 hours of surgery.[18]

While nationally recognized consensus does not exist regarding case cancellation, many centers consider cancelling elective surgery for patients with hyperglycemia of 300–350 mg/dL or higher. Our patient had a blood sugar of 320 mg/dL, so consideration of rescheduling surgery might be entertained. However, an elevated glucose level should not be the only factor dictating a case cancellation the morning of surgery. Several other issues need to be taken into account. One is the proposed surgery (such as an inpatient procedure where poor diabetes control could lead to postoperative infection or delayed wound healing vs. an ambulatory procedure). Another is whether this morning glucose elevation is due to temporarily altering the patient's outpatient regimen (stopping the oral antidiabetics and altering the dose of long-acting insulin the night before surgery) which could explain the glucose level in an otherwise controlled diabetes. Last, a determination should be made of whether the glucose elevation represents a hyperglycemic state such as DKA or HHS, which would make a clinician inclined to canceling an elective procedure.

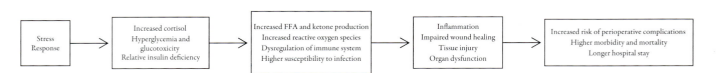

Figure 29.1 Relationship between stress hyperglycemia and postoperative outcomes.
Adapted from Figure 1 in Clement et al. Management of diabetes and hyperglycemia in hospitals. *Diabetes Care*. 2004 Feb;27(2):553–591.

PREPARING THE PATIENT FOR ANESTHESIA AND SURGERY

Attention must be paid to preoperative hydration status. Osmotic diuresis due to hyperglycemia increases risk of dehydration for patients with DM. Oral medications may also cause diarrhea and result in dehydration. If the patient shows signs of dehydration, IV infusion of isotonic crystalloid solution is warranted. Dextrose-containing solutions should be avoided when hyperglycemia is already present.

Acutely hyperglycemic patients may require insulin therapy, and all patients with type 1 diabetes must never be without insulin or ketoacidosis may ensue. Either IV or SQ insulin may be administered. Rapid-acting insulin to correct for hyperglycemia is the norm as sliding scale insulin has fallen out of favor.[30] Institutions should implement perioperative and inpatient insulin order sets that are based on attention to basal, correction, and prandial needs. Insulin sensitivity dictates patient response. Factors influencing insulin sensitivity include renal function, type and duration of diabetes, age, BMI, presence of nonalcoholic fatty liver disease (NAFLD), ethnicity, and physical activity.[31,32] Insulin requirements will tend to be reduced if there is renal impairment in the postoperative period. Insulin-naïve patients tend to require less insulin and should be dosed accordingly given risk of hypoglycemia.

Conversely, patients may require administration of glucose-containing solutions if hypoglycemia is present.

CARBOHYDRATE LOADING IN PREPARATION FOR SURGERY AS PART OF ENHANCED RECOVERY PROTOCOLS

A relatively recent phenomenon in perioperative care is the creation of enhanced recovery after surgery (ERAS) protocols. These protocols have demonstrated improved postsurgical outcomes in certain settings. Frequently these protocols involve more liberal oral intake on the day of surgery, including the patient drinking a carbohydrate-rich drink as soon as 2 hours before surgery. The purpose of the carbohydrate-rich drink is to avoid entering a catabolic state. Insulin sensitivity has been shown to increase in patients who consume carbohydrate-rich fluids preoperatively[33], and patients undergoing major abdominal surgery have shorter hospital length of stay.[34] However, preoperative carbohydrate loading does not appear to reduce postoperative complication rates.[35]

Most trials of carbohydrate loading have excluded patients with DM, but small studies have been conducted and have shown that the use of carbohydrate-rich drinks may be safe if given 3 hours before surgery[36] While this is promising, we recommend caution in carbohydrate-loading patients who have diabetes and show signs on gastroparesis or other autonomic neuropathy. There are currently no widely validated algorithms for managing potential hyperglycemia associated with ERAS protocols. Insulin may play a role, but further investigation is needed.

MANAGEMENT OF PERIOPERATIVE MEDICATIONS

Multiple oral and injectable medications are used in the treatment of DM. There is insufficient evidence regarding alterations to perioperative dosing of most oral antihyperglycemic agents and noninsulin injectable medications. It is recommended to hold metformin on the day of surgery for patients at high risk of lactic acidosis perioperatively (e.g., with liver or kidney failure or receiving intravenous contrast). Metformin could be continued on the day of surgery for ambulatory procedures because it does not cause hypoglycemia and the risk of lactic acidosis is negligible.[29,37] Another two classes of oral medications merit special considerations: the GLP1 agonists and the sodium glucose cotransport (SGLT2) inhibitors. Concerns with GLP1 agonists pertain to their ability to delay gastric emptying and whether an aspiration risk is present in patients taking these agents, especially when the dose was recently increased. There is definite perioperative glycemic benefit to continuing them in patients with diabetes.[38-40] The American Society of Anesthesiologists (ASA) very recently published guidance cautioning regarding the "full stomach" risk with GLP1 agonist and recommends holding the daily dosed GLP1 given on the day of surgery and the weekly dosed GLP1 a week prior to procedure.[41] The SGLT 2 inhibitors continued perioperative can lead to euglycemic DKA therefore it is recommended to hold them starting 3–4 days prior to surgery.[37] The remainder of other oral diabetes medications should generally be held the morning of surgery[19] (Table 29.2).

Hospitals and ambulatory surgery centers (ASCs) may have preexisting protocols regarding the management of preoperative insulin regimen adjustments, and we recommend adherence to local standards. A framework for perioperative insulin management is found in Table 29.3.

CHOICE OF INSULIN FOR MANAGEMENT OF HYPERGLYCEMIA

Given the pharmacokinetics and metabolism of noninsulin diabetes medications, rapid-acting insulin (either SQ or IV) is generally used to correct for hyperglycemia in the perioperative period. In the setting of glucose toxicity, if IV insulin is indicated, regular insulin should be used given its short half-life. Patients with type 1 diabetes should never be without basal insulin because ketoacidosis can ensue.

CONTINUOUS SUBCUTANEOUS INSULIN THERAPY (INSULIN PUMPS)

Insulin pumps are increasingly being utilized in the inpatient setting and are recommended by the recent Endocrine Society guidelines to be continued rather than changed to SQ basal bolus insulin.[20] The primary consideration in making such a decision is who will operate the device. If the patient will have altered consciousness for 1–2 hours, continued insulin pump use could be considered. If the patient will not be able to operate the insulin pump for more than

Table 29.2 PERIOPERATIVE MANAGEMENT OF ORAL ANTIHYPERGLYCEMIC MEDICATIONS

MEDICATION CLASS	EXAMPLES	ADMINISTRATION BEFORE DAY OF SURGERY	ADMINISTRATION ON MORNING OF SURGERY	ADDITIONAL CONSIDERATIONS
Alpha-glucosidase inhibitors	Acarbose, Miglitol	Continue	Hold	—
Biguanides		Continue	Hold	In patients without contraindications and with preserved renal function (GFR[a] >50 mL/min) undergoing ambulatory surgeries for which no more than one meal is expected to be omitted, non-interruption may be acceptable.
DPP-4 inhibitors		Continue	Hold	For patients undergoing ambulatory surgeries for which no more than one meal is expected to be omitted, noninterruption may be acceptable.
GLP-1 agonists		Continue[b]	Hold	Before day of surgery: For GI surgeries or when concern for nausea, vomiting, or gut dysfunction, consider holding weekly dose within 7 days before surgery. Day of surgery: If weekly dose is due on morning of surgery, delay until later in day after surgery is complete.
Insulin secretogogues (sulfonylureas, glinides)	Glipizide, glyburide, glimepiride repaglinide, nateglinide	Continue	Hold	—
SGLT-2 inhibitors	Dapagliflozin, canagliflozin, empagliflozin, ertugliflozin	Hold	Hold	Canagliflozin, dapagliflozin, and empagliflozin should each be discontinued at least three days before scheduled surgery. Ertugliflozin should be discontinued at least four days before scheduled surgery.
Thiazolidinediones	Pioglitazone	Continue	Hold	—

[a]DPP-4, dipeptidyl peptidase-4; GFR, glomerular filtration rate; GLP-1, glucagon-like peptide-I; SGLT-2, sodium glucose co-transporter 2.
[b]See additional considerations.
From Pfeifer et al. Mayo Clin Proc. 2021 Jun;96(6):1655–1669.

this timeframe, either another expert operator should be available or an alternative insulin management used. Use of "hybrid closed-loop" insulin pumps (conventional insulin pumps communicating and adjusting insulin delivery based on a continuous glucose monitor value) in this setting are subject to the same caveats. In addition, when used intraoperatively, several principles should be followed. The pump should be positioned so that the current from the monopolar cautery (frequently used intraoperatively) to the grounding pad does not cross the device, it should be easily accessible to the anesthesiologist, and the infusion site should not interfere with the surgical site. Similar principles apply to the continuous glucose monitor (part of the hybrid closed loop system), which should be placed ideally more than 24 hours prior (to ensure accuracy) in a noncompressible, easily accessible site. Values from the continuous glucose monitors can be used to guide intraoperative insulin therapy as long as they are confirmed with point-of-care glucose testing, which currently remains standard of care.

CONCLUSION

- DM is a chronic secondary diagnosis, impacting care for millions of surgical patients.
- Long-standing DM contributes to development of micro- and macrovascular complications, all of which can affect short- and long-term perioperative risk.
- A thorough DM-specific history can aid in the preoperative assessment and optimization of patients undergoing surgery.
- Patients with DM require individualized preoperative education addressing diabetes-specific medication needs and postoperative care prior to scheduling elective surgery.
- Patients taking insulin to manage their diabetes must adjust their regimen to avoid significant hypo- or hyperglycemia preoperatively.

Table 29.3 **PERIOPERATIVE INSULIN MANAGEMENT**

MEDICATION CLASS	EXAMPLES	ADMINISTRATION BEFORE DAY OF SURGERY	ADMINISTRATION ON MORNING OF SURGERY	ADDITIONAL CONSIDERATIONS
Insulin, intermediateacting		Continue[b]	Continue[b]	Decrease dose by 50% on morning of surgery and consider 25% dose reduction on evening before surgery
Insulin, long-acting	Glargine, detemir, degludec	Continue[b]	Continue[b]	Administer 60%–80% of usual dose the evening before surgery (or the morning of surgery, if normally taken in the morning) in those with type 2 diabetes and those prone to hypoglycemia
Insulin, premixed	Human NPH/regular 70/30; insulin lispro protamine/lispro 75/25	Continue	Hold	
Insulin, pump	Regular, aspart, lispro, glulisine	Continue	Continue[b]	Continue basal infusion at 100% of usual rate and do not provide boluses
Insulin, short-/rapidacting		Continue	Hold	May use on the morning of surgery for urgent treatment of hyperglycemia
Insulin, U-500		Continue	Continue[b]	Reduce dose on morning of surgery based on patient's blood glucose and risk factors for hypoglycemia

[a]NPH, neutral protamine Hagedom.
[b]See additional considerations.
From Pfeifer et al. Mayo Clin Proc. 2021 Jun;96(6):1655–1669.

- Single, point-of-care capillary fingerstick testing on day of surgery is an inadequate data point on which to decide whether to safely proceed with elective surgery.
- HbA1c testing is vital to informing the global risk of glycemia on perioperative outcomes and recovery; it is generally agreed to target a HbA1c of less than 8% when possible prior to elective surgeries.
- Rapid-acting insulin can be used to treat perioperative hyperglycemia in a patient otherwise optimized for surgery.

REVIEW QUESTIONS

1. A 65-year-old man with T2DM for 22 years and debilitating osteoarthritis is scheduled for elective right total knee replacement (TKR). His HbA1c 1 month prior to procedure is 9.8%. What is the appropriate next step in his preoperative care?

   a. Proceed with elective TKR as planned.
   b. Immediately begin basal/bolus insulin therapy.
   c. Expedited visitation to an endocrinologist or PCP to optimize glycemic control
   d. Repeat HbA1c testing now and check a fasting serum glucose

The correct answer is c.

For TKR it is recommended to have an HbA1c of less than 8%, therefore the patient's diabetes control should be optimized before surgery.

2. A 72-year-old female patient with long-standing T2DM complicated by mild chronic kidney disease and nonproliferative diabetic retinopathy (NPDR) is scheduled for an elective right carpal tunnel release. Perioperatively, the patient is at greatest risk for

   a. Hyperglycemia.
   b. Acute renal failure.
   c. Difficult airway intubation.
   d. Hypotension.

The correct answer is c.

Patients with DM may develop limited joint mobility (also known as cheiroarthropathy), which is due to glycosylation of collagen tissues. Common manifestations include short stature and tight waxy skin, which may make venipuncture more difficult. If the joints involved include the temporomandibular joint, the atlantooccipital joint, or the cervical spine, endotracheal intubation may be challenging.

3. A 31-year-old female patient with type 1 diabetes arrives to OR holding for an elective carpal tunnel repair. She complains of nausea and vague abdominal pain since the early morning. Which of the following is immediately indicated?

   a. Check a fingerstick blood glucose and give correction insulin.

- b. Order 1 L of normal saline hydration.
- c. Cancel the case and discharge the patient to home.
- d. Send STAT chemistries and urine to assess for ketoacidosis.

The correct answer is d.

Hyperglycemia accompanied by nausea, vomiting, and abdominal pain could signal the onset of DKA.

4. A morbidly obese 52-year-old man with long-standing T2DM is preparing for elective sleeve gastrectomy. His diabetes is controlled on multiple daily insulin injections (basal/bolus therapy) along with metformin and a glimepiride. Prior to scheduling his bariatric surgery, the surgical team should instruct the patient to

- a. Contact his endocrinologist for preoperative medication instructions leading up to surgery.
- b. Hold all oral diabetes agents on the morning of scheduled sleeve gastrectomy.
- c. Take half the usual dose of his long-acting insulin on the night prior to surgery.
- d. Stop his diabetes medications upon initiating the preop bariatric liquid diet 2 weeks prior to surgery.

The correct answer is a.

Given than diet is altered in the weeks leading up to bariatric surgery with transition to a high-protein, low-carbohydrate diet, alteration of the antidiabetes medication regimen is likely. One should consider endocrinology input.

5. Which of the following statements is true regarding ERAS protocols in people with diabetes?

- a. ERAS has been shown to improve outcomes in patients with diabetes undergoing elective surgery.
- b. Patients with diabetes should not be included in ERAS protocols given risk of hyperglycemia.
- c. Patients with diabetes should receive a low-carbohydrate drink 2 hours preoperatively to improve postoperative outcomes.
- d. ERAS has not yet been well-validated in patients with diabetes; use should be based on clinical judgment on a case-by-case basis.

The correct answer is d.

Outcomes for patients undergoing carbohydrate loading as part of an ERAS protocol in patients with diabetes have not shown clear benefit. It has fallen out of favor in some institutions.

6. A 47-year-old female patient with a 25+ pack year smoking history and long-standing, uncontrolled T2DM is referred for elective femoropopliteal bypass surgery. Her preoperative HbA1c is 12.4%. She is referred to a local endocrinologist for assistance with glycemic control. After initial visitation with the endocrinologist, the patient checks her sugars four times daily and starts a regimen of multiple daily insulin injections. Three months later, her HbA1c has dropped to 9.5%. Her fingerstick log reveals fasting sugars in the low 100s and prepandial numbers in the 130s to 140s. Which of the following is true regarding her planned surgery?

- a. She should further delay her surgery until her HbA1c drops below 8%.
- b. HbA1c will lag behind her improved fingerstick glucose numbers; she is optimized for surgery.
- c. Surgery team should check a fructosamine level prior to considering elective surgery.
- d. The patient should be started on insulin pump therapy to better optimize preoperative glycemic control.

The correct answer is b.

Hemoglobin A1c reflects control of the disease over the previous 3 months rather than recent glucose values. Consideration might be given to fructosamine, which reflects shorter-term control.

7. Which of the following statements is most accurate regarding continuous SQ insulin infusion (insulin pump) therapy in patients undergoing urgent surgical intervention?

- a. SQ insulin infusion sites should be removed preoperatively, especially if they interfere with the sterile surgical field.
- b. All patients with an insulin pump should receive an IV insulin infusion in the perioperative period to prevent ketosis.
- c. Endocrinology consultation should be obtained urgently to determine appropriateness of pump continuation during surgery.
- d. Insulin pumps will automatically control blood sugar perioperatively.

The correct answer is a.

When an emergency procedure is planned in a patient wearing an insulin pump, it is best practice to transition to an insulin infusion, especially if the infusion site interferes with the surgical location.

8. Which of the following procedures is most impacted by poor perioperative glycemic control?

- a. Cholecystectomy.
- b. Coronary artery bypass grafting.
- c. Knee arthroscopy.
- d. Sleeve gastrectomy.

The correct answer is b.

There are a wealth of data on poor outcomes in cardiac surgery patients with poorly controlled glucose levels. Tighter glycemic targets should be considered in these patients.

9. In patients with diabetes, which covariable has the greatest impact on insulin sensitivity in the postoperative period?

- a. Renal function.
- b. PO status.
- c. Preoperative HbA1c.
- d. Disease duration.

The correct answer is a.

Patients with impaired renal function or low BMI, or insulin-naive patients require less insulin for hyperglycemia correction.

10. Which of the following patients is most at-risk for developing hypoglycemia unawareness?

    a. A 19-year-old female with T1DM on insulin pump.
    b. A 47-year-old male with T2DM for 15 years on oral agents.
    c. A 27-year-old pregnant female with gestational diabetes.
    d. A 67-year-old male with T1DM for 41 years on multiple insulin injections.

The correct answer is d.

Patients with long-standing T1DM can develop hypoglycemia unawareness in the setting of repeated episodes of hypoglycemia.

REFERENCES

1. CDC. National diabetes statistics report. https://www.cdc.gov/diabetes/php/data-research/?CDC_AAref_Val=https://www.cdc.gov/diabetes/data/statistics-report/index.html
2. Ahlqvist E, Storm P, Käräjämäki A, et al. Novel subgroups of adult-onset diabetes and their association with outcomes: A data-driven cluster analysis of six variables. *Lancet Diabetes Endocrinol*. 2018 May;6(5):361–369.
3. ElSayed NA, Aleppo G, Aroda VR, et al. 2. Classification and diagnosis of diabetes: Standards of care in diabetes—2023. *Diabetes Care*. 2023 Jan 01;46(Suppl 1):S19–S40.
4. American Diabetes Association. Peripheral arterial disease in people with diabetes. *Diabetes Care*. 2003 Dec;26(12):3333–3341.
5. Vinik AI, Casellini C, Parson HK, Colberg SR, Nevoret ML. Cardiac autonomic neuropathy in diabetes: A predictor of cardiometabolic events. *Front Neurosci*. 2018;12:591.
6. Holman RR, Paul SK, Bethel MA, Matthews DR, Neil HA. 10-Year follow-up of intensive glucose control in type 2 diabetes. *N Engl J Med*. 2008 Oct 09;359(15):1577–1589.
7. Wackers FJ, Young LH, Inzucchi SE, et al. Detection of silent myocardial ischemia in asymptomatic diabetic subjects: The DIAD study. *Diabetes Care*. 2004 Aug;27(8):1954–1961.
8. Vinik AI, Maser RE, Mitchell BD, Freeman R. Diabetic autonomic neuropathy. *Diabetes Care*. 2003 May;26(5):1553–1579.
9. Vinik AI, Ziegler D. Diabetic cardiovascular autonomic neuropathy. *Circulation*. 2007 Jan 23;115(3):387–397.
10. Miller JD, Richman DC. Preoperative evaluation of patients with diabetes mellitus. *Anesthesiol Clin*. 2016 Mar;34(1):155–169.
11. Burgos LG, Ebert TJ, Asiddao C, et al. Increased intraoperative cardiovascular morbidity in diabetics with autonomic neuropathy. *Anesthesiology*. 1989 Apr;70(4):591–597.
12. van den Boom W, Schroeder RA, Manning MW, Setji TL, Fiestan GO, Dunson DB. Effect of A1C and glucose on postoperative mortality in noncardiac and cardiac surgeries. *Diabetes Care*. 2018 Apr;41(4):782–788.
13. Park J, Oh AR, Lee SH, et al. Associations between preoperative glucose and hemoglobin A1c level and myocardial injury after noncardiac surgery. *J Am Heart Assoc*. 2021 Apr 06;10(7):e019216.
14. Orasanu G, Plutzky J. The pathologic continuum of diabetic vascular disease. *J Am Coll Cardiol*. 2009 Feb 03;53(5 Suppl):S35–S42.
15. Spijkerman AM, Dekker JM, Nijpels G, et al. Microvascular complications at time of diagnosis of type 2 diabetes are similar among diabetic patients detected by targeted screening and patients newly diagnosed in general practice: The Hoorn screening study. *Diabetes Care*. 2003 Sep;26(9):2604–2608.
16. Fleisher LA, Fleischmann KE, Auerbach AD, et al. 2014 ACC/AHA guideline on perioperative cardiovascular evaluation and management of patients undergoing noncardiac surgery: A report of the American College of Cardiology/American Heart Association Task Force on Practice Guidelines. *Circulation*. 2014 Aug 1;130(24):2215–2245.
17. Nathan DM, Kuenen J, Borg R, et al. Translating the A1C assay into estimated average glucose values. *Diabetes Care*. 2008 Aug;31(8):1473–1478.
18. ElSayed NA, Aleppo G, Aroda VR, et al. 6. Glycemic targets: Standards of care in diabetes – 2023. *Diabetes Care*. 2023 Jan 01;46(Suppl 1):S97–S110.
19. ElSayed NA, Aleppo G, Aroda VR, et al. 16. Diabetes care in the hospital: Standards of care in diabetes – 2023. *Diabetes Care*. 2023 Jan 01;46(Suppl 1):S267–S278.
20. Korytkowski MT, Muniyappa R, Antinori-Lent K, et al. Management of hyperglycemia in hospitalized adult patients in non-critical care settings: An Endocrine Society clinical practice guideline. *J Clin Endocrinol Metab*. 2022 Jul 14;107(8):2101–2128.
21. Underwood P, Askari R, Hurwitz S, Chamarthi B, Garg R. Preoperative A1C and clinical outcomes in patients with diabetes undergoing major noncardiac surgical procedures. *Diabetes Care*. 2014;37(3):611–616.
22. Lopez LF, Reaven PD, Harman SM. Review: The relationship of hemoglobin A1c to postoperative surgical risk with an emphasis on joint replacement surgery. *J Diabetes Complications*. 2017 Dec;31(12):1710–1718.
23. Kwon S, Thompson R, Dellinger P, Yanez D, Farrohki E, Flum D. Importance of perioperative glycemic control in general surgery: A report from the Surgical Care and Outcomes Assessment Program. *Ann Surg*. 2013 Jan;257(1):8–14.
24. Umpierrez GE, Isaacs SD, Bazargan N, You X, Thaler LM, Kitabchi AE. Hyperglycemia: An independent marker of in-hospital mortality in patients with undiagnosed diabetes. *J Clin Endocrinol Metab*. 2002 Mar;87(3):978–982.
25. Frisch A, Chandra P, Smiley D, et al. Prevalence and clinical outcome of hyperglycemia in the perioperative period in noncardiac surgery. *Diabetes Care*. 2010 Aug;33(8):1783–1788.
26. Duggan EW, Carlson K, Umpierrez GE. Perioperative hyperglycemia management: An update. *Anesthesiology*. 2017;126(3):547–560.
27. Clement S, Braithwaite SS, Magee MF, et al. Management of diabetes and hyperglycemia in hospitals. *Diabetes Care*. 2004 Feb;27(2):553–591.
28. Davis G, Fayfman M, Reyes-Umpierrez D, et al. Stress hyperglycemia in general surgery: Why should we care? *J Diabetes Complications*. 2018 Mar;32(3):305–309.
29. Joshi GP, Ankichetty SP, Gan TJ, Chung F. Society for Ambulatory Anesthesia consensus statement on preoperative selection of adult patients with obstructive sleep apnea scheduled for ambulatory surgery. *Anesth Analg*. 2012 Nov;115(5):1060–1068.
30. Umpierrez GE, Smiley D, Zisman A, et al. Randomized study of basal-bolus insulin therapy in the inpatient management of patients with type 2 diabetes (RABBIT 2 trial). *Diabetes Care*. 2007 Sep;30(9):2181–2186.
31. Akwo EA, Sahinoz M, Alsouqi A, Siew ED, Ikizler TA, Hung AM. Effect modification of body mass index and kidney function on insulin sensitivity among patients with moderate CKD and healthy controls. *Kidney Int Rep*. 2021 Nov;6(11):2811–2820.
32. Najjar SM, Caprio S, Gastaldelli A. Insulin clearance in health and disease. *Annu Rev Physiol*. 2023 Feb 10;85:363–381.
33. Wang ZG, Wang Q, Wang WJ, Qin HL. Randomized clinical trial to compare the effects of preoperative oral carbohydrate versus placebo on insulin resistance after colorectal surgery. *Br J Surg*. 2010 Mar;97(3):317–327.
34. Awad S, Varadhan KK, Ljungqvist O, Lobo DN. A meta-analysis of randomised controlled trials on preoperative oral carbohydrate treatment in elective surgery. *Clin Nutr*. 2013 Feb;32(1):34–44.
35. Amer MA, Smith MD, Herbison GP, Plank LD, McCall JL. Network meta-analysis of the effect of preoperative carbohydrate loading on recovery after elective surgery. *Br J Surg*. 2017 Feb;104(3):187–197.
36. Gustafsson UO, Nygren J, Thorell A, et al. Preoperative carbohydrate loading may be used in type 2 diabetes patients. *Acta Anaesthesiol Scand*. 2008 Aug;52(7):946–951.

37. Pfeifer KJ, Selzer A, Mendez CE, et al. Preoperative management of endocrine, hormonal, and urologic medications: Society for Perioperative Assessment and Quality Improvement (SPAQI) consensus statement. *Mayo Clin Proc.* 2021 06;96(6):1655–1669.
38. Hulst AH, Visscher MJ, Godfried MB, et al. Liraglutide for perioperative management of hyperglycaemia in cardiac surgery patients: A multicentre randomized superiority trial. *Diabetes Obes Metab.* 2020 Apr;22(4):557–565.
39. Polderman JAW, van Steen SCJ, Thiel B, et al. Perioperative management of patients with type-2 diabetes mellitus undergoing non-cardiac surgery using liraglutide, glucose-insulin-potassium infusion or intravenous insulin bolus regimens: A randomised controlled trial. *Anaesthesia.* 2018 Mar;73(3):332–339.
40. Besch G, Perrotti A, Mauny F, et al. Clinical effectiveness of intravenous exenatide infusion in perioperative glycemic control after coronary artery bypass graft surgery: A phase II/III randomized trial. *Anesthesiology.* 2017 Nov;127(5):775–787.
41. Joshi GP, Abdelmalak BB, Weigel WA, et al. American Society of Anesthesiologists consensus-based guidance on preoperative management of patients (adults and children) on glucagon-like peptide-1 (GLP-1) receptor agonists. June 29, 2023. Available at: https://www.asahq.org/about-asa/newsroom/news-releases/2023/06/american-society-of-anesthesiologists-consensus-based-guidance-on-preoperative. Accessed May 27, 2024.

30.

PHEOCHROMOCYTOMA AND MEN SYNDROMES

Zyad J. Carr, Andrea Farela, and Adriana D. Oprea

STEM CASE AND KEY QUESTIONS

A 55-year-old woman with a history of irritable bowel syndrome, gastroesophageal reflux disease (GERD), anxiety, multiple small bowel obstructions post several lysis of adhesions surgeries, and an adrenal mass presented for an outpatient colonoscopy for recurrent constipation. She is taking no outpatient prescription medications. Preoperative evaluation (including review of systems) on the day of the procedure is unremarkable, other than a slightly elevated blood pressure of 142/96 with a heart rate of 86.

During the colonoscopy under moderate sedation with propofol, the blood pressure spikes to 221/126 and subsequently 232/129, which prompts abandonment of the procedure.

Could the blood pressure spikes be related to the adrenal mass?

What workup is recommended for patients with an incidentally found adrenal mass? Any specific hormonal tests? Imaging studies?

The patient is scheduled to follow-up with her primary care doctor who orders hormonal testing. The serum metanephrines come back elevated at greater than 10 times the normal levels. The patient is diagnosed with a pheochromocytoma and referred to an endocrinologist for medical optimization and to an endocrine surgeon for surgical resection.

What is pheochromocytoma? What other types of adrenal tumors are there?

What other conditions can be associated with the presence of a pheochromocytoma?

What medical treatment is recommended prior to pheochromocytoma resection? Any specific agents? What is the optimal duration of therapy? What are the goals of medical optimization?

The patient is placed on the lowest-dose doxazosin by the endocrinologist who plans to reassess the blood pressure values weekly and adjust the dose. The patient is scheduled for an open adrenalectomy in 3 weeks, and the endocrine surgeon refers the patient for a pre-surgical evaluation visit prior to adrenalectomy.

What preoperative workup is indicated prior to an adrenalectomy for pheochromocytoma resection?

In addition to standard preoperative laboratory tests, is an ECG indicated? What would you expect to see?

Should additional cardiac testing be considered? What would trigger additional tests, and what tests would you order?

How is the preoperative evaluation different for patients with pheochromocytoma versus patients with other hormonally active adrenal adenomas or a nonfunctioning adenoma?

During your preoperative evaluation visit, the endocrinologist's evaluation suggests that there is concern for multiple endocrine neoplasia (MEN) syndrome because the patient's family members have been diagnosed with medullary thyroid cancer.

What are the MEN syndromes? How many types are there?

What comorbidities should you be concerned about in different types of MEN? Is additional workup indicated preoperatively?

What are perioperative concerns pertaining to different comorbidities?

One week prior to adrenalectomy, you receive a from the concerned endocrinologist, stating that the patient had several syncopal events and subsequent emergency room visits. They are concerned that the patient may not tolerate alpha blockade.

Should the patient be transitioned to a different antihypertensive medication? If so, what would be your choices?

Is it paramount for the patient to be alpha-blocked prior to adrenalectomy for pheochromocytoma? What are the perioperative implications if alpha blockade is not possible?

The patient presents for open adrenalectomy. The blood pressure in the holding area is 152/96 and the patient is anxious regarding the upcoming procedure.

Would you proceed with the adrenalectomy? What pharmacological or nonpharmacological interventions would you use to decrease the blood pressure preoperatively?

What anesthetic plan would you propose to the patient? Would there be advantages to a thoracic epidural placement for postoperative pain control in addition to general anesthesia?

What surgical techniques are available for adrenalectomy, and what are their advantages and drawbacks?

What would the anesthesia induction plan entail? Any anesthetics you should avoid? Any of them offering specific advantages/disadvantages?

Are you planning to place an arterial line? Would you place it pre- or post-induction? How about intravenous access? A pulmonary artery (PA) catheter? Additional monitoring necessary?

The patient receives midazolam and is placed on a dexmedetomidine infusion at 0.4 mcg/kg/h. A preinduction arterial line is placed, and general anesthesia is induced with propofol, fentanyl, and rocuronium.

What are the critical portions of the procedure, and what would you have prepared to treat hemodynamic instability?

Any specific adjuncts you could use to blunt the sympathetic surge during surgical manipulation?

What would you expect to encounter after vein isolation? Any specific preparations for that?

The adrenalectomy proceeds uneventfully except for mild blood pressure swings, and the surgeon plans to admit the patient to the regular ward.

Would you agree with this decision? Should all pheochromocytoma patients be admitted to the ICU postoperatively?

What problems would you expect to see immediately postoperatively, and how would you address them?

DISCUSSION

INTRODUCTION

PPGLs are derived from chromaffin cells from neural crest tissue and are responsible for catecholamine production. Pheochromocytomas (PCC) originate from adrenal tissue, and paragangliomas (PGL) are derived from extra-adrenal ganglia. The overall incidence of PPGL is low, and fewer than 2,000 cases are diagnosed each year in the United States.[1] Pheochromocytoma commonly associated with the MEN type 2 (MEN2) syndrome, with symptoms present in 50% of MEN2 patients.[2] PGLs are commonly found in the head and neck, are parasympathetically active, and usually hormonally inactive. Some PGLs, often categorized as *extra-adrenal pheochromocytomas*, are retroperitoneal, and the vast actively secrete catecholamines.

PRESENTING SYMPTOMS

Patients with symptomatic PPGLs may present with paroxysmal sympathomimetic symptoms such as excessive sweating, palpitations, tachycardia, tremor, or headache although 50% of patients will be asymptomatic. Remarkably, 20–30% of PPGLs are incidentally detected on abdominal imaging for other indications.[3]

Furthermore, most patients do not have the classic symptom triad of episodic headache, sweating, and tachycardia. Rarely, pheochromocytoma crisis may occur and is manifest with refractory hypertension, altered mental status, and hyperthermia. Other, more nuanced symptoms include orthostatic hypotension, visual disturbances related to papilledema, or stress-induced cardiomyopathy. Rare symptoms may include intra-adrenal bleeding, hemoptysis, and even hypoglycemia.[4,5] Glucose intolerance is one of the major complications of pheochromocytoma, and more than half of patients may have evidence of hyperglycemia or overt diabetes mellitus, mediated by excessively stimulated gluconeogenesis and glycogenolysis.[6,7] Patients with associated hyperparathyroidism may have symptoms of fatigue, excessive thirst, constipation, anorexia, and elevated serum calcium or parathyroid hormone levels.

DIAGNOSIS

Due to the variability of clinical presentation, initial workup for PPGLs is contingent on the confirmation of excessive catecholamine production with either plasma or urinary screening followed by locus identification using imaging modalities. Many clinicians utilize plasma free metanephrines, rather than traditional 24-hour urinary metanephrine testing due to availability and high sensitivity, but it is limited by its lower specificity.[8,9] Initial imaging studies include CT or MRI. If no mass is visualized, further imaging with iobenguane I-123 scintigraphy or fludeoxyglucose-positron emission tomography (PET) may be performed. 68-Ga DOTA-0-Phe1-Tyr-3 octreotate PET is a reserved option for detection of metastatic disease (Figure 30.1).

PREOPERATIVE MANAGEMENT

Definitive surgical management of PPGLs is contingent on excellent preoperative medical management. Resection of pheochromocytoma remains a high-risk surgical due to the possibility of tumor-mediated sympathetic storming resulting in hypertensive crises and potentially lethal ventricular dysrhythmias. Preoperative medical therapy has two primary goals: control of refractory hypertension and intravascular volume expansion. First-line therapy remains selective (e.g., prazosin, doxazosin) or nonselective (e.g., phenoxybenzamine) alpha-adrenergic blockade for a minimum of 7 days prior to surgical intervention.[10] Nonselective alpha-adrenergic blockade is superior to selective in reducing the risk of intraoperative hypertension in one recent study but is used rarely

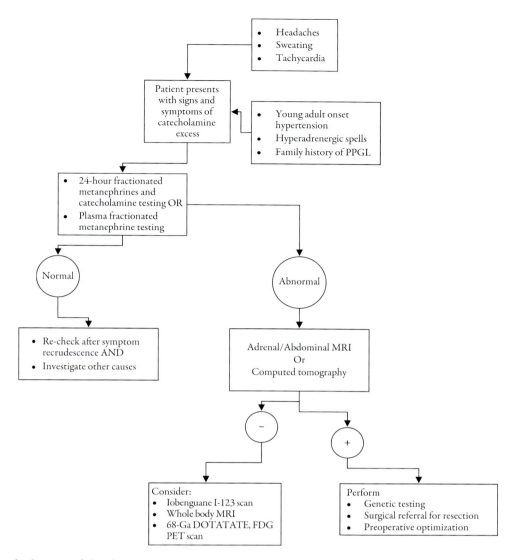

Figure 30.1 Algorithm for diagnosis of pheochromocytoma.
From Young WF. Pheochromocytoma: 1926–1993. In: *Trends in Endocrinology and Metabolism*, volume 4, Elsevier Science, Inc. (1993) pg. 122.

in clinical practice.[11] If long-term pharmacological therapy is indicated, as in patients with metastatic pheochromocytoma, selective alpha-adrenergic antagonism may be favored due to a lower incidence of side effects and reduced cost. Combined alpha and beta adrenergic blockade has been successfully utilized to prepare patients for surgery but only after initial selective alpha-adrenergic blockade has been instituted.[12] The traditional concept of delaying beta-1 and -2 adrenergic receptor blockade until adequate peripheral alpha-adrenergic receptor blockade occurs is due to the concern for a paradoxical rise in blood pressure caused by unopposed alpha-1 adrenergic activation without the salutary benefit of beta-2 adrenergic receptor-mediated vasodilation. Although emphasis on adequate preoperative blood pressure control has been long considered standard of care, Shimmack and colleagues found surprisingly little support in the scientific literature in favor of aggressive alpha-adrenergic blockade, although they did not find strong evidence to abandon it. The arguments against alpha-adrenergic blockade center around the risks for serious side effects associated with alpha-adrenergic blockade in the perioperative time period, particularly hypotension.[13] PPGL patients suffer from high rates of postoperative hypotension, and patients with prolonged hypotension have a higher rates of complications, intensive care admissions, and mechanical ventilation.[14]

In addition, clinicians should be aware of the potential for acute decompensated failure from the administration of beta-adrenergic blockade in patients with unrecognized catecholamine cardiomyopathy. Second-line agents to improve blood pressure control include calcium channel antagonists. The favored calcium channel antagonists are the dihydropyridines, with preferential vasodilatory properties and limited chronotropic and ionotropic effects on the heart. Their use allows focused targeting of the profound peripheral vasoconstriction observed in patients with catecholamine-secreting tumors without the negative inotropic effects observed with beta blockers effects on cardiac output. Catecholamine synthesis inhibition (e.g., metyrosine) is reserved for treatment of patients with refractory hypertension or metastatic disease and may result in more intraoperative hemodynamic instability.[15] Metyrosine, a tyrosine hydroxylase inhibitor, is also associated with numerous adverse effects such as extrapyramidal reactions, diarrhea, confusion, eosinophilia, and hypersensitivity reactions. Corticosteroids, norepinephrine reuptake inhibitors, and tricyclic antidepressants should be avoided as these may precipitate release of catecholamines. The modified Roizen criteria are utilized to determine adequate control prior to surgical correction and include an absence of blood pressure measurement of greater than 160/90 for 24 hours prior to surgical intervention, resolution of orthostatic hypotension, resolution of ECG changes, and no more than one premature ventricular contraction per 5-minute interval.[16] More recently, the Endocrine Society recommends a preoperative blood pressure of 130/80 before pheochromocytoma resection.[17] Dietary sodium supplementation and high oral fluid intake are also traditionally recommended to correct the volume depletion inherent to these patients, however new findings have challenged this concept. Kong et al. examined PPGL patients treated with traditional preoperative IV hydration protocols compared with PPGL patients who were not and found no difference in perioperative hemodynamics or improved in-hospital complications.[18] Preoperative workup should include ECG, CBC, and electrolytes. Patients with evidence of poor functional status should proceed for transthoracic echocardiography (TTE). Further cardiac workup should be dictated by symptomatology. Outpatient preoperative management of pheochromocytoma is acceptable when compared to inpatient optimization.[19]

INTRAOPERATIVE MANAGEMENT

Advancements in preoperative management have facilitated the intraoperative care of PPGL patients during surgical resection. Core requirements for safe intraoperative care include invasive blood pressure monitoring, adequate IV access, and an armamentarium of vasopressors and vasodilators. Transesophageal echocardiography (TEE) may be indicated in patients with preexisting cardiac disease and, rarely, PA catheterization may be indicated. Patients with chronic catecholamine excess–associated cardiomyopathy may have ECG abnormalities (37%), coronary artery disease (26%), or a prolonged QT interval (16%). Disturbances of contractility, mitral valve insufficiency or significant vasospasm-induced myocardial ischemia are also relatively common, and TEE may be useful in monitoring these conditions.[20] Advances in laparoscopic approaches have resulted in improved outcomes, but complex resections may require open surgical techniques where regional anesthesia may prove beneficial.[21,22] Combined epidural-general anesthesia in this patient population was found to be effective in reducing a postoperative complications.[22]

Anesthesia care may be categorized into induction and pre- and post-resection phases. Induction of anesthesia and subsequent endotracheal anesthesia induces a substantial sympathetic stress response in humans and may result in myocardial ischemia, hypertension, and cardiac arrhythmia.[23] There is no definitive therapy to reduce this stress response but lidocaine pretreatment, beta blockers, and narcotics may reduce the risk of adverse events. Furthermore, this sympathetic stress response may be severely exaggerated in patients with PPGLs, resulting in a sustained hypertensive crisis. Therefore, selection of induction agents should aim to anticipate and minimize this eventuality. Pre-induction anxiolysis with short-acting benzodiazepines may be indicated on transport to the operating room. A post-induction arterial line is then established once the patient is adequately anesthetized. Ketamine, an intravenous NMDA antagonist, is avoided due to its sympathomimetic properties, but volatile anesthetics, such as sevoflurane, or IV anesthetics, such as propofol, have favorable properties for both induction and maintenance of general anesthesia.

The pre-resection phase is highlighted by the risk of hypertensive episodes related to surgical stimulation. Hemodynamic stability in the pre-resection phase is enhanced by a sympatholytic approach using remifentanil, dexmedetomidine, and intraoperative smooth muscle relaxation using magnesium sulfate.[24,25] Dexmedetomidine, an alpha-2 agonist, stimulates presynaptic alpha-2 adrenoreceptors and inhibits further release of norepinephrine. By reducing heart rate and vascular tone, it is a theoretically ideal anesthetic adjunct for this surgical population. Remifentanil is a potent opioid analgesic with a rapid onset and recovery time, making it a useful anesthesia adjunct in cases with fluctuating surgical stimulation. In addition, two IV vasodilators are commonly used to prevent hypertensive crises. Nitroglycerin, a potent IV venodilator with a rapid on- and offset is an acceptable medication for the prevention or treatment of hypertensive crisis. Magnesium sulfate has been utilized as a vasodilator because its mechanism of blocking calcium-mediated smooth muscle relaxation has been found effective in reducing hypertensive episodes associated with PPGLs[25] (Table 30.1).

The post-resection phase is characterized by the risk of catecholamine-resistant shock after surgical vein isolation and ligation. First-line therapy remains phenylephrine or norepinephrine. Alternative strategies include the administration of vasopressin, a V_1 receptor agonist that promotes peripheral arteriolar vasoconstriction; milrinone, a phosphodiesterase III inhibitor with cardiac inotropic and lusitropic effects, both may be effective adjuncts for the treatment of this phenomenon.[26,27] Many PPGL patients may have impaired glucose metabolism and insulin resistance resulting in intraoperative blood glucose swings. Close intraoperative monitoring and permissive levels of less than 180 mg/dL are recommended because aggressive intraoperative treatment may result in postoperative hypoglycemia.

POSTOPERATIVE MANAGEMENT

Diligent postoperative care of PPGL resection patients is mandated since the postoperative time period can be fraught with

Table 30.1 SELECT DRUGS IN PHEOCHROMOCYTOMA AND PARAGANGLIOMA RESECTION

DRUG CLASS	REPRESENTATIVE MEDICATION(S)	MECHANISM OF ACTION	DURATION OF ACTION	PERIOPERATIVE INDICATION	PERIOPERATIVE ADVERSE EFFECTS
PREOPERATIVE MANAGEMENT					
Alpha-1 antagonist	Prazosin, Doxazosin	Peripheral vasodilation	10–24 hours	Preoperative BP control	Orthostatic hypotension, palpitations
Alpha-1,2 antagonist	Phenoxybenzamine	Peripheral vasodilation	3–4 days	Preoperative BP control	Orthostatic hypotension, reflex tachycardia
Beta-1-selective antagonist	Atenolol	Inhibits cardiac and vascular smooth muscle sympathetic stimulation	12 hours	Preoperative BP control	Bradycardia, hypotension
Dihydropyridines (Ca^{2+} channel blocker)	Amlodipine	Peripheral vasodilation	24 hours	Preoperative BP control	Reflex tachycardia, peripheral edema
Tyrosine 3-monoxygenase inhibitor	Metyrosine	Inhibits catecholamine synthesis	2–3 days	Preoperative BP control	Tremor, diarrhea, sedation
INTRAOPERATIVE MANAGEMENT					
Benzodiazepine	Midazolam	Gamma aminobutyric acid (GABA) agonist; sedation	1–6 hours	Anxiolysis	Excessive sedation, postoperative delirium
Opioid	Remifentanil, fentanyl	Mu-opioid receptor agonism: analgesia	Remifentanil: 3–4 minutes Fentanyl: 30–60 minutes	Analgesia	Remifentanil: truncal rigidity, tachyphylaxis Fentanyl: respiratory depression, serotonin syndrome
Alpha-2 agonist (highly selective)	Dexmedetomidine	Alpha-2 antagonism; peripheral vasodilation, locus coeruleus noradrenergic inhibition, sedation	6 minutes	Anesthetic adjunct	Bradycardia, hypotension
Nitrates	Nitroglycerin	Pro-drug of nitric oxide; peripheral vasodilation	2–3 minutes	Intraoperative hypertension	Hypotension, reflex tachycardia
Antidiuretic hormone	Vasopressin	V1 receptor agonism; ↑ arteriolar vascular tone V2 receptor agonist: ↑ water permeability at renal tubule.	Vasopressor effect: 15 minutes Antidiuretic effect: 1–2 hours	Intraoperative hypotension Refractory shock	Arrhythmias, bradycardia, hyponatremia, right heart failure
Catecholamine	Norepinephrine	Alpha-1 and Beta-1 agonism: peripheral, splanchnic vasoconstriction	5–10 minutes	Intraoperative hypotension	Excessive vasoconstriction, reflex bradycardia, arrhythmia

A wide of variety of vasoactive drugs may be exploited in the preoperative and intraoperative hemodynamic management of PPGL manipulation and resection. Hemodynamic management requires careful preoperative drug selection and titration to prevent intraoperative hemodynamic crisis. In addition, thoughtful anticipation of the different hemodynamic sequelae of the surgical procedure results in improved hemodynamic stability.

BP, blood pressure; Ca^{2+}, calcium; V1, Arginine vasopressin receptor subtype 1; V2, Arginine vasopressin receptor subtype 2.

---

potential complications. Major complications include postoperative bleeding, persistent vasoplegia requiring vasopressor support, or refractory hypertension from inadequate surgical resection. Rebound hyperinsulinemia may result in profound hypoglycemia and requires close blood glucose observation. Postoperative hypertension may be a result of inadequate surgical resection, metastatic PPGLs, or residual effect of intraoperative vasopressors. Close blood pressure monitoring with aggressive antihypertensive treatments may be necessary to treat this condition. Postoperative hypotension may be triggered by PPGL resection and the resultant loss of circulating catecholamines or by persistent phenoxybenzamine-related alpha-1 blockade causing persistent vasodilation. The hemodynamic compromise may be partially explained by PPGL adrenoreceptor desensitization and the sudden absence of previously high plasma catecholamines.[28] Management begins with an assessment of volume responsiveness and IV fluid challenge and progressively escalates to vasopressors to maintain normotension. Thirty percent of patients required administration of vasoactive substances in the postoperative period, but postoperative bleeding complications appear uncommon.[29] Postoperative arrhythmias are not uncommon, and treatment should follow current cardiac guidelines. Sinus tachycardia is the most common postoperative arrhythmia, and the workup should include assessment for common underlying causes: pain, under-resuscitation, or medication effect. A high index of suspicion of new arrhythmia should be present and prompt clinicians to have a low threshold to obtain serial ECG and cardiac enzymes to rule out myocardial ischemia. Symptoms of myocardial ischemia may be atypical in presentation during the postoperative period. Congestive heart failure may be considered, particularly if the patient has preoperative echocardiography suggestive of systolic or diastolic left ventricular dysfunction. Secondary adrenocortical insufficiency may occur in patients with bilateral PPGL resection, and a random cortisol level may be helpful in gauging the need for corticosteroid supplementation. Given the risk for numerous potential adverse events, the consensus recommendation is that postoperative care should be performed in the ICU. However, at least one study has suggested that hemodynamically stable postoperative patients may be admitted to non-ICU wards without increased risk.[30] ICU stays appear to be short (1.5 ±1.6 days), making the benefits of mandatory ICU admission unclear.[31]

MULTIPLE ENDOCRINE NEOPLASIA SYNDROMES

MEN syndromes comprise various combinations of benign and sometimes malignant tumors of endocrine glands. The designation "multiple" refers to the possibility of developing tumors in multiple endocrine glands or multiple tumors in the same gland. Some of these tumors may represent a challenge for the anesthesiologist during the perioperative period given their potential to produce abnormalities capable of altering hemodynamics, and unmask potentially life-threatening electrolyte and hormonal imbalances.

MEN can be grouped in two broad types: *MEN type 1 or Wermer syndrome*, a rare autosomal dominant disorder that consists of tumors of the parathyroid, pancreatic islet cells, and pituitary gland.

MEN type 2 can be divided in three clinical subtypes, which are all inherited in an autosomal dominant fashion.

1. *MEN 2A or Sipple's syndrome* makes up approximately 60–90% of all MEN2 cases and includes medullary thyroid carcinoma (MTC) in 95% of cases, pheochromocytoma in approximately 50%, and parathyroid adenomas causing hyperparathyroidism in about 20–30%.

2. *MEN 2B, Wagenmann-Froboese syndrome, or mucosal neuroma syndrome* represents only about 5% and comprises associations of pheochromocytoma, medullary thyroid cancer, and mucosal neuromas.

3. *Familial medullary thyroid cancer* (FMTC) is the only variant that involves only one gland and constitute 5–35% of MEN 2 cases.[32]

PERIOPERATIVE MANAGEMENT

It is of utmost importance to characterize the type of MEN syndrome prior to elective surgery to determine its implication for anesthetic management.

Given the common overlap of MEN syndrome, a thorough evaluation of electrolyte and hormonal abnormalities is warranted.

Preoperative characterization of baseline volume status and cardiovascular and hemodynamic parameters is also important. The most problematic entity for the anesthesiologist is aforementioned pheochromocytoma, but other conditions may have potential impact on patient's outcomes; hypercalcemia from parathyroid tumors, hypocalcemia from MTC, hypoglycemia from insulinomas, carcinoid crisis from gastrointestinal tract neuroendocrine tumors, and hypercortisolism from pituitary neoplasms.[33]

SPECIFIC CONDITIONS

Parathyroid Tumors

Primary hypercalcemia, low serum phosphate, and elevated parathyroid hormone are the main manifestations. The clinical symptomatology is diverse and may include moderate to severe dehydration, tachycardia, polyuria, anorexia, vomiting, extreme weakness lethargy, and psychiatric signs and symptoms. These patients will require excision of the affected parathyroid gland to correct the biochemical abnormalities.

Perioperative management revolves mainly around monitoring calcium levels. A shortened QT interval and a prolonged PR interval detected on ECG can be indicative of elevated serum calcium, which may reduce the threshold for anesthesia-related cardiac dysrhythmia. Hypercalcemia may cause an unpredictable response to neuromuscular blocking agents, and these should be carefully titrated and monitored with neuromuscular monitoring to avoid potential respiratory compromise from residual muscular blockade.

Interventions to lower plasma concentrations of calcium include diuresis with normal saline hydration to enhance renal calcium excretion, followed by the addition of loop diuretics such as furosemide. Preoperatively, IV mithramycin or bisphosphonates have been used to rapidly lower life-threatening hypercalcemia. Patients may be prone to osteoporosis, necessitating careful operating table positioning to avoid pathological fractures.

Commonly cited postoperative complications include bleeding, recurrent laryngeal nerve injury, and metabolic abnormalities such as hypocalcemia, hypophosphatemia, hypomagnesemia, and hypokalemia. Uncontrolled bleeding, can cause development of hematoma that can cause life-threatening compromise of the airway. Recurrent laryngeal nerve injury, depending on whether it is unilateral or bilateral, partial or complete, can cause a range of symptoms from hoarseness or stridor to complete airway obstruction. Metabolic abnormalities can be catastrophic if not closely monitored and aggressively corrected. The most common is transient mild hypocalcemia that can cause neuromuscular irritability, seizures, and laryngeal spasms. Therefore, close postoperative electrolyte monitoring is important.[34]

These postoperative complications also apply to patients undergoing thyroidectomy for medullary thyroid carcinoma.

Pancreatic Islet Cell Tumors

Insulinomas and gastrinomas are the two most common tumors that have implications for the anesthesiologist. Profound secondary hypoglycemia can occur due to tumor-mediated insulin hypersecretion and symptoms may appear when plasma glucose falls below 50 mg/dL. Low serum glucose levels may present with a catecholaminergic response which include anxiety, tremor, nausea, hunger, diaphoresis, palpitations, or neuroglycopenia (headache, lethargy, diplopia, dizziness, seizures, and, when severe, confusion or even coma).

Medical management of insulinomas include diazoxide and somatostatin analogues like octreotide. It is recommended to continue these medication through the morning of surgery. The patient should also receive a continuous infusion of 10% dextrose during the fasting period.

Clinical manifestations of hypoglycemia may be masked under general anesthesia and a strategy for close intraoperative blood glucose monitoring of blood glucose levels to avoid any neurological sequelae. Additional intraoperative strategies for cerebral protection include methods to decrease the cerebral metabolic oxygen consumption and maintenance of normocarbia.

Postoperatively, hyperglycemia often occurs, and is a useful indicator of adequate tumor resection. Close glucose monitoring should be continued until levels normalize.[33]

Gastrinoma is a gastrin-releasing endocrine tumor responsible for Zollinger-Ellison syndrome, a syndrome characterized by peptic ulcer disease, diarrhea, and esophageal reflux. Two main intraoperative considerations need to be acknowledged: hypovolemia and electrolyte abnormalities. Commonly, hypokalemia and metabolic alkalosis are produced secondary to the typical profuse, watery diarrhea associated with this condition, and the loss of large fluid volumes from gastric hypersecretion. In addition, the commonly observed gastric hypersecretion may predisposes the patient to aspiration events and warrants rapid-sequence induction to reduce the risk of pulmonary aspiration. Antacid prophylaxis with proton pump inhibitors and H_2-receptor antagonists should be maintained until surgery.[35]

Carcinoid Tumors

Most carcinoids associated with MEN (69%) are of foregut origin (thymus, bronchus, stomach, and duodenum). Carcinoids are more commonly associated with MEN type 1 than MEN type 2. These tumors release biochemical mediators that lead to carcinoid syndrome, and may precipitate perioperative hemodynamic instability. The three most important mediators released are serotonin, histamine, and kinins.

Carcinoid syndrome may commonly present with hypotension, hypertension, cutaneous flushing, bronchoconstriction, diarrhea, and carcinoid heart disease.

The patient's baseline cardiovascular status, volume status, electrolyte abnormalities, bronchospasm, or hyperglycemia should be assessed and treated if possible, prior to surgery. Invasive arterial monitoring should be established prior to the induction of anesthesia. Histaminergic or catecholaminergic drug should be avoided during induction of anesthesia.

Benzodiazepine premedication can reduce stress-induced catecholamine release.[36] Sympathomimetic and histaminergic drugs such as ketamine, morphine, meperidine, atracurium, and pancuronium are avoided. For induction, propofol may be the optimal sedative-hypnotic, since it blunts laryngeal reflexes to intubation and does not cause histamine release.

Intraoperative carcinoid crisis presents with hyper- or hypotension, bronchospasm, hypoglycemia, cardiac dysrhythmias, or heart failure. It is more likely to happen during induction, tracheal intubation, surgical stimulation, or after use of drugs that cause histamine release. Hypertension can be treated by increasing depth of anesthesia or administration of negative inotropes. Intraoperative hypotension may be optimally treated with vasopressin.

Octreotide has become the drug of choice for control of symptoms of carcinoid syndrome and carcinoid crisis. Bronchospasm can be treated with inhaled beta agonists, which, are not contraindicated.[36]

Due to residual effects of mediators or presence of previously undetected metastases, close postoperative monitoring is indicated.

Pituitary Tumors

Anterior pituitary tumors are part of MEN 1 syndrome, and abnormal secretion of human growth hormone (HGH) is the most relevant to anesthesiologists. HGH may precipitate acromegaly, and consequently, craniofacial abnormalities that can predispose to a difficult airway. These patients generally have prognathism, enlarged nose and lips, dental malocclusion, and enlarged tongue, epiglottis, and lower jaw. A thorough physical examination of the airway and early preparation of alternative airway management tools aids in reducing the risk of unanticipated difficult airway.

In summary, MEN syndromes may create unique challenges for the anesthesiologist. Careful preoperative evaluation, watchful intraoperative monitoring that continues into the postoperative period, awareness of perioperative complications and timely management will be crucial to achieve good outcomes.

CONCLUSION

- PPGLs are neuroendocrine-derived tumors that may have significant hormonal activity.
- PPGLs are often associated with familial syndromes such as MEN2, neurofibromatosis type 1, and von Hippel-Lindau syndrome.
- Patients may be asymptomatic or may present with symptoms of paroxysmal headache, flushing, sweating, and tachycardia.
- Diagnosis is performed with urinary or plasma metanephrine measurement. a CT, MRI, or scintigraphy are used to locate the metabolically active tumor.
- Close preoperative blood pressure management, usually with selective or nonselective alpha blockade, must be instituted prior to surgical resection.
- Preoperative optimization, aggressive intraoperative hemodynamic monitoring, and close postoperative monitoring will result in favorable clinical outcomes.
- Newfound uses for well-known medications such as magnesium, phosphodiesterase III inhibitors, and vasopressin may further improve clinical outcomes.

REVIEW QUESTIONS

1. The following signs and symptoms are consistent with a pheochromocytoma *except*

    a. Hypertension.
    b. Panic attacks.
    c. Hypoglycemia.
    d. Palpitations.
    e. Sweating.

The correct answer is c.

Patients with symptomatic PPGLs may present with paroxysmal sympathomimetic symptoms such as excessive sweating, palpitations, tachycardia, tremor, or headache although 50% of patients will be asymptomatic. Rarely, pheochromocytoma crisis may occur and is manifest with refractory hypertension, altered mental status, and hyperthermia.

2. The Roizen criteria for optimization prior to pheochromocytoma resection include all *except*

    a. A blood pressure measurement of less than 160/90 for 24 hours prior to surgical intervention.
    b. Resolution of orthostatic hypotension.
    c. Blood pressure of less than 130/80 before surgical resection.
    d. Resolution of ECG changes.
    e. No more than one premature ventricular contraction per 5-minute interval.

The correct answer is c.

The Endocrine Society guidelines recommend a blood pressure level of less than 130/80 before surgical resection; all others are part of the Roizen criteria.

3. During pheochromocytoma resection all the following anesthetic agents are safe *except*

    a. Ketamine.
    b. Propofol.
    c. Lidocaine.
    d. Fentanyl.
    e. Rocuronium.

The correct answer is a.

Ketamine, due to its sympathomimetic effects, should be avoided during the pheochromocytoma resection.

4. All these medications can be safely used during carcinoid crisis *except*

    a. Octreotide.
    d. Albuterol.
    c. Ephedrine.
    d. Vasopressin.
    e. Ketamine.

The correct answer is c.

Sympathomimetics can potentiate carcinoid crisis and therefore are relatively contraindicated.

REFERENCES

1. Beard CM, Sheps SG, Kurland LT, Carney JA, Lie JT. Occurrence of pheochromocytoma in Rochester, Minnesota, 1950 through 1979. *Mayo Clin Proc*. 1983 Dec;58(12):802–804.
2. Pomares FJ, Cañas R, Rodriguez JM, Hernandez AM, Parrilla P, Tebar FJ. Differences between sporadic and multiple endocrine neoplasia type 2A phaeochromocytoma. *Clin Endocrinol (Oxf)*. 1998 Feb;48(2):195–200.
3. Kopetschke R, Slisko M, Kilisli A, et al. Frequent incidental discovery of phaeochromocytoma: Data from a German cohort of 201 phaeochromocytoma. *Eur J Endocrinol*. 2009 Aug;161(2):355–361.
4. Lambrecht A, Inglis JM, Young R. Abdominal pain with intra-adrenal bleeding as an initial presentation of pheochromocytoma. *BMJ Case Rep*. 2021 Jan 11;14(1):e237975.
5. Endo Y, Kitago M, Shinoda M, et al. Extra-adrenal pheochromocytoma with initial symptom of haemoptysis: A case report and review of literature. *BMC Surg*. 2021 Jan 6;21(1):13.
6. Elenkova A, Matrozova J, Vasilev V, Robeva R, Zacharieva S. Prevalence and progression of carbohydrate disorders in patients with pheochromocytoma/paraganglioma: Retrospective single-center study. *Ann Endocrinol (Paris)*. 2020 Feb;81(1):3–10.
7. Abe I, Islam F, Lam AK-Y. Glucose intolerance on phaeochromocytoma and paraganglioma—The current understanding and clinical perspectives. *Front Endocrinol*. 2020;11:593780.
8. Pacak K. Preoperative management of the pheochromocytoma patient. *J Clin Endocrinol Metab*. 2007 Nov;92(11):4069–4079.
9. Procopiou M, Finney H, Akker SA, et al. Evaluation of an enzyme immunoassay for plasma-free metanephrines in the diagnosis of catecholamine-secreting tumors. *Eur J Endocrinol*. 2009 Jul;161(1):131–140.
10. Lenders JW, Duh QY, Eisenhofer G, et al. Pheochromocytoma and paraganglioma: An endocrine society clinical practice guideline. *J Clin Endocrinol Metab*. 2014 Jun;99(6):1915–1942.

11. Kong H, Li N, Yang XC, Nie XL, Tian J, Wang DX. Nonselective compared with selective α-blockade is associated with less intraoperative hypertension in patients with pheochromocytomas and paragangliomas: A retrospective cohort study with propensity score matching. *Anesth Analg*. 2021 Jan;132(1):140–149.
12. Fang F, Ding L, He Q, Liu M. Preoperative management of pheochromocytoma and paraganglioma. *Front Endocrinol (Lausanne)*. 2020;11:586795.
13. Schimmack S, Kaiser J, Probst P, Kalkum E, Diener MK, Strobel O. Meta-analysis of α-blockade versus no blockade before adrenalectomy for phaeochromocytoma. *Br J Surg*. 2020 Jan;107(2):e102–e108.
14. Kong H, Li N, Tian J, Li XY. Risk predictors of prolonged hypotension after open surgery for pheochromocytomas and paragangliomas. *World J Surg*. 2020 Nov;44(11):3786–3794.
15. Butz JJ, Weingarten TN, Cavalcante AN, et al. Perioperative hemodynamics and outcomes of patients on metyrosine undergoing resection of pheochromocytoma or paraganglioma. *Int J Surg*. 2017 Oct;46:1–6.
16. Roizen MF, Hunt TK, Beaupre PN, et al. The effect of alpha-adrenergic blockade on cardiac performance and tissue oxygen delivery during excision of pheochromocytoma. *Surgery*. 1983 Dec;94(6):941–945.
17. Lenders JW, Duh QY, Eisenhofer G, et al. Pheochromocytoma and paraganglioma: An endocrine society clinical practice guideline. *J Clin Endocrinol Metab*. 2014 Jun;99(6):1915–1942.
18. Kong H, Yang JN, Tian J, et al. Preoperative intravenous rehydration for patients with pheochromocytomas and paragangliomas: Is it necessary? A propensity score matching analysis. *BMC Anesthesiol*. 2020 Nov 30;20(1):294.
19. Witteles RM. Safe and cost-effective preoperative preparation of patients with pheochromocytoma. *Anesth Analg*. 2000;91(2):302–304.
20. Kassim TA, Clarke DD, Mai VQ, Clyde PW, Mohamed Shakir KM Catecholamine-induced cardiomyopathy. *Endocr Pract*. 2008 Dec;14(9):1137–1149.
21. Fu SQ, Wang SY, Chen Q, Liu YT, Li ZL, Sun T. Laparoscopic versus open surgery for pheochromocytoma: A meta-analysis. *BMC Surg*. 2020 Jul 25;20(1):167.
22. Li N, Kong H, Li SL, Zhu SN, Wang DX. Combined epidural-general anesthesia was associated with lower risk of postoperative complications in patients undergoing open abdominal surgery for pheochromocytoma: A retrospective cohort study. *PLoS One*. 2018;13(2):e0192924.
23. Khan FA, Ullah H. Pharmacological agents for preventing morbidity associated with the haemodynamic response to tracheal intubation. *Cochrane Database Syst Rev*. 2013 Jul;3(7):Cd004087.
24. Livingstone M, Duttchen K, Thompson J, et al. Hemodynamic stability during pheochromocytoma resection: Lessons learned over the last two decades. *Ann Surg Oncol*. 2015 Dec;22(13):4175–4180.
25. Lord MS, Augoustides JG. Perioperative management of pheochromocytoma: Focus on magnesium, clevidipine, and vasopressin. *J Cardiothorac Vasc Anesth*. 2012 Jun;26(3):526–531.
26. Hylton DJ, Minot PR, Mihm FG. Another role for angiotensin II: Vasopressin-refractory shock after pheochromocytoma resection: A case report. *A A Pract*. 2020 Jan 15;14(2):54–57.
27. Nagamine Y, Nishinarita R, Mizutani K, Goto T. [The use of arginine vasopressin and phosphodiesterase III inhibitor for circulatory shock after the resection of a massive adrenal pheochromocytoma]. *Masui*. 2016 Jun;65(6):624–627.
28. Mamilla D, Araque KA, Brofferio A, et al. Postoperative management in patients with pheochromocytoma and paraganglioma. *Cancers (Basel)*. 2019 Jul 3;11(7):936.
29. de Fourmestraux A, Salomon L, Abbou CC, Grise P. Ten year experience of retroperitoneal laparoscopic resection for pheochromocytomas: A dual-centre study of 72 cases. *World J Urol*. 2015 Aug;33(8):1103–1107.
30. Papachristos AJ, Cherry TJ, Nyandoro MG, et al. Bi-national review of phaeochromocytoma care: Is ICU admission always necessary? *World J Surg*. 2021;45(3):790–796.
31. Fang AM, Rosen J, Saidian A, et al. Perioperative outcomes of laparoscopic, robotic, and open approaches to pheochromocytoma. *J Robot Surg*. 2020 Dec;14(6):849–854.
32. Moo-Young TA, Traugott AL, Moley JF. Sporadic and familial medullary thyroid carcinoma: State of the art. *Surg Clin North Am*. 2009 Oct;89(5):1193–1204.
33. Grant F. Anesthetic considerations in the multiple endocrine neoplasia syndromes. *Curr Opin Anaesthesiol*. 2005 Jun;18(3):345–352.
34. Malhotra S, Sodhi V. Anaesthesia for thyroid and parathyroid surgery. *Cont Educ Anaesth Crit Care Pain*. 2007;7(2):55–58.
35. Dougherty TB, Cronau LH. Anesthetic implications for surgical patients with endocrine tumors. *Int Anesthesiol Clin*. 1998;36(3):31–44.
36. Fernandez-Robles C, Carr ZJ, Oprea AD. Endocrine emergencies in anesthesia. *Curr Opin Anaesthesiol*. 2021 Jun 01;34(3):326–334.

PART IV

WOMEN'S HEALTH

31.

PREGNANT PATIENT FOR NON-OBSTETRIC SURGERY

Nayema K. Salimi and Kristen L. Fardelmann

STEM CASE AND KEY QUESTIONS

A 27-year-old woman arrives to a community hospital emergency department complaining of increased right upper quadrant abdominal pain associated with nausea and vomiting, especially after meals. She is in 9/10 pain and has not been able to tolerate solid food for the past 24 hours. Her vital signs are notable for a heart rate of 121 beats per minute, blood pressure of 149/83 mmHg, respiratory rate of 24 breaths per minute, and temperature of 101.1°F. Her abdomen is tender to palpation with guarding and negative for rebound tenderness. Elevations in her liver function tests (LFTs) and white blood cell count are found on laboratory evaluation. Abdominal ultrasound reveals the presence of gallstones, pericholecystic fluid, and gallbladder wall thickening. She is diagnosed with acute cholecystitis, and the surgical service is recommending a laparoscopic cholecystectomy.

When is a screening pregnancy test indicated prior to surgery?

As part of the evaluation for abdominal pain, the patient received a urine pregnancy test which was found to be positive. On further inquiry, the patient reports a history of abnormal menses and has not had a menstrual cycle in at least 4 months. She denies knowledge of her pregnancy and has not received prenatal care.

What is the appropriate next step in the preoperative evaluation for the pregnant patient?

What requirements are expected of an institution to provide care to this patient population?

The obstetric team affiliated with the community hospital is consulted for evaluation and reveals that they do not provide 24-hour in-house coverage. Additionally, there is only a Level I neonatal ICU (NICU) available, capable of basic newborn care and unable to accept a preterm infant.

Is it appropriate to delay surgery in a pregnant patient?

The surgeons discuss the risks, benefits, and alternative options of medical management, endoscopic intervention, and surgery with the patient. Based on the severity of the patient's symptoms, it is decided that the patient does indeed warrant surgical intervention. Given her gestational age and lack of available obstetric services, the patient is transferred to a tertiary care center for further obstetric and surgical management. IV fluid administration and antibiotic treatment are initiated prior to transfer. Further medical management includes acetaminophen, antiemetics, pain control with opioid medications, and a NPO order.

On arrival at the tertiary care facility, the patient is met by the obstetric team who performs an ultrasound and dates her at approximately 27 weeks gestational age. The NICU team is notified of her arrival and plans for anticipatory care. She continues to endorse 7/10 right upper quadrant abdominal pain despite analgesics. Her heart rate is 108 bpm, blood pressure is 139/64 mmHg, and respiratory rate is 22 breaths per minute. The patient is counseled on the risks, benefits, and alternatives of the operation and consents for a laparoscopic cholecystectomy.

What kind of monitoring is recommended during the perioperative period?

What are the pros and cons of continuous intraoperative fetal monitoring?

The obstetrician recommends continuous fetal heart rate (FHR) monitoring in the preoperative, intraoperative, and postoperative phases of care. The patient is counseled on the risk of preterm delivery and is given one dose of betamethasone preoperatively. After discussion with obstetrics and neonatology, the patient consents to emergency cesarean delivery in the setting of persistent fetal distress.

You will be the staff anesthesiologist for this case and are working with a junior resident who is not familiar with obstetric patients. When discussing your anesthetic plan, you are asked the following questions:

How do you counsel the patient on her risks of surgery and anesthesia during pregnancy?

What medications would you avoid in pregnancy?

Are there any additional monitors that you would need?

During your assessment, the patient denies any significant past medical or surgical history, has no known drug allergies, and reports an exercise tolerance of greater than 4 metabolic equivalents (METS). She denies any prior anesthetics and does not have a family history of complications with anesthesia. She does, however, endorse motion sickness. She has not taken any food or drink by mouth in at least 8 hours and continues to note abdominal pain and mild nausea. On physical examination, she is 5′6″ and weighs 102 kg with a BMI of 36.3 kg/m². She has a 2/6 holosystolic murmur heard best at the left upper sternal border without radiation, and her breath sounds are diminished at the bases. Her airway evaluation reveals a Mallampati Class II score, interincisor distance of greater 3 fingerbreadths, and full range of motion of her neck. An 18-gauge peripheral IV is present in her right antecubital fossa. Her hematocrit is 36%. Risks, benefits, and alternatives are discussed, and consent is obtained for general anesthesia (GA).

Preoperatively, the patient is given aspiration prophylaxis with sodium citrate, famotidine, and metoclopramide. Prior to anesthetic induction, sequential compression devices are placed on her lower extremities for deep vein thrombosis prophylaxis. Following preoxygenation, GA is induced with a rapid-sequence induction.

What implications do the physiologic changes of pregnancy have on her anesthetic plan?

Following induction, a size 6.5 mm endotracheal tube (ETT) is placed and secured at 21 cm at the lip. An orogastric tube is placed, and intermediate acting neuromuscular blocking (NMB) agent is administered. You intentionally hyperventilate the patient to maintain an end tidal carbon dioxide ($EtCO_2$) between 30 and 32 mmHg. She is afebrile and tachycardic with a heart rate of 100 bpm and blood pressure is 108/53 mmHg. Fetal heart rate tracing remains reassuring throughout induction.

Soon after incision, a trocar is placed, and the abdomen is insufflated to a pressure of 15 mmHg. Within moments, the patient becomes bradycardic to 40 bpm and hypotensive with a systolic pressure of 70 mmHg. The labor and birth nurse announces a decrease in the FHR.

How do you troubleshoot acute hypotension after insufflation?

What physiologic changes are associated with pneumoperitoneum?

You immediately communicate with the surgical team and request desufflation of the abdomen. The patient's hemodynamics restabilize with desufflation and administration of ephedrine. The FHR tracing is reassuring after a transient bradycardic episode associated with maternal hypotension. The patient is repositioned with a wedge under her right hip to obtain adequate left uterine displacement and a 500 cc bolus of crystalloid solution is administered. Insufflation is reattempted slowly to a maximum pressure of 10 mmHg. The patient's hemodynamics are stable, and the FHR tracing is reassuring.

As the case progresses, the surgeons note significant adhesions that are making the procedure technically challenging to perform laparoscopically. A small area of bleeding is noted during mobilization of the gallbladder. The patient's hemodynamics remain stable, and the FHR remains reassuring. Hemostasis is subsequently achieved, the abdomen is desufflated, and the surgeons begin to suture the incisions. The estimated blood loss is 400 cc. Total IV fluid administration is 1,700 cc. Intraoperative analgesia includes 1,000 mg IV acetaminophen, 100 mcg IV fentanyl and 0.8 mg IV hydromorphone.

How would you approach emergence and reversal of NMB for this patient?

Sugammadex is administered, and adequate reversal of NMB is noted. On emergence, the patient's systolic blood pressure increases to 160 mmHg. The patient is extubated uneventfully. In the PACU, the patient is alert and oriented, reporting 3/10 abdominal pain. Her blood pressure remains mildly elevated at 142/89 mmHg. The FHR remains reassuring. Postoperative laboratory evaluation is notable for continued elevations in her LFTs and a hematocrit of 29%.

What must remain on the differential for a pregnant patient with abnormal LFTs and hypertension?

What are the diagnostic criteria for pre-eclampsia?

As the patient is readying for discharge to her inpatient room, she becomes unresponsive and is witnessed to have twitching of her facial muscles that progresses to tonic-clonic movements. The anesthesia team is notified. The team initiates 100% oxygen via facemask, and her seizure breaks prior to administration of medications. After regaining consciousness, the patient appears confused and slow to respond. The surgical, obstetric, and NICU teams are called to the bedside and are concerned for eclamptic seizure. The FHR monitor is replaced and found to be reassuring.

How do you manage eclamptic seizures?

The patient's mental status returns to baseline. She is treated with a magnesium sulfate load followed by an infusion and admitted to the high-risk obstetric service for further management.

DISCUSSION

Non-obstetric surgery has been estimated to occur in 0.7–2% of all pregnancies.[1,2] However, the true occurrence is thought to be even higher due to the prevalence of unrecognized pregnancies at the time of surgery and the high incidence (20–30%) of early pregnancy loss.[3] When assessing all surgical procedures (obstetric and non-obstetric) in pregnancy, a retrospective analysis of 1.6 million pregnancies in Denmark from 1996 to 2015 found the incidence to be 6.4%.[2] The most common non-obstetric surgical interventions performed during pregnancy are abdominal procedures (appendectomy and cholecystectomy) followed by dental, nail/skin, orthopedic, gynecologic, ENT, perianal, and breast procedures.[1,2] In a retrospective study that analyzed 2,000 pregnant patients from the American College of Surgeons National Surgical Quality Improvement Program who underwent non-obstetric surgery, the prevalence of composite major postoperative complications was 5.8% and 30-day postoperative maternal mortality was 0.25%.[4] Risk factors for postoperative complications include increased age, preoperative systemic infection, New York Heart Association class III–IV, American Society of

Anesthesiologists (ASA) classification IV or V, preoperative comorbidities, and increasing operative time.[4]

ROUTINE PREGNANCY TESTING

In 2012, the ASA Taskforce on Preanesthesia Evaluation stated, "Pregnancy testing may be offered to female patients of childbearing age and for whom the result would alter the patient's management."[5] Mandatory routine pregnancy testing is not recommended for all patients in the preoperative period.[6] Surgical procedures which have the potential for creating fetal harm, including those involving the uterine cavity, those that may alter uterine blood flow (including cardiac and vascular procedures), and procedures which may introduce fetal teratogens such as radiation, are recommended to have preoperative pregnancy testing.[6] For other cases, pregnancy testing should be offered to patients if the knowledge of such results would impact a patient's medical management. Laparoscopic intra-abdominal procedures are considered of indeterminant risk to the fetus.[6] Screening for urine beta human chorionic gonadotropin (hCG) of greater than 25 IU/L is a sensitive and specific marker for pregnancy 14 days after fertilization.[6] Correlation with serum hCG may be necessary in specific clinical scenarios.[6,7]

Of women who are routinely screened, 0.15–2.2% are found to have a positive pregnancy test.[7] The incidence of pregnancy in a cohort of 2,056 women of childbearing potential presenting for ambulatory surgery was 0.3% leading to 100% cancellation or postponement of surgical intervention.[8] The possibility of false-negative and false-positive tests should be considered as the results have potential social, medical, and medico-legal implications for the patient, embryo/fetus, and physicians.[7,9,10]

From a medico-legal standpoint, caution should be taken to ensure that the results of a urine pregnancy test are reviewed, if ordered, and appropriately revealed to the patient.[6,11] The failure to check the results and document the risk of miscarriage may pose negative medico-legal consequences for the anesthesiologist.[6,7,11] Ultimately, it is the patient's right to decide if they desire to have a pregnancy test performed. The patient has an ethical right to patient autonomy, informed consent, beneficence, and nonmaleficence.[6] Ideally, the patient receives counseling on risks, benefits, and alternatives to preoperative pregnancy testing and the potential risks of surgery and anesthesia on maternal and fetal outcomes if pregnant.[6] Recommendations include development of education pamphlets for improved shared decision-making and institutional protocols for preoperative pregnancy screening.[6]

PREOPERATIVE EVALUATION OF THE PREGNANT PATIENT

The preoperative evaluation includes a thorough history and physical exam focusing on anesthesia history, past medical history, past surgical history, functional status, allergies, medications, family history, and social history.[5] An obstetric history should be obtained, including a history of prior pregnancies and current gestational age. Specific inquiry for common obstetric diagnoses should be performed, including hypertensive disorders of pregnancy, gestational diabetes, gestational thrombocytopenia, coagulation abnormalities, and use of anticoagulation.[12] The physical exam should concentrate on the maternal airway, cardiovascular and lung exam, BMI, and vital signs.[5,12] Routine laboratory evaluation in the healthy pregnant patient undergoing low-risk surgery is not warranted.[12] Routine type and screen are not recommended unless the procedure or clinical scenario is associated with high risk of hemorrhage.[12] Evaluation of platelet count is necessary in the pregnant patient with hypertension as part of the diagnostic evaluation for preeclampsia or hemolysis, elevated liver enzymes, and low platelet count (HELLP) syndrome.[12–14]

Preoperative obstetric consultation is recommended for all pregnant patients scheduled for non-obstetric surgery by the American College of Obstetricians and Gynecologists (ACOG) and ASA.[15] During consultation, the obstetrician should evaluate the well-being of the mother and fetus, consider the administration of corticosteroids in viable pregnancies at premature gestational ages, and determine appropriate perioperative venous thromboembolism prophylaxis.[15] Furthermore, obstetricians and anesthesiologists should discuss the risks, benefits, and alternatives of surgery and anesthesia during pregnancy and should obtain informed consent.[15] Consultation in the preoperative period provides an opportunity to discuss intraoperative FHR monitoring with the surgical team, obstetric nursing staff, anesthesiologists, obstetricians, and neonatologists. Finally, preoperative consultation provides the opportunity to discuss the potential for intervention in the setting of intraoperative fetal distress of a viable fetus.[15] Informed consent may include neonatology consultation to discuss the outcomes of an infant born at a particular gestational age as emergent cesarean delivery is considered for all viable fetuses with persistent distress on fetal monitoring.

TIMING OF NON-OBSTETRIC SURGERY DURING PREGNANCY

Emergent surgery should never be delayed due to the potential for adverse outcomes in mother and fetus.[4,15] In contrast to emergent surgery, it is recommended to delay elective surgery in pregnancy until after delivery.[15] In fact, delay of elective surgery should be considered until about 6 weeks postpartum, at which time most maternal physiologic changes in pregnancy are back to their pre-pregnancy baseline. As in our case, multidisciplinary consultation may benefit the pregnant patient who meets medical necessity for an urgent procedure to optimize maternal and fetal well-being prior to intervention, create a multidisciplinary perioperative plan, and provide counseling to the patient. For patients at advanced gestational ages, consideration may be given to preprocedural delivery of the fetus by cesarean section to minimize exposure to anesthetic agents.

Historically, the second trimester was thought to be the safest time for surgery due to concerns regarding teratogenicity and pregnancy loss in the first trimester and preterm labor in the third trimester.[16,17] However, available evidence reveals the first trimester is the most common period for surgical interventions followed by the second trimester and then the third trimester.[2]

In a retrospective cohort study from the American College of Surgeons' National Surgical Quality Improvement Program that propensity-matched females 1:1 with nonpregnant women undergoing the same operations, there was no statistical difference in 30-day mortality rates or overall morbidity.[18] Prevalence of major postoperative complications following non-obstetric surgery in pregnancy is low.[4]

However, evidence should be noted for pregnant patients with appendicitis as it may be associated with significant adverse maternal and fetal outcomes, especially when delays in surgical intervention are reviewed. When compared to the nonpregnant patient, the pregnant patient with appendicitis is at higher risk of sepsis, appendicitis with peritonitis, bowel obstruction, postoperative pneumonia, postoperative infection, and length of stay of greater than 3 days.[19] For patients with appendicitis with perforation, the rate of fetal loss was reported at 10.9% compared to 2.6% in appendicitis without perforation.[20]

Adverse maternal and fetal complications are also seen with delays of care in other surgical pathologies. Analyzing surgical trends between 2003 and 2015, the timing of surgical intervention after admission for acute cholecystitis in the pregnant patient significantly shortened, and each day surgery was delayed was associated with an increase in maternal and fetal complications.[21] When compared to medical management, Cheng et al. found that laparoscopic cholecystectomy was associated with significantly lower rates of preterm labor, preterm delivery, abortion, antepartum hemorrhage, and amniotic infection.[21] A study by Kuy et al. also revealed higher rates of adverse maternal and fetal complications when biliary disease in pregnancy was managed nonoperatively compared to cholecystectomy.[22]

INSTITUTIONAL RESOURCES FOR NON-OBSTETRIC SURGERY

When contemplating maternal transfers of care, the capabilities of the institution must be considered including its access to resources (imaging techniques, blood product availability, laboratory testing, etc.), the level of expertise of the obstetric and neonatal teams, and the availability of supportive services (obstetric anesthesiologists, subspecialty surgical services, and critical care medicine). Criteria for levels of maternal care have been proposed to standardize systems and minimize maternal and fetal morbidity and mortality.[23] Currently, there are four proposed designated levels of care: basic care (level I), specialty care (level II), subspecialty care (level III), and regional perinatal healthcare centers (level IV).[23]

Non-obstetric surgery in pregnancy should occur at an institution with the following services and resources[15]:

- An obstetric clinician with surgical privileges at the institution should be involved in the care of the patient.
- If fetal monitoring is planned:

- An individual qualified in FHR pattern interpretation should be available.
- The obstetrician involved in the patient's care should have cesarean delivery privileges and be readily available.
- Neonatal and pediatric services should be readily available to provide resuscitation at the gestational age of the fetus.

PATIENT COUNSELING

In recent years, non-obstetric surgery in pregnancy has garnered significant national attention. In 2016, the Food and Drug Administration (FDA) issued a warning regarding anesthetic agents and their use in pregnant patients.[24] Specifically, the FDA reported that repeated or lengthy exposure (>3 hours in duration) to GA or sedative medications in pregnant women during the third trimester may affect the neurocognitive and behavioral development of the child.[24] The FDA outlined the requirement for the following commonly administered medications to state this warning on their labels: desflurane, sevoflurane, isoflurane, halothane, propofol, etomidate, ketamine, methohexital, pentobarbital, lorazepam injection, and midazolam injection or syrup.[24] In response, the ACOG disseminated an update to the Committee Opinion on Non-Obstetric Surgery During Pregnancy in collaboration with the ASA. In particular, the update includes the following statements: "No currently used anesthetic agents have been shown to have any teratogenic effects in humans when using standard concentrations at any gestational age. There is no evidence that in utero human exposure to anesthetic or sedative drugs has any effect on the developing fetal brain; and there are no animal data to support an effect with limited exposures less than 3 hours in duration."[15]

A meta-analysis of 65 animal studies evaluating the effects of GA during pregnancy on neurocognitive development of the fetus revealed that GA during pregnancy impaired learning and memory and also resulted in neuronal injury in all models irrespective of anesthetic drugs administered and timing of exposure to agents.[25] Limitations to the application of study findings in humans included risk of bias, exposure of anesthetics at greater than 1 minimal alveolar concentration (MAC), with a duration of more than 3 hours, occurrence of multiple exposures, lack of surgical pathology/intervention, conduct and monitoring of anesthesia below current clinical standards in humans, and inability to translate exposure risk for animal species with significantly different brain development compared with humans.[25] Furthermore, respiratory depression, hypoxemia, and hypercarbia were likely and are known to impair neurocognitive function and cause neuronal apoptosis.[25] In contrast to animal studies, compelling evidence supporting neurocognitive dysfunction in humans after exposure to anesthetic agents is lacking. Translational value is limited as most non-obstetric surgical procedures in pregnancy last less than 3 hours and repeated exposure to anesthesia is rare.

In 2021, Ing et al. presented the only study to date supporting a potential neurocognitive effect of prenatal exposure to anesthesia in humans.[26] This observational cohort study compared children in Australia (Raine Study) with prenatal exposure to GA (n = 22) between 1989 and 1992 to children without exposure (n = 2002) using six neuropsychological and behavioral tests including the Child Behavioral Checklist (CBCL).[27] There were no statistically significant differences in outcomes related to language, cognition, motor function, or total CBCL score.[27] There was a statistical difference in externalizing behavior on the CBCL.[27] The CBCL is a screening tool that is not particularly sensitive.[26] It is important to note that the difference in externalizing behavior found using the Likert scoring system of the CBCL is not associated with any diagnosis, and the clinical relevance of these findings, if any, is unclear.[26] This study was unable to adjust for several significant confounding variables such as maternal smoking and stressful life events during pregnancy that are known contributors to increased externalizing behavior scores.[26]

In 2023, Bleeser et al. presented the largest study to date analyzing neurodevelopmental outcomes after prenatal exposure to anesthesia during maternal surgery.[28] Between 2001 and 2018, exposed cases (n = 129) and matched controls (n = 453) were compared for global executive function, total psychosocial issues, mental health diagnoses, and internalizing and externalizing behavior problems with the CBCL.[28] Prenatal exposure to GA was not associated with clinically meaningful impairments in neurodevelopmental outcomes, including no significant differences between total CBCL, internalizing behavior on the CBCL, and externalizing behavior on the CBCL.[28]

When considering the potential impact of surgical and anesthetic exposure to neurocognitive fetal outcomes, it is important to note the experience of the fetal surgery population.[26] In a prospective, randomized trial, the Management of Myelomeningocele Study (MOMS) compared prenatal (antepartum) versus postnatal fetal myelomeningocele repair in a healthy maternal population.[29] Antepartum repair during fetal surgery in pregnancy includes exposure to several agents identified by the FDA as potentially harmful to the neurocognitive and behavioral outcomes of the fetus.[30] During fetal surgery, maternal and fetal anesthetic management includes administration of anesthetic agents such as propofol and sevoflurane at 1–3 MAC for likely more than 3 hours duration.[30] Although limitations in assessing this population exist, when independent experts compared the prenatal versus postnatal repair patients at 12 months, 30 months, and 5.9–10.3 years of age, no statistical difference in neurocognitive or behavioral outcomes was found.[29,31,32]

The evidence is overall reassuring, and concerns related to adverse neurodevelopment outcomes in recent publications should not change our current clinical practice or limit access to interventions for patients who require surgery during pregnancy.

In addition to concerns related to neurocognitive and behavioral outcomes, historical hesitance in providing surgical interventions in the pregnant patient has focused on the risk of teratogenicity, miscarriage, stillbirth, and preterm labor.[1,16,17,33] Of note, several limitations to the application of available literature to current patient management and counseling exist. Limitations include the retrospective nature of the literature; the pooling of different disease pathologies, surgical interventions, and anesthetic techniques in single analyses of outcomes; the use of outdated imaging, surgical, and anesthetic techniques in data analysis; the comparison of pregnant patients undergoing surgical procedures to the general healthy pregnant population; and the insufficient reporting on perinatal outcomes.[33] Most importantly, a majority of the available literature neglects to compare outcomes in pregnant patients who receive medical management versus surgical intervention within the same disease pathology.[33] The contribution of the stress related to disease pathology, surgical intervention, and anesthetic technique to outcome measures is difficult to discern. Despite the potential concerns related to anesthetic exposure in pregnancy and the previously mentioned limitations in the literature, it remains essential that surgery and anesthesia are provided to the pregnant patient when medically necessary.

When counseling patients, there is insufficient evidence to support a difference in the rate of early pregnancy loss due to surgery during the first trimester in comparison to the rate of miscarriage in the general population.[33] Nonelective indications for surgery may include factors which themselves may be associated with pregnancy loss (e.g., potential for sepsis or shock). In addition, there is insufficient evidence to suggest that non-obstetric surgery, especially in the third trimester of pregnancy, may increase the risk of preterm labor or preterm birth.[33] A systemic review of preterm birth in patients receiving non-obstetric surgical interventions found a preterm birth rate of 8.2%, compared to 10–12% in the general obstetric population of the United States.[20,33] Despite these findings, patients should still be counseled on the symptoms of preterm labor such as abdominal pain, changes in vaginal discharge, pelvic or lower abdominal pressure, constant dull low backache, frequent contractions, and ruptured membranes.

PHYSIOLOGIC CHANGES IN PREGNANCY AND THE ANESTHETIC IMPLICATIONS

Pregnancy is associated with a multitude of physiological changes that impact just about every organ system. The following is a focused list of relevant changes that occur with pregnancy[34]:

- Cardiac output increases as early as 5 weeks gestation to a maximum of about 50% by the end of the second trimester. This change in cardiac output is a result of increases in heart rate (25%) and stroke volume (25%). Additional increases in cardiac output are observed in labor and in the immediate postpartum period.

- Increases in ejection fraction, myocardial contractility, left ventricular end-diastolic volume, and left ventricular enlargement are seen.

- Systemic vascular resistance decreases in early pregnancy, reaching a nadir at 20 weeks gestation, and subsequently increasing during late gestation.

- There is no change in capillary wedge pressure, central venous pressure, or pulmonary arterial diastolic pressure.
- A benign flow murmur can be heard at the left sternal border because of increased vascular volume and dilation of the tricuspid annulus.
- Increased cardiac output supplies the uterus, kidneys, and extremities with the term gravid uterus receiving about 700mL/min of blood flow.
- After 20 weeks gestation, the gravid uterus creates aortocaval compression when lying supine.
- There is an increase in oxygen consumption and CO_2 production.
- Functional residual capacity decreases by the fifth month of pregnancy.
- FEV_1, FEV_1/FVC, flow-volume loop, closing capacity, and vital capacity are unchanged.
- Minute ventilation increases primarily as a result of increased tidal volume resulting in respiratory alkalosis with metabolic compensation and a pH of 7.44.
- PaO_2 increases to between 100 and 105 mmHg.
- $PaCO_2$ decreases to about 30 mmHg.
- There is an increase in glomerular filtration rate and creatinine clearance.
- Maternal plasma volume increases greater than the increase in red blood cell volume leading to a dilutional anemia with normal hemoglobin level of 11.6g/dL.
- Pregnancy is a state of accelerated, but compensated intravascular coagulation and patients are at increased risk of clot formation.
- Thrombocytopenia is common in pregnancy with etiologies including gestational thrombocytopenia (exaggerated normal effect of pregnancy), hypertensive disorders of pregnancy, or idiopathic thrombocytopenia. Platelet aggregation increases.
- The baseline leukocyte count increases during pregnancy.
- Gastric emptying is not altered during pregnancy, but there is a decrease in lower esophageal sphincter tone, leading to an increase in gastroesophageal reflux.
- Despite increased volume of distribution and increased plasma volume, there is a decrease in plasma albumin concentration.
- Levels of plasma cholinesterase decrease.
- The MAC is decreased; however, this does not necessarily correlate to decreased inhaled anesthetic requirements.

The anesthetic implications of these changes can be seen in Figure 31.1.

THE OBSTETRIC AIRWAY

Compared to the general population, notable differences in the obstetric airway exist including nasopharyngeal mucosal vascular engorgement and edema resulting in friable tissue. The Mallampati score increases during pregnancy.[35] The incidence of failed tracheal intubation in the obstetric population was previously estimated at 2.6 per 1,000 GAs, with a maternal mortality rate secondary to failed intubation of 2.3 per 100,000 GAs for cesarean section.[36] Interestingly, in an observational study of only 3,115 obstetric patients with almost 60% of the cohort having a BMI of 25 kg/m^2, the incidence of failed intubation was found to be 1 in 370 for cesarean section and 1 in 188 for non-cesarean surgery.[37] In 2022, Reale et al. presented a multicenter, retrospective cohort study of more than 14,000 patients utilizing data from the Multicenter Perioperative Outcomes Group (MPOG) that revealed a risk of difficult intubation of 1:49 and a risk of failed intubation of 1:808 during GA for cesarean section.[38] Risk factors for difficult airway in the obstetric population include increased BMI; Mallampati score of III or IV; receding mandible, short thyromental distance, or small hyoid-to-mentum distance; limited jaw protrusion; limited mouth opening; cervical spine limitations; short neck; increased neck circumference; and protruding maxillary incisors.[38–40]

Preparation for the obstetric airway occurs in the preoperative setting. With the known decrease in lower esophageal tone associated with pregnancy, a fasting period for solid foods of at least 6–8 hours and clear liquids of 2 hours is recommended in addition to consideration of preoperative nonparticulate antacid prophylaxis, H_2- receptor antagonists, and metoclopramide.[12] The Obstetric Anaesthetists' Association and Difficult Airway Society has developed a difficult airway algorithm for the obstetric patient.[41] Due to rapid desaturation in pregnancy, adequate preoxygenation is essential. Key considerations for airway management in pregnancy include adequate patient positioning, use of cricoid pressure, rapid-sequence induction, adequate NMB, access to adequate sugammadex doses (16 mg/kg), and access to video laryngoscopy, supraglottic airway devices, and cricothyrotomy kits.[41]

PLACENTAL TRANSFER OF MEDICATIONS AND FETAL RISK

Passive diffusion, carrier-mediated cellular uptake and efflux, and transcytosis are the mechanisms for molecule and drug transfer across the placenta.[42] Medications (including many commonly used anesthetics such as inhaled anesthetics, propofol, methohexital, and phenobarbital) that rapidly diffuse across the placenta are placental blood flow-dependent.[42] Placental transfer of medications is based on molecular weight, charge, protein binding, lipophilicity, and concentration gradient.[42,43] Tetro et al. describes, "The intensity and duration of fetal effects of drugs depend [on] the dose taken by the mother, maternal and fetal pharmacokinetics, and individual factors such as pharmacogenetics, concurrent disease states, and concomitantly taken medications."[42] In pregnancy, alterations in drug bioavailability, distribution, clearance, and

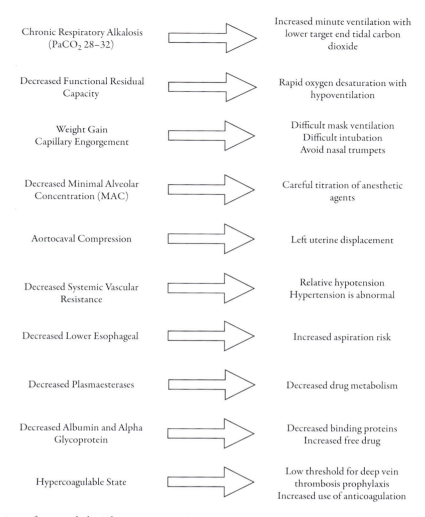

Figure 31.1 Anesthetic implications of maternal physiology.

half-life occur due to physiologic changes.[43] Furthermore, the placenta is physiologically active and is involved in drug metabolism.[43]

In 2015, the US FDA ruled that the current pregnancy classification categories (A–D and X) used since 1979 would be phased out by a new classification system known as the Pregnancy and Lactation Labeling Rule.[44] The change was intended to help healthcare professionals and patients with shared decision-making on the risks and benefits of medication use during pregnancy and breastfeeding periods.[44] In the former classification system, most commonly used anesthetic agents were classified as Category B (propofol, ketamine, ondansetron, metoclopramide, cefazolin, lidocaine, oxycodone, acetaminophen) or C (etomidate, succinylcholine, rocuronium, ephedrine, phenylephrine, sodium citrate, fentanyl, sufentanil, remifentanil, morphine, hydromorphone, ibuprofen, and ketorolac).[43,45] Category B indicated that animal studies did not suggest harm to the fetus, however, no well-controlled studies in humans exist. Category C indicated a lack of well-controlled human studies and either a lack of available animal studies or adverse effects to the fetus were suggested in animal studies.

ANESTHETIC AND SEDATIVE AGENTS IN PREGNANCY

At clinically administered doses, teratogenesis in humans has not been associated with any commonly used anesthetic agents.[46] Mazze et al. analyzed 5,405 procedures in 720,000 pregnant women and found no increase in congenital malformations during prenatal maternal surgery.[47] A systematic review of maternal and fetal outcomes during non-obstetric surgery in pregnancy by Cohen-Kerem et al. found no statistically significant increase in birth defects.[20]

Despite the lack of labeling support and study evidence in pregnancy, medications including propofol, succinylcholine, non-depolarizing NMB agents, inhaled anesthetics, fentanyl, morphine, and hydromorphone have a long history of safe use in the pregnant population.[45] The administration of appropriate medications to achieve adequate hypnosis, pain relief, hemodynamic stability, and surgical environment is essential during non-obstetric surgery to maximize maternal and fetal well-being. Regional anesthetic techniques should be considered to minimize the risks of GA exposure when possible. Although a thorough discussion of each anesthetic agent is out of the scope of this chapter, specific medications and their use in pregnancy will be noted below.

Benzodiazepines

Benzodiazepine use in pregnancy has gathered attention due to a potential association with its use and cleft lip.[48,49] However, no human studies have found a teratogenic effect with a single dose of midazolam during anesthesia.[46] Although some authors recommend avoiding use of midazolam in the first trimester, risk versus benefit should be considered on a case-by-case basis in a shared decision-making model as significant stress may also be associated with adverse maternal and fetal outcomes.[43,50]

Nitrous Oxide

Retrospective human studies that rely on voluntary self-reporting of outcomes have shown an association between nitrous oxide with spontaneous abortion, infertility, and decreased birth weight.[46] In a study of three Swedish healthcare registries that included 5,405 operations with more than 50% of cases performed under GA with nitrous oxide, findings suggested an increase in low-birth-weight and very-low-birth-weight infants but no increase in congenital malformations or stillbirths compared to the general population.[47] Many animal studies supporting teratogenic effects of nitrous oxide have used significant doses for prolonged periods of time.[46] Further studies are needed to assess the neurotoxic effects of nitrous oxide in pregnancy.

Muscle Relaxants and Reversal Agents

Succinylcholine and non-depolarizing NMB agents do not readily cross the placenta. However, case reports on the use of neostigmine in combination with glycopyrrolate in the pregnant patient indicate the potential for clinically significant fetal bradycardia after administration.[51] It is believed that neostigmine crosses the placenta to a greater extent than glycopyrrolate leading to unopposed, nonselective anticholinesterase activity that increases acetylcholine activity at the cardiac muscarinic receptors with resultant fetal bradycardia.[51] Atropine is known to readily cross the placenta.

Sugammadex is an alternative medication to reverse steroidal non-depolarizing NMB. When compared to neostigmine, advantages of sugammadex include rapid and complete antagonism of non-depolarizing NMB with a minimal side-effect profile.[52,53] The Society for Obstetric Anesthesiology and Perinatology's (SOAP) consensus statement on the use of sugammadex in pregnancy recommends avoiding it in early pregnancy due to concerns that it can bind progesterone—a necessary hormone for maintenance of pregnancy.[54] It is also recommended to use sugammadex with caution in patients who are near term or recently delivered due to the unknown effects on lactation.[54] Additionally, all women of childbearing age should be warned of the potential that sugammadex may interfere with hormonal contraception and are recommended to use additional barrier or nonhormonal contraceptive for 1 week after administration.[54]

There is insufficient evidence to support the use of any particular medication or combination of medications to reverse non-depolarizing NMB in the pregnant population. Decisions should be made on a case-by-case basis in a shared decision-making model.

With the known risk of difficult airway and failed tracheal intubation in the obstetric population, rapid-sequence induction with high-dose rocuronium has the potential to optimize the patient for intubation.[36,38] In a cannot intubate, cannot ventilate scenario, the risk of high-dose rocuronium administration is significant. Due to its predictable, rapid recovery of deep NMB, the use of sugammadex is recommended in this clinical scenario at any gestational age.[52,54]

FETAL MONITORING

Intraoperative FHR monitoring recommendations are dependent on gestational age, ability to access monitoring site during the procedure, ability to perform emergent cesarean delivery, and other patient specific factors.[15] Continuous or intermittent FHR monitoring may be utilized to improve fetal well-being through maternal interventions such as optimized left uterine displacement, adequate oxygenation, and sufficient hemodynamic stability. FHR changes are expected with the use of specific anesthetic medications and techniques. For example, opioids may reduce the baseline heart rate by 10–25 bpm and decrease variability.[55,56]

If the fetus is previable, the ACOG recommends pre- and post-procedure FHR assessment.[15] Although the ACOG recommends continuous FHR monitoring for viable fetuses where there is a potential for emergent cesarean delivery for fetal indications,[15] the argument has been made that continuous monitoring may be useful even in previable gestations as a marker of intraoperative fetal compromise and a trigger to improve maternal conditions.[33] Delivery of the viable fetus may be warranted in the setting of persistent fetal distress unresponsive to maternal interventions. After discussion of the potential maternal and neonatal morbidity and mortality associated with fetal delivery at the current gestational age, maternal preference and consent regarding desire for emergent cesarean delivery versus no intervention in the setting of fetal distress should be ascertained and documented by the obstetric and neonatal teams prior to surgery.[55]

LAPAROSCOPY DURING PREGNANCY

The application of laparoscopy as a surgical technique for non-obstetric surgery in pregnancy has increased over the past 20 years, most notably as a result of the 2007 and 2011 recommendations from the Society of American Gastrointestinal and Endoscopic Surgeons.[2,21,57] The recommendations state that pregnant patients with indicated acute abdominal pathology requiring surgical intervention qualify for laparoscopic treatment at any gestational age or trimester.[57] Furthermore, as in the nonpregnant patient, the pregnant patient benefits from the advances of laparoscopic techniques, including their association with less postoperative pain and ileus, decreased length of stay, and faster recovery to baseline function.[57] Specific considerations regarding use of laparoscopy in pregnancy include risks for uterine and fetal trauma, increased maternal carbon dioxide and fetal acidosis, decreased uteroplacental perfusion secondary to increased intra-abdominal pressure, decreased maternal cardiac output, and aortocaval compression.[58] When performing laparoscopic surgery during pregnancy, surgical planning must include safe placement of the trocars with the position of the gravid uterus and its displacement of abdominal structures.

In a recent study of almost 24,000 pregnant patients with acute cholecystitis from the National Inpatient Sample between 2003 and 2015, laparoscopic interventions (59.6%) were most common followed by nonoperative medical management (36.3%) and open cholecystectomy (4.2%).[21] A meta-analysis of laparoscopy versus open surgical intervention for symptomatic cholelithiasis during pregnancy found that laparoscopic techniques are associated with lower rates of fetal, maternal, and surgical complications.[59]

PREECLAMPSIA AND ECLAMPSIA: DIAGNOSIS AND MANAGEMENT

Preeclampsia is a systemic disorder of pregnancy characterized by endothelial dysfunction with multisystem involvement (see Table 31.1) and significant implications for maternal and fetal morbidity and mortality.

Table 31.1 **SYSTEMIC FEATURES OF PREECLAMPSIA**

Central nervous system	Severe headache, visual disturbance, hyperreflexia, coma, seizure, intracerebral hemorrhage, PRES
Airway	Decreased tracheal diameter 2/2 capillary engorgement → pharyngolaryngeal/subglottic edema
Cardiac	Increased SVR and afterload, decreased cardiac output, left ventricular diastolic dysfunction → HTN + intravascular depletion → heart failure, peripartum cardiomyopathy
Pulmonary	Diastolic dysfunction, endothelium dysfunction, decreased oncotic pressure → pulmonary edema → acute hypoxemic respiratory failure
Renal	Decreased GFR → oliguria, hyperuricemia and renal failure
Hepatic	Increased liver function tests → liver failure RUQ pain → subscapular hemorrhage, hematoma, infarction, capsular rupture → intra-abdominal bleeding
Hematologic	Coagulopathy → thrombocytopenia, HELLP, DIC
Obstetric	Intrauterine growth restriction Placental abruption Postpartum hemorrhage Fetal demise

DIC, disseminated intravascular coagulopathy; GFR, glomerular filtration rate; HELLP, hemolysis, elevated liver enzymes, and low platelet count; HTN, hypertension; RUQ, right upper quadrant; SVR, systemic vascular resistance.

The ACOG has identified the following as diagnostic criteria for preeclampsia[14]:

- New-onset hypertension at least 4 hours apart most commonly after 20 weeks gestation (prior to 20 weeks gestation, elevations in blood pressure are most commonly due to chronic hypertension)
  - Hypertension criteria: systolic blood pressure >140 mmHg or diastolic blood pressure >90 mmHg
- And proteinuria diagnosed with either:
  - Urine protein/creatinine ratio >0.3
  - Urine dipstick protein of 2+
  - 24-hour urine protein collection value of >300 mg
- In the absence of proteinuria, new-onset hypertension associated with new onset of any of the following criteria:
  - Platelet count <100 × 10^9/L
  - Serum creatinine concentration >1.1 mg/dL or a doubling of baseline serum creatinine concentration in the absence of underlying renal disease
  - Impaired liver function: elevated liver transaminases to twice the upper limit of normal concentrations, severe persistent right upper quadrant or epigastric pain not explained by another diagnosis
  - Pulmonary edema
  - New-onset headache unresponsive to medications and not explained by another diagnosis
  - Visual disturbances

In our case, the patient had persistent elevations in her blood pressure and elevation of her liver function tests which were attributed to her pain and acute cholecystitis but may have been multifactorial. Patients with preeclampsia are at risk of developing multiorgan dysfunction including eclampsia, HELLP syndrome, disseminated intravascular coagulopathy (DIC), pulmonary edema, and intracerebral hemorrhage. The management of preeclampsia is determined by severity and gestational age.[14] Obstetricians must balance the risk of progressive disease with neonatal growth and fetal lung development.[14] Fetal and maternal surveillance with close symptomatic monitoring, blood pressure control, and frequent fetal assessment are recommended.[14]

Eclampsia is defined as new-onset tonic-clonic seizure in the absence of other etiology for seizure.[60] The incidence of eclampsia in developed countries is between 1.6 and 10 per 10,000 deliveries.[60] The acute care of an eclamptic seizure includes lateral decubitus maternal positioning, placement of padding for maternal safety, maintenance of airway patency, provision of supplemental oxygenation via facemask, and continuous assessment for aspiration.[60] Emergent intubation is not indicated unless airway patency or oxygenation is compromised.[60]

Medication management of seizure activity includes magnesium sulfate bolus of 6 g over 15–20 minutes followed by an infusion of 2 g/hour in patients with adequate renal function.[60] Lorazepam may be indicated for second-line treatment.[60] Approximately 20–38% of women do not exhibit hypertension or proteinuria before an eclamptic seizure episode.[14] Eclampsia should be high on the differential for any pregnant patient who presents with altered mental status. In preeclamptic patients, magnesium sulfate has been shown to halve the risk of eclampsia and likely decreases maternal mortality.[61] Magnesium has the additional benefits of decreasing placental abruptions and providing fetal neuroprotection, however, magnesium levels must be closely monitored due to concerns for toxicity.[61]

CONCLUSION

- Non-obstetric surgery occurs in up to 2% of all pregnancies in the United States and most commonly involves abdominal and orthopedic procedures.

- Medically necessary surgery in the pregnant patient should never be delayed due to concerns for the stress of surgery and anesthesia because delaying care is associated with significant maternal and fetal morbidity and mortality.

- A multidisciplinary approach to care including experts in surgery, obstetrics, anesthesia, and neonatology provides the framework to optimize maternal and fetal outcomes.

- Patients must be counseled on the risks, benefits, and alternatives of surgical intervention during pregnancy. Evidence comparing medical management versus surgical management for surgical specific pathologies is growing.

- The most significant components of intraoperative care include the maintenance of maternal oxygenation, acid-base balance, and hemodynamic stability.

- Fetal monitoring with a FHR before and after the procedure is recommended at a minimum for both viable and previable pregnancies. The decision to perform continuous intraoperative FHR monitoring, and what to do in case of a non-reassuring fetal assessment, should be discussed with the patient preoperatively.

- No commonly used anesthetic agent has been shown to have negative effects on neurocognitive development or teratogenicity at any gestational age.

- Pregnancy-specific conditions must remain in the differential for any patient who presents for non-obstetric surgery in pregnancy.

REVIEW QUESTIONS

1. According to the ASA Taskforce on Preanesthesia Evaluation, which of the following procedures are thought to have a high risk of fetal harm and should warrant a preoperative pregnancy test?

   a. Total abdominal hysterectomy.
   b. Laparoscopic appendectomy.
   c. Ankle open reduction internal fixation.
   d. Laparoscopic ovarian cystectomy.

   The correct answer is a.

   Surgical procedures which have the potential for creating fetal harm, including those involving the uterine cavity, those that may alter uterine blood flow (including cardiac and vascular procedures), and procedures which may introduce fetal teratogens such as radiation, are recommended to have preoperative pregnancy testing.[6] Laparoscopic intra-abdominal procedures are at indeterminant risk.[6]

2. A 38-year-old woman is getting an endoscopic retrograde cholangiopancreatography for severe abdominal pain, thought to be due to gallstone pancreatitis. She declines a preoperative urine pregnancy test. What is the best way to handle the situation?

   a. Proceed without any further action
   b. Obtain a serum hCG level without her consent
   c. Refuse to perform the procedure until pregnancy is ruled out
   d. Discuss the potential risks of anesthesia on the developing fetus and the potential of pregnancy loss with the patient and document the conversation and her decision to decline pregnancy testing.

   The correct answer is d.

   Ultimately, it is the patient's right to decide if she desires to have a pregnancy test performed. Ideally, the patient receives counseling on risks, benefits, and alternatives to preoperative pregnancy testing and the potential risks of surgery and anesthesia on maternal and fetal outcomes if pregnant.[6] This discussion should be documented in the chart for medicolegal purposes.

3. When counseling a patient on the risks of surgery and anesthesia on the developing fetus, all the following are true *except*

   a. None of the commonly used anesthetic medications is a known teratogen, at any gestational age.
   b. There is no evidence that short durations of anesthesia cause neurocognitive dysfunction in the developing fetus.
   c. Elective surgery should be postponed until after delivery.
   d. Surgical pathologies in pregnant patients should be medically managed due to the risk of surgery and anesthesia to the growing fetus.

   The correct answer is d.

   Although elective surgeries should be delayed until at least 6 weeks postpartum when the physiologic changes of pregnancy have subsided, there may be more harm done to the health of the mother, and subsequently the fetus, if emergency surgery is postponed.

4. A 21-year-old at 34 weeks gestational age presents to the emergency department with sharp right lower quadrant abdominal pain and is diagnosed with appendicitis. She is

scheduled for a laparoscopic appendectomy. Continuous fetal monitoring is planned during the procedure. All the following personnel should be notified of her planned procedure and immediately available *except*

   a. Someone capable of performing neonatal resuscitation and the appropriate level of NICU care.
   b. An obstetrician who has privileges in the institution in case of cesarean section.
   c. Someone qualified and skilled in interpreting fetal monitoring.
   d. An obstetric anesthesiologist to supervise the case.

The correct answer is d.

This patient is having laparoscopic abdominal surgery during her third trimester. Since the decision is made to use continuous monitoring, the resources needed to act upon non-reassuring FHRs and undergo an emergency cesarean section should be immediately available. This includes someone qualified in the interpretation of fetal monitoring, an obstetrician with cesarean delivery privileges in the hospital, and a NICU that can care for an infant of the fetus's gestational age at a minimum. In an ideal situation, an obstetric-trained anesthesiologist would be present for any high-risk non-obstetric surgery, however, it is not a requirement for delivery. Given the high incidence of non-obstetric surgery during pregnancy, non-obstetric trained anesthesiologists should also be familiar with the physiologic changes of pregnancy and their anesthetic implications. Furthermore, they should be familiar with fetal monitoring and the potential for emergent cesarean delivery.

5. A 19-year-old woman at 13 weeks gestational age is undergoing a laparoscopic cholecystectomy and has received rocuronium intraoperatively. The procedure has ended, and she currently has 2/4 twitches on a train-of-four monitor. All of the following medications are appropriate for reversal of her neuromuscular blockade, except?

   a. Sugammadex.
   b. Glycopyrrolate and neostigmine.
   c. Atropine and neostigmine.
   d. None of the above.

The correct answer is a.

This patient still has residual neuromuscular blockade as evidenced by her train-of-four ratio and requires reversal prior to extubation. Sugammadex should be used with caution in women who are early in pregnancy as it binds progesterone and may impact the progression of pregnancy.[54]

6. You are working with a medical student who asks you, "Why are pregnant patients at a higher risk of aspiration?" All the following are true of pregnant patients who are at term gestation *except*

   a. Decreased gastric emptying.
   b. Decreased lower esophageal sphincter tone.
   c. Upward displacement of the stomach due to the gravid uterus.
   d. Esophageal peristalsis is slowed.

The correct answer is a.

Pregnant patients do not have delayed gastric emptying during pregnancy, although gastric emptying is delayed during labor.[34]

7. A 24-year-old woman who is 32 weeks pregnant arrives to clinic with a blood pressure of 156/98. On review of her vitals, she has had multiple blood pressures that have been greater than 140/90 over the past 12 weeks. Which of the following labs does not aid in the diagnosis of preeclampsia?

   a. Urine protein/creatinine ratio.
   b. D-dimer.
   c. Serum creatinine.
   d. Liver function tests.

The correct answer is b.

Pregnancy is a hypercoagulable state and is known to cause elevations in D-dimer levels.[34] The diagnosis of preeclampsia includes a multisystem assessment of central nervous system, cardiovascular, renal, hepatic, and hematologic involvement. Proteinuria is a diagnostic criterion of the disease and can be diagnosed with a 24-hour urine collection and 2+ urine dipstick, or more commonly, with a urine protein/creatinine ratio.[14] Serum creatinine aids in the diagnosis of renal dysfunction and in determining magnesium dosing for management.[14]

8. Which of the following is not a potential complication of preeclampsia?

   a. Intracerebral hemorrhage.
   b. Lower extremity neuropathy.
   c. Fetal growth restriction.
   d. Pulmonary edema.

The correct answer is b.

Neuropathy is not one of the nervous system manifestations of preeclampsia.[14]

REFERENCES

1. Balinskaite V, Bottle A, Sodhi V, et al. The risk of adverse pregnancy outcomes following nonobstetric surgery during pregnancy: Estimates from a retrospective cohort study of 6.5 million pregnancies. *Ann Surg.* 2017;266:260–266.
2. Rasmussen AS, Christiansen CF, Uldbjerg N, et al. Obstetric and non-obstetric surgery during pregnancy: A 20-year Danish population-based prevalence study. *BMJ Open.* 2019;9:e028136.
3. Wilcox AJ, Weinberg CR, O'Connor JF, et al. Incidence of early loss of pregnancy. *N Engl J Med.* 1988;319:189–194.
4. Erekson EA, Brousseau EC, Dick-Biascoechea MA, et al. Maternal postoperative complications after nonobstetric antenatal surgery. *J Matern Fetal Neonatal Med.* 2012;25(12):2639–2644.
5. American Society of Anesthesiologists. Practice advisory for preanesthesia evaluation: An updated report by the American Society of Anesthesiologists Task Force on preanesthesia evaluation. *Anesthesiology.* 2012;116(3):522–538.
6. American Society of Anesthesiologists Committee on Quality Management and Departmental Administration. Pregnancy testing prior to anesthesia and pregnancy. Adopted by the ASA House of Delegates on October 26, 2016. http://www.asahq.org/quality-and-practice-management/standards-guidelines-and-related-resources/pregnancy-testing-prior-to-anesthesia-and-surgery
7. Jackson SH. Preoperative pregnancy testing in adults. *ASA Monitor.* 2018;82(11):24–27.

8. Manley S, de Kalaita G, Joseph NJ, et al. Preoperative pregnancy testing in ambulatory surgery. *Anesthesiology*. 1995;83:690–693.
9. Kahn RL, Stanton MA, Tong-Ngork S, et al. One-year experience with day-of-surgery pregnancy testing before elective orthopedic procedures. *Anesth Analg*. 2008;106(4):1127–1131.
10. Bodin SG, Edwards EF, Roy RC, et al. False confidences in preoperative pregnancy testing. *Anesth Analg*. 2010;110:256–257.
11. Wheeler M, Cote CJ. Preoperative pregnancy testing in a tertiary care children's hospital: A medico-legal conundrum. *J Clin Anesth*. 1999;11:56–63.
12. American Society of Anesthesiologists. Practice guidelines for obstetric anesthesia: An updated report by the American Society of Anesthesiologists Task Force on Obstetric Anesthesia and the Society for Obstetric Anesthesia and Perinatology. *Anesthesiology*. 2016;124:270–300.
13. US Preventive Services Task Force. Screening for preeclampsia: US Preventive Services Task Force recommendation statement. *JAMA*. 2017;317(16):1661–1667.
14. American College of Obstetricians and Gynecologists. Gestational hypertension and preeclampsia. ACOG Practice Bulletin, Number 222. *Obstet Gynecol*. 2020;135(6):e237–e260.
15. American College of Obstetricians and Gynecologists. Nonobstetric surgery in pregnancy. ACOG Committee Opinion No. 775. *Obstet Gynecol*. 2019;133:e285–e286.
16. Visser BC, Glasgow RE, Mulvihill KK, et al. Safety and timing of nonobstetric abdominal surgery in pregnancy. *Dig Surg*. 2001;18:409–417.
17. American College of Obstetricians and Gynecologists. Nonobstetric surgery during pregnancy. Committee Opinion No. 696. *Obstet Gynecol*. 2017;129:777–778.
18. Moore HB, Juarez-Colunga E, Bronsert M, et al. Effect of pregnancy on adverse outcomes after general surgery. *JAMA Surg*. 2015;150(7):637–643.
19. Abbasi N, Patenaude V, Abenhaim HA. Management and outcomes of acute appendicitis in pregnancy-population-based study of over 7000 cases. *BJOG*. 2014;121:1509–1514.
20. Cohen-Kerem R, Railton C, Oren D, et al. Pregnancy outcome following non-obstetric surgical intervention. *Am J Surg*. 2005;190(3):467–473.
21. Cheng V, Matsushima K, Sandhu K, et al. Surgical trends in the management of acute cholecystitis during pregnancy. *Surg Endosc*. 2020. doi:10.1007/s00464-020-08054-w.
22. Kuy S, Roman SA, Desai R, et al. Outcomes following cholecystectomy in pregnant and nonpregnant women. *Surgery*. 2009;146(2):358–366.
23. American College of Obstetricians and Gynecologists and the Society for Maternal-Fetal Medicine. Obstetric care consensus: Levels of maternal care. *Obstet Gynecol*. 2019;134(2):e41–e55.
24. US Food and Drug Administration. FDA Drug Safety Communication: FDA Review Results in New Warnings about Using General Anesthetics and Sedation Drugs in Young Children and Pregnant Women. FDA; 2016. http://www.fda.gov/Drugs/DrugSafety/ucm532356.htm
25. Bleeser T, Van Der Veeken L, Fieuws S, et al. Effects of general anaesthesia during pregnancy on neurocognitive development of the fetus: A systematic review and meta-analysis. *Br J Anaesth*. 2021;126(6):1128–1140.
26. Fardelmann K, Gaiser R. Does anesthesia and surgery during pregnancy really affect learning and behavior in the offspring: The holy grail in anesthesiology research. *Anesth Analg*. 2021;133(3):592–594.
27. Ing C, Landau R, DeStephano D, et al. Prenatal exposure to general anesthesia and childhood behavioral deficit. *Anesth Analg*. 2021;133:595–605.
28. Bleeser T, Devroe S, Lucas N, et al. Neurodevelopmental outcomes after prenatal exposure to anaesthesia for maternal surgery: A propensity-score weighted bidirectional cohort study. *Anaesthesia*. 2023;78:159–169.
29. Adzick NS, Thom EA, Spong CY, et al. A randomized trial of prenatal versus postnatal repair of myelomeningocele. *N Engl J Med*. 2011;364:993–1004.
30. Hoagland MA, Chatterjee D. Anesthesia for fetal surgery. *Pediatric Anesthesia* 2017;27:346–357.
31. Farmer DL, Thom EA, Brock JW, et al. The management of myelomeningocele study: Full cohort 30-month pediatric outcomes. *Am J Obstet Gynecol*. 2018;218:256.e1–13.
32. Houtrow AJ, Thom EA, Fletcher JM, et al. Prenatal repair of myelomeningocele and school-age functional outcomes. *Pediatrics*. 2020;145(2):e20191544.
33. Tolcher MC, Fisher WE, Clark SL. Nonobstetric surgery during pregnancy. *Obstet Gynecol*. 2018;132:395–403.
34. Kacmar RM, Gaiser R. Physiologic changes of pregnancy. In: Chestnut DH, Wong CA, Tsen LC, et al., eds. *Chestnut's Obstetric Anesthesia*. 6th ed. Elsevier; 2020:13–37.
35. Pilkington S, Carli F, Dakin MJ, et al. Increase in Mallampati score during pregnancy. *BJA*. 1995;74:638–642.
36. Kinsella SM, Winton AL, Mushambi MC, et al. Failed tracheal intubation during obstetric general anaesthesia: A literature review. *IJOA*. 2015;24:356–374.
37. Odor PM, Bampoe S, Moonesinghe SR, et al. General anaesthetic and airway management practice for obstetric surgery in England: A prospective, multicentre observational study. *Anaesthesia*. 2021;76(4):460–471. doi:10.1111/anae.15250
38. Reale SC, Bauer ME, Klumpner TT, et al. Frequency and risk factors for difficult intubation in women undergoing general anesthesia for cesarean delivery: A multicenter retrospective cohort analysis. *Anesthesiology*. 2022;136:697–708.
39. Rocke DA, Murray WB, Rout CC. Relative risk analysis of factors associated with difficult intubation in obstetric anesthesia. *Anesthesiology*. 1992;77:67–73.
40. Quinn AC, Milne D, Columb M, et al. Failed tracheal intubation in obstetric anaesthesia: 2 Yr national case-control study in the UK. *BJA*. 2013;110(1):74–80.
41. Mushambi MC, Kinsella SM, Popat M, et al. Obstetric Anaesthetists' Association and Difficult Airway Society guidelines for the management of difficult and failed tracheal intubation in obstetrics. *Anaesthesia*. 2015;70:1286–1306.
42. Tetro N, Moushaev S, Rubinchik-Stern M, et al. The placental barrier: The gate and the fate in drug distribution. *Pharm Res*. 2018;35(4):71.
43. Ansari J, Carvalho B, Shafer SL, et al. Pharmacokinetics and pharmacodynamics of drugs commonly used in pregnancy and parturition. *Anesth Analg*. 2016;122:786–804.
44. US Food and Drug Administration. Pregnancy and Lactation Labeling (Drugs) Final Rule. http://fda.gov/drugs/labeling-information-drug-products/pregnancy-and-lactation-labeling-drugs-final-rule
45. Carvalho B, Wong CA. Drug labeling in the practice of obstetric anesthesia. *Am J Obstet Gynecol*. 2015;212(1):24–27.
46. Briggs GG, Freeman RK, Towers CV, et al. *Drugs in Pregnancy and Lactation: A Reference Guide to Fetal and Neonatal Risk*. 11th ed. Wolters Kluwer; 2021.
47. Mazze RI, Kallen B. Reproductive outcome after anesthesia and operation during pregnancy: A registry study of 5405 cases. *Am J Obstet Gynecol*. 1989;161(5):1178–1185.
48. Safra MJ, Oakley GP. Association between cleft lip with or without cleft palate and prenatal exposure to diazepam. *Lancet*. 1975;306(7933):478–480.
49. Dolovich LR, Addis A, Regis Vaillancourt JM, et al. Benzodiazepine use in pregnancy and major malformations or oral cleft: Meta-analysis of cohort and case-control studies. *BMJ*. 1998;317:839–843.
50. Tearne JE, Allen KL, Herbison CE, et al. The association between prenatal environment and children's mental health trajectories from 2 to 14 years. *Eur Child Adolesc Psychiatr*. 2015;24:1015–1024.
51. Clark RB, Brown MA, Lattin DL. Neostigmine, atropine, and glycopyrrolate: Does neostigmine cross the placenta? *Anesthesiology*. 1996;84:450–452.
52. Richardson MG, Raymond BL. Sugammadex administration in pregnant women and in women of reproductive potential: A narrative review. *Anesth Analg*. 2020;130:1628–1637.
53. Keating GM. Sugammadex: A review of neuromuscular blockade reversal. *Drugs*. 2016;76:1041–1052.

54. Willet AW, Butwick AJ, Togioka B, et al; Society for Obstetric Anesthesia and Perinatology Ad Hoc Task Force. Statement on sugammadex during pregnancy and lactation. 2019. https://www.soap.org/assests/docs/SOAP_Statement_Sugammadex_During_Pregnancy_Lactation_APPROVED.pdf.
55. McCurdy RJ. Intraoperative fetal monitoring for nonobstetric surgery. *Clin Obstet Gynecol.* 2020;63(2):370–378.
56. Petrie RH, Yeh SY, Murata Y, et al. The effect of drugs on fetal heart rate variability. *Am J Obstet Gynecol.* 1978;130(3):294–299.
57. Pearl J, Price R, Richardson W, et al. Guidelines for diagnosis, treatment, and use of laparoscopy for surgical problems during pregnancy. *Surg Endosc.* 2011;25:3479–3492.
58. Bauchat JR, Van de Velde M. Nonobstetric surgery during pregnancy. In: Chestnut DH, Wong CA, Tsen LC, et al., eds. *Chestnut's Obstetric Anesthesia.* 6th ed. Elsevier; 2020:368–391.
59. Sedaghat N, Cao AM, Eslick GD, et al. Laparoscopic versus open cholecystectomy in pregnancy: A systematic review and meta-analysis. *Surg Endosc.* 2017;31:673–679.
60. Bartal MF, Sibai BM. Eclampsia in the 21st century. *Am J Obstet Gynecol.* 2022;226(2S):S1237–S1253.
61. Altman D, Carroli G, Duley L, et al.; Magpie Trial Collaborative Group. Do women with pre-eclampsia, and their babies, benefit from magnesium sulphate? The Magpie Trial: A randomised placebo-controlled trial. *Lancet.* 2002;359:1877–1890.

32.

OLDER PRIMIGRAVIDA WITH TWIN PREGNANCY FOR ELECTIVE CESAREAN DELIVERY

Evan Jin, Sangeeta Kumaraswami, and Garret Weber

STEM CASE AND KEY QUESTIONS

A 45-year-old African American woman, 5′ 2″ inches tall and weighing 170 kg (BMI 68) is 27 weeks pregnant. She is having dichorionic twins. She has had three prior cesarean deliveries, and her last pregnancy was more than 10 years ago. She has a history of insulin-dependent diabetes and obstructive sleep apnea (OSA). She gives a history of smoking cigarettes for the past 2 years or so. She has a history of preeclampsia in two prior pregnancies and is on low-dose aspirin during this pregnancy. Her only other medication is methadone, which she takes for opioid use disorder due to prior substance abuse. Recently she has had increasing shortness of breath and is unable to climb a flight of stairs. She also has had to use two pillows at night to sleep. She also refuses a blood transfusion.

What are the considerations for gravid patients who are of advanced maternal age (AMA)?

The patient is evaluated in the preoperative anesthesia clinic in close communication with her obstetrician. She is counseled on complications associated with AMA. She recalls a discussion regarding AMA and associated risks during genetic counseling. Anesthetic implications of a repeat cesarean delivery are discussed.

What are the risk factors associated with multiple gestations?

The patient asks about vaginal delivery. It is explained that an increased risk of complications exists in pursuing an expectant delivery after three prior cesarean deliveries. She is counseled on potential timing of a scheduled delivery in the third trimester and risk of bleeding with likelihood of intra-abdominal adhesions, given her three prior cesarean deliveries. She is also given a referral to a cardiologist.

What are the hypertensive disorders of pregnancy?

When seen in the cardiologist's office, the patient is noted to have a blood pressure of 140/90 mm Hg. This is similar to the blood pressure in the obstetrician's office during the past two visits. She has no protein in her urine. She is diagnosed with gestational hypertension and is started on labetalol with a plan for blood pressure monitoring as an outpatient. An echocardiogram is done which demonstrates an ejection fraction of 40%. She is then diagnosed with peripartum cardiomyopathy. She is counseled on fluid restriction and started on furosemide. Over the next few weeks her symptoms are gradually found to improve.

What are the preanesthetic considerations for diabetic patients during pregnancy?

She is seen again in the preoperative anesthesia clinic ahead of her cesarean delivery. She reveals that her diabetes was diagnosed at age 9 and that she is currently on a basal long-acting insulin glargine and short-acting insulin lispro. Glucose determinations have guided adjustments in diet and insulin therapy. Her last HbA1c was 7.5 and her blood sugars range from 100 to 200 mg/dL daily. The patient is explained about NPO requirements prior to elective surgery with a fasting requirement of 8 hours and only non-carbohydrate clear liquids up to 2 hours prior to surgery. She is given instructions regarding adjustment of her insulin doses prior to surgery.

What are the cultural considerations for preoperative obstetric anesthetic care?

The patient expresses initial concern regarding anesthetic options during her delivery. She reports that she was told by a family member that epidurals may cause permanent paralysis. Her church and friends have told her that it is best to have a natural delivery without any anesthesia. She also reports a negative experience in the past, as described below.

What is peripartum cardiomyopathy?

The anesthetic plan and the benefits and risks of neuraxial and general anesthesia are explained to the patient. She expresses anxiety secondary to a difficult neuraxial placement with her past deliveries. She is reassured that experienced anesthesiologists will be part of her care team. The safety and benefits of neuraxial techniques for anesthesia for her cesarean delivery are reiterated. Since she has a history of cardiomyopathy, preoperative invasive monitoring is discussed including potential central venous access for vasoactive medications and arterial cannulation for continuous blood pressure monitoring. The need for postpartum thromboprophylaxis is also discussed.

What are the risk factors for peripartum bleeding?

The patient undergoes ultrasonography followed by placental MRI. She is found to have a placenta previa and a placenta percreta with invasion of bladder serosa. A multidisciplinary meeting is held to schedule a plan for delivery at 34 weeks gestation. A tentative plan is established for placement of an epidural catheter and invasive vascular access (central venous access and radial arterial cannulation) preoperatively and an interventional radiology consultation for preoperative placement of bilateral internal iliac artery stents and intraoperative angiographic arterial embolization. Surgery consultation is also requested for perioperative resuscitative endovascular balloon occlusion of the aorta (REBOA) and urology is consulted for placement of ureteral stents. The tentative plan is for patients to receive a surgical anesthetic via the epidural for the delivery of the fetus and then conversion to general anesthesia (GA) if hysterectomy is done.

What are the ethics of refusal of blood products?

When discussing the intraoperative risks, the patient promptly states that her religion (Jehovah's Witness) explicitly prohibits blood transfusions. She shares a list of products that she will not accept. She states that she would rather die than receive a blood transfusion even in the case of a life-threatening hemorrhage. After a detailed discussion, all products acceptable to her are documented in the medical record. An iron infusion is ordered due to her anemia.

What are the risk factors for difficult neuraxial placement?

The initial attempt at epidural placement at the L4–L5 interspace is unsuccessful. The anatomical landmarks are unable to be palpated due to her morbid obesity. The patient is repositioned and ultrasonography is used to guide epidural placement. A longer Tuohy epidural needle is also employed given the increased depth of placement, and the epidural is successfully placed. A dural puncture epidural (DPE) technique is used to confirm placement. A spinal anesthetic is avoided due to concerns regarding her cardiomyopathy and changes in hemodynamics. The epidural catheter is loaded slowly and incrementally with local anesthetic, achieving a surgical level of anesthesia within 15 minutes.

What are the implications of obesity to the parturient?

The epidural is working optimally, right internal jugular central venous access and radial artery cannulation is completed, and preoperative internal iliac artery balloon catheters are placed by the interventional radiology team. The cesarean delivery is done under epidural anesthesia and twins are delivered. Due to a plan for hysterectomy, a preparation is now made for GA. She is preoxygenated and a rapid-sequence induction is done. Initial attempts at intubation are unsuccessful with direct laryngoscopy and video laryngoscopy. A second anesthesiologist is called for help. A laryngeal mask airway is placed in the interim to ventilate the patient. Endotracheal intubation is done with a flexible bronchoscope using the laryngeal mask airway as a conduit.

What are the implications of OSA in the pregnant patient during the postpartum period?

Increased bleeding is encountered intraoperatively. Tranexamic acid is administered and the intraoperative cell salvage system is used to transfuse the patient's own blood. She remains hemodynamically stable, and the hysterectomy is completed without complications. The patient is extubated and transferred to the PACU. She receives epidurally administered preservative-free morphine with a plan in place for postoperative monitoring for respiratory depression. A dilute local anesthetic solution is also continuously administered through the indwelling epidural catheter for postoperative pain relief. She is seen to be falling asleep with intermittent desaturation to the 80s on pulse oximetry. She is placed on noninvasive ventilation (continuous positive airway pressure) without further episodes of oxygen desaturation. She is started on a postoperative thromboprophylaxis regimen with a plan to remove the epidural catheter the following day.

What is the postpartum pain management plan for an opioid-tolerant patient with a history of substance use disorder?

The following morning her epidural catheter is removed. A few hours later she is seen for a postanesthetic evaluation. She reports severe incisional pain as well as back pain. She is concerned regarding additional opioids upon discharge causing a relapse in her substance use disorder. She receives an ultrasound-guided truncal block. Acetaminophen and NSAIDs are administered on a regular "round-the-clock" basis, with a plan to use opioids as "rescue" analgesics. Her daily dose of methadone is continued. The patient is discharged on the third postoperative day. She only required one oral oxycodone dose for severe breakthrough incisional pain. A follow-up plan is initiated and coordinated with her outpatient methadone maintenance program.

DISCUSSION

ADVANCED MATERNAL AGE

Pregnancy at an AMA is becoming increasingly common. AMA has traditionally been defined as 35 years or older, with some referring to it as 40 years or older. Recently a category of "very advanced maternal age" has also been described for women older than 45–50 years.[1] AMA is associated with a higher risk of adverse outcomes with a linear trend evident for each 5-year increase in maternal age beyond 34 years.[2] Older women experience a higher rate of spontaneous abortions and ectopic pregnancies, with increased chromosomal abnormalities and congenital anomalies in offsprings.[3] Placental abnormalities including abruptio placenta and placenta previa are also higher.[4] They are more likely to experience labor dystocia, be delivered by cesarean, and have an increased risk of maternal death.[5,6] Perinatal morbidity is also higher in the AMA population with increased low birth weight and preterm delivery observed.[7]

TRIAL OF LABOR AFTER CESAREAN DELIVERY AND VAGINAL BIRTH AFTER CESAREAN DELIVERY

Cesarean delivery is the most common major surgical procedure performed worldwide. While the rate of cesarean delivery varies by country, it remains 30–32% in the United States.[8]

Women with previous cesarean deliveries may deliver vaginally in subsequent pregnancies. Women attempting a trial of labor after cesarean delivery (TOLAC) have a 60–80% probability of vaginal birth after cesarean delivery (VBAC), with likelihood being based on demographic and obstetric characteristics.[9] Factors that predict successful VBAC include previous vaginal birth, younger maternal age, spontaneous labor, and nonrecurrent indication for previous cesarean (e.g., breech). Predictors of failed TOLAC include augmented or induced labor, gestational age greater than 40 weeks, maternal obesity, increasing maternal age, Black or Hispanic race, and fetal macrosomia of greater than 4,000 g.[10] The outcome that most commonly increases risk of maternal morbidity and mortality is uterine rupture. This risk increases with the number of previous uterine incisions.[11] Uterine rupture refers to separation of a uterine scar resulting in fetal compromise and maternal hemorrhage, requiring emergency cesarean delivery or postpartum laparotomy. The term should not be confused with *uterine scar dehiscence*, which is an asymptomatic uterine wall defect that does not result in fetal compromise or maternal hemorrhage.[10] In women who have undergone one prior cesarean delivery, the risk for uterine rupture among non-laboring women is about 1.6 per 1,000, the risk increases three-fold to 5.2 per 1,000 among women in spontaneous labor, and it increased five-fold to 7.7 per 1,000 in those undergoing induction of labor.[12] The most common sign of uterine rupture is fetal bradycardia which is present in nearly 70% of cases and may be preceded by a non-reassuring fetal heart tracing,[13] Other signs and symptoms include abdominal pain (7–10%), vaginal bleeding (3–5%), hemodynamic instability (5–10%), and recession of the presenting part (5%).

Women with one or two previous low-transverse cesarean deliveries and without contraindications to vaginal birth are candidates for a trial of labor. Data regarding the risk of attempting TOLAC with more than two previous cesarean deliveries are limited. Women with a twin pregnancy and one previous low-transverse cesarean delivery who are otherwise candidates for a twin vaginal delivery may be candidates for TOLAC. Contraindications to planned TOLAC include previous classic or T-shaped incision or extensive transfundal uterine surgery, previous uterine rupture, medical or obstetric complications that preclude labor and vaginal delivery, and inability to perform an emergency cesarean delivery because of unavailable surgeon, anesthesiologist, or operating room staff.[10]

The availability of optimal pain control using neuraxial analgesia may encourage more women to choose TOLAC.[14] Neuraxial analgesia does not decrease the likelihood of successful VBAC.[13] Effective analgesia should not be expected to mask the signs or symptoms of uterine rupture because the most common sign of rupture is fetal heart tracing abnormalities. Patients should be counseled preoperatively regarding early neuraxial catheter placement to provide rapid access to safe surgical anesthesia.

MULTIPLE GESTATIONS

The incidence of multiple gestations has been increasing rapidly over the past 30–40 years.[15] The increased incidence in multifetal gestations has been attributed to a shift toward an older maternal age at conception, when multifetal gestations are more likely to occur naturally, and an increased use of assisted reproductive technology, which are more likely to result in multifetal gestations.[16]

Twin pregnancies are classified as monozygotic or dizygotic according to whether one or two separate ova are fertilized. They are then divided according to the number of placenta (monochorionic for one, dichorionic for two) and also classified by the number of amniotic sacs (monoamniotic and diamniotic). Only monozygotic twins have the possibility of sharing one placenta (monochorionic) or sharing one amniotic sac (monoamniotic).[15] One placenta giving blood supply to two fetuses can result in a complication known as *twin-to-twin transfusion syndrome*. In this syndrome, the twins develop a vascular connection between each other. One twin ends up donating blood to the other twin. The donor twin develops fetal growth restriction and anemia while the recipient twin develops volume overload. This occurs in about 10–15% of monochorionic diamniotic pregnancies and can lead to fetal death.[16]

Multiple gestation accelerates and may exaggerate the physiologic changes of pregnancy.[16] Women with twin pregnancies were found to have a 10% increase in cardiac output compared to women with singleton pregnancies.[17] An increase in the number of fetuses also results in increased upward pressure on the diaphragm leading to a further decrease in functional residual capacity (FRC). Greater uterine size displaces the stomach cephalad, and, with a decreased competence of the lower esophageal sphincter, there is an increased risk of aspiration.[18] The plasma volume is also more in twin pregnancies, which would increase the dilutional anemia already found in normal pregnancies.

Medical complications such as hyperemesis, hypertensive disorders of pregnancy, and gestational diabetes mellitus (DM) are more common with multifetal gestations, resulting in increased maternal morbidity and mortality. The increased uterine distension may increase the likelihood of uterine atony and significantly increase blood loss during pregnancy.[18] Multiple gestations are associated with a higher incidence of abnormal presentations due to the need to accommodate two or more fetuses within the uterine cavity. Multifetal gestations are also associated significantly with spontaneous preterm birth resulting in increased infant morbidity and mortality.[16]

Patients with multiple gestations should plan to deliver in a setting where an emergency operative delivery can be performed immediately. Most obstetricians will favor cesarean delivery for all patients with three or more fetuses and for twin pregnancies where twin A has a breech or shoulder presentation.[16] Most obstetricians will allow for a trial of labor if both twins have a vertex presentation. When twin A has a vertex presentation and is delivered vaginally, the obstetrician must make a decision about the method of delivery of twin B. If twin B had a nonvertex position, options would include external cephalic version followed by resumption of labor, internal podalic version and total breech extraction, or cesarean delivery.[18]

Early epidural analgesia should also be discussed preoperatively to allow for optimal analgesia and flexibility for any subsequent anesthetic and surgical needs. Pharmacological aspiration prophylaxis should be administered, and large-bore IV access should be planned due to an increased risk for peripartum hemorrhage.

HYPERTENSIVE DISORDERS OF PREGNANCY

These disorders encompass a range of conditions that include chronic hypertension, gestational hypertension, preeclampsia, and eclampsia (Table 32.1). Up to 50% of women with gestational hypertension eventually develop proteinuria or other end-organ dysfunction consistent with the diagnosis of preeclampsia, and this progression is more likely when the hypertension is diagnosed before 32 weeks of gestation.[19] The risk of developing preeclampsia is highest if a woman has a personal history of preeclampsia in previous pregnancies (seven-fold increase). Other risk factors include maternal age of older than 40 years, multiple gestation, diabetes, obesity, and chronic hypertension. Nevertheless, most cases of preeclampsia occur in healthy women with no obvious risk factors.[20]

Hypertensive disorders of pregnancy complicate approximately 5–10% of pregnancies and continue to be among the leading causes of maternal death, predominantly from hemorrhagic stroke, complications of seizures, and peripartum cardiomyopathy. Because of disruption of cerebral autoregulation in preeclampsia, preeclamptic women are at a higher risk for intracranial bleeding at much lower blood pressures (>155 mm Hg).[21] If severe hypertension (>160/110 mm Hg) is encountered, a repeat measurement should be obtained every 5 minutes for 15 minutes. If two severe blood pressures are obtained within 15 minutes, immediate treatment should be started. Treatment with first-line agents such as IV labetalol or hydralazine and oral short-acting nifedipine should be initiated within 30–60 minutes to decrease the risk of maternal stroke. The objective of treatment is to achieve blood pressures in the range of 140–150/90–100 mm Hg while avoiding an overcorrection of blood pressure that compromises uteroplacental blood flow.[20] Second-line interventions include continuous infusions of nicardipine, esmolol, or even sodium nitroprusside in extreme emergencies.

The incidence of eclampsia is reported to be 1 in 2,000–3,500 pregnancies, with more than 90% of cases occurring after 28 weeks gestation.[20] The common underlying insult is acute severe hypertension causing vasogenic edema and leading to encephalopathy and seizures. Commonly reported symptoms include persistent occipital or frontal headache, blurred vision, photophobia, right upper quadrant or epigastric pain, or altered mental status. Magnesium sulfate is the most effective agent for preventing eclampsia. A 4 g loading dose is given over 15–20 minutes, followed by a 2 g/hour infusion. Ten percent of patients will have a second seizure while on magnesium so an additional bolus of 2 g over 3–5 minutes can be administered. The use of magnesium for eclamptic seizure prophylaxis is also recommended for women with severe features.

Primary prevention of preeclampsia can be initiated with daily aspirin therapy during the late first trimester for women with a history of preeclampsia with severe features who presented prior to 34 weeks gestation in a previous pregnancy.[22] Delivery is recommended at 34 weeks gestation for preeclampsia with severe features, at 37 weeks in the absence of severe features, and urgently in the setting of eclampsia. Deteriorating maternal or fetal status may necessitate delivery at earlier gestations. Point-of-care ultrasound including echocardiography and lung imaging is a useful tool to guide fluid therapy. Since preeclampsia is often associated with intravascular depletion, fluid management is typically restrictive. Ultrasound may also

Table 32.1 CLASSIFICATION OF THE HYPERTENSIVE DISORDERS OF PREGNANCY

Chronic hypertension: Hypertension (systolic blood pressure >140 or diastolic blood pressure >90) diagnosed before pregnancy or before 20 weeks gestation	Gestational hypertension: New-onset hypertension diagnosed after 20 weeks of gestation without proteinuria or evidence of end-organ damage	Preeclampsia without severe features: New-onset hypertension after 20 weeks with proteinuria, but no evidence of end-organ damage

Preeclampsia with severe features:
New-onset hypertension after 20 weeks of gestation with[a]:
Severe range blood pressure (systolic blood pressure >160, diastolic blood pressure >110)
OR
End-organ damage:
Thrombocytopenia with platelets <100
Serum creatinine >1.1 or doubling of baseline
Transaminitis: Twice normal or persistent right upper quadrant pain
Pulmonary edema
New-onset headache or visual symptoms

[a]The following are diagnostic criteria for preeclampsia with severe features. The presence of one of these features establishes the diagnosis, but more than one may be present.

be used to assess airway and gastric volume (to identify who is at greater risk of aspiration) and detect intracranial hypertension (detection of changes in the optic nerve sheath diameter that occurs with preeclampsia).[20]

If the obstetric team is committed to delivery, an early neuraxial catheter should be recommended to allow for both labor analgesia and surgical anesthesia. However, patient choice, lack of time, or coagulopathy may preclude its use.[23] Concerns with GA include the difficult airway that may be exaggerated in preeclampsia, acute increase in blood pressure from direct laryngoscopy with risk of intracranial hemorrhage, and potentiation of the action of neuromuscular blocking agents by magnesium. Placement of a preinduction arterial line for continuous blood pressure monitoring and administration of pharmacologic agents such as esmolol, nitroglycerin, and remifentanil before intubation should be considered to closely monitor the blood pressure and blunt the hemodynamic response in severe cases.

The acronym "HELLP," characterized by hemolysis, elevated levels of liver enzymes, and a low platelet count, was coined in 1982 to describe a variant of preeclampsia. However, a substantial fraction of women with HELLP syndrome do not have hypertension or proteinuria. The platelet count can fall precipitously in HELLP syndrome. Thrombocytopenia can also be a part of preeclampsia-related endothelial dysfunction.[23] The admission platelet count is an excellent predictor of subsequent thrombocytopenia. If the platelet count is less than 100,000/mm^3, further coagulation studies may be useful. If undergoing induction of labor, serial platelet counts every 6 hours may be useful to detect declining platelet counts. The main concern is the risk of development of spinal-epidural hematoma following neuraxial anesthesia and includes both catheter placement and removal. For platelet counts of greater than 70,000/mm^3, it is reasonable to proceed with a neuraxial procedure if clinically indicated.[24] If the platelet count is between 50,000 and 70,000/mm^3 then an assessment of risk-benefit ratio would guide decision-making. Women with a platelet count less than 50,000/mm^3 are at a significantly increased risk of bleeding, and this may preclude the administration of neuraxial anesthesia. Viscoelastic monitors of coagulation may also be useful in the decision-making about neuraxial block administration. Platelet function analysis is also helpful in these patients. However, the actual ability of both to predict the risk for epidural hematoma requires further study. Platelet transfusions are recommended in preeclampsia for active bleeding or to improve the platelet count to 50,000mm^3 before cesarean delivery. However, platelet transfusion is not recommended to facilitate neuraxial anesthesia in these patients. In addition to transfusion-related risks, they may be less effective in these patients, likely due to platelet consumption.

OBESITY

Obesity is defined as having a BMI of greater than 30 kg/m^2. The World Health Organization defines three grades of obesity: class I (BMI 30.0–34.9 kg/m^2), class II (BMI 35.0–39.9 kg/m^2, and class III (BMI ≥40 kg/m^2 or greater). The prevalence of class III obesity among women of reproductive age has significantly increased in recent years.[25] The American College of Obstetrics and Gynecology (ACOG) recommends a formal antepartum anesthesiology consultation for obese women.[26]

Obesity contributes to reducing the already-decreased FRC found in all pregnant women. This further increases the likelihood of desaturation during periods of apnea.[25] Morbidly obese women also have increased left ventricular mass on echocardiogram versus nonobese controls.[27] Obesity has an additive effect on the increased plasma volume and cardiac output during pregnancy. Morbidly obese patients are at higher risk of pulmonary aspiration of gastric contents.

Obesity is associated with a significantly increased incidence of maternal, fetal, and neonatal complications. These include hypertensive disorders of pregnancy, gestational diabetes, thromboembolic complications, dysfunctional labor, shoulder dystocia, fetal macrosomia, operative vaginal delivery, and neonatal death.[25] Labor progresses more slowly with increasing BMI.[27] There is a higher risk of poor uterine contractility and failed medical induction of labor in obese parturients. A four-fold increase in the risk of cesarean delivery has been seen in parturients with a BMI of greater than 40 kg/m^2 compared with parturients of normal weight.[28] Obesity also increases the overall risk of death during pregnancy.

An appropriate-sized blood pressure cuff must be used for noninvasive blood pressure measurements. IV access may be challenging, and ultrasound guidance may be required. If peripheral venous cannulation is unsuccessful, central venous cannulation may be necessary.[25] Specialized bariatric equipment including appropriately-sized beds and operating tables should be available. Additional staff and the availability of specialized devices like air-inflated mats should be available for positioning and transfer of these patients.[29,30]

Early administration of neuraxial analgesia is recommended given the increased likelihood of cesarean delivery and increased risk of GA. The quality of the epidural block should be assessed, and the catheter should be replaced if not providing optimal analgesia. There is an increased risk for failed epidural labor analgesia and need for catheter replacement with increasing BMI.[29] Technical difficulties in placement should be expected. Providers may experience difficulty in palpating the spinous processes and identifying the midline. There may be an increased needle insertion depth required to reach the epidural space which may inadvertently create a needle path that starts in the midline but unintentionally diverts laterally. The presence of fat pockets may give the provider a false loss of resistance outside the epidural space.[25]

Periprocedurally one can overcome some of these challenges with ultrasound guidance.[31] One can identify the midline, the desired interspace, and measure the depth to the epidural space. Use of ultrasound has been shown to reduce the number attempts required to access the epidural space.[24] Soft tissue compression with the ultrasound probe can result in underestimation of the depth of the epidural space in obese patients. A novel ultrasound device that uses neuraxial pattern-recognition software to identify depth and midline is currently available (Accuro, Rivanna Medical, Charlottesville,

VA). In one study of 47 patients, it was shown to have high first-pass success rates.[32]

When compared to the epidural technique, the combined spinal-epidural (CSE) technique offers the advantage of confirmation of the correct location of the epidural needle when backflow of cerebrospinal fluid is observed through the spinal needle.[25] The dural-puncture epidural technique is a modification of the CSE technique with a similar advantage. Epidural catheters placed using the CSE technique have a higher success rate. Spinal anesthesia alone may result in an insufficient duration of surgical anesthesia for a cesarean section in a patient with severe obesity.

All morbidly obese women undergoing cesarean delivery should be placed in a ramped position with left uterine displacement, irrespective of the anesthetic technique. This optimizes the patient position for mask ventilation, laryngoscopy, and endotracheal intubation.[25] Advanced airway equipment should be readily available. Preoperative discussion with the surgical team regarding the type of incision (vertical or horizontal and involved dermatomes) and positioning of the panniculus is necessary. The use of a neuraxial double-catheter technique has been described for vertical supraumbilical abdominal incisions.[30] This involves use of a lumbar spinal catheter or CSE technique combined with a lower thoracic epidural catheter that can be used both intra- and postoperatively. The plan for retraction of the panniculus should be discussed because hemodynamic and respiratory compromise, and fetal compromise are risks with cephalad retraction.

Morbidly obese patients may be at significant risk for OSA. Pregnancy-related changes like nasal mucosal edema can both worsen preexisting OSA or lead to the development of OSA.[33] The combination of obesity, OSA, GA, and opioid administration may increase the risk for opioid-induced respiratory depression.[25] Following administration of neuraxial morphine, respiratory monitoring is suggested for high-risk patients with comorbidities or with risk factors that predispose them to respiratory depression.[34] In the presence of preoperative risk factors such as cardiopulmonary or neurological comorbidities, morbid obesity, known or suspected OSA, chronic opioid use or abuse, hypertension and magnesium administration, or perioperative risk factors such as GA, administration of concomitant sedating medications (benzodiazepines, magnesium), IV opioid administration, and a desaturating event in PACU, the respiratory rate and sedation assessments (q1h for 12 hours; q2h for 12–24 hours) as well as additional monitoring modalities such as pulse oximetry and capnography are recommended.

Morbidly obese patients are also at particular risk for venous thromboembolism (VTE). VTE is one of the leading causes of maternal mortality in the United States. The peripartum period is a hypercoagulable state. Cesarean delivery, particularly when complicated by postpartum hemorrhage or infection and the presence of medical factors such as obesity, hypertension, heart disease, preeclampsia, and multiple gestation, greatly increase risk.[35] For patients undergoing cesarean delivery with additional risk factors for thromboembolism, post-cesarean thromboprophylaxis should be administered. Multidisciplinary coordination is necessary when patients are on a thromboprophylaxis regimen with indwelling neuraxial catheters to reduce the risk of spinal-epidural hematoma.[36]

DIABETES MELLITUS

DM affects about 8% of people worldwide. Pregnant women may have either a preexisting diagnosis of DM (pregestational) or develop DM over the course of their pregnancy (gestational).[37] DM complicates 7% of all pregnancies, with a large proportion being gestational.[38] Pregestational DM is associated with an increase in preterm labor and delivery. It is important to screen for DM because uncontrolled hyperglycemia in pregnancy can lead to serious complications like fetal macrosomia and fetal death. DM can also lead to an increase in shoulder dystocia.[37]

Screening for DM occurs at 24–28 weeks gestation. It involves either a one- or two-step test.[38] The test is done during the late-second or early-third trimester stage because it is believed that placental hormone secretion at this time causes increased insulin resistance.[38] Women who develop gestational DM are first instructed to try diet and exercise for blood sugar control. Pharmacological therapy with oral hypoglycemic agents such as metformin or the sulfonylureas glipizide or glibenclamide may be initiated if the lifestyle changes are not clinically effective. If this does not work, the mainstay treatment is insulin.[39] Patients with multiple gestations may have an even higher insulin requirement than singleton patients.[40] The recommended blood sugar parameters for women with pregestational or gestational DM are a fasting sugar of less than 95 mg/dL and a 1-hour postprandial sugar of less than 140 mg/dL. The goal is to prevent the development of complications such as diabetic retinopathy and nephropathy.[38,39] These goals also help avoid the harmful effects of hyperglycemia to the fetus.

For patients in preterm labor, the administration of beta agonists like terbutaline for tocolysis and corticosteroids for lung protection can cause hyperglycemia and may even precipitate diabetic ketoacidosis in type 1 diabetics. Maternal insulin requirements decrease with the onset of labor, increase again during the second stage of labor, and decrease markedly during the early postpartum period. Diabetic patients should undergo close monitoring of their blood sugars throughout the labor course.[37]

IV glucose and insulin infusion during the peripartum period should be titrated to maintain a maternal blood glucose concentration of 70–90 mg/dL.[37] For patients presenting for a scheduled cesarean delivery, ACOG recommends continuing long-acting insulin (e.g., glargine) the night before.[39] This recommendation is different from the general preoperative recommendations which typically recommend a dose reduction in long-acting insulin the evening prior to surgery.[41] If the patient takes long-acting insulin medication twice daily and has a normally scheduled dose on the morning of surgery, one can consider dose reduction to prevent hypoglycemia. It is also recommended to hold any short-acting prandial insulin doses as the patient will be fasting (NPO).[41,42]

Long-standing diabetics may develop gastroparesis and may have an even greater risk of aspiration than a nondiabetic parturient.[37] Assessment of the airway is essential due to development of the stiff-joint syndrome, in which diabetic patients have difficulty in extending their neck. Patients with known cardiovascular autonomic dysfunction from DM are also at risk of increased vasopressor use during GA.[37] Neonates are at risk of hypoglycemia, which likely results from the sustained fetal hyperinsulinemia in response to chronic intrauterine hyperglycemia.[37]

PERIPARTUM CARDIOMYOPATHY

Peripartum cardiomyopathy is the development of heart failure in the last month of pregnancy or within 5 months of delivery. A small subset of patients present during the second or third trimesters. Other causes of heart failure should be excluded, and the absence of other recognizable cardiac disease before the last month of pregnancy should be verified.[43] Echocardiographic diagnostic criteria include reduced ejection fraction (≤45%), fractional shortening (≤30%) or both, and end-diastolic dimension of greater than 27 mm/m² body surface area. It affects 1 in 1,000–4,000 live births in the United States and is associated with age older than 30 years, African race, multiparity, multiple gestation, hypertension, and preeclampsia. The etiology remains unclear. Proposed mechanisms include viral myocarditis, an abnormal immune response, or an increase in prolactin secretion.[44]

Most women present with signs and symptoms of heart failure, including orthopnea and paroxysmal nocturnal dyspnea. These symptoms can be confused with those of normal pregnancy, especially during late gestation, a fact that often leads to a missed or delayed diagnosis and to underestimation of the incidence of this condition.[45]

Management of peripartum cardiomyopathy is largely limited to the same neurohormonal antagonists used in other forms of cardiomyopathy, and currently no proven peripartum disease-specific therapies exist. Treatment is focused, as with other forms of systolic failure, on controlling volume status, neutralizing maladaptive neurohormonal responses, and preventing thromboembolic and arrhythmic complications.[44] Diuretics and nitrates are the agents of choice for volume control, although caution is required if used before delivery to avoid hypotension and impaired uterine perfusion. Neurohormonal blockade with angiotensin-converting enzyme (ACE) inhibitors or angiotensin receptor blockers (ARBs) can be used postpartum but are contraindicated during pregnancy. Beta blockade should be considered and is likely safe during pregnancy. Critically ill patients with signs of low cardiac output or refractory pulmonary edema may require inotropes, an intra-aortic balloon pump or ventricular assist devices.[44,45]

ANTEPARTUM AND POSTPARTUM HEMORRHAGE AND THE PLACENTA ACCRETA SPECTRUM

In the United States, hemorrhage accounts for 11.4% of pregnancy-related deaths.[12] Causes of antepartum hemorrhage include placenta previa, placental abruption, uterine rupture, and vasa previa. In placenta previa, the placenta covers the cervix. It presents classically as painless vaginal bleeding. Risk factors include AMA, multiparity, and previous cesarean delivery. Placental abruption is the separation of the placenta from the uterine wall. Risk factors include AMA, multiparity, preeclampsia, substance use, and trauma. Complications include hemorrhagic shock with possibility of hemorrhage concealed behind the placenta, coagulopathy, and fetal compromise.[12] Preanesthetic evaluation for patients with antepartum hemorrhage should include airway examination and intravascular volume assessment. Availability of cross-matched blood should be ensured. Large-bore IV access and blood product preparation is essential.

The choice of anesthetic technique depends on the urgency for delivery and the degree of maternal hypotension.[12] Neuraxial anesthesia is preferred in stable patients with adequate intravascular volume status and normal coagulation studies. GA is sometimes necessary when presented with urgent cesarean delivery that is accompanied by unstable maternal status, a severely non-reassuring fetal status, or both. Vasa previa occurs when the fetal blood vessels traverse the fetal membranes, covering the internal cervical os. Ruptured vasa previa is a true obstetric emergency.

The ACOG defines postpartum hemorrhage as blood loss greater than or equal to 1,000 mL, or blood loss accompanied by signs or symptoms of hypovolemia within 24 hours of birth.[46] Uterine atony is the most common cause of severe hemorrhage.[47] Conditions associated with uterine atony include cesarean delivery; induced, augmented, or prolonged labor; multiple gestation; high parity; AMA; hypertension; and diabetes.

Other causes of postpartum hemorrhage include genital trauma, retained placenta, uterine inversion, and placenta accreta spectrum. Retained placenta is failure to deliver the placenta completely within 30 minutes of delivery of the infant. The severity of bleeding can be life-threatening, requiring transfusion. Uterine inversion is a rare event defined as the turning inside-out of all or part of the uterus. The hemorrhage and consequent hemodynamic instability may be worsened by concurrent vagal reflex-mediated bradycardia. Historically, the shock is considered to be out of proportion to the blood loss in these patients.[12] Immediate replacement of the uterus, and discontinuation of uterotonics until the uterus is replaced, is indicated. Nitroglycerin may be administered for uterine relaxation. GA may also become necessary especially in unstable patients. In cases of severe uterine atony, in addition to oxytocin, additional uterotonic agents such as methylergonovine and/or carboprost should be considered, if not contraindicated.

Placenta accreta is defined as a placenta that in whole or in part invades the uterine wall and is inseparable from it. The incidence is increasing because of the higher overall cesarean delivery rate.[48] Three types of placenta accreta occur and together are referred to as *placenta accreta spectrum* (previously called *morbidly adherent placenta*). *Placenta accreta vera* involves the adherence of the basal plate of the placenta directly to the myometrium without a decidual layer in between. In *placenta increta*, the chorionic villi invade the uterine myometrium. *Placenta percreta* involves invasion of the placenta through myometrium into the serosa and surrounding organs like the bladder. The presence of previous cesarean delivery and placenta previa significantly increases risk of placenta accreta spectrum. Following diagnosis, it is recommended to do a planned preterm cesarean delivery and hysterectomy with the placenta left in situ because any attempts to remove it may initiate hemorrhage. Surgery at 34 weeks gestation is recommended, given the increased risk of bleeding with increasing gestational age.

Major blood loss should be anticipated during the procedure. As the uterus cannot contract with the placenta adherent to it, there is uncontrolled uterine bleeding. Any unintended incision into placental tissue will also cause great amounts of bleeding. Blood loss can be between 1.5 and 8 L though blood loss upward of 25 L has been reported.[48,49] Strategies to minimize blood loss and decrease transfusion requirements include preoperative insertion of internal iliac artery balloon catheters. Placement of these catheters is also controversial as complications could include disruption of the vasculature and lower extremity ischemia. Current recommendations for use of these catheters include those with unresectable placenta percreta or those who decline blood products.[50] REBOA is another minimally invasive technique using a balloon catheter to temporarily occlude large vessels in support of hemorrhage control. Prophylactic use of this modality has been suggested for these cases.[12,51]

The preoperative anesthetic plan should include a plan for transfusion therapy. Patients with placenta accreta spectrum should be managed only in facilities with multidisciplinary specialists and a well-staffed blood bank. Access to massive transfusion protocols enables delivery of blood products to the operating room in fixed ratios. Transfusion therapy guided by viscoelastic monitoring rather than using a fixed ratio may reduce the overall amount of administered blood products. Care must be taken to avoid hypothermia, acidosis, and hypocalcemia. Obstetric hemorrhage may be associated with accelerated factor consumption, especially fibrinogen.[12] Coagulopathy may be out of proportion to blood loss because of rapid consumption of fibrinogen. Aggressive early resuscitation with packed red cells, plasma, cryoprecipitate, and platelets should be planned, along with use of fibrinogen concentrate if necessary. The administration of tranexamic acid should be planned as it decreases blood loss and transfusion risk without increasing rates of thromboembolism.[52] The use of intraoperative cell-saver technology in obstetric anesthesia is gaining acceptance. Concerns do exist, however, that blood cell salvage may precipitate amniotic fluid embolism and cause maternal–fetal anti-D alloimmunization. Data suggest that a low risk exists when a leukocyte depletion filter is used.[47] Anti-RhD immunoglobulin should be administered to prevent the occurrence of Rhesus isoimmunization in those Rhesus-negative mothers who have receive cell-salvaged blood.[53]

JEHOVAH'S WITNESS PATIENTS

The care of Jehovah's Witness parturients presents many ethical, medical, and legal concerns as many patients refuse allogeneic blood transfusions on religious grounds. This refusal is a constitutionally protected right that has been recognized by the United States.[53] These patients will typically reject transfusion of primary blood components (whole blood, packed red cells, white cells, platelets, and plasma). Some products that may be acceptable include red cell fractions (hemoglobin-based substitutes), white cell fractions (interferons, interleukins), plasma fractions (albumin, immunoglobulin, clotting factors), and natural clotting factors (prothrombin complex concentrate, factor VII concentrate). Although most refuse allogeneic blood transfusion and preoperatively stored autologous blood, they accept almost all other forms of medical treatment.

A multidisciplinary approach is recommended to facilitate coordination of care. Patients should be interviewed in a noncoercive environment and assumptions regarding individualized care and patient preferences should not be made. Verification of acceptable treatments and documentation of patient's wishes is essential. High-dose recombinant erythropoietin in combination with supplemental iron and folate has been used effectively in Jehovah's Witness patients during pregnancy and the postpartum period to enhance hemoglobin synthesis. Clinicians should be aware that erythropoiesis-stimulating agents may increase risk of thrombosis. Acceptance of fluid resuscitation with crystalloid and colloid volume expanders (albumin) should be confirmed.

A discussion regarding use of blood conservation techniques such as intraoperative blood cell salvage and acute normovolemic hemodilution is also essential.[47,53] Some Jehovah's Witnesses may consent to the use of these techniques, viewing them as extensions of their circulatory system. Other Witnesses might require that the withdrawn blood be maintained in a circuit that is in continuous contact with their body. Therefore, care should be taken to maintain a closed-circuit continuous flow system. Similarly, an epidural blood patch may be done in these patients using a closed-circuit system.

Surgical techniques to minimize blood loss should be discussed preoperatively. These include surgical expertise in techniques, use of hemostatic devices such as electrocautery, physical occlusion of bleeding vessels, and use of minimally invasive approaches and early consideration for hysterectomy. Phlebotomy should be limited, and appropriate use of pharmacological agents that reduce blood loss such as uterotonics, desmopressin, and tranexamic acid should be considered.

RACIAL AND ETHNIC DISPARITIES

The two most well-known disparities in obstetric anesthesia are the decreased utilization of neuraxial labor analgesia by Hispanic and Black women and the decreased utilization of neuraxial anesthesia and thus increase in GA in Black women for cesarean deliveries.[54]

A study in 2004 found that, in Medicaid claims in Georgia in 1998, 60% of Caucasian women were given labor neuraxial analgesia versus 50% of Black women and 35% of Hispanic women.[54] Another study at an academic center in the United States found that 85% of non-Hispanic Caucasian women received labor neuraxial analgesia versus 67% of Black women and 51% of Hispanic women.[54] With regards to decreased neuraxial anesthesia and increased GA for cesarean deliveries, a study of 50,947 cesarean deliveries in the United States showed that African American women had the highest odds of receiving GA. The rates were 11.3% for African Americans, 5.2% for Caucasians, and 5.8% for Hispanics.[55]

Additionally, Black women have a higher risk of severe maternal morbidity (a term that encompasses diagnoses like eclampsia, thrombotic embolism, and need for mechanical ventilation).[56] The maternal mortality rate of Black women is four times higher compared to Caucasians.[55]

Common reasons for refusing neuraxial analgesia or anesthesia include a distrust and fear of paralysis and back pain and fixed ideations that women must cope with labor pain nonmedically. It is hypothesized that these reasonings may be more pervasive in Hispanic and possibly Black patient populations. Additionally, providers may have both explicit and implicit biases. In a study in Israel, it was suggested that providers may view women of different races or ethnicities of having less pain than they may actually have.[57] Additionally, women of minority groups may seek out midwives who may suggest that they avoid neuraxial blocks. Language barriers and poor access to hospitals with 24-hour anesthesia services may be additional challenges.[54] Suggested solutions include providing educational materials in the patient's native language, either in-person or through the internet. Preoperative counseling and education may also be beneficial. Additionally, increasing workforce diversity can also help both providers and patients to gain a better understanding of the challenges that minority women face when presenting to a labor and delivery unit.[56]

SUBSTANCE USE DISORDER

A history of opioid use disorder and smoking may be encountered when caring for obstetric patients. The prevalence of opioid use disorders among people aged 20–34 has doubled from 1998 to 2011.[58] Pain management can be particularly challenging in these patients. Preanesthetic assessment should include developing a mutually agreeable strategy for pain management with appropriate goals for pain intensity scores. Questions regarding their substance use disorder should be asked in a respectful and nonjudgmental manner.[58] Chronic opioid requirements or pharmacological maintenance therapy should be continued throughout the hospitalization and postpartum period, with additional therapies for acute pain management. The precise dose of methadone must be confirmed, because improper dosing can result in inadequate analgesia, withdrawal phenomena, or life-threatening overdose. Any methadone or buprenorphine dose adjustments must be done in consultation with the prescribing physicians.

Whenever feasible, neuraxial anesthesia should be utilized in patient with chronic pain. Opioid requirements will likely be higher in these patients. Mixed opioid agonist/antagonist drugs (e.g., nalbuphine is commonly used for labor analgesia or opioid induced pruritus) should likely be minimized as they may precipitate withdrawal. Options for nonopioid multimodal pain management should be discussed. A plan for multimodal therapy that includes neuraxial morphine and truncal nerve blocks should be initiated.[59] Postoperatively, patients should be managed with scheduled doses of acetaminophen and nonsteroidal anti-inflammatory agents, if no medical contraindication exists.

In 2016, about 7.2% of pregnant women smoked tobacco. Smoking is associated with increased rates of placenta previa, placental abruption, and fetal growth restriction.[60] Smoking is a risk factor for several perioperative complications including respiratory sequelae and impaired wound healing. Anesthesiologists can play a vital role in smoking cessation when assessing these patients preoperatively. The "Ask-Advise-Refer" approach involves asking patients about their smoking history, advising them to quit based on its harmful health effects, and referring them to "quitline" services. Even brief encounters can be effective for smoking cessation. Patients should be counseled that even brief smoke-free intervals are beneficial.[61] Smoking cessation and counseling should be offered at every preoperative visit and at any point during gestation.

REVIEW QUESTIONS

1. A 32-year-old G3P2 woman at 36 weeks gestation presents to the labor and delivery unit in labor with a blood pressure of 144/96 on two separate measurements an hour apart. She received her prenatal care at an outside hospital, and the obstetrics team is calling for her previous records. Her 24-hour urine protein is currently being collected. Her initial laboratory values come back and all her values are within normal limits except for a creatinine of 1.4. What hypertensive disorder of pregnancy does this patient have?

   a. Gestational hypertension.
   b. Preeclampsia without severe features.
   c. Preeclampsia with severe features.
   d. Chronic hypertension.

   The correct answer is c.

   The patient has preeclampsia with severe features due to the elevated blood pressure (SBP >140, DBP >90) and end-organ dysfunction as shown by the elevated serum creatinine (Cr >1.1). The patient does not need to have evidence of proteinuria to have preeclampsia with severe features. The presence of end-organ dysfunction excludes the diagnosis of gestational hypertension and chronic hypertension.[20]

2. A 42-year-old G7P3 woman at 26 weeks gestation presents for her preoperative clinic appointment. She has a BMI of 24 and a history of exercise-induced asthma. Which of the following events is *most* likely increased in this patient?

   a. Peripartum transfusion.
   b. Failed epidural.
   c. Prolonged labor.
   d. Postoperative pneumonia.

   The correct answer is a.

   AMA is associated with placental abnormalities including placenta previa.[4] Failed epidural, prolonged labor, and postoperative pneumonia are not specifically increased in a patient with AMA.

3. A 35-year-old woman presents for VBAC to the labor and delivery suite after extensive preoperative planning regarding her birthing plan. She is counseled on the risk of uterine rupture. Which of the following is the *most* common presenting sign or symptom of uterine rupture?

   a. Abdominal pain.
   b. Vaginal bleeding.
   c. Fetal bradycardia.
   d. Recession of the presenting part.

The correct answer is c.

Fetal bradycardia is present in nearly 70% of cases and may be preceded by a non-reassuring fetal heart tracing. It is the most common sign of uterine rupture. Other signs and symptoms include abdominal pain (7–10%), vaginal bleeding (3–5%), hemodynamic instability (5–10%), and recession of the presenting part (5%).[13]

4. A 37-year-old G5P3 woman presents at 26 weeks with twin gestation. Which of the following pregnancy related conditions is the patient *most* at risk for?

   a. Pre-eclampsia.
   b. Chorioamnionitis.
   c. Peroneal neuropathy.
   d. Migraine.

The correct answer is a.

Multiple-gestation pregnancies are significantly associated with hypertensive disorders of pregnancy such as preeclampsia.[18] The other conditions may occur during the perioperative and peri-labor period but are not specifically increased in twin gestation pregnancies.

5. A 39-year-old woman at 25 weeks gestation presents with increasing shortness of breath and generalized edema. She requires two pillows at night to sleep. She is diagnosed with peripartum cardiomyopathy. Which of the following medications is most likely acceptable for her at this point?

   a. Lisinopril.
   b. Furosemide.
   c. Valsartan.
   d. Warfarin.

The correct answer is b.

Generally, the initial treatment for peripartum cardiomyopathy includes sodium restriction and the use of loop diuretics which are acceptable during pregnancy. While ACE/ARB inhibitors have a role in the management of heart failure outside of pregnancy, they are incompatible with pregnancy and contraindicated.[44,45] Furthermore, while anticoagulation is generally indicated for cardiomyopathy, warfarin is contraindicated due to its teratogenicity.

6. A 38-year-old woman who is at 27 weeks gestation and is 150 kg and has a BMI of 55 presents for her preoperative anesthesia evaluation. Which of the following is *least* likely associated with her underlying obesity?

   a. OSA.
   b. Difficult neuraxial placement.
   c. Difficult airway.
   d. Spinal headache.

The correct answer is d.

Obesity during pregnancy is associated with increased risk for the parturient in multiple domains. There is an increased risk of OSA, which often requires close monitoring with continuous pulse oximetry and capnography when long-acting opioids are used (e.g., spinal morphine). Both the placement of a neuraxial block (e.g., epidural) and airway management including endotracheal intubation may prove to be extremely challenging in the obese parturient.[29,33,34] It is unlikely that the obese parturient is at a higher risk of a spinal headache.

7. A 37-year-old woman with a twin gestation pregnancy presents to the preoperative evaluation clinic in anticipation for a scheduled repeat caesarian section. She has a history of pregestational diabetes with an HbA1c of 9.8. Which of the following is *least* likely to increase perioperatively in the parturient?

   a. Aspiration risk.
   b. Neonatal hypoglycemia.
   c. Preoperative insulin sensitivity.
   d. Vasopressor requirements under GA.

The correct answer is c.

During pregnancy and especially in the late second/early third trimester, the insulin requirements increase and there is a decreased insulin sensitivity (increased resistance) requiring a larger dose. Pregestational diabetes increases the risk in the parturient of aspiration due to autonomic dysfunction and impaired gastric motility in addition to the baseline increased aspiration risk in the nondiabetic parturient. There may also be an increased vasopressor requirement while under GA due to the autonomic dysfunction as well. Furthermore, the neonate may have an increased insulin level due to chronic hyperglycemia in utero resulting in hypoglycemia at birth.[37–39]

8. A 33-year-old woman presents for preoperative OB anesthesia evaluation. She is scheduled for a C-section and has a history of diagnosed placenta accreta. She has had three prior caesarian deliveries. Despite counseling regarding risks of hemorrhage, she adamantly refuses all transfusion on religious grounds. She states that she is a Jehovah's Witness and her religion explicitly prohibits any blood transfusion. What is the *most* acceptable approach in the management of this point?

   a. Explain the risk of life-threatening hemorrhage and that blood transfusion is compulsory.
   b. Avoid blood transfusion and prepare a list of acceptable resuscitative agents preoperatively.
   c. Attempt to dissuade the patient of her beliefs and explain that transfusion is a must.
   d. Refuse to take care of the patient and call the hospital risk management/legal division.

The correct answer is b.

Patients have the autonomy to refuse blood products even if the situation of life-threatening hemorrhage. Alternative options such as closed-circuit cell saver and acceptable resuscitative agents should be discussed. There is a well-established legal precedent for the patient's right to refusal.[53] The other choices are not indicated and not the best practice in the care of such patients.

9. A 27-year-old Hispanic woman presents for preoperative evaluation for elective C-section. Which of the following is *most* accurate regarding racial disparities in obstetric anesthetic care?

   a. Hispanic women have similar outcomes to Caucasian women.
   b. Neuraxial use is equal among women from different ethnic backgrounds.
   c. Hispanic women have decreased utilization of neuraxial anesthesia.
   d. Hispanic patients have less pain during labor and operative deliveries.

The correct answer is c.

It has been well established that racial disparities exist in the realm of obstetric care. Hispanic and Black women have both decreased utilization of neuraxial anesthesia for both labor and operative deliveries.[54–56] This has implications for postoperative outcomes and risks associated with increased GA for C-section. The other choices do not reflect the harsh reality of health disparities that many face in obstetric management. Additional education and diversity in the workplace are some of the proposed solutions to improve the care provided.

10. A 31-year-old woman presents 3 days before scheduled repeat C-section for a preoperative evaluation. She has a history of asthma and morbid obesity and smokes approximately 1 pack per day despite prior counseling at multiple times during the pregnancy regarding smoking cessation. Which of the following is the *most* appropriate advice to give the patient at this point?

   a. Since it is less than 4 weeks prior to surgery patient should not quit until postoperatively.
   b. Offer smoking cessation counseling, support, and the benefits of quitting at any time.
   c. Inform the patient that she is intentionally harming herself and the baby without remorse.
   d. Since she is not AMA, her risk is not high and she can continue smoking if desired.

The correct answer is b.

Smoking cessation should be offered at any point during gestation. While reduced complication rates are seen quitting more than 4 weeks preoperatively, the benefits clearly outweigh the risks to quitting and patients should continue to be offered support, encouragement, and options for quitting even days prior to surgery. There is no increase in pulmonary complications even in patients who quit shortly before surgery. Patients should be given motivational interviewing using an "Ask-Advice-Refer" approach for behavioral change.[60,61]

REFERENCES

1. Fitzpatrick KE, Tuffnell D, Kurinczuk JJ, Knight M. Pregnancy at very advanced maternal age: A UK population-based cohort study. *BJOG*. 2017;124:1097–1106.
2. Callaghan WM, Berg CJ. Pregnancy-related mortality among women aged 35 years and older, United States, 1991–1997. *Obstet Gynecol*. 2003;102:1015–1021.
3. Rouse CE, Eckert LO, Babarinsa I, et al. Spontaneous abortion and ectopic pregnancy: Case definition & guidelines for data collection, analysis, and presentation of maternal immunization safety data. *Vaccine*. 2017;35(48 Pt A):6563–6574.
4. Martinelli KG, Garcia EM, dos Santos Neto ET, da Gama SGN. Advanced maternal age and its association with placenta praevia and placental abruption. *Cad Saude Publica*. 2018;34 (2):e00206116.
5. Waldenstrom U, Ekeus C. Risk of labor dystocia increases with maternal age irrespective of parity: A population-based register study. *Acta Obstet Gynecol Scand*. 2017;96:1063.
6. Cleary-Goldman J, Malone FD, Vidaver J, et al. Impact of maternal age on obstetric outcome. *Obstet Gynecol*. 2005;105(5Pt 1):983–990.
7. Richards MK, Flanagan MR, Littman AJ, Burke AK, Callegari LS. Primary cesarean section and adverse delivery outcomes among women of very advanced maternal age. *J Perinatol*. 2016;36(4):272–277.
8. Clapp MA, Barth WH. The future of cesarean delivery rates in the United States. *Clin Obstet Gynecol*. 2017;60:829–839.
9. Hawkins JL. The anesthesiologist's role during attempted VBAC. *Clin Obstet Gynecol*. 2012;55:1005–1013.
10. Chestnut DH. Trial of labor and vaginal birth after cesarean delivery. In: Chestnut DH, Wong CA, Tsen LC, et al., eds. *Chestnut's Obstetric Anesthesia: Principles and Practice*. 6th ed. Elsevier Saunders; 2020:409–421.
11. Caughey AB, Shipp TD, Repke JT, Zelop CM, Cohen A, Lieberman E. Rate of uterine rupture during a trial of labor in women with one or two prior cesarean deliveries. *Am J Obstet Gynecol*. 1999;181:872–876.
12. Banayan JM, Hofer JE, Scavone BM. Antepartum and postpartum hemorrhage. In: Chestnut DH, Wong CA, Tsen LC, et al., eds. *Chestnut's Obstetric Anesthesia: Principles and Practice*. 6th ed. Elsevier Saunders; 2020:901–936.
13. Bucklin BA. Vaginal birth after cesarean delivery. *Anesthesiology*. 2003;99:1444–1448.
14. The American College of Obstetricians and Gynecologists. *Vaginal Birth After Cesarean Delivery*. American College of Obstetricians and Gynecologists; 2019.
15. Martin JA, Hamilton BE, Osterman MJ. Three decades of twin births in the United States, 1980–2009. *NCHS Data Brief*. 2012;(80):1–8.
16. Committee on Practice Bulletins—Obstetrics; Society for Maternal–Fetal Medicine. Practice bulletin no. 169: Multifetal gestations: Twin, triplet, and higher-order multifetal pregnancies. *Obstet Gynecol*. 2016;128:e131–e146.
17. Kuleva M, Youssef A, Maroni E, et al. Maternal cardiac function in normal twin pregnancy: A longitudinal study. *Ultrasound Obstet Gynecol*. 2011;38:575–580.
18. Hawkins JA. Abnormal presentation and multiple gestation. In: Chestnut DH, Wong CA, Tsen LC, et al., eds. *Chestnut's Obstetric Anesthesia: Principles and Practice*. 6th ed. Elsevier Saunders; 2020:822–839.
19. American College of Obstetricians and Gynecologists. Practice bulletin no. 222: Gestational hypertension and preeclampsia. *Obstet Gynecol*. 2020;135:e237–e260.
20. Siddique MM, Banayan JM, Hofer JE. Pre-eclampsia through the eyes of the obstetrician and anesthesiologist. *Int J Obstet Anesth*. 2019;40:140–148.
21. van Veen TR, Panerai RB, Haeri S, et al. Cerebral autoregulation in different hypertensive disorders of pregnancy. *Am J Obstet Gynecol*. 2015;212(513):e511–517.
22. Bujold E, Roberge S, Lacasse Y, et al. Prevention of pre-eclampsia and intrauterine growth restriction with aspirin started in early pregnancy: A meta-analysis. *Obstet Gynecol*. 2010;116:402–414.

23. Dyer RA, Swanevelder JL, Bateman BT. Hypertensive disorders. In: Chestnut DH, Wong CA, Tsen LC, et al., eds. *Chestnut's Obstetric Anesthesia: Principles and Practice*. 6th ed. Elsevier Saunders; 2020:840–878.

24. Bauer ME, Arendt K, Beilin Y. The Society for Obstetric Anesthesia and Perinatology Interdisciplinary consensus statement on neuraxial procedures in obstetric patients with thrombocytopenia. *Anesth Analg*. 2021:1–14.

25. Habib AS, D'Angelo R. Obesity. In: Chestnut DH, Wong CA, Tsen LC, et al., eds. *Chestnut's Obstetric Anesthesia: Principles and Practice*. 6th ed. Elsevier Saunders; 2020:1190–1206.

26. American College of Obstetricians and Gynecologists. Practice Bulletin No. 156: Obesity in pregnancy. *Obstet Gynecol*. 2015;126:e112–e126.

27. Buddeberg BS, Fernandes NL, Vorster A, et al. Cardiac structure and function in morbidly obese parturients: An echocardiographic study. *Anesth Analg*. 2019;129(2):444–449.

28. Cedergren MI. Non-elective caesarean delivery due to ineffective uterine contractility or due to obstructed labour in relation to maternal body mass index. *Eur J Obstet Gynecol Reprod Bio*. 2009;145:163–166.

29. Kominiarek MA, Zhang J, Vanveldhuisen P, Troendle J, Beaver J, Hibbard JU. Contemporary labor patterns: The impact of maternal body mass index. *Am J Obstet Gynecol*. 2011;205(3):244.e1–8.

30. Taylor CR, Dominguez JE, Habib AS. Obesity and obstetric anesthesia: Current insights. *Local Reg Anesth*. 2019;12:111–124.

31. Young B, Onwochei D, Desai N. Conventional landmark palpation vs. preprocedural ultrasound for neuraxial analgesia and anaesthesia in obstetrics—a systematic review and meta-analysis with trial sequential analyses. *Anaesthesia*. 2021;76:818–831.

32. Seligman KM, Weiniger CF, Carvalho B. The accuracy of a handheld ultrasound device for neuraxial depth and landmark assessment: A prospective cohort trial. *Anesth Analg*. 2018;126(6):1995–1998.

33. Dominguez JE, Krystal AD, Habib AS. Obstructive sleep apnea in pregnant women: A review of pregnancy outcomes and an approach to management. *Anesth Analg*. 2018;127(5):1167–1177.

34. Bauchat JR, Weiniger CF, Sultan P, et al. Society for Obstetric Anesthesia and Perinatology consensus statement: Monitoring recommendations for prevention and detection of respiratory depression associated with administration of neuraxial morphine for cesarean delivery analgesia. *Anesth Analg*. 2019;129:458–474.

35. American College of Obstetricians and Gynecologists. Practice Bulletin No. 196 Summary: Thromboembolism in pregnancy. *Obstet Gynecol*. 2018;132:243–248.

36. Leffert L, Butwick A, Carvalho B, et al. The Society for Obstetric Anesthesia and Perinatology consensus statement on the anesthetic management of pregnant and postpartum women receiving thromboprophylaxis or higher dose anticoagulants. *Anesth Analg*. 2018;126:928–944.

37. Wissler RN. Endocrine disorders. In: Chestnut DH, Wong CA, Tsen LC, et al., eds. *Chestnut's Obstetric Anesthesia: Principles and Practice*. 6th ed. Elsevier Saunders; 2020:1056–1087.

38. American College of Obstetricians and Gynecologists. Practice Bulletin No. 190: Gestational diabetes mellitus. *Obstet Gynecol*. 2018;131(2):e49–e64.

39. American College of Obstetricians and Gynecologists' Committee on Practice Bulletins – Obstetrics. ACOG Practice Bulletin No. 201: Pregestational diabetes mellitus. *Obstet Gynecol*. 2018;132(6):e228–e248.

40. Callesen NF, Ringholm L, Stage E, Damm P, Mathiesen ER. Insulin requirements in type 1 diabetic pregnancy: Do twin pregnant women require twice as much insulin as singleton pregnant women? *Diabetes Care*. 2012;35(6):1246–1248.

41. Duggan EW, Carlson K, Umpierrez GE. Perioperative hyperglycemia management: An update [published correction appears in *Anesthesiology*. 2018 Nov;129(5):1053]. *Anesthesiology*. 2017;126(3):547–560.

42. Joshi GP, Chung F, Vann MA, et al. Society for Ambulatory Anesthesia consensus statement on perioperative blood glucose management in diabetic patients undergoing ambulatory surgery. *Anesth Analg*. 2010;111(6):1378–1387.

43. Vidovich MI. Cardiovascular diseases. In: Chestnut DH, Wong CA, Tsen LC, et al., eds. *Chestnut's Obstetric Anesthesia: Principles and Practice*. 6th ed. Elsevier Saunders; 2020:987–1032.

44. Dennis AT. Heart failure in pregnant women: Is it peripartum cardiomyopathy? *Anesth Analg*. 2015;120:638–643.

45. Arany Z, Elkayam U. Peripartum cardiomyopathy. *Circulation*. 2016;133:1397–1409.

46. American College of Obstetricians and Gynecologists. Practice Bulletin No. 183 summary: Postpartum hemorrhage. *Obstet Gynecol*. 2017;130:923–925.

47. Tsen LC, Bateman BT. Anesthesia for cesarean delivery. In: Chestnut DH, Wong CA, Tsen LC, et al., eds. *Chestnut's Obstetric Anesthesia: Principles and Practice*. 6th ed. Elsevier Saunders; 2020:568–626.

48. Belfort MA, Shamshirsaz AA, Fox KA. The diagnosis and management of morbidly adherent placenta. *Semin Perinatol*. 2018;42:49–58.

49. Feldman JB, Kumaraswami S. Cesarean hysterectomy in a parturient with morbidly adherent placenta complicated by postoperative ischemic stroke secondary to vertebral artery dissection: A case report. *A A Pract*. 2019;12:9–14.

50. Belfort MA; Society for Maternal-Fetal Medicine Publications Committee. Placenta accreta. *Am J Obstet Gynecol*. 2010;203:430–439.

51. Ordonez CA, Manzano-Nunez R, Parra MW, et al. Prophylactic use of resuscitative endovascular balloon occlusion of the aorta in women with abnormal placentation: A systematic review, meta-analysis, and case series. *J Trauma Acute Care Surg*. 2018;84:809–818.

52. WOMAN Trial Collaborators. Effect of early tranexamic acid administration on mortality, hysterectomy, and other morbidities in women with post-partum haemorrhage (WOMAN): An international, randomised, double-blind, placebo-controlled trial. *Lancet*. 2017;389:2105–2116.

53. Mason CL, Tran CK. Caring for the Jehovah's Witness parturient. *Anesth Analg*. 2015;121:1564–1569.

54. Lange EMS, Rao S, Toledo P. Racial and ethnic disparities in obstetric anesthesia. *Semin Perinatol*. 2017;41:293–298.

55. Butwick AJ, Blumenfeld YJ, Brookfield KF, Nelson LM, Weiniger CF. Racial and ethnic disparities in mode of anesthesia for Cesarean delivery. *Anesth Analg*. 2016;122:472–479.

56. Lee A, Leffert L. Gloving up for the fight against racial and ethnic disparities in obstetric care. *J Clin Anesth*. 2020;67:109988.

57. Sheiner EK, Sheiner E, Shoham-Vardi I, Mazor M, Katz M. Ethnic differences influence care giver's estimates of pain during labor. *Pain*. 1999;81:299–305.

58. Leffert L. Substance use disorders. In: Chestnut DH, Wong CA, Tsen LC, et al., eds. *Chestnut's Obstetric Anesthesia: Principles and Practice*. 6th ed. Elsevier Saunders; 2020:1248–1273.

59. Sutton CD, Carvalho B. Optimal pain management after cesarean delivery. *Anesthesiol Clin*. 2017;35(1):107–124.

60. American College of Obstetricians and Gynecologists. Committee Opinion, Number 807: Tobacco and nicotine cessation during pregnancy. *Obstet Gynecol*. 2020;135(5):e221–e229.

61. Wong J, An D, Urman RD, et al. Society for Perioperative Assessment and Quality Improvement (SPAQI) consensus statement on perioperative smoking cessation. *Anesth Analg*. 2020;131(3):955–968.

PART V

SURGICAL CONSIDERATIONS

33.

MINIMALLY INVASIVE SURGERY AND OTHER ELEMENTS OF ENHANCED RECOVERY PROTOCOLS

Lesley Bennici, Morgane Factor, Sunitha M. Singh, and Ana Costa

STEM CASE AND KEY QUESTIONS

A 46-year-old woman with a history of ovarian cancer is scheduled for a robotic hysterectomy and bilateral salpingo-oopherectomy. Her past medical history is relevant for obesity and bilateral deep vein thromboses diagnosed 3 months ago. She was treated with apixaban. The patient arrives at the preoperative testing clinic for presurgical laboratory work and preoperative evaluation. After you perform a thorough history and physical exam, the patient asks what type of anesthesia she will receive and its risks.

What do you say to the patient?

You explain that she will undergo general anesthesia with an endotracheal tube as she needs to be immobile throughout the surgery with ventilation and oxygenation well controlled while in steep Trendelenburg position.

The patient is concerned about her history of bilateral deep vein thromboses (DVT) and blood thinner use. How will you manage her risk of venous thromboembolism (VTE)?

Due to her history of bilateral DVTs, this patient is at increased risk for perioperative venous thromboembolism despite having completed treatment with apixaban. You perform a careful history regarding any persistent symptoms and timing of the patient's last dose of apixaban, and you review the latest hematology note. Using a scoring system such as the Caprini Score for venous thromboembolism, you determine that this patient's comorbidities (history of DVT, obesity) and type of surgery (>45 minutes, robotic) place her at high risk (4.0%) for perioperative VTE. You recommend perioperative bilateral sequential compression devices placed before induction as well as subcutaneous unfractionated heparin.

The patient arrives for surgery and reveals she had a carbohydrate drink 6 hours prior to her surgery.

Would you make her wait 8 hours to be NPO prior to her surgery?

You are assigned to also care for her during her surgery after evaluating her in the preoperative clinic. After reiterating your anesthetic plan, she tells you that she has been reading on the internet and is concerned about being nauseated after surgery.

How would you explain her risk of postoperative nausea and vomiting (PONV)?

You calculate an simplified score of 3 indicating approximately a 60% 24-hour risk of PONV. However, this patient's risk for PONV is increased since she is having a gynecological procedure and the surgery may take a few hours given the fact that it is a robotic procedure in an obese patient.

She asks if you can do anything to help prevent PONV this during surgery. How would you answer her? What changes would you make to your anesthetic plan?

You tell her that she will receive several antinausea medications and her anesthesia will be provided "through the vein," avoiding volatile anesthesia gases to decrease her risk for PONV. In addition, you are planning a multimodal analgetic technique with IV lidocaine and IV acetaminophen.

After the induction of general anesthesia and endotracheal intubation, what procedures would you perform prior to allowing the surgeon to start?

As robotic surgeries present positioning challenges for the perioperative team, you place two IV lines in addition to standard American Society of Anesthesiologists (ASA) monitoring. The physical dimensions of the robot make it necessary to tuck the patient's arms to facilitate the surgeon's proximity to the patient. This prevents you from having access to the patient's upper extremities during the surgery, therefore twitch monitors cannot be applied on the forearm, and you ensure well-working IV access prior to tucking the arms.

Prior to the start of surgery, how will the patient be positioned, and what considerations are warranted in the prevention of position injuries?

The stirrups for lithotomy are cushioned to avoid injury to the lower extremities, the arms and hands are placed on cushions and tucked, fingers are protected from getting entrapped in the break of the operating room table when the lower portion is lowered allowing for the surgeon to have access to the pelvis, and the face is protected with a foam pillow to prevent injuries from surgical instruments.

After surgical incision and insufflation of the peritoneum, the ventilator alarms due to elevated peak airway pressures. What is the issue, and what measures will you take at this point?

Together, pneumoperitoneum and steep Trendelenburg positioning lead to an increase in intra-abdominal pressure leading to decreased functional residual capacity (FRC), increased physiologic dead space, greater ventilation/perfusion mismatch, decreased pulmonary compliance, and increased airway pressures. You ensure proper placement of the endotracheal tube (confirmed with bilateral breath sounds being present) and perform recruitment maneuvers consisting of giving a large-volume breath held over a few seconds to provide persistently increased airway pressures and expand collapsed alveoli. The settings on the ventilator are adjusted to provide smaller tidal volumes at higher respiratory rates, thus decreasing the maximum peak airway pressure.

Two hours into the surgery, both the end-tidal CO_2 and oxygen saturation decrease, and the patient becomes hypotensive. What is the inciting event? What are you going to do to resuscitate the patient?

In the setting of a pneumoperitoneum and an abrupt decrease in the end-tidal CO_2, a venous air embolus is the first item on the differential diagnosis. Although uncommon, venous air emboli occur during laparoscopic and robotic surgeries and can be catastrophic. As air becomes entrained in the right side of the heart, typically the right atrium, blood is no longer able to flow between the heart chambers as the entrained air creates an air lock and halts circulation. The patient is positioned in left lateral decubitus with the head down to promote the air lock to float to the upper aspect of the right atrium and not impede flow of blood to the right ventricle. A central line is immediately placed to aspirate air from the venous circulation while vasopressors are started. Despite attempts, cardiovascular collapse soon ensues necessitating advanced cardiac life support (ACLS) and cardiothoracic surgery is called to evaluate for further interventions. While waiting for the cardiothoracic surgeon, the patient regains hemodynamic stability and the collective decision is to proceed with the surgery. Due to difficult anatomy and difficult surgical visualization secondary to obesity and intraoperative bleeding, the surgery lasts 6 hours. You notice at the end of the case that the patient has slid up in the bed due to the steep Trendelenburg, and her face is swollen.

What are some things you would be concerned about postoperatively with such a prolonged surgical time?

Facial edema following prolonged steep Trendelenburg positioning is concerning for airway edema and potential respiratory difficulties following extubation. Once the surgery is finished, you position the patient in reverse Trendelenburg position, perform a leak test, which is positive, and proceed with extubating the patient. Despite your choice of anesthetic and attempts to avoid PONV (administered intravenous dexamethasone and ondansetron intraoperatively), the patient is nauseated in PACU.

Do you have any concerns regarding post discharge nausea and vomiting (PDNV)? Is this different than PONV?

As the patient is experiencing PONV in the PACU, you prescribe a rescue antiemetic medication from a different class compared to the antiemetic medications she received as prophylaxis. Her nausea resolves, and she is discharged home later in the day.

DISCUSSION

POSITIONING AND PHYSIOLOGIC CONSIDERATIONS FOR PATIENTS UNDERGOING ROBOTIC HYSTERECTOMY

Anesthetic management for robotic hysterectomy requires many specific considerations. The primary considerations are the physical and physiologic disturbances of surgical positioning, increased risk of PONV, risks of prolonged surgery time, and desire for same-day discharge.

As discussed in the questions above, patients need to be positioned in lithotomy and steep Trendelenburg with arms tucked at the sides during a robotic hysterectomy. This prevents the anesthesiologist from having access to the upper extremities for intraoperative placement of lines and monitors, increases risk of nerve and crush injury, and often causes major physiologic disturbance. Some anesthesiologists may choose to place an arterial line prior to positioning especially if blood draws are needed during the case, such as blood glucose measurements, arterial blood gases, hemoglobin concentration, and coagulation studies.

Two providers are necessary to lift and abduct the legs at the same time to avoid strain on the lumbar spine. Special attention must be paid to the fingers to avoid crush injury as they may get trapped in the moving portion of the operating room table when the bottom part of the bed is lowered. If arms are tucked too tightly and without appropriate padding, there is also the risk of injury to nerves of the upper extremity. Lithotomy position requires that the hips be flexed and lower extremities raised and abducted in stirrups, putting the patient at risk for common peroneal and saphenous nerve injury if appropriate padding is not ensured. The common peroneal nerve is the most common lower extremity injury in surgeries requiring lithotomy position for extended periods of time. The most effective way to prevent a common peroneal nerve injury is to utilize padded, cushioned stirrups and avoid making them too tight around the patient's lower extremities. It is important to avoid hip hyperflexion, so as not to increase the risk of injury to the femoral and lateral femoral cutaneous nerves. Hyperabduction of the legs may injure the obturator nerve. The sciatic nerve is at risk for stretch injury if the hips are hyperflexed, hyperabducted, or excessively externally rotated in lithotomy.[1] The duration of the lithotomy position is extremely important as patients in this position for longer than 2 hours are at a higher risk for neuropathies.[2] As robotic hysterectomies can sometimes be lengthy operations, it is also important to note that increased surgical time increases the risk of neuropathy.

In addition to potential nerve injuries, the lithotomy position causes physiologic changes, such as increased venous return when the legs are elevated, the cephalad displacement of the diaphragm leading to reduced lung compliance, and exacerbation of existing back pain at the lumbar spine. Furthermore, lithotomy may cause decreased perfusion of the elevated extremities leading to decreased sensation and potential ischemia as well as compartment syndrome.[3] Physiologic disturbances are common with prolonged robotic surgeries in steep Trendelenburg positioning. Table 33.1 presents a summary of these physiologic disturbances by organ system.

Difficulties with mechanical ventilation are one of the most challenging aspects of the anesthetic management for robotic hysterectomies. Steep Trendelenburg positioning can lead to right mainstem intubation, increased peak airway pressures, ventilation-perfusion mismatch, atelectasis, aspiration, pulmonary edema, and pneumothorax. This requires careful preoperative consideration with regard to a patient's body habitus because obesity can exacerbate many of these issues, as well as a patient's comorbid pulmonary issues. If a patient has a high BMI or poor lung function preoperatively, it may be wise to discuss with the surgical team whether an open surgical approach is feasible. Intraoperatively, peak airway pressures can often be managed by utilizing a strategy that includes increased respiratory rate, decreased tidal volumes, and permissive hypercapnia. Most anesthesiologists will attempt to keep the peak airway pressure below 40 cm H_2O. Adding some positive end-expiratory pressure (PEEP) to the ventilator settings can also help to keep small alveoli open.

Additionally, should the end tidal CO_2 abruptly drop at any point, the rare but fatal complication of venous air embolism should always be considered and treated, as outlined in the stem question.

Increased risk of PONV associated with robotic gynecologic surgery is a rather important consideration since it can lead to patient distress and dissatisfaction postoperatively, as well as delayed discharge to home. Severe PONV can also lead to a prolonged PACU or hospital stay, thereby increasing hospital costs. Identification of at-risk patients and providing appropriate prophylaxis is key in preventing PONV. There are many risk factors for PONV. They can be divided into two groups—patient-specific risk factors and surgery-specific risk factors. Patient-specific factors for adults include female sex, a history of PONV or motion sickness, nonsmoking status, and young age. Surgery-specific risk factors associated with a higher incidence of PONV include laparoscopic, bariatric, and gynecological surgery. Cholecystectomy has also been shown to be associated with an increased risk of PONV. Length of surgery also affects the risk for PONV, with longer surgeries being associated with more PONV than shorter surgeries. Box 33.1 shows a summary of patient-specific risk factors associated with PONV.

Once risk factors have been identified, patients can be assigned a simplified Apfel score to estimate the incidence of PONV.[4] This score is solely based on four risk factors: female sex, nonsmoking status, history of PONV and/or motion sickness, and use of postoperative opioids. By assigning a score from 0 to 4 based on how many risk factors a patient has, PONV can be reduced at an institutional level due to guide prophylaxis and therapy. Strategies for reducing risk of PONV include administration of at least two pharmacologic antiemetic medications intraoperatively for PONV prophylaxis. The most commonly used combination antiemetic prophylaxis in practice is the 5HT3 receptor antagonist, ondansetron, towards the end of the case

Table 33.1 PHYSIOLOGIC DISTURBANCES FROM PROLONGED ROBOTIC SURGERY IN STEEP TRENDELENBURG POSITIONING

Central nervous system	Cerebral edema, hypothermia
Peripheral nervous system	Upper and lower extremity nerve injuries (compression, stretching, ischemia)
Ophthalmic	Corneal abrasion, retinal tear/detachment, ischemic optic neuropathy
Cardiovascular	Bradycardia, ischemic changes on ECG, myocardial infarction
Respiratory	Mainstem intubation, atelectasis, ventilation perfusion mismatch, aspiration, pulmonary edema, pneumothorax
Renal	Acute kidney injury, oliguria
Gastrointestinal/hepatobiliary	Acute liver injury
Vascular	Deep vein thrombosis, compartment syndrome, rhabdomyolysis
Musculoskeletal	Cervical and lumbar strain, pressure lesions, contusions/ecchymoses
Edema	Subcutaneous emphysema, chemosis/conjunctival edema, facial edema, airway edema

Box 33.1 POSTOPERATIVE NAUSEA AND VOMITING (PONV) RISK FACTOR SUMMARY IN ADULTS

Female sex
Younger age
History of motion sickness or prior PONV
Nonsmoker
Type of surgery (ex/ robotic/laparoscopic, gynecologic)
Duration of anesthesia/surgery (hours)
Use of general anesthesia instead of regional anesthesia
Use of volatile anesthetics (dose-dependent) and nitrous oxide (duration-dependent) instead of total intravenous anesthesia
Administration of postoperative opioids (dose-dependent)

and the corticosteroid, dexamethasone, at the beginning of the case. Premedication with the NK1 receptor antagonist, aprepitant, should also be considered preoperatively. Additional considerations pertain to minimizing perioperative administration of opioids, using multimodal analgesia, and using regional anesthetic techniques when available and appropriate. Dexmedetomidine and/or lidocaine infusion intraoperatively allow for less intraoperative opiate use and less subsequent PONV. Intraoperative use of IV acetaminophen is also useful to reduce opiate use and the incidence of PONV. The use of propofol infusions as part of total IV anesthesia protocols instead of volatile agents results in less nausea. Other factors that can be optimized to help reduce PONV are to ensure that the patient is adequately hydrated intraoperatively to maintain euvolemia. Also, reversing paralysis using sugammadex instead of neostigmine and glycopyrrolate may be beneficial.

Patients at high risk for PONV should be identified preoperatively and steps should be taken to minimize that baseline risk. Box 33.2 summarizes the steps to reduce baseline PONV risk.

In the event the patient experiences PONV, treatment guidelines recommend[5]

1. The use of multimodal prophylaxis in patients with one or more risk factors.

2. 5-HT3 receptor antagonists (ondansetron is most commonly used). Side effects include slight QTc prolongation, headache, elevated liver enzymes, and constipation.

3. NK1 receptor antagonists (aprepitant) are more efficacious for postoperative vomiting rather than nausea and are more efficacious than ondansetron. These agents reduce incidence of vomiting on both postoperative day 1 and 2.

4. Corticosteroids (dexamethasone is most commonly used). Dose ranges between 4 and 10 mg. Data support the early dosing of dexamethasone at the beginning of a case rather than at the end for prevention of PONV. Given in a single dose, dexamethasone 4 mg IV does not have adverse effects on wound healing, produces only mild glucose elevation, and does not results in increased postoperative bleeding or cancer recurrence.

5. Antidopaminergics

    1. *Droperidol*: Effective but its use has significantly declined following a black box warning by the US Food and Drug Administration (FDA) of sudden cardiac death in doses greater than 25 mg. Antiemetic doses can result in mild QTc prolongation comparable to ondansetron. Effect on QTc when drugs are combined is same as each agent alone.

    2. *Haloperidol*: Not approved for use as antiemetic. Side effects include QTc prolongation, increased sedation.

    3. *Metoclopramide*: Uncertain antiemetic efficacy.

6. The antihistamine diphenhydramine is effective for PONV prophylaxis but optimal dosing, timing, and side-effect profile are unclear.

7. Anticholinergic (e.g., scopolamine patch) can be applied preoperatively or evening before. Onset of effect is 2–4 hours. Adverse events are generally mild, most commonly visual disturbances, dry mouth, and dizziness.

8. Gabapentinoids (gabapentin and pregabalin) given 1–2 hours before surgery decrease PONV and can also reduce pain severity, total morphine consumption. Disadvantages include sedation, visual disturbances, dizziness, and headache.

9. Midazolam.

10. Ephedrine has an effect for 3 hours postoperatively when administered near the end of surgery.

11. Fluids to achieve adequate hydration by minimizing perioperative fasting time and maintaining clinical euvolemia.

12. Carbohydrate loading.

PDNV is different from PONV in that patients experience nausea and vomiting after discharge from the hospital, which often presents a challenging problem since the antiemetics available need to be taken orally. Severe PDNV can lead to an emergency room visit and/or a hospital readmission. Therefore, anesthesiologists should be diligent in identifying a patient's risk for PONV, utilizing a multimodal strategy to prevent PONV, minimizing factors known to cause PONV, and aggressively treating PONV.

ENHANCED RECOVERY AFTER SURGERY PRINCIPLES

Surgical stimulation and manipulation cause the body to enter a catabolic state which can be associated with increased morbidity and delayed recovery.[6] Surgical stress can cause increased insulin resistance, impaired coagulation,

---

Box 33.2 **STEPS TO REDUCE BASELINE POSTOPERATIVE NAUSEA AND VOMITING (PONV) RISK**

Utilize multimodal analgesic techniques (IV acetaminophen, alpha-2 agonists)
Minimize intraoperative and postoperative opioids
Avoid volatile anesthetics
Avoid nitrous oxide administration for >1 hour
Utilize propofol for induction and maintenance of anesthesia
Utilize sugammadex instead of neostigmine for reversal of neuromuscular blockade
Provide adequate intravenous hydration

gastrointestinal dysfunction, and pulmonary complications. Enhanced recovery after surgery (ERAS) programs are multi-disciplinary, perioperative care pathways that aim to maintain normal physiology and achieve early recovery after surgical procedures. As such, ERAS pathways combine evidence-based best practice to diminish the effects of physiologic stress and improve the rehabilitation of surgical patients.[7]

The concept of ERAS was first described in the 1990s and has been well-studied within the realm of colorectal surgery. As a result, these programs are widely practiced in major surgery and are shown to improve postsurgical outcomes.[8,9] The implementation of ERAS for open and minimally invasive benign gynecologic and gynecologic oncology surgeries has been quite promising.

ERAS programs comprise several elements through the perioperative period to optimize and reduce variability in care, reduce the surgical stress response, and promote an early return to baseline function. The cornerstones of an enhanced recovery pathway include preoperative counseling, select bowel preparation, multimodal and opioid sparing approaches to pain management, utilization of minimally invasive surgical techniques, maintenance of normothermia, goal-directed fluid management, and promotion of postoperative recovery strategies (e.g., early mobilization, implementation of diet, and appropriate thromboprophylaxis).[10–15] Key elements of an ERAS gynecological pathway are described in Table 33.2.

ERAS pathways are initiated at the initial preoperative visit. Patient diaries and handouts are encouraged to facilitate patient education and engagement. These comprehensive booklets are very useful for illustrating the goals of ERAS, setting expectations, and answering common questions (e.g., How will my pain be managed?). With an ERAS pathway, patients are empowered to be active participants in their care.[16] Identification of tobacco and alcohol use during the preoperative period is incredibly important since smoking and alcohol cessation have both been proven to minimize complication rates and improve patient outcomes. Additionally, increased BMI and obesity, diabetes, sleep apnea, and anemia are other important patient factors that should be recognized preoperatively to plan for appropriate perioperative management.[17]

Prolonged preoperative fasting depletes liver glycogen stores, impairs glucose metabolism, and increases insulin resistance. The adverse effects of this physiologic cascade are well described. ERAS pathways recommend avoiding prolonged fasting and dehydration by providing complex carbohydrate (CHO) clear liquids to patients preoperatively. By reducing preoperative thirst as well as postoperative insulin resistance, there is an overall reduction in hospital length of stay as well as enhanced patient satisfaction associated with these beverages.[18] Carbohydrate loading routines vary across pathways, but they typically include at least one 12 oz beverage containing 50 g of a complex carbohydrate (i.e., maltodextrin). There is a lack of consensus for providing complex CHO beverages to patients with diabetes mellitus (DM). However, the available evidence reports that complex CHO drinks can be given to patients with DM without increased risk for intra- and postoperative hyperglycemia or surgical complications.[19] Additionally, there is no anesthetic contraindication to the intake of clear fluids up until 2 hours before surgery. Studies have shown that this does not increase gastric content, reduce gastric fluid pH or increase overall complication rates.[20–22]

Intraoperative anesthetic management and postoperative pain control are important aspects of any ERAS pathway. Opioid administration has been associated with impaired bowel function, decreased mobility, increased risk of PONV, and increased risk of pulmonary complications. All these delay recovery and negatively affect the patient's experience. Additionally, the prevalence of opioid use disorder in the population at large has been an important factor in the development of multimodal, opioid-sparing pain management strategies.

Pre-medication with acetaminophen and gabapentin decreases total narcotic requirement while improving postoperative pain scores and patient satisfaction. Ketorolac, an NSAID, also decreases postoperative pain without increasing postoperative bleeding risk.[23] Neuraxial anesthetic techniques should be used judiciously to avoid limiting mobility while decreasing postoperative pain and opioid requirement. Regional anesthesia techniques, such as the transversus abdominis plane (TAP) block, can also reduce postoperative opioid consumption but may have a limited role with a minimally invasive surgical technique.[24] Intraoperative anesthetic management often employs a total IV anesthesia, opioid-sparing technique to avoid volatile gases which can lead to PONV and impaired bowel function. Postoperative opioid consumption can be decreased via the use of scheduled gabapentin, acetaminophen, and NSAIDs.

Standardized care pathways such as ERAS have been consistently shown to reduce postoperative analgesic requirement, facilitate an early return of bowel function and ambulation, reduce postoperative length of stay, decrease complication and readmission rates, and improve patient satisfaction Moreover, the use of an ERAS pathway has not been found to increase readmission rates, reoperation rates, or overall mortality.[25] A significant amount of primary outcomes related to ERAS effectiveness has been concentrated on examining the clinical benefits within comparable cohorts. However, recent studies in colorectal and gynecologic oncology patients show ERAS pathways may also promote health equity.[26,27] Several factors contribute to surgical health disparities (e.g., patient, provider, geography, access). Reducing variability in care by standardizing patient optimization and delivery of care may eliminate inequalities and implicit biases, thus working to close the gaps in healthcare. Within an ERAS pathway, it is unclear whether specific elements are more impactful than others. However, the most successful ERAS pathways are ones in which multiple components are executed. Given the potential for improved outcomes, the implementation of ERAS pathways should be strongly considered by institutions.

Table 33.2 **ENHANCED RECOVERY AFTER SURGERY (ERAS) PRINCIPLES**

ELEMENTS OF AN ERAS PATHWAY

PHASE		INTERVENTION	GOAL
Preoperative	Surgery and Pre-Operative/Pre-Admission Clinics	Identify/Label ERAS patients	Inform perioperative care team
		Patient education and counseling about ERAS pathway, surgery, and recovery expectations	Empower patients; set expectations
		Bowel preparation up to 5 days prior (ex/ polyethylene glycol)	Avoid unnecessary dehydration
		Risk optimization and malnutrition screening	Improve immune function
		Preoperative fasting with patient NPO for regular diet after midnight, clear liquids allowed until 2 hours prior to induction of anesthesia	A metabolically fed state better equips patients for surgical stress, aligns with ASA guidelines
		Carbohydrate loading with administration of 20 ounces carbohydrate and electrolyte containing clear liquid drink, 2 hours prior to induction of anesthesia	A metabolically fed state better equips patients for surgical stress
	Pre-Surgical Area	PONV prophylaxis using multimodal approach	Anti-emetics reduce PONV, facilitates oral intake & recovery
		Fluid management via peripheral IV insertion without additional IV fluid administration	Goal directed fluid therapy is associated with reduced complications (cardiac, wound infections, LOS)
		Multimodal pain management with administration of non-opioid pain medications such as PO acetaminophen, celecoxib, gabapentin	Preventive analgesia, improved post-operative pain, decreased opioid use & side effects
		Venous thromboprophylaxis with sequential compression devices + subcutaneous heparin or enoxaparin	Reduce risk of DVT
Intraoperative		Antibiotic administration before skin incision	Reduce risk of SSIs
		Minimally invasive surgery	Reduce post-operative pain and complications, decrease surgery time and associated risks
		Avoid long-acting sedatives. Anesthetic induction often includes NMDA antagonists such as IV ketamine	Facilitate rapid awakening
		Opioid sparing strategies: Epidural/Spinal/TAP Blocks	Reduce post-operative pain and complications; minimize opioid use
		Multimodal pain management with IV lidocaine and IV ketamine infusions in addition to regional anesthesia techniques	Reduce post-operative pain and improve return to GI function
		Fluid management to maintain euvolemia	Goal directed fluid therapy is associated with reduced complications (cardiac, wound infections, LOS)
		Minimize OGT/NGT	Facilitates early return to oral nutrition and ambulation.
		Maintain normothermia	Maintaining normal body temperature is associated with a reduction in SSIs
Postoperative		Venous thromboembolism with sequential compression devices + subcutaneous heparin or enoxaparin	Reduce risk of blood clots
		Control PONV using 2–3 classes of anti-emetics	Facilitate oral intake, speeds recovery
		Multimodal pain management with administration of PO acetaminophen, ibuprofen, and non-opioid pain medications. PO opioid medication use should be minimized	Scheduled MMA minimizes opioid use & side effects, facilitates mobility & recovery
		Early mobility with patient out of bed to chair on night after surgery and patient ambulating 3 times per day beginning POD#1	Improves recovery with goal to early discharge home
		Early feeding with clear liquids in recovery on POD#0, soft diet on POD#1 and transition to regular diet as tolerated	Improves recovery with goal to early discharge home
		Early discharge as soon as patient is ambulating, tolerating a regular diet, and has pain control with oral medications	Improves patient satisfaction

ASA, American Society of Anesthesiologists; DVT, deep vein thrombosis; ERAS, enhanced recovery after surgery; LOS, length of stay; MMA, multimodal analgesia; NGT, nasogastric tube; NMDA, N-methyl-D-aspartate; OGT, oral gastric tube; POD, postoperative day; PONV post operative nausea and vomiting; SSI surgical site infection; TAP transversus abdominus plane.

CONCLUSION

- Robotic hysterectomies present multiple challenges to the anesthesiologist.
- Prolonged surgery duration increases the risk for complications.
- Steep Trendelenburg can lead to difficulties in mechanical ventilation, position injuries, and other adverse events.
- Young women are at an increased risk for PONV.
- PONV risk factors should be identified preoperatively, and the anesthesiologist should utilize PONV prophylaxis aggressively in patients at a higher risk for PONV.
- PONV treatment guidelines emphasize multimodal use of antiemetic medications and reduction of opioid use.
- ERAS pathways benefit patients in various ways.

REVIEW QUESTIONS

1. After undergoing a 7-hour robotic hysterectomy, a patient complains of numbness on the lower extremities leading to foot drop. What is the most common lower extremity nerve to be injured during prolonged surgeries in the lithotomy position?

   a. Sciatic nerve.
   b. Femoral nerve.
   c. Saphenous nerve.
   d. Common peroneal nerve.

   The correct answer is d.

   The common peroneal nerve is the most common lower extremity injury in surgeries requiring lithotomy position for extended periods of time. The most effective way to prevent a common peroneal nerve injury is to utilize padded, cushioned stirrups and avoid making them too tight around the patient's lower extremities.

2. During the surgery, the anesthesiologist notices both the end-tidal CO_2 and blood pressure decrease acutely. At that point, the robot is already docked, the patient's abdomen is insufflated, and the patient is in steep Trendelenburg. What is the most likely etiology of the acute decrease in end-tidal CO_2 and blood pressure?

   a. Acute blood loss.
   b. Anaphylaxis.
   c. Venous air embolism.
   d. Main-stem intubation.

   The correct answer is c.

   The most common cause of a decrease in both blood pressure and end tidal CO_2 is venous air embolism. Anaphylaxis and acute blood loss manifests as hypotension and main-stem intubation as hypoxia but with no change in end tidal CO_2.

3. After the surgeon insufflated the abdomen as the patient was in steep Trendelenburg, the anesthesiologist noticed the ventilator registering high peak pressures and small tidal volumes. The oxygen saturation remained 96% on 50% FiO_2. What is a likely cause of these ventilatory changes?

   a. Right main-stem intubation.
   b. Bronchospasm.
   c. Laryngospasm.
   d. Pneumothorax.

   The correct answer is a.

   Mainstem intubation is a common complication of steep Trendelenburg positioning paired with abdominal insufflation, resulting in a slow decrease in $ETCO_2$.

4. The anesthesiologist identifies the patient as high risk for PONV and administers aprepitant preoperatively and dexamethasone and ondansetron intraoperatively. The patient reports nausea in the PACU. As per current guidelines, what is the best next step to treat her nausea?

   a. Administer a second dose of ondansetron.
   b. Administer a second dose of dexamethasone.
   c. Administer droperidol.
   d. Administer IV fluids.

   The correct answer is c.

   Current guidelines recommend a third antiemetic from a different class than the ones administered intraoperatively to be given in the PACU for PONV rescue.

5. The surgeon reports excessive bleeding intraoperatively and makes the decision to convert the surgery from a robotic hysterectomy to an open hysterectomy. The operating room team is aware that the consent clearly stated the possibility of converting the robotic surgery to an open surgery. Considering the patient being at a higher risk for PONV, what is the best mode of analgesia to treat her pain prior to emergence from anesthesia?

   a. Administer much higher doses of narcotics.
   b. Perform TAP blocks.
   c. Write for an IV patient-controlled analgesia medication.
   d. Infiltrate local anesthetic into the incision.

   The correct answer is b.

   Minimizing narcotic contributes to preventing PONV. For an open incision, a regional anesthesia technique is indicated to minimize postoperative pain. In this case, as an open procedure was not initially planned, a TAP block may be appropriate to decrease perioperative narcotic use.

6. The patient is under a GYN ERAS pathway. Which of the following does not violate NPO guidelines for anesthesia?

   a. Consumption of 20-ounce carbohydrate drink 2 hours prior to induction of anesthesia.
   b. Consumption of crackers 2 hours prior to induction of anesthesia.
   c. Consumption of coffee with cream 2 hours prior to induction of anesthesia.
   d. Consumption of a half-gallon of water 1 hour prior to induction of anesthesia.

The correct answer is a.

A carbohydrate load administered 2 hours prior to anesthesia induction does not violate the latest ASA guidelines on preoperative fasting and is consistent with ERAS principles.

7. The surgery unexpectedly takes 12 hours with the patient in steep Trendelenburg and lithotomy for most of that time. At the end of the surgery, the anesthesiologist notices the patient's face is edematous. What is a recommended practice prior to extubation in this situation?

   a. Perform a cuff leak test.
   b. Check the position of the endotracheal tube with a fiberoptic scope.
   c. Administer more narcotics.
   d. Remove the sequential compression device.

The correct answer is a.

Airway edema is a concern with prolonged Trendelenburg positioning, and a cuff leak test should be performed prior to extubation.

REFERENCES

1. Wieslander CK, Boreham MK, Phelan J, Schaffer JI, Corton MM. Video: Avoiding nerve injury during gynecologic surgery. *J Pelvic Med Surg*. 11:S54. doi:10.1097/01.spv.0000179338.89281.62
2. Warner MA, Warner DO, Harper CM, Schroeder DR, Maxson PM. Lower extremity neuropathies associated with lithotomy positions. *Anesthesiology*. 2000 Oct;93(4):938–942. doi:10.1097/00000542-200010000-00010. PMID: 11020742
3. Breyer K, Roth S. Patient positioning and associated risks. *Miller's Anesthesia*. 34:1079–1112.e6.
4. Apfel CC, Läärä E, Koivuranta M, Greim CA, Roewer N. A simplified risk score for predicting postoperative nausea and vomiting: Conclusions from cross-validations between two centers. *Anesthesiology*. 1999 Sep;91(3):693–700. doi:10.1097/00000542-199909000-00022. PMID: 10485781
5. Gan TJ, Belani KG, Bergese S, et al. Fourth consensus guidelines for the management of postoperative nausea and vomiting. *Anesth Analg*. 2020 Aug;131(2):411–448. doi:10.1213/ANE.0000000000004833
6. Kehlet H, Wilmore DW. Evidence-based surgical care and the evolution of fast-track surgery. *Ann Surg*. 2008;248:189–198.
7. Kalogera E, Dowdy SC. Enhanced recovery pathway in gynecologic surgery: Improving outcomes through evidence-based medicine. *Obstet Gynecol Clin North Am*. 2016;43:551–573.
8. Singh SM, Liverpool A, Romeiser JL, et al. Types of surgical patients enrolled in enhanced recovery after surgery (ERAS) programs in the USA. *Perioper Med*. 2021;10:12. https://doi.org/10.1186/s13741-021-00185-5
9. Joliat GR, Ljungqvist O, Wasylak T, et al. Beyond surgery: Clinical and economic impact of enhanced recovery after surgery programs. *BMC Health Serv Res*. 2018;18:1008. https://doi.org/10.1186/s12913-018-3824-0
10. Miralpeix E, Nick AM, Meyer LA, et al. A call for new standard of care in perioperative gynecologic oncology practice: Impact of enhanced recovery after surgery (ERAS) programs. *Gynecol Oncol*. 2016;141:371–378.
11. Modesitt SC, Sarosiek BM, Trowbridge ER, et al. Enhanced recovery implementation in major gynecologic surgeries: Effect of care standardization. *Obstet Gynecol*. 2016;128:457–466.
12. Nelson G, Kalogera E, Dowdy SC. Enhanced recovery pathways in gynecologic oncology. *Gynecol Oncol*. 2014;135:586–594.
13. Yoong W, Sivashanmugarajan V, Relph S, et al. Can enhanced recovery pathways improve outcomes of vaginal hysterectomy? Cohort control study. *J Minim Invasive Gynecol*. 2014;21:83–89.
14. Kalogera E, Bakkum-Gamez JN, Jankowski CJ, et al. Enhanced recovery in gynecologic surgery. *Obstet Gynecol*. 2013;122:319–328.
15. Chapman JS, Roddy E, Ueda S, Brooks R, Chen LL, Chen LM. Enhanced recovery pathways for improving outcomes after minimally invasive gynecologic oncology surgery. *Obstet Gynecol*. 2016;128:138–144.
16. Varadhan KK, Neal KR, Dejong CH, Fearon KC, Ljungqvist O, Lobo DN. The enhanced recovery after surgery (ERAS) pathway for patients undergoing major elective open colorectal surgery: A meta-analysis of randomized controlled trials. *Clin Nutr*. 2010;29:434–440.
17. Myers K, Hajek P, Hinds C, McRobbie H. Stopping smoking shortly before surgery and postoperative complications: A systematic review and meta-analysis. *Arch Intern Med*. 2011;171:983–989.
18. Lassen K, Soop M, Nygren J, et al. Consensus review of optimal perioperative care in colorectal surgery: Enhanced Recovery After Surgery (ERAS) group recommendations. *Arch Surg*. 2009;144:961–969.
19. Robinson KN, Cassady BA, Hegazi RA, Wischmeyer PE. Preoperative carbohydrate loading in surgical patients with type 2 diabetes: Are concerns supported by data? *Clinical Nutr ESPEN*. 2021 Oct 1;45:1–8. https://doi.org/10.1016/j.clnesp.2021.08.023 https://doi.org/10.1016/j.clnesp.2021.08.023
20. Nelson G, Altman AD, Nick A, et al. Guidelines for pre- and intraoperative care in gynecologic/oncology surgery: Enhanced Recovery After Surgery (ERAS(R)) Society recommendations—Part I. *Gynecol Oncol*. 2016;140:313–322.
21. American Society of Anesthesiologists. Practice guidelines for preoperative fasting and the use of pharmacologic agents to reduce the risk of pulmonary aspiration: Application to healthy patients undergoing elective procedures: An updated report by the American Society of Anesthesiologists Task Force on Preoperative Fasting and the Use of Pharmacologic Agents to Reduce the Risk of Pulmonary Aspiration. *Anesthesiology*. 2017;126:376–393. doi:https://doi.org/10.1097/ALN.0000000000001452
22. Steinberg AC, Schimpf MO, White AB, et al. Preemptive analgesia for postoperative hysterectomy pain control: Systematic review and clinical practice guidelines. *Am J Obstet Gynecol*. 2017;217:303–313.e6.
23. Gobble RM, Hoang HL, Kachniarz B, Orgill DP. Ketorolac does not increase perioperative bleeding: A meta-analysis of randomized controlled trials. *Plast Reconstr Surg*. 2014;133:741–755.
24. El Hachem L, Small E, Chung P, et al. Randomized controlled double-blind trial of transversus abdominis plane block versus trocar site infiltration in gynecologic laparoscopy. *Am J Obstet Gynecol* 2015;212(182):e1–e9.
25. Scheib SA, Thomassee M, Kenner JL. Enhanced recovery after surgery in gynecology: A review of the literature. *J Minim Invasive Gynecol*. 2019 Feb;26(2):327–343.
26. Alimena S, Fallah P, Stephenson B, Feltmate C, Feldman S, Elias KM. Comparison of Enhanced Recovery After Surgery (ERAS) metrics by race among gynecologic oncology patients: Ensuring equitable outcomes. *Gynecol Oncol*. 2023 Apr;171:31–38. PMID: 36804619 doi:10.1016/j.ygyno.2023.02.005
27. Marques IC, Wahl TS, Chu DI. Enhanced recovery after surgery and surgical disparities. *Surg Clin N Am*. 2018;98(6);1223–1232. PMID: 30390854 doi:10.1016/j.suc.2018.07.015

34.

BLOOD CONSERVATION

Seth Perelman and Christian Mabry

STEM CASE AND KEY QUESTIONS

A 67-year-old man presents emergently to the operating room for colon resection for a bleeding rectal tumor. The patient was transferred directly to the operating room from the emergency department. He presented to the emergency department earlier that day because of an episode of syncope at home. The patient had been feeling light-headed with episodes of dizziness, predominately after standing, for about 5 days. Three hours before his syncopal episode, he noticed bright red blood in his stool.

The patient only has a history of hypertension treated with an angiotensin-converting enzyme inhibitor. He is 5′ 11″ tall with a weight of 85 kg.

During the preoperative interview, the clinician discovers that the patient is a Jehovah's Witness. He will not accept transfusion of any blood or blood products but will accept nonblood alternatives. His most recent complete blood count shows a hemoglobin of 8.8 g/dL and hematocrit of 26.3%. His heart rate is 92 beats/minute with a blood pressure of 109/51 mm Hg. His heart rate increases to 107 beats/minute and blood pressure decreases to 89/40 mmHg upon standing.

What types of anemia are there?

The World Health Organization defines anemia as hemoglobin levels less than 12 g/dL for women and less than 13 g/dL for men, although there is some debate about whether gender should be a factor in this definition.[1] Several different types of anemia exist, with iron deficiency anemia and anemia of chronic inflammation being the most common.[2] Iron deficiency is a major nutritional burden on our healthcare system and plays an important role in the anemia seen in an estimated 2 billion people worldwide.[2,3] The exact definition of iron deficiency anemia is controversial, however, most institutions use a combination low hemoglobin in the presence of low ferritin and low transferrin saturation (see Table 34.1). A low reticulocyte-hemoglobin level can also be the sole diagnostic tool for iron deficiency anemia. Since transferrin saturation can be determined through an equation using total iron binding capacity and transferrin level (in mg/dL), low iron stores can be calculated when transferrin saturation is not available.

As the name suggests, chronic inflammation plays a key role in the second most common type of anemia. This inflammation can be from infection, chronic kidney disease, cancer, or tissue injury that releases proinflammatory cytokines.[4] In this condition, iron stores are adequate but there is an inability to deliver this iron to the bone marrow.[4] This is reflected as high serum ferritin along with low serum transferrin saturation. Hepcidin is the principal hormone responsible for inhibiting mobilization of iron stores in chronic inflammation.[5] Thus, hepcidin is elevated in anemia of chronic inflammation, leading to a functional iron deficiency.[2]

This patient is displaying many of the common signs and symptoms of anemia with the most likely etiology being iron deficiency anemia from acute on chronic blood loss. Given this patient's history, however, the possibility of a multifactorial anemia should also be considered. Further lab work that focuses on iron stores, red blood cell (RBC) mass, other nutritional deficiencies, and major organ dysfunction will help make the diagnosis.

What are the general indications for a blood transfusion in any patient?

RBCs contain hemoglobin molecules, each of which can carry up to four oxygen molecules.[4] Decreasing RBC mass constitutes anemia; the degree of anemia and the impairment of tissue oxygenation are one indication for packed RBC (PRBC) transfusion.[11] Tissue oxygenation, however, should not be the sole parameter to determine when to transfuse PRBCs. At a physiologic level, transfusions should occur with the goal of increasing whole body oxygen delivery (DO_2) and at the same time increasing oxygen consumption (VO_2).[12] One without the other will create a mismatch and an inability to maximize tissue oxygenation. Thus, the ability to increase oxygen consumption should be considered when contemplating a blood transfusion.

Madjdpour and Spahn argue that a whole-body oxygen extraction ratio should be a predominant variable in any transfusion algorithm.[12] There is tremendous physiological reserve for oxygen extraction, and a severe drop in hemoglobin can be overcome by increasing the extraction ratio.[12] Even hemoglobin levels as low as 3 g/dL can be tolerated because of the body's ability to use dissolved oxygen for consumption.[13] Up to 74% of oxygen consumption can come from this dissolved oxygen, up from less than 2% when breathing ambient air during normal conditions.[13]

The most common clinical indication for RBC transfusion is symptomatology. As with this patient, a thorough history and physical exam can strongly rule in or rule out anemia as the etiology of a patient's symptoms even before

Table 34.1 VARIOUS DEFINITIONS OF IRON DEFICIENCY ANEMIA

REFERENCE	FERRITIN (NG/ML)	TRANSFERRIN SATURATION (%)
Auerbach M et al.[6]	Ferritin <15 alone *or* <15–25 *and*	<15
Muñoz M et al.[7]	<30 alone	
Shander A et al.[8]		<20 alone
Guinn NR et al.[9]	<100 *and* *or*	<20 <20 alone
Injectafer (ferric carboxymaltose) package insert[10]	≤100 alone *or* <300 *and*	<30

any lab work is done. This patient is tachycardic, borderline hypotensive, and reports positional symptoms that indicate inadequate cerebral oxygenation. As a general rule, clinical judgment should be the predominant factor when deciding to transfuse. The presence or absence of cardiopulmonary disease, the volume and speed of blood loss, and ability to stop the bleeding vessel should all be considered. Although some authors have suggested a specific number as a transfusion threshold, our belief is that each individual patient should be assessed independently with no specific lab value as the transfusion trigger.

Other components of whole blood have different indications outside of tissue oxygenation. Platelets are generally given, in the setting of thrombocytopenia or platelet dysfunction, to control acute, ongoing coagulopathy or to prevent suspected future bleeding.[14] Plasma is primarily used to reverse a coagulopathy. Plasma contains all coagulation proteins and can emergently reverse the effects of warfarin or replace a specific factor concentrate if it is unavailable.[14] Massive transfusion protocols typically include plasma in their algorithm as part of a balanced blood component replacement measure. In bleeding patients with either a lack of factor VIII, von Willebrand factor, or fibrinogen, cryoprecipitate can be given.[15] Cryoprecipitate has the additional advantage of minimizing volume replacement as most units contain less than 50 mL of fluid.[15]

Due to patient autonomy and the Jehovah's Witness religious doctrine that prevents the acceptance of allogenic blood, this patient is not a candidate for a blood transfusion. Thus, maximizing tissue oxygenation here will involve only non-blood alternatives. If possible, the clinician must have a clear and detailed discussion with the patient concerning his preferences and document this in the medical record appropriately. Each Jehovah's Witness might have varying opinions about what is acceptable or not acceptable or how the blood products must be handled. This places the responsibility on the clinician to gather this information before proceeding to the operating room.

What are some of the risks of proceeding to the operating room with this patient?

If this patient's symptomatology and anemia are not addressed, he is at high risk for hemodynamic instability upon induction and maintenance of general anesthesia. This is because almost all medications given for induction and maintenance of anesthesia cause peripheral vasodilation and hypotension. Venous blood will pool in the extremities, reflexive vasoconstriction will be blunted, and profound hypotension, possibly unresponsive to treatment, could ensue. If the hypotension is severe and prolonged enough, the ultimate fear is that there will be a decrease in oxygen delivery to the myocardium leading to ischemia and possibly fatal arrhythmias.

Even if the myocardium is able to sustain contractility in this scenario, the clinician should also be concerned about decreased perfusion to the other major organs. Anemia, hypotension, and decreased organ perfusion can also lead to acute kidney injury, hepatic failure, pulmonary insufficiency with prolonged intubation, acidosis and electrolyte abnormalities, and cerebral ischemia and infarction. These concerns warrant the need for multiple large IV lines and an arterial line for beat-to-beat blood pressure monitoring and efficient laboratory test draws as well as postoperative intensive care monitoring.

Given the direct transfer to the operating room, the clinician has limited time to adequately prepare this patient for surgery. One of the first steps would be to return the patient to a euvolemic status as quickly as possible. Crystalloids should be given as quickly as possible. A pressure bag can help expedite this fluid delivery. If proper IV access is in place, large volumes of crystalloid can be given in a short period of time. An alternative to crystalloids is the fractionated blood component albumin.[16] In this patient, however, the acceptance of albumin should be discussed as it is likely considered a "minor fraction," and each individual Jehovah's Witness will likely have specific opinions about its use.[17]

Simultaneous, multidisciplinary perioperative blood management strategies will be the most effective means of minimizing the risk associated with bringing this patient to the operating room. While euvolemia is being established, minimizing further blood loss during the surgery is essential. Techniques such as cell salvage (washing and reinfusing any blood lost during the procedure), arterial tourniquets (not possible in this example), or permissive hypotension could be used.[18] In addition, optimizing the patient's tolerance to anemia with supplemental oxygen via an endotracheal tube, paralysis, cooling, or hyperbaric therapy could also be considered.[18]

What is the preoperative cardiac risk assessment for this patient having noncardiac surgery?

The three most common preoperative risk assessment tools are the 2014 American College of Cardiology and American Heart Association (ACC/AHA) Guideline on Perioperative Cardiovascular Evaluation and Management of Patients Undergoing Noncardiac Surgery; the American College of Surgeons National Surgical Quality Improvement Program Surgical Risk Calculator; and the National Surgical Quality Improvement Program Myocardial Infarction or Cardiac Arrest.[19] Each of these calculators attempts to predict a patient's risk for a major adverse event during the perioperative period. While the ACC/AHA guidelines focus on the complication risk during admission, the other two calculators expand this time frame to include the 30 days after surgery as well. Each uses a set of known or suspected diagnoses as factors that increase or decrease a patient's risk. The idea behind these calculators is that the clinician will attempt to modify these factors in the preoperative, intraoperative, or postoperative period to decrease the overall risk.

Although different criteria exist for each calculator, the overall theme centers around preexisting major organ insufficiency (cardiovascular, renal, pulmonary, endocrine, etc.) and the complication risk of the proposed procedure. As with many criteria in medicine, this tool categorizes the risk as low, intermediate/average, or high. For those procedures deemed to be intermediate/average or high, hopefully an intervention can or will be done to recategorize the patient to a lower risk. Since each calculator uses different criteria, this patient has slightly different risk assessments for this surgery depending on the calculator used. Most clinicians would consider him to have above average risk for any complication given the emergent nature of the procedure, the necessity to violate the peritoneum during the surgery, and his preexisting anemia. This anemia is causing hemodynamic distress as he has developed tachycardic to keep up with the metabolic demand.

What can be done emergently to better optimize the patient from a hemodynamic perspective?

As mentioned, the initial management of this patient should focus on volume replacement as quickly as possible. This bleeding tumor has caused hypovolemia which should be quickly replaced with crystalloid or colloid, ideally started in transport to the hospital or by the emergency department upon admission. Without a history of heart failure or renal failure, it is unlikely that large boluses of fluids will cause congestive heart failure or pulmonary edema so the clinician should infuse fluids liberally during the initial assessment. Multiple large-bore IV access should be established quickly and used to replace multiple liters as soon as possible. If peripheral access is not available or not sufficient, a central line can be placed to aid in this resuscitation.

While fluid replacement occurs, pharmacologic support with a vasoactive medication like ephedrine or phenylephrine can be given to temporarily maintain hemodynamic stability. Bolus injections or a continuous drip are options until the source of the bleed and hemodynamic lability are identified and treated. Although not directly used for treatment, arterial line insertion is commonly performed as well to allow for second-by-second blood pressure monitoring as well as to allow easy laboratory draws. Access to immediate and accurate information about this patient's changing blood pressures will be vital to monitor his response to treatment until the surgeon can definitively stop the bleeding. It will also allow for accurate assessment of blood pressure if permissive hypotension is deemed necessary. The clinician must be conscious, however, to use pediatric tubes for lab draws and minimize blood draws. Iatrogenic phlebotomy is the most common cause of anemia in hospitalized patients and overuse could be life-threatening in this patient.

If the patient did not present emergently, what other options would be available to him?

If this were not an emergent surgery and active bleeding was not a concern, the healthcare team would have other options available to optimize this patient before his surgery. Ideally, a time frame of more than 21 days would allow for maximum benefit for most preoperative treatments. Some hospitals have instituted preoperative anemia clinics, run by anesthesiologists or licensed independent practitioners, that use a combination of IV iron treatments and subcutaneous erythropoietin as a way to enhance the body's physiologic response to anemia.

Anemia has multiple etiologies, so establishing this diagnosis is the first step of any preoperative anemia clinic. Iron studies (ferritin, transferrin level, transferrin saturation, iron level, and total iron binding capacity) should be part of the regular preoperative labs (which includes a CBC) for any patient with a known or suspected history of anemia or who is scheduled for a procedure with a moderate risk of significant blood loss (>500 mL). Preferred IV agents, such as ferric carboxymaltose, ferric derisomaltose, or iron dextran, can replete total iron stores with one or two separate infusions, each lasting approximately 15–30 minutes. Due to low molecular weight, many of the newer preparations have significantly less side effects and shorter infusion times when compared to older formulations like iron gluconate or high-molecular-weight iron dextran. Ideally, the patient is not scheduled for surgery for at least 1 week after the infusion to allow for maximum hemoglobin increase. In addition to increasing RBC mass, iron repletion in itself has a wide range of benefits. These situations differ considerably from nonsurgical patients because of the time-sensitive nature of the preoperative period. IV iron repletion has in many instances replaced oral iron since enteral iron repletion can take months to work effectively and has many poorly tolerated side effects.

For urgent procedures in an iron deficient, anemic patient, a combination of SQ erythropoietin and IV iron can be used. Erythropoietin is a natural hormone made by the renal system that increases RBC production. These situations, however, require appropriate deep vein thrombosis prophylaxis in the preoperative period due to the increased risk of clotting with erythropoietin treatment.

Some patients may have a functional iron deficiency. Anemia of chronic inflammation will increase the patient's ferritin, may not respond to IV iron alone, and may require erythropoietin supplementation and treatment of the underlying chronic disease.

In addition to pharmacologic treatments, elective surgery in a Jehovah's Witness patient will give the clinicians adequate time to establish what blood products the patient will or will not accept. This autonomy is paramount when treating a Jehovah's Witness. The patient should not be rushed or persuaded to choose any one option. If he or she feels more comfortable discussing the subject with their family or Church leaders, then the blood product options should be printed out in simple language to be discussed and decided on at a future date. A patient blood management (PBM) coordinator or liaison has been very beneficial in discussing these matters of conscience with the patient.

What is the physiology of anemia as well as the perceived efficacy and limitations of PRBC transfusion?

Anemia is defined as a reduction in the number of circulating RBCs. We rely on indices such as hemoglobin (Hgb), hematocrit (Hct), and RBC count since the measurement of blood volume in relation to RBC mass is not generally available. Limitations of these indices are that they are all concentrations, dependent on RBC mass and plasma volume. If the RBC mass and plasma volume are decreased, as in acute hemorrhage, normal values for Hgb and Hct may be present initially. For instance, a pregnant patient in her third trimester has an expanded plasma volume so may have a low Hgb or Hct. This is despite having an increased RBC mass. The signs and symptoms associated with anemia are varied, complex, and dependent on a multitude of factors. These factors include the chronicity of the anemia, the volume status of the patient, and the oxygen demands of the patient. All of these factors must be considered prior to transfusing an anemic patient, and it is often difficult to separate the symptoms associated with volume depletion from those of acute anemia.

The ultimate goal in the management of anemia is the avoidance of ischemia and a disruption of the balance between global oxygen (O_2) delivery (DO_2) and global oxygen consumption (VO_2). The ratio of (VO_2/DO_2) is the O_2 extraction ratio; in healthy individuals, the global DO_2 exceeds global VO_2 by a factor of two- to four-fold, allowing for a significant safety margin.[20] In the setting of an inadequate O_2 supply to meet the cellular O_2 requirements, tissue ischemia will ensue.

Moderate anemia in the absence of hypovolemia is usually well tolerated with an absence of associated symptoms because of this wide safety margin between DO_2 and VO_2. In varying degrees of anemia, despite a marked decrease in O_2 delivery, VO_2 is maintained (Figure 34.1).[20] This occurs with acute normovolemic anemia in a healthy patient. Beyond a critical value, the so-called critical DO_2 ($DO_{2\ CRIT}$), VO_2 decreases, tissue hypoxia develops, and VO_2 is dependent on DO_2.[20]

Physiologic compensatory mechanisms to maintain DO_2 in the setting of normovolemic anemia or hypoperfusion include an increase in oxygen extraction from a baseline of 25% to a maximum of 60%.[21] This compensatory mechanism alone can maintain adequate DO_2 to a Hgb concentration of 8–9 g/dL in a resting healthy individual.[2] Anemia below this level will elicit a compensatory physiologic response. This manifests as an increased cardiac output (stroke volume multiplied by heart rate), increased sympathetic response, increased oxygen unloading to cells due to increased RBC concentrations of 2,3-diphosphoglycerate (DPG), and increases in plasma volume from the redistribution of blood flow.[22] Overall, these compensatory mechanisms can maintain oxygen delivery in a resting healthy individual to Hgb concentrations as low as 5 g/dL.[23] As basal cardiac output increases, symptoms of anemia are manifested clinically by fatigue, dyspnea, and tachycardia. Individual variability in the manifestation of anemia will depend on the level of exertion and the presence of underlying cardiac disease. More severe anemia (supply-dependent O_2 consumption) may lead to altered consciousness and potentially life-threatening complications such as myocardial infarction, arrhythmia, and shock. All of these signs and symptoms of anemia are aggravated in the setting of hypovolemia.

Historically, the treatment for these anemia-associated symptoms was to transfuse the patient when these signs and symptoms arose. However, the realization of the risks associated with transfusion—namely, infectious risks, immunomodulatory risks, and risks of volume overload—have tempered this historical doctrine of maintaining a Hgb of at least 10 g/dL.

Global DO_2 is determined by cardiac output (CO) and arterial oxygen content (CaO_2):

$$DO_2 = CO \times CaO_2$$

DO_2 is in mL/min, CO in L/min, and CaO_2 in mL/dL.

CaO_2 is the sum of the hemoglobin-bound form of oxygen and physically dissolved oxygen in plasma:

$$CaO_2 = (SaO_2 \times 1.34 \times [Hb]) + (0.03 \times PaO_2)$$

The hemoglobin-bound oxygen is the product of the arterial oxygen saturation (SaO_2, in %), the oxygen-carrying capacity of hemoglobin (1.34, in mL/g), and the hemoglobin concentration ([Hgb], in g/dL), and dissolved oxygen is the product of the plasma oxygen dissolution coefficient at body temperature (0.003, in mL/(dl mm Hg)) and the partial pressure of oxygen in arterial blood (PaO_2, in mm Hg).[20]

The recognition of the risks of allogeneic transfusion, as well an understanding of the physiologic compensatory mechanisms of anemia, has led to the realization that other options are available for the management of anemia. Transfusion is just one option and should be reserved for unstable patients with an active bleed. Stable patients, even with moderate or severe anemia, should be managed with a focus on their tolerance to this anemia. Expansion of intravascular volume to allow

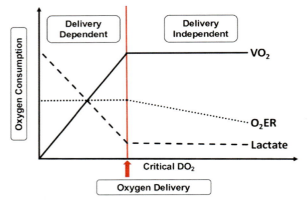

Figure 34.1 VO_2–DO_2 relationship. At a critical threshold of DO_2 ($DO_{2\ CRIT}$), VO_2 begins to fall rapidly. The body responds by extracting more oxygen in cases of decreased DO_2. Once DO_2 drops below the critical threshold cellular metabolism becomes anaerobic with the subsequent production of lactate.
Modified from Madjdpour C. *Best Pract Res Clin Anaesthesiol*. 2007;21:163–171.

the compensatory cardiovascular response to preserve oxygen transport should be the first action taken by the clinician.[24]

In recent years, the efficacy of transfusion has been questioned. While it is clear that the efficacy of transfusion is greatest in those who are hemodynamically unstable with active bleeding, it is often difficult to assess the efficacy of transfusion in the stable patient.[25] It has been more than 18 years since the Transfusion Requirements in Critical Care (TRICC) trial, which was the first major randomized clinical trial to show that a restrictive transfusion strategy (Hgb 7–9 g/dL) is as effective and possibly a superior strategy to a liberal transfusion strategy (Hgb 10–12 g/dL).[26] These findings have been corroborated by other large randomized controlled trials and epidemiological studies, and it is clear that patients who receive any blood transfusions, as well as an increasing number of transfusions, have a higher incidence of morbidity and mortality.[27–29]

Several studies have looked at the relationship between transfusion, DO_2, and VO_2 in critically ill patients. While the Hgb value universally increases indicating an increase in DO_2, the positive effects on VO_2 have been inconsistent. The primary goal of allogeneic transfusion is not necessarily to increase the Hgb, a value that often dictates practice, but to increase oxygen delivery and hence tissue oxygenation. In a review of allogeneic transfusions and oxygen kinetics, the authors identified only 5 out of 14 studies where an increase in Hgb and DO_2 was associated with an increase in VO_2.[30] Explanations proposed to explain this inconsistency include the absence of tissue hypoxia and the lack of DO_2/VO_2 dependency in some patients, the effect of the "storage lesion" of blood, changes of allogeneic blood and impaired microcirculatory O_2 unloading, and decreased levels of 2,3 DPG with a leftward shift of the oxyhemoglobin curve.

While allogeneic blood transfusion is clearly life-saving in certain clinical scenarios, its clinical efficacy is inconsistent in many clinical studies. Clinicians must attempt to identify which patients will benefit from a transfusion and in which patients the risk outweighs the benefit. Observations from Jehovah's Witness patients who decline blood transfusions for religious reasons have shown that morbidity and mortality do not occur until the Hgb drops to very low levels and that evidence of tissue ischemia may not arise until Hgb levels drop below 7 gm/dL.[31] In one case report of a Jehovah's Witness patient in whom VO_2 and DO_2 were measured, a DO_2 critical level was achieved at a Hgb of 4 g/dL.[32] Only once this Hgb level was achieved did DO_2 become insufficient enough for VO_2 to decrease.[32] What is clear from an understanding of the physiology of anemia is that the treatment of anemia and determination of the elusive Hgb trigger is not a one-size-fits-all scenario. Many patients will tolerate a Hgb of 7 g/dL and some patients (e.g., significant cardiovascular disease) may require a higher Hgb. Additionally, one must consider that the Hgb value is a laboratory value prone to measurement errors and is dependent on the patient's volume status.[33]

The main factors to consider in the decision to transfuse the anemic patient are whether the anemia is acute or chronic. In the acute anemic surgical patient, the primary factors to consider include the baseline Hgb, the extent of blood loss, volume status, and the presence of comorbidities that may impair the ability to tolerate anemia. The consideration of all these factors makes a discrete Hgb value elusive despite the existence of clinical practice guidelines from various medical societies.[34] Published guidelines (Table 34.2) generally agree that most patients with a Hgb of 6–7 g/dL may benefit from a transfusion, while patients with a Hgb greater than 10 m/dL likely will not benefit from a transfusion. Thus, in the absence of acute myocardial infarction or cerebrovascular ischemia, postoperative transfusion may be inappropriate for patients with a hemoglobin level of greater than 7 g/dL Other clinical practice guidelines have refuted a transfusion "trigger" alone since the literature is insufficient to define a discrete transfusion trigger and an appropriate transfusion should be based on the individual assessment of the patient's clinical status.[35]

Specifically, what are the Jehovah's Witness's beliefs regarding blood transfusions?

Jehovah's Witness are a Christian group with greater than 8 million members worldwide and greater than 1.2 million members in the United States.[36] A major tenet requires abstinence from blood transfusion based on the literal interpretation of multiple Biblical passages.

> Genesis 9:4: But flesh with the life thereof, *which is* the blood thereof, shall ye not eat.
>
> Leviticus 17:10: And whatsoever man *there be* ... that eateth any manner of blood; I will even set my face against that soul that eateth blood, and will cut him off from among his people.
>
> Deuteronomy 12:23: Simply be firmly resolved not to eat the blood, because the blood is the soul and you must not eat the soul with the flesh.[37]

Nonadherence to these beliefs may risk ostracism and possibly excommunication from church membership. While this major tenet of blood abstinence is a religious belief, not a medical decision, it is erroneous to assume that all Jehovah's Witness members adhere to this tenet.[38] Based on their religious beliefs, members of the Jehovah's Witness faith do not accept blood products categorized as "primary components," which includes RBCs, white blood cells, plasma, or platelets as well as autologous blood products donated preoperatively. However, autologous blood products, such as cell salvage and acute normovolemic hemodilution (ANH), that are removed and remain in a continuous circuit connected to the donor may be acceptable. Additionally, minor blood fractions, which may include cryoprecipitate, albumin, factor concentrates, and hemostatic agents, may be acceptable and are considered matters of conscience, dependent on the patient's own personal values. Because of differences in personal values that may conflict with the strict adherence to blood abstinence, it is important to ask all Jehovah's Witness patients their personal informed preferences in private, to remove the possibility of coercion from family members or church members. Individual

Table 34.2 TRANSFUSION GUIDELINES BY MEDICAL SOCIETIES

TRANSFUSION GUIDELINES BY MEDICAL SOCIETIES	RBC USUALLY INDICATED	RBC RARELY INDICATED	EQUIVOCAL	FACTORS TO CONSIDER	TARGET POPULATION
CAP (1998)	Hb<6g/dl	Hb > 10g/dl	Hb 6–10g/dl	Peripheral tissue oxygenation, clinical signs & symptoms, Hb, extent/rate of bleeding	General
ASA (2006)	Hb<6gldl	Hb > 10g/dl	Hb 6–10g/dl	Ischemia, extent/rate of bleeding. volume status, factors for hypoxia complications	Perioperative
STS (2007)	Hb<6g/dl (Hb<7g/dl in postoperative patients and higher if risk of end-organ ischemia)	Hb > 10g/dl		Age, severity of illness. cardiac function, ischemia. extent/rate of blood loss, Hb, SvO_2	Cardiac surgery
SCCM (2009)	Hb<7g/dl if ventilated, trauma or stable cardiac disease Hb<8g/dl in acute coronary syndrome)	Hb > 10g/dl		Volume status. shock, duration, extent of anemia, cardiopulmonary parameters	Critically ill
AABB (2012)	Hb≤7gldl in critically ill patients, Hb≤8 g/dl in surgical patients or patients with pre-existing cardiovascular disease when symptoms are present		Patients with acute coronary syndrome	Hb levels as well as symptoms (chest pain, orthostatic hypotension, unresponsive tachycardia, heart failure)	Hospitalized.
BCSH (2013)	Hb≤7g/dl, target range 7–9gldl	Hb > 9g/dl		Specific co-morbidities or acute illnesses may modify clinical decision-making (sepsis, traumatic brain injury, ischemic heart disease)	hemodynamically stable
NICE (201S)	Hb<7g/dl			Major hemorrhage, acute coronary syndrome, need for regular blood transfusions for chronic anemia	Critically ill

Note: CAP: College of American Pathologists; ASA: American Society of Anesthesiologists; STS: Society of Thoracic Surgeons; SCCM: Society of Critical Care Medicine; AABB: American Association of Blood Banks; BCSH: British Committee for Standards in Haematology; NICE: National Institute for Health and Care Excellence.

Adapted from Shander A. *Blood Transf.* 2013;11:193–202.

Jehovah's Witness patients may approach this ban on transfusion differently, and there may be significant variability on which blood products or derivatives they may accept or decline. Because of this variability, an advance directive clearly itemizing which blood products, derivatives, or autotransfusion techniques may be acceptable are paramount to the proper and respectful care of the Jehovah's Witness patient (Table 34.3). Generally, most Jehovah's Witness patients abide by these principles[39,40]:

1. They will generally not accept whole blood or any of its four major components: RBCs, platelets, white blood cells, and plasma.

2. Some accept blood fractions (e.g., albumin, coagulation factors, prothrombin complex concentrates (PCCs), factor VIIa, cryoprecipitate, thrombin) as determined by individual discretion.

3. Autologous blood transfusion is generally unacceptable unless the blood is in a continuous closed loop that circulates back into the patient so that blood remains in continuity with the body (e.g., hemodialysis, cardiopulmonary bypass, ANH).

How should the informed consent process for a Jehovah's Witness be performed?

Adult patients with decision-making capacity may refuse certain aspects of medical care as long as they are informed of the relative risks of their decision. This refusal includes life-saving interventions. This respect for patient autonomy is a cornerstone of the ethical and legal values of Western medicine, placing the emphasis of the preservation of quality of life, rather than the preservation of "life." Respecting the autonomous wishes of the Jehovah's Witness patient, thereby honoring their spiritual beliefs, prioritizes their belief in a good spiritual

Table 34.3 SUMMARY OF JEHOVAH'S WITNESSES PRODUCTS ACCEPTABILITY

PERMITTED	*POTENTIALLY* PERMITTED (REQUIRES CONFIRMATION)	PROHIBITED (REQUIRES CONFIRMATION)
Crystalloids	[a]Albumin	Whole blood
IV/PO iron, vitamin C, vitamin B_{12}, folic acid	Immunoglobulins	Packed red blood cells
tranexamic acid, aminocaproic acid	[b]Factor concentrates	Fresh frozen plasma
Desmopressin acetate (DDAVP)	Cell Saver	Platelets
	[a]Erythropoeitin (EPO), [a]Darbepoeitin	Preoperative autologous blood donation
	Cryoprecipitate	
	Hemoglobin-based oxygen carriers (HBOCs)	

[a]In patients who do not accept albumin, albumin-containing products must also be avoided including erythropoietin under brand names Procrit and Epogen; albumin-free products include erythropoietin alfa-epbx (Retacrit) and darbepoeitin (Aranesp).

[b]Factor concentrates include four-factor prothrombin complex concentrate (Kcentra), activated prothrombin complex concentrate (FEIBA), and recombinant factor VIIa (Novoseven).

existence even after death. This is an example of beneficence, a core value in medical ethics.

The Jehovah's Witness patient may have an advance directive expressly indicating which blood therapies are refused and which component therapies and blood conservation strategies are acceptable. These documents are helpful in developing care plans to respect and honor the patient's values. In addition to an advance directive, a healthcare facility should have its own distinct consent form to guide the care of the bloodless patient. In either instance, for patients who have decision-making capacity there should an attempt to validate that the patient is informed of the risks of his decision and that his decision was made objectively without coercion. Utilizing the support of the Hospital Liaison Committee, comprised of local Jehovah's Witness ministers, can also help create an acceptable care plan for the Jehovah's Witness patient.

Ideally, a standardized bloodless transfusion consent form or worksheet would clearly document the patient's wishes regarding blood component refusal and acceptable transfusion alternatives and blood conservation modalities. As discussed earlier, while most Jehovah's Witness patients will not accept the major blood fractions (RBC, platelets, and plasma), the acceptance of minor fractions is a conscientious decision based on their personal beliefs. These "minor fractions," or fractionated blood components, include cryoprecipitate, PCCs, concentrated clotting factors, and albumin, among others. Some of these potentially objectionable fractions (albumin, thrombin) may be present in topical hemostatic agents or as part of a recombinant product (albumin in erythropoietin). Additionally, other medical therapies and blood conservation strategies such as hemodilution, hemodialysis, cardiopulmonary bypass, apheresis, and cell salvage should be clearly discussed and documented. Some of the modalities may require the creation of a closed continuous circuit, so that the blood is never completely separated from the patient.

A review of 705 Jehovah's Witness (Table 34.4) patients at a major PBM hospital revealed that the vast majority of Jehovah's Witness patients accepted minor fractions and

Table 34.4 TREATMENT MODALITIES (PRODUCT/PROCEDURE) ACCEPTANCE IN 705 JEHOVAH'S WITNESS PATIENTS

PRODUCT/TREATMENT/PROCEDURE	ACCEPT	REFUSE
Albumin (blood fraction)	93.9%	6.1%
Erythropoietin (contains albumin)	94.9%	5.1%
Immune Globulins (blood fraction)	93.7%	6.3%
Clotting factors (plasma-derived fractions)	91.2%	8.8%
Fractional agents derived from platelets, plasma or Hgb	92.6%	7.4%
Topical tissue adhesives, hemostatics (blood fractions)	93.3%	6.7%
Cryoprecipitates (blood fraction)	86.3%	12.4%
Intraoperative acute normovolemic hemodilution* (ANH)	96.9%	3.1%
Intraoperative cell salvage* (CS)	97.1%	2.8%
Postop cell salvage* (CS)	96.5%	3.5%
Cardiopulmonary bypass (CPB)	97.1%	2.5%

* Extracorporeal circulation is a closed continuous system without blood storage From Shander A. Personal Communication. In; Emeritus Chief Department of Anesthesiology, Critical Care and Hyperbaric Medicine. Englewood Hospital and Medical Center, Englewood, NJ. Adjunct Clinical Professor of Anesthesiology, Medicine and Surgery, Icahn School of Medicine at Mount Sinai, NY. Clinical Professor of Anesthesiology Rutgers Medical School, NJ.

continuous closed-loop blood conservation strategies and therapies (personal communication Aryeh Shander, Emeritus Chief Department of Anesthesiology, Critical Care and Hyperbaric Medicine. Englewood Hospital and Medical Center, Englewood, NJ).

Without an informed discussion and documentation of the patient's wishes, valuable therapy may be withheld, or

Table 34.5 MODEL OF CONSENT FOR JEHOVAH'S WITNESS PATIENTS

Bloodless Medicine and Surgery Program: Treatment Option Checklist
I _____ decline blood transfusions. I decline whole blood, red blood cells, white blood cells, platelets or plasma under any circumstances. I decline transfusion of blood or any of its major components even if a doctor believes I need a transfusion to preserve my health or my life. I fully understand and accept the risks involved in declining blood transfusions. I have been given information about alternatives to transfusion. These alternatives include non-blood volume expanders and other non-blood management alternatives listed below. All of my questions have been answered.
With regard to the following treatment options, I have put my initials next to those that are acceptable to me: Bloodless Medicine and Surgery Program Treatment Option Checklist

PRODUCT OR TREATMENT INVOLVING MINOR FRACTIONS OF BLOOD	ACCEPT	DECLINE
Albumin (protein extracted from plasma): Used as a blood volume expander. Also used in medications. Examples: Erythropoietin (Epo), Procrit and Neupogen		
Immune Globulins (proteins extracted from plasma): Used in medications to provide immunity, improve immune response to infections. Examples: Intravenous Immunoglobulins (IVIG), and for Rh incompatibility (Rhogam)		
Clotting factors (various proteins extracted from plasma): Used to stop active bleeding. Example: Prothrombin Complex Concentrate (PCC), Factor VII		
Cryoprecipitate (various proteins extracted from plasma): Used to stop active bleeding.		
Topical hemostatic agents (Various proteins extracted from plasma or animal derived sources): Used to stop bleeding. Examples: Tisseel, Gelform, BioGlue, Fibrin Glue and Autologous Platelet Gel		
Cryo Reduced Plasma		
Interferons (protein extracted from white cell): Used for cancer treatments and viral infections. Examples: Roferon-A and Intron A		
Procedure or Treatment Involving the Use of My own Blood	Accept	Decline
Cell Salvage ("cell-saver"): Patient's blood is retrieved, filtered and returned in a closed loop process during or after surgery.		
Hemodilution: (ANH) Specific amounts of the patient's blood are removed when surgery begins, diverted to bags and replaced with non-blood volume expander. Blood is then returned in a continuous system during or at the end of surgery.		
Hemodialysis: Patient's blood is filtered through a machine to clean it. This is done when there is insufficient kidney function.		
Heart-Lung machine: Patient's blood is directed to a cardiopulmonary bypass pump that oxygenates and returns the blood to patient during cardiovascular surgery.		
Tagging or Labeling: Patient's blood is combined with radioactive material to mark (tag) the red cell then mixed for several minutes and returned via vein. Often used to locate site of internal bleeding.		
Epidural Blood Patch: Patient's blood is removed from vein and injected into spinal membrane to seal a spinal fluid leak.		
Other Procedures	Accept	Decline
Non-organ tissue transplantation		
Bone transplantation		

therapy may be administered without the patient's consent. A PBM worksheet facilitates and standardizes care across the whole continuum of patient care while honoring the Jehovah's Witness patient's beliefs.[41] A sample template worksheet and consent are shown in Table 34.5.

Advance directives, living wills, or transfusion refusal forms are ethically and legally recognized as the patient's own voice.

The respect for patient autonomy extends for future healthcare decisions that may arise if a patient becomes incompetent, and these advance directives should be honored under those circumstances. If a patient lacks competency but has verbally expressed their wishes before losing decision-making capacity, their wishes should be honored unless there is serious doubt of the patient's capacity at the time of his expressed wishes. A medical ethics consultation may help to clarify the situation. If the patient without decision-making capacity never clearly expressed his wishes, then a hierarchy for surrogate decision-making should be followed, which may vary from state to state. The legal and ethical role of the surrogate is to speak the values of the patient when they were known, even if these values conflict with the surrogate's values. If the patient never expressed their wishes and currently lacks decision-making capacity, then decisions should be based on the patient's best interests, taking into account standard medical practice and the patient's current medical condition. This scenario may arise in emergency situations, when a patient may not be able to express their wishes and an advance directive may not be available.[42]

Explain the concept of patient autonomy in regard to the refusal of medical therapies.

A paternalistic medical ethical framework existed before the 20th century, whereby the physician, not the patient, determined what was in the patient's best interest. These decisions were usually based on the preservation of life. During the 20th century, however, a cultural as well as legal shift led to patient autonomy playing a predominant role in determining a physician's actions. This shift in decision-making from physician to patient, with a reliance on the preservation of "quality" of life, led to the process of informed consent becoming a cornerstone of patient autonomy and Western medical ethics.

Informed consent can be examined in the context of the four basic medical ethical principles of Beauchamp and Childress:

1. *Respect for autonomy*: Respecting a patient's decision-making capacity
2. *Nonmaleficence*: Avoiding harm
3. *Beneficence*: "Doing good," balancing benefits against risk
4. *Justice*: Distributing benefits, risks, and costs fairly[43,44]

Respect for patient autonomy acknowledges that competent patients may make decisions regarding their own healthcare issues even when they are against recommended medical treatment. Informed consent and the corollary, informed refusal, allows competent adults to choose among treatments based on their values, goals, beliefs, and priorities for the future. When a patient refuses life-sustaining therapy it is the duty of the physician to discern whether the patient has decision-making capacity. The patient must be able to understand the nature of the procedure; the risks, benefits, and alternatives; and the probable outcomes of both acceptance and refusal of the recommended therapy.

In the case of the Jehovah's Witness patient, the consequences of refusing a life-saving blood transfusion must be made clear to the patient so that they are "informed." A physician, desiring to benefit the patient, may want to provide a blood transfusion based on the principle of "beneficence," believing that it is of clear medical benefit. However, when properly and compassionately informed, the patient is free to choose whether to accept the transfusion based on a desire to live or to refuse the transfusion based on his religious convictions regarding the acceptance of blood transfusions, even if his choice would result in death as a predictable outcome. The principle of "nonmaleficence" applies here since the avoidance of spiritual harm is valued by respecting the patient's decision.

What are the legal considerations in the competent adult patient in terms of withholding life-saving treatment?

While legal decisions are not always synonymous with ethical principles, a review of legal precedents provides insight into the shift in medical ethics from a paternalistic viewpoint to an emphasis on patient autonomy. As early as 1914, in *Schloendorff v. Society of New York Hospital*, the courts determined that "Every human being of adult years and sound mind has a right to determine what shall be done with his own body" and that an operation without consent constitutes medical battery.[45] However, in the early 1960s, forced transfusion of a Jehovah's Witness patient was allowed based on the ruling that their faith did not forbid a forced transfusion, only a consensual one.[46] Over the past 40 years the courts have upheld the rights of adult Jehovah's Witness patients to refuse life-saving transfusions and have rejected earlier legal precedents. These rights are based on the constitutional guarantees of the right to privacy and noninterference based of the 14th Amendment. Additionally, the landmark cases of Karen Ann Quinlan and Nancy Cruzan, where the courts upheld the rights of surrogate decision-makers to discontinue life-sustaining medical therapy, further supported the durability of patient's constitutional rights. In 1990, the Congress passed the Patient Self-Determination Act of 1990, requiring healthcare clinicians to inform patients of their rights regarding decisions concerning their own medical care, specifically ensuring the patient's right to accept or refuse medical care in addition to dictating their future care by means of an advance directive or living will should they become incapacitated.[47]

The patient's wife says she wants her husband to have a blood transfusion, if necessary. How should the healthcare team handle this situation?

Physicians demonstrate respect for a competent patient's autonomy by accepting their informed decisions, even when their decision may be in direct conflict with what is medically indicated. Without respect for informed refusal, the concept of informed consent would be invalidated. An essential role of the responsible physician is to determine the patient's capacity to refuse or consent for treatment, since a consent is not valid unless the patient is capable of making medical decisions. Determining capacity is a clinical judgment based on the patient's cognitive and physical functioning and the complexity, risks, and possible repercussions of the medical treatment at hand.[48]

As Derse states: "Medical decision-making capacity is present when the patient is able to understand information about the medical condition and its consequences, to reason and deliberate about the various choices, to make a choice consistent with his or her values and goals, to communicate this choice to the physician, and to maintain this choice consistently over time."[49]

In this particular case, the patient is an adult with decision-making capacity, and, as long as his decision is well informed, it must be honored and accepted regardless of the wife's objections.

This informed discussion should ultimately occur in an environment free from potential coercive influences since decisions expressed in front of family members or friends may be different from decisions expressed in private. The intent of a private discussion should not be to convince a Jehovah's Witness patient to accept blood, which in itself may be coercive, but instead used as an opportunity to ensure that the patient's wishes are expressed and honored. In legal cases, life-saving treatment against a competent patient's wishes has resulted in suits for battery, medical negligence, and lack of informed consent.

An emergency situation may create limitations in determining decision-making capacity, but an emergency situation does not invalidate a competent adult's decision. However, pathophysiological conditions may alter decision-making capacity, and, in an emergency situation, when a patient's wishes are not evident and there is no surrogate decision-maker, immediate intervention may proceed without informed consent to prevent death or serious morbidity. The "emergency exception" is based on the presumption that the preservation of life would be the choice made by a reasonable person.[50]

Is the clinician obligated to take care of this patient?

Physicians may express that to withhold life-saving treatment may violate their own moral principles and that withholding a life-saving blood transfusion or not administering CPR would be in conflict with their own personal beliefs. However, physicians are granted significant societal privilege through their social contract with their patient, which places the moral interests of a competent adult above their own moral interests. Physicians are aware of their moral obligations to patients and are often able to avoid specific patient circumstances that may violate their own personal beliefs. However, the very integrity of medical ethics would be violated if physicians routinely superseded their patient's moral rights. A patient's right to informed, autonomous decision-making is a cornerstone tenet of medical ethics, and physicians are facilitators of this social contract. Often, these conflicts can be avoided with proper planning within the anesthesia department, and alternative options can be offered to the clinician that would still ensure appropriate patient care. Under these circumstances the physician can ethically remove himself from patient care, allowing another physician without any moral objections to provide care. Unfortunately, emergency situations may arise where "opting out" is not an option, and the physician is obligated to provide ethically directed care in accordance with the patient's values and not impose his own personal beliefs on the patient.[51]

CONCLUSION

- A rapidly bleeding patient who presents emergently to the operating room creates a unique challenge for the healthcare team because the usual process of informed consent and explanation of the risks of benefits of the procedure as well as the risks and benefits of the patient's wishes is limited.

- RBC and blood product infusions are the mainstay of treatment in most patients with severe anemia showing signs of end-organ ischemia.

- Jehovah's Witness are patients who generally refuse "major" blood products because of religious doctrine. The use of "minor" blood fractions is unique to each individual and should be discussed in detail so the clinician does not run the risk of medical assault by violating a patient's wishes.

- The implementation of a PBM program, which addresses the management of all patients, including "bloodless" patients like the Jehovah's Witness community, can coordinate the fluid management strategy with the beliefs of the patient before an acute event occurs.

REVIEW QUESTIONS

1. All of the following are clinical indications for a blood transfusion, *except*

   a. Volume resuscitation in a stable hypovolemic patient.
   b. Hemodynamically unstable patient following a postpartum hemorrhage.
   c. Postoperative cardiac surgical patient with a Hgb 6 g/dL.
   d. An 80-year-old tachycardic, hypotensive patient with a GI hemorrhage and a Hgb of 7 g/dL.

   The correct answer is a.

   A stable hypovolemic patient should be resuscitated with crystalloid or colloid solutions. Transfusion should be considered in all other scenarios.

2. A Jehovah's Witness patient is scheduled for an elective mitral valve repair and is found to have a Hgb of 11.3 g/dL on preoperative testing. All of the following are incorrect, *except*

   a. Obtain iron studies and manage the anemia preoperatively.
   b. Proceed with planned surgery since patient is asymptomatic.
   c. Try to convince patient to accept a transfusion if needed.
   d. Obtain consent for transfusion from spouse while patient is undergoing surgery.

   The correct answer is a.

   This patient is anemic by definition, and cardiac surgery is generally associated with major blood loss. In a Jehovah's Witness patient, in an elective situation, preoperative optimization of anemia is paramount.

3. Jehovah's Witness will generally accept all of the following blood components or blood conservation techniques, *except*

   a. Acute normovolemic hemodilution in a closed-loop configuration.
   b. Cell salvage in a closed-loop configuration.

c. Platelets.
d. PCC.

The correct answer is c.

Jehovah's Witness patients do not accept any blood components (RBCs, platelets, FFP) but may accept fractions (albumin, PCC).

4. Advance directives, living wills, and transfusion refusal forms are

   a. Ethically and legally recognized as the patient's own voice.
   b. Valid only for 1 year.
   c. Are invalidated if the patient becomes incapacitated.
   d. Always requires a medical ethics consultation.

The correct answer is a

Advance directives, living wills, and transfusion refusal forms represent the voice of the patient even when incapacitated and are valid permanently.

5. Informed consent is based on the following principles, *except*

   a. Respect for autonomy.
   b. Beneficence.
   c. Nonmaleficence.
   d. Physician's determination of what's best for the patient.

The correct answer is d.

A physician's beliefs should not interfere with patient's autonomy.

6. The following statements regarding iron deficiency anemia (IDA) are true, *except*

   a. IDA is one of several causes of anemia.
   b. IDA is a major burden on our healthcare system.
   c. Preoperative IDA is an independent predictor of morbidity and mortality.
   d. Risks of preoperative IDA are ameliorated with transfusion of RBCs.

The correct answer is d.

The treatment for IDA is oral or IV iron, not RBC transfusion.

REFERENCES

1. Khusun H, Yip R, Schultink W, Dillon DH. World Health Organization hemoglobin cut-off points for the detection of anemia are valid for an Indonesian population. *J Nutr*. 1999;129(9):1669–1674.
2. Ellermann I, Bueckmann A, Eveslage M, et al. Treating anemia in the preanesthesia assessment clinic: Results of a retrospective evaluation. *Anesth Analg*. 2018 Jun 25. doi:10.1213/ANE.0000000000003583
3. Steinbicker AU, Muckenthaler MU. Out of balance-systemic iron homeostasis in iron-related disorders. *Nutrients*. 2013;5(8):3034–3061.
4. Adamson Jehovah's Witness. Iron deficiency and other hypoproliferative anemias. In: Jameson J, Fauci A, Kasper D, Hauser S, Longo D, Loscalzo J, eds. *Harrison's Principles of Internal Medicine*. 19th ed. McGraw-Hill; 2014. http://accessmedicine.mhmedical.com.ezproxy.med.nyu.edu/content.aspx?bookid=1130&sectionid=79731112
5. Lawson T, Ralph C. Perioperative Jehovah's Witnesses: A review. *Brit J Anaesth*. 2015;115(5):676–687.
6. Auerbach M, Adamson JW. How we diagnose and treat iron deficiency anemia. *Am J Hematol*. 2016 Jan;91(1):31–38.
7. Muñoz M, Acheson AG, Auerbach M, et al. International consensus statement on the peri-operative management of anaemia and iron deficiency. *Anaesthesia*. 2017;72:233–247.
8. Shander A, Goodnough L, Javidroozi M, et al. Iron deficiency anemia—Bridging the knowledge and practice gap. *Transfus Med Rev*. 2014;28:156–166.
9. Guinn NR, Guercio JR, Hopkins TJ, et al. How do we develop and implement a preoperative anemia clinic designed to improve perioperative outcomes and reduce cost? *Transfusion*. 2016;56:297–303.
10. Injectafer. Package insert. Vifor International. 2013. https://injectafer.com/prescribing-information-portlet/getDocument?product=IF&inline=true
11. Silver BJ. Anemia. In: Carey WD, ed. *Current Clinical Medicine*. 2nd ed. Saunders Elsevier; 2010:577–583.
12. Madjdpour C, Spahn DR. Allogeneic red blood cell transfusions: Efficacy, risks, and alternatives and indications. *Brit J Anaeth*. 2005;95(1):33–42.
13. Habler OP, Kleen MS, Hutter JW, et al. Hemodilution and intravenous perflubron emulsion as an alternative to blood transfusion: Effects on tissue oxygenation during profound hemodilution in anesthetized dogs. *Transfusion*. 1998;38:145–155.
14. Kluckman M, Stern E, Reeves L. Hematologic emergencies. In: Stone CK, Humphries RL, eds. *CURRENT Diagnosis & Treatment: Emergency Medicine*. 8th ed. McGraw-Hill; 2017. http://accessmedicine.mhmedical.com.ezproxy.med.nyu.edu/content.aspx?bookid=2172&sectionid=165067275
15. Dzieczkowski J, Anderson KC. Transfusion biology and therapy. In: Jameson J, Fauci A, Kasper D, Hauser S, Longo D, Loscalzo J, eds. *Harrison's Principles of Internal Medicine*. 19th ed. McGraw-Hill; 2014. http://accessmedicine.mhmedical.com.ezproxy.med.nyu.edu/content.aspx?bookid=1130&sectionid=79731112
16. Jorgenson TD, Golbaba B, Guinn N, Smith CE. The case for a standardized blood transfusion consent form. *ASA Monitor*. 2017;81(6):48–50. http://monitor.pubs.asahq.org/pdfaccess.ashx?url=/data/journals/asam/936264/
17. Watchtower. Blood Fractions and Surgical Procedures. In: *Keep Yourselves in God's Love*. Watchtower Bible and Tract Society of New York; 2016:215–218.
18. Lawson T, Ralph C. Perioperative Jehovah's Witnesses: A review. *Br J Anaesth*. 2015;115(5):676–687.
19. Glance LG, Faden E, Dutton RP, et al. Impact of the choice of risk model for identifying low-risk patients using the 2014 American College of Cardiology/American Heart Association perioperative guidelines. *Anesthesiology*. 2018 Jul 12. doi:10.1097/ALN.0000000000002341. [Epub ahead of print]
20. Madjdpour C, Spahn DR. Allogeneic red blood cell transfusion: Physiology of oxygen transport. *Best Pract Res Clin Anaesthesiol*. 2007:21(2):163–171.
21. Jones J. Transfusion in oligemia. In: Mollison PL, Engelfriet CP, Contreras M, eds. *Blood Transfusion in Clinical Medicine*. 8th ed. Blackwell; 1987:41–67.
22. Goodnough LT, Levy JH, Murphy MF. Concepts of blood transfusion in adults. *Lancet*. 2013 May 25;381(9880):1845–1854.
23. Weiskopf RB, Viele MK, Feiner J, et al. Human cardiovascular and metabolic response to acute, severe isovolemic anemia. *JAMA*. 1998;279(3):217.
24. Madjdpour C, Spahn DR, Weiskopf RB. Anemia and perioperative red blood cell transfusion: A matter of tolerance. *Crit Care Med*. 2006;34(5 Suppl):S102–S108.
25. Vincent JL, Sakr Y, De Backer D, Van der Linden P. Efficacy of allogeneic red blood cell transfusions. *Best Pract Res Clin Anaesthesiol*. 2007;21(2):209–219.
26. Hebert PC, Wells G, Blajchman MA, et al. A multicenter, randomized, controlled clinical trial of transfusion requirements in critical care. *N Engl J Med*. 1999; 340:409–417.

27. Bush RL, Pevec WC, Holcroft JW. A prospective, randomized trial limiting perioperative red blood cell transfusions in vascular patients. *Am J Surg.* 1997 Aug;174(2):143–148.
28. Vincent JL, Baron JF, Reinhart K, et al. ABC (Anemia and Blood Transfusion in Critical Care) Investigators: Anemia and blood transfusion in critically ill patients. *JAMA.* 2002:25;288(12):1499–1507.
29. Corwin HL, Gettinger A, Pearl RG, et al. The CRIT study: Anemia and blood transfusion in the critically ill: Current clinical practice in the United States. *Crit Care Med.* 2004:32(1):39–52.
30. Hebert PC, Van der Linden P, Biro G, Hu LQ. Physiologic aspects of anemia. *Crit Care Clin.* 2004:20(2):187–212.
31. Carson JL, Noveck H, Berlin JA, Gould SA. Mortality and morbidity in patients with very low postoperative Hb levels who decline blood transfusion. *Transfusion.* 2002;42(7):812–818.
32. van Woerkens EC, Trouwborst A, van Lanschot JJ. Profound hemodilution: What is the critical level of hemodilution at which oxygen delivery-dependent oxygen consumption starts in an anesthetized human? *Anesth Analg.* 1992 Nov;75(5):818–821.
33. Shander A, Kim TY, Goodnough LT. Thresholds, triggers, or requirements: Time to look beyond the transfusion trials. *J Thorac Dis.* 2018:10(3):1152–1157.
34. Goodnough LT, Levy JH, Murphy MF. Concepts of blood transfusion in adults. *Lancet.* 2013 May 25;381(9880):1845–1854.
35. National Blood Authority. Patient blood management guideline: Module 2 – Perioperative. https://www.blood.gov.au/system/files/documents/pbm-module-2.pdf
36. Jehovah's Witness. How many of Jehovah's witnesses are there worldwide? https://www.jw.org/en/jehovahs-witnesses/faq/how-many-jw-members/
37. Jehovah's Witness. Why don't Jehovah's witnesses accept blood transfusions? https://www.jw.org/en/jehovahs-witnesses/faq/jehovahs-witnesses-why-no-blood-transfusions/
38. Jabbour N, Bramstedt KA. *Transfusion Free Medicine and Surgery.* 2nd ed. Wiley Blackwell; 2014:22–23.
39. Scharman CD, Burger D, Shatzel JJ, et al. Treatment of individuals who cannot receive blood products for religious or other reasons. *Am J Hematol.* 2017;92:1370–1381.
40. Singh Jassar A, Ford PA. Cardiac surgery in Jehovah's Witness patients: Ten-year experience. *Ann Thorac Surg.* 2012;93:19–25.
41. Jorgenson, TD, Golbaba B, Guinn NR, Smith CE. When blood is not an option: The case for a standardized blood transfusion consent form. *ASA Monitor.* 2017 June;81(6).
42. Jabbour N, Bramstedt KA. *Transfusion Free Medicine and Surgery.* 2nd ed. Wiley Blackwell; 2014: 21–22.
43. Beauchamp TL, Childress JF. *Principles of Biomedical Ethics.* 7th ed. Oxford University Press; 2013.
44. West JM. Ethical issues in the care of Jehovah's Witnesses. *Curr Opin Anesthesiol.* 2014;27:170–176.
45. *Schloendorff v Society of New York Hospital,* 105 N. E. 92 (N.Y. 1914).
46. *Raleigh Fitkin-Paul Morgan Memorial Hospital v Anderson,* 42 N. J. 421 (1964).
47. 101st Congress. H.R. 4449. Patient Self Determination Act of 1990. (1989–1990).
48. Moskop JC. Informed consent in the emergency department. *Emerge Med Clin North Am.* 1999;17(2):327–340.
49. Derse AR. What part of "no" don't you understand? Patient refusal of recommended treatment in the emergency department. *Mt Sinai J Med.* 2005;72(4):221–227.
50. Cooper S. AMA journal of ethics. *Virtual Mentor.* 2010:12(6):444–449.
51. American Society of Anesthesiologists. *Ethical Guidelines for the Anesthesia Care of Patients with Do Not Resuscitate Orders or Other Directives that Limit Treatment.* 2009. https://www.asahq.org/For-Members/Standards-Guidelines-and-Statements.aspx

PART VI

ETHICS AND SHARED DECISION-MAKING

35.

WHEN DNR STANDS IN THE OR

WHO BENEFITS? WHO DECIDES?

Joseph F. Kras

STEM CASE AND KEY QUESTIONS

A 63-year-old man with Parkinson's disease and chronic leg pain secondary to peripheral vascular disease is scheduled for placement of a spinal cord stimulator under monitored anesthesia care (MAC). He states that "If I go while I'm under, just let me go."

How do you respond to this statement?

The patient's wife explains that the patient has had a long history of debilitating leg pain from peripheral vascular disease. Over the past 2 years he has developed rapidly progressing Parkinson's disease which has added to his general debility and dissatisfaction with his life. The hope with the spinal cord stimulator is that his leg pain will decrease enough to allow him greater mobility. The patient had a temporary spinal cord stimulator placed in the office with a good response. When you ask the patient directly what his thoughts on the matter are, he responds "If I die let me go. All of you doctors just want your money, anyway."

Does the patient have a lethal condition? Does he have a right to demand to be DNR?

Further attempts at engaging the patient in conversation are not very productive. The patient cannot specify what condition has necessitated him getting the spinal cord stimulator, nor can he relate his medical history in any detail. He does say that he wants the operation and is consistent in saying that he wants to continue to be DNR.

Does the patient have the ability to decide for himself whether he is DNR or not? What are the elements of decisional capacity?

The patient's wife is much more communicative than the patient and asks and answers questions appropriately. She states that the patient has repeatedly stated that his current quality of life was unacceptable to him, and thus he wished to be DNR. When asked to act as a surrogate for her husband, however, she was reluctant to take on that responsibility and asked that you involve their adult son and daughter in the conversation. The children are not there, so you decide to first discuss the situation with the surgeon before calling the children.

The surgeon, Dr. Cutter, says that he always suspends DNR orders on his patients.

How do you reply?

Does a surgeon have the right to demand that the patient rescind their DNR orders in order to have surgery?

After much discussion with the surgeon, he agrees to discuss the matter with the son and daughter. You call the son and daughter on the phone, and they insist on coming in to discuss the matter in person. The son insists on following what his father said and continuing the DNR perioperatively. The daughter (who lives out of town) does not want her father to die and suggests that he is only saying he wants to be DNR because he is depressed.

Which child gets to be the surrogate for the patient? Does it matter that the son is 2 years older?

You undertake a detailed discussion of options for the anesthetic with the children and the wife and the risks and benefits of each option. Similarities and overlap between resuscitation and anesthesia are discussed, as well as possible options short of a complete DNR. Finally, after about 30 minutes of discussion, the wife, son, and daughter agree that if the patient arrests and it looks like he can recover to the level that he had going into the operation, he should continue to be resuscitated. However, if he arrests and he looks like he will not do well postoperatively, then resuscitation should be stopped.

Is what the family described a possible option? How do you decide when to stop resuscitation in this instance?

The surgeon initially stuck to his position of wanting the DNR fully rescinded but now agrees to abide by what the family wants. You do also, and so the case proceeds. Typically, this case is done under light to medium sedation with the patient in the prone position. Unfortunately, the patient has become a bit more agitated, going on about how if anything goes wrong he's going to sue and then relating how he is just done with living. Because of his current state the case is done under a general anesthetic. He does well, there are no events, and he and his family are all satisfied afterward.

There were two surgical cases with two different surgeons to follow in that room. Neither one is particularly happy with having been delayed. You receive an email later that day from administration asking you why you were late starting your case today.

DISCUSSION

A patient coming to the OR with a DNR order remains one of the more problematic situations in medicine. It is a situation with ethical, moral, and sometimes legal implications, as well as logistical problems. An individual's wish to not be resuscitated comes into direct conflict with the physician's duty to care for that patient to the best of their ability. To fully understand how these orders affect the patient (and their medical team) we need to have an understanding of the history of resuscitation as well as the history of orders to limit treatment.

HISTORY OF CPR AND DNR ORDERS

Peter Safar first combined artificial respiration with chest compressions to form the basis of modern cardiopulmonary resuscitation (CPR) in 1959. He himself (with James Elam) discovered the efficacy of opening the airway via tilting the head back and protruding the jaw as necessary, while Knickerbocker had serendipitously discovered that when pushing on paddles placed on the chest an arterial waveform was produced.[1] Calibrated vaporizers were not available in operating rooms, and halothane was known to produce pulselessness. Therefore, this technique of resuscitation from the iatrogenic induction of severe hypotension quickly became very popular in the operating room setting and also spread to other areas of the hospital. By the 1970s, CPR was being utilized in out-of-hospital settings, even being taught to lay people. It soon became the expected norm that any patient whose heart had stopped would have CPR performed on them.

Concurrent with the rise of CPR was the rise of ICUs and mechanical ventilators in hospitals. These first started appearing during the 1950s polio epidemics but became much more widespread during the 1960s.[2] We had won World War II, the economy was going gangbusters, and we were getting ready to send a man to the moon. Why couldn't we conquer disease and put off death to some indefinite future? Unfortunately, reality did not quite live up to the (implied) promise of conquering disease and death through technological advances. Certainly, some patients were able to get back to the same level of existence and independence they had before, but many more experienced either a markedly decreased level of functioning or getting "stuck" on life support, relegated to a slow death in the ICU. Many found this unacceptable, not wanting to be resuscitated if it meant spending long amounts of time on a ventilator in the ICU and then either dying or being sent to a nursing home. Doctors experienced distress at resuscitating people who were terminally ill or otherwise so severely debilitated that their physicians thought CPR to be wholly inappropriate. They developed a number of means of preventing inappropriate resuscitation through practicing "slow codes," "chemical codes," or passing on orders to caregivers not to resuscitate either verbally or through marking charts with purple dots.[3]

The 1970s saw the rise of the "patient's rights" movement, where the public rebelled against the prevalent paternalism of physicians and demanded that patients be able to make their own decisions regarding their healthcare. They wanted their autonomy respected in all decisions, including whether they were to be resuscitated or not. The American Medical Association (AMA) was the first organization to call for a formal entry into the patient's chart directing that they not be resuscitated.[4]

There were also legal cases and governmental actions that affected how a patient's resuscitation status was addressed. Karen Ann Quinlan was a 21-year-old woman who lapsed into a persistent vegetative state after drinking alcohol and taking Valium while on a crash diet. She was maintained on a ventilator and feeding tube. In 1976, the New Jersey Supreme Court decided that the constitutional right to privacy extended into the ability to refuse continued invasive ventilation.[5]

Court cases in both California and Massachusetts in 1986 upheld a patient's right to refuse feeding tubes even if it meant that the patient would die.[6] Another case that dealt with the patient's and their representative's rights to refuse treatment was the Nancy Cruzon case. Nancy Cruzon was a 25-year-old who crashed her car and landed face down in the water. She, too, ended up in a persistent vegetative state after being resuscitated by paramedics. Several years later her parents requested the removal of her feeding tube, which the state of Missouri did not want to grant because this would cause her death. The state said that they needed "clear and convincing evidence" of the patient's wishes before removing the tube. Vague statements about not wanting to be a vegetable would not suffice. The US Supreme Court heard its first "right to die" case in 1990 and upheld the State of Missouri's right to demand such evidence. This led to the rise of *advance directives* being written, such that patients could convey their wishes to their future caretakers.[7] In 1983, the President's Commission for the Study of Ethical Problems in Medicine and Biomedical and Behavioral Research published a report detailing how medical treatments could be ethically withheld.[8] By 1989, withholding nonbeneficial treatments in terminal patients after the consent of the patient or their representative was commonplace,[9] and in 1990 Congress passed the Patient Self-Determination Act, which required all healthcare institutions to inform patients of their right to refuse or accept medical care, as well as their right to execute a written advance directive.[10] The patient had been firmly placed in the driver's seat.

DNR IN THE OR

The Patient Self-Determination Act should have cleared everything up. Patients' rights do not stop at the door to the OR. According to that law patients should have the right to refuse any intervention, including resuscitation in the OR. Unfortunately, that was not translated into practice in the near term and continues to be problematic in many places more than 30 years later. In a 1993 survey, 37% of surgeons and 60% of anesthesiologists assumed that a DNR order would be automatically suspended during surgery.[11] Anecdotally and experimentally, this has been shown to still be a problem during the 21st century.[12,13]

Truog pointed out this discrepancy in the anesthesia literature in 1991,[14] recommending that all such DNR orders be approached individually and compassionately by surgeons and anesthesiologists rather than by blanket policies. The American Society of Anesthesiologists (ASA) issued an ethical guideline in 1993 advocating that all DNR orders undergo "required reconsideration" before the patient proceed to the OR. This guideline was last revised in 2013, and last reviewed in 2018.[15] The American College of Surgeons (ACS) issued their own statement in 1994 (latest revision in 2013) which stated, "Policies that lead either to the automatic enforcement of all DNR orders or to disregarding or automatically cancelling such orders do not sufficiently support a patient's right to self-determination,"[16] and the Association of Operating Room Nurses (AORN) also uses similar language in their statement.[17] The concept of not only allowing for patients to choose which modalities of resuscitation they would allow but, alternatively, also to agree with their physicians how resuscitation should or should not proceed based on what goals the patient was trying to achieve was introduced in a paper by Truog, Waisel, and Burns in 1999.[18] So-called *goal-directed resuscitation* has the potential to align much more closely with a patient's wishes but is also much harder for a team to implement.

POSSIBLE BENEFIT TO PATIENTS CONTINUING DNR TO THE OR

There are many reasons that a patient may be DNR. They may be in the end stages of a terminal disease, where resuscitation may give them a bit of longevity but no cure to their underlying disease. Similarly, they may have a significant burden of chronic disease which may not be terminal but nevertheless renders their quality of life unacceptable to them. In either instance, they may be in need of or elect to have an operative procedure. Such procedure may be to facilitate their discharge from the hospital to a long-term facility (such as a tracheostomy or percutaneous feeding tube) or may be to relieve symptoms caused by their underlying disease (such as relieving an obstructed bowel). However, while they may wish to proceed with surgery, they may also wish to not be resuscitated should they arrest in the OR. This wish may stem from not wanting to be left stuck on machines for the rest of their life or a consideration that a death under anesthesia is not such a bad way to die. Most people prefer to either die at home or in an inpatient hospice, not in an ICU.[19]

Our medical system and serious disease conspire to rob patients of many things—their independence, vitality, dignity, and their autonomy. It is incumbent on us to do all that we can to maintain their dignity and autonomy while they are under our care. Blanket policies that suspend a patient's DNR order serve to undermine both goals.

Patients are individuals, and their goals are theirs alone. They may wish to be resuscitated only if it is most likely that they will return to their present state of independence. Alternatively, they may judge some increased dependence to be acceptable as long as it is most likely that their cognition and ability to interact with others is intact. Or they may be unwilling to undergo the extra pain that follows chest compressions and defibrillation. Many patients who come to the OR with an existing DNR are moderately to severely frail. In those who are frail, 95% will die in the hospital, and, of those who survive to discharge, 83% will go to a long-term care facility.[20] Whatever their individual reasons, policies that are put in place should support the patient's goals whenever possible.

POSSIBLE BENEFITS TO SURGEONS AND ANESTHESIOLOGISTS IN SUSPENDING DNR IN THE OR

The OR is a place where people come to get things fixed. Surgeons, anesthesiologists, and the rest of the perioperative team are focused on doing things to fix the patient, not on allowing them to die. The OR is also a dynamic environment where surgical and pharmacologic interventions are constantly being applied to the patient in the interest of curing them and maintaining physiologic stability. It is possible that these interventions may result in situations where a short course of resuscitation is necessary, especially when operating on older and debilitated patients. To stand by and "do nothing" in such a situation is antithetical to the nature of both surgeons and anesthesiologists. Neither wish to feel like they killed the patient by not countering the last action that occurred just prior to the patient arresting.

Much of anesthetic care is mirrored in resuscitation. Airway control, artificial ventilation, and administering vasoactive drugs are all part and parcel of a routine anesthetic as well as resuscitation.

Unless a patient is having a procedure done under strict local anesthetic there will need to be a discussion about what modalities will be utilized during the anesthetic that are contrary to a "full" DNR order. Of course, such a nuanced discussion will need to start with exploring the patient's present and future goals and how those fit with having surgery and anesthesia. If not discovered initially, many "what if" questions will need to be explored. These will include such things as "What if I'm not able to wean you from the ventilator at the end of the case?", "What if your blood pressure gets so low that I need to do chest compressions in order to circulate the drugs to restore your blood pressure?", "What if your heart goes into a temporary abnormal rhythm that it needs to be shocked out of?", "If we take you back to the ICU on a ventilator, how much time are you willing to endure that?" "Would your answer change if you were slowly improving over that time frame?", and "What decrease in function physically and mentally is consistent with your goals?" These discussions necessarily take much longer than the standard preop informed consent discussions, and, unfortunately, many times are not pursued prior to the day of surgery. And time during the day in an OR environment is a very precious commodity.

Patients who have a DNR are at greater risk of 30-day mortality after surgery. The perioperative team may question whether the benefits outweigh the risk of undergoing an operation if the patient is more likely to die in the short term.[21] Surgeons are somewhat unique in feeling they form a "covenant" with their patients to "get them through, no matter what," which precludes discussion of what to do if things go badly.[22] Additionally, surgeons also commonly feel that they obtain "surgical buy in" from patients without specifically discussing resuscitation options with patients, and, in this discussion, the patient implicitly gives surgeons permission to continue doing what the surgeon thinks is best for their survival, including suspending DNR.[23]

CLARIFYING THE DNR ORDER, INCLUDING PROCEDURE AND GOAL-DIRECTED LIMITS

When changing the patient's DNR status for surgery (rescinding it in part or in toto) there needs to be a change recorded in the part of the chart where code status is specified as well as, ideally, an accompanying progress note detailing the discussion held with the patient. Such a progress note is very helpful in lending depth and avoiding confusion as patients are taken care of by multiple practitioners over the span of days and even over several hours. As referenced above, one may agree with patients to modify their code status either by a checklist method of what is acceptable to the patient or by recording how the patient felt various options for resuscitation fit with their goals, thus empowering their surgeon and anesthesiologist to decide at the time whether and how to proceed if their heart stopped. Table 35.1 illustrates one example of how a code status might be modified.

An additional consideration when modifying an existing DNR order is specifying when such modification is to end, if ever. This will vary depending on the planned procedure and expected postop course and should be included in the progress note accompanying the code status change.

BARRIERS TO A PERIOPERATIVE DNR ORDER

The OR environment conspires against properly discerning and respecting a patient's choices for such "peripheral matters" such as their code status. Ideally one should have a detailed discussion of code status with each patient who comes to the OR. This is impossible to do in the current environment. If one knows ahead of the surgical date that the patient has an existing DNR or has a serious enough disease burden and/or a long and difficult enough case being treated, then one can either visit the patient in-house prior to the OR date, contact them by phone or internet audiovisual connection, and/or possibly also get input from their primary care physician about their disease course and what discussions have occurred up to that point addressing their resuscitation wishes.

Unfortunately, patients' surgical date, time, and OR assignment often change, which may change the anesthesia team that will be taking care of them. Many times one only finds out as the patient is being evaluated in the preop holding area that the patient wishes to continue their DNR to the OR. At this point the production pressure inherent to this setting greatly works against addressing this issue properly.[24] The patient will be lucky if they have one family member present, and their decisional capacity may be limited because of their disease state, anxiety, pain, drug effects, cognitive dysfunction, and lack of hearing aids or glasses. If they are a foreign-language speaker then interpretation of their values, goals, and choices will be more difficult, even with the assistance of a professional language interpreter.

Physicians and patients both have difficulty discussing issues of death and failure, especially in the context of the immediate preop period.[25] It is best to remind patients that the goal is to honor their wishes and that the best way to do so is by having a discussion with them before anything untoward happens because such a conversation may be impossible later. Such conversations are also "gifts" to their loved ones because it relieves them of the burden of making what are felt to be "life or death" decisions for someone else as well as the accompanying guilt that they may have made the wrong choice.

UNILATERAL DNR DURING PANDEMICS AND OTHER DISASTERS

Given the burden that the COVID-19 pandemic has had on health systems all over the world, it is prudent to mention that there are times when the ethics of a situation change. In the usual situation, it is the tension and balance between the autonomy of the patient to control what does and does not happen to them balanced against the physician's autonomy to practice how they feel is medically appropriate (beneficence) that governs decisions whether and how to modify a patient's DNR order. This balance is heavily weighted to decide on what a patient wants as opposed to their physician wants because the patient bears the most significant burdens from any decision.

During pandemics and other disasters this calculus may be changed as medical systems become overwhelmed and struggle to treat patients with normal as well as extraordinary medical needs. In such cases, the needs of the community are also factored into the mix under the principle of justice (or fairness). In such times, the patient's ability to receive a palliative surgery may be limited, and, depending on their overall disease state and the availability of ICU beds, their ability to determine their own code status may also be limited. In such cases, it is incumbent on the healthcare system to have clear policies in place beforehand and to have absolute transparency to all patients about what those policies are.

Table 35.1 **SAMPLE ADDENDUM TO CODE STATUS**

Option 1 Full resuscitation	The patient desires that ALL possible measures be utilized in the event of respiratory or cardiac arrest
Option 2 Limited resuscitation: Procedure-directed resuscitation	The patient refuses the following resuscitative measures (a checklist follows which lists the procedures the patient refuses) Note: checking intubation automatically checks off chest compressions and defibrillation
Option 3 Limited resuscitation: Goal-directed resuscitation	The patient only wishes to be resuscitated IF the following goals are most likely being supported (list of patient goals follows)
Option 4 DNR	The patient REFUSES ALL resuscitative measures, no matter the reason underlying the respiratory or cardiac arrest

DECISIONAL CAPACITY AND SURROGACY

As mentioned above, several factors may temporarily or permanently rob a person of their ability to make their own decisions. *Decisional capacity* is the ability of a patient to make a particular decision at a particular point in time. A patient may be judged not able to make a complex medical decision but may at the same time retain the capacity to make a less complex decision, such as who they would want to designate to speak on their behalf. Often psychiatric, psychological, or ethics consultations are sought to help in determining a patient's decisional capacity. However, any physician can (and should) be making most of these decisions. Indeed, the patient's attending physicians are in the best position to put such evaluations into the context of the decisions at hand. Box 35.1 details the basic elements involved in whether a patient has decisional capacity.

If a patient has lost capacity temporarily (due to sundowning, drugs, or other factors) and the decision is not urgent, then the best way to approach this is to wait or work toward the patient regaining capacity so that they can decide for themselves. On the other hand, if a decision is needed urgently or a patient cannot be returned to having capacity, then a suitable surrogate to speak for the patient must be found. State laws vary somewhat on who can speak for the patient as well as what decisions can and cannot be made by the surrogate.[26] If a patient has a legal guardian appointed for them, then that person is the one who makes all decisions, whether you as their physician feel the patient has decisional capacity or not. If a patient does not have capacity, it is preferable for a patient to have designated a surrogate through a durable power of attorney for healthcare form (or other similarly named equivalent legal forms) prior to them losing decisional capacity. As has been mentioned, in some cases, a patient may lack the capacity to make complex medical decisions but still retain the capacity to name a surrogate. If they have lost all capacity, then a surrogate is sought to speak for the patient. Many states have a specific order of surrogacy by statute, which usually starts with a spouse, followed by adult children, parents, and adult siblings. Members of the same class (e.g., siblings) are treated in a similar fashion. Some states do not specify a specific order. In any case, one is seeking a person who knows the patient, interacts with them on a regular basis, and is willing to make decisions on the basis of what that person would have wanted.

Box 35.1 **DECISIONAL CAPACITY**

Elements of Decisional Capacity

Able to Communicate a basically consistent Choice
Able to Understand their medical condition(s), AND have insight into how these conditions affect them
Able to Understand the risks and benefits of options offered to them (including the option of no treatment)
Able to manipulate information in a somewhat Rational and Consistent Fashion

WHAT TO DO WHEN CONFLICTS ARISE

Patients are usually reluctant to disagree with their doctors, so when they do so (even in an indirect fashion) then it is important that their concerns be explored and their questions answered. Although it can take a bit of time, open-ended statements such as "That's an interesting statement; please tell me more what you mean by that" can both show your concern for their viewpoint as well as help you to understand where the area of conflict lies. Having conversations with patients prior to the day of surgery is preferable because patient anxiety is higher on the day of surgery.[27]

Whenever there are high-stakes decisions being made there are certain to be instances of conflict arising. This conflict may be between the medical team and the family, between members of the medical team, or between family members. In addressing conflicts between the medical team and the patient (or their surrogate), every effort should be made to not have them deteriorate to requiring a decision by the courts system. A process termed "shared decision-making," where both parties contribute their expertise (the physician(s) on the medical aspects, the patient/surrogate on their values as they apply) is usually preferable for solving such conflicts.[28] In some instances, several discussions will be necessary to resolve conflict, but, in most instances of conflict over perioperative DNR status, a single 5- to 10-minute discussion is all that is necessary. Of course, if the patient does not have decisional capacity and family members are disagreeing among themselves, then more time might be needed.

In the instance where an anesthesiologist feels they cannot comply with a patient's wish to remain DNR, then American Society of Anesthesiologists Guidelines state that "When an anesthesiologist finds the patient's or surgeon's/proceduralist's limitations of intervention decisions to be irreconcilable with one's own moral views, then the anesthesiologist should withdraw in a nonjudgmental fashion, providing an alternative for care in a timely fashion."[29] Respect for the patient and their values—always remembering who has the most to lose in the decision and above all remembering to listen to the patient—goes a long way toward resolving and avoiding conflicts.

CONCLUSION

- The DNR order is the only order in medicine that prevents treatment and is often initiated by the patient or their surrogate.
- DNR refers to resuscitation only, *not* to limiting any other therapy.
- Patient's rights do not end at the door to the OR.
- A patient's goals and the surgical team's goals are not necessarily the same.
- A DNR order must be reviewed and any modification agreed upon by the patient and their physicians prior to proceeding to surgery.

- A "limited resuscitation" code order may be limited by specific procedures or by patient goals.
- There are significant barriers to implementation of ethical reconsideration of DNR orders perioperatively.

REVIEW QUESTIONS

1. Possible advantage(s) that may accrue to the patient who maintains a (modified) DNR perioperatively is/are

   a. May avoid pain of cracked ribs.
   b. May avoid being resuscitated to a functional state lower than preoperatively.
   c. May avoid being discharged to a long-term care facility
   d. May die under anesthesia rather than in an ICU.
   e. Answers a, b, and c.
   f. All of the above.

   The correct answer is f.

   Several possible advantages accrue to a person who is able to continue some form of her DNR perioperatively, the chief one being that their autonomy as a human is respected. Rather than having a "one size fits all" policy, each person is considered as an individual, with individual wants and needs.[14,18] These can include wanting to avoid the physical pain that follows resuscitation, the burden of ending up "on machines" in an ICU, or ending up in a long-term facility rather than being discharged back home. Although not suicidal, many patients may prefer a peaceful death under anesthesia rather than a long, drawn out one in an ICU.[24]

2. How should anesthesiologists address DNR in the OR?

   a. DNR is automatically suspended perioperatively until the patient leaves the PACU.
   b. DNR is automatically suspended for the OR, PACU, and until the surgeon feels the acute recovery is over.
   c. Patients are informed that DNR must be suspended for the OR and PACU.
   d. DNR is not automatically suspended.

   The correct answer is d.

   The ASA "Ethical guidelines for the anesthesia care of patients with do-not-resuscitate orders or other directives that limit treatment"[15] state that policies that automatically suspend DNR orders do not sufficiently address a patient's right to self-determination and that communication is essential among all involved parties.

3. The main ethical principle supporting continuing DNR orders perioperatively is

   a. Beneficence.
   b. Autonomy.
   c. Nonmaleficence.
   d. Fairness.

   The correct answer is b.

   The 1970s saw the start of the "patient's rights" movement, where patients wrested control of their medical care from their doctors. This was supported by a number of court cases[5-7] as well as by the 1990 Patient Self Determination Act.[10]

4. The main ethical principle supporting physicians wishing to suspend DNR perioperatively is

   a. Beneficence.
   b. Autonomy.
   c. Nonmaleficence.
   d. Fairness.

   The correct answer is a.

   A physician's reluctance to continue DNR orders perioperatively is rooted in many factors, including knowing that CPR in the OR is more successful than in other places in the hospital,[24] the knowledge that many aspects of resuscitation are part and parcel of normal anesthetic care,[14] and the knowledge that the OR is a goal-directed area where patients come with a specific problem that the team is there to fix. Thus, it is the physician's striving to do the best thing for their patient (beneficence) that underlies their desire to suspend the DNR.

5. If the anesthesiologist has a moral reason they feel they cannot comply with a patient's wish to proceed with a DNR in place, they should

   a. Do the case, code the patient if needed, and not tell the patient unless asked.
   b. Do the case, code as needed, and tell the family only standard anesthetic interventions were done.
   c. Cancel the case.
   d. Withdraw from the case and arrange for someone else to do it.

   The correct answer is d.

   In the majority of instances, we should comply with a patient's wishes for their DNR status. They are the ones who have the most to lose. The ASA Guidelines state, however, "When an anesthesiologist finds the patient's or surgeon's/proceduralist's limitations of intervention decisions to be irreconcilable with one's own moral views, then the anesthesiologist should withdraw in a nonjudgmental fashion, providing an alternative for care in a timely fashion."[29]

6. The best time for the anesthesiologist to discuss code status with the patient is

   a. Never: the surgeon knows the patient best, so we should just go with that.
   b. In the preop area, so we are sure we know their current wishes.
   c. Some time prior to the day of surgery.
   d. After they are sedated, so they aren't as nervous about it.

   The correct answer is c.

   Because of the nature of scheduling and lack of emphasis on its importance, most discussions of a patient's preexisting DNR status end up taking place in the preoperative area. This is less than ideal, given the production pressure that exists in this arena and the heightened anxiety patients experience just prior to proceeding to the OR.[27] It is imperative that a shared discussion take place, though, so "Better late than never." It is preferable, though, that discussions of code status take place in a quiet area when there is no time crunch.

7. The American College of Surgeons Statement says that the best approach to perioperative DNR is

   a. Individualized, with final authority resting with the surgeon.
   b. There is no ACS policy.
   c. A policy of "required reconsideration" of existing DNR orders.
   d. Automatic suspension of DNR for 30 days.

The correct answer is c.

Thirty-day mortality statistics for individual surgeons (and anesthesiologists) are reported to the Center for Medicaid and Medicare Services (CMS). In patients having large, complicated procedures, suspending their DNR for 30 days may make sense. However the ACS Statement on the subject does not address this and instead says that the best approach is a policy of required reconsideration of existing DNR orders.[16]

8. Which of the following is *not* an element of decisional capacity?

   a. Able to describe the risks and benefits of options offered to them.
   b. Being awake and oriented × 3.
   c. Able to communicate a consistent choice.
   d. Able to manipulate information in a rational manner.

The correct answer is b.

Many practitioners confuse a patient's being oriented to their surroundings with them possessing decisional capacity. Patients can, indeed, be somewhat disoriented (or even have some psychosis) as long as it does not interfere with their ability to understand the proposed procedure, the risks and benefits of proceeding and any alternatives, and be able to manipulate such information in a rational manner and communicate a somewhat consistent choice to their practitioner (Box 35.1).

9. Options for an existing DNR order include

   a. Modifying the order, specifying which resuscitative measures would be allowed.
   b. Suspending the order, specifying that full resuscitation measures would be allowed.
   c. Modifying the order, specifying that resuscitation should be carried out only if it would be congruent with certain specified goals.
   d. All of the above.

The correct answer is d.

For a procedure that will be done under local anesthetic or very light sedation, it is possible that a DNR can be maintained as is. Once a patient is given any more than minimal sedation it may be necessary to modify an existing DNR order in some fashion. For example, if a patient is going to have general anesthesia, then it is almost always necessary for the patient to consent to placement of a breathing tube. If strong anesthetic drugs are being used, then it makes sense that the anesthesiologist be allowed to use similarly strong drugs to counteract their effects.

It may or may not make sense for a patient to allow themselves to undergo chest compressions and countershock therapy. Whether or not they do so may depend on their personal goals and values, and modifying their code status such that resuscitation be directed in terms of those goals and values may make more sense than a checklist of specific procedures to be allowed or disallowed.[18]

10. Advantages that may accrue to the anesthesiologist or surgeon by suspending a perioperative DNR include

    a. Being able to honor their commitment to do "everything they can" for the patient.
    b. Being able to treat iatrogenic causes of respiratory or cardiac arrest.
    c. Being able to do "what they usually do" instead of figuring out if what they are doing conforms to the patient's goals.
    d. Answers a and b only.
    e. All of the above.

The correct answer is e.

The OR is a unique environment that is very goal-directed. Surgeons and anesthesiologists both usually "feel better" if they are doing everything they can to "save" a patient.[22,23] Suspending a DNR is consistent with this. There are also multiple moments in any surgery and anesthetic procedure where normal interventions may result in abnormal responses in patients. Practitioners feel better if they are able to counteract these responses and correct the situation. Finally, although using a "goal-directed" resuscitation plan may most fully honor a patient's wishes, it can be cumbersome to operationalize such a plan in the heat of the moment.[18]

REFERENCES

1. Safer P. From control of airway and breathing to cardiopulmonary—Cerebral resuscitation. *Anesthesiology*. 2001;95:789–791.
2. Grenvik A, Pinsky M. Evolution of the intensive care unit as a clinical center and critical care medicine as a discipline. *Crit Care Clin*. 2009;25:239–250.
3. Burns JP, Edwards J, Johnson J, Cassem NH, Truog RD, Do-not-resuscitate order after 25 years. *Crit Care Med*. 2003;31:1543–1550.
4. American Heart Association: Standards and guidelines for cardiopulmonary resuscitation (CPR) and emergency cardiac care (ECC): Medicolegal considerations and recommendations. *JAMA*. 1974;227(Suppl):864–866.
5. *Re Quinlan*. 70 N. J. 10; 355 A.2d 647 (NJ 1976).
6. Mathews MA. Suicidal competence and the patient's right to refuse lifesaving treatment. *Calif. L. Rev.* 1987;75:707–758.
7. *Re Cruzan v Director, Missouri Department of Health*. 497 U. S. 261 (1990).
8. President's Commission for the Study of Ethical Problems in Medicine and Biomedical and Behavioral Research. *Deciding to Forego Life-Sustaining Treatment. A Report on the Ethical, Medical,*

and Legal Issues in Treatment Decisions. US Government Printing Office; 1983.
9. Luce J, White D. A history of ethics and law in the intensive care unit. *Crit Care Clin.* 2009;25:221–237.
10. La Puma J, Orentlicher D, Moss R. Advance directives on admission clinical implications and analysis of the Patient Self-Determination Act of 1990. *JAMA.* 1991;266:402–405.
11. Clemency MV, Thompson NJ. "Do Not Resuscitate" (DNR) orders in the perioperative period: A comparison of the perspectives of anesthesiologists, internists, and surgeons. *Anesth Analg.* 1994;78(4):651–658.
12. Rome L, Rothenberg D. 2012 March 17. The Cool Hand Luke syndrome: Failure to communicate the preoperative do not resuscitate (DNR) order. Case report presented at the Midwest Anesthesia Residents Conference, Chicago.
13. Waisel D, Simon R, Truog R, Baboolal H, Raemer D. Anesthesiologist management of perioperative do-not-resuscitate orders: A simulation-based experiment. *Sim Healthcare.* 2009;4(2):70–76.
14. Truog RD. Do-not-resuscitate orders during anesthesia and surgery. *Anesthesiology.* 1991:74:606–608.
15. American Society of Anesthesiologists. Statement on the ethical guidelines for the anesthesia care of patients with do-not-resuscitate orders or other directives that limit treatment. Reaffirmed 2018 Oct 17. http://www.asahq.org/~/media/sites/asahq/files/public/resources/standards-guidelines/ethical-guidelines-for-the-anesthesia-care-of-patients.pdf
16. American College of Surgeons. Statement on advance directives by patients: "Do not resuscitate" in the operating room. 2014 Jan 1. http://www.facs.org/fellows_info/statements/st-19.html
17. Association of Perioperative Registered Nurses. Perioperative care of patients with do-not-resuscitate or allow-natural-death orders. AORN position statement. Reaffirmed April 2014. https://www.aorn.org/-/media/aorn/guidelines/position-statements/posstat-patients-dnr.pdf
18. Truog R, Waisel D, Burns J. DNR in the OR: A goal-directed approach. *Anesthesiology* 1999:90:289–295.
19. Higginson I, Sen-Gupta G. Place of care in advanced cancer: A qualitative systematic literature review of patient preferences. *J Palliat Med.* 2000;3:287–300.
20. Fernando SM, McIsaac DI, Rochwerg B, et al. Frailty and associated outcomes and resource utilization following in-hospital cardiac arrest. *Resuscitation.* 2020;146:138–144.
21. Brovman EY, Walsh EC, Burton BN, et al. Postoperative outcomes in patients with a do-not-resuscitate (DNR) order undergoing elective procedures. *J Clin Anesth.* 2018;48:81–88.
22. Cassell J, Buchman TG, Streat S, et al. Surgeons, intensivists, and the covenant of care: Administrative models and values affecting care at the end of life—Updated. *Crit Care Med.* 2003;31(5):1551–1559.
23. Schwarze ML, Redmann AJ, Alexander GC, Brasel KJ. Surgeons expect patients to buy-in to postoperative life support preoperatively: Results of a national survey. *Crit Care Med.* 2013;41(1):1–8.
24. Waisel DB, Burns JP, Johnson JA, Hardart GE, Truog RD. Guidelines for perioperative Do-not-resuscitate policies. *J Clin Anesth.* 2002;14:467–473.
25. Burkle CM, Keith M Swetz KM, Armstrong MH Keegan MT. Patient and doctor attitudes and beliefs concerning perioperative do not resuscitate orders: Anesthesiologists' growing compliance with patient autonomy and self determination guidelines. *BMC Anesthesiology.* 2013;13(2):1–7. http://www.biomedcentral.com/1471-2253/13/2
26. Pope, TM. Legal fundamentals of surrogate decision making. *Chest.* 2012;141(4):1074–1081.
27. Mitchell M. Patient anxiety and modern elective surgery: A literature review. *J Clin Nursing.* 2003;12:806–815.
28. Chandrakantan A, Saunders T. Perioperative ethical issues. *Anesthesiol Clin.* 2016;34:35–42.
29. American Society of Anesthesiologists. Statement on ethical guidelines for the anesthesia care of patients with do-not-resuscitate orders or other directives that limit treatment. Reaffirmed 2018 Oct 17. https://www.asahq.org/standards-and-guidelines/ethical-guidelines-for-the-anesthesia-care-of-patients-with-do-not-resuscitate-orders-or-other-directives-that-limit-treatment

36.

INFORMED CONSENT

DO WE REALLY DO THIS CORRECTLY?

Stephen Harden and Nicholas Sadovnikoff

STEM CASE AND KEY QUESTIONS

An 81-year-old man with an unknown past medical history is brought to the hospital by helicopter as a full trauma after a fall from 25 feet. Prior to arrival, it is reported that he struck his head and had a transient loss of consciousness. On arrival, he is alert and complaining of severe back pain and right-sided chest pain. He is hemodynamically unstable after 2 L of IV fluid. During the evaluation, it is discovered that he has minimal sensation or movement from his chest to his toes. A chest x-ray reveals multiple right-sided rib fractures and a right pneumothorax. The patient becomes increasingly tachypneic and confused. He is then intubated for hypoxia, and a right-sided chest tube is placed for the pneumothorax. He is started on a vasopressor for ongoing hypotension. After a negative FAST exam, the patient is transported to the CT scanner for further evaluation. He is found to have a displaced T5 burst fracture with retropulsion into the spinal cord. Neurosurgery is consulted and recommends an emergent decompression and fusion. The on-call anesthesiologist is notified and seeks informed consent for anesthesia.

What are the basic components of informed consent?

The basic components of informed consent, as described by Beauchamp and Childress in their primer, *Principles of Biomedical Ethics*,[1] are

1. *Threshold elements*: Competence, decision-making capacity, and voluntariness

2. *Informational elements*: Disclosure, recommendation, and understanding

3. *Consent elements*: Decision and autonomous authorization

The threshold elements exist to provide a framework for initiating the consent process. The roles of competence and decision-making capacity have similar goals, namely to ensure that the consenting party possesses the cognitive integrity to understand the information, process the information, and make an autonomous decision. The two words are often used interchangeably but they have different definitions. *Decision-making capacity* is determined by an individual's ability to understand the nature and consequences of their decisions and behaviors at a specific moment in time. In a medical context, a patient may have decision-making capacity if he or she can demonstrate understanding of the information, manipulate the information, and then arrive at an autonomous, voluntary choice. Decision-making capacity is assessed and determined by qualified healthcare professionals.

On the other hand, *competence* is a legal concept. It is determined by the court system alone. If a patient is legally declared incompetent, there will be an appointed surrogate decision-maker, which may be a family member, attorney, or someone else. However, if a physician declares a patient to lack decision-making capacity, he or she effectively functions as a "gatekeeper," as described by Beauchamp and Childress,[1] to a declaration of incompetence. While not legally declaring a patient to lack competence, a physician may pursue consent for an intervention from a surrogate decision-maker if the patient is found to lack the capacity to fully appreciate and understand the intended procedure.

Voluntariness is an element that describes a decision that is made freely, without coercion, including by means of force, fraud, deceit, duress, or any other constraints. This is rooted in the ethical principle of respect for personal autonomy and is described at length by the Nuremberg Code.[2] The principle of autonomy states that an individual is free to make decisions absent from the interference of others. The principle of voluntariness requires that a decision specifically be made in the absence of coercive influence, specifically of other people. Other examples of coercion include threats, guilt, enticements, and bribes. Of note, the presence of an aggressive or debilitating disease, psychiatric disorder, or an addiction are not considered to be coercive.

This element creates conflict for the physician. How does one make a strong recommendation without being perceived as being unbiased, or worse, coercive? Physicians are and should be biased by years of education, training, and experience, and it is allowable to make strong recommendations as such. Influence through coercion—that is, by threats of force, harm, or abandonment—clearly violates the element of voluntariness in most situations. However, persuasion by appealing to facts and reason are permissible and should be welcomed into an informed consent discussion. Manipulation is another form of influence that includes lying, withholding key information, providing false information regarding alternatives, tone of voice, framing of options as negative instead of positive, and appealing to personal desires, biases, or institutional culture. Lastly, a very strong recommendation that does not violate the principle of voluntariness to one patient may in fact produce undue influence on a more vulnerable patient, thus violating the principle of voluntariness.

The informational elements include disclosure of necessary material information, recommendation of a plan, and demonstration of understanding of the disclosed information and recommendation. In one sense, disclosure is the most important and essential element in informed consent. This comes from the legal context of civil litigation that focuses on physicians as agents of disclosure, particularly of specific risks of certain treatments or procedures. On the other hand, the disclosure of material information is less about protection from liability and more about providing the necessary information to ensure a patient makes a well-informed, autonomous choice. In fact, the element of disclosure specifically provides the basis for sufficient decision-making by a patient. As discussed in Beauchamp and Childress,[1] there are five key pieces to adequate disclosure:

1. All facts a patient would consider material when deciding to consent or not to a procedure or treatment,
2. All information the physician deems to be material to the procedure or treatment,
3. A professional recommendation,
4. A description of the purpose of consent, and
5. A description of the limits of consent.

The element of recommendation returns again to the concern of coercion. As described previously, a physician may indicate passionately their belief that a particular treatment, procedure, or other course of action is best for the patient. However, this preference should not be enforced with coercion, including threats of abandonment or otherwise limiting full care. Furthermore, a physician must not manipulate any facts regarding a patient's particular predicament to unduly influence a decision. As discussed previously, this can be a difficult position for a physician. The ability to differentiate between persuasion and manipulation is a challenging skill to develop. In most physician–patient relationships, the physician holds a position of power due to a greater wealth of knowledge. This position demands discernment and thoughtful reflection. At all times, a physician's recommendation is just that, and not a predetermined course of action. Any patient's choice to not follow that recommendation is to be honored and respected.

The element of understanding is closely linked to the element of decision-making capacity. A patient must be able to articulate a clear understanding of the nature of a procedure, its potential risks and benefits, and the possible consequences of any decision. The element of understanding is a fluid concept that may change with increased medical complexity. For example, a patient with clear decision-making capacity can have confusion or misconceptions regarding a specific procedure in the context of complex medical information. Importantly, simply describing the risks and benefits of a procedure to a patient is clearly insufficient. A patient must be able to recapitulate the relevant information and indicate comprehension of the risks and benefits both of consenting to a procedure and of declining a procedure.

Lastly, a patient must make a decision with autonomous authorization. Once the patient has reached a decision, it must be clearly, explicitly, and unambiguously stated and then meticulously documented. Furthermore, a detailed documentation of the entire consent process and discussion is warranted, particularly in cases of high-stakes decisions, such as a particularly risky surgery. Attention should be given to all of the above elements in the documentation.

Furthermore, the patient's autonomous wishes should be clearly documented. During situations with high stakes or if there is controversy, the condition under which the patient consents *or refuses* should be documented; namely, that the patient was free from all coercive influences and clearly has decision-making capacity.

Are there different standards of disclosure?

The standards for determining the content of a disclosure discussion have evolved to include three positions, partially due to legal considerations. They include the reasonable-physician standard, the reasonable-patient standard, and the particular-patient standard.

The *reasonable-physician (or professional practice) standard* is an early concept that asks what material information a *reasonable physician* in a given community would provide to a patient regarding a proposed intervention. As society has moved to a position of more patient autonomy and shared decision-making, this standard has become increasingly viewed as paternalistic.

The shift to general acceptance of the concepts of shared decision-making and patient autonomy has led to the development of the *reasonable-patient (or reasonable person) standard*. The reasonable physician standard, as described above, asks what a physician in a given situation would consider adequate information. On the other hand, the reasonable patient standard asks what a hypothetical, otherwise *reasonable patient* would consider adequate information for a given situation.

Basing a standard on what information a "reasonable patient" would determine to be adequate creates a problem because there is a vast spectrum of the level of detail a particular patient actually wants to hear. Therefore, the *particular-patient (or subjective person) standard* was created to allow a physician to adjust the level of detail to match their *particular patient's* desire to know. This is appealing because it inherently allows a physician to accommodate individual patient's individual wishes. However, it results in a loose standard and has therefore not been adopted by the courts. Physicians therefore continue to provide more information than is really wished for, fearing accusations of withholding information, particularly the possibilities of complications or less than optimal outcomes. The particular-patient standard is allowable and can be followed, but it is imperative for the physician to ensure that all questions are fully answered and that the details of the discussion are carefully documented.

The patient in this scenario is sedated and intubated and therefore does not have capacity to consent to any intervention.

His spouse is available, so the anesthesiologist approaches her to obtain consent.

In the event that a patient cannot consent to an intervention, who should provide consent, and how is that determined?

First, it should be determined that the patient is in fact incapacitated or otherwise determined to be incompetent. If this is the case, then a surrogate decision-maker should be identified if appropriate. According to Beauchamp and Childress,[1] a surrogate decision-maker must possess the qualifications of competence, adequate knowledge and information, emotional stability, and a commitment to the incompetent patient's interests that is free of coercion and conflicts of interest. Importantly, the surrogate decision-maker must be acting to represent the autonomous wishes of the patient. Representation of the patient's known wishes may not be viewed, at least by some, as acting in the patient's best interest. However, honoring the patient's known autonomous wishes, as expressed through a surrogate decision-maker, takes precedent over acting in what might be considered as being in the patient's best interest. In the absence of an *advance directive*, which could legally designate any individual as the surrogate decision-maker, the patient's closest family, including spouse, siblings, parents, and adult children, becomes the first choice as a surrogate. Determination of the individual legally authorized surrogate decision-maker rests ultimately with each state's laws. A family member must meet the above qualifications to act as surrogate. The term "family" has many problems because it is imprecise and increasingly anachronistic. For example, the patient's closest relative by traditional definitions (or as determined by state law) may be personally distant or even estranged. If any family member is determined to be acting in conflict to a patient's documented autonomous wishes, in ignorance of the details, or in bad faith, the physician should seek to disqualify them from making decisions.

The role of the physician cannot be overstated when in discussion with surrogate decision-makers. The physician must seek to guide the surrogates through often-difficult decisions. It is important to provide adequate information while also gracefully maintaining a patient's dignity. Furthermore, the physician should seek to help surrogates see rapid changes in a patient's condition. This unburdens the surrogates from the difficult decision at hand and helps guide them through the process.

Lastly, the courts play a role as a final decision-maker. The courts provide a mechanism to appoint a legal guardian absent the family if there is reason to suspect the surrogate decision-makers in place (i.e., the family) are not acting in accordance with the patient's autonomous wishes or best interest. As previously described, the courts may also legally declare a patient or surrogate decision-maker as competent or incompetent.

What must be discussed when consenting for anesthesia?

Anesthesia professionals must first distinguish consent for anesthesia from consent for surgery. While it is true that consenting to most surgical procedures implies some consent to some form of anesthesia, the situation is more complex. A separate consent process for anesthesia emphasizes the anesthesiologist's role in providing care to the patient. Furthermore, especially for inherently high-risk surgical procedures, it disentangles the risks of surgery from the risk of anesthesia. Anesthesia professionals, including anesthesiologists, nurse anesthetists, anesthesiology assistants, and other qualified healthcare providers who work directly with these anesthesia professionals (e.g., a physician assistant or nurse practitioner in a preoperative clinic) are uniquely qualified to describe the benefits of various forms of anesthesia as well as each anesthetic's material risks.

A discussion for consent must include a disclosure of pertinent material risks of the recommended anesthesia and its reasonable alternatives. According to the American Society of Anesthesiologists (ASA) Manual on Professional Liability,[3] material risks should include both common events with no long-term consequences as well as rare events that may result in significant morbidity or mortality. Based on survey results of anesthesiologists, common risks of general anesthetics include oral or dental damage, sore throat, hoarseness, postoperative nausea and vomiting, drowsiness, and urinary retention. Severe risks include awareness during surgery, postoperative vision loss, aspiration, respiratory failure, organ failure, malignant hyperthermia, drug reactions, and lastly, the risks of failure to recover from the anesthetic, coma, and death. This is not a comprehensive list but includes most common and rare but serious complications.

The anesthesiologist appropriately discusses all material risks of general anesthesia, informing the surrogate there is no alternative for this procedure. The patient's surrogate expresses concerns regarding the use of trainees during the surgery. She states she knows someone that had a bad experience with a resident many years ago.

What should be disclosed regarding who participates in the patient's care?

Legally, this varies by state. Some states require one to disclose all persons who may be expected to participate in the care of the patient during the intervention. Whether legally required or not, all persons involved in the care of a patient should generally be disclosed. This may include attending anesthesiologists, resident anesthesiologists, nurse anesthetists, student nurse anesthetists, anesthesiology assistants, anesthesiology assistant students, and medical students. In this situation, the surrogate should be reassured that a provider with appropriate education and experience will always be providing care to the patient, albeit sometimes in a direct supervisory role.

The surrogate decision-maker consents to proceed with anesthesia for the necessary surgery. The patient undergoes an emergent T4–T6 decompression with a T3–T7 posterior fusion. The surgery lasts several hours and is complicated by hemorrhage requiring transfusion of blood. He also has a period of hypotension during a particularly rapid period of bleeding. Postoperatively, the patient is transported to the surgical ICU intubated but otherwise in stable condition. On postoperative day 1, he is weaned from the ventilator and successfully extubated. Over the next 2 days, the patient begins to show signs of acute renal failure. The nephrology team is consulted for consideration for renal replacement therapy. However, the patient makes it very clear that he does not want dialysis of any kind, stating, "I don't want to rely on machines the rest of my life." Renal replacement therapy is deferred. Later that evening, the patient develops progressive delirium. The next day, his son informs his nurse that he has consumed "several" beers every night for as long as he can remember. At this point, the delirium has progressed and is multifactorial in the setting of acute illness, alcohol withdrawal, and uremia. However, he continues to have moments of clarity where he adamantly refuses dialysis.

How should decision-making capacity be assessed?

Capacity to make decisions in the context of acute medical illness can by a very dynamic process that requires ongoing assessment. It is true that no one particular test exists to determine who has capacity and who does not have capacity. In the context of delirium and other rapidly reversible medical conditions (e.g., drug withdrawal, transient ischemic attack, intoxication, sedative effects, seizure, etc.), it must be assessed frequently, as the patient's capacity may change by the hour. This differs from chronic conditions, including severe intellectual disability, dementia, and untreated psychosis. Furthermore, a patient does not need to possess full capacity in all aspects of life. He or she must only be able to demonstrate capacity to make a judgment about a particular medical intervention, in this case dialysis. Generally, if the patient cannot understand the consequences of his choice to refuse dialysis in this acute setting—namely, the progression of uremia—it would be acceptable to consent the surrogate decision-maker while still actively treating other causes of delirium.

Occasionally, the process of obtaining informed consent can present anesthesiologists with an ethical challenge that they are unable to resolve readily. If time permits, it may be prudent to have a psychiatrist evaluate a patient's decision-making capacity in cases where this is unclear or in cases where a patient's surrogate decision-maker appears to disagree with the patient's wishes. Furthermore, institutional ethics resources often provide a consultation service to provide experience and expertise in helping to resolve concerns. These services should be consulted whenever appropriate.

The patient's surrogate decision-maker consents for dialysis. The patient receives continuous renal replacement therapy and treatment for likely alcohol withdrawal. His delirium slowly resolves, and he is transitioned to hemodialysis. He is transferred to the floor for ongoing nutritional support, physical therapy, and hemodialysis. One evening, he has a sudden respiratory decompensation. He is urgently transferred back to the ICU. An anesthesiologist is called to the bedside, and the patient is emergently reintubated.

Are there situations in which the needed informed consent is less strict or even not necessary?

In general, true emergency situations, such as the respiratory failure experienced in our example case, do not need to adhere to the same strict standards of obtaining informed consent as elective interventions. This implied consent is predicated on the assumption that patients would want life-sustaining treatment. If practical, an anesthesiologist should pursue an abbreviated form of the consent process. However, this is often not possible, as in situations where the patient is decisionally incapable, has no immediately available surrogate decision-makers, and has no clear documentation regarding life-sustaining maneuvers. To be clear, the expectation for the anesthesiologist in this situation is to pursue full resuscitative care, *even to a patient who otherwise might have declined such care on an elective basis*. If it is later clarified that the patient had expressly not wanted aggressive medical care, life-sustaining resuscitative therapies can then be discontinued. However, the alternative of choosing not to resuscitate a patient always has one clear outcome. For this clear reason, it is recommended and prudent to pursue initial life-sustaining interventions until all facts about the patient's wishes are known.

The patient is now intubated and mechanically ventilated. He is again delirious and appears very anxious at times. He has a very weak cough, but his overall respiratory status appears to improve with regular suctioning. The critical care physician decides he is as optimized as possible and extubates the patient. At first, the patient appears well but continues to have a very weak cough. Over the next day, he becomes increasingly tachypneic and hypoxic. He is told that reintubation is imminent. He is clearly delirious but adamantly refuses intubation, stating, "I never wanted to live like this." His spouse and adult children are at the bedside. They agree with unanimity that intubation is the right thing to do. However, the patient's daughter notes that the patient has in fact stated many times in the past that he would never want to live in a wheelchair.

What is the next step when a family disagrees with the patient's wishes?

The answer is two-fold. First, note the severity of the consequences of this decision: namely, life or death. If time permits, the patient's capacity should have an evaluation by a psychiatrist. If available, an urgent ethics consultation may be sought to help mediate the situation and lay the ethical foundation for decision. If time does not permit (e.g., the patient's condition is deteriorating too quickly), then the prudent decision is to preserve life and again intubate the patient until further details and questions can be addressed. As addressed previously, aggressive interventions can always be discontinued.

The anesthesiologist called to the bedside explains to the family the need for reintubation. The family understands the procedure, why it is necessary, and its risks, and they consent to the procedure. The patient is quickly intubated without complication. Over the next several days, he fails to wean from the ventilator. The general surgeon on service is consulted for a tracheostomy. The day before the procedure, an advance practice nurse (APRN) who works with the anesthesiologists at the hospital comes by to assess the patient and consent for the anesthesia the following day.

Who should physically consent a patient for a procedure or other intervention?

As discussed in a recent publication in the *New England Journal of Medicine*,[4] healthcare occurs in an increasingly team-based system. The publication editorializes about a recent malpractice case regarding the language of consent in Pennsylvania (*Shinal v. Toms*[5]). The majority ruled that the physician was liable because he was not the specific healthcare provider to actually obtain informed consent. Notably, the surgeon did discuss the procedure, its risks, and their alternatives at length while in consultation with the patient. Furthermore, he documented the details of this discussion. However, he did not personally execute the duty of informed consent, as the language of the law in Pennsylvania specifies, when the patient returned to the clinic some time after the initial consultation. Another provider obtained the consent when the patient returned to the office at another date. This ruling has led in Pennsylvania to the cumbersome process of informed consent only being executed by the attending physician in charge of a particular intervention. At this time, this has not been applied in other states. The authors of the editorial strongly argue in opposition to the ruling, instead encouraging a more practical approach, as outlined here. First, they propose providing structural support to ensure all who participate in informed consent discussions have the right training and tools to faithfully execute the consent process. Second, they suggest that all attending physicians speak directly with the patient prior to any procedure to ensure that all questions have truly been answered and that the patient is comfortable going forward with the procedure. This allows modern medicine to continue using the efficient team-based approach and also provides the direct physician–patient relationship that is expected.

The tracheostomy occurs without complication. The patient is slowly weaned from the ventilator over the next week. His delirium completely resolves. He eventually is discharged to a rehabilitation facility to continue physical therapy for his spinal cord injury. He makes steady progress with his recovery, and his tracheostomy site is decannulated. While at the facility, the patient requests and obtains an order to "Do Not Resuscitate, Do Not Intubate." One day, the patient falls from bed and suffers an open distal radius fracture. He is transported to the hospital for evaluation. The orthopedic surgeon recommends an open reduction and internal fixation. The anesthesiologist suggests a nerve block to help with pain after surgery.

What additional risks should the anesthesiologist address regarding a nerve block?

In accordance with the ASA Manual on Professional Liability,[3] the "common risks" should include prolonged numbness and failure of the technique. The "rare but severe risks" should include bleeding, infection, nerve damage, persistent weakness or numbness, seizures, coma, and death. Other specific risks should be tailored to the individual regional technique or block. For example, neuraxial techniques have the added risks of postdural puncture headache and backache.

The anesthesiologist discusses a brachial plexus perineural block with the patient, to which he consents. He also discusses the potential need for general anesthesia. The patient appears upset, revealing that the surgeon told him that his DNR/DNI order would be reversed for the procedure, per hospital policy.

The DNR/DNI order is automatically reversed for the operating room, right?

Much controversy surrounds the issue of DNR/DNI orders for surgical procedures. Not surprisingly, the ASA has published guidelines[6] regarding this dilemma. According to the ASA guidelines, simply reversing the DNR/DNI orders for a procedure or operation would fail to address a patient's right to self-determination. Instead, they recommend reviewing the DNR/DNI order with the patient or surrogate whenever possible. This allows clarification or modification of the goals of resuscitation in the context of a procedure that requires anesthesia. It is imperative to explain that some actions (e.g., intubation or use of vasopressors) may be necessary for the safety of the patient during an operation but would be considered resuscitative in other situations. One of three alternative routes may be taken:

1. *Full resuscitation*: This allows for all resuscitative measures to be used during the immediate acute-care setting.
2. *Limited resuscitation with regard to certain procedures only*: This allows for the anesthesiologist to employ certain procedures (e.g., intubation) that may be necessary for the operation without employing other procedures (e.g., chest compressions, electrical defibrillation, etc.).
3. *Limited resuscitation with regards to the patient's goals and values*: This allows for the anesthesiologist and surgeon to use clinical judgment to determine what is appropriate for the patient in the context of *both* the situation of the procedure *and* the patient's goals. This effectively gives permission to treat rapidly reversible complications and not treat complications that would lead to irreversible, permanent results.

This conversation should be thoroughly documented in the chart by the anesthesiologist. Furthermore, it should be clarified when these perioperative resuscitative efforts should revert to the previously documented goals, namely "DNR/DNI." The ASA recommends[6] this time point to be either discharge from the PACU or when the effects of anesthesia or sedatives have subsided. Of note, the American College of Surgeons (ACS) and Association of Operating Room Nurses (AORN) have also published similar guidelines[7,8] consistent with the ASA guidelines.

The anesthesiologist readdresses the patient's wishes for resuscitation in the operating room. The patient asks the anesthesiologist to use clinical judgment during the operation, but he very frankly states he does not want to be dependent on a ventilator for any period of time after the surgery. The anesthesiologist performs a dense perineural brachial plexus block and administers moderate sedation for the surgery. The surgery has no complications, and the patient recovers quickly in the PACU.

Suppose the patient had another medical complication that made his situation suddenly more complex. For example, what should happen if the patient developed an ST-elevation myocardial infarction in the PACU? Does the increased medical complexity affect a patient or surrogate's understanding in the process of informed consent?

As described above, one of the key elements of informed consent is understanding. Namely, a patient or surrogate must be able to articulate an understanding of the nature of the procedure, its potential benefits and risks, and the possible consequences of the decision. The conditions of an emergent high-stakes decision may introduce confusion and limit understanding. Even otherwise competent persons with clear decision-making capacity can have a lack of understanding in the context of new, complex medical information. If a patient or surrogate cannot indicate comprehension of risks and benefits of a proposed intervention, then they do not satisfy informational elements of informed consent. Furthermore, it is acceptable to calibrate the degree of cognitive integrity of an individual to the gravity of the decision. For example, a relatively healthy individual may consent to anesthesia for a minor procedure, even if he or she possessed some cognitive impairment. A patient with similar cognitive impairment may be unable to consent to a procedure with high stakes (e.g., an open abdominal aortic aneurysm repair in a patient with severe renal dysfunction). If there is any doubt about patient understanding, the anesthesiologist should consider a psychiatry consult to help with capacity assessment. Furthermore, the ethics consultative service may be utilized, as previously described.

Are there any problems with this framework of informed consent?

The framework of using threshold, informational, and consent elements to obtain informed consent works well in many situations, particularly when a physician–patient relationship truly exists. However, there are multiple caveats to this approach.

First, the physician–patient dyad is often actually a myriad. Medical care is increasingly complex and increasingly reliant on a team-based approach. A patient may present for a complex surgery involving multiple surgeons with multiple assistants. Furthermore, a patient may be under significant influence from family and friends, some of whom may be at the bedside in the preoperative area. The consent process is more likely to involve a conversation involving multiple parties, often with similar but varying interests.

Second, assessment of competence is imprecise. As illustrated above, there are varying situations where a patient may be deemed competent for one procedure but not for another, depending on the gravity of the situation.

Third, confirmation of voluntariness is challenging. As described above, a physician must ensure the consent is truly free of coercion, including undue influence from the physician. This is another dynamic concept that varies from patient to patient.

Fourth, disclosure is subject to legal scrutiny. Disclosure has at least three approaches. The particular-patient standard is probably the most patient-centric approach. However, in light of legal scrutiny and a litigious culture, most physicians will follow some variation of the reasonable-physician standard and reasonable-person standard, fearing liability if a material risk is not disclosed.

Fifth, recommendation can be viewed as paternalistic. Emphasis is increasingly placed on the principle of autonomy with regards to medical decision-making. Physicians may find it challenging to make recommendations, sometimes passionately, without becoming paternalistic or even coercive.

Sixth, confirmation of understanding can be subjective. Understanding changes with medical complexity and acuity of illness. This clearly creates a spectrum of understanding for most patients. It becomes a subjective judgment to discern when a patient transitions from understanding the risk and benefits of a simple procedure to failing to understand those of a more complex procedure.

Lastly, the consent may fall to surrogates. Even if the consent itself is clear, surrogate decision-making can present many challenges. Firstly, surrogates are rarely held to the same standards of rigorous assessment of competence and voluntariness. Second, the surrogate may not actually know the patient's wishes. Third, the surrogate may know the patient's wishes, but may not actually follow those wishes. Fourth, the surrogate may not actually understand the medical issues at hand. Lastly, the surrogate may be skeptical or mistrustful of the medical team's intentions.

DISCUSSION

The process of obtaining informed consent from a patient before a planned intervention is an essential process conducted between the patient and the physician performing the intervention, including anesthesiologists. Anesthesiologists are unique in that most patients have already consented to a surgical or other interventional procedure, the performance of which requires anesthesia. There are many fundamental components of the informed consent process, and it is imperative for all physicians to have a firm grasp of them.

Anesthesiologists are placed in a rather unique position when it comes to the consent process. In the overwhelming majority of cases, the anesthesiologist must obtain "consent" from a patient who has already consented to a surgical procedure. In many institutions, the consent for anesthesia is even explicitly included in the surgical consent form. Since essentially no patients would choose to have surgery without anesthesia, the discussion between an anesthesiologist and the patient is focused almost entirely on the material risks and benefits of any anesthetic procedures and techniques that may be used and not on the decision to actually have anesthesia.

While most anesthesiologists spend an overwhelming majority of clinical time in the operating room, the anesthesiologist's role is of course not limited to just the perioperative environment. Anesthesiologists also play vital roles in ICUs, labor and birth units, pain clinics, and preoperative clinics. Anesthesiologists also often play a role on emergency response teams with chief roles in airway management or resuscitative efforts. It is therefore vital for the anesthesiologist to fully grasp the informed consent process. In the case presented in this chapter, the anesthesiologist must apply the components of the informed consent process during a variety of different clinical situations, including elective procedures, high-risk procedures, emergencies, and situations without an immediately clear answer.

The process of informed consent functions as an extension of a major concept of medical ethics, the respect for autonomy. The concept fundamentally holds that an individual patient has the right to decide what will or will not be done to them (the "consent" component). Furthermore, the patient's decision must be made in the context of being as fully educated as possible about the nature of his or her medical condition and the respective risks and benefits of choosing to either undergo or decline the proposed intervention (the "informed" component). This is a simplistic approach, and the details of each patient's individual circumstances often lead to multiple questions that must be explored.

- Is the patient making the decision of his or her own free will, without any undue influence or coercion?
- Does the patient comprehend the relevant information with which he or she is being furnished?
- Does the patient possess the necessary mental capacity to process the information, understand the stakes, and make a reasoned decision in that moment?
- Is the information being provided to the patient thorough and without bias?
- Has the patient been presented with the material risks and benefits of all the alternatives to the proposed procedure, including doing nothing?

In *Principles of Biomedical Ethics*, Beauchamp and Childress[1] lay a foundation from which to best understand the process of informed consent. They divide the informed consent process into three categories of fundamental components: threshold elements, informational elements, and consent elements, as listed below:

Threshold elements (preconditions)

- Competence
- Decision-making capacity (to understand and decide)
- Voluntariness (in deciding)

Informational elements

- Disclosure (of material information)
- Recommendation (of a plan)
- Understanding (of disclosure and recommendation)

Consent elements

- Decision (in favor a plan)
- Autonomous authorization (of the chosen plan)

This is not an exhaustive framework, but it does cover most considerations in a standard informed consent process, even if complicated.

Threshold elements are the preconditions that must be present to proceed with a meaningful and appropriate consent process to take place. The patient must be competent, have decision-making capacity, and make the decision voluntarily.

Decision-making capacity is the ability for a patient to understand the information, process the information, manipulate the information, and make an autonomous decision. *Competence* is very similar but is technically a legal classification that is determined by a court of law. In the context of a consent process, the distinction is largely irrelevant. A patient either does or does not have the necessary cognitive function to participate in the consent process for a given procedure. Of note, it is widely accepted that the degree of cognitive integrity necessary to consent may be calibrated to the gravity of the decision. In other words, mild cognitive impairment is acceptable when the stakes are low but not when the stakes are high. If there is uncertainly, evaluation by a psychiatrist may be used to assess capacity.

Voluntariness is a more narrow extension of autonomy. It implies the absence of coercion, specifically by other people. Patients whose decisions are influenced by other people through such mechanisms as threat, enticement, or guilt may be influenced to forgo voluntariness, thus voiding the validity of an informed consent process. Note that although conditions such as debilitating or aggressive disease, psychiatric disorders, and addictions may affect decision-making, they are not considered coercive in this situation. A distinction must be made between coercion and recommendation. A physician is expected to recommend, and even strongly advocate for, a certain course of action. This is not viewed as coercion unless the physician threatens the patient with undue consequences, such abandonment, should the recommendation be rejected.

Informational elements refer to the content and quality of the information provided to a patient in the course of obtaining consent as well as to how the patient comprehends that information. The components include multiple standards of disclosure, recommendation, and understanding.

The *disclosure* is a description of the proposed medical intervention along with a review of the expected benefits, potential material risks, and alternative interventions. This is a notably troublesome term because the word "disclosure" often implies the revealing of information that has previously been withheld or even concealed. Furthermore, "disclosure" is also the term used in the context of providing patients with information about adverse consequences or unintended complications that have occurred as result of a medical treatment or procedure. However, in the context of the consent process, the word "disclosure" is a proactive description of potential risks or complications of a proposed intervention. There are three major standards of disclosure that evolved over several decades: the reasonable-physician standard, the reasonable-patient standard, and the particular-patient standard.

The reasonable-physician (or professional practice) standard is one of the earliest concepts of disclosure and describes what a *reasonable physician* in a given community would provide to a patient regarding the risks of a proposed intervention. Not surprisingly, this standard has increasingly become viewed as paternalistic as the movement toward patient autonomy and shared decision-making has gained momentum.

Conversely, the reasonable-patient (or reasonable person) standard shifts the focus from what the physician would consider adequate information to what a hypothetical *reasonable patient* would consider adequate information. This concept is increasingly accepted as the concepts of shared decision-making and patient autonomy have gained general acceptance.

Lastly, the particular-patient (or subjective person) standard allows the physician to adjust the level of detail furnished to that individual's desire to know. This accommodates the reality that, among "reasonable patients," there is a vast spectrum of the level of detail that patients actually wish to hear. This is appealing because it is the most patient-centered approach. However, it is a relatively loose concept and has not been adopted by the courts. Therefore, physicians generally impose more information on their patients than the patients really wish to receive out of fear of being accused of withholding information regarding he possibility of complications or unsuccessful outcomes. Certainly, the general principle of the particular-patient standard may be followed, but the physician must ensure that all of the patient's questions are answered and should carefully document the extent of the content of the discussion.

The recommendation is a designation of a preferential course of action made by the physician. Importantly, this is not "coercive." Physicians may passionately indicate their belief that a particular course of action is most desirable for the patient, but they should not enforce this preference by threats of abandonment or other means of coercion. The physician should also avoid manipulation of the facts of a particular patient's predicament to influence the decision. The distinction between persuasion and manipulation may at times be difficult to discern. Generally, the physician is in a position of power, being in possession of the greater wealth of knowledge.

The element of understanding is similar to decision-making capacity, but it has a more narrow definition. A patient consenting or declining a procedure should be able to articulate an understanding of the nature of the procedure, its potential benefits and risks, and the possible consequences of the decision. A patient may have already met the precondition (or threshold element) of adequate decision-making capacity. However, the conditions under which high-stakes decisions are made may introduce confusion. Furthermore, persons with clearly demonstrated decision-making capacity can exhibit confusion or misconceptions while receiving complex medical information. A patient must be able to recapitulate the information presented. Notably, simply describing the risks and benefits to a patient is insufficient. A patient must be able to indicate their comprehension of those risks and benefits.

Lastly, the consent elements include a decision as well as autonomous authorization. Once a patient has arrived at a decision, it must be clearly and unambiguously stated and meticulously documented. If it is a high-stakes decision, then a detailed documentation of the consent process is warranted, with attention to all of the previously described considerations. Furthermore, the documentation should reflect the patient's autonomous wishes. Again, if it is a high-stakes decision, it may be valuable to document the conditions pertaining to the patient's autonomy, namely the absence of coercive influences and the confirmation of decisional capacity. It cannot be overstated that the patient's autonomous wishes to consent to or refuse a proposed medical intervention, when determined to have decision-making capacity, must be honored.

It is important to understand the historical medico-legal considerations of the process of informed consent. Since the 1950s, a number of medico-legal decisions have been characterized by a progressive emphasis on the rights of the individual patient. An important manifestation of this trend is seen in the growth and development of legal attention to the importance of the principles of informed consent. The former standard of obtaining *assent*, the agreement of a patient to have a procedure, has been replaced by the legal expectation of obtaining *consent*, the autonomous, informed authorization by a patient to have a procedure, which is described throughout this chapter.

This progression has occurred principally through three court cases: Salgo, Natanson, and Canterbury.[9-11] These cases constitute the legal evolution of the principles of informed consent. In 1957, the California court first used the phrase "informed consent" in *Salgo v. Trustees of Leland Stanford Hospital*.[9] In the case, Salgo became paraplegic after translumbar aortography. He had not been informed of the risks of the procedure. The court thus ruled for the need for "intelligent" consent by requiring the physician to discuss the risks, benefits, and alternatives of a procedure to the patient.

In 1960, *Natanson v. Kline*[10] began to define what information should be told to the patient to actually fulfill the requirement of informed consent. Natanson had severe radiation burns after the use of cobalt radiation therapy, a new technology. Though some disclosure of risks had taken place, the court held that the disclosure was inadequate. Furthermore, this case introduced the professional practice standard, as described earlier.

In 1972, *Canterbury v. Spence*[11] refined further the legal standard of what material information should be disclosed in a consent discussion. Canterbury became quadriplegic after a laminectomy. He then sued, claiming that he should have been informed about the low but finite likelihood of the significant complication of paralysis. The surgeons fulfilled the professional practice (reasonable physician) standard, but the court held that the disclosure was insufficient and, in the decision, generated the reasonable-person standard, as described earlier, which requires a physician to disclose the information that the hypothetical "reasonable patient" would consider important in making a decision to consent to an intervention.

Importantly, the two most powerful protections available to physicians in the medicolegal context are (1) the provision of a thorough and compassionate discussion of the risks and benefits of the proposed procedures with the patient, allowing time for all questions to be answered and (2) meticulous documentation of said discussions in the medical record.

Lastly, a few unique situations deserve some discussion. Same-day surgeries, preoperative evaluation clinics, emergency situations, and cases with multiple providers present challenges to the consent process, and anesthesiologists must be aware of these issues.

With the growth of same-day surgery and preoperative evaluation clinics over the past two decades, the practitioner who performs the preoperative evaluation and obtains informed consent is often not the anesthesiologist who will be actually providing anesthesia. Furthermore, in a same-day surgery setting, a patient may not even meet the anesthesiologist or participate in an informed consent discussion until minutes before the scheduled surgery. In this case, the rushed atmosphere may compromise the process. Anesthesiologists must be aware of this issue and develop organizational, institutional, and personal steps to minimize their impact on the informed consent process.

In emergency situations, the requirements for obtaining informed consent become less strict. Implied consent in these situations is predicated on the assumption that patients want life-sustaining treatment. If practical, anesthesiologists should attempt a consent process. However, in many emergencies, the patient is decisionally incapable and no surrogate decision-maker is available. In this situation, the expectation is to provide full resuscitative care, as previously described. It is prudent to favor life-sustaining treatments until all facts about the patient's wishes are known.

It is increasingly the case that patents are cared for more by a team of providers than by one individual. The consent process should make this as transparent as possible, with hospital policies and consent forms reflecting this reality. Some complex procedures have multiple teams of surgeons (e.g., cancer surgeries with lengthy free flap reconstructions) and may have multiple anesthesiologists. Again, this should be made explicitly clear to the patient.

Anesthesiologists are uniquely positioned in the process of informed consent. The vast majority of patients have already consented to surgery and therefore implicitly agreed to anesthesia. This leaves the focus on the anesthetic options and their relative risks and benefits. However, anesthesiologists are not absolved from having an awareness and understanding of the fundamental ethical principles of informed consent. Anesthesiologists play crucial roles throughout the hospital and may seek informed consent outside the immediate perioperative setting. Furthermore, all anesthesiologists are moral agents with a responsibility to the overall well-being and autonomous preferences of their patients. Institutional ethics consultative services are becoming increasingly available and may provide valuable assistance and guidance when complicated ethical issues arise. Lastly, to better understand the legal informed consent standards in their particular practice location, it is prudent for anesthesiologists to consult their institution's attorneys, personal attorneys, and local medical organizations.

CONCLUSION

- The basic components of informed consent are threshold elements (competence, decision-making capacity, and voluntariness), informational elements (disclosure, recommendation, and understanding), and consent elements (decision and autonomous authorization).

- The physician plays an important role as a "gatekeeper" to a declaration of incompetence.

- Physicians must seek to make strong recommendations without causing undue influence or coercion. Furthermore, physicians must ensure that external sources of coercive influence are eliminated when a decision is made.

- Adequate disclosure includes the facts a patient would consider material, the facts the physician would consider material, a recommendation, a description of the purpose of consent, and a description of the limits of consent.

- There are three standards of disclosure: the reasonable-physician standard, the reasonable-patient standard, and the particular-patient standard.

- If a patient is incapacitated or otherwise determined to be incompetent to make medical decisions, a surrogate decision-maker should be identified and possess the following qualifications: competence, adequate knowledge and information, emotional stability, and a commitment to the patient's interests that is free of coercion and conflicts of interest.

- The material risks of anesthesia must be distinguished from the risks of the surgery or procedure. Material risks should include common risks as well as rare but severe risks.

- In the context of acute illness, decision-making capacity is a dynamic process that must be assessed frequently.

- In the setting of ethical challenges that cannot be readily resolved, institutional ethics resources may be considered whenever appropriate and available.

- During an emergency with no immediately available surrogate decision-maker, the expectation is to pursue full resuscitative care. This can be discontinued once the patient's wishes have been clarified.

- Orders for DNR/DNI should be readdressed with the patient or surrogate decision-maker whenever presenting for a procedure requiring anesthesia.

REVIEW QUESTIONS

1. A 42-year-old man presents for an open reduction and internal fixation of a tibial plateau fracture. The anesthesiologist reviews the patient's medical history and consents him for general anesthesia. Which of the following is a key component of disclosure?

    a. A discussion of the common risks of general anesthesia.
    b. A discussion of the rare but serious risks of general anesthesia.
    c. A discussion of the alternatives of general anesthesia.
    d. All of the above.

The correct answer is d.

Disclosure is one of the informational elements of informed consent. There are five key parts to adequate disclosure:

   1. All facts a patient would consider material when deciding to consent or not to a procedure or treatment,

2. All information the physician deems to be material to the procedure or treatment,
3. A professional recommendation,
4. A description of the purpose of consent, and
5. A description of the limits of consent.

The anesthesiologist should always deem common risks, rare but serious risks, and possible alternatives as material information that should be discussed as part of the disclosure when seeking informed consent for anesthesia.

2. An elderly woman with lung cancer presents for an open thoracotomy and left upper lobectomy. The anesthesiologist strongly recommends an epidural for postoperative analgesia. The patient expresses concern about the safety of an epidural. The anesthesiologist tells her, "I'll do what I can, but you will probably have a lot of pain without the epidural." This risks violating which of the following elements of informed consent?

a. Voluntariness.
b. Competence.
c. Autonomous authorization.
d. Decision.

The correct answer is a.

Voluntariness is a component of the threshold elements. It requires that decisions be made by a patient that are free of coercion, including by means of force, fraud, deceit, duress, or other constraints. It also means the physician must make recommendations that are free of threats of force, harm, and abandonment. By appealing to the threat of uncontrollable pain, the anesthesiologist may place undue influence on the patient and risk violating the principle of voluntariness.

3. A 38-year-old woman has a past medical history of a cerebral arteriovenous malformation (AVM) complicated by an intracranial hemorrhage 1 year ago with associated neurological deficits, including mild intellectual disability and word-finding difficulties. The patient now presents for a complex AVM resection with significant risk of morbidity. The patient recently consented to anesthesia for an MRI for preoperative imaging. The patient struggles to recapitulate the risks of anesthesia for this much more complex intervention. Which of the following elements may not be satisfied for informed consent to take place?

a. Recommendation.
b. Understanding.
c. Decision-making capacity.
d. Disclosure.

The correct answer is b.

Understanding is another component of the informational elements. It is closely linked to the element of decision-making capacity. It essentially requires a patient to be able to clearly articulate a clear understanding of the nature of the proposed procedure, its potential risks and benefits, and the possible consequences of any decision. Importantly, understanding is a fluid concept that may change with increasing medical complexity.

4. A very nervous 21-year-old man presents for an appendectomy for acute appendicitis. The anesthesiologist reviews his medical history and begins to explain the risks of general anesthesia. The patient suddenly cuts off the anesthesiologists, stating, "Do whatever you have to do. You can knock me out but I don't want to know anything." Which of the following standards of disclosure would the anesthesiologist be following if she tailored her disclosure of risks of anesthesia to this patient's request?

a. Reasonable-physician standard.
b. Particular-patient standard.
c. Reasonable-patient standard.
d. None of the above.

The correct answer is b.

There are three basic standards of disclosure: the reasonable-physician standard, the reasonable-patient standard, and the particular-patient standard.

The reasonable-physician standard asks what material a reasonable physician in a given community would provide to a patient. The reasonable-patient standard, on the other hand, asks what a hypothetical reasonable patient in a given community would consider adequate information. Lastly, the particular-patient standard allows the physician to adjust the level of detail to match their particular patient's desire to know. While this is the most patient-centered approach, it is a loose standard, has not been adopted by the courts, and may leave a physician open to litigation if certain material risks were not adequately disclosed.

5. A 54-year-old woman with a history of schizoaffective disorder, mild intellectual disability, and tonsillar cancer presents with a fracture of the neck of her right femur after falling down some stairs. Three years ago, she had radiation of her head and neck, which was complicated by severe osteoradionecrosis requiring mandibulectomy with free flap reconstruction. Her intubation note describes three attempts at an awake intubation with a flexible video laryngoscope. On examination, the patient is noted to have trismus. The anesthesiologist begins to consent the patient for neuraxial anesthesia because of concerns about the airway. The patient demands general anesthesia, stating, "I had a spinal 30 years ago when I had a C-section and it was the worst experience of my life. Just put me to sleep!" The anesthesiologist is concerned she does not understand the serious risks of general anesthesia given her extremely high-risk airway and baseline cognitive deficits. What is the next best step?

a. Respect the patient's wishes and proceed with general anesthesia.
b. If available, consult psychiatry to assist with an assessment of capacity.
c. Consult with the hospital ethics committee.
d. Get a second opinion with a more senior colleague.
e. Answers b, c, and d.

The correct answer is e.

As previously discussed, the element of understanding is closely linked to decision-making capacity. A patient must be able to recapitulate the relevant information and indicate comprehension of the risks and benefits of consenting to a procedure and of declining a procedure. To have decision-making capacity, a patient must be able to arrive at an autonomous, voluntary choice after fully demonstrating understanding of the relevant information presented. In a situation of high acuity and high medical complexity, some patients may be unable to demonstrate enough understanding to possess decision-making capacity. If time permits, it is prudent to consult a psychiatrist for decision-making capacity as well as any available institutional ethics resources. It may also be helpful to obtain a second opinion from a senior colleague if available.

6. A frail 94-year-old man who lives alone is involved in a motor vehicle accident. He is unconscious at the scene and is transported by ambulance to the hospital. In the trauma bay, he is noted to be disoriented and combative. During evaluation, he develops progressive respiratory distress, which quickly deteriorates to hypoxemic respiratory failure and cardiac arrest. There are no family members present. What is the best next step?

    a. Defer cardiopulmonary resuscitation because the patient is too frail.
    b. Proceed with full resuscitative efforts.
    c. Attempt to locate and contact the patient's family to determine his wishes.
    d. Answers b and c.

The correct answer is d.

In emergency situations, the process of informed consent is less strict and not necessary. If practical, an abbreviated form of the consent process may be pursued. However, in many emergency situations, the patient is incapable of making decisions and a surrogate is not immediately available. If the patient's wishes are unknown, it is the expectation to go forward with full resuscitative care while attempting to contact a surrogate decision-maker. Life-sustaining interventions can always be discontinued if discovered after the fact to not be in line with the patient's previously stated goals of care.

7. Decision-making capacity is generally regarded as a dynamic process that may change with rapid changes in medical condition. True or false?

    a. True.
    b. False.

The correct answer is a.

Decision-making capacity is a fundamental component of the threshold elements of informed consent. As previously described, it is an ability to understand one's decision and its consequences at that moment in time. In the context of acute illness and medical care, this can be a very fluid, dynamic process. A patient who otherwise has decision-making capacity may lack capacity when delirious, intoxicated, or under the influence of sedatives or anesthetics. The physician must frequently assess for decision-making capacity and function as a gatekeeper to a declaration of incompetence. Importantly, competence is strictly a legal concept. It is determined by the court system alone. If a court declares an individual to be incompetent, it must appoint a surrogate decision-maker, which may be a family member, attorney, or someone else.

REFERENCES

1. Beauchamp T, Childress J. *Principles of Biomedical Ethics*. 7th ed. Oxford University Press; 2013.
2. The Nuremberg Code (1947). *Br Med J*. 1996;313:1448.
3. ASA Committee on Professional Liability. *Manual on Professional Liability*. American Society of Anesthesiologists; 2010:8–9.
4. Fernandez Lynch H, Joffe S, Feldman E. Informed consent and the role of the treating physician. *N Engl J Med*. 2018;378(25):2433–2438.
5. *Shinal v. Toms*, 162 A.3d 429 (PA. 2017).
6. American Society of Anesthesiologists. Statement on the ethical guidelines for the anesthesia care of patients with do-not-resuscitate orders or other directives that limit treatment. 2013.
7. American College of Surgeons. Statement on advance directives by patients: "Do not resuscitate" in the operating room. *Bull Am Coll Surg*. 2014;99(1):42–43.
8. AORN. *AORN Position Statement on Perioperative Care of Patients with Do-Not-Resuscitate or Allow-Natural-Death Orders*; 2014.
9. *Salgo v. Trustees of Leland Stanford Hospital*, 154 P.2d 560 (Cal. App 1957).
10. *Natanson v. Kline*, 350 P.2d 1093 (Kan. 1960).
11. *Canterbury v. Spence*, 464 F.2d 772 (D. C. Cir. 1972).

37.

CAN I REFUSE TO ANESTHETIZE THIS PATIENT?

Jeanna D. Blitz

STEM CASE AND KEY QUESTIONS

A 71-year-old man presents to the preoperative evaluation clinic in preparation for femoral-popliteal bypass surgery. The surgery is scheduled for 4 days from now.

You meet the patient and learn that his past medical history is significant for severe chronic obstructive pulmonary disease (COPD), morbid obesity, obstructive sleep apnea (OSA), atrial fibrillation, coronary artery disease (CAD) status post multiple cardiac stents, congestive heart failure (CHF), peripheral vascular disease (PVD), significant gastroesophageal reflux disease (GERD), hypothyroidism, hypercholesterolemia, and benign prostatic hypertrophy. The patient hands you his medication list (Table 37.1).

Upon questioning, he reports a half-block exercise tolerance due to dyspnea with exertion, as well as claudication in his lower extremities. You ask him how many pillows he sleeps on at night and he replies "a stack." He attributes this to both his orthopnea and the fact that when he is at less than 45 degrees upright, he experiences severe regurgitation that is not well controlled on his reflux medications. He is nonadherent with his continuous positive airway pressure (CPAP) therapy for his sleep apnea. He notes that he needs to get up several times at night to urinate and that taking the CPAP mask off and putting it back on is cumbersome; he also feels the CPAP therapy makes his reflux symptoms worse.

His past surgical history includes several prior cardiac catheterizations with placement of cardiac stents (in 1998, 2008, and 2019) and a laparoscopic cholecystectomy in 2013. His only known allergy is to pineapple. He presently smokes 1 pack of cigarettes per day (he has a 60 pack-year smoking history) but does not drink alcohol.

What is this patient's American Society of Anesthesiologist (ASA)'s Physical Classification (ASA-PS) score?

This patient is an ASA-PS 3, given his severe systemic diseases. While the ASA score is useful for communicating the patient's current health status, it is an example of a risk scale and not a specific prediction of an individual patient's risk when used alone. The current version of the ASA-PS classification system (Table 37.2) was published after a revision process by the ASA Committee on Economics and Professional Affairs.[1]

The surgery will be performed by the chief of vascular surgery. According to his consult note in the patient's medical record, the surgery is not urgent but is clearly indicated. The patient reports that he approached this surgeon to perform the surgery because they have been long-time neighbors. The patient desires the surgery to alleviate his severe leg pain and to be free of opioid pain medication, given what he has heard in recent news stories related to the dangers of the opioid crisis.

His social support system is poor. He is a retired art history professor who lives alone in an apartment complex and rarely has the opportunity to see his two grown children who live on the other side of the country. He has difficulty traveling due to his limited mobility and occasionally misses medical appointments for this reason.

On physical exam, you note that he is 65 inches tall and weighs 253 pounds (BMI = 42). He is sitting with his hands on his thighs, hunched forward and coughing up creamy beige sputum throughout the exam. He has poor dentition, and his airway exam reveals a Mallampati class 3 airway, with good mouth opening, a large tongue and a thick neck, and very limited neck extension. Auscultation of his heart and lungs reveals diffuse rhonchi and a 2/6 systolic murmur. The patient's room air saturation is noted to be 94%. His heart rate is 77 beats per minute and irregular, and his blood pressure is 162/98.

What details of his history and physical exam are you most concerned about? Which of these details are potentially modifiable prior to proceeding with surgery?

The patient exhibits several factors associated with an increased risk of developing postoperative pulmonary complications such as respiratory failure, pneumonia, prolonged ventilator use, and/or stay in the ICU. These risk factors include his age, BMI, current smoking status, COPD, poor functional status, ASA-PS score of 3, and the proposed plan for general endotracheal anesthesia.[3] An additional concern is his nonadherence with CPAP therapy for his OSA. Long-untreated sleep apnea may result in significant pulmonary and cardiac complications due to chronic exposure to hypoxemia. Sequelae of chronic OSA include hypertension, atrial fibrillation, myocardial infarction, stroke, pulmonary hypertension, the development of metabolic syndrome, and decreased quality of life due to daytime somnolence.

This patient's functional status is also extremely poor, most likely from a combination of his PVD and pulmonary and cardiac conditions. Poor functional status has been demonstrated to be an independent predictor of increased risk of mortality and major morbidity in the perioperative period. As such, it is included in several risk prediction tools

Table 37.1 **DAILY MEDICATION LIST**

Levalbuterol nebulizer 8 times daily	Apixaban 5 mg twice daily
Theophylline 200 mg/day	Clopidogrel 75 mg/day
Tiotropium bromide 2 puffs daily	Cilostazol 100 mg twice daily
Levothyroxine 112 mcg/day	Aspirin 325 mg/day
Pantoprazole 40 mg/day	Digoxin 125 mcg/day
Sucralfate 1 g three times daily	Oxycodone/acetaminophen 5 mg/325 mg every 6 hours
Fluticasone spray as needed	Diltiazem 240 mg/day
Potassium 20 mEq daily	Losartan 25 mg/day
Finasteride 5 mg/day	Furosemide 60 mg/day
Silodosin 4 mg every evening	Atorvastatin 40 mg every evening

Table 37.2 **DEFINITIONS OF AMERICAN SOCIETY OF ANESTHESIOLOGISTS PHYSICAL STATUS (ASA PS)**[2]

ASA PS	DESCRIPTION
I	A normal healthy patient
II	A patient with mild systemic disease
III	A patient with severe systemic disease
IV	A patient with severe systemic disease that is a constant threat to life
V	A moribund patient who is not expected to survive without the operation
VI	A declared brain-dead patient whose organs are being removed for donor purposes

Used with permission from the American Society of Anesthesiologists. ASA Physical Status Classification System (asahq.org).

such as the American College of Surgeons National Surgical Quality Improvement Program (NSQIP) calculator and the National Surgical Quality Improvement Program Myocardial Infarction or Cardiac Arrest calculator (MICA) and forms the basis of the ASA-PS score assignment.[2,4,5] His poor functional status, when combined with his significant cardiac history, raises concern about his perioperative risk even further. His uncontrolled GERD is concerning, given his inability to lie flat due to regurgitation; this may increase his risk of aspiration. Finally, another concern is this patient's poor social support system, which may lead to a prolonged length of hospital stay, increase his risk of readmission after discharge, and may result in the need for discharge to a skilled nursing facility.

Of the factors noted above, the timing of the surgery, reinstitution of his CPAP therapy, improvement of his poorly controlled hypertension, his current tobacco use, and potential alternatives to a general endotracheal anesthetic are potentially modifiable. His productive cough is concerning for a current COPD exacerbation; delay of surgery in favor of treatment of his exacerbation and potentially even initiation of a prehabilitation program of exercise may be of benefit. Prehabilitation has been demonstrated to improve outcomes in high-risk patients prior to surgery[6]; however, given the patient's current claudication symptoms, this may not be an option for our particular patient. This patient's nonadherence with his CPAP mask must be addressed. Reinitiation of his CPAP use prior to surgery may improve his postoperative respiratory outcomes. His lack of support system should be addressed. It is to the patient's benefit to have him undergo a social work assessment to create a plan for his postoperative care and disposition prior to proceeding with the surgery.[7] Finally, there is an opportunity to better control his hypertension.

How would you counsel him regarding his current smoking habit? What if surgery were tomorrow?

The impact of smoking on perioperative morbidity and mortality may be significantly underrated. Smokers are at a 40% increased odds of 30-day mortality as well as 30–100% increased odds of morbidity related to surgical site infection, unplanned intubation, pneumonia, sepsis, length of stay, and a higher utilization of postoperative ICU services. This is attributed to decreased macrophage function, a reduction in coronary flow reserve, and vascular endothelial dysfunction. Patients should be counseled to quit smoking at any time prior to surgery, including the day before. Benefits of smoking cessation are seen within 12 hours: carbon monoxide and cyanide levels decrease and lower nicotine levels improve vasodilatation and oxygen delivery and utilization, resulting in improvement in wound healing.[8]

What preoperative tests will you require the patient to have to proceed with the surgery? Can you justify how the results of the tests you have ordered will influence the patient's perioperative outcomes?

The ASA published a Practice Advisory for the Preanesthesia Evaluation.[9] In the document, the task force recommends that preoperative tests should not be ordered routinely; rather, they should be performed on a selective basis for the purposes of guiding or optimizing perioperative management. The Practice Advisory emphasizes that a thorough preoperative history and physical exam are the most important components of the preanesthesia evaluation and should guide any preoperative lab testing and workup. It is also important to note that it is not recommended to repeat test results that are present in the medical record within 6 months of surgery provided there has been no significant change in the patient's medical history. The task force also recognized that, in older patients or those with multiple cardiac risk factors, ECG abnormalities may be more frequent; therefore, age alone is no longer considered an indication for a preoperative ECG. Although tests such as pulmonary function testing (PFTs), chest radiograph, and arterial blood gas may confirm clinical suspicions or qualify the severity of the pulmonary disease, they should be obtained only in selected patients where knowledge of the result of the test will change perioperative management. PFTs and hypercarbia are not accurate predictors of post-procedural complications, and only 2% of chest x-ray (CXR) abnormalities discovered on preoperative examination led to a change in management in a systematic review.

Given that this is a high-risk surgery on a patient with multiple comorbidities including OSA, atrial fibrillation, CAD, CHF, and poor functional status, a preoperative CBC, basic metabolic panel, and ECG are appropriate. Review of an echocardiogram within the past 2 years (in the absence of significant clinical change) may also be useful in this patient.

He has had a CBC and comprehensive metabolic profile within the past 2 months; results are within normal limits, with the exception of a creatinine level of 1.6 (glomerular filtration rate [GFR] is 43 mL/min/1.73 m^2). His ECG reveals atrial fibrillation. An echocardiogram report from 9 months ago revealed a low-normal left ventricular ejection fraction, but the left ventricular filling pattern is consistent with impaired relaxation. There is mild right atrial dilatation and right ventricular enlargement. The patient has not undergone a stress test in more than 7 years.

You contact the patient's pulmonologist from another nearby academic institution to discuss the extent of the patient's pulmonary disease. She offers to send you the results of his most recent PFTs, as well as a CXR that was performed within the past 3 months. His PFTs reveal severe expiratory airflow limitation with an FVC of 120% predicted and an FEV$_1$/FVC of 47%. Flows show no improvement with bronchodilator. His diffusion capacity is moderately reduced. The chest radiography report includes the following line: "aspiration PNA remains a consideration." Along with the medical records, she includes a consultation letter stating that the "severity of the patient's pulmonary disease, poor pulmonary function and chronic productive cough put this patient at extremely high risk for pulmonary complications including respiratory failure and pneumonia." She writes that the patient is "too high a risk for anesthesia" and "will not clear him" for the proposed surgery.

Are you willing to go against the pulmonologist's written recommendations that the patient not undergo this surgery?

A preoperative discussion with this patient's pulmonologist, cardiologist, or other providers with whom he has an enduring relationship is valuable when creating the perioperative optimization plan for this patient. It should be emphasized that the goal of the discussion with other providers lies in the ability to capture a robust, detailed patient history and gain an understanding of the patient's physical status over time; by contrast, a written "clearance" note by other providers in most cases offers little additional value or medico-legal protection.[10] Prior studies even found that preoperative consultations provided by physicians who are *not* specifically trained in perioperative medicine are associated with increased hospital stay and postoperative mortality.[11,12] It is important to consult with our medical colleagues when a specific question arises related to the perioperative management of the patient; however, we must also keep in mind that we are not asking permission from the patient's medical doctors to proceed with surgery and anesthesia but rather engaging them as partners in a model of shared decision-making. While preoperative PFTs and a CXR are not clearly indicated for this patient, review of any relevant preexisting test results is an important component of a thorough preanesthesia evaluation.[9] Ultimately, the decision regarding whether to proceed with surgery is the patient's. The patient has the right to a discussion exploring his goals related to surgery and to be informed of the risks and benefits of the proposed operation.[13]

What is this patient's perioperative risk?

The perioperative mortality rate for patients assigned an ASA-PS score of 3 is reported to be 1.8–4.3%, and up to 23% for an ASA 4 patient.[14] However, it is important to note that to truly predict this patient's global perioperative risk, the ASA-PS score cannot be used alone. A risk prediction tool such as the NSQIP calculator must be used.[4] The patient's global perioperative risk is a combination of surgical risk and individual patient physical status risk, and each risk factor may not be simply additive: certain medical conditions, such as chronic kidney disease and anemia, act as "risk multipliers" in the perioperative period. Other conditions are inextricably linked: patients with significant PVD are likely to also have cardiac or cerebrovascular disease, increasing their risk of major adverse cardiac and cerebrovascular events. Furthermore, peripheral vascular surgery is considered high risk for the development of major adverse cardiac events (MACE) including death and myocardial infarction due to the inherent severity of the surgery. Prior risk scores such as the Revised Cardiac Risk Index (RCRI) substantially underestimate cardiac risk in patients presenting for vascular surgery. The Vascular Study Group of New England (VSGNE)[15] developed a risk index specifically to accurately assess risk related to vascular surgery. A specific risk scoring tool for each type of vascular surgery is available online.[16] Using the online risk scoring tool specific to infra-inguinal bypass, this patient has a predicted risk of postoperative myocardial infarction of 2% if his preoperative stress test results are abnormal. Without the benefits of recent (within past 2 years) results of this test, his estimated risk is reported as 1.3%. VSGNE also includes a separate risk prediction tool to predict postoperative pulmonary complications; the factors used to calculate risk include BMI, GFR, age, tobacco use, history of CHF, COPD, functional status, type of surgery, urgency of procedure, transfer from home versus skilled facility, and need for dialysis. Application of this risk predictor for our patient reveals a risk of 6.2% for developing postoperative pneumonia or respiratory failure.

The NSQIP calculator may be used to predict a patient's risk of a multitude of serious complications compared to the average patient's risk. Inputting our hypothetical patient's information into this model reveals that he is at higher risk than the average patient in all categories measured, including mortality (1.2%), pneumonia (2.9%), cardiac complications (3.2%), readmission (16.8%), and discharge to a skilled nursing facility (25%) (Figure 37.1).

You call the surgeon to discuss your assessment of this patient's perioperative risk and to devise a perioperative plan to see him through surgery and the recovery period safely. He agrees to a meeting with you and the patient. The surgeon reassures the patient that this is a very simple procedure and

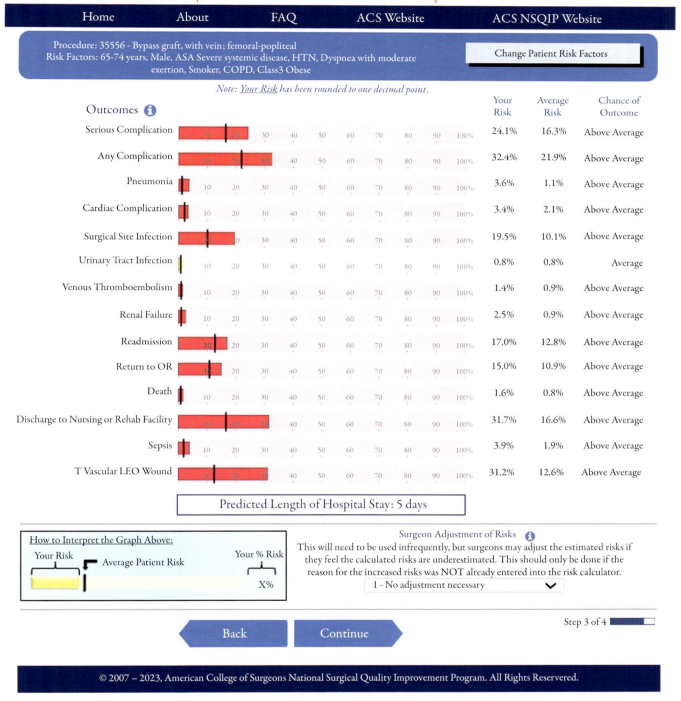

Figure 37.1 American College of Surgeons National Surgical Quality Improvement Program (NSQIP) Risk Calculator report for our hypothetical patient.
Used with permission https://riskcalculator.facs.org/RiskCalculator/

that he does not anticipate any of these complications. He informs you that he performs this surgery under "light anesthesia" "all the time" and that he just wants you to make sure that the patient "won't cough" while he is operating.

How do you respond to the surgeon? Is there anything else that you would like to discuss with him?

You address the pulmonologist's assessment and concerns with the patient and the surgeon. You also point out that the patient is unable to lie supine due to dyspnea, a chronic cough, and regurgitation of gastric contents. The surgeon is not concerned by this, pointing out that the patient underwent a cardiac catheterization procedure as recently as 4 years ago and was able to tolerate lying supine. Furthermore, he is concerned that if the PVD is left untreated, the patient may eventually require emergency surgery, which he feels would put the patient at even greater risk than undertaking an elective approach. When you ask, he notes that a percutaneous transluminal angioplasty is not an option. Given that the plan is for the patient to remain on his antiplatelet and anticoagulant medications, you inform the patient that he is not a candidate for neuraxial block with light sedation and that the plan would be to proceed with a general endotracheal anesthetic, despite his increased risk.

You emphasize to the patient that there are significant risks associated with proceeding with surgery at this time. You note that the information gained from a preoperative stress test would help you better determine his risk of postoperative cardiac complications including heart attack and death, and you recommend that he undergo this test. The patient refuses your recommendation, noting that he does not want a stress test, asking "what's the point?" He tells you that he has already gone through multiple cardiac catheterizations and placement of stents and it was a terrible experience because he was "forced" to lie supine—a position that he cannot tolerate due to his dyspnea and symptoms of regurgitation. Furthermore, his perception is that the prior cardiac stent procedures have not improved his health status appreciably. He says he doesn't want any further cardiac interventions and would rather risk a heart attack to have this surgery.

In response to your recommendations that he begin a smoking cessation program, he reports that he is not ready to quit and that he uses smoking to help him cope with his constant pain related to his PVD. He shares that once he is able to undergo the fem-pop bypass and his leg pain improves, he plans to wean off of his opioid pain medications, quit smoking, and begin a walking program to improve his functional status. A significant part of his desire for surgery is because he believes it will reduce his pain and allow him to wean off of his long-term opioids, which he is worried about becoming dependent on.

Furthermore, he notes that his serious regurgitation prevents him from using his CPAP mask as recommended. He again insists that his preference is to proceed with the vascular surgery in his current condition, albeit at higher risk.

You believe that your recommendations for a preoperative stress test and optimization of his pulmonary status are important and would impact the patient's perioperative management and outcomes. Can you refuse to anesthetize this patient and prevent him from proceeding with surgery?

Patient autonomy is one of the major principles of medical ethics. Patients have the right to consent to or refuse treatment. This patient wants the procedure and appears to understand the associated risks.

Informed consent requires the presence of three elements: voluntariness, adequate information, and the capacity to decide.[17] The patient has made a voluntary decision to proceed with surgery. While his constant pain may be considered a coercive factor, his desire to wean off opioid medication and improve his functional status by treating his PVD can be viewed as rational reasons to proceed. His reasons reflect an appropriate understanding and realistic goals for the proposed surgery. He has clearly expressed his desire to proceed with surgery without additional testing or optimization without coercion, and he articulated rational reasons. Furthermore, he has been given all the information he needs to make an informed decision. Elements of an informed decision include an assessment of *risk*, knowledge of the *benefits* of the surgery, and the *alternatives* to the proposed treatment that are available.

Although we cannot quantitate his specific risk without the further testing that he does not want, he understands that he is at higher risk than the average patient who has this surgery. He has articulated the *benefits* of femoral-popliteal bypass surgery, including a reduction in his leg pain. Finally, he is aware that the alternative to this surgery is conservative therapy. He has been clear that the conservative approach is not offering him the pain relief and quality of life that he wants.

Although it is possible for a patient's decision-making capacity to become clouded by opiate use, this does not appear to be the case in this scenario. Given that the elements required for informed decision-making are present, we must conclude that the patient is giving informed consent to proceed with this high-risk surgery at increased risk. Refusing to anesthetize him would violate this patient's autonomy.[10]

Ultimately, the patient proceeds to surgery. He undergoes an uneventful right femoral-popliteal arterial bypass under a general endotracheal anesthetic including standard monitors and an arterial line. The patient's discharge home is delayed by his inability to urinate postoperatively, difficulty with pain management, and lack of a support system at home to assist with his recovery, but he is eventually discharged on postoperative day 5.

Was this patient's visit to the preoperative clinic warranted?

We can make the case that, in patients with a high burden of preexisting comorbidities or unfavorable social determinants of health, a well-coordinated preoperative evaluation clinic visit will add value with regard to improving clinical outcomes, fostering shared decision-making, and decreasing unnecessary resource utilization. In the case of this patient, although he refused the recommendations of the preoperative medicine specialist, the visit afforded his care team the ability to plan for his case and ensure that the patient's decision to proceed with surgery was informed and free from coercion.

DISCUSSION

Current reform of our national healthcare delivery system includes a movement toward cost-effective, coordinated care with an emphasis on comparative effectiveness research. With this paradigm shift comes tremendous opportunity for anesthesiologists. As Drs. Grocott and Pearse proclaimed in a 2012 editorial in the *British Journal of Anaesthesia*, "Perioperative medicine is the future of anaesthesia, if our specialty is to thrive."[18] As leaders of the perioperative team, our goals are several-fold: risk stratification and medical optimization, facilitation of communication among all members of the interdisciplinary team (including the patient), and patient education. In patients with increased perioperative risk related to preexisting comorbidities, their social situations, or a low level of health literacy, an in-person preoperative evaluation clinic visit will likely facilitate achieving shared perioperative goals including obtaining true informed consent.

Anesthesiologists have earned the right to view themselves as the "patient's protector" throughout the perioperative period due to the specialty's long-lived commitment to patient safety. However, our desire to protect the patient from adverse outcomes must be balanced with the patient's goals and desires. The current focus on including the patient in the decision-making process requires that we understand the primary principles of medical ethics. These include *patient autonomy*, *beneficence* (promoting good), *nonmaleficence* (avoiding harm), and *justice* (giving to each that which is his due).[13,17] An informed decision-making process includes the application of these key principles in a 2-step approach:

An Evidence-Based Assessment of Perioperative Risk

Overall risk is a combination of surgical risk, risk-related to the patient's comorbidities and physical status, and risk related to social and behavioral health issues such as smoking status, support system, stability of home life, access to nutrition, and psychological state.[19] The need exists for an entirely objective index of a patient's health status that incorporates *all* domains that impact a patient's perioperative outcomes. In the absence of one gold standard to assess overall risk, several risk predictors and screening tools may need to be combined to present a complete picture of risk to the patient. Well-validated risk prediction tools, such as the VSGNE and ACS NSQIP, may be combined with a frailty assessment tool,[20] the Brief Health Literacy Assessment tool,[21] or the pain catastrophization score[22] as indicated.

It is important that risk stratification occur in the context of presenting potential opportunities for the patient to mitigate the risk. For example, the American Heart Association guidelines for risk assessment prior to noncardiac surgery[23] recommend that preoperative stress testing is indicated for this patient whose calculated risk of MACE is greater than 1% *only if* the results will change our management. The results of the stress test may influence our recommendations for risk reduction strategies including preoperative adjustment of his medications (beneficence); however, it can be argued that we may also take the approach of assuming that the patient's stress test will be positive and thus tailor the anesthetic plan accordingly.

Obtaining Informed Consent

The principle of patient autonomy acknowledges that patients have the right to consent to or refuse treatment. The three elements of consent are voluntariness, adequate information, and the capacity to act.[13] This patient is voluntarily requesting the procedure. The information that he must be given to make an informed choice includes

1. The *risk* of proceeding with the proposed surgery and anesthetic. The discussion and presentation of risk should extend beyond risk of death and morbidity to include a discussion of the possibility of discharge to a skilled nursing facility and the potential loss of independence (whether temporary or permanent), as well as any other risks that are relevant to the patient's desired goals and other factors that the patient has identified as most important to him.

2. The *benefits* of the fem-pop bypass must also be clearly articulated to him. A discussion of the benefits facilitates the setting of expectations for the perioperative course and allows us to address any potential goal misalignment related to the proposed benefits versus the patient's perception of what the surgery will accomplish.

3. The *alternative* forms of treatment, including conservative therapy, and opting to forego any further treatment.

If these three elements are achieved, we should conclude that he has given his informed consent. Refusing to anesthetize him would violate his autonomy in this particular clinical scenario.

Finally, an assessment of the patient's capacity to act must occur. A patient is deemed to have capacity when he has the ability to communicate a choice, understand the information necessary to make the decision, appreciate the implications of the choice, and weigh options and consequences of the potential decision.[24]

Under what circumstances can a physician refuse to treat a patient? The answer to this question hinges on the ability to establish ethical grounds for the refusal of care and whether or not a doctor–patient relationship already exists. If no prior relationship between the physician and patient exists, the physician is not required to initiate care, except in an emergency.[10] However, it is unethical for physicians to refuse to initiate care based on a bias against patients with specific characteristics or demographics. If a prior relationship does exist and the physician wishes to divorce herself from the patient's care, she must give the patient adequate notice and assist in finding another physician who is equally or more qualified to assume care of the patient. If transfer of care to another equally qualified physician does not occur, the physician can be accused of patient abandonment, which is illegal.[10]

Physicians have a moral duty to provide healthcare. The anesthesiologist in this clinical scenario is employed by the hospital where this patient has presented for treatment, and they have been assigned to provide a professional service for him. In this case, the surgeon and the patient have already agreed to accept the substantial surgical risk for the benefit of pain relief and better function. The anesthesiologist may not be able to refuse to participate in the patient's care solely on the grounds of "riskiness" if all elements of informed consent are present. On the one hand, anesthesiologists may only decline to treat a patient if they have a religious or moral objection to the proposed procedure.[10] On the other hand, a medical professional cannot be forced to provide care that they judge unsafe, below the professional standard for safe care, or harmful to the patient because providing care under these circumstances would violate the ethical principle of nonmaleficence.[13] However, this argument must exist separate from the desire to avoid a lawsuit in the event of an adverse outcome.[10]

While the anesthesiologist may not refuse to care for this patient on the grounds of increased risk alone, they have the responsibility to inform the patient about opportunities to mitigate his risk and educate the patient about behavioral changes that will impact his long-term health in order to fulfill the ethical principle of justice. Personally relevant, pre-hospital education can be used to motivate patients, thus increasing optimization, reducing length of stay, and adjusting patient expectations about surgical outcome.[25] Additionally, patients who participate in decision-making may have higher satisfaction and improved engagement and adherence with health recommendations.[26] Often, the perioperative period represents a window of opportunity when patients may be most receptive to making behavioral and health changes that extend beyond the perioperative period. For example, smoking cessation counseling during the preoperative clinic visit has significant impact on both short- and long-term quit rates.[27,28]

The anesthesiologist also has a responsibility to both the patient and institution to provide care that is not wasteful of resources or that exposes the patient to additional test-related risk due to false positives and follow-up interventions. This would violate the ethical principle of nonmaleficence. When a patient is refusing further preoperative testing, the physician must respect the patient's decision unless it would clearly lead to care that was futile or substandard by professional guidelines.[13] Another potential way that a patient may be exposed to harm through preoperative testing is related to the financial cost incurred by the test as well as the financial and physical cost of any complications that occur. As Hug articulated in his Rovenstine memorial lecture: "We need to separate what we can do from what we should do."[29] Physicians are ethically obligated to abide by the patient's decision to refuse treatment no matter how strongly we disagree with their decision; otherwise, we physicians risk violating laws that exist to protect the patient from what could be considered abuse, battery, or coercion.[30] Our goal is to provide our patients with a shared decision-making process rooted in the principles of medical ethics and informed by evidence. The proposed perioperative plan should be designed to maximize potential benefits and minimize potential harm in accordance with the patient's own values. While there is no agreed upon method for resolving conflicts between two or more ethics principles, each decision should be made within the context of the given case.[31]

CONCLUSION

- Goals of the preoperative patient evaluation include risk stratification and medical optimization, facilitation of communication among all members of the interdisciplinary team, care coordination, and patient education.

- The primary principles of medical ethics are patient autonomy, beneficence (promoting good), nonmaleficence (avoiding harm), and justice (giving to each that which is his due).

- An informed decision-making process must include an evidence-based assessment of perioperative risk and the obtaining of informed consent.

- The elements required for consent are voluntariness, adequate information, and the capacity to act.

- The principle of patient autonomy acknowledges that patients have the right to consent to or refuse treatment.

- Physicians may refuse to provide care only if a doctor–patient relationship does not already exist, except in an emergency.

- Physicians cannot be forced to provide care that they judge to be below the professional standard for safe care or harmful to the patient because this would violate the ethical principle of nonmaleficence.

- Physicians have a responsibility to inform the patient about their risk as well as opportunities to mitigate risk, in order to fulfill the ethical principle of justice.

REVIEW QUESTIONS

1. Predictors of postoperative pulmonary complications include

   a. Current cigarette use.
   b. BMI of 30 or higher.
   c. COPD.
   d. All of the above.

   The correct answer is d.

   Other risk factors for the development of postoperative pulmonary complications include CHF; age; poor functional status; low albumin levels; ASA-PS score 3 or higher; intrathoracic, upper abdominal, or surgery on the head and neck; and proposed general endotracheal anesthesia.

2. Patients who are current cigarette smokers should be advised to

   a. Quit smoking preoperatively, regardless of surgical time frame.
   b. Quit only if surgery is more than 2 weeks away.
   c. Quit only if surgery is more than 4 weeks away.
   d. Quit only if date of surgery is more than 8 weeks away.

   The correct answer is a.

   Patients should be counseled to quit smoking at any time prior to surgery, including the day before. Benefits of smoking cessation are seen within 12 hours: carbon monoxide and cyanide levels decrease and lower nicotine levels improve vasodilatation and oxygen delivery and utilization, resulting in improvement in wound healing. An increase in quit rate up to

1 year postoperatively after exposure to preoperative smoking cessation counseling is also possible.

3. Examples of a risk prediction tool include

   a. NSQIP calculator.
   b. ASA-PS score.
   c. RCRI score.
   d. Brief Health Literacy assessment tool.

The correct answer is a.

The ACS NSQIP calculator is an example of a risk prediction tool; it is capable of providing a risk profile specific to each individual patient. The other options listed are examples of a risk scale (ASA-PS score), risk score (RCRI), and a screening tool (Brief Health Literacy tool).

4. The *best* example of the principle of nonmaleficence is

   a. Treating all patients equitably.
   b. Avoiding routine preoperative testing without clinical indication.
   c. Not offering alternative procedures that are deemed high risk.
   d. Promoting good health through patient-centered health coaching.

The correct answer is b.

Providing equitable treatment to all patients represents the principle of justice. Not offering alternatives associated with risk violates the elements required to obtain informed consent as well as the principle of patient autonomy. Promotion of good health represents beneficence.

5. To provide informed consent, the following must be present (select all that apply):

   a. The risk of proceeding with the proposed surgery and anesthetic.
   b. The benefits of proceeding with the proposed surgery and anesthetic.
   c. The alternatives to the proposed treatment, including conservative therapy and opting to forego any further treatment.
   d. Capacity to act.

The correct answer is a, b, c, and d.

Elements required for consent are voluntariness, adequate information about both the perioperative risks and benefits, and the capacity to act.

REFERENCES

1. Sweitzer BJ. Three wise men (x2) and the ASA-physical status classification system. *Anesthesiology*. 2017 Apr;126:577–578.
2. American Society of Anesthesiologists. Statement on ASA physical status classification system. 2014 Oct. https://www.asahq.org/standards-and-guidelines/asa-physical-status-classification-system
3. Johnson RG, Arozullah AM, Neumayer L, et al. Multivariable predictors of postoperative respiratory failure after general and vascular surgery: Results from the patient safety in surgery study. *J Am Coll Surg*. 2007;204:1188–1198.
4. American College of Surgeons. Surgical risk calculator. https://riskcalculator.facs.org/RiskCalculator/
5. Gupta PK, Gupta H, Sundaram A, et al. Development and validation of a risk calculator for prediction of cardiac risk after surgery. *Circulation*. 2011;124(4):381.
6. Banugo P, Amoako D. Prehabilitation. *BJA Educ*. 2017;17(12): 401–405.
7. Hoel AW, Zamor KC. Transitions of care and long-term surveillance after vascular surgery. *Semin Vasc Surg*. 2015 Jun;28(2):134–140.
8. Wong J, et al. Short-term preoperative smoking cessation and postoperative complications: A systematic review and meta-analysis. *Can J Anaesth*. 2012;59:268–279.
9. American Society of Anesthesiologists Task Force. Practice advisory for preanesthesia evaluation: An updated report by the American Society of Anesthesiologists Task Force on preanesthesia evaluation. *Anesthesiology*. 2012 Mar;116(3):522–538.
10. ASA syllabus on ethics: Informed consent. https://pubs.asahq.org/monitor/article-abstract/81/5/50/5926/Ethics-Resources?redirectedFrom=fulltext
11. Wijeysundera DN, Austin PC, Beattie WS, Hux JE, Laupacis A. Outcomes and processes of care related to preoperative medical consultation. *Arch Intern Med*. 2010;170:1365–1374.
12. Beckerleg W, Kobewka D, Wijeysundera D, Sood MM, McIsaac DI. Association of preoperative medical consultation with reduction in adverse outcomes and use processes of care among residents of Ontario, Canada. *JAMA Int Med*. 2023 May; 183(5):470–478.
13. Van Norman, G. Preoperative testing: Ethical challenges, evidence-based medicine and informed consent. In: Jericho BG, ed., *Ethical Issues in Anesthesiology and Surgery*. Springer International; 2015:17–31.
14. Morgan GE Jr, Mikhail MS, Murray MJ. Clinical Anesthesiology. 3rd ed. McGraw Hill; 2002:156–159.
15. Bertges DJ, Neal D, Schanzer A, et al. The vascular quality initiative cardiac risk index for prediction of myocardial infarction after vascular surgery. *J Vasc Surg*. 2016 Nov;64(5):1411–1421.
16. QxMD. Estimate peri-operative risk around the time of vascular surgery using vascular quality initiative risk calculators. https://qxmd.com/vascular-study-group-new-england-decision-support-tools
17. Beauchamp T, Childress J. *Principles of Biomedical Ethics*. 7th ed. Oxford University Press; 2013.
18. Grocott MPW, Pearse RM. Perioperative medicine: The future of anaesthesia? *Br J Anaesth*. 2012;108(5):723–726.
19. Magnan, S. *Social Determinants of Health 101 for Health Care: Five Plus Five. NAM Perspectives*. Discussion paper. National Academy of Medicine; 2017. doi:10.31478/201710c
20. Darvall JN, Loth J, Bose T, et al. Accuracy of the Clinical Frailty Scale for perioperative frailty screening: A prospective observational study. *Can J Anaesth*. 2020 Jun;67(6):694–705.
21. Chew LD, Bradley KA, Boyko EJ. Brief questions to identify patients with inadequate health literacy. *Fam Med*. 2004;36(8):588–594.
22. Sullivan MJL. *The Pain Catastrophizing Scale: User Manual*. McGill University; 2009.
23. Fleisher LA, Fleischmann KE, Auerbach AD, et al. ACC/AHA Guideline on perioperative cardiovascular evaluation and management of patients undergoing noncardiac surgery: A report of the American College of Cardiology/ American Heart Association Task Force on practice guidelines. *J Am Coll Cardiol*. 2014 Dec 9;64(22):e77–137.
24. Appelbaum PS. Clinical practice: Assessment of patients' competence to consent to treatment. *N Engl J Med*. 2007;357:1834–1840.
25. Martindale RG, Deveney CW. Preoperative risk reduction: Strategies to optimize outcomes. *Surg Clin N Am*. 2013;93:1041–1055.
26. Yoon RS, Nellans KW, Geller JA, Kim AD, Jacobs MR, Macaulay W. Patient education before hip or knee arthroplasty lowers length of stay. *J Arthroplasty*. 2010;25:547–551.
27. Zaki A, Abrishami A, Wong J, et al. Interventions in the preoperative clinic for long term smoking cessation: A quantitative systematic review. *Can J Anaesth*. 2008;55:11–21.

28. Wong J, Abrishami A, Yang Y, et al. A perioperative smoking cessation intervention with varenicline: A double-blind, randomized, placebo-controlled trial. *Anesthesiology*. 2012;117:755–764.
29. Hug CC Jr. Rovenstine lecture: Patient values, Hippocrates, science, and technology: What we (physicians) can do versus what we could do for the patient. *Anesthesiology*. 2000;93(2):556–564.
30. Van Norman GA, Palmer SK. The ethical boundaries of persuasion: Coercion and restraint of patients in clinical anesthesia practice. *Int Anesthesiol Clin*. 2001;39(3):131–143.
31. Jonsen A, Siegler M, Winslade W. *Ethics*. 7th ed. McGraw-Hill Medical; 2010.

38.

DIFFICULT CONVERSATIONS

Laura J. Ostapenko and Katherine A. Hill

STEM CASE AND KEY QUESTIONS

A 65-year-old woman was recently hospitalized with cholecystitis. Upon presenting to the emergency department with abdominal pain for the past 2 weeks, she was found to have fever, tachycardia, and hypotension along with right upper quadrant ultrasound findings of a thickened gallbladder wall surrounded by pericholecystic fluid. After broad-spectrum antibiotic therapy and fluid resuscitation, she continued to need vasopressor therapy to treat her hypotension. Blood cultures demonstrated bacteremia. Given her clinical picture, the general surgery team did not offer a cholecystectomy for source control of her cholecystitis. Instead, the acute care surgery team recommended a consult to interventional radiology (IR) for placement of a percutaneous cholecystostomy drain.

What is shared decision-making? What are clinical scenarios in which clinicians should employ shared decision-making prior to making a recommendation?

The cholecystostomy drain was successfully placed by IR. Over the next days, her clinical status improved, and she was ready for discharge on oral antibiotics with the cholecystostomy drain in place. At discharge, she was given an appointment for follow-up in the acute-care surgery outpatient clinic. She was told that at that appointment she would discuss how to further manage the percutaneous cholecystostomy tube.

What are common structured communication tools used to facilitate medical decision-making? What are their common elements?

The patient arrived for her outpatient follow-up appointment with acute-care surgery. She tells the nurse who roomed her that she does not want to have surgery because she is worried about her heart, but she also "hates this darn tube," and she continues to have postprandial episodes of pain. The acute-care surgeon reviews her imaging, which shows a thickened and contracted gallbladder indicative of chronic cholecystitis and cholelithiasis; biliary nuclear imaging shows that the cystic duct remains obstructed. The surgeon pauses to consider, as this does not look like a routine laparoscopic cholecystectomy.

How can a clinician prepare for a medical decision-making conversation?

After a review of the patient's post-hospital course and a physical exam, the surgeon sits down to discuss treatment options with her.

The surgeon says, "I'm glad we got you through that hospitalization, but we should talk about what's next. Would it be ok to summarize where things are with your gallbladder? You had life-threatening gallbladder inflammation, or cholecystitis, that we needed to treat with that tube and antibiotics, rather than surgery, because of how unstable you were. Now, you still have gallstones and what looks like chronic inflammation of your gallbladder. The most definitive way to improve your symptoms, remove the tube, and prevent further episodes is a surgery to remove the gallbladder. For you, I think there's a higher chance of an open procedure, but I would still start by trying a laparoscopic approach." The surgeon goes on to describe the operation, its risks, and the typical postoperative course.

The surgeon and patient agree to move forward toward surgery. The surgeon tells the patient that the next step is for the patient to be referred to the hospital's preoperative clinic. The preoperative clinic will help the patient prepare for surgery.

What elements of a shared-decision-making conversation can you identify in what the surgeon said? What suggestions do you have that could have made it better?

When the preoperative clinic receives the referral, a nurse does a chart review and finds an echocardiogram from 5 years ago that reports mild-moderate pulmonary hypertension with recommendation for yearly cardiology follow-up. However, this follow-up did not occur. Prior to the patient's preoperative clinic appointment, an echocardiogram is ordered to assess the patient's current heart structure and function. The echocardiogram shows normal right ventricular structure and function but likely moderate-severe pulmonary hypertension based on a tricuspid regurgitant jet.

How can a clinician reframe a conversation in the setting of new medical information? What do you feel as you approach a difficult conversation?

At her preoperative clinic appointment, the patient sits down with an anesthesiologist. After reviewing the patient's medical record, interviewing the patient, and performing a clinical examination, the anesthesiologist discusses treatment options with the patient in the setting of this new clinical information. Using structured communication tools, the anesthesiologist sets the stage for the conversation, assures a shared medical context, and clarifies the patient's values in the setting of the new shared medical context.

What might the anesthesiologist say to set the stage? How might he assure a shared medical context?

The anesthesiologist suggests a conversation to talk about the echocardiogram results as well as the patient's health overall and what those things mean for upcoming surgery. The anesthesiologist also asks whether anyone else ought to be part of the conversation and ensures a quiet room without interruptions. With the patient's permission to proceed, the anesthesiologist conveys that the patient's echocardiogram showed worsening pulmonary hypertension, or high blood pressure in the lungs, which affects the way the heart works. This means that upcoming surgery is more risky, especially as the surgeon's plan is to attempt a laparoscopic approach. The patient is understandably dismayed and asks, "What do you mean? Am I going to die? Are you cancelling my surgery? I can't believe this!"

What strategies can the anesthesiologist use to address these questions? Do you think the patient is asking for more cognitive information or expressing an emotional response?

After effectively responding to the patient's emotion, they both pause. The patient says, "Ok, so what should I do about surgery?"

What questions can the anesthesiologist ask to clarify the patient's values? What are some recommendations that could be offered depending on different values she might have?

The anesthesiologist asks for more information regarding the patient's hopes and fears about the surgery and finds out that the patient really despises the cholecystostomy tube, the way it feels, and taking care of it. She hates the way she feels after she eats and can't stand the thought of being sick anymore. About 10 years ago, she underwent surgery and radiation for breast cancer and has continued her regular surveillance visits and imaging. Regarding that experience, she says, "Well, it wasn't fun, but I got through it." She values being physically independent and wants to be able to enjoy her time at the beach with her family, about 6 months from now.

Given this information, the anesthesiologist says, "It sounds like your current state is definitely not tolerable for you, and you've been someone willing to go through a lot of medical care, engage with doctors and hospitals, to maintain your health and your independence." The patient agrees with this and asks for a recommendation on how to proceed.

The anesthesiologist recommends, based on these values, that they work toward proceeding with surgery. They plan together to further assess and optimize the patient's pulmonary hypertension preoperatively by referring the patient to a pulmonary hypertension specialist. They also plan together to talk with the surgeon about foregoing a laparoscopic approach and planning for an open cholecystectomy to minimize operative time and anesthesia risks. The patient is pleased and agrees with this plan, and the anesthesiologist reaches out to the surgeon by phone to discuss it.

How could the anesthesiologist summarize their conversation when they are relaying this information back to the surgeon?

The anesthesiologist says, "I saw your patient today. My goal is to support you in treating her gallstone disease. We talked about her values—she definitely can't tolerate her life the way it is, and she wants her gallbladder to be removed. I want to facilitate that while minimizing her risks from anesthesia. Unfortunately, her echocardiogram showed worsening pulmonary hypertension. I worry that laparoscopic surgery would be higher risk for her than an open surgery. I wonder if the procedure could be done open, in order to decrease her operating room time and avoid laparoscopic surgery. What do you think?" The surgeon asks some clarifying questions about her risks with pneumoperitoneum/laparoscopy and ultimately agrees, especially since they also thought a laparoscopic cholecystectomy for her, if possible at all, might be complex.

Identify ways that structured communication tools can be used in interdisciplinary conversation to achieve consensus.

Four weeks later, the patient presents for surgery. She undergoes open cholecystectomy without complications and is discharged from the hospital on postoperative day 4. Her abdominal complaints are resolved, and she establishes care with a pulmonary hypertension specialist. The surgeon continues to refer complex patients to the anesthesiologist for preoperative assessment due to their thoughtful and values-based approach.

DISCUSSION

Clinicians make clinical care recommendations in almost every encounter. In the perioperative period, surgeons often make recommendations regarding medical management or surgical intervention. Anesthesiologists often make recommendations on a particular anesthetic approach. When should shared decision-making be employed prior to making these recommendations?

Given time and resource limitations, shared decision-making could most benefit patients faced with a consequential clinical perioperative decision. Some perioperative decisions are not highly consequential, such as deciding to use one local anesthetic over another in a peripheral nerve block in an otherwise healthy patient. In some cases, a decision is not offered to a patient: resection is not offered for pancreatic cancer that has metastasized. The supposition that shared decision-making is most useful for patients facing consequential clinical perioperative decisions is mirrored in the fact that much of the research on physician–patient communication has been done in the setting of caring for patients with serious illness.[1] Oncology and palliative medicine have pioneered structured communication tools for difficult conversations.[2-4]

Multiple studies have found that clinicians find these conversations stressful.[5,6] The source of this stress on clinicians is multifactorial: worries about disrupting the physician–patient relationship, responding to patient emotions, or responding to their own emotions.

Some worries have not been substantiated in the research. Research on patient response to conversations about prognosis has found that the physician–patient relationship may be strengthened through these conversations.[7] Other studies indicate that when physicians engage in difficult discussions with patients, often about prognosis, those patients are overall more satisfied with their care.[8]

Another source of stress particular to the perioperative setting is that these conversations often take place without a previously established physician–patient relationship. Research demonstrates that as the duration of a physician–patient relationship increases, prognostic accuracy actually decreases.[9] It may be the newcomer to the clinical scenario who can prognosticate most accurately and thus have a much-needed conversation about the realities of that person's perioperative care.

The communication tools pioneered for shared decision-making can be applied more broadly to any "difficult conversation." A "difficult conversation" can be defined as any conversation in which emotionally laden information is presented, discussed, and processed. This broad definition allows inclusion of conversations with diverse goals (delivering feedback, coming to a treatment decision, making a recommendation) and between participants in a diverse set of roles (clinician, patient, learner, teacher, colleague).

PERIOPERATIVE CONVERSATIONS: SETTING THE STAGE

Setting the stage for a difficult conversation is the first step. To have a productive conversation, a clinician must gather the following: people, time, and information.

- *People*: If a patient says, "My wife helps me make all these decisions," then it is no good having a conversation without the patient's wife in the room. In some situations, it may be necessary to have a colleague—such as the surgeon or the oncologist—in the room to have a productive conversation.

- *Time*: Perioperative medicine specialists often comment: "The preop bay on the day of surgery is not the place to have a conversation about whether to cancel the surgery." Difficult conversations in the surgery clinic or preoperative clinic are a gift to the patient and perioperative colleagues. However, it is also true that sometimes a conversation needs to be had, even if it is a bad time.

- *Information*: Two concerns that fall under this topic are having enough information for a productive conversation and being able to match the information presented to the patient's information preferences.
  - *Enough Information*: It is difficult to have a conversation about the risks of surgery and anesthesia in a patient with pulmonary hypertension if the results of their right heart catheterization aren't back yet. Sometimes, the results of a test are needed for a productive conversation.
  - *The Form of Information*: Some patients want medical terminology and medical reasoning, and some patients don't. It is important to ask about information preferences and give the patient a choice.[10,11] The following questions can be helpful: "Some patients like the 10,000-foot view, like looking out the window of an airplane. Some patients like every little detail, like being on the ground and turning over every stone. Which sounds more like you?"

- If there isn't "enough" people, time, and information, the conversation may need to be delayed!

PERIOPERATIVE CONVERSATIONS: WHAT SHOULD BE COVERED?

The American College of Surgeons National Surgical Quality Improvement Program (ACS NSQIP) and the American Geriatrics Society (AGS) have established guidelines for best practices for both preoperative assessment and perioperative management of the geriatric surgical patient.[12,13] Because these patients are a population at higher risk for complications, these guidelines can be helpful for any patient considered "high risk" or where a "difficult conversation" might be indicated.

Capacity: Capacity is a prerequisite for shared decision-making. Decision-making capacity has four criteria:

- The patient can indicate his or her treatment choice.
- The patient understands the relevant information being conveyed.
- The patient acknowledges his or her medical condition, options, and likely outcomes.
- The patient can reason about treatment options.

The physician should confirm this by asking the patient to describe his or her medical condition in their own words and the options and indications for surgery. Even if a patient has capacity, a patient may prefer to share or delegate decision-making. Asking "Is there someone else that we should include in this discussion?" is a way to support patient preference and autonomy.[12]

Clarifying treatment goals and making a treatment plan: Multiple communication frameworks exist for this cornerstone of shared decision-making. Most can be divided into four key steps:

1. Agreeing on the medical context,
2. Responding to emotion,
3. Clarifying values in the setting of that medical context, and
4. Making a recommendation.

Below, two communication frameworks are explored in detail. Making sure that the treatment goals and plan are communicated to the relevant providers is an essential and often overlooked follow-up to the actual conversation with the patient.[12,13]

Advance Directives: Ask about any existing advance directives and encourage the patient to complete one if they do not already have one. Designate a healthcare proxy or surrogate decision-maker and document this in the medical chart.

Preexisting Do Not Resuscitate (DNR) or Do Not Intubate (DNI) orders should prompt a "required reconsideration" by the patient and healthcare team preoperatively to discuss which resuscitation procedures might be encountered, which are essential to the success of the procedure, or which are non-essential and may be refused.[13]

COMMUNICATION FRAMEWORKS

Multiple communication frameworks have been published to facilitate clinician–patient communication within a difficult conversation. Examples include Ariadne Labs's Serious Illness Conversation Guide, SPIKES, and REMAP.[2–4] While SPIKES and REMAP are explained in detail below, all of these frameworks share the same four key steps: agreeing on the medical context, responding to emotion, clarifying values in the setting of that medical context, and making a recommendation.

SPIKES

The SPIKES cognitive map was developed by Rob Buckman and Walter Baile and includes six steps, labeled by the letters of the mnemonic device: Set-up, Perception, Invitation, Knowledge, Emotion, and Summary.[2] See the steps outlined in Table 38.1.

REMAP

REMAP was developed by Anthony Back, James Tulsky, and Robert Arnold as a guide for "goals of care" conversations. It is also a mnemonic, which includes five steps: Reframe the Information, Expect Emotion, Map Patient Values, Align with Values, and Propose a Plan. Of note, the steps in REMAP of "Expect Emotion" and "Align with Values" are key places for the clinician to pause and reflect to the patient that either emotional response or information offered has been recognized and understood.[3]

In perioperative care, difficult conversations also occur when managing postoperative complications or conveying intraoperative findings. See Table 38.2 for an example of how to use REMAP when discussing postoperative care with a patient's family member.

RESPONDING TO EMOTION

Both of these frameworks, as well as others in the literature, emphasize responding to emotion. When emotions arise in difficult conversations, it is often a sign that the clinician is doing the important work of actually having the difficult conversation. If patients do not experience emotion during a difficult conversation, it may mean that the clinician has not effectively conveyed the consequential perioperative decision that needs to be made.

Previous work in serious illness care has emphasized that patients provide clinicians with "empathetic opportunities" to respond to emotion.[14–18] Yet clinicians often respond to a patient's "emotion cue" with information, without acknowledging the emotion.[16]

The mnemonic NURSE details five categories of statements/questions that can be used to acknowledge and respond to emotion, called in some research "empathic continuers."[16,17,19,20] Table 38.3 details the mnemonic and examples of each of the five categories.

It's important to note that different people may respond differently to the same statement or question. For example, a possible response to "I see the sadness in those tears" is "I'm not sad. I've lost all hope." At first glance, this response may seem like a failure: the patient has disputed the clinician's statement. In actuality, the patient has given the clinician a gift: the patient has named their own emotion as "hopeless." The conversation can now continue, addressing the emotion of hopelessness.

While responding to patient emotions can be difficult, it is important to again emphasize *emotion means the clinician is doing the job of having the difficult conversation.*

Table 38.1 SPIKES FRAMEWORK FOR DIFFICULT CONVERSATIONS

		DEFINITION	EXAMPLE
S	Set-up	Prepare for the conversation, including environment and people who need to be present (for both the patient and the clinician team)	Ensure a private space, ask whether the patient would like others present (or on the phone), allow adequate time for the conversation
P	Perception	Ask what the patient understands	"What have you been told already about your risks for surgery?"
I	Invitation	Ask whether the patient wants information about their health, and how much information they prefer?	"Would it be ok for me to summarize my understanding of the operation in light of your current health?"
K	Knowledge	Convey information in small chunks, without jargon. Consider using foreshadowing.	"Unfortunately, your lung disease is severe, and that means putting you on a breathing machine for surgery has high risks for you."
E	Emotion	Notice and recognize emotion in response to the information given.	"I know this isn't what you were hoping for. I wish this surgery were more straightforward for you."
S	Summary	Restate what's been discussed and next steps.	"You've told me avoiding getting 'stuck' on a ventilator is the most important thing. Given your risks, I'd recommend not moving forward with this operation and looking for non-surgical ways to manage your hernia discomfort."

Table 38.2 **REMAP FRAMEWORK FOR DIFFICULT CONVERSATIONS**

		DEFINITION	EXAMPLE
R	Reframe	Assess the patient's understanding and provide new information. Place details into a bigger picture – give a "headline."	What have the doctors told you so far? ... That's correct, your father has a life-threatening abdominal infection. That means that in the operating room, we weren't able to complete the surgery due to how unstable he became. He'll be brought to the ICU with a temporary dressing on his abdomen. We'll try to stabilize his heart and vital signs, and plan to return to surgery tomorrow."
E	Expect Emotion	Look for verbal or nonverbal emotional responses. Attending to emotion often needs to occur multiple times in a conversation.	"This is so unexpected. Nobody could blame you for being overwhelmed and afraid for him."
M	Map values	Step back to explore the patient's values before discussing choices – what matters most, and what concerns are there for the future?	"I wonder, if your father could hear all this, what he might say about it? What would be most important to him? Had he ever seen family or friends go through something like this?"
A	Align	Verbally reflect back what you hear from the patient, sometimes this includes contradiction or ambivalence. Use reflections to hypothesize what the patient means.	"It sounds like he knew going in, that the surgery was an emergency and was risky given his health. He was always willing to go through a lot to try to get more time with his family and grandchildren."
P	Propose a Plan	Make a recommendation based on patient values. Choose the options that you believe have the best chance to attain the patient's goals.	"Could I make a recommendation? I think given what you've told me about your father, that we should do everything possible to stabilize him and return to surgery tomorrow. If, in the coming days it looks like he may not survive, or may not be able to interact with his family, then we should talk again about whether continuing all this aggressive ICU care makes sense for him."

Table 38.3 **NURSE STATEMENTS**

		DEFINITION	EXAMPLE
N	Name	Name the emotion.	"Based on that statement, I take that you are frustrated right now." "I see your tears; I see the sadness."
U	Understand	Normalize and acknowledge, stop short of claiming to understand everything.	"I can't imagine how hard it could be to hear this news." "Based on what you've told me, I can imagine that this news is really surprising."
R	Respect	Praise and recognize the patient's or family's effort.	"I see how hard you've worked to take care of yourself." "I see how much you've tried to shield your family from your illness."
S	Support	Commit to caring for them.	"We are going to see you through this surgery." "We are here to help you understand and make a decision based on this information."
E	Explore	Ask what they mean.	"Can you tell me more about what those tears mean?"

INTERDISCIPLINARY COMMUNICATION: MAKING A RECOMMENDATION

After employing a communication framework and formulating a treatment plan, the plan still needs to be communicated to relevant clinicians. This is an essential—but often overlooked—part of having difficult conversations.

A new treatment plan can be difficult for other clinicians to understand or accept. Prior to discussing a treatment plan recommendation, it is important to ensure a shared understanding of the medical situation. Treatment plans often change when the medical situation changes: a new cancer diagnosis, a new finding on echocardiography. Once there is a shared understanding of the situation, formulate a recommendation using the three-step structured communication tool for making a recommendation: Wish-Worry-Wonder (Figure 38.1).

- *Wish*: A wish statement is an opportunity to align with another person's values, intentions, or goals. This aligning statement allows that the next statement—the "worry"—may be something that colleagues can align against, like a team facing a challenge.[14]

- *Worry*: A worry statement reframes the current situation by introducing a challenge.

- *Wonder*: This is the place to "float" a recommendation. It's a nudge for a clinical colleague to put the pieces together themselves.

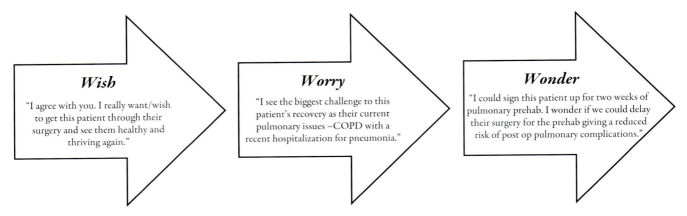

Figure 38.1 The Wish-Worry-Wonder framework for difficult conversations.

After making an initial recommendation ("wonder" statement), the colleague may express a different perspective. Wish-Worry-Wonder can be repeated. Wish: continue to align with the colleague's perspective, acknowledging shared goals. Worry: express your concerns about the alternate plan. Wonder: suggest other paths forward to achieve the shared goals.

TROUBLE SPOTS AND WHERE TO GO FOR HELP

There are circumstances when the following occurs:

- You aren't able to reach a "shared understanding" of the medical information with the patient and family.
- Strong emotion arises and cannot be diffused enough to proceed with eliciting values or planning next steps.
- The patient or family is ambivalent, seems at a loss in how to proceed or does not agree with any of the treatment options.

In these cases, one consideration is pausing the conversation for that day and asking about planning for an additional visit. Other options are to offer to include other family members or support people or to consider arranging a multidisciplinary meeting in person or (less preferably) by phone, together with the various specialists involved. Alternatively, one could consider what other communication or "difficult conversation" resources may be available, such as the following:

- Palliative care (or supportive care) consultation
- Online communication skills resources:
  - https://www.vitaltalk.org/
  - https://www.instituteforhumancaring.org/Resources.aspx
  - https://www.ariadnelabs.org/serious-illness-care/

CONCLUSION

- Shared decision-making can be challenging in the perioperative care setting for a variety of reasons; having a practiced conversation framework can be helpful.
- Frameworks most commonly have four parts: agreeing on the medical context, responding to emotion, clarifying values in the setting of that medical context, and making a recommendation.
- Anticipate emotional responses and attend to the emotion before providing more cognitive information. Emotion means you are doing the important work of having the conversation.
- Use similar communication tools, such as Wish-Worry-Wonder, to convey the patient's values and treatment plan with other providers involved in his or her care.

REVIEW QUESTIONS

1. Which of the following is true regarding perioperative difficult conversations?

   a. Patients are distressed by hearing serious medical news. Therefore, having difficult conversations is likely to damage the patient–physician relationship.
   b. The clinician who has known the patient the longest can prognosticate most accurately.
   c. If a patient has a DNI order, the patient has already made a decision about intubation. Therefore, intubation should not be discussed as part of their perioperative plan.
   d. Optimizing the setting sometimes means including other specialists, such as the patient's surgeon or oncologist.

   The correct answer is d.
   Regarding choice a, studies have shown that having difficult conversations does not damage the patient–physician

relationship, and, in contrast, those patients are overall more satisfied with their care. Unlike in choice b, studies also show that as the duration of physician–patient relationship increases, prognostic accuracy actually decreases. If a patient has a DNI order, as in choice c, national guidelines recommend a pre-operative "required reconsideration" by the patient and their healthcare team regarding treatment limitations during the procedure. Choice d is correct, where optimizing the setting includes having the right people, such as other specialists if needed.

2. Which of the following is true about communicating with patients?

    a. Patients always want to hear medical information in as much detail as possible.
    b. Most structured communication frameworks share similar components.
    c. A "difficult conversation" requires that the patient have a terminal illness.
    d. Communication principles are specific to the patient–physician relationship and cannot be applied to communication within the interdisciplinary team.

The correct answer is b.

Patients do not always want medical information in great detail, in contrast to a, and we recommend asking about information preferences prior to difficult conversations. Regarding choice c, a "difficult conversation" can be defined as any conversation in which emotionally laden information is presented, discussed, and processed, and this allows application of communication principles to multiple settings, including conversations between members of the interdisciplinary team (unlike d). Choice b is correct, in that most structured communication frameworks share four similar components: agreeing on the medical context, responding to emotion, clarifying values in the setting of that medical context, and making a recommendation.

3. Which of the following is an important component of most difficult conversation frameworks, including SPIKES and REMAP?

    a. Setting.
    b. Document your conversation.
    c. Respond to emotion.
    d. Map patient values.

The correct answer is c.

Regarding choice a, setting is included in the "S" of SPIKES, for Set-up, but is absent from REMAP. Documentation (choice b) is part of other frameworks such as the Serious Illness Conversation Guide, but is absent from SPIKES and REMAP. Mapping patient values (d) is part of REMAP but not explicitly listed in SPIKES. Choice c is correct as SPIKES and REMAP (as well as other frameworks) include an emphasis on recognizing and responding to emotion.

4. Which of the following is an example of an effective NURSE statement?

    a. "The echo showed that your pulmonary hypertension has become severe."
    b. "We should talk about whether surgery is the right option for you."
    c. "I understand exactly how you feel."
    d. "I can't imagine how scary it is to hear this."

The correct answer is d.

Choice a provides medical information but does not fall into a NURSE category of empathic responses. Choice b is a transition statement indicating wanting to make a plan. Choice c. is an empathic response, but, within the NURSE categories, the "U" for understand contains a caution against stating that you understand exactly what someone else is experiencing. Choice d is correct and is a more effective way to form an "Understand" statement without claiming to understand everything.

5. Which of the following is *not* an essential part of setting the stage for a difficult conversation?

    a. Setting aside time for the conversation.
    b. Ensuring that the relevant people are present.
    c. Finding a room with soft lighting and comfortable chairs.
    d. Gathering the relevant medical information.

The correct answer is c.

Setting the stage includes having the necessary people (choice b), time (choice a), and information (choice d). Although a private and comfortable space (choice c) can be optimal, this is not essential for having difficult conversations. These conversations often occur in a variety of less-than-ideal settings throughout the hospital, clinic, or other environments of medical care. The content of the conversation (with people, time, and information) is more essential to setting the stage than the external environment.

6. In assessing capacity, which of the following patient responses would prompt concern and follow-up?

    a. "I understand my condition from 10,000 feet, but I don't like to get into details."
    b. "I'm having trouble making a choice. I see the risks and benefits of both options."
    c. "I know you say I have cancer, Doc. But I don't believe that."
    d. "When I was young, I never thought anything bad could happen. Now I don't know."

The correct answer is c.

In assessing capacity, there are four criteria: the patient (1) is able to indicate a choice; (2) understands the relevant information; (3) acknowledges the medical condition, the options, and their likely outcomes; and (4) can reason about these options. Choice c is correct and prompts the most concern about capacity because the patient does not acknowledge their medical condition. Choice a expresses an information preference, which does not exclude capacity. Choice b conveys ambivalence or uncertainty about the options, but does not indicate an inability to reason about the options. Choice d indicates worry about the future and perhaps a change in risk aversion over time, neither of which exclude capacity.

7. Which of the following pairing correctly explains the step in "Wish-Worry-Wonder"?

    a. Wish: Express the patient's hopes and dreams for the future.

    b. Worry: List all of the medical concerns with the current plan.

    c. Wonder: Float a recommendation, nudging a clinical colleague toward a new course of action.

The correct answer is c.

Regarding choice a, a "wish" statement is an alignment of the goal or value between participants in the conversation. This may sometimes include the patient's hopes and dreams, but not always. The "worry" (b) introduces a challenge to that goal, but does not exhaustively list all medical concerns. Choice c is correct, where one "wonders" in order to recommend a possible course of action.

REFERENCES

1. Smith RC, Hoppe RB. The patient's story: Integrating the patient- and physician-centered approaches to interviewing. *Ann Intern Med.* 1991 Sep 15;115(6):470–477. doi:10.7326/0003-4819-115-6-470
2. Baile WF, Buckman R, Lenzi R, Glober G, Beale EA, Kudelka AP. SPIKES: A six-step protocol for delivering bad news: Application to the patient with cancer. *Oncologist.* 2000;5(4):302–311. doi:10.1634/theoncologist.5-4-302
3. Childers JW, Back AL, Tulsky JA, Arnold RM. REMAP: A framework for goals of care conversations. *J Oncol Pract.* 2017 Oct;13(10):e844–e850. doi:10.1200/jop.2016.018796
4. Daubman BR, Bernacki R, Stoltenberg M, Wilson E, Jacobsen J. Best practices for teaching clinicians to use a serious illness conversation guide. *Palliat Med Rep.* 2020;1(1):135–142. doi:10.1089/pmr.2020.0066
5. Christakis NA, Iwashyna TJ. Attitude and self-reported practice regarding prognostication in a national sample of internists. *Arch Intern Med.* 1998 Nov 23;158(21):2389–2395. doi:10.1001/archinte.158.21.2389
6. Ptacek JT, McIntosh EG. Physician challenges in communicating bad news. *J Behav Med.* 2009 Aug;32(4):380–387. doi:10.1007/s10865-009-9213-8
7. Fenton JJ, Duberstein PR, Kravitz RL, et al. Impact of prognostic discussions on the patient-physician relationship: Prospective cohort study. *J Clin Oncol.* Jan 20 2018;36(3):225–230. doi:10.1200/JCO.2017.75.6288
8. Heyland DK, Allan DE, Rocker G, et al. Discussing prognosis with patients and their families near the end of life: Impact on satisfaction with end-of-life care. *Open Med.* 2009 Jun 16;3(2):e101–e110.
9. Christakis NA, Lamont EB. Extent and determinants of error in doctors' prognoses in terminally ill patients: Prospective cohort study. *BMJ.* 2000 Feb 19;320(7233):469–472. doi:10.1136/bmj.320.7233.469
10. Ahalt C, Walter LC, Yourman L, Eng C, Pérez-Stable EJ, Smith AK. "Knowing is better": Preferences of diverse older adults for discussing prognosis. *J Gen Intern Med.* 2012 May;27(5):568–575. doi:10.1007/s11606-011-1933-0
11. White DB, Evans LR, Bautista CA, Luce JM, Lo B. Are physicians' recommendations to limit life support beneficial or burdensome? Bringing empirical data to the debate. *Am J Respir Crit Care Med.* 2009 Aug 15;180(4):320–325. doi:10.1164/rccm.200811-1776OC
12. Chow WB, Rosenthal RA, Merkow RP, et al. Optimal preoperative assessment of the geriatric surgical patient: A best practices guideline from the American College of Surgeons National Surgical Quality Improvement Program and the American Geriatrics Society. *J Am Coll Surg.* 2012 Oct;215(4):453–466. doi:10.1016/j.jamcollsurg.2012.06.017
13. Mohanty S, Rosenthal RA, Russell MM, Neuman MD, Ko CY, Esnaola NF. Optimal perioperative management of the geriatric patient: A best practices guideline from the American College of Surgeons NSQIP and the American Geriatrics Society. *J Am Coll Surg.* 2016 May;222(5):930–947. doi:10.1016/j.jamcollsurg.2015.12.026
14. Quill TE, Arnold RM, Platt F. "I wish things were different": Expressing wishes in response to loss, futility, and unrealistic hopes. *Ann Intern Med.* 2001 Oct 2;135(7):551–555. doi:10.7326/0003-4819-135-7-200110020-00022
15. Back AL, Arnold RM. "Isn't there anything more you can do?": When empathic statements work, and when they don't. *J Palliat Med.* 2013 Nov;16(11):1429–1432. doi:10.1089/jpm.2013.0193
16. Suchman AL, Markakis K, Beckman HB, Frankel R. A model of empathic communication in the medical interview. *JAMA.* 1997 Feb 26;277(8):678–682.
17. Tulsky JA, Arnold RM, Alexander SC, et al. Enhancing communication between oncologists and patients with a computer-based training program: A randomized trial. *Ann Intern Med.* 2011 Nov 01;155(9):593–601. doi:10.7326/0003-4819-155-9-201111010-00007
18. Back AL, Arnold RM. "Yes it's sad, but what should I do?" Moving from empathy to action in discussing goals of care. *J Palliat Med.* 2014 Feb;17(2):141–144. doi:10.1089/jpm.2013.0197
19. Back A, Arnold RM, Tulsky JA. *Mastering Communication with Seriously Ill Patients: Balancing Honesty with Empathy and Hope.* Cambridge University Press; 2009:x.
20. Portenoy RK, Bruera E. *Topics in Palliative Care.* Oxford University Press; 1997:v.

PART VII

MISCELLANEOUS

39.

THIS PATIENT HAS 17 ALLERGIES: INCLUDING "GENERAL ANESTHESIA"

Debra D. Pulley

STEM CASE AND KEY QUESTIONS

A 52-year-old woman presents to the preoperative clinic in preparation for a thyroidectomy to remove a multinodular goiter. Before you see her, the nurse tells you she has 17 allergies—including "general anesthesia."

What information about the allergy needs to be obtained from the patient or medical record? What is the difference between an allergy and an adverse reaction?

You review what the nurse obtained from the patient. You make note of each reaction. You tell the patient that you have reviewed her allergy list and she will not be exposed to the majority of her allergens, but you need to discuss five of her allergies.

1. *Allergy to "all opioids."* She says she has severe nausea and vomiting. You ask her which ones she has been given and if she has had problems with other opioids. She tells you it has been mainly with pills she takes by mouth. She tells you she did not have any nausea or vomiting with the last surgery. You tell her that pain after removal of the thyroid gland is usually not that great, but, in case she does need pain medication, you will prescribe what she has tolerated before.

2. *Allergy to epinephrine.* She says it caused her heart to race and she felt as though she was going to die. She tells you this happened at the dentist's office and was told it was because of epinephrine. You explain to her that epinephrine naturally occurs in the body and can be lifesaving. You explain her reaction was probably related to some of the drug going directly into the blood instead of near the nerve. You add that if she needs epinephrine, you will give it to her.

3. *Allergy to local anesthetics.* She states she had a seizure when they did a block. She does not want it to happen again. You explain to her that when local anesthetics are given close to a nerve, some of the drug can be absorbed into the bloodstream and can cause a seizure, similar to what happened with the epinephrine. You add that she may get some local anesthetics during the surgery to help with pain.

4. *Allergy to general anesthesia.* She says after an operation she woke up in the ICU. They told her that her tongue had swollen. She really did not understand what happened. A friend told her tongue swelling can be an allergic reaction. You tell her you will obtain her records to see what happened and will call her once you have reviewed them.

5. *Allergy to cefotetan.* She says cefotetan caused her to get hives and she felt ill at the time. She was given medicine to help. She was told that she is allergic to cefotetan and should never have it again. You tell her that antibiotics are usually not needed for routine thyroidectomy. If she does need antibiotics, she will not be given cefotetan due to her past allergic reaction.

What is the differential diagnosis for tongue swelling intraoperatively? What is the incidence of perioperative immediate hypersensitivity reactions? What is the pathophysiology of anaphylaxis? When would you refer a patient to an allergist?

You are able to get all the information you need after requesting additional medical records. You call the patient and tell her that you discovered she actually had direct injury to her tongue and the surgical team was concerned she might not breath well immediately after the surgery. She was intentionally kept asleep until her tongue partially healed. There was no allergy involved, and you will give her similar anesthetic drugs including a combination of medicines to reduce nausea and vomiting. She is pleased with your plan and thanks you for explaining. You then amend the allergy documentation in her record. About 2 weeks later, she calls the surgeon to say that she has been having trouble swallowing meat. A computed tomography (CT) scan is ordered.

What are the indications of imaging the neck/airway in patients with goiters? What are the symptoms/signs of hyperthyroidism? When would you cancel surgery due to hyperthyroidism? What are the symptoms/signs of hypothyroidism? When would you cancel surgery due to hypothyroidism? What complications can occur after a thyroidectomy?

A CT scan shows her trachea is deviated to the left, but there is no tracheal compression. You plan for a potential difficult airway but are able to intubate using video laryngoscopy. After extubation, there is no serious sign of recurrent laryngeal nerve damage. In the PACU, there is no evidence of neck hematoma and no stridor from acute hypocalcemia.

DISCUSSION

DEFINITIONS AND DOCUMENTATION OF ADVERSE DRUG REACTIONS

When making medical decisions it is important to know of past harmful reactions. However, documentation and reporting of these adverse reactions/allergies can be inaccurate and potentially lead to harm.[1] Unfortunately, consensus guidelines for documentation are lacking or have been ignored. Adverse reactions are unintended or undesirable effects that are possibly related to a drug administration, whereas an allergic reaction is an overreaction of the immunologic system in response to exposure to an allergen (also known as *hypersensitivity reaction*). In 2022, a work group from the Adverse Reactions to Drug, Biological, and Latex Committee of the American Academy of Allergy, Asthma, and Immunology provided examples of how to document reactions and gave the following recommendations to improve the allergy section of electronic health records.[2]

- Standard terminology/definitions across all areas of healthcare delivery
- Anyone who documents allergies needs formalized training on accurate documentation (across all levels of education)
- Reconfiguration of the "allergy" section of the electronic health record (EHR) to separate adverse reactions into different categories (e.g., drug, contact, food, other)
- Adverse drug reactions should be further divided into patient-reported, patient preferences, patient with a specific predisposition, and immunologically mediated hypersensitivity/allergy
- Include in documentation specific name, date noted (date of reaction), reaction, reaction type, severity, and free text details
- Clinicians should review and amend documentation as needed (see example in Table 39.1).

Table 39.1 EXAMPLE OF AMENDMENT OF ALLERGY DOCUMENTATION

PRIOR TO ALLERGY EVALUATION	FOLLOWING ALLERGY EVALUATION
Drug: Amoxicillin	Drug: Amoxicillin
Date Noted: 1990	Date Noted: 1990
Reaction: Hives	Reaction: Hives
Type: Allergy/HSR	Type: Allergy/HSR
Severity: Moderate	Severity: Moderate
Free text: "Hives occurred 48 hours after start of 10 day course treated with antihistamines at age 5, reported by patient's mother. Has avoided all beta-lactams since that time."	Free text: "Hives occurred 48 hours after start of 10 day course treated with antihistamines at age 5, reported by patient's mother. Has avoided all beta-lactams since that time. *Negative skin testing and drug challenge 03/10/2020, see Dr. Lisban's Allergy note*"

Adapted from Guyer AC, et al.[2]

PATIENTS WITH PREVIOUS ADVERSE REACTIONS SUGGESTIVE OF ALLERGY

An assessment needs to be done preoperatively to determine if referral to an allergist is needed for patients who present with anaphylaxis especially if the causative agent has not been determined.[3]

Tongue swelling can occur perioperatively from a number of factors. Trauma or pressure injury from insertion of oral airways, laryngeal mask airways, laryngoscopes, transesophageal echocardiography probes, and surgery can produce associated swelling of the tongue. Swelling can also occur from positioning, from surgery near the airway or affecting venous drainage, a hypersensitivity reaction, and angioedema. It is important to manage the airway to ensure adequate oxygenation and ventilation. Additionally, it is also important to know the likely cause because that can potentially lead to additional treatment to prevent further deterioration. Angioedema is extravasation of local plasma causing nonpitting, nondependent swelling, and it is often asymmetric. It can be mast cell-mediated, commonly associated with urticarial and hypotension via an immunoglobulin E (IgE)-mediated hypersensitivity reaction, but it can also be kinin-related (as in angiotensin-converting enzyme [ACE] inhibitors) (see Figure 39.1).[4] Figure 39.2 shows a treatment approach to angioedema.[4]

When a patient has a reported penicillin allergy, frequently alternative antibiotics are used which may not be as effective. A study published in 2018 showed this practice increased the odds of developing a surgical site infection by 50%.[5] Studies have shown that half of antibiotic allergies are to penicillin, but patients frequently do not remember which type of penicillin they were given. In many cases, the reaction was a rash, and it was a long time ago. Cross-reactivity between beta-lactam antibiotics is due to side-chain similarities. Cefazolin does not share

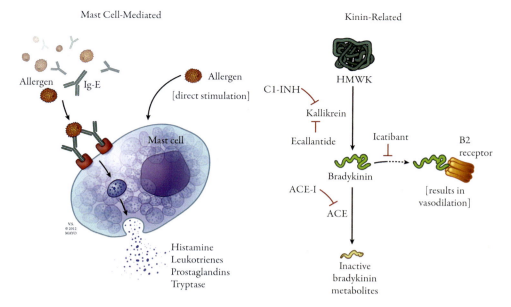

Figure 39.1 Pathophysiology of angioedema.
Reprinted with permission from Barbara DW, et al.[4]

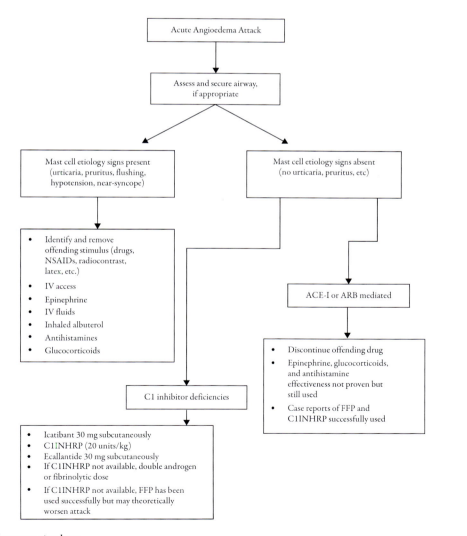

Figure 39.2 Management of acute angioedema.
Reprinted with permission From Barbara DW, et al.[4]

structural R1 side-chain similarities with penicillin and may be given safely in cases of a previous reaction with mild symptoms.[6]

PERIOPERATIVE ANAPHYLAXIS

The World Allergy Organization defines anaphylaxis as a serious allergic reaction that is rapid in onset and might cause death.[7] The list of criteria that must be met was recently shortened to require only one of the two criteria. The first criterion is acute onset of illness (minutes to several hours) with simultaneous involvement of skin/mucosa and at least one of the following (respiratory or circulatory compromise or severe gastrointestinal symptoms). The second criterion is acute onset of hypotension, bronchospasm, or laryngeal involvement after exposure to a known allergen. In the operating room, there are many potential causes for respiratory issues and hypotension (e.g., endotracheal tube [ETT] malpositioning, pulmonary edema, transfusion related acute lung injury [TRALI], overdose of anesthetic drugs, cardiogenic shock, hemorrhage, pulmonary embolism, tension pneumothorax, vasovagal, sepsis, etc.)[8,9] Table 39.2 shows the Modified Ring and Messmer Classification for grading severity of anaphylaxis.[9]

Anaphylaxis can be mediated immunologically (e.g., IgE, immune complex/complement) or nonimmunologically (sudden mast cell or basophil degranulation in the absence of immunoglobulins) (see Figure 39.3).[10] The importance of knowing the mechanism is that an IgE-mediated allergen may be amenable to desensitization in some cases. Unfortunately, the exact mechanisms by which an agent causes anaphylaxis may not be well understood.

Table 39.2 MODIFIED RING AND MESSMER GRADING

GRADE	CLINICAL SIGNS
I	Skin, mucosal signs, or both: general erythema, extensive urticarial, or both
II	Moderate multiorgan involvement: skin, moderate hypotension, tachycardia, bronchospasm or gastrointestinal symptoms
III	Life-threatening mono- or multiorgan involvement: severe bronchospasm, life-threatening hypotension, tachycardia or bradycardia
IV	Cardiac (usually PEA) or respiratory arrest (may not have cutaneous signs until perfusion has been restored)

From Garvey LH, et al.[9]

The most commonly implicated agents for perioperative anaphylaxis are antibiotics and neuromuscular blocking agents. Chlorhexidine, dyes, and sugammadex are also commonly implicated. Latex is less often implicated due to safety measures since the 1990s to lessen exposure in the perioperative environment. Other agents identified include alpha-galactosidase, gelatins, allogeneic blood products, hypnotics, opioids, radiocontrast media, and local anesthetics.[8]

Perioperative anaphylaxis requires prompt recognition and early treatment with epinephrine and resuscitation fluids to prevent further deterioration. After stabilization, blood level tryptase can be obtained 30 minutes to 2 hours to see if it is elevated (indicative of IgE mediation).[8] In addition, a baseline tryptase level must be obtained. Patients with systemic

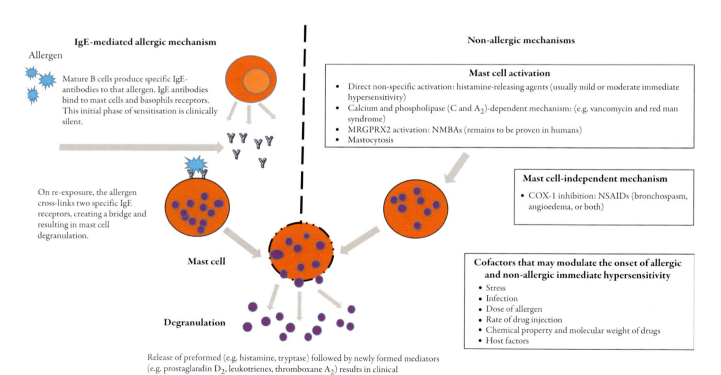

Figure 39.3 Pathophysiology of anaphylaxis.
Reprinted with permission from Dewachter P, et al.[10]

mastocytosis and hereditary alpha-tryptasemia can have elevated baseline levels. A recent study reported a ratio of greater than 1.685 (acute tryptase/baseline) is more likely to be anaphylaxis while maximizing sensitivity and specificity with the acute level taken within 4 hours of the event.[11] Follow-up is important to determine future risks especially if the agent has not been identified. Referral to an allergist may be useful, and, in some cases, desensitization may be possible.[8]

THYROIDECTOMY AND THYROID DISEASES

Thyroidectomy is surgical resection of the thyroid gland (total or partial). Indications include symptomatic benign disease (nodule/goiter), concern for malignancy, and hyperthyroid conditions.[12] Symptoms of compression include dysphagia, globus sensation (sensation of lump in the throat), positional dyspnea, or hoarseness. Overall, thyroidectomy is considered a low-risk surgery (0.2% in total thyroidectomy).[13] Due to close proximity, injury can occur to the recurrent laryngeal nerve (unilateral or bilateral). Postoperatively, the patient may be hoarse or have stridor/respiratory distress requiring intubation. Intraoperatively, there are various methods of recurrent laryngeal nerve monitoring including ETTs with integrated electrodes. Additional causes of respiratory distress can occur requiring additional measures besides supportive and include swelling from cervical hematoma or hypocalcemia.[14] Preoperative assessment should include thyroid function studies and ultrasound imaging. If the patient has compression symptoms, cross-sectional imaging should also be performed.

Hyperthyroidism can be caused by overproduction of thyroid hormone by the entire gland (Grave's disease), nodules/goiter, thyroiditis, or exogenous thyroid hormone administration. Symptoms and signs are shown in Box 39.1.[15] Patients with untreated or poorly controlled hyperthyroidism undergoing nonthyroid surgery should have elective surgery delayed until euthyroid due risk of perioperative thyroid storm.[16]

Hypothyroidism can be caused by autoimmune disease (e.g., Hashimoto's thyroiditis), partial/total thyroidectomy, radiation treatment, medications (e.g., amiodarone),

---

Box 39.1 **SYMPTOMS AND SIGNS OF HYPERTHYROIDISM**

Increased appetite, weight loss, heat intolerance
Anxiety, depression, disturbed sleep, hyperactivity, emotional lability
Fatigue, weakness, tremor, brisk reflexes, muscle wasting
Palpitations, peripheral edema, tachycardia, atrial fibrillation, hypertension, heart failure
Goiter, neck enlargement, eyelid retraction
Shortness of breath, dyspnea
Hypercoagulability
Nausea, loose stools, frequent bowel movements

Adapted from Wiersinga WM, et al.[15]

Box 39.2 **SYMPTOMS AND SIGNS OF HYPOTHYROIDISM**

Weight gain, cold intolerance, hair loss
Impaired memory, depression, dementia
Hoarseness of voice, neuropathy, ataxia
Bradycardia, diastolic dysfunction, prolonged QT, abnormal T wave
Goiter, periorbital edema
Hypoventilation
Thrombosis or coagulopathy
Delayed gastric emptying, constipation

Adapted from Chaker L, et al.[17]

---

infiltrative disorders (e.g., sarcoidosis), or pituitary disorders. Symptoms and signs are shown in Box 39.2.[17] Patients with severe hypothyroidism (myxedema coma, severe symptoms, free thyroxine <0.5 ng/dL) should have elective surgery delayed until the hypothyroidism has been treated.[18]

CONCLUSION

- Opportunities exist to improve documentation of adverse reactions especially in electronic health records.
- Anaphylaxis is a life-threatening complication requiring immediate treatment.
- After perioperative anaphylaxis, identification of the offending agent is important to elucidate, and the patient may need referral to an allergist especially if the cause is not clinically obvious.
- Evidence supports safe use of cefazolin in patients with a reported penicillin allergy.
- Overall, thyroidectomy is a safe surgery, but life-threatening complications can occur. Awareness and preparation is important to reduce morbidity/mortality.

REVIEW QUESTIONS

Choose the best answer.

1. Which statement is true about perioperative anaphylaxis?

    a. Mortality rate is estimated at 15%.
    b. Grade III severity is when cardiac arrest occurs.
    c. Anaphylaxis is only caused by IgE mediated activation of mast cells.
    d. Mast cell degranulation releases mediators such as histamine, tryptase, serotonin, prostaglandins, and platelet activated factor.

    The correct answer is d.
    Mortality rate varies across countries (1.4–6%). Grade IV severity is when cardiac arrest occurs. Activation can occur via other mechanisms besides IgE.[8]

2. Of the list below, which agent is most frequently reported as the cause in perioperative hypersensitivity reactions?

   a. Local anesthetics.
   b. Latex.
   c. Alpha-gal.
   d. Chlorhexidine.

The correct answer is d.

Chlorhexidine is commonly implicated along with antibiotics and neuromuscular blocking agents. The incidence of latex hypersensitivity reactions has markedly decreased over the years.[8]

3. Which of the following statements about food allergies is false?

   a. Protamine can be used in patients with seafood allergy.
   b. Gelatin colloids and gelatin-containing glues should be avoided in patients with alpha-gal allergy.
   c. Propofol cannot be used in patients with an egg allergy.
   d. Avoid latex exposure in patients with food allergy to banana, kiwi, chestnuts, and avocado.

The correct answer is c.

Propofol can be used in patients with an egg allergy.[8]

4. Which of the following statements is not true about the thyroid gland?

   a. Symptoms/signs of hyperthyroidism include tachycardia, heat intolerance, and weight loss.
   b. Symptoms/signs of thyrotoxicosis/thyroid storm can include fever, tachycardia, and can lead to cardiogenic shock, multiple organ failure, and death.
   c. Myxedema coma is complication of severe hypothyroidism leading to altered mental status, bradycardia, multiple organ failure, and death.
   d. Thyroid storm does not occur in patients with mild hyperthyroidism.

The correct answer is d.

It is difficult to predict preoperatively who will go into thyroid storm.[15–17]

5. Which of the following statements concerning the recurrent laryngeal nerve (RLN) is not true?

   a. Risk of temporary or permanent vocal cord dysfunction varies based on factors such as age, thyroid size, extent of dissection, and surgeon experience.
   b. Calcium channel blockers may improve recovery of transient RLN dysfunction.
   c. The RLN controls all intrinsic muscles of the larynx.
   d. Repositioning of the endotracheal tube can result in gain of a lost signal.

The correct answer is c.

RLN controls all intrinsic muscles of the larynx except for the cricothyroid muscle, which is innervated by the external branch of the superior laryngeal nerve.[14]

REFERENCES

1. Blumenthal KG, Park MA, Macy EM. Redesigning the allergy module of the electronic health record. *Ann Allergy Asthma Immunol.* 2016 Aug;117(2):126–131. doi:10.1016/j.anai.2016.05.017
2. Guyer AC, Macy E, White AA, et al. Allergy electronic health record documentation: A 2022 Work Group Report of the AAAAI Adverse Reactions to Drugs, Biologicals, and Latex Committee. *J Allergy Clin Immunol Pract.* 2022 Nov;10(11):2854–2867. doi:10.1016/j.jaip.2022.08.020
3. Dewachter P, Kopac P, Laguna JJ, et al. Anaesthetic management of patients with pre-existing allergic conditions: A narrative review. *Br J Anaesth.* 2019;123(1):e65–e81. doi:https://doi.org/10.1016/j.bja.2019.01.020
4. Barbara DW, Ronan KP, Maddox DE, Warner MA. Perioperative angioedema: Background, diagnosis, and management. *J Clin Anesth.* 2013 Jun;25(4):335–343. doi:10.1016/j.jclinane.2012.07.009
5. Blumenthal KG, Ryan EE, Li Y, Lee H, Kuhlen JL, Shenoy ES. The impact of a reported penicillin allergy on surgical site infection risk. *Clin Infect Dis.* 2018 Jan 18;66(3):329–336. doi:10.1093/cid/cix794
6. Hermanides J, Lemkes BA, Prins JM, Hollmann MW, Terreehorst I. Presumed β-lactam allergy and cross-reactivity in the operating theater: A practical approach. *Anesthesiology.* 2018;129(2):335–342. doi:10.1097/aln.0000000000002252
7. Cardona V, Ansotegui IJ, Ebisawa M, et al. World allergy organization anaphylaxis guidance 2020. *World Allergy Organ J.* 2020 Oct;13(10):100472. doi:10.1016/j.waojou.2020.100472
8. Tacquard C, Iba T, Levy JH. Perioperative anaphylaxis. *Anesthesiology.* 2023 Jan 1;138(1):100–110. doi:10.1097/ALN.0000000000004419
9. Garvey LH, Dewachter P, Hepner DL, et al. Management of suspected immediate perioperative allergic reactions: An international overview and consensus recommendations. *Br J Anaesth.* 2019;123(1):e50–e64. doi:https://doi.org/10.1016/j.bja.2019.04.044
10. Dewachter P, Savic L. Perioperative anaphylaxis: Pathophysiology, clinical presentation and management. *BJA Educ.* Oct 2019;19(10):313–320. doi:10.1016/j.bjae.2019.06.002
11. Mateja A, Wang Q, Chovanec J, et al. Defining baseline variability of serum tryptase levels improves accuracy in identifying anaphylaxis. *J Allergy Clin Immunol.* 2022 Mar;149(3):1010–1017 e10. doi:10.1016/j.jaci.2021.08.007
12. Patel KN, Yip L, Lubitz CC, et al. Executive summary of the American Association of Endocrine Surgeons guidelines for the definitive surgical management of thyroid disease in adults. *Ann Surg.* Mar 2020;271(3):399–410. doi:10.1097/SLA.0000000000003735
13. Bhattacharyya N, Fried MP. Assessment of the morbidity and complications of total thyroidectomy. *Arch Otolaryngol Head Neck Surg.* 2002 Apr;128(4):389–392. doi:10.1001/archotol.128.4.389
14. Patel KN, Yip L, Lubitz CC, et al. The American Association of Endocrine Surgeons guidelines for the definitive surgical management of thyroid disease in adults. *Ann Surg.* 2020 Mar;271(3):e21–e93. doi:10.1097/SLA.0000000000003580
15. Wiersinga WM, Poppe KG, Effraimidis G. Hyperthyroidism: Aetiology, pathogenesis, diagnosis, management, complications, and prognosis. *Lancet Diabetes Endocrinol.* 2023;11(4):282–298. doi:https://doi.org/10.1016/S2213-8587(23)00005-0
16. de Mul N, Damstra J, Nieveen van Dijkum EJM, et al. Risk of perioperative thyroid storm in hyperthyroid patients: A systematic review. *Br J Anaesth.* 2021 Dec;127(6):879–889. doi:10.1016/j.bja.2021.06.043
17. Chaker L, Bianco AC, Jonklaas J, Peeters RP. Hypothyroidism. *Lancet.* 2017 Sep 23;390(10101):1550–1562. doi:10.1016/S0140-6736(17)30703-1
18. Himes CP, Ganesh R, Wight EC, Simha V, Liebow M. Perioperative evaluation and management of endocrine disorders. *Mayo Clin Proc.* 2020 Dec;95(12):2760–2774. doi:10.1016/j.mayocp.2020.05.004

40.

NONVERBAL AUTISTIC 30-YEAR-OLD FOR FULL MOUTH DENTAL REHABILITATION WITH MALIGNANT HYPERTHERMIA

Jonathan Bacon and Ralph Epstein

STEM CASE AND KEY QUESTIONS

A 30-year-old man with autism is scheduled to undergo wisdom teeth extractions and full mouth dental rehabilitation under general anesthesia (GA) at a community hospital. He is 6′ 3″ and weighs 100 kg. The day prior to treatment, the anesthesiologist notices that the chart is flagged for "extremely combative behavior" and "autism." No additional information is included in the electronic medical record (EMR). In anticipation of an uncooperative patient, the anesthesiologist contemplates an oral sedative prescription to be taken by the patient at home, prior to arrival.

What are the goals of pre-hospital sedation for a combative patient?

As many as 30% of special needs patients require the use of physical restraint to facilitate anesthetic induction.[1] This introduces a host of safety issues for both the patient and anesthesia team along with ethical concerns surrounding restraint. Oral premedications have traditionally been used in pediatric anesthesiology. They aim to decrease anxiety, improve parental separation, and mask acceptance prior to induction of anesthesia. However, in the combative special needs population, oral premedication serves primarily as behavior modification to bridge a safe anesthetic induction. When a pre-hospital sedative is required, the role of these medications is to relax the patient sufficiently to accept direction, exit the car, and enter a presurgical setting without resistance and with minimal assistance. They intend to facilitate safe arrival of the patient, transfer of care, and induction of anesthesia. Pre-hospital sedatives are reserved for only the most combative patients who would not tolerate oral premedication or intramuscular (IM) injection within the presurgical setting.

What pharmacological properties would be desirable in a pre-hospital, oral sedative for a combative patient with autism?

Pre-hospital oral sedatives must be judiciously selected to preserve respiratory drive and maintain pharyngeal muscle tone to prevent respiratory depression, hypoventilation, and obstruction, respectively. Medications administered at home must also preserve consciousness and protective airway reflexes. They must have a low bioavailability range and a wide therapeutic index. For the combative, special needs patient, the oral agent selected should ideally exhibit sympatholytic properties to attenuate the fight or flight response, which is commonly encountered in presurgical settings with these patients.[1-3] It should be understood that many of our commonly used oral premedications, such as midazolam, ketamine, and dexmedetomidine, would be contraindicated for administration at home.

Which medication class would be a wise choice for pre-hospital oral sedation in a combative patient with autism?

Alpha-2 agonists are an excellent option for home administration in a combative patient with autism. They are safe when prescribed for long-term use in this population and effectively decrease hyperactivity and impulsivity.[4,5] Side effects are typically drowsiness and fatigue, which are desirable characteristics in a pre-hospital sedative. They demonstrate minimal hypoventilatory effects and preserve the ventilatory response to CO_2.[6] The most commonly implemented alpha-2 agonists in clinical practice are clonidine, tizanidine, dexmedetomidine, and guanfacine. Clonidine and tizanidine have a long track record of safety when prescribed orally and have been used for decades in the treatment of multiple conditions. Most notably, they have treated hypertension, anxiety, attention deficit disorder (ADD)/attention deficit hyperactivity disorder (ADHD), chronic pain, myofascial pain, postoperative shivering, and spasticity secondary to CNS disorders and cerebral palsy.[7]

In recent years, intravenous (IV) dexmedetomidine has been used to prevent emergence delirium in children and prevent generalized delirium in pediatric and adult intensive care unit (ICU) patients.[8,9] It is currently gaining popularity for procedural sedation and awake intubations and has the demonstrated advantage of decreased airway secretions.[10] Furthermore, alpha-2 agonists significantly decrease monitored anesthesia care (MAC) requirements,[11,12] making them particularly attractive for anesthesiologists. When taken orally, they demonstrate limited variability in their bioavailability. This leads to a more predictable drug, which is desirable for any pharmacological agent, but especially when administered in an unmonitored setting. The range of bioavailability for enteral clonidine, dexmedetomidine, and tizanidine is 88–96%,[13] 12–20%,[14] and 20–34%,[15,16] respectively.

Literature supports a significantly altered stress response to perioperative procedures including venipuncture in patients with special needs and autism.[2,3] This can lead to increases in heart rate, other injurious behavior, aggression, and unanticipated adverse perioperative events. Autistic patients also demonstrate abnormal levels of circulating neurotransmitters when compared to neurotypical controls. Specifically, plasma norepinephrine (NE) concentrations have been shown to be elevated in the ASD population.[17] It is therefore reasonable to conclude that alpha-2 agonists, which decrease production, secretion, and reuptake of NE, may be effective in their management. By decreasing circulating NE, alpha-2 agonists may attenuate the fight-or-flight response and combativity that are often triggered by an unfamiliar, perioperative environment.

Explain the specific mechanisms by which alpha-2 agonists modulate sedation and pain in the central and peripheral nervous systems.

Alpha-2 agonists modulate both central and peripheral nervous systems. Their action is mediated through receptor subtypes 2A, 2B, and 2C. While subtypes 2A and 2C predominate centrally, subtype 2B tends to exert its action peripherally. All three subtypes are G protein-coupled receptors, which inhibit adenyl cyclase resulting in decreased levels of cAMP. This causes increased K$^+$ efflux and decreased Ca^{++} influx through Ca^{++}-activated channels leading to hyperpolarization of the cell and a suppression of nerve firing. This produces various effects in different regions of the nervous system.

The central sedative effects of alpha 2-agonists are primarily exerted within the locus coeruleus in the brainstem. The locus coeruleus is the principal site of NE production in the brain. Therefore, when alpha-2 agonism causes suppression of neurotransmission within the locus coeruleus, the result is decreased production and secretion of NE. This is mediated through the alpha-2A and alpha-2C receptor subtypes. Decreased circulating NE levels are then responsible for the central sedative effects of these medications. In the periphery, reduced NE levels lead to decreases in heart rate and blood pressure. Agonism at the alpha-2B receptor acts to directly decrease vasomotor tone, which also contributes to a decrease in systemic vascular resistance. Bradycardia is mediated via the alpha-2A receptor subtype by inhibiting the cardioaccelerator nerves and through vagomimetic action.[18]

The analgesic effects of alpha-2 agonists are mediated in the dorsal horn of the spinal column where agonism decreases the release of substance P and glutamate. Glutamate is the primary excitatory neurotransmitter of the nervous system, and substance P is a neurotransmitter chiefly involved in the neurotransmission of pain and inflammation. Following a noxious stimulus, nociceptive neurons transmit action potentials via primary afferent nerve fibers to laminae I and II of the dorsal horn in the spinal cord. Signal transduction is typically carried out by specialized C and A delta fibers. Upon arrival of these signals, substance P and glutamate are released. This activates postsynaptic receptors within the spinothalamic tract, leading to the perception of pain within the thalamus. Consequently, by decreasing the release of substance P and glutamate, the perception of pain is decreased, resulting in the analgesic effect associated with these medications.[19]

Are there any options for treatment of oversedation induced through alpha-2 agonism?

Atipamezole is a selective alpha-2 antagonist that has been shown to rapidly reverse both the sympatholytic and sedative effects of alpha-2 agonists in a dose-dependent fashion in human studies.[20,21] It exists predominantly in veterinary medicine and is approved and marketed in the US and several European countries for the reversal of medetomidine. Medetomidine is a racemic mixture of the pharmacologically active dextrorotatory enantiomer dexmedetomidine and the pharmacologically inactive levorotary enantiomer levomedetomidine. It is currently not approved for use in humans. Similar to other reversal agents, the provider must be cognizant of the deleterious effects of rapid reversal of the analgesia, sedation, and sympatholytic activity provided by alpha-2 agonists. One study demonstrated a 10-fold increase in plasma NE concentrations following rapid administration of atipamezole.[21]

Which oral alpha-2 agonist should be selected for pre-hospital sedation in this patient?

Tizanidine is an excellent alpha-2 agonist selection for this patient. It is preferred over clonidine because it has less effect on blood pressure and heart rate[6,22] and offers a shorter duration of action, which should expedite time to discharge. Tizanidine has also demonstrated a wide therapeutic index, which is particularly important for drugs administered at home. While typical oral dosages range from 2–6 mg, it is safe in doses as high as 36 mg/day.[23] Common side effects at these doses are somnolence, xerostomia, and fatigue.

Tizanidine takes 1 hour to reach peak plasma levels following oral administration.[22] Consequently, peak sedation should coincide nicely with arrival and hospital admission. Tizanidine also has the additional benefit of being formulated in both a tablet and a capsule. Caretakers can crush the tablet and mix the powder into a beverage of choice for the patient. Compounding pharmacies can also make this in an elixir formulation.

Currently, there are no clinical guidelines for dosing of pre-hospital tizanidine for sedation in the combative ASD population. Therefore, recommendations are based on the authors' experience with this population over several years. The authors have used tizanidine as follows:

- 20–40 kg: 8 mg tizanidine
- 40–70 kg: 12 mg tizanidine
- >70 kg: 16 mg tizanidine

The following is a clinical example of the efficacy of tizanidine administered preoperatively: an 85 kg aggressive autistic patient was seen in the author's private office on a Friday for evaluation of a loose crown. Upon leaving the office, the patient threw his caretaker, who weighed more than 100 kg, into the wall located in the lobby (see Figure 40.1).

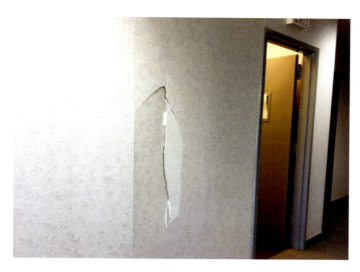

Figure 40.1 Dental office lobby wall damage from patient with autism aggressively pushing his caregiver during visit for evaluation.

The patient in our case example returned on Monday after taking tizanidine 16 mg, 45 minutes prior to arrival. Upon arrival, the autistic patient sat in a wheelchair located in the waiting room and allowed the dentist anesthesiologist to administer an IM admixture of ketamine and midazolam.

Unfortunately, the anesthesiologist was unable to reach the patient's group home to prescribe the pre-hospital oral sedative. Subsequently, the patient arrived at the hospital on the day of surgery and refused to exit the car. He was accompanied by his two parents, along with two aides from the group home in which he resides. The anesthesiologist was notified and an interview with the parents was initiated while the patient remained in the car with his caretakers. The parents confirmed that the patient was NPO since 10:00 p.m. yesterday. The patient was wearing noise-canceling headphones and was repeatedly clasping his hands together while rocking in his seat. Drool was noted on his chin.

In anticipation of an uncooperative patient, the anesthesiologist considers an IM ketamine injection. What dosages have proven efficacious in this population?

Ketamine is the most popular agent for IM injection in the special needs population. It offers a rapid onset of analgesia, amnesia, dissociation, and modest immobility. When administered intramuscularly, its bioavailability is approximately 93%.[24] It takes effect within 3–4 minutes[25] and its duration of action is 20–30 minutes.[26] While many textbooks propose doses of 8–10 mg/kg for effective sedation, most literature supports that these doses are general anesthetic doses. In fact, doses of IM ketamine ranging from 4 to 11 mg/kg have produced GA.[24]

It is important to make the distinction between doses used for GA and those needed as a bridge to successful induction. Using IM ketamine as a single agent to induce and maintain GA is rarely the objective with a combative patient. Rather, sufficient relaxation for mask placement or gaining IV access is the goal. It is for this reason that ketamine use, as a bridge agent to induction, more closely resembles its use for procedural sedation than for GA. Ketamine has proved efficacious for procedural sedation in IM doses as low as 2–2.5 mg/kg in healthy children.[27–30]

However, in patients with excited delirium, 5 mg/kg has proved effective in minimizing agitation and aggressive behavior.[31–35] Hence, the practitioner must weigh the benefits of immobility and sedation with the sequelae of increasing doses and prolonged recovery. The proper dose for combative ASD patients likely falls somewhere between 2.5 and 5 mg/kg when used as a singular bridge agent for successful induction. These doses may be lowered if adjunctive agents are combined with the ketamine. All providers should understand that ketamine produces analgesia in IM doses as low as 0.5–1 mg/kg and impairs memory in IM doses as little as 0.25–0.5 mg/kg.[24]

Which adjunctive medications are occasionally combined with IM ketamine? Explain the rationale behind these additions.

Benzodiazepines are occasionally combined with ketamine for several reasons. Primarily, they decrease the incidence of dysphoria and are superior to other drug classes in this respect.[36] Benzodiazepines lessen the stark, phenotypic expression of ketamine that is observed when ketamine is administered as a single agent. Namely, distant gaze and uninhibited vocalizations can be reduced by co-administration of benzodiazepines. While these stark effects may be unremarkable for anesthesia professionals, family members can often become overwhelmed when witnessing their loved one in a dissociative state. Diazepam and midazolam have been studied extensively, and both effectively attenuate this dysphoric response.[36–39] When compared with one another, midazolam seems to produce slightly less dysphoria.[37]

Dexmedetomidine has also proved effective when combined with ketamine in an IM injection. This combination is particularly beneficial because the effects of each medication are balanced by the other. Specifically, the tachycardia and sialorrhea associated with ketamine are counteracted by the bradycardia and antisialagogue effects of dexmedetomidine. The authors have used this combination successfully in a ratio of ketamine 3.0 mg/kg mixed with dexmedetomidine 1.0 mcg/kg as a bridge to induction of GA. However, this admixture should be avoided in patients taking guanfacine or other alpha-2 agonists because severe and persistent bradycardia may occur.[40,41]

Other agents that are periodically combined with ketamine include glycopyrrolate and atropine. These medications are used to attenuate sialorrhea induced by ketamine. Unfortunately, both atropine and glycopyrrolate are poorly absorbed via the IM route. They achieve peak plasma concentrations roughly 30 minutes[42,43] following injection, and their antisialagogue effect corresponds with this peak.[44] Hence, the utility of antimuscarinic drug administration for this purpose is questionable. The anesthesia provider may likely achieve a faster antisialagogue effect by obtaining IV access and administering the drug via the IV route.

Our case example patient seemingly calmed, and the parents were able to coax him out of the car with a promise of breakfast. Hospital admission was swiftly completed, and the patient was moved to a presurgical holding unit. The anesthesiologist was able to continue gathering data regarding the patient's medical history, which included GA for dental rehabilitation at age 12, with no complications, and GA for dental rehabilitation at age 17, notable for an episode of malignant hyperthermia (MH).

ANESTHETIC HISTORY

Following induction of the patient's second GA, he rapidly developed a hypermetabolic state consistent with MH. The condition was swiftly diagnosed and treated by the anesthesia team. The patient responded favorably to dantrolene, cooling measures, and diuretics. He remained under observation in the pediatric ICU for 72 hours and was discharged to home in stable condition with no residual complications. Due to the remote location of MH testing centers and poor patient cooperation, a muscle biopsy was never performed to confirm MH diagnosis.

What is the incidence of malignant hyperthermia? Which subsets of the population are more susceptible to malignant hyperthermia?

MH occurs in 1:100,000 adult anesthetics and 1:30,000 pediatric anesthetics.[45] On average, patients develop MH on their third anesthetic exposure, after 1–2 previous uneventful exposures to triggering agents.[46] Accordingly, all providers should recognize that a negative MH history does not ensure freedom from vulnerability. Patient subsets who are more susceptible to MH include males (2:1), patients with central core disease (CCD), and patients with myopathies including multi-minicore disease (MmD), central nuclear myopathy, King-Denborough syndrome, STAC3 (Native American) myopathy, and congenital myopathy with cores and rods.[46–48]

FAMILY HISTORY

The patient's family history is notable for his father's coronary artery disease, status post myocardial infarction at age 41 and three-vessel coronary artery bypass graft (CABG) and type 2 diabetes mellitus (T2DM). His mother also has T2DM.

PAST MEDICAL HISTORY

The parents and aides report a vague medical history with autism diagnosed at age 3 and ADHD diagnosed at age 6. Doctors were considering a schizophrenia diagnosis during puberty due to his aggressive behavior, but the matter was not pursued. Since adolescence, he has had no major medical interventions, surgeries, or hospitalizations, except for the MH episode. According to his aides, he attends yearly check-ups via the group home's physician. However, at these appointments he does not allow blood draws, nor does he permit the doctor to approach him or listen to him with a stethoscope. He is extremely sedentary while at his group home and remains in his room the majority of the day.

Given the patient's history and inability to assess metabolic equivalents (METS), is further preoperative testing indicated prior to GA?

This patient does not require additional testing prior to GA according to the 2014 American College of Cardiologists (ACC)/American Heart Association (AHA) Guideline on Perioperative Cardiovascular Evaluation and Management of Patients Undergoing Non-Cardiac Surgery.[49] It should be noted that family history has no influence on patient risk assessment prior to surgery. Family history is taken to infer susceptibility to MH, pseudocholinesterase deficiency, and coagulopathies.

However, a number of surgical and patient factors are important when deciding whether the patient warrants further evaluation prior to surgery. First, it must be determined whether the surgery is elective or emergent. All emergency surgeries should proceed without further testing as the risk to life and limb is too great and time-sensitive to warrant further workup. In this case, the patient is presenting for a nonemergent, elective surgery. Therefore, additional testing would be warranted in certain situations.

Next, the risk of major adverse cardiac events (MACE) must be determined using the patient history and type of surgery. In this example, the patient is presenting for dental rehabilitation and wisdom teeth extractions, which is deemed a low-risk surgery. The Revised Cardiac Risk Index (RCRI) or American College of Surgeons National Surgical Quality Improvement Program (NSQIP) calculators can be used to discern the patient's overall risk of MACE during the perioperative period.[50]

In this circumstance, the patient's risk of MACE using either calculating system is determined to be low (<1%). Therefore, there is no need to evaluate the patient's functional status using METS. In fact, given the patient factors and type of surgery, there is class III evidence supporting no benefit to further evaluation prior to this patient's surgery. Consequently, the patient should proceed to surgery without further testing.

MEDICATIONS

The patient is receiving risperidone, dextroamphetamine/amphetamine, clonidine, fluoxetine, clozapine, multivitamin, and fish oil.

Discuss the drug classification and mechanism of action of risperidone. What are important anesthetic considerations regarding this medication?

Risperidone is classified as a second-generation (atypical) antipsychotic medication. It is the most commonly prescribed atypical antipsychotic for children and adolescents.[51,52] Other notable members of this class include ziprasidone, quetiapine, and clozapine. Risperidone is prescribed for the treatment of conduct disorders, including oppositional defiant disorder (ODD) and disruptive behavior. In autistic patients, it aims to lessen irritability and aggression.

Second-generation antipsychotics act by antagonizing dopamine and serotonin at the D_2 and $5\text{-}HT_{2A}$ receptors, respectively.[53] For this reason, they are also referred to as serotonin-dopamine antagonists. These medications demonstrate decreased neuroleptic and metabolic side effects when compared to first-generation medications such as haloperidol, droperidol, and chlorpromazine. That being said, the anesthesia provider should still be cognizant of the possibility of neuroleptic malignant syndrome (NMS). Risperidone-induced NMS has been cited extensively in the literature.[54–57]

Atypical medications may also precipitate extrapyramidal reactions including akathisia, Parkinsonian symptoms, and tardive dyskinesia. Consequently, anesthesiologists should avoid medications with antidopaminergic effects. These include, but are not limited to, metoclopramide, haloperidol, and droperidol, which are often used for adjunctive postoperative nausea and vomiting (PONV) therapy. Risperidone may also induce hypothermia by inhibiting peripheral vasoconstriction via alpha-adrenergic antagonism.[58] This typically occurs upon initiation of the drug.

What condition does clozapine treat? Explain side effects that would be of significance to the anesthesia provider.

Clozapine is a second-generation (atypical) antipsychotic used to treat schizophrenia and schizoaffective disorder. It is the only medication approved by the US Food and Drug Administration (FDA) to manage suicidal behavior in patients with schizophrenia and has been shown to decrease mortality.[59] Clozapine causes less extrapyramidal symptoms than other atypical antipsychotics. However, due to a myriad of additional side effects, it is reserved exclusively for treatment-resistant schizophrenia when other antipsychotics have proved unsuccessful. The anesthesia provider should understand that clozapine use implies a psychiatric history, which in the ASD population is usually synonymous with a history of aggression.

Clozapine is unique because of its ability to precipitate agranulocytosis, which occurs in roughly 1% of individuals.[60,61] It is also known to induce cardiovascular side effects including myocarditis in 1% of patients. Orthostatic hypotension, tachycardia, and dyslipidemia have also been reported.[61] These signs typically present within the first month of use. While most antipsychotics cause dry mouth, clozapine produces hypersalivation.[62] It can lower the seizure threshold and is associated with an increased risk of gastric hypomobility.[60,63] Clozapine can also cause hypothermia when therapy is first initiated. This is likely a result of peripheral vasoconstriction via alpha-adrenergic antagonism.[58]

Discuss the drug classification and mechanism of action for fluoxetine. What are some important anesthetic considerations regarding these drugs?

Fluoxetine is classified as a second-generation antidepressant medication in the selective serotonin reuptake inhibitor (SSRI) family. It is used to treat obsessive compulsive disorder (OCD) and lessen restrictive and repetitive behavior in autistic patients. Other prominent members of this family include paroxetine, sertraline, citalopram, and escitalopram. These medications selectively inhibit the 5-hydroxytryptamine transporter in the CNS leading to elevated serotonin levels across the synaptic cleft.[64] In contrast, classical antidepressants such as monoamine oxidase inhibitors (MAOIs) and tricyclic antidepressants (TCAs) are nonselective. They influence multiple drug targets and therefore demonstrate greater toxicity and side effects when compared to second-generation medications.

SSRIs can precipitate a host of drug interactions and physiologic derangements. Most notably, SSRIs can increase bleeding and inhibit a variety of cytochrome oxidase systems including CYP 1A2, 2C9, 2D6, and 3A4.[65] As such, they may increase plasma concentrations of drugs that depend on these systems for clearance. Some noteworthy examples include warfarin, midazolam, theophylline, and type 1 antiarrhythmic agents such as lidocaine, procainamide, and phenytoin. The anesthesia provider should anticipate additional medications that might be influenced and titrate accordingly.

SSRIs induce bleeding through their influence on serotonin. Serotonin plays a prominent role in clot formation. It is transported and released by platelets following endothelial injury. When released, it increases platelet aggregation[66] and causes vasoconstriction of injured blood vessels, thereby initiating the clot. However, patients on SSRIs have a high proportion of their serotonin bound up in the synaptic cleft. Therefore, less is available for platelet aggregation, which explains the mechanism for increased bleeding with these medications.[67] This bleeding risk is synergistically amplified with the concomitant use of NSAIDs. The addition of NSAIDs to SSRIs has demonstrated a 15-fold increase in upper GI bleeding from baseline.[67] As such, it may be prudent to avoid NSAIDs in these patients. Yet clinically significant surgical bleeding has not been demonstrated.

As SSRIs augment serotonin levels within the CNS, anesthesia providers should be particularly aware of *serotonin syndrome*. Medications that prevent presynaptic uptake of serotonin, such as tramadol, meperidine, pentazocine, fenfluramine, and dextromethorphan, should be avoided. SSRIs have also been known to cause the syndrome of inappropriate antidiuretic hormone (SIADH) in the elderly, although the mechanism is incompletely understood.[68,69] Discontinuation of SSRI medications can induce withdrawal and produce symptoms such as agitation, irritability, and sweating. For this reason, SSRIs should be continued throughout the perioperative period.[64]

The medical history of our patient is completed, and an IM injection is prepared. The anesthesiologist programs the infusion pumps and considers physiologic irregularities and medical comorbidities that may be common in ASD patients.

What are some common medical comorbidities associated with autism?

Autistic patients are more prone to concomitant neurodevelopmental and behavioral disorders. It is estimated that 70% of patients with ASD have at least one concomitant psychological disorder, while 40% have been diagnosed with two or more. Most notably, anxiety, ADHD, and ODD occur in approximately 30% of individuals with autism.[70] Furthermore, as many as 75% of these patients have intellectual disability.[70] Schizophrenia and sleeplessness occur at rates 10 times that of the general population. Accordingly, the prudent anesthesiologist should anticipate these commonalities and use that knowledge to better empathize with the patient and family.

The prevalence of seizure disorder is significantly elevated in the ASD population. Roughly 30% of autistic patients have a seizure disorder compared with only 2–3% of the general population.[71] Most autistic patients suffer from generalized tonic-clonic seizures (88%).[70] However, research has demonstrated that subclinical epileptiform activity may be present in as many as 82% of autistic patients,[72] even in the absence of a diagnosed disorder. For this reason, the anesthesia provider must remain attentive as seizure activity could present with subtlety.

GI disorders disproportionately affect patients with ASD at a rate of approximately 11%,[73] while GI symptoms may exist in as many as 91% of children with ASD. Reflux esophagitis, gastric and intestinal inflammation, and carbohydrate malabsorption have been evidenced endoscopically and histologically.[74] Symptoms such as diarrhea, gaseousness, bloating, abdominal pain, and stool impaction are extremely common and have been shown to occur at significantly greater rates when compared with age-matched siblings.[75] It is hypothesized that GI abnormalities are grossly underappreciated and underdiagnosed in this population. The anesthesia provider should understand that unrecognized symptoms could partly explain the abundance of behavioral problems encountered in this population. In addition, autistic patients are at an elevated risk of mortality secondary to pulmonary complications, specifically pneumonia. This risk seems to correlate with an increasing degree of intellectual disability.[76]

What physiological abnormalities may be seen in autistic patients?

Autistic patients may express a variety of physiological abnormalities when compared to neurotypical individuals. Generally, autonomic dysregulation is evidenced by heightened baseline sympathetic activity with decreased parasympathetic activity. In one investigation, reduced cardiac parasympathetic activity was demonstrated in children with autism.[77] Other studies have observed abnormalities in skin conductance and pupillary light reactivity, suggesting dysregulation of the NE-mediated sympathetic nervous system.[78]

Multiple investigations have evidenced a diminished respiratory sinus arrhythmia in ASD patients.[79] As sinus arrhythmia acts as a surrogate for parasympathetic tone,[80] its diminution suggests a decrease in parasympathetic control. Vagal nerve stimulation has also exhibited success in treating some aspects of ASD, lending credence to the theory that overabundant sympathetic tone may contribute to unwanted symptoms. In summary, it appears as though autistic patients demonstrate not only a heightened baseline sympathetic tone, but also decreased parasympathetic control.

Autistic patients also exhibit immune dysfunction. Multiple studies have evidenced an association between immune dysregulation and severity of autism symptoms. Research has demonstrated increased plasma cytokines in ASD patients. This increase is correlated with increasingly negative behaviors.[81] Furthermore, as many of these elevated cytokines are pro-inflammatory mediators, an inflammatory etiology is suggested.[82,83] To support this assertion, treatment with IV immunoglobulin (IVIG), NSAIDs, and other immune modulators, which decrease circulating cytokines, have been shown to decrease symptoms.[84–86] In conclusion, there is an association between immune abnormalities, inflammation, and severity of ASD symptoms.[87]

Autistic patients are prone to inborn metabolic disturbances. Mitochondrial dysfunction exists in as many as 7.2% of individuals with autism compared with only 0.01% of the general population.[88] Research has evidenced impairment of electron transport chain complexes causing disturbances in energy production. It has also shown alterations in oxidation-reduction reactions, which can generate reactive oxygen species (ROS). It is proposed that oxidative stress imposed by ROS is what, in part, contributes to ASD. Elevations in markers of oxidative stress and reductions in antioxidants have supported this assertion.[89] Glutathione is a marker for protection against oxidative stress and is shown to be decreased in autistic patients.[90]

Folate metabolism and methylation pathways are frequently abnormal in ASD patients. Of note, methylenetetrahydrofolate reductase (MTHFR) gene polymorphisms are more common in autistic patients. One investigation found homozygous MTHFR deficiencies in 23% of patients with autism.[91] The homozygous genotype is significant for anesthesiologists because it can lead to elevated homocysteine levels and folate trapping following nitrous oxide administration. Complications including myelopathy, peripheral neuropathy, hemiparesis, and death have occurred.[91]

In one instance, an infant with unknown MTHFR deficiency expired following two general anesthetics with nitrous oxide. The autopsy demonstrated cerebral atrophy and severe demyelination secondary to elevated homocysteine levels and decreased methionine. These findings are consistent with other deaths following nitrous oxide administration to unknown homozygous individuals. In the majority of these cases, dietary B_{12} levels were critically low, making the patient particularly susceptible to the irreversible inhibition of B_{12} by nitrous oxide. Case reports have been limited to the pediatric population, suggesting vulnerability in younger patients[92] (Figure 40.2).

For our case example, multiple staff members are called on to assist the anesthesiologist with induction. The patient is lightly restrained but does not demonstrate aggressive behavior. An IM admixture of ketamine 400 mg (4 mg/kg) and midazolam 5 mg (0.05 mg/kg) is administered to the patient in the presurgical unit. Five minutes following the injection, the patient is sufficiently sedated and wheeled to the operating room without incident. Upon transfer to the operating room table, increased secretions are noted by the anesthesiologist. Suction is attempted but the patient's jaw remains rigid and his mouth is unable to be opened. Consequently, suctioning is abandoned and oxygen is applied via facemask. Although access appears difficult, IV cannulation is attempted by a senior resident in the dorsum of the left hand. Upon entering the skin, the patient retracts his hand slightly and emits a single cough. The anesthesiologist quickly notices a lack of air exchange and is unable to ventilate with positive pressure. A preliminary working diagnosis of total laryngospasm is made. A Larson maneuver is performed and positive pressure is applied, but to no avail.

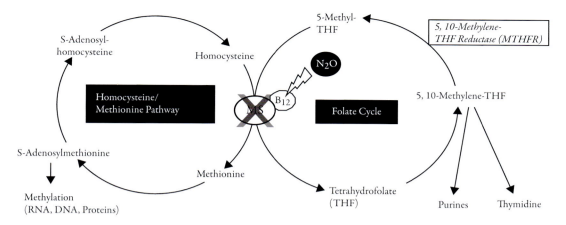

Figure 40.2 Inhibition of methionine synthase (MS) by nitrous oxide (N_2O) occurs at a critical juncture of two pathways: the folate cycle and the remethylation of methionine from homocysteine. Nitrous oxide oxidizes the cobalt atom of vitamin B12 (cobalamin), thereby inactivating vitamin B12 as a necessary cofactor for methionine synthase function. The subsequent accumulation of 5-methyl-tetrahydrofolate due to inactive methionine synthase is called "folate trapping."
THF, tetrahydrofolate.
From Nagele P, Zeugswetter B, Wiener C, Burger H, Hüpfl M, Mittlböck M, Födinger M. Influence of methylenetetrahydrofolate reductase gene polymorphisms on homocysteine concentrations after nitrous oxide anesthesia. *Anesthesiology*. 2008;109(1):36–43. doi:10.1097/ALN.0b013e318178820b.

What are some novel options for the treatment of laryngospasm without IV access in a patient with MH?

One option to consider is IM rocuronium. Its bioavailability exceeds 80%, and peak plasma concentrations are reached in 13 minutes.[93] While studied exclusively in infants and children, it has been shown to adequately provide muscular relaxation and tracheal intubating conditions. In one investigation, IM rocuronium injection to the deltoid, dosed at 1 mg/kg in infants and 1.8 mg/kg in children, produced complete neuromuscular blockade in approximately 8 minutes.[94] In a similar study, these same doses achieved intubating conditions in as little as 3 minutes.[95]

What remains unknown is at what point prior to attainment of proper intubating conditions that a laryngospasm would break sufficiently to allow adequate oxygenation and ventilation. As neuromuscular recovery begins 60–90 minutes following IM administration, this approach should be reserved for emergencies or longer-duration procedures.[93] Alternative IM paralytics including atracurium, mivacurium, and pancuronium have produced slower blockade and therefore are not recommended.[96–98]

Another unique alternative in this situation is the administration of topical local anesthetic to break the laryngospasm. This has been performed via transtracheal injection, nebulizer, and atomization via laryngeal tracheal atomizer (LTA). Transtracheal lidocaine has been used effectively to treat post-extubation stridor in 1 minute at doses of approximately 1.5 mg/kg. Nebulized 2% lidocaine has also demonstrated complete resolution of post-extubation partial laryngospasm. Atomized 2% lidocaine has been shown to decrease post-extubation laryngospasm and stridor when applied prior to emergence.[99] The topical approach has also proved effective in treating laryngospasm in cats. Notably, higher concentrations of lidocaine (5% and 10%) provided significantly longer protection against laryngospasm than did 2% solutions.[100]

In our case, help is summoned. Shortly thereafter, the patient's oxygen saturation starts to fall. The anesthesiologist administers 100 mg (1 mg/kg) of IM rocuronium (50 mg/5 mL in each vastus lateralis). Meanwhile, the senior resident is once again instructed to attempt IV cannulation, which is successful with a 22-gauge catheter. Positive-pressure ventilation is applied by the anesthesiologist and is effective in increasing the saturation to 98%. A cricothyrotomy was considered, but due to the improved saturation the surgical intervention was abandoned.

Infusions of propofol and remifentanil are initiated, along with the administration of 100 mcg of fentanyl. A nerve stimulator is placed over the ulnar nerve. After 5 minutes, 1:4 twitches is recorded. The patient is easily intubated with a grade 1 view. Dental and oral surgical treatment ensues and is completed in 2.5 hours. At the completion of the procedure, 4:4 twitches are noted at the ulnar nerve. Nonetheless, neuromuscular blockade is definitively reversed with 200 mg (2 mg/kg) of IV sugammadex.

Minutes later, the patient meets extubation criteria and is extubated on the operating room table. Upon transfer from table to stretcher, the patient becomes combative and begins thrashing and violently swinging his arms. The anesthesiologist administers 25 mcg (0.25 mcg/kg) of IV dexmedetomidine which effectively relaxes the patient within 30 seconds. The patient is then transported to the PACU, recovered, and discharged without incident.

DISCUSSION

There is a paucity of data regarding anesthetic management of the combative patient with autism. Lack of staff knowledge regarding ASD patients and their specific needs is not only inconvenient, but has also contributed to adverse outcomes in the medical arena.[101–103] The aim of this chapter is to offer a comprehensive review of ASD for the anesthesia provider. It is intended to promote thought regarding anesthetic scenarios that may arise when treating these patients through a review of some current literature and a discussion of novel pharmacologic approaches. By investigating physiological differences, comorbidities, medications, and unusual scenarios, the reader will be better prepared to treat combative patients, ASD patients, and patients with special needs in the future. The ensuing discussion is intended to expand on and supplement the information provided above.

A 2009 study sought to understand the experiences of both caregivers and hospital staff surrounding hospital admissions for patients with special needs. Interestingly, while the delivery of medical care was perceived as satisfactory, the social aspects of these admissions were deemed inadequate.[104] Lack of staff knowledge regarding the specific challenges faced by these families was cited as one of the primary themes needing improvement. In particular, adherence to routines and comfort in familiar surroundings were underappreciated by hospital personnel.[104]

Accordingly, the unpleasant nature of the presurgical environment is likely underestimated in the ASD population. Administration of a pre-hospital sedative could improve the patient experience by offering sedation during a heightened time of distress. While neurotypical individuals may exhibit elevated anxiety in anticipation of entering an operating room, ASD patients may demonstrate similar or increased anxiety in anticipation of entering the unfamiliar presurgical setting. For this reason, a pre-hospital oral sedative should be considered.

Pre-hospital sedation can offer the additional benefit of safety to healthcare workers providing care for combative patients. Paramedics and emergency medical technicians (EMTs) have pioneered pre-hospital sedation. Through pharmacologic intervention, they have allowed for the safe arrival, admission, and assessment of patients by emergency physicians. Commonly used agents include droperidol, haloperidol, diphenhydramine, and ketamine. Unfortunately, these pre-hospital sedatives are administered intramuscularly and therefore cannot be performed by family members or aides. Studies have demonstrated adverse events with all of these agents when administered in the field. Common observations include hypersalivation, vomiting, emergence reaction, laryngospasm, and need for intubation.[105–107] Accordingly, this approach requires advanced training and an extensive allocation of resources, which are beyond the scope of this discussion.

The risk that combative patients pose to healthcare workers may also be underappreciated. Although rare, assault and death have occurred at the hands of combative patients.[108] In a large investigation, 8% of fatalities for EMTs in the line of duty were due to assault by hostile patients. Furthermore, a disproportionate number of assault victims were female. While the risk of injury that combative patients pose to anesthesia providers has not been quantified, anecdotal evidence supports the validity of this threat. As such, premedication may be essential to the safety and well-being of providers.

Oral pre-hospital sedation for combative patients must be distinguished from oral premedication use in the presurgical setting. The latter has been covered extensively in the literature. In contrast, pre-hospital oral sedation has different objectives and is rarely explored by scholarly publications. Furthermore, it should be understood that many of our commonly used presurgical oral sedatives would not be indicated for administration at home. Some key examples include midazolam, ketamine, and dexmedetomidine.

Midazolam is the most commonly used perioperative premedication in anesthesia. It is also the most commonly used oral premedication in children. However, it would be a poor choice for oral premedication prior to hospital admission. Benzodiazepines have demonstrated paradoxical responses in patients with ASD.[109,110] This is believed to be due to altered function at the level of the gamma aminobutyric acid (GABA)–benzodiazepine receptor interface. They induce laxity of oropharyngeal musculature leading to an increased incidence of obstruction.[111–116] Specifically, genioglossal muscle tone is reduced, causing the tongue to migrate posteriorly. Therefore, while midazolam is an excellent oral sedative for the monitored presurgical setting, it is contraindicated for home administration.

Furthermore, the pharmacokinetic profile of oral midazolam is not favorable for home premedication. Midazolam has demonstrated an incredibly wide bioavailability range, which makes it inherently unpredictable. The bioavailability has been reported to be as little as 9% to as much as 71%, with roughly 35–50% being the average bioavailability found in most investigations.[117,118] This discrepancy is namely due to extreme variability in the intestinal and hepatic CYP3A4 enzyme system. Midazolam has a short duration of action and peak effect. In adults taking 20–40 mg of oral midazolam, peak blood levels were reached in as little as 15 minutes for the majority of subjects.[119] If administered at home, peak drug effect would likely occur prior to the patient's arrival at the hospital, therefore negating its utility. Ironically, while peak effect of oral midazolam occurs quite rapidly, it has been shown to significantly increase length of stay following surgery.[120]

Oral ketamine is another agent that has been used extensively in the special needs population. For presurgical sedation of ASD patients, 6–7 mg/kg has proved efficacious.[121] Unlike midazolam, it does not produce laxity of oropharyngeal musculature[112] and is favored for its bronchodilatory properties and ability to maintain spontaneous respiration. However, ketamine is a dissociative anesthetic and a potent stimulator of oral and tracheobronchial secretions.[122] The risk of anesthetic staging and laryngospasm, albeit remote,[123] cannot justify its use in the doses required for this purpose. The risk of aspiration secondary to loss of protective reflexes poses another complication with ketamine.

Oral dexmedetomidine is becoming more popular as an oral premedication in pediatric and special needs patients. However, it has not been studied sufficiently to advocate home administration at this time. Currently, it is effective and safe for procedural sedation in enteral doses up to 5 mcg/kg.[124,125] At these doses, it also provides a significant analgesic effect when compared to lower oral doses. Following oral administration, the onset of sedation begins in 25 minutes and takes approximately 2 hours to reach peak effect.[14]

Dexmedetomidine is formulated as a liquid suspension with an unpleasant flavor, making PO administration difficult in some patients. There are also concerns with prehospital administration as dispensing is difficult and the potential for bradycardic and hypotensive effects in an unmonitored setting are too great. As time to peak effect is quicker and delivery mechanism is more convenient, tizanidine remains preferable to dexmedetomidine for pre-hospital sedation.

Unfortunately, it is often difficult for providers to prescribe pre-hospital oral sedatives for special needs patients. A myriad of obstacles exists including communication breakdown with caretakers, lack of family resources, and patient refusal. Alternatively, provider discomfort and lack of preparation can present additional barriers to administration. Nonetheless, combative ASD patients will require sedation to allow the induction of anesthesia. This often comes in the form of an IM ketamine injection. As such, strong consideration should be given to adjunctive agents, namely midazolam. Midazolam will lower the total ketamine required to achieve sedation and prevent dysphoria. This may greatly expedite patient recovery, especially for brief procedures.

The IM dose of midazolam to prevent dysphoria is unknown. However, IV doses of 0.05–0.07 mg/kg have been effective for this purpose.[37,38] As the bioavailability of IM midazolam is 87%,[11] IM doses of approximately 0.05 mg/kg would likely produce similar results. Another IM adjunct that may prevent ketamine dysphoria is dexmedetomidine. While it has not been investigated for this purpose, the authors of this chapter have found it to improve separation and prevent dysphoria when 0.1 mcg/kg is combined with 3 mg/kg of IM ketamine as an admixture. In a recent study, this admixture proved safe, effective, and performed comparably to IM ketamine and midazolam.[40]

It should be understood that IM midazolam, when administered alone, is a poor sedative agent for the special needs population. In doses as high as 0.4 mg/kg, IM midazolam did not sufficiently relax patients for suturing in the emergency department (ED). The majority of these patients still had to be restrained.[126] Therefore, midazolam should only be considered as an adjunctive agent to complement ketamine.

Provider experience and comfort play a considerable role when managing combative autistic patients. Because general anesthesiologists infrequently treat this population, the provider may be less practiced in oral and IM approaches. Lack of IV access upon commencement of anesthesia may add an additional layer of unease for the practitioner. It is therefore essential for each provider to become familiar with the available options to achieve a successful anesthetic induction.

A final consideration when treating combative ASD patients is the inability to conduct preoperative assessment. This greatly limits the anticipatory abilities of the anesthesiologist. Stress is amplified by poor cooperation, which necessitates unusual induction techniques. Consequently, perilous situations can arise quickly and unexpectedly, especially concerning airway management. These hazards are compounded by lack of IV access during the induction of anesthesia.

All in all, the anesthetic management of combative autistic patients can prove incredibly challenging yet equally rewarding. With communicative ability diminished, the anesthesia provider must look to alternative approaches to deliver safe anesthesia. Through continuous rehearsal of unfamiliar scenarios, one can improve reaction speed and improve patient outcomes. By understanding inherent differences and effective management strategies, the autism community can be better served by anesthesia providers today and in the future.

CONCLUSION

- ASD patients are more likely to require GA, and the prevalence of this condition is increasing.

- Pre-hospital sedation can improve safety and satisfaction of care for combative autistic patients.

- Alpha-2 agonists provide ideal pharmacologic properties for use in a combative patient with autism.

- Adjunctive agents, namely benzodiazepines and dexmedetomidine, should be considered when administering IM ketamine.

- Psychotropic and antidepressant medications can produce a myriad of side effects and physiologic derangements which the anesthesiologist should review.

- ASD patients are more prone to psychological disorders, seizures, and gastrointestinal disease.

- ASD patients have increased sympathetic tone, decreased parasympathetic tone, and are more prone to immune and metabolic dysfunction.

- Topical lidocaine and IM rocuronium can be utilized to break a laryngospasm in MH patients without IV access.

REVIEW QUESTIONS

1. Alpha-2 agonists induce analgesia in the dorsal horn of the spinal column by decreasing the release of which substances?

   a. NE and substance P.
   b. Substance P and serotonin.
   c. NE and glutamate.
   d. Substance P and glutamate.

   The correct answer is d.

   Nociceptive signals are carried by C and A delta fibers to the dorsal horn of the spinal column. Upon arrival of these signals, substance P and glutamate are released. This activates postsynaptic receptors within the spinothalamic tract leading to the perception of pain within the thalamus. However, alpha-2 agonists decrease the release of substance P and glutamate thereby leading to reduced pain sensation.[19]

2. Which form of seizure is most common in autistic patients?

   a. Tonic-clonic seizures (grand mal).
   b. Absence seizures (petit mal).
   c. Atonic seizures.
   d. Myoclonic seizures.

The correct answer is a.

The prevalence of seizure disorder is significantly elevated in the ASD population. Roughly 30% of autistic patients have a seizure disorder compared with only 2–3% of the general population.[71] Most autistic patients have generalized tonic-clonic seizures (88%).[70]

3. Susceptibility to MH is increased in which population?

   a. Females.
   b. Patients with multiple sclerosis.
   c. Patients with central nuclear myopathy.
   d. Patients with demyelinating disease.

The correct answer is c.

Patient subsets that are more susceptible to MH include males (2:1), patients with CCD, and patients with certain myopathies including multi-minicore disease (MmD), central nuclear myopathy, and King-Denborough syndrome.[46,47]

4. Homozygous MTHFR deficiency is more common in ASD patients and leads to elevated levels of which substance?

   a. Glutathione.
   b. Methionine.
   c. Homocysteine.
   d. Arginine.

The correct answer is c.

The homozygous MTHFR deficiency genotype is significant because it can lead to elevated homocysteine levels and folate trapping following nitrous oxide administration. Complications including myelopathy, peripheral neuropathy, hemiparesis,[91] and death have occurred.[91] In one instance, an infant with unknown MTHFR deficiency expired following two general anesthetics with nitrous oxide. The autopsy demonstrated cerebral atrophy and severe demyelination secondary to elevated homocysteine levels and decreased methionine. These findings are consistent with other deaths following nitrous oxide administration to unknown homozygous individuals.

5. The antisialagogue effect of IM glycopyrrolate coincides with its peak plasma concentration and occurs approximately

   a. 20 minutes following administration.
   b. 30 minutes following administration.
   c. 40 minutes following administration.
   d. 50 minutes following administration.

The correct answer is b.

Both atropine and glycopyrrolate are poorly absorbed via the IM route. They achieve peak plasma concentrations roughly 30 minutes[42,43] following injection, and their antisialagogue effect corresponds with this peak.[44]

6. Which dose of IM rocuronium has produced effective intubating conditions in children in approximately 3 minutes?

   a. 0.6 mg/kg.
   b. 1.8 mg/kg.
   c. 2.4 mg/kg.
   d. 3.2 mg/kg.

The correct answer is b.

In one investigation, IM rocuronium injection to the deltoid, dosed at 1 mg/kg in infants and 1.8 mg/kg in children, produced complete neuromuscular blockade in approximately 8 minutes.[94] In a similar study, these same doses achieved intubating conditions in as little as 3 minutes.[95]

7. Which of the following drug classes has demonstrated paradoxical reactions in autistic patients?

   a. Benzodiazepines.
   b. Imidazopyridine hypnotics.
   c. Dexmedetomidine.
   d. Long-acting opioids.

The correct answer is a.

Benzodiazepines have demonstrated paradoxical responses in patients with ASD.[109,110] This is believed to be due to altered function at the level of the GABA–benzodiazepine receptor interface.

8. SSRI medications cause all of the following *except*

   a. Increased bleeding.
   b. SIADH.
   c. Inhibition of CYP 1A2.
   d. Agranulocytosis.

The correct answer is d.

SSRIs have been known to cause SIADH in the elderly, although the mechanism is incompletely understood.[68,69] They inhibit a variety of cytochrome oxidase systems including CYP 1A2, 2C9, 2D6, and 3A4.[65] As such, they may increase plasma concentrations of drugs that depend on these systems for clearance. Furthermore, SSRIs induce bleeding by decreasing the amount of serotonin available to participate in platelet aggregation.[67] Last, clozapine is unique in its ability to precipitate agranulocytosis, which occurs in roughly 1% of individuals on this medication.[60,61]

9. Which of the following is *not* a proposed mechanism for some of the behaviors associated with ASD?

   a. Reactive oxygen species.
   b. Gastrointestinal disease.
   c. Parasympathetic dominance.
   d. Immunological dysfunction.

The correct answer is c.

Gastrointestinal disorders disproportionately affect patients with ASD and symptoms may exist in as many as 91% of children with ASD. It is hypothesized that GI abnormalities are grossly underappreciated and may contribute to symptoms of ASD.[75] Research has also evidenced impairment of electron transport chain complexes in ASD patients. This causes disturbances in energy production[88] and alteration of oxidation-reduction reactions which can generate ROS. It is proposed that oxidative stress imposed by ROS is what, in part, contributes to ASD.[88,89] Additionally, autistic patients exhibit immune dysfunction. Multiple studies have evidenced an association between immune dysregulation and severity of autism symptoms.[81] Autonomic dysregulation is fundamental to ASD. It is evidenced by heightened baseline sympathetic activity with decreased parasympathetic activity.[77–80]

REFERENCES

1. Seo KS, Shin TJ, Kim HJ, et al. Clinico-statistical analysis of cooperation and anesthetic induction method of dental patients with special needs. *J Korean Dent Soc Anesthesiol*. 2009;9:9–16.
2. Tordjman S, Anderson GM, Botbol M, Brailly-Tabard S, Perez-Diaz F, et al. Pain reactivity and plasma β-endorphin in children and adolescents with autistic disorder. *PLoS One*. 2009;4(8):129–141.
3. Bronsard G, Botbol M, Tordjman S. Aggression in low functioning children and adolescents with autistic disorder. Scott JG, ed. *PLoS One*. 2010;5(12):e14358. doi:10.1371/journal.pone.0014358
4. Scahill L, McCracken JT, King BH, et al. Research Units on Pediatric Psychopharmacology Autism Network. Extended-release guanfacine for hyperactivity in children with autism spectrum disorder. *Am J Psychiatr*. 2015;172(12):1197–1206.
5. Handen BL, Sahl R, Hardan AY. Guanfacine in children with autism and/or intellectual disabilities. *J Dev Behav Pediatr*. 2008;29(4):303–308.
6. Weerink MAS, Struys MMRF, Hannivoort LN, Barends CRM, Absalom AR, Colin P. Clinical pharmacokinetics and pharmacodynamics of dexmedetomidine. *Clin Pharmacokin*. 2017;56(8):893–913. doi:10.1007/s40262-017-0507-7
7. Giovannitti JA, Thoms SM, Crawford JJ. Alpha-2 adrenergic receptor agonists: A review of current clinical applications. *Anesth Prog*. 2015;62(1):31–38. doi:10.2344/0003-3006-62.1.31
8. Shukry M, Clyde MC, Kalarickal PL, Ramadhyani U. Does dexmedetomidine prevent emergence delirium in children after sevoflurane-based general anesthesia? *Pediatr Anesth*. 2005;15:1098–1104.
9. Su X, Meng ZT, Wu XH, et al. Dexmedetomidine for prevention of delirium in elderly patients after non-cardiac surgery: A randomised, double-blind, placebo-controlled trial. *Lancet*. 2016 Oct 15;388(10054):1893–1902. 10.1016/S0140-6736(16)30580-3
10. Tobias JD. Dexmedetomidine and ketamine: An effective alternative for procedural sedation? *Pediatr Crit Care Med*. 2012;13:423–427.
11. Pharmacology of pediatric anesthesia. In: Davis PJ, Cladis FP, Motoyama EK, eds., *Smith's Anesthesia for Infants and Children*. 8th ed. Elsevier; 2011:206–208.
12. Wajima Z, Yoshikawa T, Ogura A, et al. Oral tizanidine, an alpha2-adrenoceptor agonist, reduces the minimum alveolar concentration of sevoflurane in human adults. *Anesth Analg*. 2002;95:393–396.
13. Frisk-Holmberg M, Paalzow L, Edlund PO. Clonidine kinetics in man—Evidence for dose dependency and changed pharmacokinetics during chronic therapy. *Br J Clin Pharmacol*. 1981;12(5):653–658.
14. Anttila M, Penttilä J, Helminen A, Vuorilehto L, Scheinin H. Bioavailability of dexmedetomidine after extravascular doses in healthy subjects. *Br J Clin Pharmacol*. 2003;56(6):691–693. doi:10.1046/j.1365-2125.2003.01944.x
15. Granfors MT, Backman JT, Laitila J, Neuvonen PJ. Tizanidine is mainly metabolized by cytochrome P450 1A2 in vitro. *Br J Clin Pharmacol*. 2004;57(3):349–353. doi:10.1046/j.1365-2125.2003.02028.x
16. Ghanavatian S, Derian A. Tizanidine. *StatPearls*. 2018 Jan. https://www.ncbi.nlm.nih.gov/books/NBK519505/
17. Lake CR, Ziegler MG, Murphy DL. Increased norepinephrine levels and decreased dopamine-β-hydroxylase activity in primary autism. *Arch Gen Psychiatry*. 1977;34(5):553–556. doi:10.1001/archpsyc.1977.01770170063005
18. Kaur M, Singh PM. Current role of dexmedetomidine in clinical anesthesia and intensive care. *Anesth Essays Res*. 2011;5(2):128–133. doi:10.4103/0259-1162.94750
19. González-Ramírez R, Chen Y, Liedtke WB, et al. TRP channels and pain. In: Emir TLR, ed. *Neurobiology of TRP Channels*. 2nd ed. CRC Press/Taylor & Francis; 2017. https://www.ncbi.nlm.nih.gov/books/NBK476120/. doi:10.4324/9781315152837-8
20. Karhuvaara S, Kallio A, Salonen M, et al. Rapid reversal of alpha2-adrenoreceptor agonist effects by atipamezole in human volunteers. *Br J Clin Pharmacol*. 1991;31:160–165.
21. Scheinin H, Aantaa R, Anttila M, et al. Reversal of the sedative and sympatholytic effects of dexmedetomidine with a specific alpha2-adrenoceptor antagonist atipamezole: A pharmacodynamic and kinetic study in healthy volunteers. *Anesthesiology*. 1998;89:574–584.
22. Miettinen TJ, Kanto JH, Salonen MA, Scheinin M. The sedative and sympatholytic effects of oral tizanidine in healthy volunteers. *Anesth Analg*. 1996;82(4):817–820.
23. Nance PW, Bugaresti J, Shellenberger K, Sheremata W, Martinez-Arizala A. Efficacy and safety of tizanidine in the treatment of spasticity in patients with spinal cord injury. North American Tizanidine Study Group. *Neurology*. 1994;44(11 Suppl 9):S44–S51; discussion S-2.
24. Zanos P, Moaddel R, Morris PJ, et al. Ketamine and ketamine metabolite pharmacology: Insights into therapeutic mechanisms. Witkin JM, ed. *Pharmacol Rev*. 2018;70(3):621–660. doi:10.1124/pr.117.015198
25. Cote CJ, Lerman J, Todres ID. *A Practice of Anesthesia for Infants and Children E-Book: Expert Consult: Online and Print*. 5th ed. Elsevier Health Sciences; 2012.
26. Craven R. Ketamine. *Anaesthesia*. 200762(Suppl. 1):48–53.
27. McGlone RG, Ranasinghe S, Durham S. An alternative to "brutacaine": A comparison of low dose intramuscular ketamine with intranasal midazolam in children before suturing. *J Accid Emerg Med* 1998;15(4):231–236.
28. Midazolam or ketamine for procedural sedation of children in the emergency department. *Emerg Med J*. 2007;24(8):579–580 doi:10.1136/emj.2007.051318
29. McGlone R, Howes M, Joshi M. The Lancaster experience of 2.0 to 2.5 mg/kg intramuscular ketamine for paediatric sedation: 501 Cases and analysis. *Emerg Med J*. 2004;21(3):290–295. doi:10.1136/emj.2002.003772
30. Hannallah RS, Patel RI. Low-dose intramuscular ketamine for anesthesia pre-induction in young children undergoing brief outpatient procedures. *Anesthesiology*. 1989 Apr;70(4):598–600.
31. Burnett A, Salzman J, Griffith K, Kroeger B, Frascone R. The emergency department experience with prehospital ketamine: A case series of 13 patients. *Prehosp Emerg Care*. 2012;16(4):553–559.
32. Ho J, Smith S, Nystrom P, et al. Successful management of excited delirium syndrome with prehospital ketamine: Two case examples. *Prehosp Emerg Care*. 2013;17(2):274–279.
33. Scheppke K, Braghiroli J, Shalaby M, Chait R. Prehospital use of i.m. ketamine for sedation of violent and agitated patients. *West J Emerg Med*. 2014;15(7):736–741.
34. Burnett A, Peterson B, Stellpflug S, et al. The association between ketamine given for prehospital chemical restraint with intubation and hospital admission. *Am J Emerg Med*. 2015;33(1):76–79.
35. Iwanicki JL, et al. Prehospital ketamine for excited delirium in the setting of acute drug intoxication. *Clin Toxicol* 2014;52:685–686.
36. Erbguth PH, Reiman B, Klein RL. The influence of chlorpromazine, diazepam and droperidol on emergence from ketamine. *Anesth Analg*. 1972;51:693–698.
37. Cartwright PD, Pingel SM. Midazolam and diazepam in ketamine anaesthesia. *Anaesthesia*. 1984;39:439–442.
38. Somashekara SC, Govindadas D, Devashankaraiah G, et al. Midazolam premedication in attenuating ketamine psychic sequelae. *J Basic Clin Pharm*. 2010;1(4):209–213.
39. Funk W, Jakob W, Riedl T, Taeger K. Oral preanaesthetic medication for children: Double-blind randomized study of a combination of midazolam and ketamine vs midazolam or ketamine alone. *Br J Anaesth*. 2000;84:335–340.
40. Guthrie DB, Boorin MR, Sisti AR, et al. Retrospective comparison of intramuscular admixtures of ketamine and dexmedetomidine versus ketamine and midazolam for preoperative sedation. *Anesth Prog*. 2021;68:3–9.
41. Guthrie DB, Epstein RH, Boorin MR, et al. A survey of dentist anesthesiologists on preoperative intramuscular sedation. *Anesth Prog*. 2022;69:17–23.
42. Ali-Melkkila T, Kaila T, Kanto J. Glycopyrrolate: Pharmacokinetics and some pharmacodynamic findings. *Acta Anaesthesiol Scand*. 1989;33:513–517.

43. Berghem L, Berghem U. Plasma atropine concentrations determined by radioimmunoassay after single-dose I.V. and I.M. administration. *Br J Anaesth*. 1980;52:597.
44. Kentala E, Kaila T, Iisalo E, Kanto J. Intramuscular atropine in healthy volunteers: A pharmacokinetic and pharmacodynamic study. *Int J Clin Pharmacol Ther Toxicol*. 1990;28:399–404.
45. Watt S, McAllister RK. Malignant hyperthermia. *StatPearls*. 2023 Jan. https://www.ncbi.nlm.nih.gov/books/NBK430828/
46. Rosenberg H, Davis M, James D, Pollock N, Stowell K. Malignant hyperthermia. *Orphanet J Rare Dis*. 2007;2:21. doi:10.1186/1750-1172-2-21
47. Rosenberg H, Pollock N, Schiemann A, Bulger T, Stowell K. Malignant hyperthermia: A review. *Orphanet J Rare Dis*. 2015;10:93. doi:10.1186/s13023-015-0310-1
48. Gurnaney H, Brown A, Litman RS. Malignant hyperthermia and muscular dystrophies. *Anesth Analg*. 2009;109:1043–1048.
49. Fleisher L, Fleischmann K, Auerbach A, et al. 2014 ACC/AHA guideline on perioperative cardiovascular evaluation and management of patients undergoing noncardiac surgery. *J Am Coll Cardiol*. 2014 Dec;64(22)e77–e137. doi:10.1016/j.jacc.2014.07.944
50. Sweitzer BJ. *Preoperative Assessment and Management*. 3rd ed. Wolters Kluwer Health; 2018.
51. Patten SB, Waheed W, Bresee L. A review of pharmacoepidemiologic studies of antipsychotic use in children and adolescents. *Can J Psychiatry*. 2012;57(12):717–721.
52. Arango C. Child and adolescent neuropsychopharmacology: Now or never. *Eur Neuropsychopharmacol*. 2011;21(8):563–564. doi:10.1016/j.euroneuro.2011.05.006
53. Horacek J, Bubenikova-Valesova V, Kopecek M, et al. Mechanism of action of atypical antipsychotic drugs and the neurobiology of schizophrenia. *CNS Drugs*. 2006;20:389–409. https://doi.org/10.2165/00023210-200620050-00004 PMid:16696579
54. Johnson D, Philip AZ, Joseph DJ, Varghese R. Risperidone-induced neuroleptic malignant syndrome in neurodegenerative disease: A case report. *Prim Care Companion J Clin Psychiatr*. 2007;9(3):237–238.
55. Ananth J, Parameswaran S, Gunatilake S, Burgoyne K, Sidhom T. Neuroleptic malignant syndrome and atypical antipsychotic drugs. *J Clin Psychiatry*. 2004 Apr;65(4):464–470.
56. Sharma R, Trappler B, Ng YK, Leeman CP. Risperidone-induced neuroleptic malignant syndrome. *Ann Pharmacother*. 1996;30:775–778.
57. Bajjoka I, Patel T, O'Sullivan T. Risperidone-induced neuroleptic malignant syndrome. *Ann Emerg Med*. 1997;30:698–700.
58. Cherryl Z, Jolien MB, Dharmindredew R, Jan DB. Hypothermia due to antipsychotic medication: A systematic review. *Front Psychiatr*. 2017;8:165–173.
59. Vermeulen JM, van Rooijen G, van de Kerkhof MPJ, Sutterland AL, Correll CU, de Haan L. Clozapine and long-term mortality risk in patients with schizophrenia: A systematic review and meta-analysis of studies lasting 1.1–12.5 years. *Schizophren Bull*. 2019 Mar 7;45(2):315–329. https://doi.org/10.1093/schbul/sby052
60. Huyse FJ, Touw DJ, van Schijndel RS, de Lange JJ, Slaets JP. Psychotropic drugs and the perioperative period: A proposal for a guideline in elective surgery. *Psychosomatics*. 2006 Jan-Feb;47(1):8–22. doi:10.1176/appi.psy.47.1.8. PMID: 16384803
61. Yuen JWY, Kim DD, Procyshyn RM, White RF, Honer WG, Barr AM. Clozapine-induced cardiovascular side effects and autonomic dysfunction: A systematic review. *Front Neurosci*. 2018;12:203. doi:10.3389/fnins.2018.00203
62. Sockalingam S, Shammi C, Remington G. Clozapine-induced hypersalivation: A review of treatment strategies. *Can J Psychiatr*. 2007;52(6):377–384.
63. Palmer SE, McLean RM, Ellis PM, Harrison-Woolrych M. Life-threatening clozapine-induced gastrointestinal hypomotility: An analysis of 102 cases. *J Clin Psychiatr*. 2008 May;69(5):759–768.
64. Kam PCA, Chang GWM. Selective serotonin reuptake inhibitors: Pharmacology and clinical implications in anaesthesia and critical care medicine. *Anaesthesia*. 1997;52:982–988.
65. Peck T, Wong A, Norman E. Anaesthetic implications of psychoactive drugs. *Continuing Education in Anaesthesia Critical Care & Pain*. 2010 Dec 1;10(6):177–181. https://doi.org/10.1093/bjaceaccp/mkq037
66. Alderman CP, Mortiz CK, Ben-Tovim DT. Abnormal platelet aggregation associated with fluoxetine treatment. *Ann Pharmacother*. 1992;26:1517–1519.
67. Saraghi M, Golden L, Hersh EV. Anesthetic considerations for patients on antidepressant therapy—Part II. *Anesth Prog*. 2018;65(1):60–65. doi:10.2344/anpr-65-01-10
68. Blacksten JV, Birt JA. Syndrome of inappropriate secretion of antidiuretic hormone secondary to fluoxetine. *Ann Pharmacother*. 1993;27:723–724.
69. Adverse drug reactions advisory. Selective serotonin reuptake inhibitors and SIADH. *Med J Austral*. 1996;164:162.
70. Taghizadeh N, Davidson A, Williams K, Story D. Autism spectrum disorder (ASD) and its perioperative management. *Paediatr Anaesth*. 2015;25(11):1076–1084. doi:10.1111/pan.12732
71. Mannion A, Leader G. Comorbidity in autism spectrum disorder: A literature review. *Res Autism Spectr Disord*. 2013;7:1595–1616.
72. Lewine J, Andrews R, Chez M, et al. Magnetoencephalographic patterns of epileptiform activity in children with regressive autism spectrum disorders. *Pediatrics*. 1999;104:405–418. 10.1542/peds.104.3.405 [PubMed] [Cross Ref]
73. Kohane IS, McMurry A, Weber G, et al. The co-morbidity burden of children and young adults with autism spectrum disorders. Smalheiser NR, ed. *PLoS One*. 2012;7(4):e33224. doi:10.1371/journal.pone.0033224
74. Horvath K, Papadimitriou JC, Rabsztyn A, Drachenberg C, Tildon JT. Gastrointestinal abnormalities in children with autistic disorder. *J Pediatr*. 1999;135:559–563. 10.1016/S0022-3476(99)70052-1
75. Horvath K, Perman JA. Autistic disorder and gastrointestinal disease. *Curr Opin Pediatr*. 2002;14:583–587. 10.1097/00008480-200210000-00004
76. Shavelle RM, Strauss DJ, Pickett J. Causes of death in autism. *J Autism Dev Disord*. 2001;31(6):569–576.
77. Ming X, Julu PO, Brimacombe M, Connor S, Daniels ML. Reduced cardiac parasympathetic activity in children with autism. *Brain Dev*. 2005;27:509–516.
78. Hirstein W, Iversen P, Ramachandran VS. Autonomic responses of autistic children to people and objects. *Proc Biol Sci Royal Soc*. 2001;268(1479):1883–1888. doi:10.1098/rspb.2001.1724
79. Patriquin MA, Scarpa A, Friedman BH, Porges SW. Respiratory sinus arrhythmia: A marker for positive social functioning and receptive language skills in children with autism spectrum disorders. *Dev Psychobiol*. 2011. doi:10.1002/dev.21002. [PubMed] [Cross Ref]
80. Porges SW. Respiratory sinus arrhythmia: An index of vagal tone. In: Orlebeke JF, Mulder G, Van Dornen LJP, eds. *Psychophysiology of Cardiovascular Control: Models, Methods, and Data*. Plenum; 1985:437–450.
81. Ashwood P, Krakowiak P, Hertz-Picciotto I, et al. () Elevated plasma cytokines in autism spectrum disorders provide evidence of immune dysfunction and are associated with impaired behavioral outcome. *Brain Behav Immun*. 2011a;25(1):40–45.
82. Li X, Chauhn A, Shiekh AM, et al. Elevated immune response in the brain of autistic patients. *J Neuroimmunol*. 2009;207(1-2):111–116. doi:10.1016/j.jneuroim.2008.12.002
83. Jyonouchi H, Sun S, Le H. Proinflammatory and regulatory cytokine production associated with innate and adaptive immune responses in children with autism spectrum disorders and developmental regression. *J Neuroimmunol*. 2001;120:170–179.
84. Plioplys AV. Intravenous immunoglobulin treatment of children with autism. *J Child Neurol*. 1998;13(2):79–82.
85. Gupta S, Aggarwal S, Heads C. Dysregulated immune system in children with autism: Beneficial effects of intravenous immune globulin on autistic characteristics. *J Autism Dev Disord*. 1996;26(4):439–452.
86. Boris M, Kaiser CC, Goldblatt A, et al. Effect of pioglitazone treatment on behavioral symptoms in autistic children. *J Neuroinflamm*. 2007;4(3). doi:10.1186/1742-2094-4-3
87. Vinet E, Pineau CA, Clarke AE, et al. Increased risk of autism spectrum disorders in children born to women with systemic lupus

erythematosus: Results from a large population-based cohort. *Arthritis Rheumatol.* 2015;67:3201–3208.
88. Ghanizadeh A, Berk M, Farrashbandi H, Alavi Shoushtari A, Villagonzalo KA. Targeting the mitochondrial electron transport chain in autism: A systematic review and synthesis of a novel therapeutic approach. *Mitochondrion.* 2013;13(5):515–519.
89. Medical Comorbidities in Autism Spectrum Disorders. 2013. International Search Report for PCT / FR2006 / 002735 dated Jul 8, 2008. International Preliminary Report on Patentability for PCT / FR2006 / 002735 dated Jun 18, 2008.
90. Ghanizadeh A, Akhondzadeh S, Hormozi M, Makarem A, Abotorabi-Zarchi M, Firoozabadi A. Glutathione-related factors and oxidative stress in autism, a review. *Curr Med Chem.* 2012;19(23):4000–4005.
91. Boris M, Goldblatt A, Galanko J, James J. Association of MTHFR gene variants with autism. *J Am Phys Surg.* 2004;9:106–108.
92. Nagele P, Zeugswetter B, Wiener C, et al. Influence of methylenetetrahydrofolate reductase gene polymorphisms on homocysteine concentrations after nitrous oxide anesthesia. *Anesthesiology.* 2008;109(1):36–43. doi:10.1097/ALN.0b013e318178820b
93. Reynolds LM, Lau M, Brown R, Luks A, Sharma M, Fisher DM. Bioavailability of intramuscular rocuronium in infants and children. *Anesthesiology.* 1997;87:1096–1105.
94. Kaplan RF, Uejima T, Lobel G, et al. Intramuscular rocuronium in infants and children: A multicenter study to evaluate tracheal intubating conditions, onset, and duration of action. *Anesthesiology.* 1999;91(3):633.
95. Reynolds LM, Lau M, Brown R, Luks A, Fisher DM. Intramuscular rocuronium in infants and children: Dose-ranging and tracheal intubating conditions. *Anesthesiology.* 1996;85(2):231–239.
96. Johr M, Can U. Pediatric anesthesia without vascular access: Intramuscular administration of atracurium (letter). *Anesth Analg.* 1993;76:1162–1163.
97. Cauldwell CB, Lau M, Fisher DM. Is intramuscular mivacurium an alternative to intramuscular succinylcholine? *Anesthesiology.* 1994;80:320–325.
98. Iwasaki H, Namiki A, Omote T, Omote K. Neuromuscular effects of subcutaneous administration of pancuronium. *Anesthesiology.* 1992;76:1049–1051.
99. Koc C, Kocaman F, Aygenc E, Özdem C, Cekic A. The use of preoperative lidocaine to prevent stridor and laryngospasm after tonsillectomy and adenoidectomy. *Otolaryngol Head Neck Surg.* 1998;118:880–882.
100. Robinson EP, Rex MA, Brown TC. A comparison of different concentrations of lignocaine hydrochloride used for topical anaesthesia of the larynx of the cat. *Anaesth Intens Care.* 1985 May;13(2):137–144.
101. Mencap. Death by indifference. 2007. http://www.mencap.org.uk/document
102. Blitz M, Britton KC. Management of the uncooperative child. *Oral Maxillofac Surg Clin North Am* 2010;22:461–469.
103. Schreiner, MS. Ingestion of liquids compared with preoperative fasting in pediatric outpatients. *Anesthesiology.* 1990.
104. Jackson Brown F, Guvenir J. The experiences of children with learning disabilities, their carers and staff during a hospital admission, *Br J Learn Disabil.* 2008;37:110–115.
105. Cole JB, Moore JC, Nystrom PC, et al. A prospective study of ketamine versus haloperidol for severe prehospital agitation. *Clin Toxicol.* 2016;54(7):556–562.
106. O'Connor L, Rebesco M, Robinson C, et al. Outcomes of prehospital chemical sedation with ketamine versus haloperidol and benzodiazepine or physical restraint only. *Prehosp Emerg Care.* 2018;0(0):1–9.
107. Burnett AM, Watters BJ, Barringer KW, Griffith KR, Frascone RJ. Laryngospasm and hypoxia after intramuscular administration of Ketamine to a patient in excited delirium. *Prehosp Emerg Care.* 2012;16:412–414. doi:10.3109/10903127.2011.640766

108. Maguire BJ, Smith S. Injuries and fatalities among emergency medical technicians and paramedics in the United States. *Prehosp Disaster Med.* 2013;28(4):376–382. Epub 2013/05/11. 10.1017/S1049023X13003555. PubMed PMID: 23659321
109. Bruining H, Passtoors L, Goriounova N, et al. Paradoxical benzodiazepine response: A rationale for bumetanide in neurodevelopmental disorders? *Pediatrics.* 2015;136(2):e539–e543.10.1542/peds.2014-4133
110. Marrosu F, Marrosu G, Rachel MG, Biggio G. Paradoxical reactions elicited by diazepam in children with classic autism. *Functional Neurology,* 1987;2:355–361.
111. Montravers P, Dureuil B, Desmonts JM. Effects of i.v. midazolam on upper airway resistance. *Br J Anaesth.* 1992;68:27–31.
112. Drummond GB. Comparison of sedation with midazolam and ketamine: Effects on airway muscle activity. *Br J Anaesth.* 1996;76:663–667.
113. Leiter JC, Knuth SL, Krol RC, Bartlett DJR. The effects of diazepam on the genioglossal muscle activity in normal human subjects. *Am Rev Respir Dis.* 1985;132:216–219.
114. Hsu TW, Chen HM, Chen TY, Chu CS, Pan CC. The association between use of benzodiazepine receptor agonists and the risk of obstructive sleep apnea: A nationwide population-based nested case-control study. *Int J Environ Res Public Health.* 2021 Sep 15;18(18):9720. doi:10.3390/ijerph18189720. PMID: 34574645 PMCID: PMC8467455
115. Ayuse T, Hoshino Y, Kurata S, et al. The effect of gender on compensatory neuromuscular response to upper airway obstruction in normal subjects under midazolam general anesthesia. *Anesth Analg* 2009;109(4):1209–1218. doi:10.1213/ane.0b013e3181b0fc70
116. Nozaki-Taguchi N, Isono S, Nishino T, Numai T, Taguchi N. Upper airway obstruction during midazolam sedation: Modification by nasal CPAP. *Can J Anaesth.* 1995;42:685–690.
117. Reed MD, Rodarte A, Blumer JL, et al. The single-dose pharmacokinetics of midazolam and its primary metabolite in pediatric patients after oral and intravenous administration. *J Clin Pharmacol.* 2001;41(12):1359–1369. doi:10.1177/00912700122012832
118. Pacifici GM. Clinical pharmacology of midazolam in neonates and children: Effect of disease—A review. *International Journal of Pediatrics.* 2014;2014:309342. doi:10.1155/2014/309342
119. Heizmann P, Eckert M, Ziegler WH. Pharmacokinetics and bioavailability of midazolam in man. *Br. J. Clin. Pharmacol.* 1983;16:43S–49S.
120. Maeda S, Tomayasu Y, Higuchi H, et al. Independent factors affecting recovery time after sedation in patients with intellectual disabilities. *Open Dent J.* 2015;9:146–149. doi:10.2174/1874210601509010146.
121. Rainey L, van der Walt JH. The anesthetic management of autistic children. *Anaesth Intensive Care.* 1998;26:682–686.
122. Haas DA, Harper DG. Ketamine: A review of its pharmacologic properties and use in ambulatory anesthesia. *Anesth Prog.* 1992;39(3):61–68.
123. Grunwell JR, Travers C, McCracken CE, et al. Procedural sedation outside of the operating room using ketamine in 22,645 children: A report from the pediatric sedation research consortium. *Pediatr Crit Care Med.* 2016;17(12):1109–1116. doi:10.1097/PCC.0000000000000920
124. Konia, MR. Oral dexmedetomidine for preoperative sedation in an adult uncooperative autistic patient. *J Clin Anesth.* 2016 Nov;34:29–31. doi:10.1016/j.jclinane.2016.03.037
125. Singh C, Pandey RK, Saksena AK, Chandra G. A comparative evaluation of analgo-sedative effects of oral dexmedetomidine and ketamine: A triple-blind, randomized study. *Pediatr Anesth.* 2014;24(12):1252–1259. doi:10.1111/pan.12493
126. McGlone R, Fleet T, Durham S, Hollis S. A comparison of intramuscular ketamine with high dose intramuscular midazolam with and without intranasal flumazenil in children before suturing. *Emerg Med J.* 2001;18(1):34–38. doi:10.1136/emj.18.1.34

41.

PATIENT WITH AAA WITH IMPLANTED SPINAL CORD (NEURO) STIMULATOR

Meredith Whitacre and Loreta Grecu

STEM CASE AND KEY QUESTIONS

A 67-year-old man with a 50 pack-year cigarette smoking history received a screening abdominal ultrasound while attending a health fair with his wife 1 month previously. He was told at the screening fair that he should see a doctor because his aorta "looks big." He presented to his family physician who repeated the ultrasound, which confirmed aneurysmal enlargement of his aorta extending above the renal arteries. He denies any significant abdominal or flank pain. His family physician subsequently refers the patient to a vascular surgeon for consideration of operative intervention.

When is repair indicated in patients with AAA?

The patient undergoes a preoperative CT scan to delineate his aortic anatomy further; the aneurysmal sac measures approximately 6 cm in width. The surgeon states that aneurysms greater than 5.4 cm warrant surgical repair due to the increased risk of rupture.[1] The surgeon proceeds to schedule the elective procedure and requests that the patient be seen in the preoperative anesthesia clinic.

What medical conditions are associated with vascular disease? What comorbidities are of concern in a patient scheduled for an open AAA repair?

The patient presents to the preoperative clinic and states that he has been diagnosed with high blood pressure, high cholesterol, and diabetes mellitus (DM). He does not know if his renal function is normal, although he thinks his primary care physician has been "watching a lab value." He denies a history of cerebrovascular accidents or transient ischemic attacks. He does report he has a history of chronic lower extremity pain, but this has improved since he had a spinal cord stimulator (SCS) placed. He also endorses that he still smokes one to two packs of cigarettes per day.

Does the patient's functional status alter his overall risk?

The patient states that he does not know how much activity would cause him to become short of breath as he mainly sits most of the day. He intermittently gets some shortness of breath but is unsure whether this is associated with an activity.

What cardiac risk factors does the patient have? What, if any, cardiac evaluation does the patient need before proceeding with the planned surgical procedure?

Considering the patient has unknown functional status, hypertension, tobacco abuse, hyperlipidemia, and DM, a preoperative ECG is obtained. In addition, a transthoracic echocardiogram demonstrates left ventricular hypertrophy and no wall motion abnormalities. Given the normal echocardiogram, the patient did not undergo a noninvasive stress test.[2]

Does the patient need to be questioned about any other social habits?

The patient endorses that he continues to smoke and that he does have an intermittently productive cough. He states that in the winter, he often must see his family physician for difficulties "breathing" associated with a cold. His physician typically provides an inhaled bronchodilator for symptomatic relief. Upon further questioning, the patient discloses that he requires the inhaler more than just with "colds." The patient also admits to drinking at least two alcoholic beverages a day, although his wife states it may be more than that. His wife is concerned that the patient continues to smoke and worries that he will "have to keep the breathing tube."

What history is essential concerning the patient's chronic pain?

The patient reports that several years ago, he was on a significant number of narcotics as well as pain adjuncts to aid with radicular pain in his left lower extremity. He was being actively followed by a chronic pain physician who was concerned with the amount of medication the patient was using without notable pain relief. The patient tried steroid injections and physical therapy and the adjunctive medications were adjusted, all with minimal pain relief. Ultimately, the patient underwent SCS placement. Since having the stimulator placed, he has been weaned off opioids but remains on gabapentin. Radiographs demonstrate stimulator leads at the level of T8–T9.

What are the different surgical approaches used to repair AAA?

Given the anatomy of the patient's aneurysm with extension above the renal arteries, he is only a candidate for open repair. This will require a large abdominal incision with clamping of the aorta.

What intraoperative monitors are important for open AAA repair? What type of IV access would be necessary?

In preparation for the operating room, the anesthesiologist discusses with the patient the need for an arterial line and a central line. The patient is also informed that additional peripheral IV lines will be inserted as well to aid with volume resuscitation. He is informed that if difficulty arises with maintaining adequate blood pressure or there are concerns for myocardial ischemia, transesophageal echocardiography may be utilized.

What blood products, if any, should be available in the operating room on the day of surgery?

Given the potential for large-volume blood loss, the patient consented to blood product administration. He also understands that a cell salvage device will be utilized throughout the case to potentially decrease the amount of allogenic transfusion required. The patient is typed and crossed and packed red blood cells as well as fresh frozen plasma are prepared for the day of surgery.

Given the presence of a SCS, is placing an epidural catheter an option? What other pain management techniques could be considered?

Abdominal procedures typically require epidural placement at approximately the T7/8–T10 level to provide adequate pain relief. Given the SCS leads are at the level of T8–T9 there is concern that damage to the leads could occur during epidural placement. The decision is made not to place an epidural catheter, and the possibility of postoperative transverse abdominal plane blocks is discussed with the patient preoperatively. The SCS is interrogated before going into the operating room and turned off. In the operating room, the monopolar electrocautery grounding pad is placed on the opposite side and as far away as possible from the generator. In preoperative holding, the patient is administered doses of gabapentin and acetaminophen. Intraoperatively, the patient is placed on ketamine, lidocaine, and magnesium infusions to aid pain control.

What portions of the procedure present challenges for the anesthetic team in managing the patient?

At the time of the aortic cross-clamp, the patient's mean arterial pressure immediately increases to above 180 mm Hg. ST elevation is noted on the ECG. A nitroglycerin infusion is initiated at a low dose and the mean arterial pressure improves. The ST elevations consequently resolve. The patient's hemodynamics are well controlled, and the surgeon states that the cross-clamp will be removed within the next 5 minutes. In anticipation of the cross-clamp releases, the nitroglycerin is turned off, and just before release, the patient is given an IV fluid bolus, 50 mEq of bicarbonate as well as 1 g of calcium. His blood pressure drops upon clamp release but quickly rebounds following additional 100 mcg of phenylephrine and 200 mL of 5% albumin solution.

Given the medical and social history of the patient, what are potential postoperative complications?

Considering his extensive smoking history, the possibility of prolonged intubation and possible tracheostomy have already been discussed with the patient and his wife preoperatively. Postoperatively, the patient remains intubated and is taken to the ICU for recovery. On postoperative day 2 the patient begins to show signs of significant agitation despite sedation. The critical care team became concerned about possible alcohol withdrawal and immediately put the patient on the Clinical Institute Withdrawal Assessment for Alcohol (CIWA) protocol utilizing benzodiazepines. With the initiation of the protocol and the addition of scheduled bronchodilators, the patient cannot be weaned from his continuous sedation. He is extubated several days later, receiving transversus abdominis plane catheters to aid with postoperative pain control. His SCS is once again interrogated on postoperative day 1, and stimulation therapy is resumed.

DISCUSSION

DEFINITION AND CLASSIFICATION OF ABDOMINAL AORTIC ANEURYSMS

AAAs are defined as an enlargement of the abdominal aorta greater than 50% of the normal aortic diameter, or greater than 3 cm in most adults (Table 41.1).[3] In males, the diameter accurately defines risk; however, in females, the aneurysm measured in centimeters indexed to body surface area is a better predictor.[4]

Abdominal aneurysms are also classified based on the complexity of their involvement of the renal arteries. The further caudad the aneurysm extends, the more complex the aneurysm. The extent of the aneurysm also plays a role in determining the surgical approach for repair. The main types of abdominal aneurysms are classified based on the aneurysm's relation to the renal arteries (Figure 41.1 and Table 41.2).[5]

If the thoracic aorta is involved, the Crawford classification is utilized to characterize the aneurysm (Figure 41.2). Crawford types two through four have an aneurysmal component with the abdominal aorta.[6,7] Thoracic aortic involvement implies extensive disease as well as a more complex surgical intervention.

EPIDEMIOLOGY AND RISK FACTORS

Males are more likely to develop aneurysmal dilation, and, in those older than 50 years, it is estimated that 4–8% have AAAs.[8] Relatives of those with an aneurysm have approximately a 20%

Table 41.1 ANEURYSMAL SIZE CLASSIFICATION

CLASSIFICATION	MEASUREMENT
Small	<4 cm
Medium	4–5 cm
Large	>5.5 cm
Very Large	≥6 cm

Adapted from Aggarwal S et al.[3]

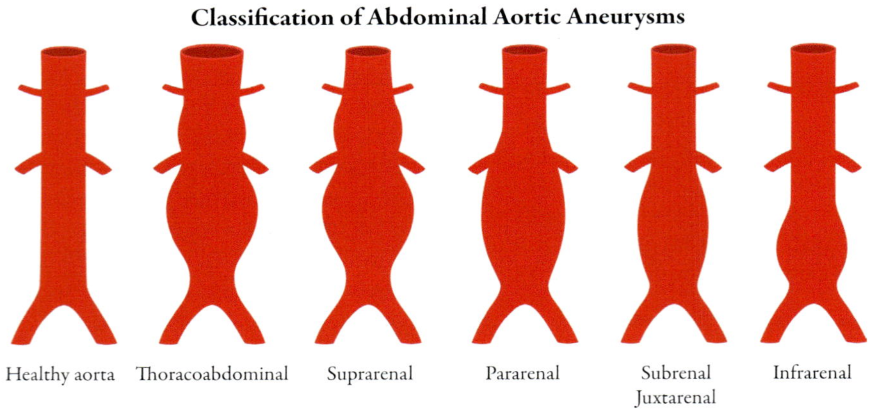

Classification of Abdominal Aortic Aneurysms

Healthy aorta Thoracoabdominal Suprarenal Pararenal Subrenal Juxtarenal Infrarenal

Figure 41.1 Abdominal aneurysms classification. Healthy abdominal aorta and abdominal aorta with various types of aneurysms.

Table 41.2 ANEURYSM LOCATION

LOCATION	DESCRIPTION
Infrarenal	Aneurysm proximal segment below the renal arteries
Juxtarenal	Aneurysm extends to the level of the renal arteries, with renal artery take off from normal aorta
Suprarenal	Aneurysm extends above the level of the renal arteries

Adapted from Chaikof EL et al.[5]

likelihood of developing an aneurysm, excluding other risk factors.[1] Though the incidence of AAAs is lower in females, they are at increased risk for rupture.[1,3]

The risk factors for developing AAA are associated with the underlying pathogenesis of aneurysmal dilation. In addition to age, cigarette smoking has been the most well-defined risk factor. One study demonstrated that smoking more than one pack per day for more than 35 years has a 12-fold increased risk of aneurysmal development.[1] Each year of smoking increases the relative risk of aneurysm development by 4%.[1] Other known risk factors include male gender, Caucasian race, atherosclerosis, hypertension, and the presence of other large artery aneurysms.[8]

The risk factors associated with rupture include current smoking, female gender, large initial aneurysm diameter, low FEV_1, increased aortic mural calcification, and elevated mean blood pressure.[1] Left unrepaired, the risk of rupture increases with aneurysm size (Table 41.3).[2]

OPERATIVE REPAIR

Indications

Patients presenting with AAAs may be asymptomatic, symptomatic, or critically ill with a ruptured aneurysm. These different presentations play a role in dictating the timing of repair. In those who are asymptomatic, the size of the aneurysm at discovery as well as the aneurysmal growth determines the need for surgical intervention. Current evidence recommends an elective repair for those with aneurysms measuring

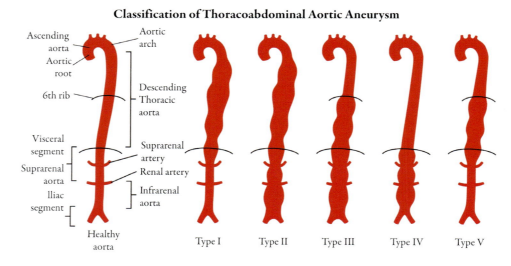

Figure 41.2 Crawford classifications of thoracoabdominal aneurysms. Healthy aorta with main parts labeled and aorta with various types of thoracoabdominal aneurysm.

Table 41.3 **RISK OF ANEURYSM RUPTURE**

ANEURYSM SIZE	RISK FOR RUPTURE (%)
<4.0 cm diameter	0
4.0–4.9 cm in diameter	0.5–5
5.0–5.9 cm in diameter	3–15
6.0–6.9 cm in diameter	10–20
7.0–7.9 cm in diameter	20–40
≥8.0 cm in diameter	30–50

Adapted from Aggarwal S et al.[3]

Table 41.4 **IMPORTANT ANATOMIC CONSIDERATIONS FOR ENDOVASCULAR AORTIC ANEURYSM REPAIR (EVAR)**

Aortic neck	Length, diameter, angle, calcification/thrombus
Aortic aneurysm	Aortic tortuosity index, aortic angle, thrombus %, aortic branch vessel involvement, pelvic perfusion
Iliac artery	Calcification, diameter & occlusive disease, iliac tortuosity index, artery angle, common iliac length, diameter

Adapted from Chaikof EL et al.[1]

greater than 5.4 cm in the absence of significant comorbidities or contraindications.[1,3] Expansion rate is another criterion used to determine if operative intervention is required. If the aneurysm expands more than 0.5 cm in a 6-month interval or greater than 1 cm in a year, then the patient should be considered for repair even if the aneurysm does not measure more than 5.4 cm.[2,9,10] Those who present with symptoms such as abdominal or back pain and no other attributable etiology are also considered for repair. In addition, patients with imaging or other clinical characteristics concerning a mycotic or inflammatory aneurysm are considered for urgent surgical intervention. A patient presenting with a ruptured aneurysm is a true emergency, in contrast to an elective repair in which time allows for adequate preoperative workup and optimization of medical comorbidities before surgical intervention.

Surgical Approach

There are two possible surgical approaches to AAAs, open and endovascular repair. Endovascular aortic aneurysm repair (EVAR) has grown in popularity, and currently, approximately 80% of patients undergo EVAR in the United States.[1] As the technology of endovascular grafts has improved including fenestrated and custom-made grafts, more patients are eligible for endovascular repair. Endovascular repair generally results in shorter operative times, decreased blood loss, and shorter hospital and ICU length of stay.[11] EVAR eliminates the hemodynamic and physiologic disturbances associated with aortic cross-clamping as well as the morbidity of a large abdominal incision. Multiple studies have confirmed a short-term decrease in mortality associated with endovascular repair, yet none demonstrates a decrease in long-term mortality.[11] The long-term complications of endovascular repair include endoleak, secondary graft rupture, and long-term cardiovascular complications. Considering the rigorous long-term surveillance, prompt intervention for endoleaks, and the improvement in overall graft durability, many vascular surgeons feel the long-term mortality data from the initial landmark trials are outdated.[9,10]

In general, endovascular repair was originally designed to treat infrarenal aneurysms, but with the subsequent advent of fenestrated grafts, the applicability has increased. Specific anatomic criteria are typically used to evaluate the appropriateness of endovascular repair. In 2018, the Society of Vascular Surgery/American Association for Vascular Surgery developed a grading scale to in determine the suitability of the patient's anatomy for endovascular repair.[1] The pertinent anatomy includes aortic neck morphology, aneurysm morphology, pelvic perfusion, and common iliac anatomy (Table 41.4).[1] Typically, patients have a CT angiogram to delineate the anatomy. Once a surgeon reviews the imaging, the decision is made as to whether the aneurysm is amenable to endovascular repair. The patient's age, functional status, renal function, and other comorbidities also play a role in the decision to proceed with endovascular repair.

In contrast to endovascular repair, which can be performed with only percutaneous access, an open repair requires a large abdominal incision using either a transperitoneal or retroperitoneal approach to obtain access to the abdominal aorta located in the retroperitoneum. Intraoperatively, aortic cross clamps are applied to exclude the diseased segment of the aorta. The cross-clamp application and release results in numerous physiologic perturbations with associated short- and long-term effects. Open repair has improved long-term outcomes and decreased long-term mortality; however, it is associated with increased length of hospital and ICU stay, days on mechanical ventilation, rates of transfusion, and anesthetic duration. Some patients may not be candidates for open intervention due to the associated perioperative physiologic stress imposed.

PREOPERATIVE EVALUATION

Based on the risk factors and pathophysiology of AAA development, patients who present for operative repair inherently have comorbidities that influence their perioperative care and outcomes. Most of the short- and long-term deaths that occur following both open and endovascular repair are a result of cardiac and pulmonary disease.[1] Coronary artery disease (CAD), chronic obstructive pulmonary disease (COPD), chronic kidney disease (CKD), hypertension, DM, and peripheral vascular disease (PVD) are all comorbidities that have the potential to influence both anesthetic management and outcomes.

Active cardiovascular conditions such as unstable angina, a recent (<1 month) myocardial infarction (MI), decompensated congestive heart failure (CHF), significant arrhythmias, or severe valvular disease warrant further evaluation before any planned operative intervention.[1] Many patients presenting for repair will not have conditions that warrant further investigation; however, they may still be at risk for perioperative major adverse cardiac events. Less than 10% of patients who have vascular surgical procedures have normal coronaries, and greater than half have advanced or severe CAD even if asymptomatic.[1,12] Underlying CAD, including asymptomatic, may manifest intraoperatively due to the stress imposed on the body from combined anesthetic and surgical factors. Routine coronary revascularization is not recommended preoperatively in patients with stable cardiac conditions; however, it is indicated in those with unstable or stable angina, myocardial ischemia, or significant left main CAD or multi-vessel disease.[1]

The patient's functional status can be a surrogate marker for cardiac and pulmonary pathology. If the patient can achieve 4 metabolic equivalents (METs) or walk up two flights of stairs without shortness of breath, then their functional capacity warrants no further workup (Table 41.5). In patients whose functional status cannot be evaluated or who are unable to achieve 4 METs without symptoms, one may consider cardiopulmonary exercise testing if they also have at least three risk factors, including mild angina, prior MI, history of CHF, DM, and CKD.[1] Recently Grant et al. evaluated different variables during cardiopulmonary exercise testing and demonstrated that multiple subthreshold values significantly reduced 3-year survival.[13] Also, prehabilitation exercise therapy before AAA repair might slightly reduce cardiac and renal complications but does not reduce 30-day mortality, pulmonary complications, need for reintervention, or postoperative bleeding.[14] Endovascular repair of aortic aneurysms appears safe in COPD patients with overall very good outcomes; optimizing patients' pulmonary status perioperatively remains an important future task.

COPD commonly coexists in patients presenting with AAAs and has been associated with increased mortality, but not with the aneurysm growth.[15,16] Another study reported that COPD may be underdiagnosed in those with AAA and highlighted the importance of pulmonary function tests (PFTs) to identify those patients.[17] Patients with a long-standing history of COPD, significant tobacco use, or inability to climb one flight of stairs are those for whom preoperative PFTs should be considered.[1] Those who are on home oxygen or patients who are already seeing a pulmonologist should be evaluated preoperatively to allow for appropriate medical optimization. Smoking cessation also plays a key role in preparing the patient for operative intervention. Patients with COPD present possible intraoperative challenges including difficulty ventilating or oxygenating, noncompliant lungs, secretions, and possible reactive airways. Postoperatively, they are at risk for prolonged intubation, COPD exacerbations, and reintubation following abdominal surgery. These complications should be discussed with the patient preoperatively. Patients with COPD should be medically optimized before surgical intervention to minimize the possibility of postoperative complications. Providing bronchodilator treatment in a preoperative holding area may benefit these patients.

CKD is another well-studied risk factor that should be identified preoperatively. It has been associated with increased mortality following aneurysm repair.[1] In patients with known moderate CKD, evidence has demonstrated that EVAR is superior to open repair despite the contrast load if anatomy is amenable; however, when the involvement of renal arteries is expected, open repair may be preferred as an alternative to renal failure requiring dialysis, which is commonly associated with worse outcome.[18] Not uncommonly, patients develop an acute kidney injury following aneurysm repair, which increases the risk of in-hospital mortality as well as the potential for worsening preexisting CKD. Several strategies are currently employed to try mitigate the postoperative decline in renal function, including preoperative hydration to achieve euvolemia and discontinuation of angiotensin-converting enzyme inhibitors or angiotensin receptor antagonists.[1,19]

Patients presenting for vascular surgery frequently have DM as a comorbidity. Although current evidence suggests that DM has a negative association with the development, expansion, and risk for rupture of AAA, DM remains an important perioperative risk factor.[20–22] DM is associated with CAD as well as PVD which raises perioperative concerns. In a prospective observational study, DM and elevated hemoglobin A1C were associated with increased risk of 6-month mortality, ICU and hospital length of stay, major adverse complications, and requirement of mechanical ventilation.[23] It is essential to address glycemic control in the perioperative period to help mitigate any postoperative complications, especially skin and soft tissue infections. Hemoglobin A1C preoperatively helps identify patients who would benefit from tighter regulation of glycemic control preoperatively. The patient's medication regimen should also be evaluated with the perioperative discontinuation of metformin on the day of surgery to decrease the risk of lactic acidosis. Holding metformin before contrast administration should also be considered due to the same concern.[24] In the setting of discontinuing oral agents for the management of DM, it becomes crucial to monitor for both hypoglycemia and hyperglycemia in the perioperative setting.

Hypertension will be frequently encountered in those presenting for AAA repair. A thorough history should be obtained about the current anti-hypertensive regimen and

Table 41.5 ACTIVITY LEVEL TO ASSESS FUNCTIONAL STATUS

ACTIVITY TOLERANCE	EXAMPLES OF ACTIVITIES
Poor (1–3 METs)	Getting dressed, light housework, eating, very slow walk
Moderate (4–7 METs)	Climbing a flight of stairs or walking uphill, running short distance, heaving housework
Good (7–10 METs)	Golfing without cart, calisthenics
Excellent (>10 METs)	Strenuous sports, jogging 10min mile or faster

Adapted from Chaikof EL et al.[1]

how well the regimen is controlling the blood pressure. One should investigate possible end-organ effects associated with chronic hypertension. It may also be helpful to note whether the patient experiences any symptoms when the blood pressure is above or below a certain threshold. Considering the rightward shift of the autoregulation curve that occurs in chronic hypertension, these patients are at increased risk for intraoperative organ hypoperfusion.[25] Knowing the patient's baseline blood pressure and pulse pressure can be helpful when managing blood pressure intraoperatively in association with aortic cross-clamp application and release. Of crucial importance is understanding that patients with hypertension are more prone to hemodynamic fluctuations that are often exaggerated intraoperatively and require vigilance about blood pressure management. One important aspect is that central blood pressure closely associated with aneurysm size and growth rate may be underappreciated, and some patients may be falsely considered normotensive.[26]

Patients with AAA and many of the associated comorbidities are often on medications that require special attention. Given the associated cardiovascular conditions, including hyperlipidemia and hypertension, these patients are often on lipid-lowering agents, aspirin, anti-hypertensives, and/or medications for the management of heart failure. Patients who are on aspirin, statins, and/or betablockers preoperatively should be continued on these medications in the perioperative period. Continuation of these medications has been associated with improved survival.[27] A beta-blocker should not be initiated in the perioperative setting and should only be administered if the patient was on the medication preoperatively because the commencement of new betablocker therapy has been associated with adverse outcomes. Other essential medications that may be encountered include antiplatelet agents and direct oral anticoagulants. Management of these medications in the perioperative period is complex, and it is vital to discern the indication for anticoagulation as well as discuss with the surgical team the need for discontinuation and the timing of resuming therapy. The timing of discontinuation of antiplatelet and anticoagulant medication may also influence the ability to perform neuraxial procedures. The American Society of Regional Anesthesia and Pain Management (ASRA) has recently updated its guidelines regarding the perioperative management of these medications and provides a valuable reference.[28]

PERIOPERATIVE CONSIDERATIONS

For AAA repair, the patient's comorbidities and the surgical approach impact decisions regarding vascular access, availability and need for blood products, arterial access, need for specialized monitoring, and postoperative analgesia. Ideally, a thoughtful discussion with the patient regarding these topics should be done in the preoperative setting. The potential complications associated with an individual patient's comorbid conditions are vital to the preoperative discourse. The options for postoperative analgesia tailored to the specific patient should also be addressed preoperatively.

The Surgical Patient with Chronic Pain

Patients with a history of chronic pain presenting for an operative procedure add another layer of complexity to the preoperative evaluation. Eliciting a thorough history of their pain, medication usage, and comorbid psychiatric conditions becomes imperative. Whether the patient consumes opioids chronically or has a SCS or intrathecal pump influences the perioperative treatment plan. Chronic pain patients are at risk for inadequate analgesia in the perioperative setting due to a variety of reasons. These patients start with and continue to have higher pain scores throughout the perioperative setting, putting them at risk for increased risk of opioid side effects.[29,30] Patients who are chronically on opioids are also likely to have opioid tolerance in addition to possible opioid-induced hyperalgesia. Opioid-induced hyperalgesia occurs as a result of the activation of pro-nociceptive pain pathways in the periphery and spinal cord—alternatively, tolerance results from the desensitization of anti-nociceptive pathways to opioids.[31] These two conditions are often difficult to distinguish clinically and often lead to increased narcotic requirements. Some centers advocate for a gradual decrease in basal narcotics ahead of the planned surgical procedure to allow for resensitization and reduced hyperalgesia.[32]

Another essential component of the preoperative visit is establishing expectations regarding the perioperative pain experience. By developing a plan tailored to the individual patient starting preoperatively and extending postoperatively, evidence has demonstrated "reduced postoperative opioid consumption, less preoperative anxiety, fewer requests for sedative medications, and shortened duration of stay after surgery."[33] Key components for perioperative management of chronic pain patients are outlined in Table 41.6.

Table 41.6 **PERIOPERATIVE PLANNING FOR CHRONIC PAIN**

PREOPERATIVE	INTRAOPERATIVE	POSTOPERATIVE
Pain history- medications, psychological, social factors	*Regional/Neuraxial*	*Acute Pain Team Involvement*
Education regarding perioperative course and pain expectations	*Multimodal medications:* Ketamine infusion	*Multimodal medications:* Consider continuation of ketamine, lidocaine, and gabapentin
Tailored analgesic plan- regional + multimodal vs multimodal	Lidocaine infusion (if not regional anesthetic)	Scheduled acetaminophen & NSAIDs (if surgically appropriate)
Continue basal narcotics & other adjunctive medications including the day of procedure	Magnesium infusion or bolus Potential addition of α_2 agonist	*Continue home analgesic regimen* (if not able to take po convert to IV equivalents)
Preoperative administration of *gabapentin and acetaminophen*	Opioid titration or infusion	*Plan for wean of increased opioid dosage* & discuss plans with patient as well as outpatient pain physician

Adapted from Khan TW, Manion S.[32]

Spinal Cord Stimulators

A subgroup of patients with chronic pain have SCS placed. The two most common indications for stimulator placement include failed back surgery syndrome and complex regional pain syndrome. In addition, patients with chronic neuropathic pain of the trunk or limbs and those with intractable low back pain are considered candidates for stimulator placement. Currently, there is an expanding field of potential uses including chronic intractable angina, PVD, visceral abdominal/pelvic pain, and peripheral nerve pain.[34] As the indications for SCSs continue to expand, the number of patients presenting for anesthetics with stimulators in place will increase. Thus, the perioperative management of these devices has become more important, although these devices don't seem to decrease overall opioid use.[35]

Spinal cord stimulation helps alleviate pain through several mechanisms. Gate control theory was the initially proposed mechanism; however, more is needed to fully explain the pain relief seen in neuropathic and other pain syndromes. Currently, both spinal and supraspinal pathways are proposed to provide analgesic benefits.[34] In ischemic pain, the SCS is thought to aid with the restoration of the balance between oxygen supply and demand. Conventionally, spinal cord stimulation involves patients trading pain for low-grade paresthesia. Several other promising modalities have been developed for pain management without associated paresthesias. High-frequency and burst stimulation are two different stimulation techniques that relieve pain with decreased or no paresthesias. Another novel technique involves dorsal root ganglion lead placement and stimulation, which allows for targeted pain treatment.[36]

SCS implantation can be achieved via a percutaneous approach or laminectomy. The electrodes ultimately sit on the dorsal column of the spinal cord within the epidural space.[34] When placed percutaneously, trial leads are typically followed by the placement of permanent leads. The anatomic location of the pain dictates the spinal level at which the electrodes are placed, with the neck and shoulder above C5 and the lower back at T8–10.

Patients who have SCS warrant special perioperative attention. Preoperatively, the stimulator should be interrogated to confirm the system remains intact and functions appropriately. Following the interrogation, the device should be programmed to the lowest possible amplitude and then turned off before induction of anesthesia for any operative procedure. The primary concern in patients with stimulators is the use of electrocautery. Current recommendations state that, when possible, bipolar cautery be used, and if monopolar cautery is required, the grounding pad should be placed as far away from the generator as possible and on the opposite side from the generator.[34] Postoperatively, the device should be interrogated once again to ensure no damage has occurred, and the stimulator is turned back on at that time. The anesthesiologist will play an essential role in coordinating device interrogation and communicating with the operative team the particular concerns regarding electrocautery.

Given the location of SCS within the epidural space, there has been some concern over whether it is feasible to place epidurals in these patients. In the obstetric literature, lumbar epidurals have been placed successfully in SCS patients. The main concern in patients presenting for abdominal procedures is that, typically, a thoracic epidural would be placed; however, this is also the most common location for SCS electrodes. Current literature is scant about the placement of epidurals above or below the level of the electrodes. Scarring within the epidural space may also make placement difficult and lead to the abnormal spread of the local anesthetic.[34] Until more evidence on this topic is available, it might be prudent to avoid thoracic epidural placement as other regional approaches may be beneficial.

PERIOPERATIVE ANALGESIA

Pain control is an essential consideration for any surgical procedure. Inadequately treated acute pain can lead to downstream negative physiologic and psychologic consequences. Adequate analgesia has been associated with decreased incidence of postoperative delirium development of chronic pain, earlier patient mobility, and improved patient satisfaction. Patients presenting for open AAA repair are at high risk for severe postoperative pain levels. These patients benefit from preoperative counseling about expectations in addition to a thorough plan to address perioperative analgesia. Depending on the individual patient's needs and other contributing factors, a combination of strategies may be necessary. Regional techniques often provide the most pain relief for patients with large abdominal incisions; nonetheless, in patients who may not be candidates for regional procedures, a multimodal approach with systemic medications can often provide adequate analgesia. Figure 41.3 outlines the potential analgesic strategies for patients having open AAA repair.

Epidural Catheters

A variety of potential regional techniques may be utilized to provide either adjunctive intraoperative analgesia or postoperative pain control. Epidurals are one of the primary analgesic options used for postoperative pain control in patients undergoing open AAA repair. Some essential contraindications to epidural placement include infection at the insertion site, coagulopathy or bleeding diathesis, and therapeutic anticoagulation if not appropriately discontinued (per the ASRA guidelines) before the planned neuraxial procedure.[28] Other relative contraindications include spinal deformity or other anatomical changes that would complicate placement, prior spinal surgery at the level of insertion, preexisting demyelinating condition, sepsis, and aortic or mitral stenosis. The potential risks associated with epidural placement include infection at the insertion site, bleeding, epidural hematoma or abscess, dural puncture with possible post-dural puncture headache, hypotension, local anesthetic toxicity, and possibly temporary or permanent nerve damage. In most cases, the benefits of epidural placement outweigh the potential risks; however, both should be discussed with patients before proceeding.

Epidural and spinal anesthesia are frequently utilized in enhanced recovery programs due to their ability to mitigate the metabolic, inflammatory, and neuroendocrine stress

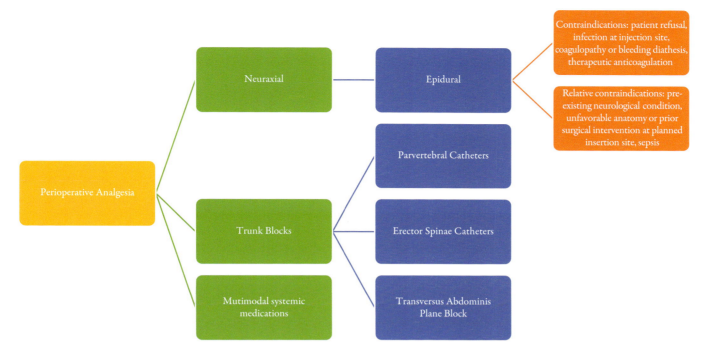

Figure 41.3 Perioperative analgesic strategies.

response.[37] In addition, epidurals may modulate sympathetic outflow leading to vasodilation and decreased afterload with resultant improvement in organ perfusion. A study published in *JAMA Surgery* noted a decrease in long-term mortality in patients undergoing open AAA repair with epidurals in place, which was attributed to a decrease in the immediate postoperative pulmonary complications, need for dialysis, and bowel ischemia in those patients who received epidural analgesia.[38] Despite the study's limitations, it is important to recognize that epidural analgesia may provide benefits beyond pain control postoperatively and warrants further investigation. Other studies have demonstrated the beneficial role epidurals play specifically in patients with COPD and open AAA repair, in large part due to decreasing the risk of postoperative pulmonary complications.[39] Given the numerous benefits associated with epidural analgesia, this option should be discussed with the patient and the surgical team in the absence of contraindications.

Paravertebral and Erector Spinae Catheters

Alternatives to neuraxial anesthesia include paravertebral and erector spinae blockade. The paravertebral block provides analgesia via local anesthetic action on the intercostal nerves, dorsal nerve branches, and the sympathetic chain as they emerge from the spinal foramina. It has been used at various institutions for thoracic procedures as an alternative to epidural, often resulting in decreased hypotension. Paravertebral catheters may be left in place for continuous infusion and placed unilaterally or bilaterally. Potential risks of placement include hemo-/pneumothorax, mediastinal puncture, epidural or intrathecal injection, and local anesthetic toxicity.[40]

Paravertebral blocks have been successfully utilized in open inguinal herniorrhaphy, open gynecologic procedures, and various other abdominal surgeries.[41] A 2018 journal article demonstrated adequate analgesia and decreased hypotension compared to an epidural in patients who had surgically placed paravertebral catheters in open AAA repair via the retroperitoneal approach.[42] Paravertebral catheters are an acceptable alternative and should be discussed preoperatively.

Erector spinae single injections and catheters are an emerging approach to blockade nerve roots with minimal risks. The local anesthetic is deposited in a plane between the erector spinal muscle and the transverse process. Local anesthetic then spreads into the paravertebral space to act on the dorsal and ventral nerve roots.[43] They are routinely placed under ultrasound guidance and have few associated risks or complications. Their use has been most notable in thoracic surgery; however, there has been recent interest in their use for abdominal procedures. A case series demonstrated adequate analgesia in 11 patients undergoing abdominal surgeries and in another case series with 4 patients who underwent laparoscopic ventral hernia repair.[43,44] Erector spinae catheters require a bilateral placement to obtain adequate an abdominal wall analgesia. Moving forward, as more data become available about their benefit in major abdominal surgery the erector spinae catheters may become a more commonly utilized regional approach.

Transversus Abdominis Plane Block

In patients who decline neuraxial or more centrally acting peripheral nerve blocks, the transversus abdominis plane (TAP) block is a potential addition to a multimodal approach for postoperative pain control. A TAP block deposits local anesthetic in a plane between the internal oblique and the transversus abdominis muscles. The afferents from T6–L1 that provide sensory innervation in the anterior and lateral abdominal wall lie with this plane and are targeted by the local anesthetic deposition.[44] Typically, a TAP block is performed under ultrasound guidance as single injections; however, leaving catheters in place is also feasible. These blocks are frequently placed in patients who were not candidates for a neuraxial procedure and have failed systemic multimodal treatment.

MULTIMODAL MEDICATIONS

Many institutions have developed a multimodal approach to postoperative pain control with the goal of decreased opioid consumption. A variety of medications can be used in a multimodal regimen, including lidocaine, ketamine, and magnesium infusions, acetaminophen, NSAIDs, gabapentin/pregabalin, and alpha-receptor agonists. Patients with a history of chronic pain, those in whom there is a concern for opioid-associated respiratory depression, or patients undergoing procedures with anticipated severe postoperative pain are those who most likely to benefit from a multimodal analgesic regimen.

Lidocaine

Lidocaine is an amide local anesthetic that can be given intravenously as an adjunct for the treatment of acute postoperative pain. The primary mechanism of action is via sodium channel blockade, thus decreasing the spontaneous transmission of pain impulses generated from injured nerve fibers and the proximal dorsal root ganglion. In addition, there is some N-methyl-D-aspartic acid (NMDA) receptors blockade. Other reported effects include decreased hyperalgesia and inflammation. Several meta-analyses have evaluated the effectiveness of IV lidocaine as a postoperative adjunct. It has been demonstrated to aid in providing acceptable pain scores and decreasing opioid consumption, postoperative nausea, and vomiting, and hospital length of stay, primarily in patients undergoing abdominal surgery.[45–47] Patients who are undergoing major abdominal surgery and do not have an epidural or regional block may benefit from IV lidocaine. In patients with underlying pulmonary disease or those sensitive to the respiratory depressant effects of systemic opioids, lidocaine infusion can be used in a multimodal approach to aid with the reduction of opioid consumption. Patients maintained on lidocaine infusion postoperatively, they should be monitored for symptoms of toxicity, including perioral numbness, metallic taste, and tinnitus, as well as more severe indicators of local anesthetic toxicity. Lidocaine levels, in addition to clinical symptoms, can also provide valuable information, with the toxicity apparent when levels reach approximately 5 mcg/mL.[47]

Ketamine

Ketamine is another IV medication that can be utilized as an adjunctive analgesic in the perioperative setting. The primary nociceptive effect of ketamine is through its inhibitory action of supraspinal NMDA receptors. However, it likely also acts on numerous other receptors, which contribute to the analgesic effect. Ketamine has been shown to effectively reduce opioid requirements when used in the perioperative setting in combination with a multimodal approach. One critical property of the medication is lack of respiratory depressant effects, which allows it to be utilized effectively in combination with other agents. Per 2018 consensus guidelines, patients who are most likely to benefit from the addition of ketamine to a multimodal regimen include those undergoing surgical procedures with anticipated significant postoperative pain, those who are at risk for opioid-related respiratory depression, and those who are opioid-tolerant or opioid-dependent.[48] Though the dose at which patients respond and can tolerate varies, the guidelines suggest an initial bolus dose of up to 0.35 mg/kg followed by an infusion with the maximum recommended dose of 1 mg/kg/hr.[48] The most notable side effect of ketamine includes hallucinations. The hallucinations may limit further up-titration of the medication if the patient finds them disturbing. Benzodiazepines and clonidine can be given following the development of hallucinations to aid in mitigating the worrisome side effects. Ketamine should not be administered to patients with severe hepatic dysfunction or severe coronary disease, nor in patients with active psychosis.

Magnesium

Magnesium infusions are more often encountered in obstetrics to treat pre-eclampsia; however, magnesium also has clinical applications for analgesia due to noncompetitive inhibition of the NMDA receptors within the spinal cord. Other proposed mechanisms include antagonism of alpha receptors and impaired calcium-mediated neuroendocrine release.[49] A meta-analysis evaluating 20 randomized controlled trials demonstrated a reduction in both early and late postoperative pain with magnesium. Magnesium infusion was also associated with decreased narcotic consumption when compared to controls. Several other meta-analyses have also demonstrated improved pain scores associated with magnesium utilization. Currently, neither a magnesium level nor a specific dosing protocol has been correlated with a reduction in opioid requirements. However, most trials have used a 30–50 mg/kg bolus dose followed by an infusion at 8–15 mg/kg for a total of 4–6 hrs. More studies are needed to define a protocol that provides maximum benefit while minimizing the risk associated with hypermagnesemia. Drowsiness, loss of deep tendon reflexes, ECG changes, prolonged neuromuscular blockade, respiratory depression, paralysis, and even cardiac arrest are possible consequences of increasing systemic magnesium levels. Magnesium may be another valuable agent to add to the armamentarium in treating postoperative pain, considering the potential physiologic perturbations that may result from hypermagnesemia.[49–51]

Other Medications

Gabapentanoids, including gabapentin and pregabalin, are frequently used as adjunctive analgesics in the perioperative setting. The precise mechanism of action for the analgesic effect of these medications is unknown. Their use in the perioperative setting is off-label, with mixed results whether they improve postoperative pain control. One meta-analysis evaluating five randomized controlled trials revealed preoperative gabapentin decreased opioid consumption in the first 24 hours postoperatively.[52] On the other hand, different studies have failed to demonstrate a clear decrease in pain scores or improved mobility after various orthopedic operations and in diabetic peripheral neuropathic pain, and even suggest that they may have cumulative sedative effects. Studies supporting the use of pregabalin are also mixed, and the results depend on the type of surgical procedure. Despite the variability in benefit, these medications may be helpful to administer proactively in the perioperative setting to aid with analgesic control, keeping in mind that a known side effect includes drowsiness or somnolence.

Alpha-agonists are another category of medications with potential benefit in treating postoperative pain. Both clonidine and the more selective dexmedetomidine have been evaluated for their efficacy in treating postoperative pain. Studies indicate that clonidine provides the most benefit when administered intrathecally or via a peripheral nerve catheter. At the same time, intraoperative administration of dexmedetomidine has been demonstrated to decrease postoperative pain and have an opioid-sparing effect.[53]

CONCLUSION

- AAA repairs require unique surgical and anesthetic planning.
- The comorbidities often associated with AAA have essential implications in the perioperative setting.
- Patients with chronic pain, especially those with SCSs, benefit from a well-thought-out perioperative analgesic plan.
- There are multiple approaches to analgesia in patients undergoing AAA repair, and these options should be discussed and tailored to fit each patient.

REVIEW QUESTIONS

1. AAAs are classified based on their relation to which of the following pairs of arteries?

    a. Iliac arteries.
    b. Renal arteries.
    c. Femoral arteries.
    d. Both b and c.

The correct answer is b.

AAAs are classified based on their relation to the renal arteries and include infrarenal, juxtarenal, and suprarenal.

2. Which comorbidity is a leading risk factor for the development of AAAs and has been associated with increased mortality?

    a. Hypertension.
    b. Diabetes.
    c. COPD.
    d. CKD.

The correct answer is c.

Patients with AAA have many significant comorbidities that affect both their anesthetic care and their overall long-term mortality. COPD has been independently associated with increased mortality in patients undergoing AAA repair.[54] It is imperative to address COPD preoperatively, which may include PFTs, pulmonology consultation, smoking cessation, and medical optimization.

3. What should be included in a preoperative evaluation in chronic pain patients undergoing AAA repair?

    a. Functional status.
    b. Pain history including medications psychological and social factors.
    c. Patient's requests for postoperative pain medications.
    d. Education regarding the perioperative course and pain expectations.
    e. Both b and d.

The correct answer is d.

Those with a history of chronic pain require a unique perioperative approach to their overall management. It is crucial in the preoperative evaluation to fully evaluate their pain history including all medications psychological and social factors in addition to educating them with regards to the perioperative plan and appropriate expectations about their pain management.[32] It is crucial to develop a well-thought-out and individualized plan for pain management. Any basal narcotics should be continued on the day of surgery.

4. Postoperative analgesic options for patients with SCS include all of the following *except*

    a. Opioid infusions.
    b. Neuraxial analgesia.
    c. Magnesium.
    d. Gabapentin.

The correct answer is b.

Opioid infusions are often appropriate for intraoperative pain management in those who do not have a functional epidural in place or are not candidates for regional anesthetic techniques. Opioid infusions are preferably avoided postoperatively in extubated patients due to the significant risk of opioid-associated respiratory depression. Potential adjunctive treatments for postoperative pain include magnesium, lidocaine, gabapentin, alpha-agonists, ketamine, and regional blocks. Neuraxial analgesia is best avoided in the case study patient with a SCS due to the risk for infection, and lead displacement; regional blocks with or without catheter placements should be attempted instead.

REFERENCES

1. Chaikof EL, Dalman RL, Eskandari MK, et al. The Society for Vascular Surgery practice guidelines on the care of patients with an abdominal aortic aneurysm. *J Vasc Surg*. 2018 Jan;67(1):2–77.e2.
2. Shalabi A. Anesthesia for vascular surgery. In: Gropper MA, Eriksson LI, Fleisher LA, Leslie K, Wiener-Kronish JP, eds. *Miller's Anesthesia*. 9th ed. Elsevier; 2020:1825–1867.
3. Aggarwal S, Qamar A, Sharma V, Sharma A. Abdominal aortic aneurysm: A comprehensive review. *Exp Clin Cardiol*. 2011 Spring;16(1):11–15.
4. Lo RC, Lu B, Fokkema MT, et al. Relative importance of aneurysm diameter and body size for predicting abdominal aortic aneurysm rupture in men and women. *J Vasc Surg*. 2014 May;59(5):1209–1216.
5. Chaikof EL, Blankensteijn JD, Harris PL, et al. Reporting standards for endovascular aortic aneurysm repair. *J Vasc Surg*. 2002 May;35(5):1048–1060.
6. Crawford ES, Crawford JL, Safi HJ, et al. Thoracoabdominal aortic aneurysms: Preoperative and intraoperative factors determining immediate and long-term results of operations in 605 patients. *J Vasc Surg*. 1986 Mar;3(3):389–404.
7. Green DB, Palumbo MC, Lau C. Imaging of thoracoabdominal aortic aneurysms. *J Thorac Imaging*. 2018;33(6):358–365.
8. Kent KC, Zwolak RM, Egorova NN, et al. Analysis of risk factors for abdominal aortic aneurysm in a cohort of more than 3 million individuals. *J Vasc Surg*. 2010 Sep;52(3):539–548.
9. Tenorio ER, Dias-Neto MF, Lima GBB, Estrera AL, Oderich GS. Endovascular repair for thoracoabdominal aortic aneurysms: Current status and future challenges. *Ann Cardiothorac Surg*. 2021 Nov;10(6):744–767.
10. Kessler V, Klopf J, Eilenberg W, Neumayer C, Brostjan C. AAA revisited: A comprehensive review of risk factors, management, and hallmarks of pathogenesis. *Biomedicines*. 2022 Jan 2;10(1):94.
11. Johal AS, Loftus IM, Boyle JR, Heikkila K, Waton S, Cromwell DA. Long-term survival after endovascular and open repair of unruptured abdominal aortic aneurysm. *Br J Surg*. 2019 Dec;106(13):1784–1793.
12. Straw S, Waduud MA, Drozd M, et al. The role of cardiopulmonary exercise testing and echocardiography prior to elective endovascular aneurysm repair. *Ann R Coll Surg Engl*. 2020 May;102(5):383–390.
13. Grant SW, Hickey GL, Wisely NA, et al. Cardiopulmonary exercise testing and survival after elective abdominal aortic aneurysm repair. *Br J Anaesth*. 2015 Mar;114(3):430–436.
14. Fenton C, Tan AR, Abaraogu UO, McCaslin JE. Prehabilitation exercise therapy before elective abdominal aortic aneurysm repair. *Cochrane Database Syst Rev*. 2021 Jul 08;7(7):CD013662.
15. Khashram M, Williman JA, Hider PN, Jones GT, Roake JA. Systematic review and meta-analysis of factors influencing survival following abdominal aortic aneurysm repair. *Eur J Vasc Endovasc Surg*. 2016 Feb;51(2):203–215.
16. Takagi H, Umemoto T. No association of chronic obstructive pulmonary disease with abdominal aortic aneurysm growth. *Heart Vessels*. 2016 Nov;31(11):1806–1816.
17. Meijer CA, Kokje VB, van Tongeren RB, et al. An association between chronic obstructive pulmonary disease and abdominal aortic aneurysm beyond smoking: Results from a case-control study. *Eur J Vasc Endovasc Surg*. 2012 Aug;44(2):153–157.
18. Plotkin A, Weaver FA, Abou-Zamzam A, et al. Risk of renal failure and death when renal arteries are involved in endovascular aortic aneurysm repair. *J Vasc Surg*. 2021 Oct;74(4):1193–1203.e3.
19. Sahai SK, Balonov K, Bentov N, et al. Preoperative management of cardiovascular medications: A Society for Perioperative Assessment and Quality Improvement (SPAQI) consensus statement. *Mayo Clin Proc*. 2022 Sep;97(9):1734–1751.
20. Takagi H, Umemoto T. Diabetes and abdominal aortic aneurysm growth. *Angiology*. 2016 Jul;67(6):513–525.
21. D'Cruz R T, Wee IJY, Syn NL, Choong A. The association between diabetes and thoracic aortic aneurysms. *J Vasc Surg*. 2019 Jan;69(1):263–268.e1.
22. Takagi H. Association of diabetes mellitus with presence, expansion, and rupture of abdominal aortic aneurysm: "Curiouser and curiouser!" cried ALICE. *Semin Vasc Surg*. 2016 Mar;29(1-2):18–26.
23. Yong PH, Weinberg L, Torkamani N, et al. The presence of diabetes and higher HbA1c are independently associated with adverse outcomes after surgery. 2018;41(6):1172–1179.
24. Pfeifer KJ, Selzer A, Mendez CE, et al. Preoperative management of endocrine, hormonal, and urologic medications: Society for Perioperative Assessment and Quality Improvement (SPAQI) consensus statement. *Mayo Clin Proc*. 2021 Jun;96(6):1655–1669.
25. Misra S. Systemic hypertension and non-cardiac surgery. *Indian J Anaesth*. 2017 Sep;61(9):697–704.
26. Rooprai J, Boodhwani M, Beauchesne L, et al. Central hypertension in patients with thoracic aortic aneurysms: Prevalence and association with aneurysm size and growth. *Am J Hypertens*. 2022 Jan 5;35(1):79–86.
27. Khashram M, Williman JA, Hider PN, Jones GT, Roake JA. Management of modifiable vascular risk factors improves late survival following abdominal aortic aneurysm repair: A systematic review and meta-analysis. *Ann Vasc Surg*. 2017;39:301–311.
28. Horlocker TT, Vandermeulen E, Kopp SL, Gogarten W, Leffert LR, Benzon HT. Regional anesthesia in the patient receiving antithrombotic or thrombolytic therapy. American Society of Regional Anesthesia and Pain Medicine Evidence-Based Guidelines (4th ed). *Reg Anesth Pain Med*. 2018;43(3):263–309.
29. Veazie S, Mackey K, Peterson K, Bourne D. Managing acute pain in patients taking medication for opioid use disorder: A rapid review. *J Gen Intern Med*. 2020 Dec;35(Suppl 3):945–953.
30. Edinoff AN, Flanagan CJ, Sinnathamby ES, et al. Treatment of acute pain in patients on naltrexone: A narrative review. *Curr Pain Headache Rep*. 2023;27(7):183–192.
31. Mercadante S, Arcuri E, Santoni A. Opioid-induced tolerance and hyperalgesia. *CNS Drugs*. 2019 Oct;33(10):943–955.
32. Khan TW, Manion S. Perioperative surgical home for the patient with chronic pain. *Anesthesiol Clin*. 2018 Jun;36(2):281–294.
33. Nafziger AN, Barkin RL. Opioid therapy in acute and chronic pain. *J Clin Pharmacol*. 2018 Sep;58(9):1111–1122.
34. Harned ME, Gish B, Zuelzer A, Grider JS. Anesthetic considerations and perioperative management of spinal cord stimulators: Literature review and initial recommendations. *Pain Physician*. 2017 May;20(4):319–329.
35. Dhruva SS, Murillo J, Ameli O, et al. Long-term outcomes in use of opioids, nonpharmacologic pain interventions, and total costs of spinal cord stimulators compared with conventional medical therapy for chronic pain. *JAMA Neurol*. 2023;80(1):18–29.
36. Verrills P, Sinclair C, Barnard A. A review of spinal cord stimulation systems for chronic pain. *J Pain Res*. 2018;9:481–493.
37. Capdevila M, Ramin S, Capdevila X. Regional anesthesia and analgesia after surgery in ICU. *Curr Opin Crit Care*. 2017 Oct;23(5):430–439.
38. Bardia A, Sood A, Mahmood F, et al. Combined epidural-general anesthesia vs general anesthesia alone for elective abdominal aortic aneurysm repair. *JAMA Surg*. 2018;151(12):1116–1123.
39. Kim TH, Lee JS, Lee SW, Oh YM. Pulmonary complications after abdominal surgery in patients with mild-to-moderate chronic obstructive pulmonary disease. *Int J Chron Obstruct Pulmon Dis*. 2016;11:2785–2796.
40. Albrecht E, Chin KJ. Advances in regional anaesthesia and acute pain management: A narrative review. *Anaesthesia*. 2020 Jan;75(Suppl 1):e101–e110.
41. Chin KJ, Versyck B, Pawa A. Ultrasound-guided fascial plane blocks of the chest wall: A state-of-the-art review. *Anaesthesia*. 2021 Jan;76(Suppl 1):110–126.
42. Jessula S, Herman CR, Kwofie K, Lee MS, Smith M, Casey P. Intraoperative insertion of paravertebral catheter for postoperative analgesia in retroperitoneal aortic aneurysm repair. *J Vasc Surg*. 2018 Apr 1;67(4):1308–1310.

43. De Cassai A, Bonvicini D, Correale C, Sandei L, Tulgar S, Tonetti T. Erector spinae plane block: A systematic qualitative review. *Minerva Anestesiol*. 2019 Mar;85(3):308–319.
44. Hemmerling TM. Pain management in abdominal surgery. *Langenbecks Arch Surg*. 2018 Nov;403(7):791–803.
45. Rekatsina M, Theodosopoulou P, Staikou C. Effects of intravenous dexmedetomidine versus lidocaine on postoperative pain, analgesic consumption and functional recovery after abdominal gynecological surgery: A randomized placebo-controlled double blind study. *Pain Physician*. 2021 Nov;24(7):E997–E1006.
46. Chu R, Umukoro N, Greer T, et al. Intravenous lidocaine infusion for the management of early postoperative pain: A comprehensive review of controlled trials. *Psychopharmacol Bull*. 2020 Oct 15;50(4 Suppl 1):216–259.
47. Weibel S, Jelting Y, Pace NL, et al. Continuous intravenous perioperative lidocaine infusion for postoperative pain and recovery in adults. *Cochrane Database Syst Rev*. 2018 Jun 4;6(6):Cd009642.
48. Schwenk ES, Viscusi ER, Buvanendran A, et al. Consensus guidelines on the use of intravenous ketamine infusions for acute pain management from the American Society of Regional Anesthesia and Pain Medicine, the American Academy of Pain Medicine, and the American Society of Anesthesiologists. *Reg Anesth Pain Med*. 2018 Jul;43(5):456–466.
49. Bugada D, Lorini LF, Lavand'homme P. Opioid free anesthesia: Evidence for short and long-term outcome. *Minerva Anestesiol*. 2021 Feb;87(2):230–237.
50. Hutchins D, Rockett M. The use of atypical analgesics by intravenous infusion for acute pain: Evidence base for lidocaine, ketamine, and magnesium. *Anaesth Intensive Care Med*. 2019 Aug 1;20(8):415–418.
51. Ghezel-Ahmadi V, Ghezel-Ahmadi D, Schirren J, Tsapopiorgas C, Beck G, Bölükbas S. Perioperative systemic magnesium sulphate to minimize acute and chronic post-thoracotomy pain: A prospective observational study. *J Thorac Dis*. 2019 Feb;11(2):418–426.
52. Tesfaye S, Sloan G, Petrie J, et al. Comparison of amitriptyline supplemented with pregabalin, pregabalin supplemented with amitriptyline, and duloxetine supplemented with pregabalin for the treatment of diabetic peripheral neuropathic pain (OPTION-DM): A multicentre, double-blind, randomised crossover trial. *Lancet*. 2022 Aug 27;400(10353):680–690.
53. Kaye AD, Chernobylsky DJ, Thakur P, et al. Dexmedetomidine in Enhanced Recovery After Surgery (ERAS) protocols for postoperative pain. *Curr Pain Headache Rep*. 2020 Apr 2;24(5):21.
54. Huber TS, Wang JG, Derrow AE, et al. Experience in the United States with intact abdominal aortic aneurysm repair. *J Vasc Surg*. 2001 Feb;33(2):304–310; discussion 10–11.

42.

PATIENT WITH PACEMAKER-DEPENDENT ICD FOR RENAL CRYOABLATION

Paula Trigo Blanco and Adriana D. Oprea

STEM CASE AND KEY QUESTIONS

A 77-year-old woman with past medical history of ischemic cardiomyopathy with moderately depressed ejection fraction (EF), complete heart block (CHB) diagnosed after several syncopal episodes, status post implantable cardioverter defibrillator (ICD) placement, and diabetes mellitus type 2 on insulin regimen presents to her primary care physician (PCP) with hematuria. The abdominal ultrasound reveals an almost isoechoic mass arising from the upper pole of her right kidney. A CT scan of her abdomen and pelvis show a solid hypodense mass on her right kidney with calcifications, as well as significant enhancement after IV contrast administration. To better delineate the surrounding soft tissues and vessels, the patient also has an MRI scan, which demonstrates no vascular invasion and confirms no nodes/liver involvement.

What is the possible etiology of this renal mass?

This renal mass might represent a benign tumor (up to 20% of enhancing small renal masses are benign) or malignant tumor (renal cell carcinoma [RCC]).[1]

What therapeutic interventions are available for RCC?

The urologist explains to the patient that both surgical partial nephrectomy and cryoablation for such small and localized renal mass are associated with similar rates of local recurrence.

What are specific preoperative considerations for this particular patient if she were scheduled to undergo a radical nephrectomy? How would you rate this patient's cardiac risk? Are there any specific cardiac tests that should be ordered preoperatively to help with risk stratification?

Upon further inquiry, the patient is able to do her activities of daily living but has dyspnea with moderate exertion. A pharmacologic stress test is ordered which reveals a large area of ischemia in the lateral territory. Upon discussion with the surgeon and anesthesiologist, the patient decides not to undergo a radical nephrectomy and to consult interventional radiology for cryoablation.

What is cryoablation? What are the main indications for cryotherapy?

Cryoablation (cryotherapy or cryosurgery) is a minimally invasive procedure that uses extremely cold temperatures to destroy tumoral tissues. It can be used to treat kidney tumors of small size and different locations within the kidney. The patient is referred to interventional radiology and anesthesia preadmission testing for consultation in anticipation of her upcoming elective cryoablation.

In addition to common preprocedural laboratory tests, what other preoperative investigations are needed?

In addition to the laboratory tests already available, a chest x-ray (CXR) is requested by the interventional radiologist, which reveals mild cardiac enlargement and an ICD in situ. The interventional radiologist inquires if there is anything he should do in regard to the patient's ICD.

How do you decide whether the patient is pacemaker-dependent or not?

The patient's history of complete heart block makes her highly likely to be pacemaker-dependent.

Are there any considerations for this patient's ICD prior to cryoablation?

The presence of an ICD in this patient is not a contraindication to cryoablation. Cryoablation is not associated with electromagnetic interference (EMI), therefore the device setting will not be altered during the procedure.

The interventional radiologist obtains a recent cardiac device interrogation (within the past 6 months) and a full report regarding her device settings, mode, and possible recent arrhythmic episodes to ensure proper functioning as well as good battery status for her pacemaker/ICD.

How would you monitor this patient?

In addition to the standard American Society of Anesthesiologists (ASA) monitors, an arterial line for invasive blood pressure measurement as well as vascular access for blood sampling, during the procedure may be useful.

What is the appropriate course of action for her ICD during the perioperative period?

This patient has an ICD, is pacing-dependent, and is undergoing cryotherapy. This freezing technique is not associated with

EMI. Therefore, the anti-tachycardia function of her ICD does not have to be inactivated and the pacemaker settings do not have to be altered preprocedurally.

DISCUSSION

INTRODUCTION

Given our aging population, the prevalence of cardiac implantable electronic devices (CIEDs) is on the rise with more than 1 million people having pacemakers (PPMs) and more than 300,000 having ICDs.[2-4] CIEDs include PPMs for the treatment of bradyarrhythmias, ICDs for management of tachyarrhythmias, cardiac resynchronization therapy (CRT) devices for systolic dysfunction with conduction delays, and implanted rhythm monitors (loop recorders).

These patients with CIEDs are frequently presenting for surgical and other interventional procedures.[5] Therefore, it is of paramount importance that anesthesia providers know how to manage these cardiac devices in the perioperative period.[6]

The majority of patients with CIEDs are evaluated yearly by their cardiologist or electrophysiologist, and their devices are interrogated on a regular basis. Perioperative considerations should be formulated by the perioperative CIED team (electrophysiologist, nurse, or technician caring for the patient's CIED) in communication with the perioperative team (surgeon, anesthesiologist, staff associated with the procedure) prior to their surgeries.[7]

INDICATIONS FOR PLACEMENT OF CIEDS

Most common indication for PPM placement is sinus node dysfunction (SND). Patients with SND present with documented symptomatic bradycardia or chronotropic incompetence, bradycardia induced by essential medical regimen, or syncopal episodes with pauses on electrophysiologic studies. In addition, severe atrioventricular (AV) node dysfunction is another indication, including complete third-degree or high-grade second-degree AV block (Mobitz II).[8,9] Other indications include syncopal events in the setting of bi- or tri-fascicular block, first-degree AV block with associated hemodynamic compromise, post myocardial infarction (when a high-degree AV block is persistent post revascularization), or for neurally mediated syncope.

Similarly, indications for ICDs can be classified into primary and secondary prevention. Patients with a prior MI and an EF of less than 35%, patients with ischemic or nonischemic cardiomyopathy and an EF of less than 35%, and patients with syncopal events in the presence of structural heart disease and ventricular arrhythmias inducible on electrophysiology studies represent the major primary prevention indications.[10-13] Additionally, patients with hypertrophic cardiomyopathy, long QT syndrome, arrhythmogenic RV, and Brugada syndrome benefit from ICD placement for prevention of sudden death. Secondary prevention implies patients have already had an episode of successfully resuscitated ventricular tachycardia (VT) or ventricular fibrillation (VF).[8,14]

CRT devices are usually indicated in patients with systolic heart failure (EF <35%) and prolonged QRS duration (>150 ms) with or without left bundle branch block. The benefits of CRT devices consist in immediate hemodynamic benefits (improved cardiac output), improved left ventricular (LV) systolic function, and the promotion of LV reverse remodeling.

PACER DEPENDENCY

One of the first steps in approaching a patient with a pacemaker or ICD/CRT (all ICD/CRT devices have pacemaker capability except subcutaneous ICD) is to determine whether the patient is pacemaker-dependent. It is generally accepted that pacemaker dependency means inadequacy or absence of intrinsic rhythm potentially resulting in bradycardia-related symptoms.[15]

In other words, pacemaker dependency is defined by how functionally dependent a patient is without pacing support. Functional dependency on pacing support may be determined based on patient's history of a syncope caused by a bradyarrhythmia requiring the pacemaker implantation, a history of CHB or AV nodal ablation that resulted in pacemaker placement, or an evaluation of the CIED that shows hemodynamic compromise when the pacing function of the CIED is temporarily disabled or programmed to the lowest programmable rate.

In addition to the patient's history and indication for device placement, dependency can be assessed from a recent device interrogation or an ECG tracing. Although no percentage of pacing guarantees pacer dependency, it is generally accepted that 100% ventricular pacing indicates a dependent scenario. Additionally, a 12-lead ECG or rhythm strip should be examined for pacing spikes. If pacing spikes are noted before most or all of either P wave or QRS complexes, then the patient should be treated as if pacemaker-dependent.

It is important to note that patients with CRT devices will present with 100% ventricular pacing on device interrogation and on the accompanying ECG. Despite that, these patients are not necessarily pacer-dependent because there is an underlying rhythm which is able to support the patient's hemodynamics.

PACEMAKER AND DEFIBRILLATOR NOMENCLATURE

CIEDs have the capability of both sensing the underlying cardiac activity as well as pacing (all CIEDs) or delivering anti-tachycardia therapy (defibrillation or anti-tachycardia pacing for ICD/CRT devices). In addition to preventing bradycardia, pacemakers are also equipped with ways of hemodynamically supporting patients during periods of stress (physical exercise, increased temperature) through a feature called *rate modulation* (responsiveness). Anesthesiologists should be familiar with the North American Society of Pacing and Electrophysiology (NASPE) and British Pacing and Electrophysiology Group (BPEG) CIED nomenclature since

> **Box 42.1** BASIC CIED INFORMATION TO BE COLLECTED
>
> *Pertinent Preoperative Information Regarding the CIED*
>
> Most recent device interrogation (within 6 months for ICD, 12 months for pacemaker)
> Device type, manufacturer, model
> Clinical indication for device placement
> Battery status
> Current programming
> Assess pacemaker dependency
> Device response to magnet placement

different modes of programming have implications in the perioperative period (Box 42.1).

Similarly, in 1993, a NASPE/BPEG defibrillator code was introduced. The four-position code describes defibrillator, arrhythmia diagnostic, and data storage capabilities. The first position of the code represents the shock chamber—none, atrium, ventricle, or dual (*O*, *A*, *V*, or *D*). The second position indicates the anti-tachycardia pacing chamber, also coded *O*, *A*, *V*, or *D*. Position three indicates the how tachyarrhythmia is detected, either with the intracardiac electrogram (*E*) or by hemodynamically (*H*). The fourth position represents the anti-bradycardia chamber (as all transvenous ICDs have also pacemaker capability).[16]

RESPONSE TO MAGNET PLACEMENT

Magnets have been historically used to help interrogate a device. In the perioperative period, they are used to prevent oversensing and inappropriate response of the CIEDs. The application of a magnet is recommended by some entities (Heart Rhythm Society [HRS] and Canadian Anesthesiologists' Society [CAS]/Canadian Cardiovascular Society [CCS]).[7,17] However, advisories and expert opinion statements caution against routine magnet use.[18–20] This is due to potential accelerated heart rate triggered by magnet placement competing with the patient's native rhythm or the risk of malignant ventricular arrhythmia due to the "R-on-T" phenomenon in the case of asynchronous pacing when there is a native rhythm.

The response to the application of a magnet over a cardiac device depends on whether it is a pacemaker or an ICD. The actual response to magnet application should be confirmed by the CIED care team during the preoperative evaluation of the device.

Most commonly, placing a magnet over the generator of a PPM results in asynchronous pacing at a fixed rate and an AV delay specific for that manufacturer (i.e., DOO, VOO, AOO). As such, all Medtronic devices will pace at a heart rate of 85 beats per minute (bpm) unless the battery is depleted. With certain manufacturers (Boston Scientific and Abbott), the device's magnet function may be disabled so that the magnet application would have no effect. It should be noted that Biotronik PPMs respond to magnets differently. The default magnet response ("Auto") of most Biotronik pacemakers consists of a brief period of asynchronous pacing (10 beats) followed by a return to the original settings at the lower rate limit. Magnet mode could be set by telemetry programming to conventional asynchronous pacing at 90 bpm or synchronous pacing continuing in original programmed mode.[21,22]

Magnet placement over a PPM generator also disables the rate modulation feature, which may be detrimental if inadvertently activated in the perioperative period.

The rate at which the PPM will pace upon magnet application will differ based on the battery life of the generator, with lower pacing rates with low battery life, which might not be sufficient to meet the patient's physiologic demands during the perioperative period.

If the patient has an ICD, the application of a magnet over the device will uniformly disable the anti-tachycardia therapy with no effect whatsoever on the pacing mode, therefore not resulting in asynchronous pacing. For patients with ICDs who are pacer-dependent and will be exposed to EMI periprocedurally, a programmer should be used to reprogram the ICD, rather than using a magnet.[20]

Placing a magnet over the device generator could have several disadvantages:

- Profound bradycardia or asystole may occur if pacing is inhibited by EMI in patients with pacer-dependent ICDs when a magnet is placed rather than using a programmer

- In obese patients, the magnet may fail to affect CIED programming.

- Patient positioning (lateral or prone) may make securing a magnet over the device generator difficult. Similarly, in certain procedures (i.e., thyroid, ENT, breast surgeries) magnet placement may compromise the sterility of the surgical field. A related issue may arise if the anesthesiologist is unable to access the magnet during the surgery and make sure it remains securely in place.

- In some patients, asynchronous pacing triggered by the magnet placement may be detrimental to the patient's hemodynamics (i.e., magnet rate of ~100 bpm characteristic for some St. Jude's or Boston Scientific devices may not be desirable in patients with coronary artery disease).

ELECTROMAGNETIC INTERFERENCE

EMI represents a malfunction of the CIED due to an electromagnetic field generated by an external source. Most commonly, during surgery, EMI is caused by the use of monopolar cautery ("Bovie").

It is currently generally accepted that EMI due to electrocautery occurs when the monopolar electrocautery is used within 15 cm (6 in) of the generator and the leads of the device.

For devices placed in the subclavian area (most common location), caution should be exercised when monopolar electrocautery is used for any procedure above the umbilicus.

For older models, where the generator is placed in the abdominal area (after cardiac surgery), the 15 cm (6 in) limit for EMI also should be observed.[20]

EMI leads to oversensing by the CIED. As such, in the case of a PPM, oversensing results in the interpretation of EMI as native cardiac activity, which leads to pacer inhibition with potential bradycardia/asystole as a result, depending on the underlying rhythm.[23-25]

When EMI occurs in the presence of an ICD, oversensing leads to interpretation of EMI by the CIED as ventricular tachycardia or fibrillation with resultant inappropriate defibrillation or anti-tachycardia therapy.

Inadvertent oversensing by the CIED in the presence of EMI can be mitigated by magnet placement or by reprogramming the device using a programmer.

Other detrimental effects of EMI include

- Damage to the CIED generator or total device failure in older devices

- Activation of the "power on reset" mode of the CIED, reverting its programming to the manufacturer-determined mode (for ICDs, defibrillation using high-energy shocks at lower heart rate limits for ventricular tachycardia, and for PPMs, pacing in a VVI only mode).[25]

- Activation of the rate responsiveness feature of PPMs or misinterpretation of EMI as atrial signals, both resulting in inappropriate tachycardia.[7]

In addition to monopolar cautery, other procedural devices can cause EMI such as radiofrequency ablation (RFA) equipment, lithotripsy (extracorporeal shock wave [ESWL] but not laser lithotripsy), transcutaneous electrical nerve stimulation (TENS) units, nerve stimulators, or MRI. Most commonly, RFA "wanding" at the end of the surgical procedures can cause EMI and reprogram a CIED.[26-32] Special situations are addressed in Table 42.1.

PREANESTHESIA EVALUATION

Prior to elective surgeries/procedures, communication between all teams involved in the patient's care should occur. Based on pertinent perioperative information, the CIED team should provide instruction for perioperative management of the devices.

The anesthesiologist is frequently called upon not only to manage the patient intraoperatively, but also to mediate communication between the surgeon and the CIED team as part of the preoperative evaluation of these patients.

Pertinent information required from the perioperative team to determine the pre/intraoperative approach consists in the type of surgery, location, whether EMI is likely present during the procedure (i.e., utilization of monopolar cautery), and the disposition plan for the patient.

The CIED team provides further information regarding the type of CIED (pacemaker vs. ICD), the indication for CIED placement, the manufacturer (e.g., Medtronic, Boston-Scientific, Abbott), adequacy of function, the remaining battery life of the device, the programming mode (i.e., DDD, VOO), whether the patient is pacemaker-dependent or not, the underlying rhythm, and its response of the device to a magnet (Box 42.1). Ideally, the CIED team will provide recommendations regarding the need to use a magnet, the need of reprogramming using a programmer, or no action.

The 2011 HRS/ASA guideline for perioperative care of patients with CIEDs recommends that any patient presenting for elective surgery who has a PPM should have an interrogation within the past 12 months, and ICDs should be evaluated every 6 months.[7]

A recent interrogation provides valuable information on the type of device, indication of placement, manufacturer, battery life, mode of programming, and pacer dependency.

When information regarding the device is not readily available during the preanesthesia evaluation, there are several ways of identifying pertinent data.

- Patient CIED identification cards usually provide helpful information regarding the manufacturer and type of device.

- Patient's old medical records (either cardiology or electrophysiology notes) are helpful.

- A call to the manufacturer (Table 42.2) can elicit valuable information.

- A recent CXR (see below) can provide clues to placement.

On patient's physical examination, pulse regularity and location of the device generator (incisional scar and palpation of the device) should assessed. A recent ECG should be available. With a few exceptions, the presence of pacer spikes in front of each QRS complex represent pacer-dependent situations.

A CXR can help identify the type of CIED (PPM vs. ICD vs. CRT device), location, and sometimes the manufacturer.[33] Presence of thick shock coil in the right ventricle, and/or in the superior vena cava is characteristic of an ICD (Figure 42.1) compared to the thin leads typical for PPMs (Figure 42.2). Similarly, the presence of a third lead in the coronary sinus characterizes a CRT device (Figure 42.3).

Twenty-four-hour technical support is available from all CIED companies (Table 42.2), and the anesthesiologist can obtain pertinent information such as device type, date of implantation, indication for placement, and behavior upon magnet application 24 hours a day.

Table 42.1 TWENTY-FOUR-HOUR TECHNICAL SUPPORT CONTACTS FOR MANUFACTURING COMPANIES

Medtronic	800-633-8766
St. Jude Medical	800-681-9293
Boston Scientific	800-227-3422
Biotronik	800-547-0394

Table 42.2 SPECIAL SITUATIONS AND ELECTROMAGNETIC INTERFERENCE RISKS

PROCEDURE	RISKS
Cardioversion	Rarely resets CIED Risk may be minimized by placing chest wall electrodes in anterior-posterior orientation with anterior pad at least 8 cm away from the CIED pulse generator CIED to be interrogated prior to discharge from PACU/unit
Intracardiac RF ablation	Same interactions as monopolar electrocautery Risk more significant risk due to the prolonged exposure to current CIED to be interrogated prior to discharge from monitored unit
Diagnostic radiation	Low risk for CIED interaction, partial CIED reset reported No preprocedure or intraprocedure precautions or interventions are recommended for CIED patients CT scanners using high radiation doses have been reported to cause CIED oversensing when the beam is directed over the generator for a prolonged exposure If syncope or near syncope during high-intensity CT scanning, the procedure should be aborted and the CIED interrogated If patients experience palpitations or chest discomfort during such imaging, the patient and the CIED should be evaluated following the procedure.
Therapeutic radiation	Most likely source of EMI to result in CIED reset to safety mode Electrical reset risk increases with the strength of the ionizing radiation employed due to the effects of scattered neutrons or protons Conventional x-ray shielding does not protect the CIED pulse generator from the effects of neutrons. Direct radiation of the CIED generator poses high risk of causing structural damage and must be avoided; generators may need to be moved out of the radiation field to prevent their becoming damage Electron beam therapy has not been reported to cause electrical reset of modern CIEDs It is recommended that a patient's CIED be interrogated before and after the first radiation therapy treatment to ensure that no interference has affected CIED function and again at the conclusion of the course of radiotherapy If radiation to the chest or high-energy photon radiation, interrogation should be performed within 24 hours of treatment
Electroconvulsive therapy (ECT)	Rarely reported to cause EMI during the electrical stimulus (brief "nonsustained VT" may be falsely detected) and 1–5 seconds of pacing inhibition is not likely to cause hemodynamic compromise. In pacer-dependent patient, prolonged seizure activity may lead to oversensing and pacer inhibition. Therefore pacer-dependent patients need to have their device reprogrammed to an asynchronous mode Patients with AICDs need to have their anti-tachycardia function disabled since seizure activity may trigger a shock due to false detection or marked sinus tachycardia approaching the VT trigger zone.
Transurethral resection of the prostate (TURP)	TURP may affect CIED function if RF energy and/or electrocautery are used EMI can be minimized by placing the cautery grounding pad on the patient's buttock or thigh and by limiting the duration of energy bursts to only a few seconds each A magnet may be placed over the CIED generator if long energy bursts become necessary
Lithotripsy	Small risk for CIED interaction Preoperative device reprogramming is not necessary Magnet should be placed over the CIED if pacing inhibition is noted and lithotripsy terminated if arrhythmias occur Rate modulation should be disabled
Endoscopy Colonoscopy	Procedures that use electrocautery (e.g., cautery of bleeding lesions, polyp resection) may cause EMI
Endoscopic retrograde cholangiopancreatography (ECRP)	ICD should be deactivated Pacer-dependent patients should have pacer reprogrammed to VOO or DOO mode
Esophagogastroduodenoscopy or capsule endoscopy	No reprogramming of CIED is necessary
Transcutaneous electrical nerve stimulator (TENS)	Can result in EMI that can affect CIEDs, thus TENS units should generally be avoided in pacer-dependent patients and those with ICDs
MRI	MRI is contraindicated in patients with CIEDs MRI can be performed in patients with MRI-ompatible CIEDs and leads, if the system has been in place for more than 6 weeks and reprogrammed (if necessary) outside of the MRI safety zone MRI-compatible pacemakers need to be reprogrammed to an asynchronous mode

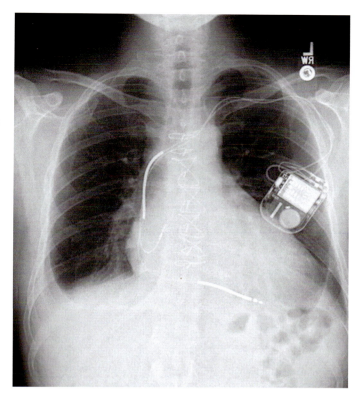

Figure 42.1 Typical appearance of an implantable cardioverter defibrillator (ICD).
Reproduced with permission from Stone ME. *Br J Anaesth*. 2011 Dec;107(Suppl 1): i16–26.

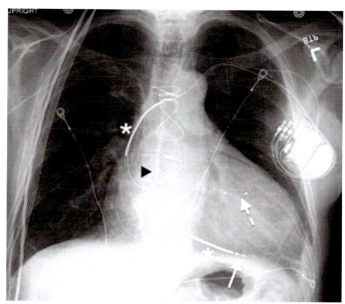

Figure 42.3 Upright frontal chest radiograph demonstrating a cardiac resynchronization therapy device: a cardiovascular implantable electronic device with supraventricular/ventricular shock coils (asterisks) and a bipolar pacing lead in the right ventricle (solid arrow), an atrial lead in the right atrium (black arrowhead), and a coronary sinus lead (dashed arrow) for biventricular pacing.
Reproduced with permission from Cronin B. *J Cardiothorac Vasc Anesth*. 2018 Aug;32(4):1871–1884.

PERIOPERATIVE ALGORITHM FOR MANAGEMENT OF CIED

Perioperative planning needs to take into account the type of device, whether EMI is likely (generally for procedures where monopolar cautery is used within 15 cm/6 in of the generator and leads of the device), and the device's response to magnet placement.

Generally speaking, procedures below the umbilicus are unlikely to affect CIED function (as long as the electrocautery pad is placed on a leg). The risk for pacing inhibition or false tachyarrhythmia detection is considered to be so low for surgical procedures performed on the lower extremities that neither reprogramming nor magnet application is considered mandatory regardless of the type of CIED (pacemaker or ICD) and regardless of pacemaker dependency (although a magnet should be available).

The use of monopolar electrocautery above the umbilicus poses greater risk of EMI and CIED interaction. In patients where EMI is anticipated and monopolar cautery is used above the umbilicus, PPMs should be reprogrammed to asynchronous pacing. A magnet can be used unless the magnet rate is undesirable (due to the patient's underlying heart pathology), the sterility of the surgical field is jeopardized, or the position of the patient during the procedure precludes it. In these latter conditions, a programmer should be used to prevent oversensing (Figure 42.4).

For patients with PPMs, it is important to disable the rate responsiveness feature either with a magnet or a programmer. Programming a PPM with a programming machine

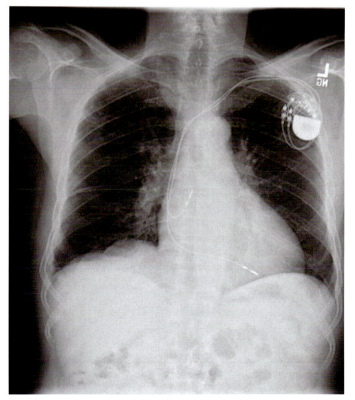

Figure 42.2 Typical appearance of a pacemaker.
Reproduced with permission from Stone ME. *Br J Anaesth*. 2011 Dec;107(Suppl 1): i16–26.

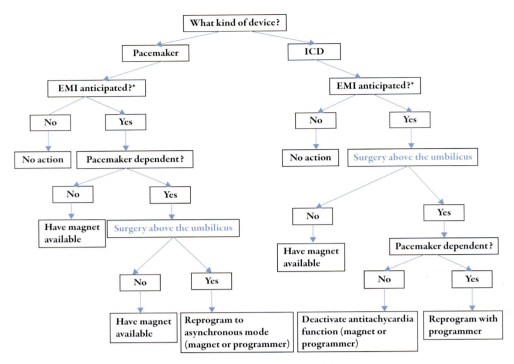

*Electrocautery used less than 15 cm (6 in) away from the generator and leads of the CIED
**For genetors placed other than in the subclavian area, please observe than 15 cm (6 in) rule for EMI

Figure 42.4 Algorithm for perioperative management of cardiac implantable electronic devices (CIEDs).

allows options that are not available with magnet application; such alternative options are important for patients who would have suboptimal cardiac function in a magnet-driven asynchronous pacing mode (i.e., if the patient's intrinsic rate increases during surgery due to pain or fever; this accelerated intrinsic rate might compete with the asynchronous pacing rate).

For those patients with ICDs undergoing surgery above the umbilicus, it is necessary to disable ICD anti-tachycardia therapy when EMI is anticipated (Figure 42.4). A magnet can be used to disable the anti-tachycardia therapy if the patient has a nondependent ICD and the positioning allows it.

For patients with dependent ICDs or if positioning precludes use of a magnet, a programmer machine should be used instead. For dependent ICDs, programming the ICD to an asynchronous pacing mode can only be accomplished with a programming machine (the pacing mode of an ICD is not affected by magnet placement). Furthermore, disabling rate-responsive pacing in an ICD can only be accomplished with a programming machine (Figure 42.4).

When a magnet or programmer is used to disable the anti-tachycardia function of the ICD, transcutaneous pacing/defibrillator pads must be placed on the patient.

One of the disadvantages of using a programming machine is the need for trained personnel, which may cause delays in the perioperative period. Nevertheless, all major CIED manufacturers have 24-hour technical support numbers for providers practicing in clinical settings without dedicated CIED teams.

INTRAOPERATIVE MANAGEMENT

For intraoperative monitoring continuous ECG is mandated. The majority of ECG monitors require configuration of high-frequency filtering to reveal pacing pulses. In addition, continuous display of pulse oximetry plethysmography and/or an invasive intra-arterial pressure waveform monitoring is also necessary throughout the perioperative period to detect mechanical systole and the presence of an adequate arterial pulse.[34]

The presence of a CIED implies being prepared for the possibility of urgent cardioversion, defibrillation, or transcutaneous pacing. Special precautions must be taken when the use of monopolar cautery (or other devices that generate EMI) is planned.[34] Transcutaneous pacing/defibrillator pads are placed on the patient to allow treatment of malignant arrhythmias. An external defibrillator with pacing capability should be immediately available.[34]

Ideal positioning of transcutaneous pacing/defibrillator pads minimizes damage to the ICD in case external defibrillation is required. The pads should never be placed directly over any CIED. For most individuals with a left-sided CIED, standard anteroposterior pad position is preferred.

Anesthetic agents do not per se affect CIED function. For patients whose CIED was placed secondary to long QT syndrome, agents that prolong the QT interval should be avoided (e.g., haloperidol, methadone, inhaled agents) due to the theoretical increased risk of polymorphic ventricular tachycardia.[35]

Several intraoperative complications should be anticipated when EMI is possible during a procedure for a patient with a CIED. If pulseless electrical activity (PEA) or hemodynamic instability occurs, it should be assumed it is due to EMI from monopolar cautery and its use should cease immediately. When the hemodynamic instability resolves, the procedure can continue using short bursts or with a magnet over a pacemaker to protect against EMI.

Should a tachyarrhythmia occur during EMI use in a patient with an ICD disabled by magnet application, the magnet should be removed to allow the CIED to defibrillate. If there is any delay in defibrillation, Zoll pads should be used for defibrillation.

To decrease the risk of EMI, the return pads must be placed such that the CIED generator and leads will not lie between the operative site and the pad to keep the current path away from the device. Moreover, the duration of monopolar electrocautery bursts should be minimized to 5 seconds or less, or, whenever possible, bipolar electrocautery should be used.[34,36,37]

POSTOPERATIVE MANAGEMENT

When the CIED settings have been altered preoperatively, the patient should remain continuously monitored in a high-acuity setting (PACU or ICU) with both ECG and pulse oximetry. The transcutaneous pacing/defibrillator pads should be left in place until the original CIED settings are restored. Also, an external defibrillator with pacing capability should remain immediately available. Postoperatively, CIEDs that were reprogrammed before surgery require reactivation of the original settings, either by removing the magnet (preoperative settings are restored) or by using a programmer (if one was used preoperatively).[34]

Postoperative interrogation of the CIED is recommended if the patient underwent emergency surgery without appropriate preoperative CIED evaluation or if there is suspicion that anti-tachyarrhythmia therapy might have been permanently disabled rather than temporarily suspended.[34]

Other approaches include recommendations from the HRS, which suggest that immediate postoperative interrogation is needed only for hemodynamically unstable patients, when a CIED is exposed to significant EMI, or after an intraoperative event (PEA, loss of capture).[7]

NEWER CIEDS AND PERIOPERATIVE MANAGEMENT

Subcutaneous ICDs have been introduced in an effort to decrease the risk of bacteremia, venous access issues, or transvenous lead fractures (Figure 42.5). While not having an anti-tachycardia pacing capability, subcutaneous ICDs can provide brief (30 seconds) anti-bradycardia therapy but only after a shock has been delivered. The response to the magnet is similar to the traditional ICDs, causing suspension of defibrillation therapy. While formal recommendations for perioperative management of subcutaneous ICDs do not exist, a magnet can be used if EMI is anticipated.[38,39]

Leadless pacemakers were also introduced to mitigate risks associated with lead placement (i.e., IV access, lead fracture, thrombosis). The Micra AV and Micra VR by Medtronic, indicated for bradycardia, provide single ventricle pacing (placed in the right ventricle) and are usually programmed in a

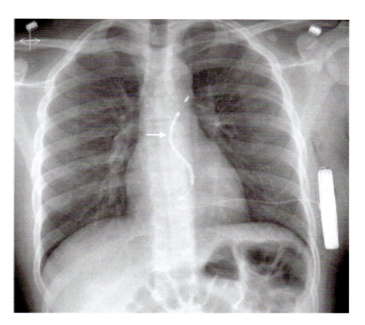

Figure 42.5 Anteroposterior chest radiograph demonstrating a subcutaneous implantable cardioverter defibrillator system in situ with the single subcutaneous electrode delineated (arrow).
Reproduced with permission from Cronin B. *J Cardiothorac Vasc Anesth*. 2018 Aug;32(4):1871–1884.

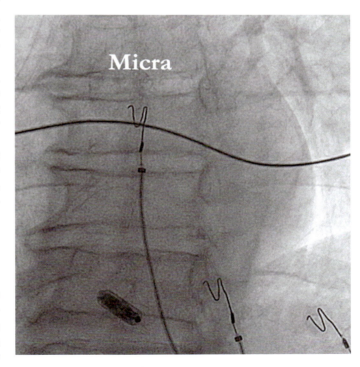

Figure 42.6 The Micra pacemaker.
Reproduced with permission from El-Chami MF. *Am J Cardiol*. 2017 Jan 1;119(1):145–148.

VVI, VVIR, VOO, OVO, VDD, VDI, ODO, or OFF pacing mode (Micra AV) and VVI, VVIR, VOO, OVO, OFF (Micra VR)[40] (Figure 42.6). The second-generation Micra AV2 has AV synchrony capability through an advanced algorithm. The drawback of the Micras is that they do not have a magnet mode, so whenever EMI is anticipated a programmer must be used.[41] Aveir is an Abbott-manufactured leadless pacemaker that can be set to VVI, VOO, OVO, and Pacing "Off" modes. If the magnet response is set to "On" and a magnet is detected by the device, the Aveir paces asynchronously (VOO mode) at 100 bpm for 5 cycles and then at a rate as a function of the battery voltage, ranging from 100 bpm at full voltage to 85 bpm at or near the recommended replacement time voltage until the magnet is no longer detected, when it will return to previously programmed parameters.[42] While the manufactures do not have recommendations for perioperative management, if one magnet does not elicit a magnet response, a second magnet may be placed on top of the first to increase the magnetic field strength, and/or different magnet may be applied.[42]

Other new devices include the Boston Scientific EMPOWER leadless pacemaker that, in conjunction with the SC-ICD can provide both anti-brady and anti-tachy therapy. Similarly, a wireless CRT device (WiSE CRT) is an endocardially placed electrode in the LV that can synchronously pace the LV in response to a signal from a traditionally placed right ventricle pacemaker.[43]

SPECIAL CONSIDERATIONS FOR CIEDS IN NON-OPERATING ROOM ENVIRONMENTS

For patients with CIEDs, several procedures performed in non-OR environment pose a risk of EMI. Gastrointestinal procedures (esophagogastroduodenoscopy, colonoscopy) usually don't involve EMI, however when cautery is used for polyp removals or during endoscopic retrograde cholangiopancreatographies (ERCPs), reprogramming of the CIED should occur in accordance with the algorithm presented earlier.

Cryotherapy ablation procedures are not associated with EMI, however radiofrequency ablation is. Recommendations for periprocedural CIED management based on the 2011 HRS guidelines are presented in Table 42.3.[7]

Table 42.3 **RECOMMENDATIONS FOR CIED MANAGEMENT FOR MRI SCAN**

MRI-CONDITIONAL DEVICE	MRI NONCONDITIONAL DEVICE
Personnel skilled in CPR, arrhythmia recognition, defibrillation, and transcutaneous pacing should be present for the procedure	A patient with an MR nonconditional CIED system can undergo MR imaging if: – there are no fractured, epicardial, or abandoned leads; – the MRI is the best test for the condition – there is an institutional protocol and a designated responsible MR physician and CIED physician
Monitoring recommended includes ECG and pulse oximetry to be continued until appropriate CIED settings are restored	An MR scan could be done immediately after implantation of a lead or generator of an MR nonconditional CIED system if clinically warranted
Personnel skilled in programming the CIED should be available	Device evaluation be performed immediately pre- and post-MRI with documentation of pacing threshold(s), P- and R-wave amplitude, and lead impedance
	A defibrillator/monitor (with external pacing function) and a manufacturer-specific device programming system should be immediately available in the holding area adjacent to the MR scanner room while an MR nonconditional CIED is reprogrammed for imaging
	Monitoring recommended includes ECG and pulse oximetry to be continued until appropriate CIED settings are restored
on	Personnel skilled in CPR, arrhythmia recognition, defibrillation, and transcutaneous pacing should be present for the procedure
	For patients with an *MR nonconditional CIED who are pacing-dependent (PM or ICD)*, it is recommended that – Personnel with the skill to program the CIED be in attendance during MR scanning – A physician with the ability to establish temporary transvenous pacing be immediately available on the premises of the imaging facility – A physician with the ability to direct CIED programming be immediately available on the premises of the imaging facility
	For patients with an MR-nonconditional CIED *who are not pacing-dependent*, it is recommended that – Personnel with the skill to program the CIED be available on the premises of the imaging facility – A physician with the ability to direct CIED programming be available on the premises of the imaging facility
	Pacing-dependent CIEDs should be programmed to an asynchronous pacing mode with deactivation of advanced or adaptive features during the MRI examination, and the pacing rate should be selected to avoid competitive pacing
	All tachyarrhythmia detections for patients with an ICD should be disabled prior to MRI
	Any resuscitative efforts and emergency treatments that involve the use of a defibrillator/monitor, device programming system, or any other MRI-unsafe equipment should be performed after moving the patient outside of Zone 4
	An MR nonconditional CIED for a nonpacing-dependent patient should be programmed to either a nonpacing mode (OVO/ODO) or to an inhibited mode (DDI/VVI), with deactivation of advanced or adaptive features during the MRI examination

CIED placement has traditionally been a contraindication to MRI. However, more recently, "MRI conditional devices" have been developed; these are implanted cardiac devices that the US Food and Drug Administration has identified as having no known hazards under specific device and MRI scanner conditions. Moreover, several studies assessed the safety of non-MRI conditional devices when certain precautions are taken.[44–46] For nonconditional MRI CIEDs, it is reasonable to perform a MRI scan if medically indicated provided that there are no fractured, abandoned, or epicardial leads. Recommendation for periprocedural management of CIEDs undergoing MRI, based on the 2017 HRS guidelines, are presented in Table 42.3.[47]

CONCLUSION

- The prevalence of patients with CIEDs is steadily on the rise.

- Knowledge of the various sources of EMI in the perioperative period is critical.

- Application of a magnet over the CIED is a feasible option. If the CIED is a pacemaker, the application of a magnet will switch to an asynchronous mode. If the patient has an ICD, the anti-tachycardia function will be disabled.

- A magnet does not affect the pacemaker function of ICDs.

- Patients with a dependent ICD undergoing surgery above the umbilicus with monopolar electrocautery must have their ICD therapy inactivated and the pacemaker mode switched to asynchronous by reprogramming the device.

- If the surgery is below the umbilicus, ICD inactivation of the anti-tachycardia function can be accomplished by applying a magnet over the cardiac device.

- If a magnet is utilized, no postoperative interrogation is needed as magnet removal results in restoration of prior settings.

- The anesthesiologist must be aware of the specific characteristics of performing these ablation procedures in a non-OR anesthesia (NORA) setting and be able to formulate a safe anesthetic plan.

- Cooperation and clear communication between the anesthesiologist and the interventional radiologist is critical for a safe and successful NORA procedure.

REVIEW QUESTIONS

1. A pacemaker with backup rate of 85 bpm is noted on the preoperative 12-lead ECG to be pacing at 59 bpm. The most likely explanation for this decrease in the pacing heart rate is

   a. Battery failure.
   b. Decreased atrial rate.
   c. Complete heart block.
   d. Bifascicular heart block.

The correct answer is a.
The anesthetic management of patient with pacemakers should include ECG monitoring. A decrease in the programmed rate of the pacemaker greater than 10% is a sign of battery failure.

2. An 82-year-old woman with syncopal episodes is found to have sick sinus syndrome and a pacemaker is implanted. Two months later she is presenting for cataract extraction. The most appropriate management of her pacemaker is

   a. Apply a magnet over the device.
   b. No action is needed.
   c. Reprogram the pacemaker to an asynchronous mode.
   d. Cancel her surgery due to the recent pacemaker implantation.

The correct answer is b.
The presence of a pacemaker does not necessarily imply the need for a magnet, since there is no EMI associated with cataract surgery. Even though the patient is most likely pacemaker-dependent, no action is needed because cataract surgery is performed without electrocautery (no EMI). Canceling this elective cataract surgery is not clinically warranted.

3. A 52-year-old man with history of alcoholic dilated cardiomyopathy had an ICD placed for primary prevention secondary to his low EF. He is now presenting for emergent exploratory laparotomy for perforated appendicitis. The most appropriate management of the ICD is

   a. Order a stress test.
   b. No action for the ICD is needed.
   c. Apply a magnet over the device.
   d. Avoid external defibrillator pads.

The correct answer is c.
This patient seems to have a non-dependent ICD (placed for primary prevention for low EF). This is an emergent surgery, and no stress test should be ordered at this point. If nothing is done regarding the ICD, there is possible EMI for the electrocautery that might interfere with the device's proper function and shock the patient inappropriately. Applying a magnet is a reasonable option, and this will disable the anti-tachycardia therapy. When a magnet is applied over the device, external defibrillator pads should be placed in case immediate defibrillation is necessary.

4. A 32-year-old woman with history of iatrogenic complete heart block suffers a viral cardiomyopathy and decision is made to implant an ICD. She is now presenting for breast lumpectomy. What is indicated regarding her ICD?

   a. Only apply a magnet over the device.
   b. Reprogram the device.
   c. No action is needed.
   d. Insert a transvenous pacemaker as a backup plan for pacing.

The correct answer is b.
This patient has a dependent ICD, and EMI due to monopolar cautery is likely during this procedure due to proximity

to the generator and leads of the device. All anti-tachycardia therapy should be disabled using a magnet or a programmer to avoid unnecessary shocks due to oversensing. However, applying a magnet over the device will not affect the pacemaker mode of the ICD. Therefore, during magnet placement, EMI may lead to severe bradycardia due to loss of pacing. Moreover, due to proximity to the surgical field, a magnet may not be appropriate even for patients with nondependent ICDs. This pacer- dependent ICD will need to be reprogrammed with a programmer. Inserting a transvenous pacemaker is an invasive technique unnecessary in this setting.

5. Sources of electromagnetic interference (EMI) can be

    a. Ultrasound waves.
    b. Ionizing radiation from CT scanning.
    c. Cryoablation.
    d. Electrocautery.

The correct answer is d.

6. A patient is scheduled to undergo elective inguinal hernia repair. He had a pacemaker placed 7 years ago for sick sinus syndrome. The most appropriate action in preparation would be to have a device interrogation available

    a. Within the past 2 years.
    b. Within the past year.
    c. Within the past 5 years.
    d. No recent interrogation is needed.

The correct answer is b.

The HRS recommends that any patient presenting for elective surgery who has a pacemaker should have an interrogation within the past 12 months, and ICDs should be evaluated every 6 months.

7. A 77-year-old patient with a DDD-R pacemaker for history of complete heart block is scheduled for a Whipple procedure. The pacemaker has been reprogrammed to the asynchronous (DOO) mode at a rate of 70 bpm for the surgery. After anesthesia induction, the patient's heart rate increases to 88 bpm with unchanged blood pressure (117/62). Which of the following actions would be most appropriate?

    a. Place a magnet over the pacemaker generator.
    b. Administer lidocaine.
    c. Administer esmolol.
    d. No action is needed.

The correct answer is c.

Pacemakers should be temporarily reprogrammed into asynchronous mode for surgery with EMI above the umbilicus, like this abdominal surgery. With the VOO and DOO modes, the possibility of an R on T phenomenon exists if the native heart rate exceeds the programmed rate or when there are frequent premature atrial (PAC) or ventricular (PVC) contractions. In the presence of PACs or PVCs, repolarization may occur at the same time the pacemaker is discharging (R wave). Placing a magnet would not affect pacer function after it has been reprogrammed. Administering IV lidocaine or changing the volatile agent will not be useful in this scenario.

Administration of esmolol will slow down the heart rate so the pacemaker will be able to "generate" the heart rate.

8. An 87-year-old patient with a subclavian-placed ICD is to undergo upper abdominal surgery that requires electrocautery. Which of the following statements is true?

    a. The electrocautery pad should be placed as close to the pulse generator as possible.
    b. ECG continuous monitoring is not necessary.
    c. Placing a magnet over the ICD will deactivate the pacing function of the ICD.
    d. Placing defibrillation pads prophylactically is required.

The correct answer is d.

The application of a magnet over a pacemaker will cause asynchronous pacing. However, magnets do not affect the pacing rate of ICDs. The electrocautery pad should be placed away from the ICD. Any time the anti-tachycardia function of an ICD is disabled, defibrillation pads should be placed prophylactically for immediate shocking capability.

REFERENCES

1. Shuch B, Amin A, Armstrong AJ, et al. Understanding pathologic variants of renal cell carcinoma: Distilling therapeutic opportunities from biologic complexity. *Eur Urol*. 2015 Jan;67(1):85–97.
2. Cleland JG, Daubert JC, Erdmann E, et al. The effect of cardiac resynchronization on morbidity and mortality in heart failure. *N Engl J Med*. 2005 Apr;352(15):1539–1549.
3. Pokorney SD, Miller AL, Chen AY, et al. Reassessment of cardiac function and implantable cardioverter-defibrillator use among Medicare patients with low ejection fraction after myocardial infarction. *Circulation*. 2017 Jan;135(1):38–47.
4. Pokorney SD, Miller AL, Chen AY, et al. Implantable cardioverter-defibrillator use among Medicare patients with low ejection fraction after acute myocardial infarction. *JAMA*. 2015 Jun 23–30;313(24):2433–2440.
5. Rozner MA, Schulman PM. Creating an anesthesiologist-run pacemaker and defibrillator service: Closing the perioperative care gap for these patients. *Anesthesiology*. 2015 Nov;123(5):990–992.
6. Allen M. Pacemakers and implantable cardioverter defibrillators. *Anaesthesia*. 2006 Sep;61(9):883–890.
7. Crossley GH, Poole JE, Rozner MA, et al. The Heart Rhythm Society (HRS)/American Society of Anesthesiologists (ASA) expert consensus statement on the perioperative management of patients with implantable defibrillators, pacemakers and arrhythmia monitors: Facilities and patient management this document was developed as a joint project with the American Society of Anesthesiologists (ASA), and in collaboration with the American Heart Association (AHA), and the Society of Thoracic Surgeons (STS). *Heart Rhythm*. 2011 Jul;8(7):1114–1154.
8. Epstein AE, DiMarco JP, Ellenbogen KA, et al. 2012 ACCF/AHA/HRS focused update incorporated into the ACCF/AHA/HRS 2008 guidelines for device-based therapy of cardiac rhythm abnormalities: A report of the American College of Cardiology Foundation/American Heart Association Task Force on practice guidelines and the Heart Rhythm Society. *J Am Coll Cardiol*. 2013 Jan;61(3):e6–e75.
9. Brignole M, Auricchio A, Baron-Esquivias G, et al. 2013 ESC guidelines on cardiac pacing and cardiac resynchronization therapy: The Task Force on cardiac pacing and resynchronization therapy of the European Society of Cardiology (ESC). Developed in collaboration with the European Heart Rhythm Association (EHRA). *Eur Heart J*. 2013 Aug;34(29):2281–2329.

10. Russo AM, Stainback RF, Bailey SR, et al. ACCF/HRS/AHA/ASE/HFSA/SCAI/SCCT/SCMR 2013 appropriate use criteria for implantable cardioverter-defibrillators and cardiac resynchronization therapy: A report of the American College of Cardiology Foundation appropriate use criteria task force, Heart Rhythm Society, American Heart Association, American Society of Echocardiography, Heart Failure Society of America, Society for Cardiovascular Angiography and Interventions, Society of Cardiovascular Computed Tomography, and Society for Cardiovascular Magnetic Resonance. *J Am Coll Cardiol*. 2013 Mar;61(12):1318–1368.

11. Moss AJ, Zareba W, Hall WJ, et al. Prophylactic implantation of a defibrillator in patients with myocardial infarction and reduced ejection fraction. *N Engl J Med*. 2002 Mar;346(12):877–883.

12. Goldberger Z, Lampert R. Implantable cardioverter-defibrillators: Expanding indications and technologies. *JAMA*. 2006 Feb;295(7):809–818.

13. Kadish A, Dyer A, Daubert JP, et al. Prophylactic defibrillator implantation in patients with nonischemic dilated cardiomyopathy. *N Engl J Med*. 2004 May;350(21):2151–2158.

14. Ponikowski P, Voors AA, Anker SD, et al. 2016 ESC guidelines for the diagnosis and treatment of acute and chronic heart failure: The task force for the diagnosis and treatment of acute and chronic heart failure of the European Society of Cardiology (ESC), developed with the special contribution of the Heart Failure Association (HFA) of the ESC. *Eur Heart J*. 2016 Jul;37(27):2129–2200.

15. Korantzopoulos P, Letsas KP, Grekas G, Goudevenos JA. Pacemaker dependency after implantation of electrophysiological devices. *Europace*. 2009 Sep;11(9):1151–1155.

16. Salukhe TV, Dob D, Sutton R. Pacemakers and defibrillators: Anaesthetic implications. *Br J Anaesth*. 2004 Jul;93(1):95–104.

17. Healey JS, Merchant R, Simpson C, et al. Society position statement: Canadian Cardiovascular Society/Canadian Anesthesiologists' Society/Canadian Heart Rhythm Society joint position statement on the perioperative management of patients with implanted pacemakers, defibrillators, and neurostimulating devices. *Can J Anaesth*. 2012 Apr;59(4):394–407.

18. Schulman PM, Rozner MA. Case report: Use caution when applying magnets to pacemakers or defibrillators for surgery. *Anesth Analg*. 2013 Aug;117(2):422–427.

19. Rooke GA, Bowdle TA. Perioperative management of pacemakers and implantable cardioverter defibrillators: It's not just about the magnet. *Anesth Analg*. 2013 Aug;117(2):292–294.

20. Stone ME, Salter B, Fischer A. Perioperative management of patients with cardiac implantable electronic devices. *Br J Anaesth*. 2011 Dec;107(Suppl 1):i16–i26.

21. Crea P, Nicotera A. Magnet response in biotronik pacemakers: Keep attention to default mode "Auto". *Pacing Clin Electrophysiol*. 2020 Jul;43(7):770.

22. Jacob S, Panaich SS, Maheshwari R, Haddad JW, Padanilam BJ, John SK. Clinical applications of magnets on cardiac rhythm management devices. *Europace*. 2011 Sep;13(9):1222–1230.

23. Mangar D, Atlas GM, Kane PB. Electrocautery-induced pacemaker malfunction during surgery. *Can J Anaesth*. 1991 Jul;38(5):616–618.

24. Godin JF, Petitot JC. STIMAREC report. Pacemaker failures due to electrocautery and external electric shock. *Pacing Clin Electrophysiol*. 1989 Jun;12(6):1011.

25. Belott PH, Sands S, Warren J. Resetting of DDD pacemakers due to EMI. *Pacing Clin Electrophysiol*. 1984 Mar;7(2):169–172.

26. McKay RE, Rozner MA. Preventing pacemaker problems with nerve stimulators. *Anaesthesia*. 2008 May;63(5):554–556; author reply 6–7.

27. Carlson T, Andréll P, Ekre O, et al. Interference of transcutaneous electrical nerve stimulation with permanent ventricular stimulation: A new clinical problem? *Europace*. 2009 Mar;11(3):364–369.

28. Seidman SJ, Brockman R, Lewis BM, et al. In vitro tests reveal sample radiofrequency identification readers inducing clinically significant electromagnetic interference to implantable pacemakers and implantable cardioverter-defibrillators. *Heart Rhythm*. 2010 Jan;7(1):99–107.

29. Plakke MJ, Maisonave Y, Daley SM. Radiofrequency scanning for retained surgical items can cause electromagnetic interference and pacing inhibition if an asynchronous pacing mode is not applied. *A A Case Rep*. 2016 Mar;6(6):143–145.

30. Molon G, Perrone C, Maines M, et al. ICD and neuromodulation devices: Is peaceful coexistence possible? *Pacing Clin Electrophysiol*. 2011 Jun;34(6):690–693.

31. Fiek M, Dorwarth U, Durchlaub I, et al. Application of radiofrequency energy in surgical and interventional procedures: Are there interactions with ICDs? *Pacing Clin Electrophysiol*. 2004 Mar;27(3):293–298.

32. Katzenberg CA, Marcus FI, Heusinkveld RS, Mammana RB. Pacemaker failure due to radiation therapy. *Pacing Clin Electrophysiol*. 1982 Mar;5(2):156–159.

33. Boyle B, Love CJ, Marine JE, et al. Radiographic identification of cardiac implantable electronic device manufacturer: Smartphone pacemaker-ID application versus X-ray logo. *J Innov Card Rhythm Manag*. 2022 Aug;13(8):5104–5110.

34. Practice Advisory for the Perioperative Management of Patients with Cardiac Implantable Electronic Devices. Pacemakers and implantable cardioverter—Defibrillators 2020: An updated report by the American Society of Anesthesiologists Task Force on perioperative management of patients with cardiac implantable electronic devices. *Anesthesiology*. 2020;132:225–252.

35. Yildirim H, Adanir T, Atay A, Katircioğlu K, Savaci S. The effects of sevoflurane, isoflurane, and desflurane on QT interval of the ECG. *Eur J Anaesthesiol*. 2004 Jul;21(7):566–570.

36. Rozner MA, Kahl EA, Schulman PM. Inappropriate implantable cardioverter-defibrillator therapy during surgery: An important and preventable complication. *J Cardiothorac Vasc Anesth*. 2017 Jun;31(3):1037–1041.

37. Ellis MKM, Treggiari MM, Robertson JM, et al. Process improvement initiative for the perioperative management of patients with a cardiovascular implantable electronic device. *Anesth Analg*. 2017 Jul;125(1):58–65.

38. Arora L, Inampudi C. Perioperative management of cardiac rhythm assist devices in ambulatory surgery and nonoperating room anesthesia. *Curr Opin Anaesthesiol*. 2017 Dec;30(6):676–681.

40. El-Chami MF, Merchant FM, Leon AR. Leadless pacemakers. *Am J Cardiol*. 2017 Jan;119(1):145–148.

41. Cronin B, Essandoh MK. Update on cardiovascular implantable electronic devices for anesthesiologists. *J Cardiothorac Vasc Anesth*. 2018 Aug;32(4):1871–1884.

42. Tang JE, Savona SJ, Essandoh MK. Aveir leadless pacemaker: Novel technology with new anesthetic implications. *J Cardiothorac Vasc Anesth*. 2022 Dec;36(12):4501–4504.

43. Kothari P, Poorsattar SP, Graul T, et al. The year in electrophysiology: Selected highlights from 2020. *J Cardiothorac Vasc Anesth*. 2021 Jul;35(7):1942–1952.

44. Nazarian S, Hansford R, Rahsepar AA, et al. Safety of magnetic resonance imaging in patients with cardiac devices. *N Engl J Med*. 2017 Dec;377(26):2555–2564.

45. Dandamudi S, Collins JD, Carr JC, et al. The safety of cardiac and thoracic magnetic resonance imaging in patients with cardiac implantable electronic devices. *Acad Radiol*. 2016 Dec;23(12):1498–1505.

46. Lowe MD, Plummer CJ, Manisty CH, Linker NJ, Society BHR. Safe use of MRI in people with cardiac implantable electronic devices. *Heart*. 2015 Dec;101(24):1950–1953.

47. Indik JH, Gimbel JR, Abe H, et al. 2017 HRS expert consensus statement on magnetic resonance imaging and radiation exposure in patients with cardiovascular implantable electronic devices. *Heart Rhythm*. 2017 Jul;14(7):e97–e153.

43.

MY FRIEND'S SON REQUESTS SURGERY FOR GYNECOMASTIA CAUSED BY THE DRUGS HE USES FOR BODYBUILDING

Adam C. Adler and Arvind Chandrakantan

STEM CASE AND KEY QUESTIONS

A 16-year-old male football player presents to the preoperative clinic with gynecomastia secondary to self-administered anabolic steroid use.

Anabolic steroid use is a common problem among professional athletes and is increasingly used in middle and high school athletics. A recent survey demonstrated an incidence of 2.7% even in middle school athletes, showing that anabolic steroid use is pervasive even at lower levels of athletics.[1,2]

The major issue is not merely the risks from steroid use, but also from concomitant agent use as well as high-risk behaviors with substances such as alcohol, tobacco, or other performance-enhancing drugs.[3]

In this case, the index patient has gynecomastia from using exogenous testosterone. Generally, testosterone is taken in the form of injectable steroids for greater potency and to avoid bioavailability issues with oral formulations. While the ideal solution is to stop abusing anabolic steroids, recidivism is common, often due to peer pressure.[4] To the contrary, when stopping exogenous hormones, issues arise due to lack of native hormone production. Since anabolic steroid use is so common in the sports world, a lot of online resources and forums have been dedicated to avoiding routine drug testing that detects the common steroid analogues in urine. This includes cycling around known test times, urine substitutions, having fake urine samples available, and having a clean friend provide a sample.[5] While this avoids a potential ban, it is ultimately the athlete who suffers from the sequelae of use, such as the patient we detail here.

What are the common patterns of anabolic steroid use?

The patterns of steroid use include, but are not limited to

1. *Cycling*: Taking multiple doses over a period of time (generally 1 week), stopping, then restarting
2. *Stacking*: Combining multiple steroids (injectable, oral).
3. *Pyramiding*: Gradually increasing the steroid dose until reaching a predetermined peak, and then tapering the dose to zero
4. *Plateauing*: Intermittent steroid substitution to avoid developing tolerance to a single steroid

What are the risks of anabolic steroid use?

Anabolic steroids affect all major organ systems, and the risks of use are not merely confined to risk of steroid use alone.

1. *Cardiovascular*: Hypertension, increased propensity for clot formation, premature atherosclerosis, myocardial infarction, cardiomyopathy
2. *Endocrine*: Gynecomastia, decreased testes size (men), facial hair growth (women), male pattern baldness, voice deepening (women), Cushing's disease (from adrenocortical suppression) and its antecedent complications
3. *Hematology*: Polycythemia
4. *Infections* (from needle hygiene): HIV/AIDS, hepatitis B and/or C, skin infections, endocarditis
5. *Hepatobiliary*: Peliosis hepatitis, hepatocellular carcinoma
6. *Musculoskeletal system*: Increased muscle growth, tendinopathies, short stature
7. *Neuropsychiatric*: Excessive rage ("roid rage"), delusional behavior
8. *Dermatology*: Acne/cyst formation, oily scalp and skin, infections at injection site.[6]

Are any concurrent drugs utilized with steroids to enhance muscle growth?

Since the objective of anabolic steroid use is to gain muscle, lose fat, and create the appearance of larger and well-defined muscles, it is unsurprising that other agents are used concurrently and often illegally. The classes of medications used in this capacity include

1. *Nonsteroid anabolics*: Include insulin and insulin-like growth factor
2. *Thermogenics*: Used to burn fat. This class of medications include caffeine (theophyllines), banned substances such as ephedra, and nontherapeutic uses of legal medications such as thyroid hormone.

3. *Diuretics*: To reduce total body water ahead of competition.

4. *Aromatase inhibitors*: To reduce estrogen-based side effects, which will be discussed in detail later

5. *Growth hormone (GH) mimetics*: Ghrelin mimetics are available online at several unregulated websites. GH and GH analogues account for the short stature side effects seen with bodybuilders. Short stature is a somewhat coveted proposition for professional bodybuilders as it is erroneously assumed to enhance muscle size. Several tall bodybuilders have done well in recent years however.[7]

Other modalities used for competition include creatine usage, which, when cycled, causes a mild but clinically insignificant increase in serum creatinine levels. High protein intake can also lead to increased serum blood urea nitrogen (BUN) level due to increased protein catabolism. NSAIDs use to facilitate muscle gains through pain blockade are also a concern, as is chronic acetaminophen usage. Inhaled albuterol use is also increasingly common, with the goal of increasing respiratory capacity to achieve a greater number of exercise repetitions, coupled with the capacity for a mild euphoria. Due to the concomitant erectile dysfunction (ED) from anabolic steroid use, many male bodybuilders also utilize sildenafil.

Concurrent use of other illicit substances, including cocaine, heroin, and opioids, may be seen.

To obtain competition weight, many bodybuilders also go through extreme fluid restriction and dieting in the days immediately preceding competition (losing "water weight") which can lead to life-threatening dehydration and rhabdomyolysis.

Therefore, a careful history is required to identify exactly which agents are being used in what context to develop an overall picture of drug use.

What is the focus of the preoperative assessment in patients who have a history of anabolic steroid use?

The preoperative assessment should start with a history and physical examination, as for any other surgery. The specific focus of the history would be on the nature of anabolic steroid use, including cycling, as well as concurrent drug utilization. The presence of parents, especially with an adolescent, may preclude a complete history of illicit drug use from being elicited. Any symptoms of end-organ damage should be solicited. These include but are not limited to

1. *Central nervous system*: Specific questioning about mood changes including wild swings and manic behavior

2. *Cardiovascular system*: Exertional dyspnea, shortness of breath, paroxysmal nocturnal dyspnea (PND), and orthopnea should be solicited. Testosterone therapy can also lead to left ventricular hypertrophy, as well as premature atherosclerosis of both coronary and noncoronary vessels. Sildenafil, which is used in the context of atherosclerotic disease, may precipitate myocardial ischemia, so asking about exertional chest pain is also important.

3. *Respiratory*: Deep vein thromboses with a higher probability of pulmonary embolism is possible, therefore questions about paroxysmal chest pain, dyspnea, and calf tenderness should be solicited. Many cases of pulmonary embolism, including fatal emboli, have been documented as a result of steroid use.[8]

4. *Renal*: Several renal consequences from acute kidney injury (AKI) to chronic renal failure (CRF)[9] have been described in anabolic steroid users. AKI can be a consequence of excessive dieting, fluid restriction, rhabdomyolysis, or diuretic use. Elective surgery should not be attempted if the patient has untreated AKI. CRF maybe a consequence of emboli (vascular), NSAID-induced nephropathy, or either directly or indirectly from other illicit drug use. Many illicit drugs have contaminants such as talc or other nephrotoxic adjuvants mixed in, which, when injected, can cause embolic kidney injury.

5. *Hepatic*: Acetaminophen is often used by professional bodybuilders and can lead to hepatic necrosis. Similarly, most concurrent agents used for bodybuilding utilize hepatic mechanisms for metabolism, leading to long-term hepatic injury and hepatic steatosis. Eliciting history involving jaundice and right upper quadrant tenderness (possibly cholelithiasis or painful stretching of Glisson's capsule) is important.

6. *Endocrine*: Manifestations of steroid use include premature male pattern baldness and decreased testes size in males.

Concomitant erectile dysfunction is also quite common, as noted earlier, leading to sildenafil use, often illicitly. Thyroid hormone or analogues of thyroid hormone are used to increase "thermogenesis" with the goal of burning fat and accentuating muscle tone and size. Both of these synthetic analogues suppress endogenous thyroid hormone and testosterone production and action.

7. *Infectious disease*: Blisters, boils, and localized abscesses from SQ injection are quite common and are often caused by local *Streptococcus* or *Staphylococcus* organisms. Since IV agents are often simultaneously utilized along with SQ injection, there is a strong possibility of needle-sharing along with those risks. These include hepatitis B or C and HIV among others.

The examination should focus on the following:

1. *Scalp*: Male pattern baldness as a sign of chronic use (see Figure 43.1)

2. *Sclera*: To look for jaundice

3. *Cardiac*: Auscultation, including an S3 gallop due to congestive heart failure (CHF)

4. *Abdomen*: Palpation of the RUQ to look for hepatomegaly

5. *Skin*: Examination of all injection sites (SQ and IV) to look for local inflammation or pustule formation

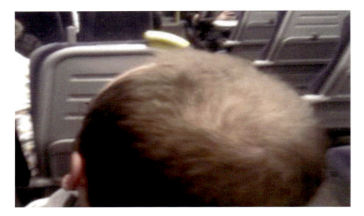

Figure 43.1 Premature male pattern baldness.

Labs to be obtained include

1. *CBC*, Chem-8 with renal function and glucose.

2. *Liver function tests* including ALT/AST and coagulation studies if hepatic disease is suspected.

3. *ECG/Echocardiogram*: To look for left ventricular hypertrophy (LVH), both drug-induced and resulting from chronically high afterload, and thrombi, as well as to assess for ischemia and function if there is evidence to suggest atherosclerotic disease or exertional dyspnea. We would suggest an initial ECG, and if there is evidence of ischemic changes and/or LVH, obtain an echocardiogram to further investigate.

4. Hepatitis B or C, HIV if concomitant IV drug use is suspected.

5. Other laboratory tests as appropriate based on history. Consider thyroid functions.

What causes gynecomastia in patients who use anabolic steroids?

Many anabolic steroids (both legal and illegal) have a high degree of aromaticity. In humans, the enzyme aromatase converts androstenedione into estrogen and estrone. The excess estrogen accounts for many of the "feminine" features seen in male bodybuilders: gynecomastia and a high-pitched voice. This conversion can be seen in Figure 43.2.

What is the treatment for gynecomastia?

First-line treatment is to cease exogeneous anabolic testosterone use. Despite this, the gynecomastia is often not reversible. Anastrozole and even tamoxifen may be utilized in this situation, although these therapies are often limited by side effects.

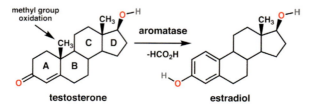

Figure 43.2 Conversion of testosterone to estradiol.

What is the surgery for gynecomastia?

Gynecomastia has two components—the tissue component and the glandular component. The tissue component often obscures the lateral aspect of the pectoralis major muscle, which is part of what drives body builders to seek surgical correction. The glandular component is cosmetically easier to excise, as the nipple often obscures the surgical incision.

In the picture to the left (figure 43.2), for example, the lateral border of the pectoralis muscle is obscured, along with glandular hypertrophy. In the picture to the right, both components have been corrected through a direct excision surgery protocol.

The surgical procedure itself is often a combination of liposuction to remove the excess fat combined with a peri-areolar incision to remove the glandular tissue to make the breasts appear symmetric and even.

What are the primary perioperative anesthetic concerns in this patient?

Hypovolemia due to dieting and fluid restriction ("cutting") remains a preoperative concern. Therefore, ensuring euvolemia prior to induction is important. The induction medications are routine. There is no contraindication to laryngeal mask airway (LMA) placement, however, given that the surgery is direct chest wall surgery, many anesthesiologists prefer to intubate with an endotracheal tube (ETT).

To ensure equality and cosmesis of both breasts, the surgeons will request steep head-up position (reverse Trendelenburg see Figure 43.3) of the bed during the procedure multiple times.

While the reverse Trendelenburg position is not maintained for long periods of time, the anesthesiologist should ensure that the patient is properly strapped down to avoid injury. Also, the ETT and circuit length should be carefully checked during positioning to avoid accidental extubation.

What are methods to prevent recurrence of gynecomastia?

As alluded to earlier, cessation of anabolic steroid use is the best method to prevent recurrence. As long as excess testosterone is present, especially in adolescence with increased aromatase presence and activity, there will be increased estrogen with all the pursuant side effects. However, many bodybuilders continue to use anabolic steroids after surgery, and therefore recurrence is common.

DISCUSSION

The most commonly used steroids are the injectable form including Deca-Durabolin (nandrolone decanoate), Durabolin (nandrolone phenpropionate), Depo-Testosterone (testosterone cypionate), and Equipoise (boldenone undecylenate; a veterinary product also known as "horse juice.")

A variety of online retailers in unregulated markets such as Mexico and Canada sell these products, as well as biopharmaceutical firms that add the specific label of "not for human use." With the ubiquity of the internet, most agents can be

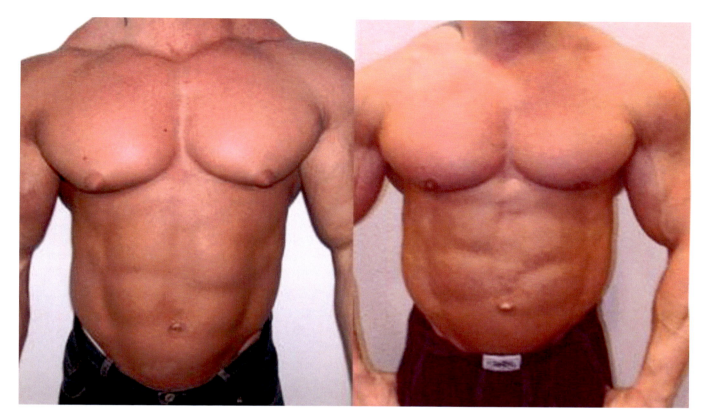

Figure 43.3 Surgery for gynecomastia.

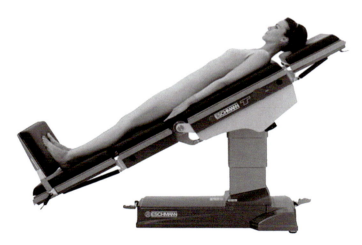

Figure 43.4 Reverse Trendelenburg position.

purchased by anyone with a cell phone and a credit card. The majority of young users (middle schoolers and adolescents) are introduced to these products by a teammate or someone in their peer group. Given the extraordinary psychological effects of the peer network, most preventative work has focused on education by figures of authority, including parents, counselors, and sports coaches.

Once injected, due to the high rate of bioavailability, most of the testosterone works on end-organ effect through multiple organ-specific mechanisms. In the musculoskeletal system, this increases muscle mass, shortens the duration for muscle recovery, and increases muscle action potential. The latter is the logic for the utilization of anabolic steroids by baseball players since hand–eye coordination is the overwhelming execution task for power hitters. Shortening the muscle action potential allows a quicker firing and allows smoother ball connection.

Exogeneous testosterone suppresses endogenous testosterone behavior and production. This leads to many of undesirable hormonal changes including decreased testis size and erectile dysfunction. In females, this contributes to facial hair growth, amenorrhea, and an androgynous body type due to suppression of endogenous estrogen.

As noted in earlier, utilization of concomitant illegal agents is a problem. Use of stimulants (e.g., amphetamines), opioids, and alcohol and tobacco is of much higher prevalence among anabolic steroid users. Other patterns of use are sport-specific. Cocaine use, both for an immediate high as well as a confidence enhancer, is common among baseball players. Marijuana dulls some of the pain effects so is much more common in contact sports (football, hockey). Tetrahydrocannabis (THC) has recently been approved for certain medical conditions in certain municipalities. However, its use in minors is highly regulated, and any positive marijuana testing in a young adult suggests illegal use.

Therefore, a patient similar to the one described in the stem case requires intensive drug testing and rehabilitation. While anabolic steroids are not psychologically addictive, many of the concomitant agents are, demanding a more holistic solution.

ANABOLIC STEROIDS • 479

CONCLUSION

- Anabolic steroid use represents the tip of the iceberg in the problematic world of adolescent competitive sports.
- A permissive (or many times drug abusive) peer culture facilitates individual coercion and use.
- Gynecomastia is very common in the male adolescent and generally resolves after puberty. However, continued or persistent signs of testosterone effect beyond the normal pubertal surge suggest exogenous use, requiring a comprehensive patient-centric approach in addition to any required surgery.

REVIEW QUESTIONS

1. Which enzyme converts testosterone into estrogen?

    a. Anhydrase.
    b. Aromatase.
    c. Alpha-hydroxylase.

The correct answer is b.
Aromatase is the enzyme which converts testosterone into estradiol.

2. An echocardiogram in a patient with chronic anabolic steroid use is most likely to demonstrate which of the following?

    a. Intracardiac thrombi.
    b. LVH.
    c. CHF.

The correct answer is b.
An echocardiogram is likely to demonstrate LVH.

3. Sharing needles among injectable steroid users puts them at risk for which of the following diseases?

    a. Hepatitis A.
    b. HIV.
    c. HLTV.

The correct answer is b.
HIV is common among needle sharers.

4. Female anabolic steroid users are likely to have which of the following side effects?

    a. High-pitched voice.
    b. Gynecomastia.
    c. Amenorrhea.

The correct answer is c.
Amenorrhea is common among female bodybuilders.

5. Which of the following bed positions is most likely to be used during gynecomastia surgery?

    a. Reverse Trendelenburg.
    b. Beach chair position.
    c. Left lateral decubitus.

The correct answer is a.
Reverse Trendelenburg is commonly used for gynecomastia correction.

6. Hypovolemia due to dietary restriction plus diuretic use will most likely contribute to which of the following on anesthetic induction?

    a. Resistant hypotension.
    b. Bradycardia.
    c. Acrocyanosis.

The correct answer is a.
Resistant hypotension is common due to fluid restriction and concomitant diuretic abuse.

7. Which of the following organisms leads to localized infections at injection sites in IV anabolic users?

    a. *Streptococcus*.
    b. *Acinetobacter*.
    c. *Pseudomonas*.

The correct answer is a.
Streptococcus is the most common skin infection in anabolic drug users.

REFERENCES

1. Nilsson S, Baigi A, Marklund B, Fridlund B. Trends in the misuse of androgenic anabolic steroids among boys 16-17 years old in a primary health care area in Sweden. *Scand J Prim Health Care*. 2001;19(3):181–182.
2. Nilsson S, Baigi A, Marklund B, Fridlund B. The prevalence of the use of androgenic anabolic steroids by adolescents in a county of Sweden. *Eur J Public Health*. 2001;11(2):195–197.
3. Malve HO. Sports pharmacology: A medical pharmacologist's perspective. *J Pharm Bioallied Sci*. 2018;10(3):126–136.
4. Vermeersch H, T'sjoen G, Kaufman JM, Vincke J. The role of testosterone in aggressive and non-aggressive risk-taking in adolescent boys. *Horm Behav*. 2008;53(3):463–471.
5. Elbe AM, Jensen SN, Elsborg P, et al. The urine marker test: An alternative approach to supervised urine collection for doping control. *Sports Med*. 2016;46(1):15–22.
6. Vorona E, Nieschlag E. Adverse effects of doping with anabolic androgenic steroids in competitive athletics, recreational sports, and bodybuilding. *Minerva Endocrinol*. 2018;43(4):476–488.
7. Goldfield GS, Woodside DB. Body image, disordered eating, and anabolic steroids in male bodybuilders: Current versus former users. *Phys Sportsmed*. 2009;37(1):111–114.
8. Vanberg P, Atar D. Androgenic anabolic steroid use and the cardiovascular system. *Handb Exp Pharmacol*. 2010;195:411–457.
9. Modlinski R, Fields KB. The effect of anabolic steroids on the gastrointestinal system, kidneys, and adrenal glands. *Curr Sports Med Rep*. 2006;5(2):104–109.

44.

PERIOPERATIVE CARE OF THE CANCER PATIENT

Cory W. Helder and Alessia Pedoto

STEM CASE AND KEY QUESTIONS

A 47-year-old female lymphoma and breast cancer survivor is presenting for preoperative evaluation for surgery on a new lung mass that is suspicious for lung cancer. On examination you hear a carotid bruit. She was initially diagnosed with lymphoma at age 19 and breast cancer at age 44. She is tentatively scheduled for a video-assisted thoracoscopic surgical (VATS) lobectomy in a month after a biopsy next week.

What is lymphoma and where can it present?

What are the treatments for lymphoma and their side effects?

Are there any long-term concerns from treatment?

The patient was diagnosed with lymphoma at age 19 after some delay, attributing her fatigue to stress from work and not having a primary care physician. Abnormal blood tests led to further testing and the eventual diagnosis of lymphoma. She was treated with systemic chemotherapy and radiation to both the mediastinum and the left supraclavicular sites. The patient remembers she was extremely fatigued and required an admission for low "blood counts" and dehydration but does not remember any issues with her heart at the time. She moved a few years later and stopped seeing her oncologist until she started screening for breast cancer.

Does her diagnosis of childhood lymphoma affect her future risk of malignancy?

What treatments exist for breast cancer?

Does the previous chemotherapy and radiation impact future treatment?

Perioperatively, how does neoadjuvant versus adjuvant therapy affect her surgical care?

The patient was diagnosed with breast cancer following a screening mammogram at age 44 when a suspicious lesion was found on her left breast. A mastectomy with axillary sentinel node biopsy was performed. The patient underwent chemotherapy a second time followed by targeted hormonal therapy. She reported receiving a different chemotherapy regimen to avoid a second exposure to some of the cytotoxic agents from her lymphoma. She did not have radiation as part of her breast cancer treatment.

She appears anxious about the risk of postoperative lymphedema. Can anything be done to minimize anxiety and risk of lymphedema?

She tells you that she cannot use her left arm for IV access or blood pressure measurements.

She has recently undergone treatment for breast cancer. What side effects of treatment might still be evident, and what medications could she still be taking?

The patient completed chemotherapy a little over a year ago and is still taking tamoxifen. She was overweight at the start of treatment but lost about 15–20 pounds, and only recently she began regaining weight. She is still fatigued at the end of most days but able to do her activities of daily living (ADLs). She was informed by her primary care physician that she is slightly anemic.

The biopsy and surgery have been scheduled, and she plans to see her oncologist and her primary care physician in advance. What counsel can you provide to prepare her for surgery, and what modifiable risk factors can her oncologist and primary care doctor help change before surgery?

Despite her moderate anemia, she is currently working but is extremely fatigued by the end of most days and, as a result, largely sedentary. Her thyroid function was checked and was normal. Laboratory tests are ordered to determine the cause of the anemia. She smokes a quarter-pack of cigarettes per day. She tried to quit during chemotherapy and succeeded in decreasing her smoking from 1 pack per day, though quitting worsened her nausea from treatment. She also tried electronic cigarettes during that period. She drinks wine most nights of the week and is slightly overweight but lost weight during chemotherapy. She was counseled about smoking and alcohol cessation in preparation for surgery. She is referred for IV iron supplementation for her anemia and is scheduled to see a nutritionist and a physical therapist next week.

What preoperative testing needs to be arranged prior to her biopsy?

Should the bruit or any of these tests delay her biopsy?

What testing needs to be arranged for her future planned lung resection, and what information can be gathered by consultation from her other clinicians?

In preparation for the lung biopsy, she is found to have a mildly impaired functional status but able to ascend a few flights of stairs. She is asymptomatic from her bruit. Common laboratory tests obtained in advance only showed anemia. A previous transthoracic echocardiogram (TTE) from her oncology treatment showed mildly decreased global function and moderately impaired relaxation without significant valvulopathies. The left ventricular function is estimated at 45–50%. The patient's left carotid artery has severe stenosis (70–80%), while mild disease is reported on the right side. A CT angiography scan of the head was performed and showed no significant intracerebral disease with adequate collaterals through the left vertebral system. Consultation with neurology and vascular surgery stated that the patient should proceed with surgery. She is started on aspirin for medical therapy. Her pulmonary function tests (PFTs) show a FEV_1 of 72% with a mild obstructive pattern and a diffusing capacity for carbon monoxide (DLCO) of 61%.

What is the importance of the biopsy before the resection, and how does her medical history change the importance of the biopsy?

The interventional radiology biopsy reveals melanoma rather than the expected lung cancer or metastatic breast cancer. This triggers her to remember a left shoulder mole removal at age 32. She had not seen her prior oncologist in several years and was told not to worry. The day she receives the results, she is scheduled for a positron emission tomography (PET) scan. No other sites of disease are identified on the scan. She is still scheduled for VATS resection of her nodule, which will now be followed by adjuvant immunotherapy.

Intraoperatively and postoperatively, what precautions should be taken for this patient based on her medical history?

The patient undergoes a left upper lobe wedge resection of her melanoma. Margins are sent intraoperatively and are free from disease. Prior to surgery the anesthesiologist places an epidural for postoperative pain management. After surgery she has a small air leak that persists for 5 days before the chest tube can be removed, delaying her recovery and discharge. In the postoperative period, she needed supplemental oxygen for 3 days. She was then discharged home with outpatient physical therapy services. After surgery she had persistent pain over her left ribs lasting weeks, which gradually improved.

What immunotherapy agents are available, and what are their indications?

She is started on ipilimumab for her metastatic melanoma after complete resection.

What toxic side effects do immunotherapy agents have?

Seven months later, she falls while walking. She is taken by her family to the hospital after being unable to bear weight on her left ankle. X-rays confirm a distal ankle fracture needing surgical repair. She is still on her immune checkpoint inhibitor. Admission laboratory tests reveal hyponatremia and hyperkalemia. The patient appears dehydrated and blames the excessive fatigue for her fall. An endocrinology consult is obtained to manage the electrolyte abnormalities, while the oncology service evaluates her prior to the operation. After her electrolytes normalize, an open reduction and internal fixation of the left ankle is performed. She is discharged with close follow-up with the endocrinologist on a steroid taper and levothyroxine supplementation. After 2 years of follow-up, there is no evidence of recurrent melanoma on her PET scan.

DISCUSSION

Cytotoxic chemotherapy, radiation, surgery, hormonal treatment, and immunotherapy agents are the mainstay of oncology treatment. Knowing what type of therapeutic protocol was used is essential for multiple reasons since malignancy can affect many organs, as in the case of lymphoma. Side effects are common during treatment, but some persist after its conclusion or develop years to decades later. Some severe examples include a second malignancy, heart failure, valvulopathy, coronary and vascular disease, venous thromboembolism, endocrinopathy, and pneumonitis. The detailed knowledge of the oncological treatment used can give the clinician insight into the severity of the disease, and, as cancer survivorship increases, patients' oncologic sequelae or the likelihood of other malignancies will continue to grow.

In the population with multiple malignancies, biopsy results carry additional importance prior to surgery, since treatment is frequently different in primary and metastatic disease. The type of the primary tumor is not easily determined on frozen specimens and may require histological stains which take days. In patients with multiple risk factors and a history of prior cancers, an unexpected diagnosis is possible and highlights the importance of both having a sound oncological plan and obtaining a diagnosis using the least invasive method possible. A comprehensive oncological history is important to guide diagnosis and preempt sequelae of prior treatments.

LYMPHOMA

Lymphoma is a malignancy of the immune system cells. It is classified as Hodgkin or non-Hodgkin lymphoma, with 85% of cases being non-Hodgkin.[1] The non-Hodgkin family represents a heterogenous group with 85–90% of cases being of B-cell origin, even though T-cell varieties exist. Lymphoma can present in any part of the body, but lymphadenopathy and splenomegaly are common. It can affect the mediastinum, liver, or bone marrow, or spread to the central nervous system depending on the type. Young women in particular are more likely to have primary mediastinal involvement of B-cell origin.[1]

LYMPHOMA TREATMENTS AND THEIR SIDE EFFECTS

Cytotoxic agents have been a mainstay of therapy for lymphoma for decades, with multiple agents given in tandem., There are many treatment strategies, based on the type of tumor, with an increasing number of targets thanks to modern genomic sequencing. CHOP-R (cyclophosphamide, doxorubicin, vincristine, prednisone, rituximab) is the primary treatment algorithm for most mature B-cell lymphomas, but some more intensive regimens are being used such as EPOCH-R (etoposide, prednisone, vincristine, cyclophosphamide, doxorubicin, rituximab) with the aim of improving survival in younger patients with more aggressive tumors. New treatments are also being developed to harness the existing immune system, such as immune checkpoint inhibitors or chimeric antigen receptor T-cell (CAR-T cell) therapy. Radiation therapy (RT) is used in conjunction with chemotherapy for bulky tumors or tumors with aggressive features.[2]

Long-term sequelae and risks are associated with these agents. The anthracycline drug doxorubicin is still included in most lymphoma and many solid tumor treatment regimens. Cardiac injury is the major drawback of anthracycline-based cytotoxic agents.[3] Cardiotoxicity is defined as *acute* if it occurs during therapy, *early* if it occurs within 1 year, or *late* if it occurs 1 or more years after therapy. While acute toxicity is rare (<1%), it tends to be characterized by conduction abnormalities and arrhythmias which typically resolve after treatment cessation. Short- and long-term toxicities are characterized by progressive left ventricular (LV) dysfunction that can lead to restrictive or dilated cardiomyopathy and congestive heart failure (CHF). Higher dose, younger patients, and female sex all increase the risk of toxicity, with a higher incidence of CHF with longer follow-up.[3] The long-term sequelae of treatment with anthracyclines places these patients at higher risk of premature atherosclerosis and coronary artery disease. According to survivorship studies, survivors of childhood non-Hodgkin's lymphoma have a 6.5-fold (confidence interval [95% CI] 2.3,14.0) risk of cardiac mortality compared to their matched peers.[4] Several current studies are aimed at reducing this risk.[3] With the growth in the number of cancer survivors, there has been an increased need for cardio-oncology specialists to monitor, prevent, and treat cardiac toxicities in this growing population. A list of common oncology treatments and their associated cardiopulmonary toxicities is found in Table 44.1.

The use of bleomycin during treatment should be investigated as part of the preoperative evaluation. The typical

Table 44.1 A LIST OF COMMON ANTINEOPLASTIC DRUGS AND TREATMENTS AND THEIR POTENTIAL CARDIOPULMONARY TOXICITIES

CLASS/DRUG	CARDIAC TOXICITY	PULMONARY TOXICITY
Anti-tumor antibiotics		
Anthracyclines	Arrhythmias, cardiac depression, dilated or restrictive	
Doxorubicin	cardiomyopathy, pericarditis, coronary artery disease,	
Daunorubicin	cardiac failure	
Bleomycin	Pericarditis, myocardial ischemia	Pneumonitis
Alkylating agents		
Cyclophosphamide	Heart block, tachyarrhythmias, CHF	
Cisplatin	Heart block, arrhythmias, CHF, myocardial ischemia	
Antibodies		
Trastuzumab	Cardiomyopathy, cardiac failure	
Rituximab	Arrhythmias	
Bevacizumab	Myocardial ischemia	
Radiotherapy	Arrhythmias, restrictive cardiomyopathy, valvulopathies, cardiac failure, coronary artery disease	Pneumonitis Pulmonary fibrosis
Immune checkpoint inhibitors	Conduction disorders, cardiomyopathy, CHF, myocarditis, pericarditis	
Anti-CTLA-4 mAb		
Ipilimumab		
Anti-PD-1 mAb		Pneumonitis
Pembrolizumab, nivolumab		
Anti-PD-L1 mAb		
Atezolizumab, durvalumab		
Microtubule-targeting agents		
Taxanes	Bradycardia/AV block, atrial and ventricular arrhythmias,	
Docetaxel	heart failure, myocardial ischemia	
Paclitaxel		
Antimetabolites		
Fluorouracil	Cardiac failure, atrial or ventricular ectopy, myocardial ischemia/infarction	

bleomycin patient is either undergoing treatment or is a survivor of non-seminoma germ cell tumors. Bleomycin can be occasionally used in some intensive chemotherapy regimens in younger patients, such as ACVBP-R[3] (doxorubicin, vindesine, cyclophosphamide, bleomycin, prednisolone and rituximab) for lymphoma. Monitoring for bleomycin pulmonary toxicity (BPT) during treatment is paramount as bleomycin is the most common chemotherapy drug responsible for pulmonary toxicity. The acute phase usually presents as dyspnea and nonproductive cough. In the short term, the DLCO can decrease but typically normalizes over the subsequent years. Acute toxicity is more common with increased doses of bleomycin (>300 units). There are many case reports of patients who received bleomycin either recently or in the distant past who subsequently developed acute lung injury in the perioperative period. Perioperative exposure to high levels of inspired oxygen (FIO_2)[5] is frequently cited as the cause. A subsequent review of cases with BPT associated the pulmonary injury with overhydration.[6] Complications are rare, so research on this topic is difficult. It is thought that lower levels of oxygen, lower bleomycin exposure, avoidance of overhydration, and a longer window since exposure are protective from developing acute lung injury. The use of the lowest FIO_2 possible to maintain a safe level of oxygen saturation is reasonable a few months after bleomycin exposure. However, extra care should be taken to avoid overhydration throughout the entire perioperative period.

RT is used frequently with both types of lymphoma and other malignancies. In particular, RT is particularly beneficial for the local control of the disease, decreasing chemotherapy doses, and improving survival in lymphoma patients with early aggressive or bulky disease.[2] However, RT carries the risk of both short- and long-term radiation toxicity. Short-term toxicities (<3 months from treatment) include fatigue, hair loss, skin changes, pneumonitis, and mucositis. Long-term toxicities are of greater consequence to the perioperative care of the oncology patient. Survivorship studies of pediatric patients receiving RT showed a relative risk (RR) of 4.3 of lung fibrosis, 6.6 of hypothyroidism, and 9.2 of thyroid carcinoma, and an increased risk of cardiac disease and valvulopathies after receiving mediastinal radiation,[4,7] Adults have a similar risk toxicity profile to the lungs and heart, such as increased risk of pneumonitis, pulmonary fibrosis, coronary artery disease, and clinically significant valvulopathies. Major cardiac event risk is increased with higher doses of radiation starting with just a few grays (Gy; unit of ionizing radiation) and with no apparent ceiling,[7] Technological advances have led to more targeted therapy to spare nearby healthy tissue,[8] and dose reduction studies are being done to minimize toxicity.[9]

CHILDHOOD LYMPHOMA AND FUTURE RISK OF MALIGNANCY

Survivors of non-Hodgkin lymphoma have a RR of 1.31 (CI: 1.29,1.34) of developing a second malignancy compared to peers after treatment. The risk is magnified in survivors of childhood lymphoma who have 4.1 times (CI: 3.1, 5.6) increase in their incidence of second malignancies,[10] this leading to a 15 times (CI: 9.6, 23.7) higher risk of death.[4] In childhood survivors, the RT-related increased risk[10,11] seems to be associated with the possible longer latency period to develop a secondary neoplasm compared to elderly survivors.[4] There is some evidence that links RT and secondary malignancies to nearby radiation fields, such as rectal cancer after pelvic or prostate RT.[7] Hodgkin lymphoma survivors after whole-body radiation seem to be at higher risk.[7,10] It is unclear if this is applicable to adults with non-Hodgkin lymphoma when RT is compared to chemotherapy alone.[12]

BREAST CANCER TREATMENTS AND THEIR TOXICITIES

Treatment options for breast cancer are diverse and involve surgery in addition to chemotherapy and radiation, hormonal, and immune therapies. In breast cancer, after chemotherapy, most patients start either anastrozole or tamoxifen for hormone-responsive variants for 5 years and trastuzumab for 1 year for HER2-positive malignancies to increase disease-free survival.

Many breast cancer regimens utilize anthracycline agents (doxorubicin, epirubicin). Alternative therapies can be chosen to avoid repeat exposure or exacerbate preexisting comorbidities. Floyd et al. reported a 10.5% incidence of CHF with a mean decrease in ejection fraction of 25% in breast cancer patients treated with a combination of anthracycline and docetaxel.[13] Trastuzumab, a HER2 targeted therapy, has been shown to increase the risk of anthracycline cardiotoxicity in breast cancer treatment.[14] This may be through dual pathways. Anthracycline cardiac toxicity causes an oxidative stress directly toxic to the myocytes, while trastuzumab affects cell signal pathways important for myocyte function.[15] Trastuzumab otherwise is generally well tolerated, with minor side effects such as diarrhea, headache, nausea, and fatigue. An anthracycline-free regimen relies on other common agents such as cyclophosphamide, docetaxel, and, in certain situations, carboplatin.[14] Cyclophosphamide is also cardiotoxic and during treatment can cause arrhythmias and heart failure, which typically resolve over 3–4 weeks.[13]

Breast cancer patients who are treated with radiation are at increased risk for long-term cardiovascular complications, especially when the left breast is affected, due to the immediate proximity of the aortic valve and many coronary vessels to the radiation fields.[16]

Tamoxifen, anastrozole, and many other hormonal agents target endocrine-sensitive breast cancers, with anastrozole being reserved for postmenopausal women. Cancer in general is associated with an increased risk of venous thromboembolism (VTE), a significant source of morbidity and mortality among cancer patients. Patients receiving chemotherapy have a several-fold increased risk of VTE compared to those not receiving chemotherapy. Tamoxifen, an estrogen modulator, also increases the risk of VTE, with a peak incidence in the first few months after initiation of treatment.[17,18] Anastrozole, an aromatase inhibitor, does not appear to have an increased risk of VTE, but it is associated with bone mineral density loss and fractures.[18]

BREAST CANCER AND SECONDARY MALIGNANCIES

Previous cancer treatment increases the risk of second malignancies. The development of solid malignancies typically has a longer latency period compared to leukemia or lymphoma after RT.[11] In this scenario, it is impossible to tell if the breast cancer was radiation-induced, but parts of the patient's breast tissue likely received more than 1 Gy of RT during her lymphoma treatment. Endometrial, ovarian, and lung cancers are the most common second malignancies.[19] After chemotherapy, the most common maintenance regimens include 5 years of anastrozole or tamoxifen for hormone-responsive breast cancer or 1 year of trastuzumab for HER2-positive malignancies. These maintenance regimens have demonstrated an increased disease-free survival.

BREAST CANCER LYMPHEDEMA

Arm precaution for lymphedema risk is variable. Most modern surgical techniques remove fewer nodes, thus decreasing the risk of postoperative lymphedema. In addition, limited literature supports typical arm precautions in the absence of a history of lymphedema, skin infections, or soft tissue infections. Several prospective cohort studies have not shown an increased risk for lymphedema in the absence of prior lymphedema or soft tissue or skin infections[20] when the blood pressure measurements or IV access were done on the surgical side. In the absence of this history, it is reasonable to use the operative arm throughout the perioperative period. Preoperative counseling of the patient should decrease any stress and concerns. In clinical practice, it is courteous to try to avoid using the arm of the axillary dissection site, if possible, but not a contraindication.

IMMUNOTHERAPY AGENTS

It has been known for a long time that the human immune system has methods to detect and eradicate tumor cells via cytotoxic CD8+ T cells. This process relies on the differentiation of T cells into CD4+ and CD8+ with the proliferation of activated T cells. For T cells to proliferate, they must bind to either a tumor cell or an antigen-presenting cell (APC) via two receptors. The T-cell receptor (TCR) binds to the major histocompatibility complex (MHC) plus a costimulatory mechanism between a T cell's CD28 receptor and the B7 protein on APCs. This triggers the proliferation of cytotoxic CD8+ T cells to attack tumor cells.

Tumor cells have developed methods to interrupt this process via inhibitory processes in the immune system. The cytotoxic T-lymphocyte associated protein 4 (CTLA-4) is a receptor on the T cell similar to CD28. It binds to B7 with higher affinity than CD28 and acts to inhibit the proliferation of T cells. Tumor cells can induce the overexpression of CTLA-4 on T cells to outcompete the CD28-B7 stimulatory signal and prevent the adaptive immune system from targeting the tumor. The immune checkpoint inhibitor ipilimumab blocks the CTLA-4 receptor on T cells, allowing for its activation and proliferation. A second target for immune checkpoint inhibitors is the programmed cell death protein 1 (PD-1) which, like CD28 or CTLA-4 on the T cells, inhibits proliferation. The PD1 receptor binds to PD-L1 or PD-L2 ligand on the surface of the tumor cells, causing inhibition. Pembrolizumab and nivolumab block PD-1 while atezolizumab, avelumab, and durvalumab affect PD-L1. Blocking CTLA-4, PD-1, and PD-L1 allows stimulation of the adaptive immune system to efficiently attack the tumor. The degree to which tumor cells express either CTLA-4 and PD-1 can predict the patient's response to these agents.[21] Immune checkpoint inhibitors have indications for unresectable melanoma, Hodgkin lymphoma, and many advanced or metastatic solid tumors (e.g., non-small cell lung [NSCLC] or colon cancer).

IMMUNOTHERAPY AGENTS' TOXICITIES

PD-L1 is not found exclusively on APCs and tumor cells. It is also found on endothelial cells, pancreatic islet cells, testes, and cardiomyocytes, leading to immune system-mediated toxicities. Immune checkpoint reactions can affect any organ but commonly affect the gastrointestinal tract causing gastritis, enterocolitis, and hepatitis, or the endocrine system. Rarer toxicities affect the heart and lungs. Twenty-four percent of patients on anti-CTLA therapy experience severe reactions needing medical treatment, delaying or possibly discontinuing therapy. This number is lower with anti-PD1 therapy, occurring in fewer than 10%.

Pituitary toxicity occurs in 10–15% of anti-CTLA therapy and in less than 1% in PD-1 therapy. Pituitary toxicity can cause hypopituitarism leading to hypothyroidism, adrenal insufficiency, and hypogonadism. Routine checking of TSH, T4, ACTH, and cortisol levels is recommended. Pituitary function does not always recover at the end of treatment, leading to lifelong hormone replacement. Patients on immune checkpoint inhibitors in the perioperative period should have an endocrinologist consult to provide specific recommendations, with a focus on electrolyte disturbances and acid-base and water homeostasis, as well as symptoms of hypothyroidism. Supplementation with a stress-dose steroid should occur as needed. Hypothyroidism can occur in 5–10% of patients, and presentation can lag up to 3 years after treatment.[22]

Fortunately, serious side effects affecting the heart and lung are rare. Cardiac toxicity affects fewer than 1% of patients and occurs during treatment. Symptoms include heart failure, conduction abnormalities, myofibrosis, and myocarditis. Treatment usually involves steroids. Severe symptoms such as elevated brain natriuretic peptide (BNP), new ECG findings, or elevated cardiac enzymes require cardiology consultation. Pneumonitis has been reported in 3–7% with PD-1 and 1.3%

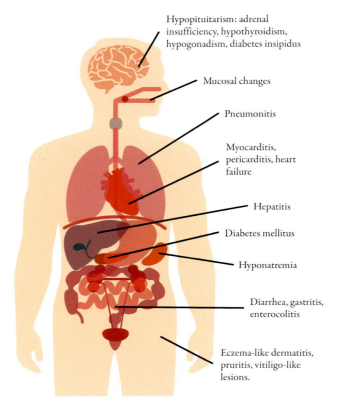

Figure 44.1 Many organs have receptors that cross-react to cause immune-related toxicities throughout the body. Figure shows affected organs and their potential toxicities.

with PD-L1 inhibitors. Pneumonitis usually presents during treatment as cough, wheeze, and dyspnea. Although pulmonary toxicity is rare, PD-1 inhibitors are used for metastatic NSCLC in patients with potentially very little pulmonary reserve. Treatment again is centered around corticosteroids.[21] Immune checkpoint inhibitors can cause pulmonary, cardiac, and endocrine pathology but show great promise in preventing disease progression and mortality for a variety of malignancies (Figure 44.1).

Cytotoxic release syndrome is a rare but potentially deadly side effect of immunotherapy that requires immediate discontinuation of treatment and supportive management.[23] The massive activation of T cells triggers the release of cytokines, which affect multiple organs. Symptoms vary from mild fever (Grade 1) to multiple organ failure (Grade 4) requiring mechanical ventilation, hemodynamic support, and high-dose steroids. This is more common with the use of CAR-T cell agents but has been described after the use of nivolumab as well.

PREOPERATIVE EVALUATION OF THE CANCER PATIENT

The preoperative evaluation of the cancer patient includes several considerations in addition to the evaluation of general medical conditions. Similarly, a comprehensive history and physical examination are necessary while keeping in mind specific effects of the cancer or its treatment in this patient population. In this patient, additional considerations are needed while undergoing thoracic surgery.

PAIN

Chronic pain is a frequent comorbid condition among cancer patients, with a prevalence of nearly 30%, with 20% of cases having a neuropathic component.[24] A subset of these patients is on chronic opioids. Taking inventory of opioid use, both short- and long-acting; non-opioid analgesic use; and the efficacy of the current regimen is useful to determine future opioid requirements during surgery. Regional analgesia can be beneficial in this population. For patients undergoing extensive procedures, their normal opioid usage should be administered in the perioperative period.

FUNCTIONAL STATUS

Fatigue is a concerning nonspecific oncologic symptom which should prompt further investigation, especially if it is persistent and affecting daily living activities. A decline in the functional status could be secondary to deconditioning, anemia, or rapid progression of disease or resulting from chemotherapy toxicity, as well as cardiac or pulmonary toxicity of prior cancer treatments. It is important to investigate endocrinopathies as possible causes (past radiation and chemotherapy increase the risk for hypothyroidism). Immunotherapy agents can also cause new endocrinopathies. Neoadjuvant or adjuvant chemotherapy, in addition to surgery, both cause a temporary decrease in functional status. There is a threshold at which a patient needs help with some or all ADLs. The further a patient is away from that threshold prior to treatment, the more likely he or she is to maintain or regain independence after oncological surgery (Figure 44.2). The preoperative period is a short window to address these medical issues to help patients both maintain ADLs and undergo full oncological treatment.

CARDIAC EVALUATION

Symptomatology as well as the temporal relationship with chemotherapy administration should be ascertained. A TTE should be obtained as part of the workup in case of exposure to multiple cardiotoxic therapies and mediastinal radiation in the presence of decreased functional capacity. Old records from previous oncology treatments might include a TTE that can be referenced. The cardiotoxic effects of prior treatments may be causing early occlusive coronary artery disease, such as the premature occlusion of the carotid artery. The current American College of Cardiologists (ACC)/American Heart Association (AHA) guidelines should apply to the oncologic patient, with the caveat of time sensitivity and limited evaluation and intervention time.[25]

PULMONARY EVALUATION

A routine pulmonary exam looking for crackles or wheezing should be performed. Additionally, exercise tolerance, respiratory

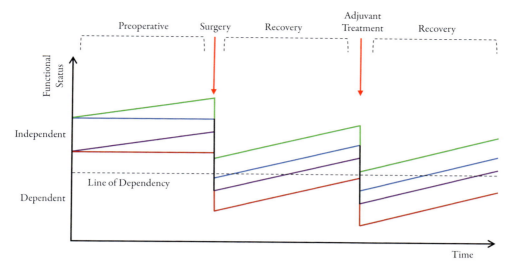

Figure 44.2 Prehabilitation is aimed at increasing a patient's health reserve before crossing the threshold or line of dependence where they will need increasing levels of support with activities of daily living (ADLs). Green and purple lines show anticipated trajectory of recovery for patients undergoing prehabilitation compared to the blue and red lines of patients not receiving prehabilitation. The blue patient spends more time requiring support with ADLs for parts of care compared to the green patient, who is independent throughout treatment. The red patient never fully recovers independence compared to the purple patient. Recovery is made more difficult due to the sequence of surgery and adjuvant treatment in quick series.

reserve, and exposure to bleomycin should be assessed. Smoking increases the risk of many types of cancer and is common among cancer patients. Counseling on the importance of smoking cessation, utilization of inhalers, and planning for nicotine replacement in the perioperative period should be done.

In this patient undergoing a lung resection, PFTs are helpful to stratify risk, counsel the patient about cardiopulmonary reserve after lung resection, and determine the maximum amount of lung tissue that can be safely removed. The lack of PFTs, however, should not preclude surgery. Clinical criteria can be used to stratify the risk of the operation, especially in nonsmokers or in active patients with limited comorbidities.[26]

A video-assisted thoracoscopic wedge resection is the standard approach for a surgical lung biopsy. Typically, peripheral wedge resections can be completed in a minimally invasive fashion, with a low risk of conversion to thoracotomy, in the absence of adhesions or prior radiation. Upper lobe resections, adhesions, FEV_1 of less than 80%, age older than 65, and Zubrod score of 2 or greater have all been used as part of predictive models for prolonged air leak, while left-sided surgery, and wedge resection can be protective.[27,28] For this reason, neuraxial analgesia should be considered and discussed at the preoperative testing if the patient has risk factors for conversion to thoracotomy or persistent air leak because this complication can increase length of stay, pain, and delay recovery. Neuraxial techniques, such as epidural or paravertebral catheters, are an effective way to manage pain, reduce splinting, and decrease adverse pulmonary events especially if the chest tube remains in place for a prolonged period.

HEMATOLOGIC CONSIDERATIONS

Anemia is pervasive in the oncological population. The prevalence of iron deficiency in patients with solid tumors is about 40%, and 33% suffer from iron deficiency anemia. Prevalence is highest for pancreatic, colorectal, and lung cancer.[29] Screening for anemia and prompt correction of vitamin and iron deficiencies can both improve fatigue and decrease the rate of transfusion. Responsiveness to treatment can help predict oncologic outcome. The prevalence of anemia increases after any chemotherapy or radiation. The combination of bone marrow suppression and inflammatory cytokine-induced iron sequestration plus chemotherapy induces malabsorption, and anorexia makes IV iron supplementation more efficacious than oral supplementation.[30] Iron deficiency is thought to be the cause of 50% of cases of anemia.[31] Bleeding, B_{12} deficiency, folate deficiency, and decreased absorption are the causes in a minority.[31] In the preoperative period, if IV iron supplementation is being considered, it is best if started early since erythropoiesis still requires 2 weeks. Erythropoietin and folate can be added to boost the effects of IV iron. The preoperative improvement of anemia is feasible, cost effective, and leads to improved outcomes in several surgical fields.[32–34] In surgical oncology, the immunomodulatory effects of transfusions on oncology outcomes is currently being debated.[35]

Additionally, screening questions should be asked about pain, erythema or edema of the legs, and any history of DVT due to the increased risk of VTE secondary to cancer and oncologic therapies. Population studies have shown that the incidence of VTE is only increasing with time. In Western cancer patients, registries show an increase in the 12-month incidence of VTE from 1% in 1997 to 3.4% in 2017.[36] Incidence appears to be even higher in patients receiving immunotherapy agents. VTE continues to be a common cause of morbidity and mortality among oncology patients.[37] As a result, a plan should be formulated to prevent VTE through the perioperative period. The ASRA guidelines should determine when to stop anticoagulation if any neuraxial procedures are planned.[38]

NEUROLOGIC EVALUATION

A carotid ultrasound is the first test done in case of a significant carotid bruit, especially if symptomatic. Significant stenosis in a young patient can be secondary to anthracycline use or high-dose radiation, especially if the field was wide enough to include the neck area. Treatment of severe stenosis is beneficial for decreasing the long-term risk of stroke but might not be prudent in the short term. As for any oncological surgical procedures, the risks and benefits of delaying surgical treatment for carotid stenting or carotid endarterectomy versus the integrity of the collateral circulation should be weighed against the speed at which the nodule is growing in conjunction with neurology, oncology, and vascular surgery. Proceeding with the biopsy may be necessary to help guide the treatment by providing additional information on how aggressive the lesion appears on pathology and the likelihood of metastasis. Medical therapy with aspirin is usually the first step in the presence of abnormal imaging.

PREHABILITATION OF THE ONCOLOGY SURGERY PATIENT

The idea of prehabilitation is aimed at increasing the patient's resilience to surgical stress by decreasing modifiable risk factors. These interventions can empower the patient to view the perioperative period as a moment to regain some control of the outcomes.[39]

The perioperative oncology period starts with two goals: obtaining adequate testing and optimizing any modifiable risk factors for surgery. Oncology cases cannot be postponed indefinitely so a risk-benefit discussion needs to take place if there is any significant delay in surgery. This window for optimization and prehabilitation is potentially longer if neoadjuvant treatment is started preoperatively. In general, efforts need to be made to address modifiable risk factors in an expedited fashion. A new diagnosis of malignancy can act as a catalyst for changes in patient behavior, and modifiable risk factors can be improved in the determined patient.

From the start of the preoperative oncology period, an effort should be made to engage and educate the patient on risks, expectations, timing, and anticipated return to normal activities. Studies have shown that psychological factors play a significant part in determining outcome, length of stay, ability to mobilize after surgery, and incidence of chronic pain. Increased anxiety predicted negative short-term operative outcomes, rate of recovery, and length of stay.[40,41] For example, depression is associated with a higher incidence of chronic pain.[40] Gillis et al. demonstrated that psychological preparation for surgery started in the preoperative period was significantly more effective at helping patients return to baseline functioning than the same intervention provided postoperatively.[42]

Smoking cessation prior to surgery is highly recommended. Upcoming surgery or the start of cancer treatment increases the success of smoking cessation programs since patients are highly motivated.[43] Persistent smoking has been linked to worsened oncological response to treatment and overall outcomes, and it negatively impacts survival.[43] The protective effect of smoking against chemotherapy-induced and postoperative nausea and vomiting[44] does not overcome the overall negative effects to the general health. The preoperative period is among the best opportunities for intervention, and patients benefit from additional resources to aid in cessation.

Smoking abstinence for more than 4 weeks has been associated with a decrease in adverse pulmonary events and infections in the postoperative period.[45,46] Preoperative smoking is associated with a RR of 2.46 (CI: 1.74, 3.48) of pulmonary complications, 2.49 (CI: 1.91, 3.26) of wound complications, and 1.6 (CI: 1.14, 2.25) of intensive care admissions.[47] Preoperative efforts to reduce smoking have been shown to decrease postoperative complications.[48] Smoking cessation even the day before surgery is beneficial, as carbon monoxide levels can normalize within 24 hours and no clear harm exists by quitting.[45] At present, little is known about the effects of electronic cigarette use in the perioperative period. However the nicotine in electronic cigarettes seems to stimulate a catecholamine release which can cause hemodynamic instability in the operative period.[49] Abstinence from marijuana 72 hours prior to surgery has been recommended. High levels of consumption have been associated with an increase in catecholamines in the perioperative period.[50]

Alcohol use has been linked to a variety of diseases including the development and recurrence of malignancies.[51] Moderate use is generally not considered a risk factor for poor perioperative outcomes, but abstinence has been shown to decrease the burden and symptoms of atrial fibrillation in patients with a history of paroxysmal atrial fibrillation after a 2-week washout period.[52] This is easily attainable in the presurgical population. Atrial fibrillation is common in many older oncology patients and is one of the main postoperative cardiac complications after thoracic noncardiac surgery. Postoperative atrial fibrillation has been shown to significantly increase the hospital length of stay and costs associated with many thoracic procedures.[53] Previous exposure to many cardiotoxic therapeutic agents may affect the onset of atrial fibrillation; however, the cumulative effect of this risk is currently unknown.

An active lifestyle prior to surgery is recommended to facilitate recovery and decrease complications. Major surgery induces a state of protein catabolism leading to further weakness. Fitness programs lasting 4–6 weeks can be accomplished in the preoperative period. Single-center randomized controlled trials for patients undergoing major surgery have shown a reduction in perioperative morbidity and improved cost effectiveness.[54,55] Several studies have shown that the benefits of aggressive preoperative physical rehabilitation can be seen in as little as 6 weeks in high-risk elderly individuals, reducing postoperative complications by 50%.[54]

Lastly, proper nutrition and avoidance of anemia are recommended by enhanced recovery after surgery (ERAS) guidelines.[56] While underweight patients (BMI <18.5 kg/m^2) are generally malnourished, a growing body of research is evaluating sarcopenic obesity. Clinically, sarcopenia is defined as lack of lean tissue mass. Sarcopenic obese patients can be normal or overweight but disproportionately lacking lean tissue and are therefore not detected by the traditional BMI metric. During chemotherapy patients tend to lose a disproportionate amount of lean tissue while losing, maintaining, or gaining adipose tissue. Aging is also associated with a replacement of lean tissue with adipose mass. Regaining lean tissue is particularly challenging in the elderly. Caloric restriction to lose adipose tissue tends to further lower lean tissue mass. Many combinations of resistance training, aerobic exercise, and high-quality supplemental protein to reach a goal intake of typically around 1.2 g/kg/day have been investigated.[57] Isoflavone supplementation appears promising in increasing lean mass in postmenopausal women.[58] There is no currently accepted best strategy, but help from a nutritionist to optimize the diet and therapy to resolve anemia are recommended. Therapy should be customized to the patient's needs, traditional diet, and access to resources. It is important to treat sarcopenic obesity since patients undergoing chemotherapy are more likely to have dose-limiting toxicities delaying or preventing completion of therapy.[59] In the surgical oncology literature, sarcopenic obesity patients undergoing gastrectomy had an odds ratio of 6.07 (CI: 1.9, 13.4) for major complications. Increased adverse events have been shown in the colorectal and hepatobiliary literature as well.[59] Unfortunately, many of the suggested treatments span more than 12 weeks to 1 year and may not be suitable for the preoperative window. However, increased physical fitness can be seen in as little as 4–6 weeks.[54,55] The benefits of even parts of a treatment program are undeniable and should be recommended independently of the time interval between the preoperative visit and surgery.

CONCLUSION

- With improvements in oncological care, there is an increasing number of cancer survivors. All patients, especially when young, have longer life expectancies and may develop second malignancies and antineoplastic toxicities.

- Cancer survivors live with the toxicities of the oncologic treatment for life. Antineoplastic toxicities can manifest at the time of treatment or can take years to decades to develop. RT toxicity has a long latency period. Anthracyclines exposure is associated with a lifetime elevated risk for cardiovascular events.

- Short-term neoadjuvant therapy toxicities often overlap with the perioperative period.

- Cardio-oncology is a growing field focused on preventing, monitoring, and treating the cardiovascular toxicities of oncology treatment and managing cardiovascular risk in patients with preexisting heart disease.

- In surgical oncology, extending the preoperative window increases the risk of cancer progression and needs to be weighed against the benefits. Despite the short window, there are many modifiable risk factors that can be addressed.

- The goal of prehabilitation is to increase the resilience of a patient before major surgery or stress and improve the patient's chances of postoperative independence. Some interventions are more effective prior to surgery than after surgery.

- Distinguishing between certain malignancies on frozen section is impossible. In surgical oncology, there must be a thorough plan for the entire perioperative period.

- Immune checkpoint inhibitors can cause pulmonary, cardiac, and endocrine pathology but show great promise in preventing disease progression and mortality for a variety of malignancies.

REVIEW QUESTIONS

1. A 77-year-old female sustained a traumatic fracture of the left ankle and left wrist. She is presenting for the open reduction and internal fixation of her left wrist. She has a history of right breast cancer, treated with a unilateral mastectomy and lymph node dissection 9 years ago followed by adjuvant chemotherapy. She has no history of lymphedema. Where should the IV access and the noninvasive blood pressure monitors be placed?

    a. IV access in the right foot; noninvasive blood pressure (NIBP) monitor on the left leg.
    b. IV access in the left antecubital; NIBP on the right arm.
    c. IV access the right arm; NIBP on right leg.
    d. IV access in the right foot and NIBP on the right leg.

    The correct answer is c.

    Several prospective cohort studies have not shown an increased risk for lymphedema in the absence of prior lymphedema or soft tissue or skin infections[20] when the blood pressure measurements or IV access were done on the surgical side. In the absence of this history, it is reasonable to use the operative arm throughout the perioperative period. Preoperative counseling of the patient should decrease any stress and concerns. In clinical practice, it is courteous to try avoiding the use of the arm of the axillary dissection site, if possible, but not a contraindication.

2. A 64-year-old woman presents with symptoms consistent with a transient ischemic attack. Which previous treatment could put her at higher risk of stroke?

    a. Prior radiation to the chest for lymphoma.
    b. Treatment with bleomycin as a child.
    c. Hormonal therapy after breast cancer for 5 years.
    d. Treatment with an immune checkpoint inhibitor for melanoma.

    The correct answer is a.

    High-dose radiation, especially if the field was wide enough to include the neck area, is a risk factor for significant carotid stenosis later in life.

3. A 68-year-old male ex-smoker has a history of melanoma 10 years ago and colon cancer 4 years ago. He presents with a peripherally located isolated lung nodule. Which procedure is he most likely to undergo?

a. Endobronchial ultrasound and biopsy for staging.
b. Video-assisted thoracoscopic excisional biopsy.
c. CT-guided needle biopsy.
d. Colonoscopy.

The correct answer is c.

In the population with multiple malignancies, biopsy results carry additional importance prior to surgery. Treatment is frequently different in primary and metastatic disease. In patients with multiple risk factors and history of prior cancers, surprises in diagnosis are possible and highlight the importance of having a sound oncological plan and obtaining a diagnosis using the least invasive method possible.

4. A 55-year-old left breast cancer survivor underwent left breast radiation 15 years ago and is now presenting with shortness of breath. Which abnormality is most likely the cause of her dyspnea?

a. Acute pulmonary embolism.
b. Aortic insufficiency.
c. Pulmonary edema.
d. Complete heart block.

The correct answer is b.

Survivorship studies of pediatric patients receiving RT showed an RR of 4.3 of lung fibrosis, 6.6 of hypothyroidism, 9.2 of thyroid carcinoma, and an increased risk of cardiac disease and valvulopathies after receiving mediastinal radiation.

5. What preoperative screening is recommended for a patient who was started on an immune checkpoint inhibitor 2 years ago?

a. Echocardiography for cardiac dysfunction.
b. Routine consultation with an endocrinologist.
c. Assessment of electrolyte levels and screening for thyroid levels.
d. Routine chest x-ray for pneumonitis.

The correct answer is c.

Pituitary toxicity due to immune checkpoint inhibitors can cause hypopituitarism leading to hypothyroidism, adrenal insufficiency, and hypogonadism. Routine checking of thyroid stimulating hormone (TSH), free thyroxine (T4), adrenocorticotropic hormone (ACTH), and cortisol levels as well as electrolytes is recommended.

6. A patient with significant weight loss and mild anemia is scheduled for surgery in 4 weeks. What is the most successful prehabilitation step prior to surgery?

a. Oral iron supplementation for iron deficiency anemia.
b. IV iron supplementation for iron deficiency anemia.
c. Physical therapy to reverse loss of lean muscle mass.
d. Alcohol cessation to decrease risk of postoperative myocardial infarction.

The correct answer is b.

Iron deficiency is thought to be the cause of 50% of cases of anemia in oncology patients. Bleeding, B_{12} deficiency, folate deficiency, and decreased absorption are the causes in a minority of patients. In the preoperative period, if IV iron supplementation is being considered, it is best if started early since erythropoiesis still requires 2 weeks.

7. A 47-year-old female is presenting for a colectomy in the late afternoon. She underwent neoadjuvant chemotherapy to decrease the size of the tumor. Her preoperative vitals are heart rate 130, respiratory rate 14, blood pressure 96/68, SpO_2 99% on room air. She underwent a bowel prep for surgery and feels dehydrated. She has suffered from fatigue ever since starting chemotherapy and has significant anxiety about surgery. What should be the next course of action?

a. Continue with surgery; the tachycardia is related to anxiety.
b. Cancel surgery and schedule a cardiac evaluation.
c. Inquire about symptoms of cardiac dysfunction, start an IV line for hydration, and obtain an ECG.
d. Consult with her oncologist about her medical history.

The correct answer is c.

Symptomatology as well as the temporal relationship with chemotherapy administration should be ascertained. The cardiotoxic effects of prior treatments may be causing early occlusive coronary artery disease, such as the premature occlusion of the carotid artery. The current ACC/AHA guidelines should apply to the oncologic patient, with the caveat of time sensitivity and limited evaluation and intervention time.

8. After left breast radiation, which vascular territory is most at risk for ischemia?

a. Left cerebral hemisphere.
b. Distal right coronary artery.
c. Left circumflex artery.
d. Distal left anterior descending artery.

The correct answer is d.

RT portends an increased risk of cardiac disease and valvulopathies after receiving treatment to the mediastinum. Adults have a similar risk toxicity profile to their lung and heart, such as increased risk of pneumonitis, pulmonary fibrosis, coronary artery disease, and clinically significant valvulopathies. Major cardiac event risk is increased with higher doses of radiation starting with just a few Gy, with no apparent ceiling.

9. Anxiety and depression in the perioperative period place patients at risk for all the following, *except*

a. Higher risk of chronic pain.
b. Risk of opioid dependence.
c. Length of stay.
d. Patient's self-reported subjective degree of physical recovery.

The correct answer is b.

Increased anxiety predicts negative short-term operative outcomes, rate of recovery, and length of stay. Depression is associated with a higher incidence of chronic pain.

REFERENCES

1. Armitage JO, Gascoyne RD, Lunning MA, Cavalli F. Non-Hodgkin lymphoma. *Lancet*. 2017;390(10091):298–310. doi:10.1016/S0140-6736(16)32407-2
2. Ng AK, Dabaja BS, Hoppe RT, Illidge T, Yahalom J. Re-examining the role of radiation therapy for diffuse large B-cell lymphoma in the modern era. *J Clin Oncol*. 2016;34(13):1443–1447. doi:10.1200/JCO.2015.64.9418
3. Scully RE, Lipshultz SE. Anthracycline cardiotoxicity in long-term survivors of childhood cancer. *Cardiovasc Toxicol*. 2007;7(2):122–128. doi:10.1007/s12012-007-0006-4
4. Mertens AC, Yasui Y, Neglia JP, et al. Late mortality experience in five-year survivors of childhood and adolescent cancer: The Childhood Cancer Survivor Study. *J Clin Oncol*. 2001;19(13):3163–3172. doi:10.1200/JCO.2001.19.13.3163
5. Haugnes HS, Oldenburg J, Bremnes RM. Pulmonary and cardiovascular toxicity in long-term testicular cancer survivors. *Urol Oncol Semin Orig Investig*. 2015;33(9):399–406. doi:10.1016/j.urolonc.2014.11.012
6. Donat SM, Levy DA. Bleomycin associated pulmonary toxicity: Is perioperative oxygen restriction necessary? *J Urol*. 1998;160(4):1347–1352. doi:10.1016/S0022-5347(01)62533-3
7. De Ruysscher D, Niedermann G, Burnet NG, Siva S, Lee AWM, Hegi-Johnson F. Radiotherapy toxicity. *Nat Rev Dis Prim*. 2019;5(1). doi:10.1038/s41572-019-0064-5
8. Illidge T, Specht L, Yahalom J, et al. Modern radiation therapy for nodal non-hodgkin lymphoma—Target definition and dose guidelines from the international lymphoma radiation oncology group. *Int J Radiat Oncol Biol Phys*. 2014;89(1):49–58. doi:10.1016/j.ijrobp.2014.01.006
9. Lowry L, Smith P, Qian W, et al. Reduced dose radiotherapy for local control in non-Hodgkin lymphoma: A randomised phase III trial. *Radiother Oncol*. 2011;100(1):86–92. doi:10.1016/j.radonc.2011.05.013
10. Friedman DL, Whitton J, Leisenring W, et al. Subsequent neoplasms in 5-year survivors of childhood cancer: The childhood cancer survivor study. *J Natl Cancer Inst*. 2010;102(14):1083–1095. doi:10.1093/jnci/djq238
11. Burt LM, Ying J, Poppe MM, et al. Risk of secondary malignancies after radiation therapy for breast cancer: Comprehensive results. *Breast*. 2018;35(2):85–94. doi:10.3857/roj.2018.00290
12. Pirani M, Marcheselli R, Marcheselli L, Bari A, Federico M, Sacchi S. Risk for second malignancies in non-Hodgkin's lymphoma survivors: A meta-analysis. *Ann Oncol*. 2011;22(8):1845–1858. doi:10.1093/annonc/mdq697
13. Floyd JD, Nguyen DT, Lobins RL, Bashir Q, Doll DC, Perry MC. Cardiotoxicity of cancer therapy. *J Clin Oncol*. 2005;23(30):7685–7696. doi:10.1200/JCO.2005.08.789
14. Harbeck N, Gnant M. Breast cancer. *Lancet*. 2017;389(10074):1134–1150. doi:10.1016/S0140-6736(16)31891-8
15. Chen J, Long JB, Hurria A, Owusu C, Steingart RM, Gross CP. Incidence of heart failure or cardiomyopathy after adjuvant trastuzumab therapy for breast cancer. *J Am Coll Cardiol*. 2012;60(24):2504–2512. doi:10.1016/j.jacc.2012.07.068
16. Belzile-Dugas E, Eisenberg MJ. Radiation-induced cardiovascular disease: Review of an underrecognized pathology. *J Am Heart Assoc*. 2021;10(18):1–10. doi:10.1161/JAHA.121.021686
17. Walker AJ, West J, Card TR, Crooks C, Kirwan CC, Grainge MJ. When are breast cancer patients at highest risk of venous thromboembolism? A cohort study using English health care data. *Blood*. 2016;127(7):849–857. doi:10.1182/blood-2015-01-625582
18. Amir E, Seruga B, Niraula S, Carlsson L, Ocaña A. Toxicity of adjuvant endocrine therapy in postmenopausal breast cancer patients: A systematic review and meta-analysis. *J Natl Cancer Inst*. 2011;103(17):1299–1309. doi:10.1093/jnci/djr242
19. Xie L, Lin C, Zhang H, Bao X. Second malignancy in young early-stage breast cancer patients with modern radiotherapy: A long-term population-based study (A STROBE-compliant study). *Medicine (Baltimore)*. 2018;97(17):e0593.
20. Asdourian MS, Skolny MN, Brunelle C, Seward CE, Salama L, Taghian AG. Precautions for breast cancer-related lymphoedema: Risk from air travel, ipsilateral arm blood pressure measurements, skin puncture, extreme temperatures, and cellulitis. *Lancet Oncol*. 2016;17(9):e392–e405. doi:10.1016/S1470-2045(16)30204-2
21. Lewis AL, Chaft J, Girotra M, Fischer GW. Immune checkpoint inhibitors: A narrative review of considerations for the anaesthesiologist. *Br J Anaesth*. 2020;124(3):251–260. doi:10.1016/j.bja.2019.11.034
22. Ryder M, Callahan M, Postow MA, Wolchok J, Fagin JA. Endocrine-related adverse events following ipilimumab in patients with advanced melanoma: A comprehensive retrospective review from a single institution. *Endocr Relat Cancer*. 2014;21(2):371–381. doi:10.1530/ERC-13-0499
23. Barker CA, Kim SK, Budhu S, Matsoukas K, Daniyan AF, D'Angelo SP. Cytokine release syndrome after radiation therapy: Case report and review of the literature. *J Immunother Cancer*. 2018;6(1):1–7. doi:10.1186/s40425-017-0311-9
24. Bouhassira D, Luporsi E, Krakowski I. Prevalence and incidence of chronic pain with or without neuropathic characteristics in patients with cancer. *Pain*. 2017;158(6):1118–1125. doi:10.1097/j.pain.0000000000000895
25. Fleisher LA, Fleischmann KE, Auerbach AD, et al. 2014 ACC/AHA guideline on perioperative cardiovascular evaluation and management of patients undergoing noncardiac surgery: A report of the American College of Cardiology/American Heart Association Task Force on Practice Guidelines. *Circulation*. 2014;130(24):2215–2245. doi:10.1161/CIR.0000000000000106
26. Boujibar F, Gravier FE, Selim J, Baste JM. Preoperative assessment for minimally invasive lung surgery: Need an update? *Thorac Cancer*. 2021;12(1):3–4. doi:10.1111/1759-7714.13753
27. Attaar A, Winger DG, Luketich JD, et al. A clinical prediction model for prolonged air leak after pulmonary resection. *J Thorac Cardiovasc Surg*. 2017;153(3):690–699.e2. doi:10.1016/j.jtcvs.2016.10.003
28. Mueller MR, Marzluf BA. The anticipation and management of air leaks and residual spaces post lung resection. *J Thorac Dis*. 2014;6(3):271–284. doi:10.3978/j.issn.2072-1439.2013.11.29
29. Ludwig H, Müldür E, Endler G, Hübl W. Prevalence of iron deficiency across different tumors and its association with poor performance status, disease status, and anemia. *Ann Oncol Off J Eur Soc Med Oncol*. 2013;24(7):1886–1892. doi:10.1093/annonc/mdt118
30. Henry DH. Parenteral iron therapy in cancer-associated anemia. *Hematology Am Soc Hematol Educ Program*. 2010;1:351–356. doi:10.1182/asheducation-2010.1.351
31. Clevenger B, Gurusamy K, Klein AA, Murphy GJ, Anker SD, Richards T. Systematic review and meta-analysis of iron therapy in anaemic adults without chronic kidney disease: Updated and abridged Cochrane review. *Eur J Heart Fail*. 2016;18(7):774–785. doi:10.1002/ejhf.514
32. Shin HW, Park JJ, Kim HJ, You HS, Choi SU, Lee MJ. Efficacy of perioperative intravenous iron therapy for transfusion in orthopedic surgery: A systematic review and meta-analysis. *PLoS One*. 2019;14(5):1–17. doi:10.1371/JOURNAL.PONE.0215469
33. Klein AA, Chau M, Yeates JA, et al. Preoperative intravenous iron before cardiac surgery: A prospective multicentre feasibility study. *Br J Anaesth*. 2020;124(3):243–250. doi:10.1016/j.bja.2019.11.023
34. Spahn DR, Schoenrath F, Spahn GH, et al. Effect of ultra-short-term treatment of patients with iron deficiency or anaemia undergoing cardiac surgery: A prospective randomised trial. *Lancet*. 2019;393(10187):2201–2212. doi:10.1016/S0140-6736(18)32555-8
35. Cata JP, Wang H, Gottumukkala V, Reuben J, Sessler DI. Inflammatory response, immunosuppression, and cancer recurrence after perioperative blood transfusions. *Br J Anaesth*. 2013;110(5):690–701. doi:10.1093/bja/aet068
36. Mulder FI, Horváth-Puhó E, van Es N, et al. Venous thromboembolism in cancer patients: A population-based cohort study. *Blood*. 2021;137(14):1959–1969. doi:10.1182/blood.2020007338

37. Khorana AA, Mackman N, Falanga A, et al. Cancer-associated venous thromboembolism. *Nat Rev Dis Prim.* 2022;8(1). doi:10.1038/s41572-022-00336-y
38. Horlocker TT, Vandermeulen E, Kopp SL, Gogarten W, Leffert LR, Benzon HT. Regional anesthesia in the patient receiving antithrombotic or thrombolytic therapy: American Society of Regional Anesthesia and Pain Medicine evidence-based guidelines (Fourth Edition). *Reg Anesth Pain Med.* 2018;43(3):263–309. doi:10.1097/AAP.0000000000000763
39. Durrand J, Singh SJ, Danjoux G. Prehabilitation. *Clin Med (Northfield Il).* 2019;19(6):458–464. doi:10.7861/clinmed.2019-0257
40. Levett DZH, Grimmett C. Psychological factors, prehabilitation and surgical outcomes: Evidence and future directions. *Anaesthesia.* 2019;74:36–42. doi:10.1111/anae.14507
41. Rosenberger PH, Jokl P, Ickovics J. Psychosocial factors and surgical outcomes: An evidence-based literature review. *J Am Acad Orthop Surg.* 2006;14(7):397–405. doi:10.5435/00124635-200607000-00002
42. Gillis C, Li C, Lee L, et al. Prehabilitation versus rehabilitation: A randomized control trial in patients undergoing colorectal resection for cancer. *Anesthesiology.* 2014;121(5):937–947. doi:10.1097/ALN.0000000000000393
43. Gritz ER, Fingeret MC, Vidrine DJ, Lazev AB, Mehta NV, Reece GP. Successes and failures of the teachable moment: Smoking cessation in cancer patients. *Cancer.* 2006;106(1):17–27. doi:10.1002/cncr.21598
44. Esra YE, Aziz Y, Zeki U, et al. Is chemotherapy-induced nausea and vomiting lower in smokers? *Int J Clin Pharmacol Ther.* 2011;49(12):709–712.
45. Carrick MA, Robson JM, Thomas C. Smoking and anaesthesia. *BJA Educ.* 2019;19(1):1–6. doi:10.1016/j.bjae.2018.09.005
46. Yoong S, Tursan d'Espaingnet E, Wiggers J, et al. WHO tobacco knowledge summaries: Tobacco and postsurgical outcomes. *Geneva World Heal Organ.* 2020:1–25.
47. Grønkjær M, Eliasen M, Skov-Ettrup LS, et al. Preoperative smoking status and postoperative complications: A systematic review and meta-analysis. *Ann Surg.* 2014;259(1):52–71. doi:10.1097/SLA.0b013e3182911913
48. Sørensen LT. Wound healing and infection in surgery. *Ann Surg.* 2012;255(6):1069–1079. doi:10.1097/sla.0b013e31824f632d
49. Feinstein MM, Katz D. Sparking the discussion about vaping and anesthesia. *Anesthesiology.* 2020;132(3):599–599. doi:10.1097/ALN.0000000000003093
50. Echeverria-Villalobos M, Todeschini AB, Stoicea N, Fiorda-Diaz J, Weaver T, Bergese SD. Perioperative care of cannabis users: A comprehensive review of pharmacological and anesthetic considerations. *J Clin Anesth.* 2019;57(March):41–49. doi:10.1016/j.jclinane.2019.03.011
51. Ratna A, Mandrekar P. Alcohol and cancer: Mechanisms and therapies. *Biomolecules.* 2017;7(3):1–20. doi:10.3390/biom7030061
52. Voskoboinik A, Kalman JM, De Silva A, et al. Alcohol abstinence in drinkers with atrial fibrillation. *N Engl J Med.* 2020;382(1):20–28. doi:10.1056/nejmoa1817591
53. Frendl G, Sodickson AC, Chung MK, et al. 2014 AATS guidelines for the prevention and management of perioperative atrial fibrillation and flutter for thoracic surgical procedures. *J Thorac Cardiovasc Surg.* 2014;148(3):e153–e193. doi:10.1016/j.jtcvs.2014.06.036
54. Barberan-Garcia A, Ubré M, Roca J, et al. Personalised prehabilitation in high-risk patients undergoing elective major abdominal surgery: A randomized blinded controlled trial. *Ann Surg.* 2018;267(1):50–56. doi:10.1097/SLA.0000000000002293
55. Tew GA, Batterham AM, Colling K, et al. Randomized feasibility trial of high-intensity interval training before elective abdominal aortic aneurysm repair. *Br J Surg.* 2017;104(13):1791–1801. doi:10.1002/bjs.10669
56. Batchelor TJP, Rasburn NJ, Abdelnour-Berchtold E, et al. Guidelines for enhanced recovery after lung surgery: Recommendations of the Enhanced Recovery after Surgery (ERAS) Society and the European Society of Thoracic Surgeons (ESTS). *Eur J Cardio-thoracic Surg.* 2019;55(1):91–115. doi:10.1093/ejcts/ezy301
57. Petroni ML, Caletti MT, Grave RD, Bazzocchi A, Aparisi Gómez MP, Marchesini G. Prevention and treatment of sarcopenic obesity in women. *Nutrients.* 2019;11(6):1–24. doi:10.3390/nu11061302
58. Aubertin-Leheudre M, Lord C, Khalil A, Dionne IJ. Six months of isoflavone supplement increases fat-free mass in obese-sarcopenic postmenopausal women: A randomized double-blind controlled trial. *Eur J Clin Nutr.* 2007;61(12):1442–1444. doi:10.1038/sj.ejcn.1602695
59. Baracos VE, Arribas L. Sarcopenic obesity: Hidden muscle wasting and its impact for survival and complications of cancer therapy. *Ann Oncol.* 2018;29(Supplement 2):ii1–ii9. doi:10.1093/annonc/mdx810

PART VIII

PACU

45.
DISCHARGE CRITERIA IN DEVELOPMENTALLY DISABLED PATIENT WITH OSA

Jonathan L. Wong and Mana Saraghi

STEM CASE AND KEY QUESTIONS

A 28-year-old overweight nonverbal man with profound developmental delay has had a decreased appetite as noted by his caregivers for the past 2 weeks. He resides in an adult care home for the developmentally disabled. The staff states he is increasingly agitated and has been hitting himself on his face for the past week. In addition, the caregivers also report a history of increasing difficulty delivering oral hygiene because the patient becomes combative on attempts to brush his teeth at night. He was evaluated by a dentist who was only able to complete a very limited oral evaluation due to the patient's developmental delay. The dentist has appointed the patient for examination under anesthesia and full mouth dental rehabilitation in the dental office. The patient's guardian states that he is healthy except for his developmental delay, and he had no anesthesia complications after his adenotonsillectomy when he was 13 years of age due to obstructive sleep apnea (OSA). However, the staff states that he snores loudly at night.

What is sleep-disordered breathing? How is it diagnosed and treated?

The patient is seen by the otolaryngologist who performed his adenotonsillectomy. A polysomnography (sleep study) is requested, but, due to the patient's developmental delay, the study could not be performed. Similarly, he was uncooperative with an attempt at a home sleep study. Because the patient was unable to cooperate, it is determined that it will be impossible to achieve any compliance with continuous positive airway pressure (CPAP). The otolaryngologist recommended no further surgical intervention at this time.

How else might you screen for OSA?

A review of the medical records from the adult care home reveals that the facility's physician has been encouraging dietary improvement and exercise due to the patient's obesity. It also appears that the physician has been following the patient for elevated blood pressure readings in the past. The anesthesiologist, concerned about the feasibility of office-based sedation, notifies the dentist that the procedure will need to be performed under general anesthesia with a definitive airway in place.

What concerns do you have for sedation and office-based anesthesia? What considerations do you have for pain management in the OSA patient?

At the anesthesiologist's request, the dentist has scheduled the patient for his procedure at an ambulatory surgical facility where the dentist has privileges. The patient is evaluated in the anesthesia preoperative assessment clinic. During a review of the medication reconciliation, the anesthesiologist noticed that the patient has been started on ibuprofen and acetaminophen with codeine "as needed for pain" by the dentist. The dentist stated that she was concerned that the patient may have increasing tooth pain. On examination, the patient can be seen rapidly pacing around the clinic, and he becomes very loud and upset when the nursing staff attempts to take him to the examination room and obtain his vital signs. The examination is unremarkable except for the fact that the patient is overweight, developmentally delayed, and would not sit still for the staff to obtain a blood pressure.

What is your anesthetic plan for induction? What are your considerations or concerns?

Given the patient's uncooperative behavior at the preoperative assessment clinic, the anesthesiologist has elected to induce the patient with an IM injection of midazolam and ketamine. The patient will then be taken to the operating room, standard ASA monitoring performed, an IV established, and the case performed under general anesthesia with a nasal endotracheal tube in place. The anesthesiologist also recommends discontinuing the preoperative acetaminophen with codeine and using a non-opioid technique. Fortunately, the facility has not administered the medications because the patient was not complaining of pain or discomfort.

What other perioperative management concerns do you have for the OSA patient? Are there any guidelines that assist in the anesthesiologist's decision-making?

The anesthesiologist would like to use an opioid-sparing technique, especially in the postoperative period. To accomplish this goal, the anesthesiologist will employ a multimodal analgesic approach using ketorolac and acetaminophen. In addition, the anesthesiologist has asked that the dentist use local anesthesia to relieve postoperative pain. The dentist has voiced concern that the patient may inadvertently "chew his lip," and that it will likely be unnecessary for routine dental rehabilitation. The anesthesiologist has also spoken with the nursing staff in the PACU, using Situation, Background, Assessment, and Recommendation (SBAR) communication and recommending that the patient be closely monitored in recovery.

What are the causes of sleep apnea/sleep-disordered breathing? How would you manage the airway in a difficult OSA patient?

The patient is induced via IM injection as planned. The injection required the assistance of several caregivers and nursing staff to provide gentle restraint and protective stabilization because the patient was particularly uncooperative as his usual daily schedule was disrupted by the NPO/dietary restrictions and interruption of his normal daily activities. As the medications take effect, the sedated patient is coaxed to the gurney. The anesthesiologist notes that the patient's airway is obstructed, suctions the airway, and provides airway support. A nasal pharyngeal airway is placed, and the patient is immediately taken to the more controlled environment of the operating room. In the operating room, monitors are placed and IV access is obtained. The anesthesiologist elected to use succinylcholine as the paralytic agent during intubation due to airway compromise. During laryngoscopy for nasal intubation, the anesthesiologist noted hypertrophic lingual tonsils, but bag mask ventilation was achieved with the nasal pharyngeal airway in place and the intubation was not difficult (Figure 45.1).

The dentist performs the dental examination and notifies the anesthesiologist that several of the molars, including the wisdom teeth, are carious and nonrestorable. Instead of performing restorations (fillings), these teeth will need surgical extraction (removal) and may cause pain and discomfort postoperatively. In addition, the dentist asks to leave ligated gauze dressings in the mouth during recovery for hemostasis.

How would you manage this patient's airway for extubation and recovery? What are your criteria for discharge from the PACU?

The dentist and anesthesiologist agreed on a long-acting local anesthetic used for trigeminal nerve blocks for postoperative pain management. The dentist also placed resorbable hemostatic dressings into the extraction sites and sutured them in place for hemostasis. Dexamethasone was administered to reduce edema of the airway from surgical extractions. In addition to the aforementioned local measures, sufficient time was allowed for the gauze to exert pressure on the extraction sites to ensure that hemostasis was achieved prior to the start of emergence from anesthesia. The patient was extubated awake with a nasal pharyngeal airway in place. The anesthesiologist also ensured that the patient was able to maintain his cardiorespiratory status on room air prior to transport to the PACU. The anesthesiologist gave a thorough report and hand-off to the supervising anesthesiologist of the PACU and the nursing staff of the intraoperative events and recovery concerns and recommendations.

Does the anesthesiologist have any guidelines to reference for determining when the patient may be discharged home? Are there any physiologic concerns for the patient after meeting criteria for discharge home?

The nasal pharyngeal airway remained in place until the patient was alert enough to remove it himself. The nursing staff weaned the patient to room air. The facility's written discharge criteria (Modified Aldrete score) were met, and the patient remained stable with no apneic or hypopnea events for an hour after the airway was removed and discharge criteria were met. Postoperative instructions were carefully reviewed with the adult care home caregivers, and the patient was discharged home without complications.

DISCUSSION

"Sleep-disordered breathing" is a term that encompasses several chronic disorders that are characterized by apnea or hypopnea during sleep. OSA is a periodic partial or complete obstruction of the airway that occurs during periods of sleep or unconsciousness. These periodic obstructions result in arterial desaturations and frequent minor ischemia-reperfusion injuries and oxidative stress. OSA is the most common form of sleep-disordered breathing.[1] Central sleep apnea (CSA) occurs due absence of ventilatory drive due to a lack of stimulatory outflow from the respiratory center located in the medulla oblongata.[2] "Mixed apneas" are individual events that begin with a lack of ventilatory drive but become obstructive.[3] "Complex sleep apnea" is a term used specifically when CSA is unmasked during titration of CPAP for OSA.[3] Sleep apnea events are defined as either *apneas*, the cessation of breathing, or *hypopneas*, a marked reduction in airflow. Apneic events are considered clinically relevant if lasting more than 10 seconds.[4]

EPIDEMIOLOGY

OSA is a very common clinical problem affecting 24% of men and 9% of women.[4] It is also well described in pediatric patients with adenotonsillar hypertrophy,[5] and there has been a rise in OSA concurrent with childhood obesity.[6] Because OSA is often asymptomatic, an estimated 82% of men and

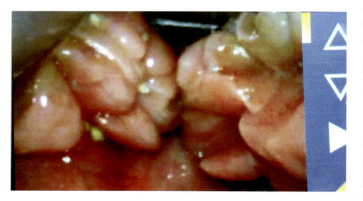

Figure 45.1 Lingual tonsils on laryngoscopy.

92% of women with moderate to severe OSA have not been diagnosed.[4]

ETIOLOGY AND PATHOGENESIS

The human pharynx should be considered a collapsible tube that lacks rigid skeletal support. The pharynx makes up the supraglottic airway and is thereby under the stress of negative pressure during normal inspiration. If the negative pressure of inspiration, in combination with any additional external forces (such as obesity), overcomes the muscle tone of the dilator muscles of the pharynx, the upper airway will collapse. Thus, both anatomic and neuromuscular factors are involved in the development of OSA.[7]

OSA is usually more pronounced during rapid eye movement (REM) sleep. This is likely due to muscle atonia that occurs during REM sleep.[8] Although it is commonly cited that the tongue is the major cause of obstruction, there is increasing literature that suggests that factors such as cross-sectional area of the pharynx, thickness and compliance of parapharyngeal muscular walls, and overall length of the pharynx may play a role.[9-13] Nevertheless, the most common factors contributing to OSA are obesity and skeletal malocclusions such as retrognathia or maxilla-mandibular hypoplasia.[7]

The repeated arousals cause fragmented sleep and cause daytime sleepiness. The repeated cycles of desaturation and reperfusion cause oxidative stress and reperfusion injuries that promote the inflammatory cascade.[14] This has also been shown to decrease parasympathetic activity and increase sympathetic activity.[15] Such pathophysiology is believed to be the root cause of the association of OSA with cardiovascular disease, cerebrovascular disease, and metabolic dysfunction. In fact, OSA is the most common condition associated with drug-resistant hypertension, with a prevalence of 64%.[16]

SYMPTOMS

Although daytime sleepiness is the principal symptom of OSA, other common symptoms include

- Loud snoring
- Choking or shortness of breath sensations during sleep
- Restless sleep
- Changes in personality
- Nocturia
- Enuresis
- Morning headaches
- Reduced libido
- Nocturnal sweating

Symptoms of children with OSA often include hyperactivity, poor academic performance and difficulty in school, inability to concentrate, and nocturnal enuresis.

DIAGNOSIS

Sleep apnea is diagnosed by polysomnography (PSG) at a sleep lab (type I). The study consists of electroencephalography (EEG), electromyography (EMG), electrooculography (EOG), ECG, oxygen saturation, respiratory effort, and airflow. Because many people are unwilling or intolerant (as in our stem case) of undergoing sleep studies at a sleep lab, efforts have been made to create portable sleep study devices. However, most of these devices have little or no evidence to support their use as a diagnostic test for OSA.[17] The polysomnography should be read and interpreted by a physician with a subspecialty and certification in sleep medicine. However, if an assessment of the severity of the patient's OSA is not present in the report, the Apnea Hypopnea Index (AHI) may be used to judge severity. The AHI tracks the average number of apneas and hypopneas, or abnormal respiratory events, per hour of sleep.[18] It is important to note that the grading criteria differ vastly between adults and children, as reflected in Table 45.1.

SCREENING

OSA is a very prevalent and often undiagnosed condition that is also associated with many common comorbidities. As such, there are numerous screening tools reported in the literature.[19,20] Four screening tools have emerged as prevalent in the practice of anesthesia. These are the Berlin Questionnaire (BQ), STOP, STOP-Bang, and the American Society of Anesthesiologists (ASA) OSA Checklist.

The BQ is a self-report instrument consisting of 10 questions organized into three categories. Although designed to screen for undiagnosed sleep apneas, it has been criticized as being difficult to memorize for practitioners and difficult for patients to answer. In addition, it has a complex scoring system that limits its usefulness for the anesthesiologist.[21]

The ASA OSA Checklist is a 14-item checklist, also spread across three categories, that was developed to assist

Table 45.1 SEVERITY OF OBSTRUCTIVE SLEEP APNEA BY THE APNEA HYPOPNEA INDEX (AHI), PEDIATRIC VS. ADULT

SEVERITY OF SLEEP APNEA	PEDIATRIC	ADULT
None	0	<5
Mild OSA	1–5	5–14
Moderate OSA	6–10	15–30
Severe OSA	>10	>30

Adult scoring should be used in patients 18 years of age and older.

Pediatric scoring should be used in patients under the age of 13.

Adolescents may use either system.

In adults, events are scored if lasting > 10 seconds. For pediatrics, the duration of event must be ≥2 missed breaths.

Adapted from Kimoff[5] and American Society of Anesthesiologists Task Force on Perioperative Management of Patients with Obstructive Sleep Apnea.[23]

anesthesiologists in identifying patients with OSA.[22,23] The ASA OSA Checklist identifies patients as being at high risk for OSA when the anesthesiologist determines that they score positive for any items across two of the three categories. The categories are (1) predisposing physical characteristics such as enlarged tonsils or high BMI; (2) history of apparent airway obstructions during sleep, including frequent or loud snoring and observed pauses in breathing; and (3) somnolence, such as fatigue despite adequate "sleep" or falling asleep in a nonstimulating environment (or at school for children). This checklist was a consensus of the ASA Task Force on Perioperative Management and has not been validated in any patient population.[4]

Due to the underdiagnosis of OSA, Chung et al. developed and validated the STOP questionnaire. The aim of the STOP questionnaire was to create a widespread and easy to use OSA screening tool for surgical patients using simple yes or no questions that patients could readily understand. Consisting of only four questions and using the acronym STOP, Chung et al. hoped that the questions would be easy and efficient to use. The questions are

S: "Do you *S*nore loudly (louder than talking or loud enough to be heard through closed doors)?"

T: "Do you often feel *T*ired, fatigued, or sleepy during daytime?"

O: "Has anyone *O*bserved you stop breathing during your sleep?"

P: "Do you have or are you being treated for high blood *P*ressure?"[24]

The STOP Questionnaire was shown to have a moderate level of sensitivity and specificity in detecting patients with OSA and was best able to screen for those patients with moderate to severe sleep apnea. Chung et al. found that by incorporating the clinical characteristics of BMI, age, neck circumference, and gender into the STOP questionnaire, the screening tool had a very high level of sensitivity and negative predictive value. The questions in "Bang" are

B: "*B*ody Mass Index (BMI) more than 35 kg/m^2?"

A: "*A*ge older than 50?"

N: "*N*eck circumference over 40 cm?"

G: "*G*ender: male?"[24]

This STOP-Bang scoring model allowed the anesthesiologist to be highly confident that the patient did not have moderate to severe sleep apnea if the patient answered yes to fewer than three items.[24]

TREATMENT

The "gold standard" in treatment for OSA is CPAP and, in severe cases, noninvasive positive pressure ventilation (NIPPV) or bi-level positive airway pressure (BiPAP). The positive airway pressure devices serve as a pneumatic splint preventing collapse of the upper airway. Not only does this keep the airway enlarged and decrease airway edema, but there is evidence that the use of CPAP increases the tone of the upper airway dilator muscles even when the CPAP is not in use.[25] Unfortunately, compliance can be a major issue with the use of these devices with as many as 50% of patients discontinuing their therapy within the first 4 weeks.[26] Additionally, lifestyle modification can play an important role as well. Modifications include weight loss; cessation of smoking, alcohol, and sedative use; and avoiding the supine position when sleeping.[7]

Due to compliance issues with CPAP, an increasing number of dental and surgical interventions claim to treat OSA. These nonventilatory methods of treatment aim at increasing the airway patency by manipulating the orofacial, nasopharyngeal, and hypopharyngeal structures. Examples include turbinectomy, septoplasty, uvulopalatoplasty, hyoid suspensions, maxillomandibular repositioning—both surgical and by means of dental prosthetics—and hypoglossal nerve stimulation. Each of these techniques has widely varying efficacy reported in the literature and at best the results are highly patient-dependent.[27] In fact, the ASA states that "a patient who has had corrective airway surgery should be assumed to remain as risk of OSA complications unless a normal sleep study has been obtained and symptoms have not returned."[23] The exception to this might be the pediatric patient who has undergone adenotonsillectomy, especially if used in combination with palatal expansion (orthodontics).[27,28]

PERIOPERATIVE CONCERNS

Guidelines for Anesthesia Providers

Anesthesia providers have multiple guidelines to consider when treating the OSA patient. The ASA has published "Practice Guidelines for the Perioperative Management of Patients with Obstructive Sleep Apnea," which received an update in 2014.[23] Practice guidelines also exist from the American Academy of Sleep Medicine,[29] the American College of Chest Physicians,[30] the Society of Ambulatory Anesthesia (SAMBA),[31] and the Society of Anesthesia and Sleep Medicine.[32,33]

Preoperative Concerns

Preoperative concerns largely focus on the screening and diagnosis of the surgical patient with OSA. This is largely due to the prevalence and underdiagnosis of OSA and the associated comorbid conditions. However, OSA has also been associated with a higher rate of postoperative morbidity and mortality, as well as difficult airways.[34–36] For ease of discussion, there are largely three types of patients whom the anesthesiologist must consider. First is the patient who has an OSA diagnosis and is compliant with therapy. Second, is the OSA patient who is either untreated or noncompliant with therapy. Third is the suspected OSA patient. There is consensus among the guidelines that one of the screening tools should be used in surgical patients to identify this third type of patient and that the patient care team should be aware of these patients and their associated postoperative complication risks.[22,23,29-31]

The anesthesiologist must also consider the use of the positive airway pressure (PAP) device in the preoperative period. For the patient who has an OSA diagnosis and is compliant with treatment, that treatment, especially PAP, should be continued. PAP therapy has been shown to reduce cardiac arrhythmias and stabilize blood pressure.[37,38] For the OSA patient who is not compliant with treatment, short-term preoperative use of PAP has also been recommended in the guidelines. Corda et al. demonstrated that even as little as 1 week of PAP therapy prior to surgery could improve pharyngeal tone and increase pharyngeal cross-sectional area.[39] Despite consensus approval for PAP, extrapolation of these physiological improvements to the perioperative patient lack sufficient evidence and warrant further research.[32] As such, it may not be cost effective or efficient for the undiagnosed OSA patient to delay surgery to undergo polysomnography and OSA treatment.

The surgeon and the anesthesiologist, as a team, recognizing the increased risk of postoperative complications, must select the venue for the procedure and the anesthesia plan. General anesthesia with a secure airway is preferred to deep sedation without a secure airway.[23] Moderate sedation may be considered and can be used in conjunction with local anesthesia and regional nerve blocks, however, the ASA Guidelines encourage the use of CPAP or an oral appliance during sedation. Unfortunately, dental procedures not only interfere with the use of such appliances, but also promote airway obstruction.

The choice of inpatient versus outpatient or ambulatory anesthesia is controversial, and there is a paucity of literature to support either option.[23,31] Nevertheless, both the ASA and SAMBA offer unvalidated decision-making tools to assist clinicians. The ASA is careful to note that their "Scoring System for Perioperative Risk from OSA: Example" is just that, an example. They recommend that the decision be made on a case-by-case basis considering factors such as "sleep apnea status, anatomical and physiological abnormalities, status of coexisting diseases, nature of surgery, type of anesthesia, need for postoperative opioids, patient age, adequacy of post discharge observation, and capabilities of the facility."[23] SAMBA has offered guidance in the fashion of a decision-making algorithm, shown in Figure 45.2[31].

Intraoperative Concerns

The anesthesiologist must consider the pharmacologic implications of the medications chosen for the anesthetic course. Although most of the literature has focused on the postoperative concerns for opioid analgesics, both with and without benzodiazepines, the anesthesiologist must also be acutely aware of the sequelae and pharmacology of the medications given during the intraoperative period.

Preoperative sedatives may be required in the developmentally delayed patient because the patient may be uncooperative,

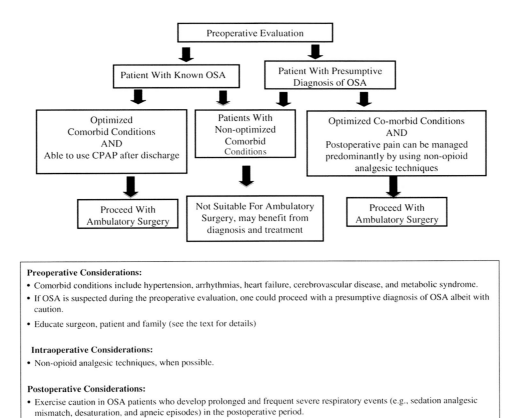

Figure 45.2 Decision-making in preoperative selection of a patient with obstructive sleep apnea scheduled for ambulatory surgery.

making IV access or even entering the operating room for induction difficult. Two common sedation techniques employ enteral benzodiazepines and IM ketamine. However, benzodiazepines and barbiturates have been shown to increase airway resistance in healthy non-OSA patients.[40] Additionally, benzodiazepines, even at a dose of 0.25 mg of triazolam, have been shown to cause obstruction and desaturations in the OSA patient.[41,42] By contrast, ketamine preserves ventilatory drive and may preserve upper airway muscular tone and patency in OSA patients and thus may be a good choice for both anesthesia and analgesia for the OSA patient.[43] It is important for the anesthesiologist to remember that these preoperative sedative techniques may have a significant impact on patient recovery and discharge.[23]

The anesthesiologist's choice of neuromuscular blockers and agents for maintenance of anesthesia has also been shown to play a role in postoperative complications. Evidence suggests that judicious use of neuromuscular blocking agents and ensuring full reversal may decrease risk for the OSA patient. However, there is insufficient evidence in the literature to guide the practitioner in the choice of neuromuscular blocking agent or the reversal of such agents.[33] Healthy (non-OSA) individuals have been shown to have greater risk of upper airway collapse even with minimal neuromuscular blockade (NMB).[44,45]

Similarly, there is insufficient evidence to guide the practitioner in the use of agents for maintenance of anesthesia.[33] In one systematic review of the literature, Ankichetty et al. found no statistically significant increase in desaturation between OSA and non-OSA patients receiving desflurane, propofol, and remifentanil for general anesthesia with a secured airway. They did observe a statistically significant increase in desaturations among patients receiving isoflurane and propofol together.[46] There is sufficient evidence to suggest that the use of propofol for procedural sedation in the OSA patient does present increased perioperative complications.[33] Although not directly related to the OSA patient, Liu et al.'s systematic review of anesthetic agents in obese patients found that desflurane followed by sevoflurane were the most favorable anesthetic agents for rapid recovery and higher postoperative oxygen saturations.[47]

There is expert consensus that general anesthesia with a secure airway is preferable to deep sedation without a secure airway. In addition, the consensus is that patients with increased risk from OSA, unless there is a medical or surgical contraindication, should be extubated awake after full reversal of NMB has been verified. A nonsupine position, such as lateral or semi-upright, is preferred for extubation and recovery.[23] For dental and oral surgical patients, the anesthesiologist and surgeon must be vigilant in ensuring that the airway is clean and clear. This includes removal of the throat pack, adequate hemostasis, and removal of all dental materials and dressings as these will further obstruct and increase airway closing pressure. Finally, there is concern of postoperative edema to the airway from surgical manipulation and, in the orthognathic patient, the possibility that the mouth will either be wired closed or fixed with elastic ligatures. In these orthognathic cases, it is imperative that the appropriate equipment

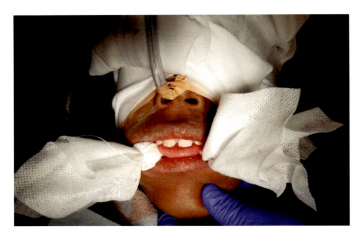

Figure 45.3 Intraoral dental dressings for extraction of teeth.

is immediately available at bedside to cut or remove these devices expeditiously and that the care team is aware of their presence and use (Figure 45.3).

Postoperative Concerns

The major postoperative concern for patients with known or suspected OSA is the potential for apneic events and subsequent desaturations which, if undetected, can lead to cerebral and myocardial infarction, arrhythmias, and even death. A multimodal analgesic approach in which opioids are reserved for severe breakthrough pain will limit the amount of opioids administered to the patient.

As discussed in the stem case, the patient was extubated fully awake with complete recovery from NMB and anesthetic agents. The patient was able to demonstrate the ability to maintain saturation on room air prior to transport to the PACU. Awake extubation is also indicated in dental and maxillofacial procedures; the patient must have recovered protective airway reflexes because the procedure itself may result in swelling and edema in the upper airway as well as the risk of residual blood and debris in the airway.[23] In the PACU, the patient should remain at least semi-upright or in the lateral decubitus position, avoiding lying completely supine, to optimize functional residual capacity and airway tone.

Multimodal analgesic techniques intercept pain pharmacologically in many different inputs along the afferent pain pathway. The use of different medications that act through differing mechanisms of action achieves analgesia synergistically while using lower doses of each drug. The adverse effects or toxicities of each medication are also reduced because adverse drug reactions are also dose-related. While many medications can intercept pain, postoperative analgesia will primarily involve local anesthetics, NSAIDs, acetaminophen (APAP), and, for severe breakthrough pain, opioids. N-methyl-D-aspartic acid (NMDA) antagonists such as ketamine and alpha-2 agonists such as dexmedetomidine play a role intraoperatively but are not appropriate for the patient who is about to be discharged to the unmonitored home environment.

Local anesthesia is at the cornerstone of analgesia in dental practice. Local anesthetics block the transmission of afferent nociceptive input from the surgical site to the central nervous system (CNS); this is accomplished by blocking sodium channels in sensory neurons and preventing propagation of action potentials. Local anesthesia is indicated in virtually all patients receiving dental care. One contraindication is an allergy to local anesthetics. Ester local anesthetics such as procaine (Novocain), tetracaine, or benzocaine have ester linkages and are hydrolyzed by tissue pseudocholinesterases. Their metabolic byproduct, para-aminobenzoic acid (PABA) results in cross-allergenicity among ester local anesthetics and with sulfonamides. Most local anesthetics used today are classified as amides, such as bupivacaine, lidocaine, and mepivacaine. Amides undergo hepatic metabolism and do not produce the metabolite PABA so cross-allergenicity with esters does not occur. A true allergy to amide local anesthetics is rare. Articaine is unique: it has both ester and amide linkages; however, hydrolysis of the ester linkage does not produce PABA.[48] The benefit of profound local anesthetic is that procedures can be completed with less pain, less sympathetic response to pain, and reduced anesthetic requirements (including less opioids) to facilitate rapid recovery with less respiratory depression.[49] Prolonged soft tissue anesthesia of the lips, cheeks, and tongue may be problematic for very young or intellectually impaired patients as they may bite this soft tissue, resulting in ulcerations of the traumatized areas. This can be avoided with strict postoperative monitoring of the patient by caretakers. In the setting of suspected or known OSA, the caregiver should be informed of the risk versus benefit of adequate postoperative analgesia using local anesthetics to reduce intraoperative and postoperative opioid requirements.

Local anesthetics have been often packaged with vasoconstrictors (such as epinephrine) to prolong the duration of anesthesia at the site of infiltration. Agonism of the alpha-1 adrenergic receptors in the oral mucosa results in vasoconstriction of the blood vessels in the area, delaying systemic absorption of local anesthesia. Some providers have mistakenly assumed that if a local anesthetic devoid of vasoconstrictor (such as 3% mepivacaine) was administered instead of 2% lidocaine with 1:100,000 epinephrine, a postoperative self-inflicted trauma such as lip biting would be avoided. However, it has been established that the duration of hard tissue anesthesia is shorter with mepivacaine, yet the duration of soft tissue anesthesia (and thus the potential for lip biting) remains the same. The danger of administering a 3% solution of mepivacaine versus a 2% solution of lidocaine is that mepivacaine is more concentrated and has a lower maximum recommended dose (MRD) (in mg/kg) than lidocaine. For a given patient and their calculated weight-based MRD, there will be a lower maximum volume of mepivacaine allowed to be administered over the surgical site before reaching the maximum recommended dose.[50,51]

Local anesthetic systemic toxicity (LAST) is a potentially serious consequence of local anesthetic overdose, but it is fortunately both rare and avoidable. Systemic toxicity is mediated by the same mechanism of action that produces the desired effects of local anesthesia—in the case of toxicity, blockage of the sodium channels in the CNS and the heart. The resulting toxidrome consists of disorientation, circumoral numbness (not just on the anesthetized side), tinnitus, seizures, arrhythmias, respiratory depression, cardiac arrest, and death.[50,52] Patients are unable to communicate the early signs of disorientation and circumoral numbness or tinnitus under general anesthesia, and the presenting sign may be one of the latter, more serious sequelae such as respiratory depression or cardiovascular collapse. Additionally, anesthesia provider must be vigilant in recording the total amount of local anesthetic administered by both the dentist as well as any IV local anesthetic administered upon anesthetic induction. The different local anesthetics act by the same mechanism of action so their toxicity is also mediated by the same mechanism of action. The toxicity is dose dependent, and once the MRD for one local anesthetic is administered, one cannot administer other local anesthetics (this includes both esters and amides).[50]

Opioid analgesics are indicated for "moderate to moderately severe pain" but should not be considered as the first-line drug of choice for postoperative pain following dental procedures and should be reserved for breakthrough pain refractory to local anesthesia, NSAIDs, and/or acetaminophen.[53] Opioids act most often on mu, delta, and kappa opioid receptors resulting in centrally mediated analgesia along with undesirable side effects such as ileus, constipation, nausea, vomiting, and respiratory depression. Opioids carry a dependence liability, and routine prescribing of opioids in excessive quantities has resulted in a prescription opioid epidemic.[54] Although medications such as acetaminophen and nonsteroidal anti-inflammatory medications (NSAIDs, such as ibuprofen) are available without a prescription, their analgesic efficacy is superior to opioids in the setting of postoperative dental pain.[55-57] Opioid efficacy is further hindered by the fact that some opioids, such as codeine and tramadol, are prodrugs; their active metabolites are morphine and o-desmethyltramadol, respectively. The metabolic activation of these drugs is contingent on the activity of the hepatic microsomal enzyme cytochrome P450 2D6 (CYP450 2D6.) Because of various inheritance patterns for the CYP450 2D6 enzyme, some individuals are rapid or poor metabolizers of codeine. It is thought that approximately 10% of the White population may be a poor metabolizer of CYP2D6 and thus be at risk of having inadequate analgesia. Conversely, patients who have the ultrarapid metabolizer phenotype are at risk for elevated blood levels of the active opioids and thus also at risk for more severe respiratory depressant effects. Furthermore, the activity of CYP2D6 enzymes can be inhibited by other medications such as celecoxib, fluoxetine, paroxetine, quinidine, and sertraline. Dexamethasone is an inducer of CYP 2D6 that can enhance the metabolic activation of these analgesic prodrugs.[55,58,59]

Studies evaluating the analgesic efficacy of NSAIDs, acetaminophen, and opioids have demonstrated that NSAIDs provide effective analgesia for dental pain.[54,56,57,60] The mechanism of action for NSAIDs reduces the propagation of inflammatory mediators, thus addressing the source of the pain. Arachidonic acid is cleaved from a damaged cell membrane by phospholipase A2. Arachidonic acid is then metabolized to prostaglandins by COX1 and COX2. Dexamethasone, a glucocorticoid, inhibits phospholipase A2 and therefore has anti-inflammatory and opioid-sparing effects.[61] The NSAIDs act by inhibiting COX1 and COX2, thus reducing the production of inflammatory mediators called prostaglandins. Some prostaglandins serve constitutive functions, such as protecting the gastrointestinal mucosa and maintaining renal blood flow and sodium and water balance. Therefore, inhibition of these prostaglandins is responsible for NSAID side effects. GI side effects can result in gastrointestinal bleeds, perforations, and ulcers—this can be problematic for patients with a history of ulcers. The bleeding risk can be potentiated by the concomitant use of other anticoagulants such as warfarin.[55] Antidepressants of the selective serotonin reuptake inhibitor (SSRI) class can also potentiate the bleeding risk of NSAIDs.[62,63] The renal side effects of NSAIDs are a concern for patients with renal disease or hypertension, and for those taking drugs that require normal renal function such as angiotensin converting enzyme (ACE) inhibitors, beta blockers, diuretics, and lithium. Even 5 days of NSAID therapy can interfere with antihypertensive medications so patients should be warned to monitor their blood pressure at home, or, in the case of lithium, they may need to have their blood lithium levels checked because lithium is a medication with a very narrow therapeutic index.[55,64-66] NSAIDs may also be contraindicated in patients with hypersensitivity to NSAIDs or aspirin, or aspirin-sensitive asthma.[49]

N-acetyl-p-aminophenol (also known as APAP, acetaminophen, or paracetamol) is another analgesic and antipyretic. Its mechanism of action is not well understood. APAP has notably less anti-inflammatory activity than NSAIDs. APAPs should not be used in patients with allergy to APAP. Hepatotoxicity is a concern with excessive consumption of APAP exceeding a maximum daily dose of 4 g.[60] While APAP does not have the same antiplatelet activity as NSAIDs, it is possible that, with acute hepatotoxicity, the production of coagulation factors may be affected. It is also possible that APAP shares a liver microsomal pathway with warfarin, and an increase in the INR may be seen. The INR should be monitored after a week of APAP therapy.[55,67,68] Many studies have demonstrated the analgesic efficacy of combinations of NSAIDs, particularly ibuprofen and APAP for postoperative dental pain. This combination can provide effective analgesia without opioids and their side effects, notably CNS and respiratory depression.[60]

It is imperative for the healthcare provider prescribing analgesics to discuss the risks, benefits, and appropriate use and storage of these very potent agents. Opioids can cause respiratory depression and carry the potential for abuse, misuse, and diversion. The patient and/or their caregiver should be given explicit instructions to monitor the patient for snoring, gasping, or any other difficulty breathing. Caretakers should be informed about the availability of naloxone, a rescue agent to reverse opioid-induced respiratory depression and loss of consciousness. Intranasal and IM formulations are available in the United States for use by laypersons. This reversal agent should be made available to OSA patients and their caregivers with instructions to administer this potentially lifesaving medication and alert emergency medical services if the patient is not breathing or not rousable.[69] The opioid analgesics should be reserved for severe breakthrough pain. The use of local anesthetic can reduce immediate postoperative pain and reduce the amount of systemic medications consumed. NSAIDs should be considered first-line drugs for postoperative analgesia because they are devoid of CNS and respiratory depression. If NSAIDs are contraindicated, APAP should be taken before taking opioids. The combination of both NSAIDs and APAP can provide synergistic analgesia prior to taking opioids.[54,60]

Discharge Criteria

The final concern for the anesthesiologist is the decision to discharge the patient to an unmonitored location such as home. The ASA Practice Guidelines have spelled out three broad goals to consider prior to discharge: (1) "Patients at increased perioperative risk from OSA should not be discharged from the recovery area to an unmonitored setting (i.e., home or unmonitored hospital bed) until they are no longer at risk of postoperative respiratory depression"; (2) "Because of their propensity to develop airway obstruction or central respiratory depression, this may require a longer stay as compared with non-OSA patients undergoing similar procedures"; and (3) "To establish that patients are able to maintain adequate oxygen saturation levels while breathing room air, respiratory function may be determined by observing patients in an unstimulated environment, preferably while asleep."[23]

The three statements from the ASA Guidelines are essentially the same goals for every patient discharged from anesthesia care, with an emphasis on the increased risk that OSA patients face. Unfortunately, the ASA Guidelines and other guidelines do not have specific recommendations to assist the anesthesiologist in determining the parameters by which an OSA patient may be safely discharged. Instead, the guidelines recommend an emphasis on the use of PAP devices when available after discharge, the education of the patient and their caregivers about OSA risks and their possible exacerbation with the use of sedatives and opioids, and the avoidance of sleeping in the supine position. Patients with undiagnosed OSA but who are positive on screening should be instructed to follow-up with their primary care physician.[22,23,30,31]

Major medical centers have attempted to institute PACU order sets and timelines (minimums of 3–4 hours of PACU observation) for discharge of the OSA patient.[22,70,71] Ankinchetty and Chung recommended those patients determined to be candidates for ambulatory surgery may be discharged if monitored for at least 60 minutes after meeting modified Aldrete criteria *and* there are no recurrent respiratory adverse events in the PACU. Recurrent respiratory adverse events were defined as oxygen desaturation less than 90%, hypopnea, apnea of greater than 10 seconds, and pain–sedation mismatches.[72] Such criteria have not been validated and have associated economic (both financial and resource) costs which may not have clinical benefit.[73]

An additional consideration is that desaturation events from OSA occur most frequently during rapid eye movement (REM) sleep. Multiple studies have shown that anesthesia and surgery cause sleep fragmentation and that "REM rebound" often occurs around the third postoperative night.[74,75] The patient is most susceptible to ischemic desaturation events during the REM cycle of sleep, and most postoperative patients will have been discharged home or be unmonitored on the hospital ward by this time. The period of REM rebound also coincides with the period in which the patient may be using opioid analgesics for acute postoperative pain management. Opioids cause a change in the ventilatory CO_2 response curve (down and to the right). The combination of opioid use at a time of increased risk for REM rebound may pose a distinct hazard for the OSA patient.

The anesthesiologist must carefully evaluate each individual patient to determine the patient's risk of postoperative complications from OSA when discharging to an unmonitored setting. The evaluation should focus on the patient's inherent risk, intraoperative factors that may exacerbate OSA, and postoperative and postsurgical course. The patient's inherent risk factors include the severity of the diagnosed or suspected OSA; the adequacy of current OSA therapy, if any; the ability to continue OSA therapy in the perioperative period; and the severity and management of other comorbid conditions. Both anesthetic and postsurgical changes must be considered as intraoperative factors that could lead to OSA-related complications. For example, upper airway surgery may cause edema or prevent the postoperative use of OSA therapeutic devices, and abdominal surgery may cause splinting that will promote upper airway collapse. Postoperative considerations include the type of and patient's response to the pain management regimen, compliance with OSA treatment, and adverse respiratory events occurring in the PACU. Another important consideration is the quality of care available at home or in other unmonitored settings as patient and their caregivers must be vigilant for the potential for complications, especially considering the use of sedatives and opioids and the timeline for adverse events during REM rebound.

The decision to discharge a patient to home or other unmonitored setting lies with the anesthesiologist. Nevertheless, a team approach with input from the surgeon, nursing, the patient, and their caregivers is necessary for individualized risk assessment. For the patient with an OSA diagnosis and who is compliant with treatment, recovery from anesthesia may take several days. However, for the undiagnosed OSA patient or the OSA patient who is noncompliant with treatment, the risks of OSA are not limited to the immediate postoperative period but the remainder of their life. Therefore, screening of the surgical patient and referral to their primary care physician is not only good anesthesia care, but good medicine.

CONCLUSION

- OSA is a very prevalent condition. Most patients with OSA are not diagnosed preoperatively.
- The use of screening tools such as the STOP-Bang model can identify patients who are likely to have moderate to severe OSA.

- The gold standard for OSA diagnosis is PSG. The gold standard for OSA treatment is PAP devices. Patients with other devices or surgical treatments should be presumed to still have OSA unless verified by PSG and currently asymptomatic.
- Patients who have OSA or are presumed to have OSA may be ambulatory surgical candidates if their medical comorbid conditions are medically optimized and they can use their CPAP, or if their pain can be managed using multimodal analgesia, predominantly without opioid analgesics.
- Current practice guidelines lack specific clinical indicators for safe discharge of the OSA patient due to an insufficient evidence base.
- The anesthesiologist, with the assistance of the surgeon and patient care team, must assess the risk for each individual patient and custom tailor discharge to an unmonitored setting based on this risk assessment.

REVIEW QUESTIONS

1. A 55-year-old, 90 kg patient is scheduled for outpatient dental extractions and alveoloplasty under nasotracheal intubated general anesthesia. The patient has a 10-year history of severe OSA for which he uses CPAP nightly. The single factor that would increase the safety of postoperative discharge is

   a. Adequate postoperative analgesia with ibuprofen.
   b. Continued use of CPAP at home.
   c. Local anesthetic block of the branches of the trigeminal nerve to reduce postoperative pain.
   d. Surgical time under 1 hour.

The correct answer is a.

Patients with OSA are at increased risk for respiratory depression secondary to postoperative opioid consumption. Therefore, it is imperative to achieve analgesia without opioids to minimize the risk of opioid-induced respiratory depression. Ibuprofen is an NSAID and respiratory depression is not a side effect. A short procedure may be painful so surgical time does not correlate with postoperative pain. A nerve block provides analgesia but will eventually resolve with time and pain will break through. Use of CPAP at home may prevent apnea secondary to obstructions, but opioid-induced depression of the respiratory drive is still possible.[76]

2. Which one of the following is *not* part of the STOP-Bang questionnaire?

   a. Daytime fatigue, sleepiness, or tiredness.
   b. Elevated blood glucose.
   c. Large neck, circumference greater than 40 cm.
   d. Obesity, a patient with a BMI of 35 or greater.
   e. Observed apnea; someone has observed the patient stop breathing while sleeping.

The correct answer is b.

While metabolic dysfunction may be associated with OSA, elevated blood glucose is not part of the STOP-Bang

Questionnaire. The questions for STOP involve Snoring, Tiredness, the Observation of apnea, and high blood Pressure. The questions in Bang concern BMI, Age, Neck circumference, and Gender.[4,24]

3. Which of the following discharge criteria should the anesthesiologist rely on when evaluating an OSA patient, whether diagnosed or undiagnosed, for discharge to an unmonitored setting?

   a. The patient meets written discharge criteria, and the patient can continue their CPAP postoperatively.
   b. The patient has been observed in PACU for more than 3 hours without complications from OSA.
   c. The patient has met modified Aldrete discharge criteria and was monitored for over an additional 60 minutes without adverse respiratory events.
   d. The patient has met written discharge criteria and is not anticipated to need more than 10 mg of oxycodone (or equianalgesic dose of oral opioids) every 4 hours for pain management.
   e. None of the above.

The correct answer is e.

Although each of the above answers has been proposed as possible criteria for discharging the OSA patient to an unmonitored setting, none of the given answers has been validated. The anesthesiologist, with the assistance of the entire patient care team, must evaluate each individual patient to assess the risk of discharging the patient to an unmonitored setting. This evaluation should include the patient's inherent risk, intraoperative factors that may exacerbate OSA, and postoperative and postsurgical course.

4. An adult developmentally delayed patient with OSA is scheduled for surgery. The patient is uncooperative in preoperative holding, has not allowed IV access, and will not cooperate for a mask induction with inhalational agents. Which of the following is the anesthesiologist's best choice for a preoperative sedative?

   a. Oral clonidine.
   b. IM injection of lorazepam.
   c. Oral midazolam.
   d. IM ketamine.
   e. Intranasal midazolam and fentanyl.

The correct answer is d.

The drug absorption via the enteral route is slow and unpredictable and could have deleterious effects in the postoperative period due to delayed absorption. Intranasal administration on an uncooperative developmentally delayed adult would be difficult due to the volume of drug that would need to be administered through a mucosal atomization device. However, more importantly, the synergistic effect of a benzodiazepine and opioid may potentiate the obstruction of OSA. Both IM drugs would be acceptable, however ketamine maintains respiratory drive and there is some evidence that it helps maintain upper airway muscular tone. Therefore, IM ketamine is the correct answer.

5. When diagnosing the severity of OSA using the AHI, which of the following is consistent with mild OSA in an adult?

   a. 0–5.
   b. 0–14.
   c. 5–14.
   d. 15–30.
   e. >30.

The correct answer is c.

In the adult patient an AHI of 0–5 is normal. However, in the pediatric patient an AHI of 0 is normal. Please refer to Table 45.1 for a review of sleep apnea severity by AHI in both the pediatric and adult patient.

6. Patients taking SSRIs and SNRIs may be at risk for bleeding through the reduction of platelet levels of serotonin. With respect to the administration of or prescription for analgesics, which drug class has the least concern for excessive bleeding in an otherwise healthy patient?

   a. Acetaminophen.
   b. Ibuprofen.
   c. Naproxen.
   d. Tramadol.

The correct answer is a.

The drug with the least concerns for bleeding or anticoagulant effects in an otherwise healthy patient is acetaminophen. Ibuprofen and naproxen are NSAIDs and their inhibition of COX-1 can result in anticoagulant effects. Tramadol is an analgesic with a mixed mechanism of action as both a mu opioid receptor agonist and an inhibitor of serotonin and norepinephrine reuptake. SSRI and SNRIs both inhibit the reuptake of serotonin in the platelet, and this contributes to an enhanced bleeding risk. The combination of NSAIDs with an SSRI or SNRI produces a synergistically increased bleeding risk.[63]

7. Which analgesic is most appropriate for a patient who is chronically taking paroxetine for depression?

   a. Codeine.
   b. Oxycodone.
   c. Tramadol.
   d. All of the above.

The correct answer is b.

Paroxetine is an inhibitor of the hepatic microsomal enzyme CYP450 2D6. Codeine and tramadol are prodrugs and rely on the enzymatic activity of CYP450 2D6 for conversion to their active metabolites, morphine and o-desmethyltramadol, respectively. Oxycodone is an active analgesic and, of the choices listed, is more appropriate for a patient chronically taking paroxetine.[63]

REFERENCES

1. Al Lawati NM, Patel SR, Ayas NT. Epidemiology, risk factors, and consequences of obstructive sleep apnea and short sleep duration. *Prog Cardiovasc Dis*. 2009;51(4):285–293. doi:10.1016/j.pcad.2008.08.001
2. Eckert DJ, Jordan AS, Merchia P, Malhotra A. Central sleep apnea. *Chest*. 2007;131(2):595–607. doi:10.1378/chest.06.2287

3. Kimoff RJ. Obstructive sleep apnea. In: V. Courtney Broaddus, Robert J. Mason, Joel D. Ernst, Tamladge E. King Jr., Stephen C. Lazarus, John F. Murray, Jay A. Nadel, Arthur S. Slutsky, eds. *Murray and Nadel's Textbook of Respiratory Medicine*. 6th ed. Elsevier/Saunders; 2016:1152–1168.
4. Chung F, Elsaid H. Screening for obstructive sleep apnea before surgery: Why is it important? *Curr Opin Anaesthesiol*. 2009;22(3):405–411. doi:10.1097/ACO.0b013e32832a96e2
5. Gozal D. Sleep-disordered breathing and school performance in children. *Pediatrics*. 1998;102(3):616–620. doi:10.1542/peds.102.3.616
6. Tripuraneni M, Paruthi S, Armbrecht ES, Mitchell RB. Obstructive sleep apnea in children. *Laryngoscope*. 2013;123(5):1289–1293. doi:10.1002/lary.23844
7. Hardinge M. Obstructive sleep apnoea. *Medicine (Baltimore)*. 2008;36(5):237–241. doi:10.1016/j.mpmed.2008.02.010
8. Rowley JA, Zahn BR, Babcock MA, Badr MS. The effect of rapid eye movement (REM) sleep on upper airway mechanics in normal human subjects. *J Physiol*. 1998;510(3):963–976. doi:10.1111/j.1469-7793.1998.00963.x
9. Schwab RJ, Pasirstein M, Pierson R, et al. Identification of upper airway anatomic risk factors for obstructive sleep apnea with volumetric magnetic resonance imaging. *Am J Respir Crit Care Med*. 2003;168(5):522–530. doi:10.1164/rccm.200208-866OC
10. McGinley BM, Schwartz AR, Schneider H, Kirkness JP, Smith PL, Patil SP. Upper airway neuromuscular compensation during sleep is defective in obstructive sleep apnea. *J Appl Physiol*. 2008;105(1):197–205. doi:10.1152/japplphysiol.01214.2007
11. Kimoff RJ. Upper airway myopathy is important in the pathophysiology of obstructive sleep apnea. *J Clin Sleep Med*. 2007;3(6):567–569.
12. Schwab RJ, Gupta KB, Gefter WB, Metzger LJ, Hoffman EA, Pack AI. Upper airway and soft tissue anatomy in normal subjects and patients with sleep-disordered breathing. Significance of the lateral pharyngeal walls. *Am J Respir Crit Care Med*. 1995;152(5):1673–1689. doi:10.1164/ajrccm.152.5.7582313
13. Jordan AS, McSharry DG, Malhotra A. Adult obstructive sleep apnoea. *The Lancet*. 2014;383(9918):736–747. doi:10.1016/S0140-6736(13)60734-5
14. Bauters F, Rietzschel ER, Hertegonne KBC, Chirinos JA. The link between obstructive sleep apnea and cardiovascular disease. *Curr Atheroscler Rep*. 2016;18(1):1. doi:10.1007/s11883-015-0556-z
15. Dempsey JA, Veasey SC, Morgan BJ, O'Donnell CP. Pathophysiology of sleep apnea. *Physiol Rev*. 2010;90(1):47–112. doi:10.1152/physrev.00043.2008
16. Pedrosa RP, Drager LF, Gonzaga CC, et al. Obstructive sleep apnea: The most common secondary cause of hypertension associated with resistant hypertension. *Hypertension*. 2011;58(5):811–817. doi:10.1161/HYPERTENSIONAHA.111.179788
17. Chesson AL, Berry RB, Pack A. Practice parameters for the use of portable monitoring devices in the investigation of suspected obstructive sleep apnea in adults. *Sleep*. 2003;26(7):907–913. doi:10.1093/sleep/26.7.907
18. Chan J, Edman JC, Koltai PJ. Obstructive sleep apnea in children. *Am Fam Physician*. 2004;69(5):1147–1154.
19. Chung F, Yegneswaran B, Liao P, et al. Validation of the Berlin Questionnaire and American Society of Anesthesiologists Checklist as screening tools for obstructive sleep apnea in surgical patients. *Anesthesiology*. 2008;108(5):822–830. doi:10.1097/ALN.0b013e31816d91b5
20. Douglass AB, Bomstein R, Nino-Murcia G, et al. The Sleep Disorders Questionnaire I: Creation and multivariate structure of SDQ. *Sleep*. 1994;17(2):160–167. doi:10.1093/sleep/17.2.160
21. Chung F. Screening for obstructive sleep apnea syndrome in the preoperative patients. *Open Anesthesiol J*. 2011;5:7–11.
22. Practice guidelines for the perioperative management of patients with obstructive sleep apnea. *Anesthesiology*. 2006;104(5):1081–1093. doi:10.1097/00000542-200605000-00026
23. American Society of Anesthesiologists Task Force on Perioperative Management of Patients with Obstructive Sleep Apnea. Practice guidelines for the perioperative management of patients with obstructive sleep apnea: An updated report by the American Society of Anesthesiologists Task Force on Perioperative Management of patients with obstructive sleep apnea. *Anesthesiology*. 2014;120(2):268–286. doi:10.1097/ALN.0000000000000053
24. Chung F, Yegneswaran B, Liao P, et al. STOP Questionnaire. *Anesthesiology*. 2008;108(5):812–821. doi:10.1097/ALN.0b013e31816d83e4
25. Fleisher KE, Krieger AC. Current trends in the treatment of obstructive sleep apnea. *J Oral Maxillofac Surg*. 2007;65(10):2056–2068. doi:10.1016/j.joms.2006.11.058
26. Zozula R, Rosen R. Compliance with continuous positive airway pressure therapy: Assessing and improving treatment outcomes. *Curr Opin Pulm Med*. 2001;7(6):391–398. doi:10.1097/00063198-200111000-00005
27. Abad VC, Guilleminault C. Treatment options for obstructive sleep apnea. *Curr Treat Options Neurol*. 2009;11(5):358–367. doi:10.1007/s11940-009-0040-6
28. Friedman M, Wilson M, Lin H, Chang H. Updated systematic review of tonsillectomy and adenoidectomy for treatment of pediatric obstructive sleep apnea/hypopnea syndrome. *Otolaryngol Neck Surg*. 2009;140(6):800–808. doi:10.1016/j.otohns.2009.01.043
29. Meoli AL, Rosen CL, Kristo D, et al. Upper airway management of the adult patient with obstructive sleep apnea in the perioperative period—Avoiding complications. *Sleep*. 2003;26(8):1060–1065. doi:10.1093/sleep/26.8.1060
30. Adesanya AO, Lee W, Greilich NB, Joshi GP. Perioperative management of obstructive sleep apnea. *Chest*. 2010;138(6):1489–1498. doi:10.1378/chest.10-1108
31. Joshi GP, Ankichetty SP, Gan TJ, Chung F. Society for Ambulatory Anesthesia consensus statement on preoperative selection of adult patients with obstructive sleep apnea scheduled for ambulatory surgery. *Anesth Analg*. 2012;115(5):1060–1068. doi:10.1213/ANE.0b013e318269cfd7
32. Chung F, Memtsoudis SG, Ramachandran SK, et al. Society of Anesthesia and Sleep Medicine guidelines on preoperative screening and assessment of adult patients with obstructive sleep apnea. *Anesth Analg*. 2016;123(2):452–473. doi:10.1213/ANE.0000000000001416
33. Memtsoudis SG, Cozowicz C, Nagappa M, et al. Society of Anesthesia and Sleep Medicine guideline on intraoperative management of adult patients with obstructive sleep apnea. *Anesth Analg*. 2018;127(4):967–987. doi:10.1213/ANE.0000000000003434
34. Gupta RM, Parvizi J, Hanssen AD, Gay PC. Postoperative complications in patients with obstructive sleep apnea syndrome undergoing hip or knee replacement: A case-control study. *Mayo Clin Proc*. 2001;76(9):897–905. doi:10.4065/76.9.897
35. Liao P, Yegneswaran B, Vairavanathan S, Zilberman P, Chung F. Postoperative complications in patients with obstructive sleep apnea: A retrospective matched cohort study. *Can J Anesth Can Anesth*. 2009;56(11):819–828. doi:10.1007/s12630-009-9190-y
36. Nagappa M, Wong DT, Cozowicz C, Ramachandran SK, Memtsoudis SG, Chung F. Is obstructive sleep apnea associated with difficult airway? Evidence from a systematic review and meta-analysis of prospective and retrospective cohort studies. Taheri S, ed. *PLoS One*. 2018;13(10):e0204904. doi:10.1371/journal.pone.0204904
37. Becker H, Brandenburg U, Peter JH, Von Wichert P. Reversal of sinus arrest and atrioventricular conduction block in patients with sleep apnea during nasal continuous positive airway pressure. *Am J Respir Crit Care Med*. 1995;151(1):215–218. doi:10.1164/ajrccm.151.1.7812557
38. Bonsignore MR. Baroreflex control of heart rate during sleep in severe obstructive sleep apnoea: Effects of acute CPAP. *Eur Respir J*. 2006;27(1):128–135. doi:10.1183/09031936.06.00042904
39. Corda L, Redolfi S, Montemurro LT, La Piana GE, Bertella E, Tantucci C. Short- and long-term effects of CPAP on upper airway anatomy and collapsibility in OSAH. *Sleep Breath*. 2009;13(2):187–193. doi:10.1007/s11325-008-0219-1
40. Eikermann M, Eckert DJ, Chamberlin NL, et al. Effects of pertobarbital on upper airway patency during sleep. *Eur Respir J*. 2010;36(3):569–576. doi:10.1183/09031936.00153809

41. Berry RB, Kouchi K, Bower J, Prosise G, Light RW. Triazolam in patients with obstructive sleep apnea. *Am J Respir Crit Care Med.* 1995;151(2):450–454. doi:10.1164/ajrccm.151.2.7842205
42. Montravers P, Dureuil B, Desmonts JM. Effects of I.V. midazolam on upper airway resistance. *Br J Anaesth.* 1992;68(1):27–31. doi:10.1093/bja/68.1.27
43. Eikermann M, Garzon-Serrano J, Kwo J, Grosse-Sundrup M, Schmidt U, Bigatello L. Do patients with obstructive sleep apnea have an increased risk of desaturation during induction of anesthesia for weight loss surgery? *Open Respir Med J.* 2010;4(1):58–62. doi:10.2174/1874306401004010058
44. Eikermann M, Vogt FM, Herbstreit F, et al. The predisposition to inspiratory upper airway collapse during partial neuromuscular blockade. *Am J Respir Crit Care Med.* 2007;175(1):9–15. doi:10.1164/rccm.200512-1862OC
45. Herbstreit F, Peters J, Eikermann M. Impaired upper airway integrity by residual neuromuscular blockade: Increased airway collapsibility and blunted genioglossus muscle activity in response to negative pharyngeal pressure. *Anesthesiology.* 2009;110(6):1253–1260. doi:10.1097/ALN.0b013e31819faa71
46. Ankichetty S, Wong J, Chung F. A systematic review of the effects of sedatives and anesthetics in patients with obstructive sleep apnea. *J Anaesthesiol Clin Pharmacol.* 2011;27(4):447. doi:10.4103/0970-9185.86574
47. Liu FL, Cherng YG, Chen SY, et al. Postoperative recovery after anesthesia in morbidly obese patients: A systematic review and meta-analysis of randomized controlled trials. *Can J Anesth Can Anesth.* 2015;62(8):907–917. doi:10.1007/s12630-015-0405-0
48. Hersh EV. Local anesthetics. In: *Oral and Maxillofacial Surgery*. 2nd ed. Saunders/Elsevier; 2009.
49. Saraghi M, Hersh EV. Three newly approved analgesics: An update. *Anesth Prog.* 2013;60(4):178–187. doi:10.2344/0003-3006-60.4.178
50. Saraghi M, Moore PA, Hersh EV. Local anesthetic calculations: Avoiding trouble with pediatric patients. *Gen Dent.* 2015;63(1):48–52.
51. Hersh EV, Hermann DG, Lamp CJ, Johnson PD, Macafee KA. Assessing the duration of mandibular soft tissue anesthesia. *J Am Dent Assoc.* 1995;126(11):1531–1536. doi:10.14219/jada.archive.1995.0082
52. Saraghi M, Hersh EV. Intranasal tetracaine and oxymetazoline spray for maxillary local anesthesia without injections. *Gen Dent.* 2017;65(2):16–19.
53. Percocet® (oxycodone and acetaminophen tablets). Package insert. Endo Pharmaceuticals; 2006. https://www.accessdata.fda.gov/drugsatfda_docs/label/2006/040330s015,040341s013,040434s003lbl.pdf
54. Hersh EV, Saraghi M, Moore PA. The prescription opioid abuse crisis and our role in it. *Gen Dent.* 2018;66(4):10–13.
55. Hersh EV, Moore PA. Adverse drug interactions in dentistry. *Periodontol 2000.* 2008;46(1):109–142. doi:10.1111/j.1600-0757.2008.00224.x
56. Edwards JE, McQuay HJ, Moore RA. Combination analgesic efficacy. *J Pain Symptom Manage.* 2002;23(2):121–130. doi:10.1016/S0885-3924(01)00404-3
57. Cooper SA, Precheur H, Rauch D, Rosenheck A, Ladov M, Engel J. Evaluation of oxycodone and acetaminophen in treatment of postoperative dental pain. *Oral Surg Oral Med Oral Pathol.* 1980;50(6):496–501. doi:10.1016/0030-4220(80)90430-2
58. Hersh EV, Moore PA. Drug interactions in dentistry. *J Am Dent Assoc.* 2004;135(3):298–311. doi:10.14219/jada.archive.2004.0178
59. Weaver JM. New FDA black box warning for codeine: How will this affect dentists? *Anesth Prog.* 2013;60(2):35–36. doi:10.2344/0003-3006-60.2.35
60. Moore PA, Hersh EV. Combining ibuprofen and acetaminophen for acute pain management after third-molar extractions. *J Am Dent Assoc.* 2013;144(8):898–908. doi:10.14219/jada.archive.2013.0207
61. Goppelt-Struebe M, Wolter D, Resch K. Glucocorticoids inhibit prostaglandin synthesis not only at the level of phospholipase A2 but also at the level of cyclo-oxygenase/PGE isomerase. *Br J Pharmacol.* 1989;98(4):1287–1295. doi:10.1111/j.1476-5381.1989.tb12676.x
62. Pinto A, Farrar JT, Hersh EV. Prescribing NSAIDs to patients on SSRIs: Possible adverse drug interaction of importance to dental practitioners. *Compend Contin Educ Dent Jamesburg NJ 1995.* 2009;30(3):142–151; quiz 152, 154.
63. Saraghi M, Golden L, Hersh EV. Anesthetic considerations for patients on antidepressant therapy—Part II. *Anesth Prog.* 2018;65(1):60–65. doi:10.2344/anpr-65-01-10
64. Lithium carbonate (tablets, capsules, oral solution). Package insert. Roxane Laboratories. 2011. https://www.accessdata.fda.gov/drugsatfda_docs/label/2011/017812s028,018421s027lbl.pdf
65. Capoten® (captopril tablets). Package insert. Par Pharmaceutical Companies; 2012. https://www.accessdata.fda.gov/drugsatfda_docs/label/2012/018343s084lbl.pdf
66. Diovan HCT® (valsartan and hydrochlorothiazide tablets). Package insert. Novartis Pharmaceuticals; 2011. https://www.accessdata.fda.gov/drugsatfda_docs/label/2011/020818s049lbl.pdf
67. Parra D, Beckey NP, Stevens GR. The effect of acetaminophen on the international normalized ratio in patients stabilized on warfarin therapy. *Pharmacotherapy.* 2007;27(5):675–683. doi:10.1592/phco.27.5.675
68. Chung L, Chakravarty EF, Kearns P, Wang C, Bush TM. Bleeding complications in patients on celecoxib and warfarin. *J Clin Pharm Ther.* 2005;30(5):471–477. doi:10.1111/j.1365-2710.2005.00676.x
69. Hendley TM, Hersh EV, Moore PA, Stahl B, Saraghi M. Treatment of opioid overdose: A brief review of naloxone pharmacology and delivery. *Gen Dent.* 2017;65(3):18–21.
70. Setaro J. Obstructive sleep apnea: A standard of care that works. *J Perianesth Nurs.* 2012;27(5):323–328. doi:10.1016/j.jopan.2012.06.005
71. Swart P, Chung F, Fleetham J. An order-based approach to facilitate postoperative decision-making for patients with sleep apnea. *Can J Anesth Can Anesth.* 2013;60(3):321–324. doi:10.1007/s12630-012-9844-z
72. Ankichetty S, Chung F. Considerations for patients with obstructive sleep apnea undergoing ambulatory surgery. *Curr Opin Anaesthesiol.* 2011;24(6):605–611. doi:10.1097/ACO.0b013e32834a10c7
73. Setaro J, Corrado T, Reinsel R, et al. Is a standard of care for patients with obstructive sleep apnea an effective tool in providing safe outcomes in PACU? *J Perianesth Nurs.* 2016;31(4):e63.
74. Knill RL, Moote CA, Skinner MI, Rose EA. Anesthesia with abdominal surgery leads to intense REM sleep during the first postoperative week. *Anesthesiology.* 1990;73(1):52–61. doi:10.1097/00000542-199007000-00009
75. Rosenberg-Adamsen S, Kehlet H, Dodds C, Rosenberg J. Postoperative sleep disturbances: Mechanisms and clinical implications. *Br J Anaesth.* 1996;76(4):552–559. doi:10.1093/bja/76.4.552
76. Dershwitz M, Walz JM. *Anesthesiology.* 7th ed. McGraw-Hill.

46.

MY PATIENT IS TWITCHING LIKE A FISH OUT OF WATER

AVOIDING THE RISKS OF RESIDUAL PARALYSIS

Ramon E. Abola

STEM CASES AND KEY QUESTIONS

A healthy 21-year-old woman presents with abdominal pain that localizes to the right lower quadrant of her abdomen. She has been nauseated for 24 hours and has been unable to eat. She has a fever of 38°C. She has a heart rate of 105, blood pressure of 117/85 and pulse oximetry (spO2) of 99% on room air. Her only medication is an oral contraceptive that she takes for birth control. She has an elevated white blood count, but the rest of her CBC is within normal limits. Her chemistry labs are within normal limits. A urine pregnancy test was negative. The CT scan of her abdomen was suggestive of appendicitis. The patient is scheduled for laparoscopic appendectomy with the general surgery service.

The patient has a postoperative nausea and vomiting (PONV) risk score of 4. She is given aprepitant preoperatively for PONV prophylaxis. During the preoperative exam, the patient appears to be in no acute distress. She is a little nervous about her upcoming surgery. She weighs 60 kg, and she has a reassuring airway exam with a Mallampati class I, good mouth opening, thyromental distance of greater than 3 finger breadths and neck full range of motion. The plan is for general anesthesia with endotracheal tube placement.

Should a rapid sequence induction be utilized when anesthetizing this patient?

If you elect to perform rapid sequence induction, will you use succinylcholine or rocuronium?

The patient is taking birth control. Should she receive any counselling with regard to anesthesia and birth control?

In the operating room, standard American Society of Anesthesiologists (ASA) monitors are placed. She is preoxygenated. Rapid sequence induction is performed using propofol and rocuronium (1.2 mg/kg). After waiting 1 minute, the patient is easily intubated with direct laryngoscopy using a Mac 3 blade and a 7.0 endotracheal tube. End-tidal carbon dioxide is confirmed, and bilateral breath sounds are heard on auscultation. The surgery proceeds uneventfully. The inflamed appendix is removed, and the surgeon closes the laparoscopy port sites. The surgery is completed in less than 1 hour. The patient is given neostigmine 4 mg and glycopyrrolate 0.8 mg for reversal of neuromuscular blockade (NMB).

When is it appropriate to give neostigmine for reversal of NMB?

What is the time to peak effect for neostigmine?

The anesthesia resident you are working with turns off the sevoflurane. Within 5 minutes, the patient opens her eyes and demonstrates spontaneous breathing with tidal volumes of 200 mL. As the patient is awake, the resident extubates her. Looking at the patient, she has a frightened look on her face. She shakes her head back and forth and tries to lift her arms but appears weak. *The patient looks like a fish out of water!* The patient is unable to lift her head, and her hand grip is weak.

What are methods to assess residual NMB? How reliable is each method?

The patient appears to have residual NMB. What should you do in this situation?

What are the differences between sugammadex and neostigmine for the reversal of NMB?

Mask ventilation is provided as a supportive measure. The patient's spO$_2$ remains 99%, however she is tachycardic with an elevated blood pressure and clearly is anxious and scared. Over the next 15 minutes, her strength continues to improve. You ask her to lift her head, and she is now able to and says "Thank Goodness! That was really scary." You transport the patient to the PACU; her vitals are within normal limits.

What are the potential complications associated with residual NMB?

The patient does well in the PACU and is discharged to the inpatient floor. Four hours later, you see that she is ambulating in the hallway and overall doing well. The patient states that she felt weak and unable to move when waking up after surgery. She said that the experience was very frightening. She is thankful now that she is better.

How would you explain to the patient what had happened?

MINI-CASE

A 50-year-old man with no medical problems presents for shoulder rotator cuff repair at an ambulatory surgery center. He weighs 80 kg. An interscalene nerve block is performed prior to surgery for postoperative pain control. The patient is given midazolam 2 mg, fentanyl 100 mcg, propofol 200 mg, and rocuronium 50 mg during anesthesia induction. The surgery proceeds uneventfully in the lateral position. The patient did not receive any additional rocuronium. It has been 2.5 hours since the beginning of the case. The patient has 4 out of 4 twitches on a train-of-four (TOF) monitor.

Should this patient receive medication for reversal of NMB?

DISCUSSION

NEUROMUSCULAR BLOCKING DRUGS

Neuromuscular blocking drugs (NMBDs) are frequently used by anesthesia providers during the perioperative period. NMBDs are utilized to facilitate endotracheal intubation and to provide surgical access in the operating room. Although NMBDs are in routine use, depth of NMB is not routinely monitored in clinical practice. Improper monitoring and inadequate reversal of NMB can result in residual NMB and weakness.

Neuromuscular Blockade Monitoring

Three methods are utilized to assess residual NMB: clinical tests, qualitative means, and quantitative means. A key measurement of residual NMB is the TOF ratio (TOFR). This ratio is the comparison of the twitch height of the fourth twitch with the first twitch on the TOF stimulation. A TOFR of greater than 0.9 demonstrates that a patient has no residual NMB.

Clinical tests, such as hand grip and head, lift are routinely employed by anesthesia providers to assess residual NMB. Unfortunately, several studies have demonstrated that volunteers and patients are able to perform a 5 second head lift with a TOFR of less than 0.5. Other clinical tests, such as leg lift, sustained hand grip, and eye opening, all can be performed with residual NMB (TOFR of less than 0.9). Essentially, clinical tests used to assess neuromuscular function cannot exclude the presence of residual paralysis unless the TOFR is less than 0.5.[1]

Qualitative monitoring describes the subjective visual or tactile assessment of a response to a peripheral nerve stimulator to assess NMB. Unfortunately, only 37% of inexperienced anesthesiologists were able to detect fade at a TOFR of 0.41–0.5. Results were similar using the double-burst stimulation method of nerve stimulation. Tactile assessment has been found to be more accurate than visual assessment but is also limited in its utility. Eighty percent of anesthesiologists were unable to detect fade when the TOFRs were between 0.51 and 0.70. Although widely available in the operating suite, the peripheral nerve stimulator as a qualitative assessment of NMB is not sufficient to detect a TOFR of greater than 0.9.[1]

A TOFR of greater than 0.4 can be measured accurately by using quantitative neuromuscular monitors. There are several methods to obtain a quantitative measure of NMB, such as mechanomyography, acceleromyography, and electromyography (EMG). Mechanomyography and acceleromyography measure movement of the thumb by the abductor pollicis in response to a stimulation of the ulnar nerve. EMG measures the signal within the abductor pollicis in response to ulnar nerve stimulation. These devices are capable of accurately calculating the ratio of the fourth twitch compared to the first twitch in a TOF stimulation. There are some limitations with these devices. Most devices require calibration at the beginning of anesthesia prior to NMDB administration, and inaccurate calibration may introduce error in the measurements. With acceleromyography, restricted movement of the thumb (i.e., patient arms are tucked) may cause inaccuracy in the device's measurements. However, quantitative measures of NMB still remain more sensitive and accurate than clinical tests or qualitative measures. Return of TOFR to greater than 0.9 would be consistent with complete reversal of NMB and should allow for extubation without residual paralysis.[1]

Residual Neuromuscular Blockade

In volunteer studies, small degrees of residual paralysis (TOFR 0.7–0.9) are associated with impaired pharyngeal function and increased risk of aspiration, weakness of upper airway muscles, and airway obstruction. Residual paralysis has also been associated with attenuation of the hypoxic ventilatory response. Patients have also reported the unpleasant subjective feeling of muscle weakness. Residual NMB has also been associated with acute respiratory events in the immediate postoperative period, delays in tracheal extubation, and an increased risk of postoperative pulmonary complications.[2]

When a patient demonstrates residual NMB, three options can be performed: (1) reintubate the patient, (2) support breathing/ventilation until recovery from NMB, or (3) administer sugammadex. Reintubation would be appropriate if the patient was hypoxic despite supportive bag mask ventilation. Reintubation may be difficult if paralysis is needed and the patient recently had received NMBD reversal. Supporting breathing and ventilation is another option that could be employed in this situation. The patient may only need a short period until they have had significant recovery from NMB. The drawback of this approach is that the patient may be aware while they are still partially paralyzed and weak, and the residual weakness may result in hypoxia, difficulty with breathing, and/or aspiration. Administration of sugammadex is also appropriate in the setting of residual paralysis from rocuronium administration with inadequate reversal with neostigmine. Sugammadex binds to any free rocuronium molecules, rendering them inactive. One would expect a TOFR of greater than 0.9 to occur within 2 minutes after giving sugammadex.

Reversal of Neuromuscular Blockade: Sugammadex Versus Neostigmine

Neostigmine is an anticholinesterase inhibitor. Reversal of NMB is accomplished by increasing the amount of acetylcholine in the neuromuscular junction. The higher proportion of acetylcholine to rocuronium after reversal provides a reversal of paralysis. Sugammadex is a cyclodextrin molecule which encapsulates a rocuronium (or other aminosteroid NMBD) compound in a 1:1 ratio. The formation of a sugammadex:rocuronium complex removes free rocuronium from circulation resulting in a reversal of NMB. The dosing for sugammadex is 2 mg/kg with a TOF count of 2, and 4 mg/kg with a post-tetanic count of 1–2. Sugammadex also binds to vecuronium but with a lower affinity than rocuronium.

Reversal of NMB with sugammadex is more rapid than with neostigmine. A comparison of reversal of rocuronium NMB found the time to achieve a TOFR greater than 0.9 was significantly shorter with sugammadex (107 seconds) compared with neostigmine (1,044 seconds).[3] A Cochrane review found that sugammadex was 10.22 minutes (6.6 times) faster than neostigmine (1.96 vs. 12.87 minutes) in reversing moderate induced paralysis. Sugammadex was 45.78 minutes (16.8 times) faster than neostigmine (2.9 vs. 48.8 minutes) in reversing deep induced paralysis.[4]

Another advantage of sugammadex is its unique ability to reverse profound NMB. In a randomized controlled trial, reversal of NMB was administered at the reappearance of 1–2 post-tetanic counts. Patients either received sugammadex 4 mg/kg or neostigmine 0.07 mg/kg with glycopyrrolate (14 mcg/kg). The mean time to recovery for a TOFR of 0.9 with sugammadex was 2.9 minutes versus 50.5 minutes with neostigmine-glycopyrrolate. Most patients (97%) who received sugammadex recovered to a TOFR of greater than 0.9 within 5 minutes after administration, whereas most neostigmine patients (73%) recovered between 30 and 60 minutes after administration.[5]

In a controlled trial by Brueckmann, patients were randomized to receive sugammadex (2 or 4 mg/kg) or neostigmine for reversal of NMB. Zero of the 74 sugammadex patients and 43% of the neostigmine patients had residual NMB at PACU admission as assessed by TOF Watch SX accelomyography. Two of the neostigmine patients had clinical signs of partial paralysis. The key finding from this study is that no patients who received sugammadex had residual NMB (TOFR of less than 0.9).[6]

Neostigmine Reversal

What is the optimal time for neostigmine reversal? The question could be better phrased to ask: How should we dose neostigmine to avoid residual NMB (TOFR less than 0.9)?

In a study by Kopman, patients who received rocuronium or cisatracurium were reversed with neostigmine (0.05 mg/kg) with glycopyrrolate (10 mcg/kg). The goal was to reverse the patients at 2 twitches, however patients received reversal with 1, 2, or 3 twitches on the TOF.

Thirty-three percent of patients in the cisatracurium group and 50% of patients in the rocuronium group had a TOFR of less than 0.9 prior to PACU transfer.[7] This study demonstrates a wide variability of efficacy with neostigmine from a TOF count of 2 where 50% of patients had a TOFR of 0.9 after 15 minutes and some had residual paralysis after 30 minutes. Neostigmine should be administered with at least a TOF count of 2 because administration prior to this is ineffective, and a patient will likely have residual paralysis during emergence and extubation. Neostigmine reversal at 4 twitches has been demonstrated to induce a more rapid return to TOFR of greater than 0.9.[8]

The time to reaching a TOFR of greater than 0.9 after reversal with neostigmine depends on the depth of NMB at the time of administration. Patients who received neostigmine 0.07 mg/kg at a TOF count of 1, 2, 3, and 4 had a median time from reversal to a TOFR of 0.9 of 28 (8.8–75), 22 (8.3–57), 15.6 (7.3–44), and 9.7 (5.1–26) minutes, respectively. At a TOF count of 4, only 55% of patients achieved TOFR of 0.9 within 10 minutes. As noted by these data, there was significant variability in neuromuscular recovery among patients.[9]

A study of extubation criteria found that anesthesia providers using quantitative neuromuscular monitoring and clinical criteria were ready to extubate patients 8 minutes after reversal with neostigmine. The mean TOFR was 0.67, and 88% of those patients who were extubated did not meet the TOFR of greater than 0.9 standard prior to extubation.[10] This suggests that, within routine clinical practice with the use of neostigmine, a significant number of patients still had residual paralysis at the time of extubation. A key lesson from this study is that reversal with neostigmine should occur well ahead of the 8 minutes observed in this study, and reversal should be even earlier if there is a lower TOF count.

Omitting Reversal of Neuromuscular Blockade

All patients who receive NMB should receive reversal to avoid residual weakness. If an anesthesiologist wishes to omit reversal of NMB, this should only be done with the use of a quantitative neuromuscular monitor. Omitting reversal should only be done when a patient has returned to a TOFR of greater than 0.9 and demonstrates no residual paralysis. For any TOFR of less than 0.9, the patient should be given a reversal agent.

RAPID-SEQUENCE INDUCTION: NEUROMUSCULAR BLOCKADE CONSIDERATIONS

Rapid-sequence induction is generally performed to minimize the risk of aspiration.[11] It should be performed in patients who are considered to have a full stomach. Examples include a patient with recent trauma who ate dinner prior to their injury, a patient with a small bowel obstruction, or a patient with an upper gastrointestinal bleed who presents with hematemesis. The general principle with rapid-sequence induction is to minimize the amount of time between when the patient is protecting their airway to when the anesthesia provider is protecting the airway with an endotracheal tube.[12]

There are multiple controversies and differences of opinions among anesthesiologists regarding the performance of rapid-sequence induction. Although beyond the scope of this chapter, here are some questions to consider.

1. Should opioids be administered as part of a rapid-sequence induction?
2. Should manual ventilation be performed prior to intubation?[13]
3. Should cricoid pressure beused during rapid sequence induction?[14]
4. What position is optimal for rapid-sequence induction? Head up? Head down?
5. What IV anesthetic should be utilized in the patient with septic shock?[15]
    a. Propofol? Etomidate? Ketamine?
    b. How significant is adrenal suppression in this patient population after receiving a dose of etomidate?[16]
6. Should rapid-sequence induction be utilized in critically ill patients?[17]

Both succinylcholine (1 mg/kg) and rocuronium (1.2 mg/kg) are appropriate choices for NMB when performing a rapid-sequence induction. The onset time for succinylcholine at 1 mg/kg (50 seconds, +/− 17 s) was similar to that in patients who received rocuronium at 1.2 mg/kg (55 seconds, +/− 14s).[18] There has been some suggestion that succinylcholine provided better intubation conditions.19 However, a randomized controlled trial (n = 1,248) of patients undergoing rapid-sequence intubation in the out of hospital setting failed to demonstrate a noninferiority of rocuronium compared with succinylcholine with regard to first-attempt endotracheal intubation success rate. The first-attempt intubation success rate was 74.6% in the rocuronium group and 79.4% in the succinylcholine group and did not meet criteria for noninferiority.[20]

One advantage of succinylcholine over rocuronium is the shorter duration of action. Succinylcholine (1 mg/kg) has a reported duration of action times from between 4–6 minutes and 10–15 minutes. Succinylcholine can be utilized for short-duration procedures where tracheal intubation is required. The short duration of succinylcholine makes it a good choice for the patient with a difficult airway. In the "cannot ventilate/cannot intubate" scenario, the rapid recovery from succinylcholine would allow the anesthesiologist to "wake up" the patient. By comparison, rocuronium (1.2 mg/kg) has a duration of action of 30–90 minutes.

The interesting question is how the introduction of sugammadex changes this concern. Sugammadex is an NMB reversal agent that forms a 1:1 complex with rocuronium. Return of spontaneous ventilation occurred earlier in a group of patients who received rocuronium (1 mg/kg) followed by sugammadex (16 mg/kg) compared to a group of patients who received succinylcholine (216 seconds vs. 406 seconds; P = 0.002).[21] The median time to 90% recovery of the first twitch on the TOF (T(1) 90%) was 168 seconds in the rocuronium-sugammadex group compared to 518 seconds in the succinylcholine group. This study suggests that rocuronium-sugammadex allowed for earlier reestablishment of spontaneous ventilation than with spontaneous recovery of succinylcholine.

SUCCINYLCHOLINE: CLINICAL CONCERNS

Succinylcholine has a large number of clinical concerns that limit the number of patients who can receive this medication.

- *Malignant hyperthermia* (MH): Succinylcholine is an MH trigger and should be avoided in patients with a personal or family history of MH.

- *Pseudocholinesterase deficiency*: Succinylcholine is metabolized by plasma butyrylcholinesterase. Patients with a deficiency in this plasma enzyme will be unable to metabolize succinylcholine and have a prolonged duration of paralysis.

- *Hyperkalemia*: Succinylcholine will increase serum potassium by 0.5–1 mEq/L after administration. However, severe hyperkalemia can occur when a patient has a denervation injury, such as a spinal cord injury, stroke, or burn. The denervation injury is associated with the increased expression of extrajunctional acetylcholine receptors. These extrajunctional receptors are outside of the neuromuscular junction and are associated with an exaggerated hyperkalemic response after succinylcholine administration.[22] Mazze described a patient who received succinylcholine 1 month after massive trauma. The serum potassium level was 3.8 mEq/L prior to receiving succinylcholine. After receiving succinylcholine, the serum potassium increased to 8.3 mEq/L and then 9.2 mEq/L at 2 and 5 minutes, respectively. The patient developed ventricular tachycardia and ventricular fibrillation.[23]

- *Myalgias*: Postoperative myalgias is a frequent occurrence in patients who had received succinylcholine. The most commonly quoted figure is approximately 50%. Succinylcholine-induced myalgia usually appears on the first day after surgery and lasts for 2–3 days. It is most commonly described as pain one might suffer after an unaccustomed degree of physical exercise and is usually located in the neck, shoulder,[24] and upper abdominal muscles.[25]

- *Black box warning in pediatrics*: Succinylcholine has a warning about its use in pediatric patients. Patients with muscular dystrophy, when given succinylcholine, may have a hyperkalemic response which can result in ventricular fibrillation and cardiac arrest. Pediatric patients may have an undiagnosed muscular dystrophy when they present to the operating room or procedural suite. Therefore, the benefit of succinylcholine must be weighed against this risk prior to use in children.[26]

- *Increased intracranial pressure (ICP)*: Succinylcholine has been associated with increased ICP in patients undergoing neurosurgery for brain tumor. Pretreatment with a low dose of non-depolarizing agent (defasciculation) theoretically may blunt the rise in ICP when using succinylcholine.[27]

- *Increased intraocular pressure (IOP)*: Succinylcholine has been associated with an increase in IOP of up to 10 mm Hg for 10 minutes. The benefits of using succinylcholine, which provides rapid, short-acting paralysis in an emergency situation where there is a risk of aspiration, need to be weighed against the risks of increasing IOP.

NEUROMUSCULAR BLOCKADE: MISCELLANEOUS TOPICS

Sugammadex and Birth Control

Although not commonly considered, several medications that a patient may receive intraoperatively could affect the efficacy of birth control. Both aprepitant and sugammadex have been identified as medications which could reduce hormonal birth control efficacy. Birth control pills are typically a combination of estrogen and progesterone like compounds. Sugammadex binds to NMBD from the steroidal class and may also bind to medications utilized for birth control. Patients of childbearing age, on birth control, should be counseled about the potential for decreased birth control efficacy and that a secondary form of non-hormonal birth control should be utilized in the immediate postoperative period. Some common perioperative antibiotics also warn about a decreased effectiveness of oral contraceptives during coadministration. More definitive data would be helpful in better understanding this potential issue, but one anesthesiologist suggests revising the anesthesia consent to contain the following general statement: "You may receive medications during your anesthetic that could interfere with the effectiveness of oral contraceptives. If you are using oral contraceptives, consider alternative methods of birth control for 7 days following your anesthetic."[28]

Residual Neuromuscular Blockade: Patient Discussion of Adverse Event

How do you disclose an adverse event to a patient or family? The key aspects of dealing with an adverse event are listening to the patient, taking time to answer and address their concerns, being truthful about the situation, and explaining how this situation will be avoided in the future. Prior to speaking with the patient, the anesthesia provider should review the details of the case and devise a plan of how they will explain what happened to the patient. Reviewing what should be said with a colleague is one strategy to prepare for this difficult conversation. With a sudden revelation of a negative experience, an appropriate initial response may be "I would like to talk to you more about this, but please give me a few minutes to fully review your case."

This scenario is similar to a patient who has had awareness under anesthesia. The patient has recall of being awake and weak with residual paralysis and that this was frightening and stressful. Opening this conversation should entail asking the patient to recount their memory of the experience and describe their concerns. It is important to understand the patient's recollection of the event prior to providing an explanation of what had occurred. Stating the facts of the events may be a prudent approach. One possible approach may be to say, "As part of your general anesthetic, we gave you a muscle relaxant medication which causes weakness but helps in performing the surgery. At the end of surgery, this muscle relaxant is reversed, but the reversal that we used was inadequate, which is why you still felt weak when waking up from anesthesia."

A few other key points to consider: (1) make sure to allot sufficient time for this conversation, (2) allow the patient to ask and have all of their questions answered, (3) plan for follow-up with the patient to answer any additional questions and address concerns, and (4) provide a plan for how this complication can and will be avoided in future surgeries.

CONCLUSION

NMB medications are frequently utilized as components of general anesthesia. Residual NMB has been associated with negative clinical outcomes. Monitoring the depth of NMB is essential to avoid residual NMB. Neostigmine or sugammadex can be utilized to reverse NMB, but they should be used in the appropriate setting with knowledge of their onset and efficacy.

REVIEW QUESTIONS

1. Which of the following measures is the most reliable to confirm that a patient has adequate reversal of NMB?

    a. Double-burst stimulus.
    b. Five-second head lift.
    c. Four twitches on the TOF.
    d. Strong hand grip.

    The correct answer is a.
    A double-burst stimulus (DBS) consists of two brief, 50 Hz tetanic bursts delivered 0.75 seconds apart. Each burst consists of three stimuli that result in two sustained muscle contractions. The DBS (D2/D1) approximates the TOFR. When quantitative monitoring is not available, the advantage of DBS over TOF is that subjectivity determined fade is more easily perceived than fade induced by TOF stimulation. However, once the TOFR exceeds 0.60, fade to DBS generally cannot be detected subjectively. Five-second head lift and hand grip are clinical tests which patients are able to perform with a TOFR of less than 0.5. The best answer to this question is TOFR, but that is not one of the choices.[29]

2. A patient on labor and delivery has a category three fetal heart tracing. She is rushed to the operating room for a stat cesarean delivery under general anesthesia. Rapid-sequence induction is performed with propofol and rocuronium. Which of the following medications will *not* prolong the effect of rocuronium?

a. Gentamicin.
b. Magnesium.
c. Propofol.
d. Sevoflurane.

The correct answer is c.

Gentamicin (an aminoglycoside antibiotic), magnesium, and sevoflurane will all potentiate the effect of neuromuscular blocking agents. Hypothermia and metabolic acidosis can also potentiate the effect of neuromuscular blocking agents.

3. A patient has undergone a total colectomy in the main operating suite. The patient received rocuronium for paralysis during the surgery which has now been reversed with sugammadex. An abdominal x-ray is performed at the end of surgery to assess for any retained foreign bodies. Prior to extubating the patient, the surgery team starts making a commotion because it appears that an x-ray detectable sponge was left inside the patient. Which medication should be given to provide paralysis for this reoperation?

a. Cis-atracurium.
b. Rocuronium.
c. Succinylcholine.
d. Vecuronium.

The correct answer is a.

In this clinical scenario, paralysis will be required for exploratory laparotomy to remove the retained foreign body. As the patient has recently received sugammadex, the clinical effects of rocuronium or vecuronium will be decreased because this new administration will bind to any free sugammadex. Succinylcholine can be given in this scenario for short duration of paralysis, but the exploratory laparotomy likely will be longer than 10–15 minutes. Cis-atracurium, as a bisbenzyltetrahydroisoquinolinium neuromuscular blocking drug, has no interaction with sugammadex and is the best choice to be utilized in this scenario.

4. A 22-year-old patient who weighs 70 kg has undergone a laparoscopic cholecystectomy. The patient received rocuronium 70 mg at the time of induction. No further rocuronium was given during the case. The case duration was 1 hour. A twitch monitor is not available. What reversal agent and dose should be utilized for this patient?

a. Neostigmine, 5 mg.
b. Neostigmine, 3.5 mg.
c. Sugammadex, 140 mg.
d. Sugammadex, 280 mg.

The correct answer is d.

Ideally, quantitative neuromuscular blocking monitoring will become a standard of care in the future with the use of TOFR. But currently it is not uncommon, based on surveys of anesthesiologists, for providers to *not* use even a qualitative monitor such as a TOF with a twitch monitor. (Don't be that person). In the absence of knowing the patient's depth of NMB, the best choice for this patient would be to receive sugammadex 4 mg/kg or 280 mg. This dose will reverse the NMB of rocuronium with a depth of at least 1 post-tetanic count. It would be expected that, after 1 hour had elapsed following a rapid-sequence dose of rocuronium, the patient should be at this level.

In clinical studies, sugammadex 2 mg/kg can also reverse rocuronium from this NMB, albeit with a slightly longer onset (~5 minutes) to reach a TOFR of greater than 0.9. However, the recommended US Food and Drug Administration dosing states that sugammadex 2 mg/kg should only be given if the patient has at least two twitches on a TOF monitor and this information is unknown without the use of a twitch monitor.

5. A patient has received succinylcholine for intubation for a cystoscopy and ureteral stent placement. No additional neuromuscular blocking agents were given. The patient has a delayed emergence from anesthesia. Which of the following should be utilized to confirm a diagnosis of pseudocholinesterase deficiency?

a. Caffeine halothane contracture test.
b. Dibucaine number.
c. Ryanodine receptor defect.
d. Twitch monitor and TOF.

The correct answer is b

The dibucaine number is the percent of pseudocholinesterase enzyme activity that is inhibited by dibucaine. The dibucaine number and the pseudocholinesterase enzyme activity results can help to identify individuals at risk for prolonged paralysis following succinylcholine. The caffeine halothane contracture test and ryanodine receptor defect are tests utilized to diagnose MH. The twitch monitor could be utilized to verify prolonged residual paralysis, but it would not confirm a diagnosis of pseudocholinesterase deficiency.

6. Which of the following patients can receive sugammadex for reversal of NMB?

a. Obstetric patient after laparoscopic cholecystectomy in the second trimester.
b. Patient with end-stage renal disease on hemodialysis.
c. Patient with cirrhosis and Child-Pugh class B liver function.
d. Patient with a chronic kidney disease and glomerular filtration rate of 20.

The correct answer is c.

The metabolic function of the liver is usually preserved until a patient has reached hepatic failure and needs a transplant. Rocuronium may be used in this patient, however cisatracurium may be a better choice for paralysis because of the hepatic impairment. Sugammadex may be utilized in patients with hepatic impairment. The sugammadex–rocuronium complex is cleared by the kidney. There are limited data on sugammadex use in pregnant women to inform on any drug-associated risks. In vitro studies indicate the sugammadex encapsulates progesterone, and the risks to fetal development have not been studied. Sugammadex is not recommended in patients with severe renal impairment (glomerular filtration rate of less than 30).

7. Which of the following adverse events are more likely to occur with the use of rocuronium?

   a. Corneal abrasion.
   b. Intraoperative awareness.
   c. Peroneal nerve neuropathy.
   d. Postoperative myalgias.

The correct answer is b.

Intraoperative awareness is often described by patients as being awake and being unable to move. Commonly, patients recount conversations or noises heard in the operating room. This unfortunate adverse event is more likely to happen with the use of NMB. In an unparalyzed patient, if the depth of anesthesia is insufficient, the patient would move and the anesthesia provider would increase the depth of anesthesia. This likely would occur below a level of awareness and recall. This is one reason why it is important to consider whether paralysis is needed for a specific surgery. Certain surgeries, such as neurosurgery or spine surgery, require paralysis because any patient movement could be catastrophic. An interesting clinical question is whether there is an increase in the rate of intraoperative awareness with the introduction of sugammadex into clinical practice. Anesthesia providers may be more liberal with their use of rocuronium as patients can now be reversed effectively from a deep blockade.

Corneal abrasion and peroneal nerve neuropathy are two adverse events that may occur in the operating room, but they are not related to the use of NMB. Postoperative myalgias are commonly reported after the use of succinylcholine but not with non-depolarizing neuromuscular blocking agents.

REFERENCES

1. Brull SJ, Murphy GS. Residual neuromuscular block: Lessons unlearned. Part II: Methods to reduce the risk of residual weakness. *Anesth Analg*. 2010;111(1):129–140.
2. Murphy GS, Brull SJ. Residual neuromuscular block: Lessons unlearned. Part I: Definitions, incidence, and adverse physiologic effects of residual neuromuscular block. *Anesth Analg*. 2010;111(1):120–128.
3. Sacan O, White PF, Tufanogullari B, Klein K. Sugammadex reversal of rocuronium-induced neuromuscular blockade: A comparison with neostigmine-glycopyrrolate and edrophonium-atropine. *Anesth Analg*. 2007;104(3):569–574.
4. Hristovska AM, Duch P, Allingstrup M, Afshari A. Efficacy and safety of sugammadex versus neostigmine in reversing neuromuscular blockade in adults. *Cochrane Database Syst Rev*. 2017;8(8):Cd012763.
5. Jones RK, Caldwell JE, Brull SJ, Soto RG. Reversal of profound rocuronium-induced blockade with sugammadex: A randomized comparison with neostigmine. *Anesthesiology*. 2008;109(5):816–824.
6. Brueckmann B, Sasaki N, Grobara P, et al. Effects of sugammadex on incidence of postoperative residual neuromuscular blockade: A randomized, controlled study. *Br J Anaesth*. 2015;115(5):743–751.
7. Kopman AF, Kopman DJ, Ng J, Zank LM. Antagonism of profound cisatracurium and rocuronium block: The role of objective assessment of neuromuscular function. *J Clin Anesth*. 2005;17(1):30–35.
8. Donati F. Residual paralysis: A real problem or did we invent a new disease? *Can J Anesth./Journal canadien d'anesthésie*. 2013;60(7):714–729.
9. Kim KS, Cheong MA, Lee HJ, Lee JM. Tactile assessment for the reversibility of rocuronium-induced neuromuscular blockade during propofol or sevoflurane anesthesia. *Anesth Analg*. 2004;99(4):1080–1085.
10. Murphy GS, Szokol JW, Marymont JH, Franklin M, Avram MJ, Vender JS. Residual paralysis at the time of tracheal extubation. *Anesth Analg*. 2005;100(6):1840–1845.
11. Sinclair RCF, Luxton MC. Rapid sequence induction. *Cont Educ Anaesth Crit Care Pain*. 2005;5(2):45–48.
12. El-Orbany M, Connolly LA. Rapid sequence induction and intubation: Current controversy. *Anesth Analg*. 2010;110(5):1318–1325.
13. Casey JD, Janz DR, Russell DW, et al. Bag-mask ventilation during tracheal intubation of critically ill adults. *N Engl J Med*. 2019;380(9):811–821.
14. Birenbaum A, Hajage D, Roche S, et al. Effect of cricoid pressure compared with a sham procedure in the rapid sequence induction of anesthesia: The IRIS randomized clinical trial. *JAMA Surg*. 2019;154(1):9–17.
15. Wan C, Hanson AC, Schulte PJ, Dong Y, Bauer PR. Propofol, ketamine, and etomidate as induction agents for intubation and outcomes in critically ill patients: A retrospective cohort study. *Crit Care Explor*. 2021;3(5):e0435.
16. Gu WJ, Wang F, Tang L, Liu JC. Single-dose etomidate does not increase mortality in patients with sepsis: A systematic review and meta-analysis of randomized controlled trials and observational studies. *Chest*. 2015;147(2):335–346.
17. Benger JR. Rethinking rapid sequence induction of anaesthesia in critically ill adults. *Lancet Respir Med*. 2019;7(12):997–999.
18. Magorian T, Flannery KB, Miller RD. Comparison of rocuronium, succinylcholine, and vecuronium for rapid-sequence induction of anesthesia in adult patients. *Anesthesiology*. 1993;79(5):913–918.
19. Tran DTT, Newton EK, Mount VAH, Lee JS, Wells GA, Perry JJ. Rocuronium versus succinylcholine for rapid sequence induction intubation. *Cochrane Database Syst Rev*. 2015(10). doi:10.1002/14651858.CD002788.pub3. Accessed 22 February 2024.
20. Guihard B, Chollet-Xémard C, Lakhnati P, et al. Effect of rocuronium vs succinylcholine on endotracheal intubation success rate among patients undergoing out-of-hospital rapid sequence intubation: A randomized clinical trial. *JAMA*. 2019;322(23):2303–2312.
21. Sørensen MK, Bretlau C, Gätke MR, Sørensen AM, Rasmussen LS. Rapid sequence induction and intubation with rocuronium-sugammadex compared with succinylcholine: A randomized trial. *Br J Anaesth*. 2012;108(4):682–689.
22. Martyn JAJ, Richtsfeld M, Warner David O. Succinylcholine-induced hyperkalemia in acquired pathologic states: Etiologic factors and molecular mechanisms. *Anesthesiology*. 2006;104(1):158–169.
23. Mazze RI, Escue HM, Houston JB. Hyperkalemia and cardiovascular collapse following administration of succinylcholine to the traumatized patient. *Anesthesiology*. 1969;31(6):540–547.
24. Murgatroyd H, Bembridge J. Intraocular pressure. *Cont Educ Anaesth Crit Care Pain*. 2008;8(3):100–103.
25. Wong SF, Chung F. Succinylcholine-associated postoperative myalgia. *Anaesthesia*. 2000;55(2):144–152.
26. Sullivan M, Thompson WK, Hill GD. Succinylcholine-induced cardiac arrest in children with undiagnosed myopathy. *Can J Anaesth*. 1994;41(6):497–501.
27. Kramer N, Lebowitz D, Walsh M, Ganti L. Rapid sequence intubation in traumatic brain-injured adults. *Cureus*. 2018;10(4):e2530–e2530.
28. Corda DM, Robards CB. Sugammadex and oral contraceptives: Is it time for a revision of the anesthesia informed consent? *Anesth Analg*. 2018;126(2):730–731.
29. Brull SJ, Kopman AF. Current status of neuromuscular reversal and monitoring: Challenges and opportunities. *Anesthesiology*. 2017;126(1):173–190.

47.

MY PATIENT IN THE PACU IS NOT MAKING ANY SENSE

Joy Steadman

STEM, KEY QUESTIONS AND DISCUSSION

The patient is a vigorous 82-year-old woman who walks a total of 5 miles a day, maintains her own lawn and garden, and does all of her own housework in a two-story home. Her past medical history is significant for hypertension since age 40, depression since her husband died 10 years ago, insomnia, osteoarthritis, and a distant history of ocular migraines. Her prior surgical history includes an open appendectomy at the age of 21, a total knee replacement at age 78, cataract surgery on both eyes, excision of a melanoma the year prior, and endometrial biopsies 2 weeks ago. All of her prior surgical interventions were done without general anesthesia. She began having dysfunctional uterine bleeding several months ago, which has become very problematic. She is using five to six "heavy-flow" menstrual pads a day. She presents for total hysterectomy using a robotic system.

Her medications are HCTZ 25 mg every morning; lisinopril 2.5 mg every morning, clonidine 0.2 mg every evening, doxepin 6 mg every evening for insomnia, fluoxetine 40 mg every morning, zaleplon 10 mg as needed for severe insomnia, and tramadol 50 mg every 12 hours as needed for severe arthritis pain.

Her vital signs are blood pressure 112/78, heart rate 85, respiratory rate 19, temperature 36.5°C, SpO_2 96% on room air, weight 52 kgs, and height 164 cm.

Her lab values are Hb 8.6, hematocrit 25.8, platelets 156,000, Na^+ 136, K^+ 4.5, Cl^- 98, Bicarb 24, blood urea nitrogen (BUN) 23, and creatinine 1.0.

The patient is willing to accept blood transfusion if required.

PREOPERATIVE

Question 1. In obtaining an informed consent, a discussion regarding delirium and postoperative cognitive dysfunction is necessary in elderly patients. What elements of her history put her at risk for delirium?

a. Insomnia

b. Ocular Migraines

c. Her age

d. Lisinopril use.

The correct answer is c.

When obtaining informed consent in the elderly, especially past age 70, discussions regarding postoperative delirium and postoperative cognitive dysfunction are important.[1] Further, understanding the nomenclature surrounding perioperative mental status issues is crucial. Evered et al. summarize much of the topic in their 2018 paper.[2] Using terms already outlined in the *Diagnostic and Statistical Manual of Mental Disorders* (DSM-5) allows frank discussions that can be deciphered correctly. Preoperative neurocognitive disorders such as depressive symptoms, Parkinson's and Alzheimer's diseases, or other types of dementia are associated with delirium. Risk factors for this patient include age, depression, and hematocrit less than 30.[3,4] Neither insomnia nor the use of lisinopril are proven risk factors. Highly functional behaviors such as distance walking and maintaining a home and garden alone suggest the patient does not suffer from dementia. Her history of ocular migraines is a specific risk for stroke but not delirium.

Question 2. Why should informed consent include the discussion of cognitive events in elderly or at-risk individuals?

a. Although such events are rare, prior discussion decreases the odds of a lawsuit.

b. Neurocognitive events can impact morbidity and mortality.

c. Arrangements for nursing home care can be made in advance.

d. The patient can cancel her surgery or get a second opinion.

The correct answer is b.

The incidence of delirium is not rare among the elderly, ranging from 3% to more than 70% depending on preoperative factors, type of surgery, and ICU stay postoperatively. One meta-analysis estimates that postoperative delirium occurs roughly 23.8% of the time.[5] While genuine informed consent can mitigate risk of tort, elderly patients may lose autonomy and require prolonged or permanent institutionalization after surgery if they suffer a significant event. Consequently, patients and their families should be advised of such issues. In the case of elective surgeries, patients may choose to cancel, but when surgical intervention is necessary, cancellation is not possible.

If alternative, less invasive means are available, patients may be inclined to pursue them in light of a truly informed consent.

Question 3. What surgical and/or anesthetic risks play a role in postoperative delirium?

  a. Regional anesthesia without adjuvants.

  b. Steep head-down position.

  c. Laparoscopic or robotic-assisted surgery.

  d. Deeper levels of general anesthesia.

The correct answer is d.

Types of surgery may influence incident delirium, with greater likelihood occurring after major surgery. Although there have been case reports of the steep head-down position causing brain edema impacting cognition and the phenomenon has been studied in terms of optic nerve sheath diameter,[6] this is not the typical cause of postoperative delirium. When comparing laparoscopic to open procedures, laparoscopic surgeries appear to decrease the incidence of delirium.[7] While discussion surrounding the use of bispectral monitoring persists, there is evidence that deep levels of general anesthesia impact the brain unfavorably. Using bispectral index monitoring to maintain lighter anesthetic levels has been shown in some small studies to decrease the likelihood of delirium and postoperative cognitive dysfunction.[8] Regional anesthesia may influence the development of postoperative cognitive dysfunction, while the use of peripheral nerve block for pain control rather than opiates may influence the development of delirium.

INTRAOPERATIVE AND PACU

The patient had multiple, dense adhesions from her open appendectomy 63 years prior, making dissection difficult and prolonged. Total surgical time was 8 hours. During the surgery, possible injury to the right ureter was suspected. The surgeon requested that intravenous dye be given to help reveal possible injury. Consequently, the patient was given 10 cc of IV methylene blue.[9] After several minutes, the patient developed hypertension and tachycardia of 211/104 and 112, respectively. Fentanyl 100 mcg was given because surgical stimulation from cystoscopy presumably caused the increase in blood pressure and heart rate. The surgeon found no evidence of ureteral injury and quickly finished the operation. The patient was extubated when she finally opened her eyes but experienced a prolonged time to awakening in the operating room. Once in the PACU, the patient was agitated, unable to appropriately answer questions, and reacted violently when nursing staff tried to examine her operative sites. Her daughter was brought to the PACU to help calm the patient. Nonetheless, the patient remained confused and belligerent, which upset the daughter greatly. For the duration of the PACU stay, periods of agitation were interspersed with lack of response to her name or to physical stimulation. The patient was unable to attend to questions regarding pain, nausea, or comfort. Her blood pressure remained elevated in the 170–180 to 100–110 range with a heart rate in the 105–115 range.

Question 4. What is *not* in the differential diagnosis of this patient's behavior?

  a. Simple emergence delirium.

  b. Cerebrovascular accident (CVA).

  c. Postoperative delirium.

  d. Acute-onset Alzheimer's.

The correct answer is d.

There is no such diagnosis of acute-onset Alzheimer's disease. The difference between emergence delirium and postoperative delirium is primarily a function of time. Emergence delirium can occur in any age group, frequently affects pediatric patients, and has a brief course. In the elderly, however, studies suggest that emergence delirium in the PACU predicts or is highly associated with ongoing delirium.[10] CVA certainly impacts cognition, and seniors with hypertension are at risk; however, CVA does not typically present with the constellation of symptoms demonstrated in this patient. Delirium specifically includes motor signs and may present as hyperactive, hypoactive, or mixed delirium, with mixed being the most common. Hypoactive delirium is the most devastating and possibly the most difficult to recognize and treat.[11] Pure hyperactive delirium is the least common but the most readily recognizable. Simple confusion includes decreased orientation and forgetfulness, but lacks any associated motor component and does not include arousal or attention disturbances. Ruling out stroke and/or increased intracranial pressure (ICP) on clinical grounds includes looking for focal signs such as facial droop, pupil asymmetry, lack of pupillary response to light, asymmetrical limb movement, ocular palsies, and papilledema. Vomiting may be a feature of increased ICP, but it also commonly occurs after general anesthesia in nonsmoking women having gynecological surgery and is not specific. There are no case reports of significant cerebral edema complicating steep head-down positioning from robotic surgery, however there are cases of ischemic optic neuropathy reported.[12] If increased ICP or stroke is strongly suspected, then emergent imaging of the brain is required.

Question 5. How can this patient's confusion state be assessed/diagnosed?

  a. There are nursing tools to help assess delirium and alert anesthesiologists.

  b. Delirium is very subjective and difficult to diagnose.

  c. Only a psychiatrist can diagnose delirium.

  d. Neuropsychiatric testing is required to make a diagnosis.

The correct answer is a.

A number of studies have used various assessment tools to detect delirium in the PACU. One study used the Richmond Agitation-Sedation Scale (RASS) along with the Confusion Assessment Method[13] in the ICU (CAM-ICU). Combining the RASS with the CAM-ICU helped nurses identify patients with delirium by the time of PACU discharge. Diagnosis using the DSM-5 criteria for delirium remains the gold standard, but requires a physician, though not necessarily a psychiatrist. Validated nursing assessment tools such as the RASS and CAM-ICU enable nursing staff to alert anesthesiologists to patients possibly developing postoperative delirium.

Although many cases of delirium will begin after the patient leaves the PACU, it remains crucial to diagnose and intervene as soon as possible. The DSM-5 criteria to diagnose delirium include disturbance of arousal/attention/focus; the disturbance is acute or rapidly developing; cognitive disturbance affects memory, language, and perceptions; the changes in arousal, focus and cognition are not better explained by a preexisting problem and are not due to a coma; and the disturbances appear temporally and directly related to exposure to medications, toxins, withdrawal, or multiple etiologies.[14]

A study comparing the CAM-ICU to the Nursing Delirium Symptom Checklist (NuDESC) suggested that neither tool was especially sensitive and may miss cases of delirium developing in the PACU.[15] The Mini-Mental State Exam has also been used to help diagnose delirium and cognitive changes, but requires familiarity with its 10 components as well as the scoring system. The 4AT is a newer test that can be found on medical calculator sites and has been validated in several different hospital settings.[16] The four A's stand for Alertness, Age, Attention (such as listing the months backward), and Acute change or fluctuating course. Other assessment methods have been described, including AWOL in the nursing literature. AWOL stands for Age, World spelled backward, Orientation, and illness (L) severity. The most important aspect of assessment is not so much which tool is used, but that PACU nurses should have reasonable familiarity with recognizing developing delirium and have some validated method of doing so.

Question 6. Why is diagnosing delirium so important, especially in the elderly?

  a. Delirium increases length of stay.

  b. Delirium is associated with increased morbidity and mortality.

  c. Delirium is associated with loss of autonomy and institutionalization.

  d. All of the above.

The correct answer is d.

A number of studies over more than two decades and encompassing different types of surgery and postoperative settings demonstrate that outcomes are poorer for patients who develop delirium. Delirium contributes to increased length of stay, increased odds of losing autonomy or becoming institutionalized after hospital discharge, and increased risk of death even months after discharge.[17,18] The diagnosis of delirium is often missed in the PACU, being attributed to residual anesthesia effects, postoperative cognitive dysfunction, or even lack of knowledge of the patient's preexisting mental status. During handoff from original caregivers to oncoming staff, preexisting mental status should be noted. Particularly in the elderly, hypoactive delirium may be mistaken for a preoperative condition, thus causing considerable delay in treatment.

Question 7. What are other perioperative risk factors for delirium in this patient?

  a. Age greater than 70.

  b. Female gender.

  c. Hemoglobin of 8.

  d. Both a and c.

The correct answer is d.

With a starting hematocrit of less than 30, additional surgical blood loss occurs. Blood retained in the removed specimen is almost always ignored by surgeons and anesthesiologists yet can comprise a significant loss in large specimens. Her history of depression, taking a non-benzodiazepine (Z-drug) for sleep, and being on tramadol are also risk factors for postoperative delirium.[19,20] Frailty was not a risk factor for this patient as evidenced by her ability to walk daily, maintain her own lawn, and perform all of her housework in a large home. Likewise, she did not appear to have preexisting dementia (not obvious by the provided history). Mild dementia may not be readily evident in the preoperative assessment unless close family members are interviewed as well. Exposure to drugs associated with postoperative delirium include inhalation agents and opiates. This patient was on tramadol prior to surgery and received fentanyl intraoperatively.

Question 8. Do you think methylene blue plays a role in this patient's "delirium?"

  a. Methylene blue is inert, so is not a problem.

  b. It treats hypotension caused by angiotensin converting enzyme I (ACEI).

  c. Methylene blue is a potent reversible inhibitor of monoamine oxidase A (MAOA).

  d. Methylene blue dose is always one vial.

The correct answer is c.

While it is true that methylene blue can treat hypotension/vasoplegia secondary to ACEI, this patient did not experience hypotension from her lisinopril, as outlined in the stem. When indigo carmine was no longer available in North America, surgeons resorted to methylene blue for a variety of purposes, including visualizing ureters during abdominal surgery. Methylene blue is not inert. It actively accepts and donates electrons, inhibiting activation of soluble guanylyl cyclase by nitric oxide. Case reports of patients developing signs and symptoms of serotonin toxicity, including delirium, highlighted the unintended consequences of delivering a monoamine oxidase inhibitor intravenously (i.e., methylene blue). Patients who are on antidepressants and those taking tramadol are at particular risk.[21] No large-scale studies have determined appropriate dosing for methylene blue, however, Verbeek et al. showed that 0.25 mg/kg was sufficient to guide identification of the ureters using near-infrared fluorescence.[22] Doses as large as 1.5 mg/kg have been used for vasoplegic syndrome with cardiac surgery. Methylene blue has a standard concentration of 10 mg/mL. Although methylene blue administration is only one of several risk factors for delirium in this patient, it is extremely important not to discount it.

Question 9. Besides evaluating the mental status, what else should be done to work up this patient?

a. Blood gases are painful and could contribute to delirium.

b. Physical exam for focal deficits, deep tendon reflexes, clonus, and hyperpyrexia.

c. CT of the head with and without contrast.

d. A chest x-ray to rule out pneumonia.

The correct answer is b.

In addition to a physical examination looking for focal neurologic signs that might indicate stroke, the patient should also be examined for abnormal deep tendon reflexes or spontaneous clonus. Brisk reflexes and clonus are associated with serotonin syndrome whereas typical postoperative delirium is not. Additionally, laboratory studies should be sent looking for electrolyte imbalances, blood gas abnormalities such as hypercarbia or significant acidosis, and postoperative anemia. For patients with delirium, the brief discomfort of obtaining labs does not outweigh the possible discovery of important laboratory findings. Hyperpyrexia can be associated with malignant hyperthermia, overtly vigorous intraoperative warming, and infectious phenomena as well as serotonin syndrome. If focal signs suggest stroke or if the patient is completely obtunded without any response, a CT of the head should be undertaken.

Question 10. What pharmacological means should be taken for treating delirium?

a. Haloperidol 5–10 mg IM should be given for postoperative delirium.

b. Dexmedetomidine infusion has been proved to cure delirium in the PACU.

c. No drug has been shown to speed up recovery from hypoactive delirium.

d. Intranasal insulin has been proved to speed recovery of delirium in very large trials.

The correct answer is c.

If there are no major laboratory abnormalities requiring treatment, pharmacological means of addressing delirium traditionally has been IV haloperidol 2–5 mg,[23] or, more recently, dexmedetomidine infusion.[24] Of note, a metanalysis of studies utilizing antipsychotics suggests that they are not useful to prevent or treat all delirium and have no impact on duration of delirium, hospital or ICU length of stay, severity of delirium, or associated mortality.[25] In a metanalysis of ICU patients, treatment with dexmedetomidine was associated with an overall reduction in prevalence but there was no statistically significant changes in length of stay, morbidity, or mortality.[25] There are no studies examining routine use of dexmedetomidine for delirium in the PACU. While hyperactive delirium is the least common subtype, it is more likely to result in patients pulling out lines, trying to get out of bed, falling, and removing catheters. For those patients, the mild sedation from low-dose IV haloperidol or a dexmedetomidine infusion may be useful.

For patients with primarily hypoactive delirium, additional sedation is unlikely to be helpful and may prolong delirium if beneficial actions cannot be undertaken, such as early mobilization. Benzodiazepines are contraindicated for use in treating delirium unless it is absolutely related to acute alcohol or benzodiazepine withdrawal. More recently, the use of intranasal insulin shows promise in treating delirium, but further study is required particularly regarding optimal dosing.[26]

While a number of studies undertaking nonpharmacological methods have attempted to prevent or treat delirium in a variety of patients, a systematic overview of methods only supports prevention of delirium in high-risk patients using multicomponent plans.[27] Such multicomponent plans require considerable resources and organization. Reorienting patients to date, time, and setting does not appear to adequately treat delirium though it does not cause harm. Helping patients mobilize early, normalize bowel and bladder functions, assisting with and maintaining adequate nutrition, non-opiate means of treating pain, and optimizing vision and hearing all appear to be beneficial in treating delirium.[28]

Constipation and urinary tract infections contribute to a higher incidence of delirium. The inability to see or hear adequately also contributes to delirium. For patients with glasses and hearing aids, it is important to reinstitute those devices as soon after surgery as possible. Early mobilization is very important in mitigating delirium as well as in helping prevent deep vein thrombosis, constipation, and pneumonia. For patients already experiencing delirium, physical and occupational therapy consults are essential. Many times, it will require more than one therapist to assist a patient experiencing delirium with mobility, self-care, feeding, etc.

Question 11. If methylene blue exposure contributed to delirium in this patient, is there any specific antidote for methylene blue or treatment for serotonin syndrome?

a. Cyproheptadine and chlorpromazine have both been used to treat serotonin syndrome.

b. Side effects of medications that treat serotonin syndrome prohibit their use.

c. Haloperidol will help with the agitation seen in serotonin syndrome.

d. Large multicenter trials show cyproheptadine to be rapidly efficacious.

The correct answer is a.

Two serotonin receptor antagonists are readily available: cyproheptadine and chlorpromazine. Cyproheptadine has been used in a number of case reports to reverse serotonin syndrome.[29] The doses described are 4–12 mg orally initially, and it takes 1–2 hours for onset. Subsequent maintenance doses can be given, not to exceed 0.5 mg/kg/day. Cyproheptadine is a first-generation antihistamine with anticholinergic properties that could contribute to sedation, confusion, and other untoward symptoms in the elderly and should only be used if the diagnosis of serotonin syndrome is most likely.

Chlorpromazine has also been used in case reports to treat serotonin syndrome, but it has side effects that include hypotension, dystonia, and tardive dyskinesia as well as sedation, tachycardia, and anxiety. Both cyproheptadine and chlorpromazine have been used in case reports, and there is a case series from 2020.[30] There are no large, multicenter trials examining their use in serotonin syndrome. Haloperidol does not specifically treat agitation in serotonin syndrome but could confound important signs such as muscle rigidity or pyrexia. Dexmedetomidine may help calm agitation, decrease hypertension, and is readily titratable but it has no specific effect on serotonin syndrome and will not help with hypoactive delirium. Cyproheptadine only comes in an oral format and may be difficult to administer in patients with delirium.

Question 12. How can anesthesiologists prevent delirium?

a. All cases of delirium can be prevented by using regional anesthesia.

b. Avoiding high-risk medications may decrease the incidence of delirium.

c. Avoiding the use of benzodiazepines always prevents delirium.

d. Cyproheptadine rapidly reverses delirium.

The correct answer is b.

In the preoperative period, eliminating high-risk medications or substances such as benzodiazepines, alcohol, or sleeping pills that contribute to delirium may be useful. However, preventing withdrawal syndromes in patients is paramount. This patient's as-needed use of tramadol suggests that she could avoid its use prior to surgery. For patients who require daily use of tramadol to control pain, it must be kept in mind that complete clearance of tramadol requires roughly 30 hours. Patients who routinely use certain sleep medications may need to wean them prior to surgery as well. Such efforts require advance preoperative assessment. Risk prediction models rarely consider adjusting preoperative medications. However, anesthesiologists are in a unique position to discuss avoiding or weaning medications prior to surgery at the preoperative planning visit.[31] For perioperative pain management, the use of non-opiate medications or regional or central neuraxial blocks helps decrease exposure to opiates. However, such techniques by themselves have not been shown to prevent postoperative delirium. While multimodal analgesia decreases opiate use, multimodal analgesia does not prevent delirium.

Melatonin may be useful as a preventative strategy but large conclusive studies are lacking.[32] Intraoperative hypotension by itself does not predict delirium; however extremely labile blood pressure appears to be related.[33] In one study, transfusion to a hemoglobin of at least 11.3 g/dL lessened the odds of developing delirium; however, this study only included 179 frail elderly patients.[34] Other studies allowing hemoglobin levels of less than 10 g/dL have not shown an increase in postoperative delirium. Specific high-risk medications that contribute to developing delirium in those seventy and older are benzodiazepines, diphenhydramine, meperidine, atypical antipsychotics, tricyclic antidepressants, and oral muscle relaxants.[35]

Question 13. What should you tell the family regarding delirium in their loved one?

a. That the delirium will rapidly pass and not impact her health.

b. That delirium is always cured with haloperidol or dexmedetomidine.

c. That the patient has serotonin syndrome, a special cause of delirium.

d. That cyproheptadine is a rapid, benign, reliable antidote.

The correct answer is c.

Disclosing that delirium may increase length of stay, morbidity, and mortality as well as the inability to gain full autonomy after hospital discharge is important. Despite preoperative consent regarding delirium, it is important to reiterate possible outcomes. Patients and families do not always remember every aspect of informed consent. Typically, delirium may resolve in days to weeks, yet it may persist in some individuals. Emphasize what measures are being taken to decrease contributing factors, as well as what role family can play in helping the patient. They can reorient her, encourage wakefulness during daylight hours, and assist with hydration and feeding if feasible. Pharmacological interventions such as haloperidol and dexmedetomidine may help in specific situations, but they are not a panacea for every case of delirium. In this specific case, administration of a medication (methylene blue) requested for a diagnostic purpose (locating ureters/checking continuity) likely precipitated her current state. Family members should be informed of the medication interaction possibly precipitating the acute delirium—particularly if evidence such as clonus, rigidity, and/or hyperpyrexia support that specific diagnosis.

Likewise, the use of an intervention like cyproheptadine should include a risk-benefit discussion since cyproheptadine can cause sedation or confusion in the elderly. All treatment decisions or interventions should be well documented, with the rationale plainly charted. In situations where hospitalists may be managing medical care while the surgical service only follows postoperative surgical implications, it behooves the anesthesiologist to discuss specific aspects of delirium with the hospitalist team.

During the PACU stay, cyproheptadine 4 mg was administered orally. The patient remained hypertensive and tachycardic. IV enalapril was administered for hypertension, aiming for a mean arterial pressure near 85, while IV metoprolol was used to lower her heart rate to less than 100 bpm. Originally, a private room on the gynecological ward was assigned for her postoperative stay.

Question 14. Should the patient go to the ICU at this point?

a. Studies show that these patients should go to the ICU because of fall risk.

b. Sleep normalization is more likely in a private room.

c. ICU nurses are better at helping with orienting patients.

d. Studies show delirium is less common in ICU patients.

The correct answer is b.

Higher-acuity beds, whether in the ICU or step-down care, offer a lower ratio of nursing care which enables closer attention to vital signs, troubleshooting hemodynamic issues or certain postoperative complications, and implementing major nursing interventions. However, the ambience of an ICU—with higher noise levels, monitors flashing/alarming, and greater ambient light overall—is more likely to sustain or lead to postoperative delirium. The incidence of delirium in the elderly requiring intensive care services is as high as 80%.[36] However, the diagnosis of delirium itself is not an indicator for higher-acuity care unless other delirium measures cannot be accomplished in a floor bed.

Postoperative delirium is a major risk factor for falling postoperatively, but preventing falls requires more than just lower ratio nursing care. ICU nurses are frequently tending to unstable patients, not merely managing fall precautions. Fall prevention includes multiple strategies such as bed alarms, sitters, avoiding sedative/hypnotics and opiates, and using physical and occupational therapists to help normalize ambulation and activities of daily living, as well as assisting patients with eating and ensuring protein ingestion is adequate. Furthermore, family members may have a greater ability to interact with patients in a private room setting rather than an ICU setting. Therefore, sending this patient to an ICU bed may not be in her interest.

Question 15. The daughter Googled postoperative delirium and notes that melatonin has been used to help normalize sleep patterns. She wants her mother to receive melatonin and has asked why it wasn't given prophylactically.

a. Read more about the use of melatonin in the treatment of delirium.

b. Order 10 mg of melatonin stat.

c. Inform the daughter that Dr. Google isn't always correct.

d. Give the patient her regular sleeping pill instead.

The correct answer is a.

It is not unusual for patients and their families to perform internet searches to learn about perioperative processes, complications, and treatment strategies. Sleep dysregulation plays a role in postoperative delirium, but a patient who develops delirium in the PACU immediately after surgery has not experienced sleep dysregulation yet. Physicians should perform a reliable search of the literature through an acceptable search engine and arrive at a properly thought-out conclusion. Melatonin prophylaxis against delirium and attempts to utilize it as treatment are not conclusive. A Cochrane database meta-analysis showed conflicting results.[37] Plasma melatonin levels are lower in the elderly experiencing delirium,[38] suggesting that supplementation may be beneficial. However, differences have been discovered between levels in hyperactive versus hypoactive delirium.

The medication ramelteon has been shown to be possibly beneficial in treating delirium in the elderly.[39] A well-conducted randomized controlled trial of more than 450 patients did not show any advantage to supplementing with 3 mg of melatonin versus placebo in preventing delirium in patients undergoing hip surgery.[40] Studies may have not discovered optimal dosing strategies in the elderly nor paired plasma melatonin levels with dosing. Therefore, one cannot derive an appropriate dose of melatonin for this patient from published trials.

Question 16. If your hospital does not have a devoted interdisciplinary program for treating or preventing postoperative delirium, how can you as the anesthesiologist advocate on behalf of this patient?

a. Tell the surgeon to order a delirium protocol.

b. Discuss what services the patient will need with the case manager.

c. Tell the nurses they need to institute delirium protocols.

d. Tell the family what strategies to use to help the patient.

The best answer is b.

While answers a, c, and d are partly correct, for comprehensive management, the case manager is best able to coordinate all required services and perform daily assessments. Traditionally, anesthesiologists might alert surgeons to an outcome, leaving it to the surgeons to handle complications. In the case of postoperative delirium, inappropriate care may worsen delirium and increase the odds of other complications, such as extrapyramidal side effects from doses of haloperidol greater than 4.5 mg/day.[41] PACU nurses should always give a complete report including outcomes like delirium, yet it is not incumbent upon nursing staff to manage delirium without physician involvement. Alerting family members to orientation strategies represents only one facet of this patient's comprehensive care. Ultimately one entity coordinating all components of delirium care and documenting in the chart is desirable and adds value to patient care.

CONCLUSION

- Altered mental status in the postoperative period is a serious medical problem.
- The elderly are particularly prone to delirium.
- The differential diagnosis includes individual patient characteristics such as frailty, age, preoperative organic brain pathology, medication interactions, thromboembolic phenomena, surgical or positioning complications, withdrawal from substances and physiologic insults such as prolonged hypotension or hypoxia.
- Length of stay, morbidity, mortality, and persistent postoperative neurocognitive dysfunction outcomes are all worse in patients who have an episode of delirium.
- There is no known reliable prevention tactics or treatment algorithms.
- Management of delirium requires an interdisciplinary approach.
- Methylene blue can precipitate serotonin syndrome.

REFERENCES

1. Benamer C, Fitzpatrick G, Ridgway P, O'Neill D. Persistent perioperative cognitive impairment: Prevention, management and sharing with patients. *Ir Med J*. 2020;113:68.
2. Evered L, Atkins K, Silbert B, Scott DA. Acute peri-operative neurocognitive disorders: A narrative review. *Anaesthesia*. 2022;77:34–42.
3. Ansaloni L, Catena F, Chattat R, et al. Risk factors and incidence of postoperative delirium in elderly patients after elective and emergency surgery. *J Br Surg*. 2010;97(2):273–280.
4. Smith PJ, Attix DK, Weldon BC, Greene NH, Monk TG. Executive function and depression as independent risk factors for postoperative delirium. *J Am Soc Anesth*. 2009 April;110(4):781–787.
5. Silva AR, Regueira P, Albuquerque E, et al. Estimates of geriatric delirium frequency in noncardiac surgeries and its evaluation across the years: A systematic review and meta-analysis. *J Am Med Dir Assoc*. 2021;22(3):613–620.
6. Colombo R, Agarossi A, Borghi B, et al. The effect of prolonged steep head-down laparoscopy on the optical nerve sheath diameter. *J Clin Mon Comput*. 2020;34:1295–1302.
7. Ito K, Suka Y, Nagai M, et al. Lower risk of postoperative delirium using laparoscopic approach for major abdominal surgery. *Surg Endoscopy*. 2019;33:2121–2127.
8. Chan MT, Cheng BC, Lee TM, Gin T; CODA Trial Group. (). BIS-guided anesthesia decreases postoperative delirium and cognitive decline. *Journal of neurosurgical anesthesiology*. 2013;25(1):33–42.
9. Manoucheri E, Cohen SL, Sandberg EM, Kibel AS, Einarsson J. Ureteral injury in laparoscopic gynecologic surgery. *Rev Obstet Gynecol*. 2012;5(2):106.
10. Sharma PT, Sieber FE, Zakriya KJ, et al. Recovery room delirium predicts postoperative delirium after hip-fracture repair. *Anesth Analg*. 2005;101(4):1215–1220.
11. Meagher DJ, Trzepacz PT. Motoric subtypes of delirium. *Sem Clin Neuropsychiatr*. 2000 April;5(2):75–85.
12. Stoffelns BM. Anterior ischemic optic neuropathy due to abdominal hemorrhage after laparotomy for uterine myoma. *Arch Gynecol Obstetr*. 2010;281:157–160.
13. Ely EW, Inouye SK, Bernard GR, et al. Delirium in mechanically ventilated patients: Validity and reliability of the confusion assessment method for the intensive care unit (CAM-ICU). *JAMA*. 2001;286(21):2703–2710.
14. The DSM-5 criteria, level of arousal, and delirium diagnosis: Inclusiveness is safer. https://bmcmedicine.biomedcentral.com/articles/10.1186/s12916-014-0141-2
15. Neufeld KJ, Leoutsakos JS, Sieber FE, et al. Evaluation of two delirium screening tools for detecting post-operative delirium in the elderly. *Br J Anaesth*. 2013;111(4):612–618.
16. Bellelli G, Morandi A, Davis DH, et al. Validation of the 4AT, a new instrument for rapid delirium screening: A study in 234 hospitalised older people. *Age Ageing*. 2014;43(4):496–502.
17. Ely E, Gautam S, Margolin R, et al. The impact of delirium in the intensive care unit on hospital length of stay. *Intensive Care Med*. 2001;27:1892–1900.
18. Inouye SK, Rushing JT, Foreman MD, Palmer RM, Pompei P. Does delirium contribute to poor hospital outcomes? A three-site epidemiologic study. *J Gen Internal Med*. 1998;13(4):234–242.
19. Gaulton TG, Wunsch H, Gaskins LJ, et al. Preoperative sedative-hypnotic medication use and adverse postoperative outcomes. *Ann Surg*. 2021;274(2):e108.
20. Brouquet A, Cudennec T, Benoist S, et al. Impaired mobility, ASA status and administration of tramadol are risk factors for postoperative delirium in patients aged 75 years or more after major abdominal surgery. *Ann Surg*. 2010;251(4):759–765.
21. US Food and Drug Administration. FDA Drug Safety Communication: Serious CNS reactions possible when methylene blue is given to patients taking certain psychiatric medications. https://www.fda.gov/drugs/drug-safety-and-availability/fda-drug-safety-communication-updated-information-about-drug-interaction-between-methylene-blue#:~:text=Most%20cases%20from%20the%20FDA%27s%20Adverse%20Event%20Reporting,doses%20ranged%20from%201%20mg%2Fkg%20to%208%20mg%2Fkg.
22. Verbeek FP, van der Vorst JR, Schaafsma BE, et al. Intraoperative near infrared fluorescence guided identification of the ureters using low dose methylene blue: A first in human experience. *J Urol*. 2013;190(2):574–579.
23. Beach SR, Gross AF, Hartney KE, Taylor JB, Rundell JR. Intravenous haloperidol: A systematic review of side effects and recommendations for clinical use. *Gen Hosp Psychiatr*. 2020;67:42–50.
24. Maldonado JR, Wysong A, Van Der Starre PJ, Block T, Miller C, Reitz BA. Dexmedetomidine and the reduction of postoperative delirium after cardiac surgery. *Psychosomatics*. 2009;50(3):206–217.
25. Nikooie R, Neufeld KJ, Oh ES, et al. Antipsychotics for treating delirium in hospitalized adults: A systematic review. *Ann Intern Med*. 2019;171(7):485–495.
26. Shpakov AO, Zorina II, Derkach KV. Hot spots for the use of intranasal insulin: Cerebral ischemia, brain injury, diabetes mellitus, endocrine disorders and postoperative delirium. *Int J Mol Sci*. 2023;24(4):3278.
27. Rohatgi N, Weng Y, Bentley J, et al. Initiative for prevention and early identification of delirium in medical-surgical units: Lessons learned in the past five years. *Am J Med*. 2019;132(12):1421–1430.
28. Thom RP, Levy-Carrick NC, Bui M, Silbersweig D. Delirium. *Am J Psychiatr*. 2019;176(10):785–793.
29. Gillman PK. The serotonin syndrome and its treatment. *J Psychopharmacol*. 1999;13(1):100–109.
30. Frye JR, Poggemiller AM, McGonagill PW, et al. Use of cyproheptadine for the treatment of serotonin syndrome: A case series. *J Clin Psychopharmacol*. 2020;40(1):95–99.
31. Parker BM, Tetzlaff JE, Litaker DL, Maurer WG. Redefining the preoperative evaluation process and the role of the anesthesiologist. *J Clin Anesth*. 2000;12(5):350–356.
32. Jaiswal SJ, McCarthy TJ, Wineinger NE, et al. Melatonin and sleep in preventing hospitalized delirium: A randomized clinical trial. *Am J Med*. 2018;131(9):1110–1117.
33. Hirsch J, DePalma G, Tsai TT, Sands LP, Leung JM. Impact of intraoperative hypotension and blood pressure fluctuations on early postoperative delirium after non-cardiac surgery. *Br J Anaesth*. 2015;115(3):418–426.

34. van der Zanden V, Beishuizen SJ, Scholtens RM, de Jonghe A, de Rooij SE, van Munster BC. The effects of blood transfusion on delirium incidence. *J Am Med Dir Assoc*. 2016;17(8):748–753.
35. 2019 American Geriatrics Society Beers Criteria Update Expert Panel: Fick DM, Semla TP, Steinman M, et al. American Geriatrics Society 2019 updated AGS Beers Criteria for potentially inappropriate medication use in older adults. *J Am Geriatr Soc*. 2019;67(4):674–694.
36. Girard TD, Pandharipande PP, Ely EW. Delirium in the intensive care unit. *Crit Care*. 2008;12:1–9.
37. Han Y, Tian Y, Wu J, et al. Melatonin and its analogs for prevention of post-cardiac surgery delirium: A systematic review and meta-analysis. *Front Cardiovasc Med*. 2022;9.
38. Shigeta H, Yasui A, Nimura Y, et al. Postoperative delirium and melatonin levels in elderly patients. *Am J Surg*. 2001;182(5):449–454.
39. Hatta K, Kishi Y, Wada K, et al. Preventive effects of ramelteon on delirium: A randomized placebo-controlled trial. *JAMA Psychiatry*. 2014;71(4):397–403.
40. de Jonghe A, van Munster BC, Goslings JC, et al. Effect of melatonin on incidence of delirium among patients with hip fracture: A multicentre, double-blind randomized controlled trial. *CMAJ* 2014;186(14):E547–E556.
41. Lonergan E, Britton AM, Luxenberg J. Antipsychotics for delirium. *Cochrane Database Syst Rev*. 2007;2.

48.

THE HR MONITOR IS ALARMING IN THE PACU

POSTOPERATIVE ARRHYTHMIAS

Avi Dobrusin and Muthuraj Kanakaraj

STEM CASE AND KEY QUESTIONS

A 63-year-old male patient with a history of obesity, hypertension, obstructive sleep apnea (OSA), and coronary artery disease (CAD) with placement of a single drug-eluting stent 5 years ago arrives in the PACU following a laparoscopic hiatal hernia repair. Suddenly, the bedside monitor begins to alarm because of tachycardia, and, upon evaluating the patient, the nurse notes an irregular pulse at a rate of 130 beats per minute (bpm) and a blood pressure of 124/76. You, as the attending anesthesiologist, are notified and come to the bedside to see the patient.

How should postoperative arrhythmias be evaluated, and what diagnostic tests are indicated?

You begin your evaluation with a focused history and physical exam. He states that he is not having any palpitations or dizziness and is just "sleepy," which you attribute to his recent anesthetic. Your exam reveals an irregular pulse, warm and well-perfused extremities, soft and mildly tender abdomen, no pedal edema, and no detectable murmur upon auscultation of his chest. You then turn your attention to his chart to review his surgical and anesthetic record. This reveals an uneventful general anesthetic, during which he only required small boluses of phenylephrine to maintain a mean arterial pressure of 70 mm Hg; he received 1.5 L of crystalloid fluid. The blood loss was estimated to be 30 mL. You also find a record of an echocardiogram from 2 months prior that demonstrated only trace mitral regurgitation, no regional wall motion abnormalities, and an ejection fraction of 65%.

You order a 12-lead ECG and ask the nurse to draw blood for a basic metabolic panel, CBC, and magnesium level. Given the patient's history of CAD, you elect to also order serial troponins. You consider performing a bedside transthoracic echocardiogram to evaluate for any functional abnormalities but defer as the patient had a very recent echocardiogram.

The ECG demonstrates an irregular rhythm with a rate of 136 bpm and absent p waves consistent with atrial fibrillation (AF) with rapid ventricular response. The patient's labs are notable for a potassium of 3.2 mmol/L and magnesium of 1.6 mg/dl.

What are the causes of postoperative AF?

Studies investigating postoperative AF have revealed that it is caused by the complex interaction of surgical, biochemical, and patient-specific factors that combine to promote the atrial ectopy and reentrant circuits that results in AF.[1] Surgical techniques, including atriotomy and use of cardiopulmonary bypass, disrupt the native cardiac conduction system and predispose patients to the development of AF. In addition, cardiopulmonary bypass can result in a systemic inflammatory response and complement activation that further increases the risk of AF.[2] High sympathetic activity in the immediate postoperative period, electrolyte derangements (hypokalemia, hypomagnesemia), and metabolic imbalance (hypoglycemia) also contribute to the development of AF. Surgical stress response activates the sympathetic nervous system and catecholamine release and increases heart rate. Hypovolemia, hypotension, anemia, trauma, and pain can also activate sympathetic system. Importantly, AF may also be a manifestation of other acute pathologies, such as sepsis, hemorrhage, and hypoxia. In these cases, identification and management of the primary cause is critical. Hypoxia causes pulmonary vasoconstriction and increase in right ventricular afterload and right atrial stretch, which could trigger AF. The patient-related factors that contribute to the development of postoperative AF include advanced age (>72 years), obesity, OSA, chronic kidney disease, hypertension, heart failure, previous myocardial infarction, left atrial enlargement, and left atrial strain.[3]

In the postoperative setting, is a rate-control or rhythm-control strategy superior?

Because the vast majority of patients with postoperative AF will convert to sinus rhythm, a rate-control strategy is generally appropriate.[4] In select patients unable to tolerate the loss of atrioventricular synchrony, rhythm control may be appropriate. You decide to administer 5 mg IV metoprolol to the patient with the goal of reducing his heart rate to between 80 and 100 bpm. The patient rapidly returns to normal sinus rhythm with a rate of 88 bpm. You then order 60 mEq potassium chloride and 2 g magnesium sulfate as you recall that electrolyte abnormalities may predispose a patient to arrhythmias.

After about 1 minute, you notice that the patient is less responsive than before and ask the nurse to repeat a set of vital signs. His blood pressure is now 68/46 and his heart rate has returned 136 bpm. You decide that your next step in managing this patient is synchronized cardioversion.

What are the indications for and risks of synchronized cardioversion?

Synchronized, direct current cardioversion is the first-line treatment for hemodynamically unstable tachyarrhythmia with a pulse. In addition, it may be considered for patients with tachyarrhythmias that are refractory to pharmacologic treatment and in those unable to tolerate the loss of sinus rhythm.

The most significant risk of cardioversion is thromboembolic events, including stroke and critical limb ischemia. While current guidelines suggest that cardioversion is safe without anticoagulation in those with AF present for less than 48 hours, recent evidence suggests that stroke risk increases as soon as 12 hours after the onset of AF.[5] In the setting of hemodynamic instability, however, anticoagulation is not feasible and should not delay electrical cardioversion. Moreover, in the postoperative period, the benefits of anticoagulation must be weighed against the risk of hemorrhage. You elect to proceed without anticoagulation.

Should patients receive sedation prior to synchronized cardioversion?

Sedative and analgesia medications are often administered prior to an elective cardioversion. However, in unstable patients, this is a more nuanced decision, as many such medications can have undesirable hemodynamic and/or respiratory effects.[6] You also recognize that oversedation may result in complications given the patient's hemodynamic status and history of OSA. Finally, you consider the patient's fasting status and are relieved to learn that the patient was appropriately fasted prior to his surgery and has not had any food or drink in the PACU.

After ensuring that airway management equipment is readily available, you administer 1 mg midazolam. The patient is then cardioverted with 100 joules. He returns to normal sinus rhythm immediately, and his blood pressure improves. He is monitored in the PACU for 2 more hours before going to the surgical step-down unit with continuous telemetry monitoring. The inpatient cardiology service is consulted and evaluates the patient the next morning.

What are the most common sequelae of postoperative AF, and what follow-up is indicated?

The attending cardiologist informs the patient that, due to the development of postoperative AF, he is at increased risk of stroke, myocardial infarction, and all-cause mortality.[7] The patient recalls that his brother has an "irregular heartbeat" and takes "blood thinners" and inquires if he similarly needs such medication. The decision of whether to pursue prophylactic anticoagulation should include consideration of a patient's medical history, propensity of AF recurrence, and risk and implications of postoperative bleeding.[4,8] With a CHA_2DS_2-$VASC_2$ score of 3, the cardiologist recommends long-term anticoagulation, and the patient agrees.[8]

The patient returns to the hospital 3 years later for an elective repair of an incisional hernia. General anesthesia was induced uneventfully, and an initial attempt was made to repair the hernia robotically; however, due to the presence of intraabdominal adhesions, the surgery was converted to an open procedure. The case proceeded without further complications, and the patient was extubated and transported to the PACU. The bedside nurse notes that the patient is becoming progressively more somnolent. His vital signs are heart rate 56 bpm with regular rate, blood pressure 118/68, respiratory rate 8, and SpO_2 93%. A nasal cannula is placed, and supplemental oxygen is administered at 3 L/pm. The patient is then re-evaluated 30 minutes later and found to be minimally responsive with shallow breathing.

What are the common causes of respiratory insufficiency in the PACU?

There are numerous potential causes of respiratory insufficiency in the postoperative period. The most common causes include opioid-induced respiratory depression, residual neuromuscular blockade, and upper airway obstruction.[9] Naloxone is administered with no change in the patient's respiratory effort. A twitch monitor is then applied and demonstrates only three twitches and no sustained tetany.

You administer 2 mg/kg of sugammadex; the patient's respiratory function improves rapidly, and his oxygen saturation begins to increase. Approximately 30 seconds later, the bedside monitor begins to alarm, displaying a heart rate of 42 bpm and a blood pressure of 98/58.

What medications used in the perioperative period are most closely associated with bradycardia?

Several medications used in the perioperative setting are associated with clinically significant bradycardia at standard therapeutic doses, including opioids, neostigmine, sugammadex, dexmedetomidine, and succinylcoline.[10] Pretreatment with an anticholinergic agent is common prior to the administration of succinylcholine or neostigmine, particularly in highly susceptible groups, such as infants and children.[11,12] Sugammadex is associated with a reduced incidence of bradycardia when compared to neostigmine.[13] Vasoconstrictive medications, such as phenylephrine, may result in baroreceptor-mediated reflex bradycardia.[14] Though the continuation of beta blockers throughout the perioperative period has been shown to decrease the rate of major adverse cardiovascular events, they also convey an increased risk of bradycardia and hypotension.[15]

As you had just administered sugammadex, you suspect that this as the cause of the patient's acute bradycardia and determine that immediate treatment is warranted.

What pharmacologic options are recommended for the treatment of bradycardia?

Anticholinergic agents, such as atropine, are the generally accepted first-line treatment for clinically significant bradycardia. Other medications that can be considered are glycopyrrolate, isoproterenol, ephedrine, dopamine, dobutamine, and theophylline.[16] In patients with a history of cardiac transplantation, atropine has been associated with a paradoxical atrioventricular block and should thus be avoided.[17,18]

You administer 1 mg atropine.[19] The patient's heart rate continues to decline, as the monitor is now reading 34 bpm.

Another blood pressure of 64/38 is obtained, and 20 mcg of epinephrine is administered with no effect on the patient's heart rate or blood pressure. The nurse asks if you would like to place pacing pads on the patient, and you agree that this would be prudent given his deteriorating clinical status.

What are the indications for transcutaneous pacing?

Transcutaneous pacing is indicated in patients with hemodynamically unstable bradycardia. It may also be considered in those who exhibit symptomatic bradycardia that is not responsive to pharmacologic therapy. Evidence does not support the use of transcutaneous pacing in cases of asystole cardiac arrest.[20]

As the pacing pads are being applied to the patient, you observe a sudden deterioration of his mental status and immediately attempt to palpate a carotid pulse. You are unable to do so and instruct the nurse to begin chest compressions. Asystole is noted on the monitor and 1 mg epinephrine is expeditiously administered to the patient. The patient is reintubated without interrupting chest compressions, and, after 2 minutes of CPR, there is a return of spontaneous circulation. The patient is started on epinephrine and propofol infusions and transported to the ICU. He is extubated the following day and discharged home 7 days later with no neurologic sequalae.

The patient returns to the hospital 4 years later for lumbar laminectomy due to worsening spinal stenosis that has been refractory to noninvasive management. Prior to surgery, he has a stress echocardiogram and repeat ECG that demonstrate normal cardiac function and no evidence of ischemia. The procedure is uneventful, although, upon arriving in the PACU, he is complaining of nausea. In accordance with the patient's postoperative orders, the nurse administers 1 mg haloperidol. Ten minutes later, the monitor begins to alarm. Glancing at the monitor you note a distinctive pattern of polymorphic ventricular tachycardia consistent with torsades de pointes (TdP).

The patient reports that he briefly felt "weak and dizzy," but the sensation passed quickly. You glance back up at the monitor and notice that the patient has returned to normal sinus rhythm.

How does the management of TdP differ between hemodynamically stable and unstable patients?

TdP may present as brief, self-resolving episodes with or without accompanying symptoms such as syncope or dizziness. In these cases, a careful review of the patient's inpatient and home medications is critical. Medications known to prolong the QTc interval should be stopped when possible and supplemental magnesium sulfate should be administered. While magnesium does not shorten the QTc interval, it has been shown to reduce the incidence of TdP, possibly by suppressing early depolarization.[21]

In unstable TdP (pulseless, hemodynamically unstable), proceed with the Advanced Cardiac Life Support (ACLS) algorithm to stabilize the patient. Administer IV magnesium. If persistent or recurrent TdP, consider transvenous pacing at 100 bpm. If transvenous pacing is not available, transcutaneous pacing can be done with sedation. Also consider giving class IB anti-arrhythmic drugs such as IV lidocaine, IV phenytoin, or IV potassium. Patient will need to be referred to an electrophysiologist for further management.[22,23]

In this stable patient, you administer 2 g magnesium sulfate and continue to monitor the patient for 2 more hours in the PACU, where he has no more episodes of TdP. You also order routine labs which demonstrate a magnesium level of 1.4 mg/dL. Upon review of his home medication list, you note that he was started on citalopram several months ago for depression and had recently been prescribed a short course of ciprofloxacin for a urinary tract infection. You then review his intraoperative anesthetic record, which reveals he received 16 mg methadone on induction and 4 mg ondansetron for postoperative nausea and vomiting prophylaxis. You believe that the combination of multiple QT-prolonging medications led to his brief episode of TdP. An ECG confirms your suspicion because the patient has a QTc of 545 ms.

What is the definition of a prolonged QTc interval?

A QTc interval greater than 450 ms in adult males or 460 ms in adult females is considered prolonged.[24] This difference is thought to be a result of the effect that sex hormones play on cardiac repolarization.[25] Based on studies of individuals with congenital long QT syndromes, a QTc of greater than 500 ms significantly increases the risk of TdP. Furthermore, for every 10 ms increase in the QTc interval, the risk of ventricular arrhythmias increases by 5–7%.[26]

Which medications commonly used in the perioperative period are known to prolong the QT interval?

Medications commonly used in the perioperative setting that may cause prolongation of the QTc interval include antiemetics (ondansetron), antipsychotics (haloperidol, droperidol), antiarrhythmics (sotalol, procainamide, amiodarone), and certain opioids (methadone).

You place a note in the patient's chart that all QT-prolonging medications should be avoided and discuss with the surgical service an appropriate time to restart his home citalopram. He is admitted to the floor with telemetry monitoring and discharged to a rehabilitation facility 4 days later.

DISCUSSION

EPIDEMIOLOGY AND PRESENTATION

Postoperative arrhythmias are common, affecting between 4–20% of patients following noncardiac surgery.[27,28] Among cardiac surgical patients, the incidence is higher, between 20% and 55%.[29] Arrhythmias most often manifest within the first 4 days following surgery.[27,30] Arrhythmias in asymptomatic patients may only be detected due to the monitoring capabilities of the PACU. Clinicians should have a high index of suspicion for deleterious arrhythmias in postoperative patients with sudden-onset symptoms such as syncope or dizziness. In contrast, more benign sinus tachycardia typically develops gradually and can be attributed to high sympathetic activity, pain, hypovolemia, or other causes.

EVALUATION AND DIAGNOSIS

In accordance with guidelines from various organizations, postoperative care should include monitoring the patients respiratory, cardiovascular, and neurologic functions.[31,32] The routine use of continuous ECG monitoring in the PACU may aid in the rapid detection of arrhythmias.

Specific consideration should be given to underlying factors that may precipitate arrhythmias in the postoperative period, such as hypovolemia, myocardial ischemia, hemorrhage, sepsis, and medication interactions (see Box 48.1). If a secondary cause is suspected, additional tests may be indicated. In cases of profound hemodynamic instability or other threats to life, immediate resuscitation should occur concurrently with diagnostic workup. The management of these secondary causes of postoperative arrhythmias is out of the scope of this chapter. Therefore, we will focus on the treatment of the arrhythmia itself, assuming that other underlying causes have been excluded.

Box 48.1 **PERIOPERATIVE RISK FACTORS FOR TACHYARRHYTHMIAS**

Extracardiac Causes

Hypoxia
Hypovolemia
Hypokalemia
Hypomagnesemia
Metabolic/Respiratory acidosis
Hypoglycemia/Hyperglycemia
Hypothermia/Hyperthermia
Shock
Sepsis
Hypervolemia
Pulmonary embolism
Pneumothorax
History of alcohol excess
History of polysubstance abuse

Cardiac Causes

Acute myocardial infarction
Myocarditis
Pericarditis

Iatrogenic

Central venous catheter/Pulmonary artery catheter misplacement
Local anesthetic toxicity
Inotropes

Surgical

Trauma
Pain
Thoracic surgery/Mediastinal manipulation
Systemic inflammatory response

From Stewart et al.[34]

MANAGEMENT OF TACHYARRHYTHMIAS

Atrial Fibrillation

Management of postoperative AF is dictated by the patient's hemodynamic stability and underlying cardiac function and can be divided into rate-based and rhythm-based approaches. Rate-control is appropriate for most patients and can be achieved with IV beta blockers or non-dihydropyridine calcium channel blockers (diltiazem or verapamil). In patients with reduced ejection fraction, IV amiodarone is recommended.[33]

The pharmacologic management of AF in patients with a history of Wolff-Parkinson-White syndrome or other ECG evidence of pre-excitation is of particular importance. In such patients, blocking or slowing conduction through the atrioventricular node may cause excessive conduction down the accessory pathway, which often has a shorter refractory period, and may lead to an increased ventricular rate and degradation of the rhythm into ventricular tachycardia or fibrillation. Therefore, drugs such as adenosine, non-dihydropyridine calcium channel blockers, and beta blockers are contraindicated.[34] In their place, procainamide or amiodarone may be used in the hemodynamically stable patient. Direct current cardioversion remains the standard for the treatment of hemodynamically unstable AF with pre-excitation.

Reentrant Supraventricular Tachyarrhythmias

Supraventricular tachyarrhythmias (SVTs) other than AF include atrioventricular nodal reentrant tachycardia (AVNRT), atrioventricular reentrant tachycardia (AVRT), and multifocal atrial tachycardia (MAT). AVNRT occurs due to the presence of multiple pathways into the atrioventricular node that conduct impulses at different speeds. In contrast, AVRT is caused by the presence of an accessory pathway, such as in Wolff-Parkinson-White syndrome, that bypasses the AV node and leads to a rapid ventricular rate.

In the general population, the initial treatment of both hemodynamically stable AVNRT and AVRT is the performance of vagal maneuvers.[35] In the immediate postoperative setting, however, these exercises may not be feasible as the patients may not be alert enough to follow instructions. If this is the case, or if vagal maneuvers are unsuccessful, adenosine is the standard first-line pharmacologic agent (see Table 48.1). The administration of adenosine also has diagnostic value as slowing conduction through the AV node will improve the ability to detect p-waves or other arrhythmias masked by the high heart rate.[35] As previously mentioned, adenosine is contraindicated in patients with a history or evidence of pre-excitation. Other agents that can be considered include IV diltiazem and verapamil.[36] Hemodynamically unstable AVNRT or AVRT should be treated with synchronized, direct current cardioversion.

MAT is defined as a narrow-complex tachycardia with at least three distinct p-wave morphologies; MAT results from presence of multiple foci of atrial activity.[35] It is associated primarily with pulmonary disease but may also occur in those patients with valvular heart disease or hypomagnesemia.[37] The management of MAT should focus on addressing the underlying

Table 48.1 PHARMACOLOGICAL MANAGEMENT OF SUPRAVENTRICULAR TACHYARRHYTHMIAS (SVTS)

SVT with narrow QRS complex

Adenosine	IV bolus 6 mg followed by 20 mL flush into a proximal vein. IV bolus 12 mg if no response in 1–2 minutes.	Facial flushing, chest pain, bronchospasm, hypotension, rarely asystole	Contraindications
			  Wolff-Parkinson-White syndrome
			  Atrial fibrillation
			  Cardiac transplant recipients
			  Cautions
			  Chronic obstructive pulmonary disease (COPD), digoxin, and verapamil

Esmolol	IV 0.5 mg kg^{-1} over 1 min, then 50–200 μg kg^{-1} min^{-1}, infusion titrated to response	Hypotension, bradycardia, heart block, bronchospasm	Cautions
			  Asthma
			  Heart failure, arteriovenous (AV) block, Ca-channel blocker treatment

Metoprolol	1–5 mg over 10 minutes		
Diltiazem	0.25 mg kg^{-1} over 2 min	Hypotension, heart block, bradycardia, negative inotropy	Cautions Heart failure, AV block, beta blocker treatment

SVT with preexcitation and refractory SVT

Amiodarone	IV 300 mg loading dose over 10 min. Followed by 900 mg over 23 hours	Hypotension, bradycardia, AV block, QTc prolongation
		Phlebitis
		Ocular, pulmonary, hepatic, hematological, neurological complications with chronic use
			Contraindications
			  Pregnancy
			  Porphyria
			  AV block
			  marked sinus bradycardia
			Cautions
			  Dilute in 5% dextrose and administer via central or a proximal central vein

From Stewart et al.[34]

---

disease as antiarrhythmic medications and cardioversion are generally ineffective. Some small studies indicate that supplemental magnesium may aid in suppressing atrial ectopy.[38]

MANAGEMENT OF POSTOPERATIVE BRADYARRHYTHMIA

Pharmacologic Management

Normotensive patients with asymptomatic bradycardia do not require immediate treatment but additional monitoring, such as telemetry, may be indicated. In those with symptomatic or severe bradycardia, immediate pharmacologic treatment is warranted. Anticholinergic medications such as atropine (0.5–1 mg) and glycopyrrolate (0.2–0.4 mg) are commonly used first-line agents. In patients unresponsive to these agents, ephedrine, epinephrine, dopamine, or isoproterenol should be considered.[16] Notably, anticholinergic medications are contraindicated in patients with a history of cardiac transplantation because of the increased risk of a paradoxical AV block in the denervated heart.[17]

Temporary Pacing

Transcutaneous or transvenous pacing is indicated in patients with hemodynamically unstable bradycardia that is refractory to pharmacologic treatment. While transcutaneous pacing is more readily available and less invasive than transvenous pacing, it is only a temporary measure and can cause thermal injury on prolonged use.[39] In addition, it may be more painful for the patient and necessitate procedural sedation similar to synchronized cardioversion. Thus, transcutaneous pacing shoulder serve only as a bridge to other pacing modalities (transvenous, epicardial, etc.).[40] All patients requiring pacing should receive a comprehensive electrophysiologic evaluation and may require placement of a permanent pacemaker.[16]

Neuraxial Anesthesia and Bradycardia

Bradycardia, and often hypotension, are common adverse effects of neuraxial anesthesia and may occur at any point in the perioperative period.[41] The physiologic mechanisms underlying this phenomenon are controversial, and multiple theories have been proposed including parasympathetic predominance following blockade of thoracic cardio-accelerator fibers and activation of the Bezold-Jarisch reflex.[42] Risk factors for neuraxial-associated bradycardia include males, baseline heart rate of less than 60 bpm, ASA physical status I, and chronic treatment with beta blockers.[41,43]

Standard pharmacologic treatments for bradycardia, including anticholinergic and sympathomimetic medications, are effective in treating neuraxial-associated bradycardia. In addition, raising the patient's legs may be beneficial as it increases preload and thus interrupts the negative chronotropic effect of the Bezold-Jarish reflex.[44]

SEQUELAE OF POSTOPERATIVE ARRHYTHMIAS

Postoperative arrhythmias are also associated with an increase in length of stay, hospital readmission rate, and healthcare costs.[30,45]

CONCLUSION

- Arrhythmias are common in the postoperative period and occur due to a constellation of surgical, biochemical, and patient-specific factors.
- The management of arrhythmias in the PACU should focus on initial stabilization, diagnostic workup, and appropriate disposition.
- While standard ACLS algorithms still apply in the postoperative setting, specific adaptations must be made to account for a patient's recent anesthetic and surgical care.
- Certain arrhythmias may be a manifestation of underlying pathologies such as hypovolemia, sepsis, or drug toxicities and must be managed accordingly.

REVIEW QUESTIONS

1. Which of the following statements about postoperative AF is false:

    a. The risk of stroke varies in proportion to baseline CHA_2DS_2VASc scores.
    b. Postoperative AF is the most common arrhythmia in the postoperative period.
    c. The incidence of stroke is higher in patients with postoperative AF following cardiac surgery than non-cardiac surgery.
    d. Postoperative AF is often considered self-limiting.

The correct answer is c.

The incidence of stroke following postoperative AF was higher after noncardiac surgery (hazard ratio [HR] 2.0; 95% confidence interval [CI], 1.7, 2.3) than cardiac surgery (HR, 1.3; 95% CI, 1.1, 1.6).[46] In one prospective series of 916 patients older than 40 years undergoing major noncardiac surgery, the frequency rate of SVT was 4%; atrial flutter and AF accounted for 63% of these arrhythmias.[47]

2. AF with ECG evidence of pre-excitation is managed with

    a. Amiodarone.
    b. Esmolol.
    c. Non-dihydropyridine calcium channel blockers.
    d. Digoxin.
    e. Adenosine.

The correct answer is a.

In patients with anterograde conduction through accessory pathways, conduction to ventricles often occurs through a combination of accessory pathways and the AV node. Slowing the conduction through the AV node will enable conduction through the accessory pathways with a short refractory period. Therefore, drugs which block AV nodal conduction can promote conduction through accessory pathways and precipitate ventricular fibrillation. Amiodarone, which is not selective for AV nodal conduction in prolonging the action potential and refractory period may be considered for AF with pre-excitation in hemodynamically stable patients.[34]

3. The following arrhythmias respond to adenosine *except*

    a. AV nodal reentrant tachycardia.
    b. Atrial fibrillation.
    c. Focal atrial tachycardia.
    d. MAT.
    e. AV nodal tachycardia.

The correct answer is d.

Adenosine terminates AV nodal tachycardia and AV nodal reentrant tachycardia. It terminates 60–80% of focal atrial tachycardia and transiently slows down ventricular rate in atrial fibrillation. Treatment of the precipitant of MAT is the priority since it is usually transient and resolves when the underlying disease process improves. It does not respond to adenosine.[34]

4. The following drugs cause prolonged QT interval *except*

    a. Methadone.
    b. Ondansetron.
    c. Haloperidol.
    d. Amiodarone.
    e. Fentanyl.

The correct answer is e.

Amiodarone and methadone are at high risk to predispose to prolonged QT interval. Haloperidol and ondansetron are at moderate risk to cause prolonged QT interval. IV ondansetron carries a higher risk than oral ondansetron.[22]

5. Magnesium exerts its anti-arrhythmic effects through the following mechanisms except:

    a. Decreased automaticity.
    b. Decreased early/delayed after depolarizations.
    c. Increased atrial and AV nodal refractory period.
    d. Decreased oxidative damage.
    e. Blocks conduction via accessory pathways.

The correct answer is d.

Magnesium is a co-factor for many ATP-mediated reactions including the control of plasma and intracellular ion transport pumps responsible for movement of sodium, calcium, potassium, and intracellular pH. As a co-factor for the Na, K-ATPase pump, it regulates the intracellular potassium levels. This helps in the modulation of automaticity and cardiac conduction pathways. The decrease in oxidative damage is responsible for its anti-ischemic effects.[48]

REFERENCES

1. Dobrev D, Aguilar M, Heijman J, Guichard JB, Nattel S. Postoperative atrial fibrillation: Mechanisms, manifestations, and management. *Nat Rev Cardiol*. 2019;16(7):417–436. doi:10.1038/s41569-019-0166-5
2. Walsh SR, Tang T, Wijewardena C, Yarham SI, Boyle JR, Gaunt ME. Postoperative arrhythmias in general surgical patients. *Ann R Coll Surg Engl*. 2007;89(2):91–95. doi:10.1308/003588407X168253
3. Qureshi M, Ahmed A, Massie V, Marshall E, Harky A. Determinants of atrial fibrillation after cardiac surgery. *Rev Cardiovasc Med*. 2021;22(2):329–341. doi:10.31083/j.rcm2202040
4. Chyou JY, Barkoudah E, Dukes JW, et al. Atrial fibrillation occurring during acute hospitalization: A scientific statement from the American Heart Association. *Circulation*. 2023;147(15):e676–e698. doi:10.1161/CIR.0000000000001133
5. Nuotio I, Hartikainen JEK, Grönberg T, Biancari F, Airaksinen KEJ. Time to cardioversion for acute atrial fibrillation and thromboembolic complications. *JAMA*. 2014;312(6):647. doi:10.1001/jama.2014.3824
6. Stronati G, Capucci A, Dello Russo A, et al. Procedural sedation for direct current cardioversion: A feasibility study between two management strategies in the emergency department. *BMC Cardiovasc Disord*. 2020;20(1):388. doi:10.1186/s12872-020-01664-1
7. AlTurki A, Marafi M, Proietti R, et al. Major adverse cardiovascular events associated with postoperative atrial fibrillation after noncardiac surgery: A systematic review and meta-analysis. *Circ Arrhythm Electrophysiol*. 2020;13(1):e007437. doi:10.1161/CIRCEP.119.007437
8. January CT, Wann LS, Calkins H, et al. 2019 AHA/ACC/HRS focused update of the 2014 AHA/ACC/HRS guideline for the management of patients with atrial fibrillation. *J Am Coll Cardiol*. 2019;74(1):104–132. doi:10.1016/j.jacc.2019.01.011
9. Karcz M, Papadakos PJ. Respiratory complications in the postanesthesia care unit: A review of pathophysiological mechanisms. *Can J Respir Ther*. 2013;49(4):21–29.
10. Hunter JM, Naguib M. Sugammadex-induced bradycardia and asystole: How great is the risk? *Br J Anaesth*. 2018;121(1):8–12. doi:10.1016/j.bja.2018.03.003
11. Mirakhur RK, Dundee JW, Clarke RSJ. Glycopyrrolate—neostigmine mixture for antagonism of neuromuscular block: Comparison with atropine—neostigmine mixture. *Br J Anaesth*. 1977;49(8):825–829. doi:10.1093/bja/49.8.825
12. Gupta B, Mishra P. A systematic review and meta-analysis of the use of succinylcholine to facilitate tracheal intubation in neonates. *Ain-Shams J Anesthesiol*. 2021;13(1):68. doi:10.1186/s42077-021-00185-z
13. Hristovska AM, Duch P, Allingstrup M, Afshari A. Efficacy and safety of sugammadex versus neostigmine in reversing neuromuscular blockade in adults. Cochrane Anaesthesia Group, ed. *Cochrane Database Syst Rev*. 2017;2017(9). doi:10.1002/14651858.CD012763
14. Jordan J, Tank J, Shannon JR, et al. Baroreflex buffering and susceptibility to vasoactive drugs. *Circulation*. 2002;105(12):1459–1464. doi:10.1161/01.CIR.0000012126.56352.FD
15. Blessberger H, Lewis SR, Pritchard MW, et al. Perioperative beta-blockers for preventing surgery-related mortality and morbidity in adults undergoing non-cardiac surgery. *Cochrane Database Syst Rev*. 2019;9(9):CD013438. doi:10.1002/14651858.CD013438
16. Kusumoto FM, Schoenfeld MH, Barrett C, et al. 2018 ACC/AHA/HRS guideline on the evaluation and management of patients with bradycardia and cardiac conduction Delay. *J Am Coll Cardiol*. 2019;74(7):e51–e156. doi:10.1016/j.jacc.2018.10.044
17. Bernheim A, Fatio R, Kiowski W, Weilenmann D, Rickli H, Rocca HPBL. Atropine often results in complete atrioventricular block or sinus arrest after cardiac transplantation: An unpredictable and dose-independent phenomenon. *Transplantation*. 2004;77(8):1181–1185. doi:10.1097/01.TP.0000122416.70287.D9
18. Wang Ji J, Ye S, Haythe J, Schulze PC, Shimbo D. The risk of adverse events associated with atropine administration during dobutamine stress echocardiography in cardiac transplant patients: A 28-year single-center experience. *J Card Fail*. 2013;19(11):762–767. doi:10.1016/j.cardfail.2013.10.002
19. American Heart Association. Algorithms. cpr.heart.org. https://cpr.heart.org/en/resuscitation-science/cpr-and-ecc-guidelines/algorithms
20. Knowlton AA, Falk RH. External cardiac pacing during in-hospital cardiac arrest. *Am J Cardiol*. 1986;57(15):1295–1298. doi:10.1016/0002-9149(86)90207-9
21. Tzivoni D, Banai S, Schuger C, et al. Treatment of torsade de pointes with magnesium sulfate. *Circulation*. 1988;77(2):392–397. doi:10.1161/01.CIR.77.2.392
22. Al-Khatib SM, Stevenson WG, Ackerman MJ, et al. 2017 AHA/ACC/HRS Guideline for Management of Patients With Ventricular Arrhythmias and the Prevention of Sudden Cardiac Death. https://www.ahajournals.org/doi/10.1161/CIR.0000000000000549#
23. American Heart Association. Highlights of the 2020 American Heart Association guidelines for CPR and ECC. https://cpr.heart.org/-/media/cpr-files/cpr-guidelines-files/highlights/hghlghts_2020_ecc_guidelines_english.pdf
24. Giudicessi JR, Noseworthy PA, Ackerman MJ. The QT interval: An emerging vital sign for the precision medicine era? *Circulation*. 2019;139(24):2711–2713. doi:10.1161/CIRCULATIONAHA.119.039598
25. Sedlak T, Shufelt C, Iribarren C, Merz CNB. Sex hormones and the QT interval: A review. *J Womens Health 2002*. 2012;21(9):933–941. doi:10.1089/jwh.2011.3444
26. Priori SG, Schwartz PJ, Napolitano C, et al. Risk stratification in the long-QT syndrome. *N Engl J Med*. 2003;348(19):1866–1874. doi:10.1056/NEJMoa022147
27. Walsh SR, Oates JE, Anderson JA, Blair SD, Makin CA, Walsh CJ. Postoperative arrhythmias in colorectal surgical patients: Incidence and clinical correlates. *Colorectal Dis*. 2006;8(3):212–216. doi:10.1111/j.1463-1318.2005.00881.x
28. Bhave PD, Goldman LE, Vittinghoff E, Maselli J, Auerbach A. Incidence, predictors, and outcomes associated with postoperative atrial fibrillation after major noncardiac surgery. *Am Heart J*. 2012;164(6):918–924. doi:10.1016/j.ahj.2012.09.004
29. Lopes LA, Agrawal DK. Post-operative atrial fibrillation: Current treatments and etiologies for a persistent surgical complication. *J Surg Res*. 2022;5(1):159–172. doi:10.26502/jsr.10020209
30. Polanczyk CA, Goldman L, Marcantonio ER, Orav EJ, Lee TH. Supraventricular arrhythmia in patients having non-cardiac surgery: Clinical correlates and effect on length of stay. *Ann Intern Med*. 1998;129(4):279–285. doi:10.7326/0003-4819-129-4-199808150-00003
31. Dobson G, Chow L, Filteau L, et al. Guidelines to the practice of anesthesia—Revised edition 2021. *Can J Anaesth*. 2021;68(1):92–129. doi:10.1007/s12630-020-01842-x
32. Updated by the Committee on Standards and Practice Parameters, Apfelbaum JL, the Task Force on Postanesthetic Care, et al. Practice guidelines for postanesthetic care: An updated report by the American Society of Anesthesiologists Task Force on postanesthetic care. *Anesthesiology*. 2013;118(2):291–307. doi:10.1097/ALN.0b013e31827773e9
33. 2020 ESC Guidelines for the diagnosis and management of atrial fibrillation developed in collaboration with the European Association for Cardio-Thoracic Surgery (EACTS) | European Heart Journal | Oxford Academic. https://www.escardio.org/static-file/Escardio/Guidelines/Documents/ehaa612.pdf
34. Stewart AM, Greaves K, Bromilow J. Supraventricular tachyarrhythmias and their management in the perioperative period. *BJA Educ*. 2015;15(2):90–97. doi:10.1093/bjaceaccp/mku018
35. Page RL, Joglar JA, Caldwell MA, et al. 2015 ACC/AHA/HRS guideline for the management of adult patients with supraventricular tachycardia. *Circulation*. 2016;133(14):e506–e574. doi:10.1161/CIR.0000000000000311
36. Dougherty AH, Jackman WM, Naccarelli GV, et al. Acute conversion of paroxysmal supraventricular tachycardia with intravenous diltiazem. IV Diltiazem study group. *Am J Cardiol*. 1992 Sep 1;70(6): 587–592.

37. Lee Scher D, Arsura EL. Multifocal atrial tachycardia: Mechanisms, clinical correlates, and treatment. *Am Heart J*. 1989;118(3):574–580. doi:10.1016/0002-8703(89)90275-5
38. Kastor JA. Multifocal atrial tachycardia. *N Engl J Med*. 1990;322(24):1713–1717. doi:10.1056/NEJM199006143222405
39. Carrizales-Sepúlveda EF, González-Sariñana LI, Ordaz-Farías A, Vera-Pineda R, Flores-Ramírez R. Thermal burn resulting from prolonged transcutaneous pacing in a patient with complete heart block. *Am J Emerg Med*. 2018;36(8):1523.e5–1523.e6. doi:10.1016/j.ajem.2018.04.038
40. Doukky R, Bargout R, Kelly RF, Calvin JE. Using transcutaneous cardiac pacing to best advantage. *J Crit Illn*. 2003;18(5):219–225.
41. Lesser JB, Sanborn KV, Valskys R, Kuroda M. Severe bradycardia during spinal and epidural anesthesia recorded by an anesthesia information management system. *Anesthesiology*. 2003;99(4):859–866. doi:10.1097/00000542-200310000-00018
42. Neal JM. Hypotension and bradycardia during spinal anesthesia: Significance, prevention, and treatment. *Tech Reg Anesth Pain Manag*. 2000;4(4):148–154. doi:10.1053/trap.2000.20600
43. Pereira IDF, Grando MM, Vianna PTG, et al. Retrospective analysis of risk factors and predictors of intraoperative complications in neuraxial blocks at Faculdade de Medicina de Botucatu-UNESP. *Braz J Anesthesiol*. 2011;61(5):568–581. doi:10.1016/S0034-7094(11)70068-X
44. Ponhold H, Vicenzi MN. Incidence of bradycardia during recovery from spinal anaesthesia: Influence of patient position. *Br J Anaesth*. 1998;81(5):723–726. doi:10.1093/bja/81.5.723
45. LaPar DJ, Speir AM, Crosby IK, et al. Postoperative atrial fibrillation significantly increases mortality, hospital readmission, and hospital costs. *Ann Thorac Surg*. 2014;98(2):527–533. doi:10.1016/j.athoracsur.2014.03.039
46. Gialdini G, Nearing K, Bhave PD, et al. Perioperative atrial fibrillation and the long-term risk of ischemic stroke. *JAMA*. 2014;312(6):616–622. doi:10.1001/jama.2014.9143
47. Hollenberg SM, Dellinger RP. Noncardiac surgery: Postoperative arrhythmias. *Crit Care Med*. 2000;28(10):N145.
48. Baker WL. Treating arrhythmias with adjunctive magnesium Identifying future research directions. *Eur Heart J Cardiovasc Pharmacother*. 2017;3(2):108–117. doi:10.1093/ehjcvp/pvw028

INDEX

For the benefit of digital users, indexed terms that span two pages (e.g., 52–53) may, on occasion, appear on only one of those pages.

Tables, figures, and boxes are indicated by an italic *t*, *f*, and *b* following the page number.

A

AAA. *See* abdominal aortic aneurysms (AAA)
abdominal aortic aneurysms (AAA), 461
  activity level to assess functional status, 456*t*
  anatomical considerations for endovascular aortic aneurysm repair (EVAR), 455*t*
  aneurysm location, 454*t*
  aneurysm size classification, 453*t*
  case and key questions, 452–53
  classification of, 454*f*
  Crawford classification of thoracoabdominal aneurysms, 453, 454*f*
  definition and classification of, 453
  endovascular aortic aneurysm repair (EVAR), 455, 455*t*
  epidemiology and risk factors, 453–54
  epidural catheters, 458–59
  ketamine, 460
  lidocaine, 460
  magnesium, 460
  multimodal medications, 460–61
  operative repair, 454–55
  paravertebral and erector spinae catheters, 459
  perioperative analgesia, 458–60
  perioperative analgesic strategies, 459*f*
  perioperative considerations, 457–58
  preoperative evaluation, 455–57
  review questions, 461
  risk of aneurysm rupture, 455*t*
  spinal cord stimulators, 458
  surgical approach, 455
  surgical patient with chronic pain, 457, 457*t*
  transversus abdominis plane block, 459–60
abdominal cancer resection
  cardiopulmonary exercise testing (CPET), 98*t*
  case and key questions, 97–100
  discussion of CPET data, 98–100
  9-panel plot, 99*f*
  See also cardiopulmonary exercise testing (CPET)
abdominoplasty, 307
ablative therapies, hepatocellular liver cancer (HCC), 17
ACC/AHA Stepwise Approach to Perioperative Cardiac Assessment, 41
achondroplasia, C-spine abnormalities, 81*t*
activity, Duke Activity Status Index (DASI), 30, 30*t*
acute coronary syndrome (ACS), 54
Acute Disease Quality Initiative and PeriOperative Quality Initiative groups, 300

acute kidney injury network (AKIN), 298–99, 299*t*, 302
  criteria for, 299*t*
  perioperative factors for, 301*f*
  perioperative management for preventing, 300–2
  Risk, Injury, Failure, Loss, ESRD (RIFLE) criteria, 298–99, 299*t*
  See also chronic kidney disease (CKD)
acute-on-chronic liver failure, 252
acute respiratory distress syndrome (ARDS), waiting period for surgery, 229
ADAPTABLE study, (Comparative Effectiveness of Aspirin Dosing in Cardiovascular Disease), 57
adrenalectomy, 333
adults. *See* geriatric assessment
advance care planning
  older adults, 126, 130
  questions to ask before surgery, 130*b*
advanced cardiac life support (ACLS), 374, 524
advance directive(s) (AD), 10–11
  perioperative conversation, 425–26
  providing consent for patient, 405
  rise of, 396
advanced maternal age (AMA), pregnancy and, 358, 359
advanced practice provider (APP), 4
adverse drug reactions
  definitions and documentation of, 434
  patients with, suggestive of allergy, 434–36
adverse reactions, difference between allergies and, 433
Adverse Reactions to Drug, Biological, and Latex Committee, American Academy of Allergy, Asthma, and Immunology, 434
AHA/ACC/ARS Guidelines for the Management of Patients with Atrial Fibrillation, 33
alcohol, substance use disorders (SUD), 72–73
alcohol use disorder (AUD)
  naltrexone for, 71–72
  postoperative opioid requirements, 75
alcohol withdrawal syndrome (AWS)
  symptoms of, 19
  treatment for, 19
allergies, 437
  adverse drug reactions, 434
  amendment of allergy documentation, 434*t*
  case and key questions, 433–34
  difference between adverse reactions and, 433
  hyperthyroidism symptoms and signs, 437*b*

hypothyroidism symptoms and signs, 437*b*
  management of acute angioedema, 435*f*
  modified Ring and Messmer grading, 436*t*
  pathophysiology of anaphylaxis, 436*f*
  pathophysiology of angioedema, 435*f*
  patients with previous adverse reactions suggestive of, 434–36
  perioperative anaphylaxis, 436–37
  review questions, 437–38
  thyroidectomy and thyroid diseases, 437
  tongue swelling, 433
alpha-agonists, abdominal aortic aneurysms (AAA), 461
Alzheimer's disease, 515
ambulatory surgical centers (ASCs), 3, 165, 218
American Academy of Allergy, Asthma, and Immunology, 434
American Academy of Otolaryngology, Head and Neck Surgery, 318
American Academy of Pediatrics (AAP), 80
American Academy of Sleep Medicine, 498
American Association of Blood Banks (AABB), transfusion guidelines, 386*t*
American Association of Retired Persons (AARP), postoperative delirium prevention, 271–72
American College of Cardiologists and American Heart Association (ACC/AHA)
  cardiac evaluation, 486
American College of Cardiology (ACC), 140
  Expert Consensus Decision Pathway for Periprocedural Management of Anticoagulation in Patients with Nonvalvular Atrial Fibrillation, 153, 157
American College of Cardiology and American Heart Association (ACC/AHA), 55
  aortic stenosis, 142
  cardiac assessment, 31*f*
  cardiac evaluation guidelines, 28
  coronary artery disease, 140
  definition of combined medical/surgical risk for proposed procedure, 140–41
  definition of surgical urgency, 140
  diagnosis of valvular disease, 142–43
  dual antiplatelet therapy (DAPT), 142
  functional capacity, 141
  Guideline on Perioperative Cardiovascular Evaluation and Management of Patients Undergoing Noncardiac Surgery, 382–83
  guidelines for perioperative cardiovascular examination, 300
  hemodynamic considerations, 144
  indications for subacute bacterial endocarditis prophylaxis, 144
  management of STEMI, 56

Perioperative Cardiovascular Evaluation and Management of Patients Undergoing Noncardiac Surgery, 58
  perioperative guidelines for heart failure, 171
  perioperative options for patients with severe aortic stenosis, 143–44
  perioperative testing algorithm for patients undergoing noncardiac surgery, 140
  point-of-care ultrasound (POCUS) images, 143*f*
  preoperative cardiac testing, 141–42
  review questions, 145–46
  subacute bacterial endocarditis prophylaxis regimens, 144
American College of Chest Physicians, 498
American College of Obstetricians and Gynecologists (ACOG), 347, 352, 355
American College of Obstetrics and Gynecology (ACOG), 362
American College of Physicians (ACP), guidelines for preoperative chest radiographs, 208
American College of Rheumatology, 79
American College of Surgeons (ACS), 16, 102–4
  DNR/DNI order, 407
  DNR orders, 396–97
  frailty score, 273
  National Surgical Quality Improvement Program (NSQIP), 126, 141, 292, 303, 346–47, 348, 382–83, 414–15, 442
  perioperative DNR, 401
  preoperative cognitive impairment, 272
American College of Surgeons National Surgical Quality Improvement Program (ACS NSQIP)
  preoperative risk calculator, 172, 416, 417*f*, 421
American College of Surgeons NSQIP Surgical Risk Calculator, 163–64
American Diabetes Association, 324, 326
  target blood glucose, 326
American Geriatrics Society (AGS), 126
  "Beers List," 127
  frailty score, 273
  preoperative cognitive impairment, 272
American Healthcare Organization (AHCA), 3
American Heart Association (AHA)
  aortic stenosis classification, 163
  case and key questions, 139–40
  guidelines, 140
  heart failure, 169
  prehabilitation, 131
  radical prostatectomy for prostate cancer, 139–40
  See also American College of Cardiology and American Heart Association (ACC/AHA)

531

American Heart Association (AHA)/
American College of Cardiology
(ACC)/Heart Failure Society of
America (HFSA)
heart failure guidelines, 169
American Heart Association (AHA)/
American Society of Anesthesiologists
(ASA)
stroke reduction considerations, 292
American Heart Association/American
College of Cardiology/Heart Rhythm
Society (AHA/ACC/HRS)
Guideline for the Management of Patients
with Atrial Fibrillation, 150
American Medical Association (AMA), 396
American Society for Anesthesiology (ASA)
classifications, 16, 24, 49
guidelines for office-based anesthesia, 165
internal cardiac defibrillator (ICD),
16, 25
Preoperative Evaluation, 49
risk stratification, 16, 24
American Society for Enhanced Recovery
and Perioperative Quality Initiative,
271–72, 274, 276
American Society of Anesthesiologists
(ASA), 3, 5, 346–47
Ask, Advice, and Refer (AAR), 212–13
blood pressure monitoring, 282
classification, 46
COVID-19 infection and mortality,
228–29
definitions of physical status, 415t
general anesthesia for seizure patients, 140
guideline for DNR orders, 396–97, 399
invasive blood pressure measurement, 464
monitoring for shoulder replacement, 196
monitoring standard, 60
monitors, 286
operating room monitors, 507
OSA Checklist, 497–98
physical classification score, 414
postoperative delirium prevention,
271–72
robotic surgeries, 373
surgical risk prediction, 253
Task Force on Perioperative Management
of Obstructive Sleep Apnea, 222,
223, 225
Taskforce on Preanesthesia Evaluation,
347, 354
transfusion guidelines, 386t
American Society of Echocardiography
(ASE), 169
American Society of Regional Anesthesia
and Pain Management (ASRA), 457
American University of Beirut (AUB),
HAS2 Cardiovascular Risk Index, 141
amphetamines, substance use disorders
(SUD), 72
anabolic steroid use, 480
case and key questions, 452–53
common patterns of, 476
conversion of testosterone to estradiol,
478f, 478
gynecomastia and, 476, 478f, 478
muscle growth, 476–77
reverse Trendelenburg position, 478, 479f
review questions, 480
risks of, 476
symptoms of end-organ damage, 477
testosterone, 478–79
See also gynecomastia
anaerobic threshold (AT)
definition, 93
determining using 9-panel plot, 110
anaphylaxis, 436

pathophysiology of, 436f
perioperative, 436–37
anemia, 16, 310
available formulations and potential risks
of IV iron, 309
case and key questions, 307
commonly used intravenous iron
formulations, 309t
definition, 381, 384
definition and implications, 307–8
etiology of, 28
evaluation of, 308f
evidence for preoperative correction
of, 308
hepcidin, 381
identification of the cause of, 308
iron deficiency anemia (IDA), 391
management of, 384
multiple etiologies, 383
patient blood management, 309–10
physiology of, 384–85
review questions, 310
role of erythropoiesis-stimulating agents,
309
safety margin between DO_2 and VO_2,
384f, 384
treatment options, 308–9
types of, 381
See also blood conservation
anesthesia
extracorporeal shock wave lithotripsy
(ESWL), 164–65
induction of, for transplanted heart, 197
informed consent for, 405
interscalene block (ISB) for shoulder
replacement, 196, 197
options offered to patient, 33–34
premature infants, 122–23
Anesthesia for Infants and Children (Smith),
312
Anesthesia Patient Safety Foundation
(APSF), 229, 238
anesthesiologists, informed consent, 408
Anesthesiology (journal), 301
anesthesiology, preoperative evaluation of
patient, 414–18
anesthesiology-run clinic
medicine clinic combined with, 5
medicine clinics separate from, 5
preoperative clinic model, 4–5
anesthetics, allergy to all local, 433
angioedema, 434
management of acute, 435f
pathophysiology of, 435f
angiotensin converting enzyme inhibitors,
heart failure treatment, 174
angiotensin II receptor blockers, heart
failure treatment, 174
angiotensin receptor-neprilysin inhibitors,
heart failure treatment, 174
antepartum hemorrhage, pregnancy and,
364–65
anticoagulation
patients' cardiac evaluation, 21–22
patient's interventional radiology
evaluation, 22–23
patient's primary care evaluation, 23
patient's pulmonary evaluation, 22
See also atrial fibrillation
anticoagulation management, evaluation, 36
antiepileptic drugs (AEDs)
enzyme induction, 265
epilepsy, 268
epilepsy treatment, 261
mechanisms of action and common side
effects for common, 262t
antigen testing algorithm

CDC, 240
COVID-19 infection, 228f
antiplatelet medications, principles of
perioperative management of, 58t
antiplatelet therapy, perioperative
management in neurosurgical patient,
59–60
aortic stenosis (AS), 28
anesthesia techniques for ESWL
procedures, 164–65
case and key questions, 162–63
etiologies of, 163
extracorporeal shock wave lithotripsy
(ESWL), 162, 164, 165
hemodynamic goals, invasive monitoring,
and anesthetic considerations, 164
overview, 163–64
performing procedures at free-standing
surgical center, 165
perioperative options for patients with
severe, 143–45
review questions, 165–66
symptoms of, 142
aortic valve replacement (AVR), 162–63
APAP (N-acetyl-p-aminophenol),
postoperative concern, 502
apixaban
indications and pharmacokinetics, 151t
interruption time, 155t
laboratory tests for, 156t
apnea(s), 496
definition, 221
premature infants, 122
See also obstructive sleep apnea (OSA)
apnea-hypopnea index (AHI), 497
diagnosis of obstructive sleep apnea
(OSA), 221, 221t
severity of obstructive sleep apnea, 497t
Appropriateness Criteria for Coronary
Revascularization, 56
Ariadne Labs's Serious Illness Conversation
Guide, 426
ARISTOLE trial, 152
Arnold, Robert, 426
arrhythmias. See postoperative arrhythmias
ascites and hepatic hydrothorax,
management in cirrhosis, 252
aspergillus, infection, 198
Association of Operating Room Nurses
(AORN)
DNR/DNI order, 407
DNR orders, 396–97
atrial fibrillation (AF), 148, 157–58
American Society of Regional
Anesthesiologists guidelines on
DOAC interruption times, 156t
annual risk of stroke, 150, 150t
anticoagulation for, 148
anticoagulation reinitiation, 157t
bridging therapy, 148, 152–54, 154t
causes of postoperative, 522
CHA_2D_2-VASc score, 150, 150t
$CHADS_2$ score, 150, 150t
common surgical procedures and risk of
bleeding, 153t
complications, 149–50
dabigatran interruption time, 155t
definition and risk factors, 149, 149t
diagnosis of, 148, 149
direct oral anticoagulant (DOAC), 148
DOACS laboratory monitoring, 155–56
evaluation, 36
factors and comorbidities, 148
invasive procedure and anticoagulants, 148
invasive procedure and warfarin, 148
laboratory tests for DOAC
monitoring, 156t

management of, 525
management of DOACS, 154–55
management of DOACS before regional
anesthesia, 155
oral anticoagulants, 148
oral anticoagulation for, 148, 150–52
oral anticoagulation indications and
pharmacokinetics, 151t
perioperative management of warfarin,
152
postoperative, 150
preoperative management, 152
rate- or rhythm-control strategy, 522
reinitiation of oral anticoagulation after
invasive procedure, 157
review questions, 158–59
rivaroxaban, edoxaban, apixaban
interruption times, 155t
sequelae of postoperative, 523
stroke risk reduction, 150–52
term, 148
thromboembolic complications, 148
treatment of, 149
work-up for, 148
attention deficit disorder (ADD), 439
attention deficit hyperactivity disorder
(ADHD), 439
autistic patient (nonverbal), 447
anesthetic history, 442
anesthetic management of combative,
445–47
case and key questions, 439–45
clozapine, 443
common medical comorbidities
associated with autism, 443–44
dental office lobby wall damage by, 441f
dexmedetomidine, 441, 446–47
family history, 442
fluoxetine, 443
folate cycle, 445f
homocysteine, 448
homocysteine/methionine pathway, 445f
inhibition of methionine synthase (MS)
by nitrous oxide, 444, 445f
ketamine, 441, 446, 447
medications, 442
midazolam, 441, 446, 447
past medical history, 442
pharmacological properties for
sedative, 439
physiological abnormalities in, 444
pre-hospital oral sedation, 439–40
review questions, 447–48
risperidone, 442–43
seizures, 447, 448
tizanidine as alpha-2 agonist, 440–41
treatment of laryngospasm without IV
access, 445
autonomy, informed consent, 408–9, 418

B
Back, Anthony, 426
back pain, smoking and, 211
back pain surgery, patient with COPD
history, 207
Baldwin Park Medical Center, Kaiser
Permanente, 20
barbiturates, substance use disorders
(SUD), 73
bariatric surgery, 307
benzodiazepine(s), 19
anesthetic and sedative agent in
pregnancy, 352
anticonvulsant, 266
autistic patient, 441
autistic patients, 448
epilepsy, 268

perioperative delirium prevention, 274
substance use disorders (SUD), 73
Berlin Questionnaire (BQ), OSA screening, 497
Bernard-Soulier syndrome, 315
Best Practice Guidelines for Postoperative Brain Health, 275
beta-2 agonists, COPD management, 209
beta blockers, heart failure treatment, 173–74
betrixaban, indications and pharmacokinetics, 151t
BioFreedom, type of bioresorbable stent (BRS), 56–57
bioresorbable stents (BRS), 56–57
  BioFreedom, 56–57
  patients undergoing PCI for ACS, 63
Biotronik, technical support contacts, 467t
biphasic response, term, 122
birth control, sugammadex and, 511
black box warning in pediatrics, succinylcholine and, 510
bleeding disorders, pediatric patients, 313–15
bleeding risk
  CHA$_2$DS$_2$-VASc versus HAS-BLED, 33, 33t
  common surgical procedures and, 152, 153t
  HAS-BLED score, 40
blood
  maximum surgical blood ordering schedule (MSBOS), 28, 29f
  storage lesion of, 385
  typing and antibody screen, 28
blood conservation, 390
  case and key questions, 381–90
  clinician obligation for patient care, 390
  emergency exception, 390
  handling spouse requests, 389–90
  informed consent process for Jehovah's Witness patients, 386–89
  Jehovah's Witness patient, 381, 383–84, 390, 391
  legal considerations, 389
  model of consent for Jehovah's Witness patients, 388t
  optimizing patient from hemodynamic perspective, 383
  options for patient before surgery, 383–84
  patient autonomy concept, 389
  physiology of anemia, 384–85
  review questions, 390–91
  risk assessment tools for noncardiac surgery, 382–83
  risks of proceeding to operating room, 382
  summary of Jehovah's Witnesses products acceptability, 387t
  transfusion guidelines by medical societies, 386t
  Transfusion Requirements in Critical Care (TRICC) trial, 385
  treatment modalities acceptance in Jehovah's Witness patients, 387t
blood glucose
  fingerstick, 323
  relationship between HbA1c and average, 325t
  See also diabetes mellitus (DM)
blood glucose control, hemoglobin A1c, 41
blood transfusion, blood loss and, 197
bone microenvironment, healthy and rheumatoid arthritis (RA), 79f
Boston Scientific, technical support contacts, 467t

bradyarrhythmias
  management of postoperative, 526–27
  neuraxial anesthesia and, 526–27
  pharmacological management, 526
  temporary pacing, 526
bradycardia
  medications in perioperative period and, 523
  pharmacologic options for treatment, 523–24
  transcutaneous pacing, 524
brain health. See perioperative brain health
brain natriuretic peptide (BNP)
  heart failure testing, 171–72
  preoperative, 43
  testing, 42
breast cancer, 481
  biopsy, 482
  immunotherapy agents, 485
  immunotherapy agents' toxicities, 485–86, 486f
  lymphedema, 485
  secondary malignancies, 485
  treatment for, 481
  treatments and toxicities, 484–85
  See also cancer patient
bridging therapy
  atrial fibrillation, 148, 152–54
  recommendations for, 154t
Brief Health Literacy Assessment, 419
British Committee for Standards in Haematology (BCSH), transfusion guidelines, 386t
British Journal of Anaesthesia (journal), 189–91, 418–19
British Pacing and Electrophysiology Group (BPEG), 465–66
bronchopulmonary dysplasia (BPD)
  diagnostic criteria for, 122t
  premature infants, 121–22
  prematurity, 117
  terminology, 121
buprenorphine
  as analgesic for OUD, 71
  approach for painful nonemergent surgery, 69
  characterization of induction, 69
  FDA for treatment of pain, 74
  maintenance dosing after surgery, 70
  options for managing in perioperative period, 69
  perioperative period and, 69
  pharmacological properties of, 67–69
  preoperative dose reduction, 69, 70f
  treatment of chronic back pain, 74
  treatment of opioid use disorder (OUD), 67
bupropion, smoking cessation, 213, 214t
business associate agreement (BAA), 9

C
Canadian Anesthesiologists' Society (CAS), 466
Canadian Cardiovascular Society (CCS), 171–72, 466
cancer
  COVID-19 infection and, 229
  risks inherent in delaying surgery, 230
cancer patient, 482, 489
  breast cancer and secondary malignancies, 485
  breast cancer lymphedema, 485
  breast cancer treatments and toxicities, 484–85
  cardiac evaluation, 486–88
  case and key questions, 481–82
  childhood lymphoma and future risk of malignancy, 484

common antineoplastic drugs, treatments, and cardiopulmonary toxicities, 483t
  functional status, 486, 487f
  hematologic considerations, 487
  immune-related toxicities throughout the body, 486f
  immunotherapy agents, 485
  immunotherapy agents' toxicities, 485–86
  lymphoma, 482
  lymphoma treatments and side effects, 483–84
  neurologic evaluation, 488
  pain, 486
  prehabilitation of oncology surgery patient, 487f, 488–89
  preoperative evaluation of, 486
  pulmonary evaluation, 486–87
  review questions, 489–90
  therapeutic protocol, 482
candida, infection, 198
cannabis, substance use disorders (SUD), 73
Canterbury v. Spence, 410
Caprini Score, venous thromboembolism, 373
capsule endoscopy, electromagnetic interference risks, 468t
carcinoid tumors, 339
cardiac allograft vasculopathy (CAV), 198
cardiac assessment, American College of Cardiology and American Heart Association (ACC/AHA), 31f
cardiac catheterization, referral for, 30–32
cardiac evaluation
  American College of Cardiologists and American Heart Association (ACC/AHA), 486
  American College of Cardiology and American Heart Association (ACC/AHA), 28
  cancer patient, 486–88
  complete blood count (CBC), 28
  Duke Activity Status Index (DASI), 30, 30t
  major adverse cardiovascular events (MACE), 28–30
  patient, 21–22
  Revised Cardiac Risk Index (RCRI), 28–29, 30t
cardiac implantable electronic devices (CIEDs), 465, 473
  anteroposterior chest radiograph demonstrating subcutaneous implantable cardioverter defibrillator system, 471f
  basic information to be collected, 466b
  electromagnetic interference, 466–67
  heart failure monitoring, 175–78
  implanted cardioverter defibrillators, 175–76
  indications for placement of, 465
  intraoperative management, 470–71
  left ventricular assist devices (LVADs), 176–78
  Micra pacemaker, 471f
  pacemaker and defibrillator nomenclature, 465–66
  pacer dependency, 465
  perioperative algorithm for management of, 469–70, 470f
  perioperative management and newer CIEDs, 471–72
  postoperative management, 471
  preanesthesia evaluation, 467
  recommendations for CIED management for MRI scan, 472t
  response to magnet placement, 466
  review questions, 473–74
  special considerations in non-operating room environments, 472–73

special situations and electromagnetic interference risks, 468t
twenty-four-hour technical support contacts for manufacturing companies, 467t
typical appearance of implantable cardioverter defibrillator (ICD), 469f
typical appearance of pacemaker, 469f
wireless hemodynamic monitoring, 178
cardiac myosin activators, heart failure treatment, 175
cardiac risk, hemoglobin A1c, 41
cardiac surgery, surgical blood order schedule, 29f
cardiac troponin (cTn)
  causes of elevated values, 54–55, 55t
  detection of elevated, 62
cardiopulmonary abnormalities
  premature infants, 120
cardiopulmonary exercise testing (CPET), 84, 86–89, 141
  abdominal cancer resection case, 97–100, 98t, 99f
  determining AT (anaerobic threshold), 93, 110
  esophagectomy case, 93–97, 94f, 94t, 95f
  laparotomy and resection case, 107–10, 107t, 108f
  neoadjuvant chemoradiotherapy case, 100–7, 100t, 101f, 102t, 103f, 104t, 105f, 106f
  review questions, 110–12
cardiorespiratory fitness, cardiopulmonary exercise testing (CPET) defining, 84, 86–89
cardiovascular mortality, procedures categorized by risk, 173t
cardiovascular system
  anabolic steroid use, 477
  smoking and nicotine pathophysiologic effects, 210
cardioversion
  electromagnetic interference risks, 468t
  indications for and risks of synchronized, 523
  sedation and, 523
CARPA (complement activation-related pseudo allergy) syndrome, 309
cataract surgery, evaluation before, 168
cefotetan, allergy to, 433
Center for Connected Health Policy, 11
Centers for Disease Control and Prevention (CDC), 19, 228
  Antigen Test Algorithm, 240
  Chinese, 233
  COVID guidelines, 240
  COVID Public Health Emergency, 232
  opioid therapy for chronic pain, 70
  prehabilitation, 131
Centers for Medicare and Medicaid Services (CMS), 10, 49, 401
central nervous system, anabolic steroid use, 477
central sleep apnea (CSA), 496
cerebrovascular accident (CVA). See stroke
cerebrovascular disease (CVD), medical risk, 141
cesarean delivery
  trial of labor and vaginal birth after, 560
  See also pregnancy and delivery
CHA$_2$D$_2$-VASc scores
  risk of perioperative thrombosis, 153
  stroke risk, 33, 33t, 43
CHADS$_2$, risk of perioperative thrombosis, 153
CHAMPION trial, 178
cheiroarthropathy, 324

INDEX · 533

chest radiograph, urgent care clinic, 26
Child Behavioral Checklist (CBCL), 348–49
Child-Pugh-Turcotte (CTP) score, 256
   surgical risk for patients with cirrhosis, 253f, 253
chronic hyperglycemia, 324
chronic kidney disease (CKD), 302
   abdominal aortic aneurysms and, 455, 456
   anemia treatment, 309
   case and key questions, 297–98
   definition and manifestations of, 298–99
   definition of, 298–302
   manifestations of, 298–302
   perioperative risks in CKD patients, 300
   preoperative evaluation of, 299–300
   review questions, 302–4
   stages of, 298t
chronic liver diseases (CLD), 250–55
   See also cirrhosis
chronic obstructive pulmonary disease (COPD), 27–28, 32, 33–34, 208–14
   abdominal aortic aneurysms and, 455, 456
   behavioral therapy, 212–13
   benefits of quitting smoking before surgery, 212
   BMI and weight loss, 38
   bupropion, 213
   cardiovascular system, 210
   case and key questions, 207–8
   characterization, 208–14
   COVID-19 infection and, 229
   electronic (e-) cigarettes, 214
   frailty and, 32–33
   gastrointestinal system, 211
   Global Initiative for Chronic Obstructive Lung Disease (GOLD) classification of patient groups, 209, 209t
   heart failure and, 169–70
   hematopoietic system, 210–11
   history of, 208
   investigations, 208
   management of acute exacerbations, 209–10
   nicotine replacement therapies, 213
   optimization of COPD patient in preparation for surgery, 210
   pathophysiologic effects of smoking and nicotine, 210–11
   pharmacotherapies for smoking cessation, 214t
   pharmacotherapy, 213–14
   preoperative management of stable, 209
   preoperative smoking cessation interventions, 212–13
   prevention and maintenance, 208
   pulmonary function testing, 41, 42
   renal system, 211
   respiratory system, 210
   reversibility of smoking induced pathologic changes, 212
   review questions, 215
   risk factors for, 35
   severity of, 208
   smoking and back pain, 211
   smoking and surgical outcomes, 211–12
   smoking cessation counseling, 209b
   treatment of, 208–9
   varenicline, 213–14
chronic renal failure (CRF), medical risk, 141
cirrhosis, 250–55
   acute-on-chronic liver failure (ACLF), 252
   ascites and hepatic hydrothorax, 252

cardiopulmonary complications of, 254
case and key questions, 249–50
clinical stages, 250–51, 255
compensated stage, 250–51
decompensated stage, 250–51
diagnosis of, 249, 251
etiology, 250
hemostasis in, 254
hepatic encephalopathy, 252
hepatorenal syndrome, 252
liver transplantation, 252
management, 251–52
nutritional status in, 254–55
preoperative evaluation in, 253–54
review questions, 255–56
scoring systems to predict postoperative mortality in, 253f, 253
screening and surveillance for high-risk gastroesophageal varices, 251
screening for liver cancer, 252
spontaneous bacterial peritonitis, 252
variceal bleeding, 251
See also elective major surgery
Cleveland Clinic, 4, 5
   Pre-Anesthesia Consultation Clinic (PACC), 5
   Pre-Anesthesia Consultation Clinic (PACC) triage questionnaire, 7
Clinical Frailty Scale (CFS), 128, 129t
Clinical Institute Withdrawal Assessment-Alcohol Scale, Revised (CIWA-Ar), 73
Clinical Risk Analysis Index (RAI-C), 128
Clinical Risk Assessment Index (RAI-C), 129t
clozapine, classification and mechanism of action, 443
coagulation
   differential diagnosis of, disorders, 315
   disorders in pediatric population, 315–17
   hemophilias, 316–17
   laboratory tests evaluating, 315
   von Willebrand disease (vWD), 315–16
   See also pediatric patient
cocaine use, 72, 479
cognitive dysfunction, anesthesia and surgery, 48
cognitive impairment, older adults, 127
College of American Pathologists (CAP), transfusion guidelines, 386t
colonoscopy, electromagnetic interference risks, 468t
colorectal surgical team
   assessment for open abdominal cancer resection, 97
   See also abdominal cancer resection
combined medical/surgical risk for proposed procedure, definition, 140–41
Committee Opinion and Non-Obstetric Surgery During Pregnancy, 348
compensated cirrhosis, 250–51
competence, informed consent, 403, 408, 409
comprehensive geriatric assessment (CGA), 126
   See also geriatric assessment
Confusion Assessment Method (CAM), 125, 275
Confusion Assessment Method for the Intensive Care Unit (CAM-ICU), 275, 516
congestive heart failure (CHF), 414
   medical risk, 141
continuous positive airway pressure (CPAP) device, obstructive sleep apnea (OSA) treatment, 218, 221, 495, 496, 498
continuous positive airway pressure (CPAP) therapy, sleep apnea, 414

conversations. See difficult conversations
coronary artery disease (CAD)
   abdominal aortic aneurysms and, 455–56
   American College of Cardiology and American Heart Association (ACC/AHA), 31f
   medical risk, 141
   patient for esophagogastroduodenoscopy (EGD)/colonoscopy, 187
   prostatectomy patient, 139
   risk factors for, 29–30, 62
   stent types, 56–57
   surgery for elderly man, 125
   surgical population, 140
   total hip arthroplasty for elderly man, 146
coronary heart disease (CHD)
   risk factors for, 62
   risk of surgery after coronary stent placement, 57–58
   types of, 54
coronary stent placement, risk of surgery after, 57–58
counseling, smoking cessation, 209b
covert stroke, 291
COVID-19 infection, 3, 239–40
   antigen testing algorithm, 228f, 228
   case and key questions, 227–32
   clinical course, 233–34
   common symptoms of infection, 228
   decision tools for delaying cancer surgery, 230
   extrapulmonary manifestations of, 234f
   guidelines for timing of surgery after, 229–30
   long-term effects of, 235–37, 236f
   morbidity and mortality from, 229
   onset, 4
   optimizing patient for endoscopic stent placement, 231–32
   pandemic course, 232–33
   PCR testing prior to surgery, 230
   perioperative considerations for current state of patient, 231
   perioperative management, 238–39
   postponing cancer surgery during, 228–29
   preoperative assessment approach, 230–31, 237–38
   protocol for preoperative assessment of COVID-19 survivors, 237t
   repeat confirmatory PCR test, 228
   review questions, 240–42
   risk factors for severe infection, 234–35, 235f
   tests for detection of infection, 227
   vaccines by Pfizer-BioNTech and Moderna, 232
   viral biology, 233
COVIDICUS multicenter randomized control trial, 231–32
CPAP. See continuous positive airway pressure (CPAP) device
CPET. See cardiopulmonary exercise testing (CPET)
CPR (cardiopulmonary resuscitation), history of DNR orders and, 396
Cruzan, Nancy, 389, 396
cryoablation, 464
cryotherapy ablation, 472
C-spine imaging
   conditions with abnormalities, 81t
   indications for lateral flexion and extensions X-rays, 81f
   review questions, 81–82
   thyroidectomies, 78
   See also rheumatoid arthritis (RA)
cultural disparities, pregnancy, 358, 365–66
cytomegalovirus (CMV), infection, 198

D
dabigatran
   indications and pharmacokinetics, 151t
   interruption time, 155t
   laboratory tests for, 156t
   US Food and Drug Administration (FDA), 150–51
decisional capacity
   DNR, 395, 399
   elements of, 399b
decision-making capacity
   assessment for informed consent, 406
   informed consent, 403, 409, 413, 418
decompensated cirrhosis, 250–51
deep brain stimulation (DBS), epilepsy treatment, 261, 265
deep brain stimulator (DBS)
   implantation for Parkinson's disease (PD), 285
   implantation of, 290
   Parkinson's disease, 282
   placement considerations, 282, 287–88
defibrillator(s)
   implanted cardioverter, 175–76
   nomenclature, 465–66
Deficit Accumulation Index, 128
delirium, 271–72
   anesthesiologist advocating for patient, 519
   definition, 271
   diagnosis of, 516
   general anesthesia and, 271
   informed consent and, 514, 515
   melatonin and, 519
   postoperative, 519
   preventing, 271
   prevention, 518
   risk factors, 516
   role of methylene blue, 516–17
   screening for, 271, 272–73
   serotonin syndrome, 518–19
   treatment of, 517
   types of post anesthetic, 272
   See also perioperative brain health; perioperative delirium prevention; post-anesthesia care unit (PACU) patient
delirium risk, surgery of older adults, 125–26
delirium risk factors, 127
   prevention strategies, 128t
depressants, substance use disorders (SUD), 72–73
dexmedetomidine, autistic patient, 439–40, 446–47
diabetes
   carbohydrate loading in preparation for surgery, 327
   choice of insulin for managing hyperglycemia, 327
   elements of preoperative, risk assessment, 325b
   epidemic, 324
   management of perioperative medications, 327
   preparing patient for anesthesia and surgery, 327
   waiting period for surgery, 229
   See also blood glucose; diabetes mellitus (DM)
diabetes mellitus (DM), 328–29
   abdominal aortic aneurysms and, 455, 456
   carpal tunnel repair, 329
   case and key questions, 323–24
   diagnostic criteria for, 324
   elective femoropopliteal bypass surgery, 330

elective sleeve gastrectomy, 330
fingerstick glucose, 323
history of type 2 DM (T2DM), 324
long-term complications and associated perioperative risk, 324
management of perioperative medications, 327, 328t
patients with limited joint mobility, 329
perioperative insulin management, 329t
pregnancy and, 358, 363–64, 367
preoperative evaluation, 324–25
review questions, 329–31
type 2 DM (T2DM), 323
diabetic ketoacidosis (DKA), 324
Diagnostic and Statistical Manual of Mental Disorders (DSM), post-operative cognitive dysfunction (POCD), 48–49
Diagnostic and Statistical Manual of Mental Disorders (DSM-5), 67
delirium criteria, 272
neurocognitive disorders, 514
diagnostic radiation, electromagnetic interference risks, 468t
difficult conversations, 424–28
anesthesiologist on echocardiogram, 424
case and key questions, 423–24
communication frameworks, 426
coverage of perioperative conversations, 425–26
interdisciplinary communication making a recommendation, 427–28
medical decision-making, 423
patient's values, 424
REMAP, 426, 429
REMAP framework for, 426, 427t
responding to emotion, 426
review questions, 428–30
setting for new medical information, 423
setting the stage for perioperative conversations, 425
SPIKES framework, 429
spikes framework for, 426, 426t
trouble spots and where to go for help, 428
Wish-Worry-Wonder framework, 430
Wish-Worry-Wonder framework for, 427–28, 428f
digoxin, heart failure treatment, 175
direct oral anticoagulant (DOAC), 148
American Society of Regional Anesthesiologists guidelines, 156t
laboratory monitoring, 155–56
laboratory tests for, 156t
management before regional anesthesia, 155
management of, 154–55
review question, 158
disasters, unilateral DNR during, 398
disclosure, informed consent, 409
disclosure standards, informed consent, 408, 412
disseminated intravascular coagulation (DIC), 315
elevated partial thromboplastin time (PTT), 315
DNR (do not resuscitate), 396–400
addendum to code status, 398t
barriers to perioperative DNR order, 398
case and key questions, 395
clarifying DNR order, 398
dealing with conflicts, 399
decisional capacity, 395
decisional capacity and surrogacy, 399
history of CPR and, 396
in operating room (OR), 396–97
possible benefits to patients continuing DNR to OR, 397

possible benefits to surgeons and anesthesiologists in suspending DNR in OR, 397–98
review questions, 400–1
surrogacy, 395, 399
unilateral DNA during pandemics and other disasters, 398
dobutamine stress echocardiography, 30
dopamine (DA/5HT), neurotransmitter, 19
Down syndrome
atlanto-axial instability (AAI) in, 80–81
C-spine abnormalities, 81t
obstructive sleep apnea (OSA), 222
pulmonary hypertension, 120
drug-eluting stent, patient with, 62, 63
dual antiplatelet therapy (DAPT), 30–32, 53, 139
ACC/AHA guidelines, 142, 145
interruption of, prior to surgery, 58–59
ischemic risk vs. bleeding risk, 32t
optimal duration of, 57
patients with history of PCI, 63
principles of perioperative management of antiplatelet medications, 58t
Duke Activity Status Index (DASI), 6–7, 30, 30t, 37, 84, 102–4, 141
functional capacity, 145, 171–77
Duke University
Preoperative Anesthesia and Surgical Screening (PASS) Clinic, 5, 11
preoperative model, 5
dysfunctional uterine bleeding (DUB), transvaginal ultrasound for, 26
dyspnea
causes of, 42
evaluation for, 26, 35
murmur and, 28
optimizing patient for surgery, 34–35, 34t
workup, 27f

E
ECGs (electrocardiograms)
anatomically contiguous ECG leads, 55t
findings during myocardial ischemia, 55–56
initial, 53, 54
non-ST elevation MIs (NSTEMI), 55
ST elevation MIs (STEMI), 55, 55t
echocardiography, 163
imaging heart failure, 171
eclampsia
definition, 353–54
diagnosis and management, 353–54
hypertensive disorder, 361–62, 361t
incidence pregnancy, 361
Edmonton Frail Scale (EFS), 128, 129t, 133, 238
edoxaban
indications and pharmacokinetics, 151t
interruption time, 155t
laboratory tests for, 156t
e-Form, electronic preoperative care pathway, 6
Elam, James, 396
elderly adults
informed consent and, 514–8
See also geriatric assessment
elective major surgery
evaluating patient for, 249–50
transverse rectus abdominus myocutaneous (TRAM) flap reconstruction, 249, 250
See also cirrhosis
elective surgery, perioperative management of antiplatelet medications, 58t
electroconvulsive therapy (ECT), 269
electromagnetic interference risks, 468t

electroencephalogram (EEG), processed, monitoring cognitive outcomes, 274
electromagnetic interference (EMI)
cardiac implantable electronic devices (CIEDs), 466–67
pacemaker and internal cardiac defibrillator (ICD), 16, 17
role of magnets for pacemakers and internal defibrillators, 17
special situations and risks, 468t
electronic cigarettes, 214
electronic medical record (EMR), 5
emergence delirium, 272
emergency situations, informed consent in, 406
Endocrine Society, 326, 327–28, 335–36
guidelines, 340
endocrine system, anabolic steroid use, 477
endoscopic retrograde cholangiopancreatography (ECRP), 472
electromagnetic interference risks, 468t
endoscopic stent placement, optimizing patient for, 231–32
endoscopy, electromagnetic interference risks, 468t
end-stage renal disease (ESRD), hemodialysis (HD) for patient, 187
Enhanced Recovery After Surgery, 133
enhanced recovery after surgery (ERAS), principles, 376–77, 378t, 380
epilepsy, 261
conditions prevalent in people with, 264t
definition of, 261
International League Against Epilepsy (ILAE) Task Force, 267t
perioperative medication management for patients with, 263b
See also seizure(s)
epinephrine, allergy to all, 433
erythropoiesis-stimulating agents (ESAs), anemia treatment, 309
esophageal adenocarcinoma. *See* neoadjuvant chemoradiotherapy
esophagectomy
cardiopulmonary exercise testing (CPET), 93, 94t
case and key questions, 93–97
discussion of, 96–97
electrocardiogram for case, 94f
9-panel plot, 95f
See also cardiopulmonary exercise testing (CPET)
esophagogastroduodenoscopy, electromagnetic interference risks, 468t
estradiol, conversion of testosterone to, 478f, 478
ethnic disparities, pregnancy, 358, 365–66
European Association of Cardio-Thoracic Surgery (EACTS), 57
European Society of Cardiology (ESC), 57, 140–41, 171–72
European Society of Clinical Nutrition and Metabolism (ESCEN), 32
evaluation and management (E&M), 10
extra-adrenal pheochromocytomas, 334

F
facilitated telemedicine visit, 8, 9t, 11
facilitated virtual visit, 8
familial medullary thyroid cancer (FMTC), multiple endocrine neoplasia (MEN) syndrome, 338
family, disagreeing with patient's wishes, 406
fat-free mass index (FFMI), 38, 40
fatty liver, 51
fetal lung development, 120–21, 121t

fetal monitoring, pregnant patient, 352
Fifth International Perioperative Neurotoxicity, postoperative delirium prevention, 271–72
fixed obstruction of the upper airway, pulmonary function test, 18f
flow-volume loops, pulmonary function test, 18f
fluoxetine, classification and mechanism of action, 443
frailty
assessment, 41
Clinical Frailty Scale (CFS), 32–33, 33t
evaluation, 38
geriatric assessment, 128
Preoperative Frailty Assessment (PFA), 32–33
screening for, 273
screening tools in preoperative setting, 129t
Frailty Index, 19–20, 128
screening tool, 19t, 25
Framingham Heart Study, 149
Fried Index, 129t
functional capacity
heart failure preoperative evaluation, 170–71
perioperative cardiac events, 141
functional capacity assessment, 43

G
gabapentanoids, abdominal aortic aneurysms (AAA), 461
gamma aminobutyric acid (GABA), neurotransmitter, 19
gastroesophageal reflux disease (GERD), 333, 414–15
lung transplant recipients, 197
premature infants, 117, 119–20
gastroesophageal varices, screening and surveillance for high-risk, 251
gastrointestinal abnormalities, premature infants, 119–20
gastrointestinal system, smoking and nicotine pathophysiologic effects, 211
general anesthesia, allergy to, 433
General Anesthesia Versus Spinal (GAS) study, premature infants, 119
general surgery, surgical blood order schedule, 29f
geriatric assessment, 125–26, 131
advance care planning, 130b, 130
approach to preoperative assessment in older adults, 126
case and key questions, 125–26
case summary, 131
cognition, mental health, and delirium, 127
components of preoperative assessment, 126–29
delirium risk factors, 128t
frailty, 128
frailty screening tools in preoperative setting, 129t
function, 127
key questions before surgery, 130t
medication review, 127–28
models of perioperative care, 131
nutrition, 128–29
prehabilitation, 130–31
review questions, 132–33
shared decision-making, 129–30
surgeries in older adults, 126
Geriatric Nutritional Risk Index (GNRI), 129, 133
Geriatric Surgery Verification (GSV), 126
Quality Improvement Program, 126

INDEX • 535

Global Initiative for Chronic Obstructive
    Lung Disease (GOLD)
  classification of patient groups, 209, 209t
  prednisolone guidelines, 210
Global Initiative for Obstructive Lung
    Disease (GOLD), 35, 38
global pandemic. *See* COVID-19 infection
glucose. *See* blood glucose
glucose intolerance, 334
glutamine, neurotransmitter, 19
goal-directed medical therapy (GDMT),
    30–32
goal-directed resuscitation, 396–97
  clarifying DNR order, 398
GoToMeeting, 9
Guidelines of the Hernia-Surge Group, 47
Gupta Myocardial Infarct or Cardiac Arrest
    (MICA), 292
Gupta Perioperative Cardiac Risk Calculator
    for Myocardial Infarction or Cardiac
    Arrest (MICA), 28
gynecological surgery, surgical blood order
    schedule, 29f
gynecomastia
  anabolic steroid use, 476
  preventing recurrence of, 478
  reverse Trendelenburg position, 480
  surgery for, 478, 479f
  treatment for, 478
  See also anabolic steroid use

H
hallucinogens, substance use disorders
    (SUD), 73–74
HAS-BLED score, 40
  surgical bleeding risk, 152
Health Insurance Portability and
    Accountability Act (HIPAA), 8–9,
    10, 11
HealthQuest (HQ) questionnaire, 6
Health Resources and Services
    Administration (HRSA), 11
heart failure
  American College of Surgeons National
    Surgical Quality Improvement
    Program, 172
  associated conditions, 169–70
  classification of, 170t
  consensus definitions for urgency of
    procedure, 173t
  considerations for minor, low-risk
    procedures, 179
  etiology and pathophysiology, 169–70
  factors predictive of perioperative
    myocardial infarction (MI) or cardiac
    arrest, 172b
  intraoperative and postoperative
    anesthetic risks in, 170
  intrinsic surgical risk, 173
  National Surgical Quality Improvement
    Program Myocardial Infarction and
    Cardiac Arrest (NSQIP MICA), 172
  New York Heart Association (NYHA)
    functional classification, 169, 169t
  preoperative evaluation, 170–72
  preoperative risk calculators, 172–73
  procedures by risk of 30-day
    cardiovascular mortality and/or
    myocardial infarction, 173t
  review questions, 180–82
  risk for perioperative cardiac death,
    nonfatal MI or nonfatal cardiac arrest,
    172b
  surgical urgency, 172–73
  systolic versus diastolic dysfunction, 169
  treatment and monitoring, 173–79
  See also pulmonary hypertension (PH)

heart failure preoperative evaluation
  assessment of functional capacity, 170–71
  brain natriuretic peptide (BNP) and
    N-terminal (NT) ProBNP, 171–72
  imaging, 171
  laboratory testing, 171–72
  preoperative examination, 170
  troponin, 172
heart failure treatment and monitoring,
    173–79
  angiotensin converting enzyme inhibitors
    and angiotensin II receptor blockers,
    174
  angiotensin receptor-neprilysin
    inhibitors, 174
  beta blockers, 173–74
  cardiac implantable electronic devices,
    175–78
  cardiac myosin activators, 175
  digoxin, 175
  implanted cardioverter defibrillators,
    175–76
  intraoperative monitoring, 175
  left ventricular assist devices, 176–78
  loop diuretics, 174
  medical management, 173–75
  mineralocorticoid receptor antagonists
    (MRAs), 174
  orthotopic heart transplantation, 178–79
  sodium-glucose cotransporter 2
    inhibitors, 174
  soluble guanylate cyclase stimulators, 175
  statins, 175
  surgical management, 178–79
  wireless hemodynamic monitoring, 178
  See also left ventricular assist devices
    (LVADs)
HeartMate II, 176
HeartMate III, 176
heart rate (HR), 93
heart rate (HR) monitor. *See* postoperative
    arrhythmias
Heart Rhythm Society (HRS), 466
  internal cardiac defibrillator (ICD),
    16, 25
heart transplant
  anesthesia in patients following, 199–200
  anesthetic medication choices, 200
  cardiopulmonary pathology of recipients,
    200
  echocardiography for patient, 196
  imaging of patient with prior, 199
  intraoperative monitor choice, 200
  neurologic complications, 199
  noncardiothoracic surgery of patient with
    prior, 199
  preoperative assessment, 199
  review questions, 201–2
  See also shoulder replacement
HeartWare HVAD, 176–77, 182
HELLP (hemolysis, elevated levels of liver
    enzymes and low platelet count)
  hypertension, 362
hematopoietic system, smoking and nicotine
    pathophysiologic effects, 210–11
hemodynamic considerations, ACC/AHA
    guidelines, 144
hemoglobin A1c (HbA1c), 323
  HbA1c as measure of glycosylation of,
    325–26
  perioperative complications and, 323
  relationship between blood glucose and,
    325t
  See also diabetes mellitus (DM)
hemophilias
  coagulation disorder, 316–17
  diagnosis and management of, 316–17

hemostasis, cirrhosis, 254
hepatic encephalopathy, 252
hepatic hydrothorax, complication of
    cirrhosis, 254
hepatic system, anabolic steroid use, 477
hepatocellular liver cancer (HCC)
  ablative therapies, 17
  interventional treatments, 17
  patient, 15
  transarterial chemoembolization (TACE)
    therapies, 17
hepatocellular liver cancer (HCC) patient,
    15
  See also perioperative surgical home
    (PSH)
hepatopulmonary syndrome (HPS),
    complication of cirrhosis, 254
hepatorenal syndrome (HRS), 252
hepcidin, anemia of chronic inflammation,
    381
hernia repair
  patient needing, 187–88
  perioperative management, 48–49
  preoperative assessment and testing, 49
  review questions, 50–51
  surgical venue, 49–50
hernia surgery, 47–48
  chronic postoperative pain, 48
  goals of elective, 47
  postoperative complications, 47–48
  symptomatic patients, 47
  techniques for repair, 47
  venue, 49–50
  See also inguinal hernia
herpes, infection, 198
hip replacement. *See* total hip replacement
    (THR)
Hospital Anxiety and Depression Scale
    (HADS), 84, 86–89
Hospital Elder Life Program (HELP), 131
Hospital Liaison Committee, Jehovah's
    Witness, 387
hyperglycemia
  choice of insulin for management of, 327
  immediate effects on perioperative risk,
    326
  perioperative management of oral
    antihyperglycemic medications, 328t
  relationship between stress, and
    postoperative outcomes, 326f
  See also blood glucose
hyperglycemic hyperosmolar state (HHS),
    324
hyperkalemia, succinylcholine and, 510
hypersensitivity reaction, 434
hypertension (HTN), 50, 51
hypertensive disorders of pregnancy, 361–62
  classification of, 361t
hyperthyroidism, 434
  symptoms and signs of, 437b
  thyroid disease, 437
hypopnea, 496
  definition, 221
hypothyroidism, 434
  symptoms and signs of, 437b
  thyroid disease, 437
hysterectomy. *See* robotic hysterectomy

I
implantable cardioverter-defibrillator
    (ICD), 168, 181, 464
  heart monitoring, 175–76
  transplantation surgery, 198
  See also cardiac implantable electronic
    devices (CIEDs)
infants. *See* premature infants
infection(s), shoulder replacement, 196, 198

infectious diseases, anabolic steroid use, 477
informed consent, 411
  advance directive, 405
  anesthesia, 405
  anesthesiologist addressing nerve block
    risks, 407
  assessing decision-making capacity, 406
  basic components, 411
  case and key questions, 403–8
  competence, 403
  decision-making capacity, 403, 406, 413
  delirium and, 514, 515
  DNR/DNI (do not resuscitate, do not
    intubate) order, 407
  elderly and at-risk individuals, 514–15
  emergency situations, 406
  family disagreeing with patient's wishes,
    406
  Jehovah's Witness patient, 386–89
  model for Jehovah's Witness patients,
    388t
  obtaining, 419–20
  participants in patient's care, 405–6
  particular-patient (subjective person)
    standard, 404
  problems in, 408
  process of obtaining, 408–11
  reasonable-patient (reasonable person)
    standard, 404
  reasonable physician standard, 404
  review questions, 411–13
  standards of disclosure, 404
  voluntariness, 403
inguinal hernia(s)
  case and key questions, 46–47
  chronic postoperative pain, 48
  complications, 46
  description of, 46
  hernia surgery, 47–48
  most common type of hernia, 47
  need for labs prior to repair, 46
  postoperative complications of hernia
    repair, 47–48
  postoperative neurocognitive
    dysfunction, 47
  preoperative urinalysis, 46
  surgery, 46
  symptoms, 46
  See also hernia surgery
inhalational agents
  seizures, 265
  seizure threshold, 265, 266t
insulin
  choice for managing hyperglycemia, 327
  continuous subcutaneous therapy
    (pumps), 327–28, 330
  perioperative management, 329t
  perioperative management of oral
    antihyperglycemic medications, 328t
internal cardiac defibrillator (ICD), 15
  functions of, 16–17
  role of magnets for, 17
International Classification of Disease, 48
International League Against Epilepsy
    (ILAE), seizure classification, 261b, 264
International Prostate Symptom Score
    (IPSS), 49–50
International Society for Heart and Lung
    Transplantation (ISHLT), 177,
    189–91
interventional radiology (IR)
  patient's IR evaluation, 22–23
  treatment procedures, 17–18
interventions, physically consenting for
    patient, 406–7
intracardiac RF ablation, electromagnetic
    interference risks, 468t

intracranial pressure (ICP), succinylcholine and, 510–11
intraocular pressure (IOP), succinylcholine and, 511
intravenous iron preparations, 34t
iron deficiency anemia (IDA), 16, 43, 308f, 310, 383, 391
　definitions of, 382t
　diagnosing, 41
　evaluation, 35
iron dextran (low molecular weight, LMW), hypersensitivity, 309, 310
iron formulations
　available, and potential risks of IV iron, 309
　commonly used intravenous, 309t
　See also anemia
ischemic heart disease (IHD), 30, 93
　preoperative evaluation of patients with, 57
　See also esophagectomy

J

JAMA Surgery (journal), 458–59
Jehovah's Witness
　beliefs regarding blood transfusion, 385–86
　blood conservation, 390, 391
　elective surgery, 383–84, 390
　Hospital Liaison Committee, 387
　informed consent process for, 386–89
　model of consent for patients, 388t
　patient, 381
　patient observations, 385
　refusal of blood products, 359, 365, 367, 368
　religious doctrine, 382
　summary of product acceptability, 387t
　treatment modalities acceptance in patients, 387, 387t
Joint Commission, 3, 49
Joint Consensus Statement on Postoperative Delirium Prevention, 271–72
Journal of the American Medical Association (JAMA), 236

K

Kaiser Permanente, Baldwin Park Medical Center, 20
Katz Activities of Daily Living (ADL) Index, 127
ketamine
　abdominal aortic aneurysms (AAA), 460
　autistic patient, 441, 446, 447
　pheochromocytoma resection, 340
kidney disease
　acute kidney injury network (AKIN), 298–99, 299t
　chronic kidney disease (CKD), 298–99, 298t
　See also chronic kidney disease (CKD)
kratom, substance use disorders (SUD), 73–74

L

lactate production, 96–97
Lancet (journal), 228–29
laparoscopy, pregnant patient, 352–53
laparotomy and resection of retroperitoneal sarcoma
　cardiopulmonary exercise testing (CPET) data, 107t
　case and key questions, 107–10
　discussion, 109–10
　9-panel plot, 108f
　See also cardiopulmonary exercise testing (CPET)

laryngeal mask airway (LMA)
　placement of, 218, 219
　premature infants, 118
　risks and benefits of removing, 219–20
Lawton Instrumental Activities of Daily Living (IADL) Scale, 127
left ventricular assist devices (LVADs), 168
　anticoagulation, 177
　currently available devices, 176
　hemodynamic considerations, 177
　intraoperative monitoring with, 177
　performance parameters and settings, 176–77
　perioperative considerations, 178
　pulsatility index (PI), 176–77
　pump flow, 176
　pump power, 176
　pump speed, 176
　See also heart failure treatment and monitoring
Legionella, infection, 198
lidocaine, abdominal aortic aneurysms (AAA), 460
lithotripsy, electromagnetic interference risks, 468t
liver. See cirrhosis
liver cancer, screening for, 252
liver cirrhosis, 17
liver disease, elevated partial thromboplastin time (PTT), 315
liver transplantation, 252
liver transplants
　demand for, 19
　list for, 24
local anesthetics, allergy to all, 433
local anesthetic systemic toxicity (LAST), 501
local anesthetic toxicity syndrome (LAST), 222
loop diuretics, heart failure treatment, 174
lung. See restrictive lung disease
lung development, stages of fetal, 120–21, 121f
lung transplant
　anesthesia in patients following, 199–200
　anesthetic medication choices, 200
　cardiopulmonary pathology of recipients, 200
　echocardiography for patient, 196
　imaging of patient with prior, 199
　immunosuppressive medications, 199
　intraoperative monitor choice, 200
　neurologic complications, 199
　noncardiothoracic surgery of patient with prior, 199
　preoperative assessment, 199
　review questions, 201–2
　SARS-CoV-2 infection and, 198, 201
　See also shoulder replacement
lupus, elevated partial thromboplastin time (PTT), 315
lymphoma, 481, 482
　antineoplastic drugs, treatments, and cardiopulmonary toxicities, 483t
　childhood, and future risk of malignancy, 484
　Hodgkin or non-Hodgkin, 482
　treatment for, 481
　treatments and side effects, 483–84
　See also cancer patient
lysergic acid diethylamide (LSD), substance use disorders (SUD), 73

M

magnesium, abdominal aortic aneurysms (AAA), 460
magnetic resonance imaging (MRI)

electromagnetic interference risks, 468t
recommendations for CIED management for MRI scan, 472t
major adverse cardiovascular events (MACE)
　categorizing patient, 42
　evaluation, 36–37
　postoperative, in patients with coronary stents, 62
malignant hyperthermia (MH), succinylcholine and, 510
malnutrition, Preoperative Nutrition Scale, 42
Management of Myelomeningocele Study (MOMS), 349
Management of Patients with Valvular Heart Disease, ACC/AHA guidelines, 143, 144
marijuana, tetrahydrocannabis (THC), 479
maximal voluntary ventilation (MVV), 93, 111–12
maximum surgical blood ordering schedule (MSBOS), 17, 29f
Mayo Postoperative Surgical Risk score (MRS), patients with cirrhosis, 253f, 253
Medicaid, 365–66
medical comorbidities, autism, 443–44
medical decision-making. See difficult conversations
Medicare, 126
　free-for-service supplement, 10
　telehealth coverage, 10
medication for opioid use disorder (MOUD), 67, 70, 71
　See also opioid use disorder (OUD)
medication management
　case and key questions, 53–54
　principles of perioperative management of antiplatelet medications, 58t
medication review, older adults, 127–28
medicine clinic
　combined with anesthesia clinic, 5
　separate from anesthesia clinic, 5
Medtronic, technical support contacts, 467t
melatonin, delirium and, 519
meningiomas
　patients with, 63
　preoperative evaluation of patients with, 59
　signs and symptoms of, 59
mental health, older adults, 127
metabolic panel, evaluation, 37
methadone
　maintenance before surgery, 75
　prescribed for opioid use disorder (OUD), 71
methylene blue
　antidote, 517–18
　role in delirium, 516–17
microwave ablation (MWA), 17
midazolam, autistic patient, 441, 446, 447
Middle East respiratory syndrome (MERS), 233
mineralocorticoid receptor antagonists (MRAs), heart failure treatment, 174
Mini-Cog, 127, 272–73, 276
Mini-Mental Status Examination (MMSE), 127, 272, 284, 285, 516
Model for End-Stage Liver Disease (MELD), 250, 253f, 253
modified Frailty Index, 128
modified Fried Index, 128
Montreal Cognitive Assessment (MoCA), 127, 284
morbidly adherent placenta, 364–65
mucopolysaccharidoses, C-spine abnormalities, 81t

Multicenter Perioperative Outcomes Group (MPOG), 350
multimodal medications, abdominal aortic aneurysms (AAA), 460–61
multiple endocrine neoplasia (MEN) syndromes, 333
　familial medullary thyroid cancer (FMTC), 338
　MEN type 1 (Wermer syndrome), 338
　MEN type 2A (Sipple's syndrome), 338
　MEN type 2B (Wagenmann-Froboese syndrome), 338
　MEN type 2 subtypes, 338
　See also PPGL (pheochromocytoma and paraganglioma)
multisystem atrophy, 284
murmur, evaluation of, 28, 41
muscarinic antagonists, COPD management, 209
muscle relaxants, anesthetic and sedative agent in pregnancy, 352
muscle relaxation, reversal, 197
myalgias, succinylcholine and, 510
myocardial infarction (MI)
　definition, 62
　Fourth Universal Definition, 54
　intraoperative monitoring of, 60
　management of postoperative, 61
　mechanism of perioperative, 60
　perioperative, 64
　procedures categorized by risk, 173t
　ST elevation, 53
　ST-elevation MI (STEMI), 54
Myocardial Infarction or Cardiac Arrest (MICA), 28–29, 141, 300
myocardial ischemia
　anatomically contiguous ECG leads, 55t
　causes of elevated cardiac troponin values, 55t
　diagnosing, 54–55
　electrocardiogram findings during, 55–56
　intraoperative monitors for, 63
　management of ST-elevation, 56
　percutaneous coronary intervention (PCI) considerations, 56

N

naltrexone
　extended-release (ER), 71–72
　knee replacement surgery and, 75
　treatment of opioid and alcohol use disorders, 71–72
Natanson v. Kline, 410
National Cancer Database, safe postponement period (SPP), 230
National Health and Nutrition Examination Survey (NHANES III), 298
National Heart, Lung, and Blood Institute, 209
National Inpatient Sample, 353
National Institute for Health and Care Excellence (NICE), transfusion guidelines, 386t
National Institutes of Health, 209
National Kidney Foundation KDOQI and DKIGO guidelines, 298
National Surgical Quality Improvement Program (NSQIP), 28–29, 47–48, 78–79, 102–4
National Surgical Quality Improvement Program Myocardial Infarction and Cardiac Arrest (NSQIP MICA), preoperative risk calculator, 172b, 172, 382–83, 414–15
necrotizing enterocolitis (NEC), 118
　premature infants, 120
neoadjuvant anthracycline chemotherapy, 107

neoadjuvant chemoradiotherapy
    CPET data after neoadjuvant therapy, 102t
    CPET data after prehabilitation, 104t
    CPET data prior to neoadjuvant therapy, 100t
    discussion, 102–7
    9-panel plot after neoadjuvant therapy, 103f
    9-panel plot after prehabilitation, 105f
    prehabilitation, 106f, 106–7
    Surgery School, 105
neostigmine
    reversal, 509
    sugammadex versus, 509
neurocognitive dysfunction (NCD), 272
    postoperative, 272, 275–76
neurodevelopment, premature infants, 118–19
neuromuscular blockade (NMB), 511
    cases and key questions, 507
    mini-case, 508
    neostigmine reversal, 509
    omitting reversal of, 509
    paralysis for reoperation, 512
    rapid-sequence induction, 509–10, 511–12
    residual, 508, 511
    reversal, 511
    reversal of, 507, 509, 512
    review questions, 511–13
    rocuronium and intraoperative awareness, 513
    succinylcholine, 512
    succinylcholine concerns, 510–11
    sugammadex and birth control, 511
    sugammadex for reversal of, 512
    sugammadex versus neostigmine, 509
neuromuscular blocking agents, 266
neuromuscular blocking drugs
    blockade monitoring, 508
    neostigmine reversal, 509
    omitting reversal of neuromuscular blockade, 509
    residual neuromuscular blockade, 508
    reversal of neuromuscular blockade, 509
neurosurgery, surgical blood order schedule, 29f
neurosurgical patient, perioperative management of antiplatelet therapy, 59–60
New England Journal of Medicine, 406–7
New Jersey Supreme Court, Quinlan case, 396
New York Heart Association (NYHA), 346–47
    functional classification for heart failure, 169, 169t, 180
nicotine replacement therapy (NRT), smoking cessation, 212, 213, 214t
nitrous oxide, anesthetic and sedative agent in pregnancy, 352
noninvasive positive pressure ventilation (NIPPV), obstructive sleep apnea, 498
non-obstetric surgery. *See* pregnant patient for non-obstetric surgery
North American Society of Pacing and Electrophysiology (NASPE), 465–66
NSAIDs, postoperative concern, 500, 501–2
Nuremberg Code, 403
nurse-run clinic, preoperative clinic model, 4
Nursing Delirium Symptom Checklist (NuDESC), 516
nutrition, 32
    European Society of Clinical Nutrition and Metabolism (ESPEN), 32
    fat-free mass index (FFMI), 38

frailty modification, 20
geriatric assessment, 128–29
screening, 40
nutritional status, cirrhosis, 254–55
Nutrition Risk Screen (NRS), 129
nutrition screening, evaluation, 37–38

O
obesity
    definition, 362
    pregnancy and, 359, 362–63, 367, 368
obesity hypoventilation syndrome (OHS), obstructive sleep apnea (OSA) coexisting with, 220
Obstetric Anaesthetists' Association and Difficult Airway Society, 350
obstructive disorder, pulmonary function test, 18f
obstructive sleep apnea (OSA), 17, 220–24, 414, 495, 496–503
    apnea-hypopnea index (AHI) for diagnosing severity of, 221t
    case and key questions, 218–20
    characterization, 220
    concerns of performing anesthesia on patient with, 218
    continuous positive airway pressure (CPAP), 495, 498
    decision-making in preoperative selection for patient, 499f
    definition, 312
    diagnosis, 221, 497
    discharge criteria, 502–3
    discharge criteria for patient with severe OSA, 220
    epidemiology, 496–97
    etiology, pathogenesis and symptoms, 220
    etiology and pathogenesis, 497
    evaluation, 37
    inpatient versus outpatient management, 222
    interventions to assist ventilation and intubation, 219
    intraoperative and postoperative considerations for patients with, 218–19
    intraoperative concerns, 499–500
    intraoral dental dressings for extraction of teeth, 500f
    laryngeal mask airway (LMA) and, 218
    lingual tonsils on laryngoscopy, 496f, 496
    medications for sedation minimizing risks, 219
    obesity and pregnancy, 363
    obesity hypoventilation syndrome (OHS) and, 220
    perioperative concerns, 498–503
    perioperative risks, 222
    postoperative concerns, 500–2
    pregnancy and, 358, 359
    preoperative concerns, 498–99
    preoperative evaluation, 221–22
    recommendations for perioperative practitioner, 223
    regional anesthesia, 222–23
    review questions, 224–25, 503–4
    risk factors for, 218
    risks and benefits of removing LMA, 219–20
    screening, 221, 495, 497–98
    severity by Apnea Hypopnea Index (API), pediatric vs. adult, 497t
    STOP-Bang questionnaire, 221b
    surgical setting for high-risk patients with severe OSA, 219
    symptoms, 497
    tonsillectomy, 312
    treatment, 221, 498

Ochsner Hospital, 20
older adults
    approach to preoperative assessment, 126
    key questions before surgery, 130t
    See also geriatric assessment
oncology surgery patient, 489, 490
    prehabilitation of, 487f, 488–89
operating room, blood risks of proceeding to, 382
operating room (OR)
    DNR (do not resuscitate) in, 396–97
    possible benefits to surgeons/anesthesiologists in suspending DNR in, 397–98
    possible benefit to patients continuing DNR to, 397
opiates, seizures, 265–66
opioid analgesics, postoperative concern, 501
opioids, allergy to all, 433
opioid use disorder (OUD), 67
    buprenorphine as analgesic, 71
    buprenorphine for treatment, 67
    chronic use contributing to poor acute pain control, 70
    diagnostic criteria for, 67, 68t
    methadone, 71
    naltrexone, 71–72, 75
    psychosocial barriers to perioperative pain management for patients with history of, 70
    review questions, 74–75
    See also substance use disorders (SUD)
optimization, 16
oral anticoagulation
    indications and pharmacokinetics, 151t
    preoperative management, 152
    reinitiation of, 157, 157t
    stroke risk reduction, 150–52
    See also atrial fibrillation
oral nutrition supplementation (ONS), 129
Organ Procurement and Transplantation Network, 198
orthopedic surgery, surgical blood order schedule, 29f
orthotopic heart transplantation
    heart failure treatment, 178–79
    immunosuppression, 179
    perioperative considerations, 179
    physiologic changes with transplanted heart, 178–79
osteoarthritis
    surgery in management, 90
    See also total hip replacement (THR)
otolaryngology surgery, surgical blood order schedule, 29f
Oxford Project to Investigate Memory and Ageing (OPTIMA), 275

P
pacemaker(s)
    nomenclature, 465–66
    pacer dependency, 465
    role of magnets for, 17
PACU. *See* post-anesthesia care unit (PACU)
pain control
    chronic opioid use and, 70
    See also opioid use disorder (OUD)
pancreatic islet cell tumors, 339
pandemics
    unilateral DNR during, 398
    See also COVID-19 infection
para-aminobenzoic acid (PABA), postoperative concern, 501
paragangliomas (PGL), 334
    See also PPGL (pheochromocytoma and paraganglioma)

parathyroid tumors, 338–39
Parkinson, James, 283
Parkinsonism-hyperpyrexia syndrome, 287
Parkinson-plus syndromes (PS), 283
Parkinson's disease (PD)
    anesthetic implications and management, 285
    anesthetic techniques, 286
    cardiovascular manifestations, 284
    case and key questions, 282–83
    cognitive manifestations, 284
    deep brain stimulator (DBS), 282
    deep brain stimulator (DBS) placement considerations, 287–88
    definition, 283
    description, 282
    diagnosis of, 283–84
    DNR and surgery, 395
    intraoperative considerations, 286, 286t
    levodopa, 284, 289
    medical management of, 284–85
    neurologic manifestations, 283–84
    pain management options, 286
    pathogenesis, 289
    pathophysiology, 283
    perioperative considerations, 286–87, 287t
    postoperative considerations, 286t, 288
    preoperative considerations, 285–86, 286t
    pulmonary manifestations, 284
    review questions, 289–90
    spinal cord stimulator, and, 395
    summary of observed non-motor symptoms, perioperative risk factors, and prevention, 287t
    surgical management of, 285–87
partial thromboplastin time (PTT), 312
    abnormal, 312
    abnormal PTT, 312
    differential diagnosis of isolated elevated PTT, 315
    risk for surgery with prolonged PTT, 312
    See also pediatric patient
patent ductus arteriosus (PDA), 118
patient blood management (PBM), 383–84
    anemia treatment, 309–10
Patient Health Questionnaire-2 (PHQ-2), 127
patient outcome, triple aim, 23, 24
Patient Self-Determination Act (1990), 389, 396
patient's rights movement, 396
    See also DNR (do not resuscitate)
PD. *See* Parkinson's disease (PD)
pediatric patient
    bleeding disorders in, 313–15
    clot formation at injury site, 314f
    coagulation disorders in pediatric population, 315–17
    differential diagnosis of coagulation disorders, 315
    differential diagnosis of isolated elevated partial thromboplastin time (PTT), 315
    hemophilias, 316–17
    laboratory tests evaluating coagulation, 315
    preoperative evaluation of, 313
    tonsillectomy, 312–13, 317
    tonsillectomy case and key questions, 312–13
    von Willebrand disease (vWD), 315–16
percutaneous coronary interventions (PCI), 62
    considerations, 56
    postoperative, 61

perioperative analgesia
  abdominal aortic aneurysms (AAA), 458–60
  epidural catheters, 458–59
  paraverbal and erector spinae catheters, 459
  transversus abdominis plane block, 459–60
Perioperative Assessment and Global Optimization (PASS-GO) program, 5
perioperative blood product management, evaluation, 35–36
perioperative brain health, 271–75
  case and key questions, 271
  delirium, 271, 272
  neurocognitive dysfunction (NCD), 272
  pathogenesis, 272
  perioperative delirium prevention, 273–75
  postoperative cognitive dysfunction (POCD), 271–72
  postoperative neurocognitive dysfunction (PNCD), 272
  review questions, 275–77
  screening for delirium and POCD/PNCD, 272–73
  screening for frailty, 273
  surgery, 275
  treatment options, 275
  See also perioperative delirium prevention
perioperative conversations
  advance directives, 425–26
  clarifying treatment goals and plan, 425
  coverage of, 425–26
  information, 425
  people, 425
  setting the stage, 425
  time, 425
  See also difficult conversations
perioperative delirium prevention
  anesthesia technique, 273
  blood pressure management, 274
  cerebral oximetry, 275
  medication strategies, 273–74
  nonpharmacologic prevention strategies, 273
  pharmacologic prevention strategies, 273
  processed electroencephalogram (EEG), 274
  ventilation, 275
  See also perioperative brain health
perioperative neurocognitive disorder (PND)
  factors increasing risk of, 48
  nomenclature, 48
Perioperative Optimization of Senior Health (POSH), 131
perioperative pain management, patients with history of opioid use disorder, 70
perioperative surgical home (PSH)
  anticoagulation, 21–23
  chronic alcohol use and liver cirrhosis affecting planned procedure, 19
  entry point for patient, 15
  explaining potential risks and complications to patient, 16
  factors and risks, 15
  fiscal concerns for implementation of, 20
  flow-volume loops, 18f
  Frailty Index, 19–20, 19t
  functions of ICDs, 16–17
  goals of, 15
  initial consults and evaluations of PSH team, 16
  internal cardiac defibrillator (ICD), 15, 16
  interventional radiologist, 17

key steps and stakeholders for, 20–21
managing cardiac pacemaker of patient, 16
medical team, 23
model, 21f, 21, 23
optimizing patient for surgery, 19–20
patient's cardiac evaluation, 21–22
patient's interventional radiology evaluation, 22–23
patient's primary care evaluation, 23
patient's pulmonary evaluation, 22
patient with hepatocellular liver cancer (HCC), 15–21
potential problems with pacemaker and intraoperative electrocautery use, 16
preoperative team of, 21
pulmonary function test, 18f
rationale for anesthesia plan, 15–16
referring patient to pulmonologist, 17
review questions, 23–25
risks, benefits and alternatives for anesthetic plan, 16
role for intraoperative and postoperative periods, 20
role of magnets for pacemakers and internal defibrillators, 17
treatment effects of procedures performed by interventional radiology (IR), 17–18
peripartum bleeding
  risk factors for, 359
  See also pregnancy and delivery
peripartum cardiomyopathy, pregnancy and, 358, 364
persistent pulmonary hypertension (PPH), 120
prematurity, 117
pheochromocytomas (PCC), 334
  algorithm for diagnosis of, 335f
  diagnosis of, 333
  extra-adrenal, 334
  MEN type 2 (MEN2) syndrome and, 334
  multiple endocrine neoplasia (MEN) syndrome and, 334
  patient diagnosis of, 333
  See also PPGL (pheochromocytoma and paraganglioma)
physical classification, ASA-PS (physical status) score, 414
physical fitness
  cardiopulmonary exercise testing (CPET) defining, 84, 86–89
  enhanced recovery after surgery (ERAS), 85, 89
physical status, definitions of, by ASA, 415t
physiological abnormalities, autistic patients, 444
pituitary tumors, 339
placenta accreta spectrum, pregnancy and, 364–65
placenta accreta vera, 364–65
placenta increta, 364–65
placenta percreta, 364–65
plasma, blood, 382
platelets, blood, 382
Pneumocystis, infection, 198
point-of-care ultrasound (POCUS), 139
  images, 143f
  imaging heart failure, 171
  valvular heart disease, 143
polysomnography, overnight sleep center, 221
portopulmonary hypertension (POPH), complication of cirrhosis, 254
positive airway pressure (PAP), obstructive sleep apnea (OSA), 499
post-anesthesia care unit (PACU)

case and key questions, 514
criteria for discharge from, 496
discharge criteria for OSA patient, 502–3
neuromuscular blockade reversal, 507
postoperative arrhythmias and, 522–24
postoperative concerns for OSA patient, 500
residual neuromuscular blockade, 507, 508
Situation, Background, Assessment, and Recommendation (SBAR), 495–96
post-anesthesia care unit (PACU) patient
  anesthesiologist advocating for patient, 519
  assessing confusion state of, 515–16
  delirium and informed consent, 514, 515
  delirium prevention, 518
  diagnosing delirium, 516
  differential diagnosis of, 515
  disclosing delirium to family, 518–19
  elderly and informed consent, 514–15
  evaluation of mental status, 517
  intraoperative, 515–19
  melatonin and delirium, 519
  methylene blue and delirium, 516–17
  methylene blue antidote, 517–18
  perioperative risk factors for delirium, 516
  pharmacological treatment of delirium, 517
  postoperative delirium, 519
  preoperative, 514–15
  serotonin syndrome, 517–18
postoperative apnea, premature infants, 122–23
postoperative arrhythmias, 527
  atrial fibrillation, 525
  case and key questions, 522–24
  causes of postoperative atrial fibrillation, 522
  epidemiology and presentation, 524
  evaluation and diagnosis, 522, 525
  management of postoperative bradyarrhythmia, 526–27
  management of tachyarrhythmias, 525–26
  perioperative risk factors for tachyarrhythmias, 525b
  pharmacological management of supraventricular tachyarrhythmias (SVTS), 526
  reentrant supraventricular tachyarrhythmias, 525–26
  review questions, 527
  sequelae of, 527
post-operative cognitive dysfunction (POCD), 271–72
  definition, 271
  general anesthesia and, 271
  incidence of, 48–49
  screening for, 271, 272–73
  term, 48
  See also perioperative brain health
postoperative delirium, 272
postoperative nausea and vomiting (PONV), 46, 51
  patient's risk of, 373
  risk factor summary in adults, 375b
  robotic hysterectomy increasing risk of, 375–76
  steps to reduce baseline risk, 375b–76b
  treatment guidelines, 376
postoperative urinary retention (POUR), 46, 49–50
postpartum hemorrhage, pregnancy and, 364–65
PPGL (pheochromocytoma and paraganglioma), 334, 340

algorithm for diagnosis of pheochromocytoma, 335f
carcinoid tumors, 339
diagnosis of, 334
intraoperative management, 336, 337t
multiple endocrine neoplasia (MEN) syndromes, 338
pancreatic islet cell tumors, 339
parathyroid tumors, 338–39
perioperative management, 338
pituitary tumors, 339
postoperative management, 336–38
preoperative management, 334–36, 337t
presenting symptoms, 334
select drugs in PPGL resection, 337t
specific conditions, 338–39
Practice Advisory for the Pre-Anesthesia Evaluation, 5, 415–16
Pre-Anesthesia Consultation Clinic (PACC)
  Cleveland Clinic, 5
  in-person visit, 9f
  triage questionnaire, 7
Pre-Anesthesia Questionnaire, 8f
preeclampsia
  diagnosis and management, 353–54
  hypertensive disorder, 361–62, 361t, 366
  primary prevention, 361–62
pregnancy and delivery
  advanced maternal age (AMA), 359
  antepartum and postpartum hemorrhage, 364–65
  case and key questions, 358–59
  cultural considerations, 358
  diabetes mellitus (DM), 363–64
  diabetic patients, 358
  gravid patients in advanced maternal age (AMA), 358
  hypertensive disorders, 358
  hypertensive disorders of, 361–62, 361t
  Jehovah's Witness patients, 365
  multiple gestations, 358, 360–61
  obesity, 362–63
  obesity implications, 359
  obstructive sleep apnea (OSA), 271, 359
  peripartum cardiomyopathy, 358, 364
  placenta accreta spectrum, 364–65
  postpartum pain management, 359
  racial and ethnic disparities, 358, 365–66
  refusing blood products, 359
  review questions, 366–68
  risk factors for multiple gestations, 358
  risk factors for neuraxial placement, 359
  risk factors for peripartum bleeding, 359
  substance use disorder, 359, 366
  trial of labor after cesarean delivery (TOLAC), 360
  vaginal birth after cesarean delivery, 360
Pregnancy and Lactation Labeling Rule, 351
pregnant patient for non-obstetric surgery, 346–54
  anesthetic and sedative agents in pregnancy, 351–52
  anesthetic implications of maternal physiology, 351f
  anesthetic plan and physiologic changes of pregnancy, 346, 349–50
  benzodiazepines, 352
  case and key questions, 345–46
  diagnostic criteria for pre-eclampsia, 346
  fetal monitoring, 352
  institutional resources for, 348
  laparoscopy during pregnancy, 352–53
  managing eclamptic seizures, 346
  muscle relaxants and reversal agents, 352
  neuromuscular blocking (NMB) agent, 346

INDEX • 539

pregnant patient for non-obstetric surgery (*cont.*)
    nitrous oxide, 352
    obstetric airway, 350
    patient counseling, 348–49
    placental transfer of medications and fetal risk, 350–51
    pneumoperitoneum and physiologic changes, 346
    preeclampsia and eclampsia, 353–54
    preoperative evaluation, 347
    review questions, 354–55
    routine pregnancy testing, 347
    systemic features of preeclampsia, 353*t*
    timing of surgery during pregnancy, 347–48
prehabilitation, older adults, 130–31
prehabilitation pathway, total hip replacement, 89
prehabilitation programs, studies and outcomes of, 87*t*
premature infants
    apnea of prematurity, 122
    bronchopulmonary dysplasia, 121–22, 122*t*
    cardiopulmonary abnormalities, 120
    case and key questions, 117–18
    definitions and epidemiology, 118
    gastrointestinal abnormalities, 119–20
    historical perspective, 118
    neurodevelopment, 118–19
    pulmonary abnormalities, 120
    regional anesthesia, postoperative apnea, and analgesic considerations, 122–23
    respiratory system development, 120–21
    retinopathy of prematurity, 119
    review questions, 123–24
    stages of fetal lung development, 121*t*
    surfactant and respiratory distress syndrome, 121
    survival rates by decades, 118*f*
Preoperative Anesthesia and Surgical Screening (PASS), Duke University, 5, 11
Preoperative Assessment and Global Optimization (PASS-GO) program, 5
preoperative cardiac testing, 141–42
preoperative clinic models, 4
    anesthesiology-run clinic, 4–5
    case and key questions, 3–4
    combined anesthesia and medicine clinic, 5
    comprehensive preoperative assessment and global optimization, 5
    nurse-run clinic, 4
    operations, 5–10
    overall triage process, 7*f*
    preoperative anesthesia and surgical screening (PASS) clinic, 5
    questionnaire, 6–8
    review questions, 10–12
    separate anesthesia and medicine clinics, 5
    telemedicine and virtual visits, 9*t*
    telephone triage, 6
    virtual visit consult, 8*f*
    virtual visits, 4, 8–10
preoperative clinics, 3
preoperative evaluation, 420
    ACS NSQIP risk calculator, 416, 417*f*, 421
    anesthesiologist advising patient, 414–18
    daily medication list, 415*t*
    defining physical status, 414, 415*t*
    evidence-based assessment of perioperative risk, 419
    impact of smoking, 415
    obtaining informed consent, 419–20
    patient's perioperative risk, 416–17
    Practice Advisory for Preanesthesia Evaluation, 415–16
    pulmonologist's written recommendation, 416
    responding to surgeon, 417–18
    review questions, 420–21
Preoperative Frailty Assessment (PFA), 32–33, 38, 39*f*, 41
Preoperative Nutrition Scale (PONS), 37
    malnutrition, 42
preoperative process, key questions for case, 3–4
preoperative prothrombin time (PT)/partial thromboplastin time (PTT), 50
preoperative testing, 38–40
    anemia, 35
    anticoagulation management, 36
    atrial fibrillation, 36
    case and key questions for, 26–35
    dyspnea, 35
    frailty, 38, 39*f*
    iron deficiency anemia, 35
    major adverse cardiovascular events (MACE), 36–37
    metabolic panel, 37
    nutrition screening, 37–38
    obstructive sleep apnea (OSA), 37
    perioperative blood product management, 35–36
    review questions, 40–43
    valvular heart disease, 36
President's Commission for the Study of Ethical Problems in Medicine and Biomedical and Behavioral Research, 396
preterm birth
    definition, 118
    historical perspective, 118*f*, 118
    See also premature infants
PREVENTT trial, iron infusion in anemic patients, 308, 310
primary care evaluation, patient's, 23
Principles of Biomedical Ethics (Beauchamp and Childress), 403, 409
proactive care of older people undergoing surgery (POPS), 131
prolonged QTc interval
    definition of, 524
    medications and, 524
prothrombin time (PT)
    definition, 315
    partial thromboplastin time (PTT), 315
pseudocholinesterase deficiency, succinylcholine and, 510
PTT. *See* partial thromboplastin time (PTT)
Public Health Emergency billing mandates, 10
pulmonary abnormalities, premature infants, 120
pulmonary arterial hypertension (PAH)
    patient with, 188
    risk of mortality in patients with, 191*t*
pulmonary artery pressure, calculation of, 189*b*
pulmonary evaluation, patient, 22
pulmonary fibrosis, 15
    See also perioperative surgical home (PSH)
pulmonary function test(s), 17, 18*f*
    benefit of, 23–24
    obstructive pattern, 24
    restrictive pulmonary disease, 24
pulmonary function testing (PFT), 41–42

referral before surgery, 27–28
pulmonary hypertension (PH)
    cases and key questions, 187–88
    classification of, 189, 190*f*
    definition of, 188
    expert consultation, 192
    fluid management, 192
    hemodynamic definition of, 188*t*
    hemodynamic support, 191–92
    inotropic support, 192
    key concepts in determining pulmonary vascular resistance, 189*b*
    management of PH crisis and acute right ventricular failure, 191–92
    mechanical circulatory support, 192
    oxygen therapy, 191
    perioperative care guidelines, 189–91
    perioperative risk assessment, 191
    review questions, 193–94
    risk of mortality in patients with, 191*t*
    symptoms and signs of, 189
    tools to assess perioperative risk in, 191*t*
    treatment of, 189
    treatment of underlying cause, 192
    vasodilator therapy, 192
    worsening of right-sided heart failure in, 192*f*

Q
quadratus lumborum blocks (QLB), 164
questionnaire, assessing perioperative process, 6–8
Question Prompt List, older adult before surgery, 129, 130*t*
Quinlan, Karen Ann, 389, 396

R
racial disparities, pregnancy, 358, 365–66, 368
radical prostatectomy, prostate cancer in older man, 139–40
radio-frequency ablation (RFA), 17
rapid eye movement (REM), obstructive sleep apnea and, 497, 502–3
rate modulation, pacemaker, 465–66
reasonable patient, informed consent, 409–10
reasonable physician, informed consent, 409
RECOVERY trial, 231–32
red blood cell (RBC), 307–8, 381
    destruction, 308
    indications for blood transfusion, 381–82
    See also anemia
renal cell carcinoma (RCC), 464
renal system(s)
    anabolic steroid use, 477
    smoking and nicotine pathophysiologic effects, 211
    See also chronic kidney disease (CKD)
respiratory distress syndrome (RDS), surfactant and, 121
respiratory exchange rate (RER), 93, 111
respiratory insufficiency, causes in PACU, 523
respiratory system
    anabolic steroid use, 477
    smoking and nicotine pathophysiologic effects, 210
respiratory system development, premature infants, 120–21, 121*t*
restrictive disorder, pulmonary function test, 18*f*
restrictive lung disease
    anesthetic implications, 288–89
    diagnosis of, 288
    etiology, 288

treatment, 288
    See also Parkinson's disease (PD)
retinopathy, premature infants, 119
reversal agents, anesthetic and sedative agent in pregnancy, 352
reverse transcriptase polymerase chain reaction (RT-PCR), SARS-CoV-2 infection, 227
Revised Cardiac Risk Index (RCRI), 28–29, 30*t*, 141, 416, 442
    patient evaluation, 42
    preoperative risk calculator, 172*b*, 172
rheumatoid arthritis (RA)
    airway, 79–81
    atlanto-axial instability (AAI), 80
    atlanto-axial subluxation (AAS), 80*f*
    atlanto-axial subluxation in patient with, 82*f*
    autoimmune disease, 78
    bone microenvironment in healthy and RA bone, 79*f*
    C-spine abnormalities, 81*t*
    C-spine involvement, 80
    disease modifying anti-rheumatic drugs (DMARDs), 79, 81
    goals of treatment, 79
    joint involvement, 79
    perioperative considerations, 79
    symptoms, 78–79
Richmond Agitation-Sedation Scale (RASS), 516
risperidone, classification and mechanism of action, 442–43
rivaroxaban
    indications and pharmacokinetics, 151*t*
    interruption time, 155*t*
    laboratory tests for, 156*t*
robotic hysterectomy
    considerations for patients undergoing, 374–76
    history of woman scheduled for, 373
    lithotomy position, 374–75
    steep Trendelenburg positioning, 374, 375, 375*t*
ROCKET AF trial, 152
rocuronium, neuromuscular blockade, 510, 513
Roizen criteria, pheochromocytoma resection, 340

S
Safar, Peter, 396
St. Jude Medical, technical support contacts, 467*t*
Salgo v. Trustees of Leland Stanford Hospital, 410
SARS-CoV-2 infection, 198
    COVID-19 global pandemic, 227
    extrapulmonary manifestations of, 234*f*
    long-term effects of, 236*f*
    lung transplantation, 198, 201
    screening, 196
    Wuhan, China, 232, 234, 235–36
    See also COVID-19 infection
scapholunate advanced collapse syndrome (SLAC), 3
    key questions for case, 3–4
Schloendorff v. Society of New York Hospital, 389
seizure(s), 264–67
    acute management in perioperative period, 266–67
    associated disorders, 264
    case and key questions, 261–64
    classifications, 261*b*

common antiepileptic drugs, mechanisms of action, and side effects, 262t
current treatment, 264–65
deep brain stimulation (DBS), 265
definition of, 261
diagnosis of, 264
diets, 265
etiology and pathophysiology, 261, 264
intraoperative considerations, 265–66
medical management, 264–65
perioperative medication management for epilepsy patients, 263b
preanesthetic evaluation, 262t
preoperative evaluation, 265
presentation, 264
review questions, 267–70
status epilepticus, 267
surgical resection, 265
vagal nerve stimulation (VNS), 265
See also epilepsy
self-expandable metal stent (SEMS), endoscopic placement of, 231
serotonin syndrome, 443
cause of delirium, 518–19
chlorpromazine and, 518
cyproheptadine, 518
treatment of, 517–18
severe acute respiratory syndrome (SARS), 233
See also COVID-19 infection; SARS-CoV-2 infection
shared decision-making, 423
geriatric assessment, 129–30, 132
Shinal v. Toms, Pennsylvania, 406–7
shoulder replacement
case and key questions, 195–98
infection signs and symptoms, 196, 198
interscalene block (ISB) as anesthetic choice for total, 196, 197
preoperative assessment for, 195
preoperative evaluation of patient, 195
Sipple's syndrome (MEN type 2A), multiple endocrine neoplasia (MEN) syndrome, 338
6-minute walk test (6MWT), 27
cardiopulmonary function, 40
men, 27
women, 27
skilled nursing facility (SNF), 20
Skype for Business, 9
sleep apnea
continuous positive airway pressure (CPAP), 414
diagnosis, 497
STOP-Bang criteria, 43
See also apnea(s); obstructive sleep apnea (OSA)
sleep-disordered breathing, 496
smoking
back pain and, 211
behavioral therapy, 212–13
benefits of quitting, before surgery, 207–8, 212
cessation counseling, 209b
COPD cause, 208
COPD treatment and cessation of, 208
counsel on, 415, 420–21
osteogenesis and wound healing, 211
postoperative cardiovascular complications, 212
postoperative respiratory complications, 211–12
pregnancy and, 368
reversibility of pathologic changes induced by, 212
surgical outcomes and, 211–12

See also chronic obstructive pulmonary disease (COPD)
Society for Ambulatory Anesthesia (SAMBA), 222, 224–25, 326
Society for Obstetric Anesthesiology and Perinatology (SOAP), 352
Society for Perioperative Assessment and Quality Improvement (SPAQI), 128
Society of Ambulatory Anesthesia (SAMBA), 498, 499
Society of American Gastrointestinal and Endoscopic Surgeons, 352–53
Society of Anesthesia and Sleep Medicine (SASM), 223, 498
Society of Critical Care Medicine (SCCM), transfusion guidelines, 386t
Society of Perioperative Assessment and Quality Improvement (SPAQI), 79
Society of Thoracic Surgeons (STS), transfusion guidelines, 386t
Society of Vascular Surgery/American Association for Vascular Surgery, 455
sodium-glucose cotransporter 2 inhibitors, heart failure treatment, 174
soluble guanylate cyclase stimulators, heart failure treatment, 175
spinal cord stimulators (SCS), 452, 453
placement of, 458
spontaneous bacterial peritonitis (SBP), 249, 252
stable ischemic heart disease (SIHD), 54
stand-alone telemedicine visit, 8, 9t
standards of disclosure, informed consent, 404–5
statins, heart failure treatment, 175
status epilepticus
International League Against Epilepsy (ILAE) Task Force, 267t
management, 267
operational definition of, 267t
presentation, 267
See also epilepsy; seizure(s)
stent types
bare metal stents (BMS), 56
coronary, 56–57
drug-eluting stents (DES), 56
steroid use. See anabolic steroid use
stimulants, substance use disorders (SUD), 72
Stony Brook University Medical Center, 4–5
STOP-Bang questionnaire, 32, 32t
criteria for sleep apnea, 43
obstructive sleep apnea (OSA), 218, 220, 222
OSA screening, 497, 498, 503–4
patient, 40
screening tool, 17, 221b
STOP questionnaire, OSA screening, 497, 498
storage lesion, blood, 385
stress testing, brain natriuretic peptide (BNP), 30
stroke, 291
anesthetic management, 292
case and key questions, 291
FAAST test, 292b
mechanisms for perioperative, 291–92
perioperative management reducing risk of, 292
review questions, 293
risk factors for perioperative, 292
timing of surgery after, 292
subacute bacterial endocarditis (SBE)
prophylaxis, 144, 145
prophylaxis regimens, 144

substance use disorders (SUD), 67
alcohol, 72–73
amphetamines, 72
barbiturates, 73
benzodiazepines, 73
cannabis, 73
cocaine, 72
depressants, 72–73
hallucinogens, 73–74
kratom, 73–74
lysergic acid diethylamide (LSD), 73
overarching principles, 72
perioperative issues in non-opioid, 72–74
pregnancy and, 359, 366
stimulants, 72
See also opioid use disorder (OUD)
succinylcholine
clinical concerns, 510–11
neuromuscular blockade, 510
sugammadex
birth control and, 511
neostigmine versus, 509
residual neuromuscular blockade, 508
reversal of neuromuscular blockade neuroblockade, 509
surfactant, respiratory distress syndrome (RDS) and, 121
surgery
CHA$_2$DS$_2$-VASc versus HAS-BLED, 33, 33t
HAS-BLED score, 40
postponement of, 33
risk after coronary stent placement, 57–58
surgery and recovery protocols
case and key questions, 373–74
enhanced recovery after surgery (ERAS) principles, 376–77, 378t
lithotomy, 374–75, 380
patients undergoing robotic hysterectomy, 374–76
postoperative nausea and vomiting (PONV), 373, 375–76
review questions, 379–80
risk factor summary for PONV in adults, 375b
steep Trendelenburg position, 373, 374, 375, 375t, 380
steps to reduce baseline PONV risk, 376b
surgical management
heart failure, 178–79
orthotopic heart transplantation, 178–79
surgical urgency
definition, 140
preoperative risk calculator, 172–73
surrogacy, DNR, 395, 399
surrogate decision-maker, informed consent, 405–6

T
tachyarrhythmias
atrial fibrillation, 525
management of, 525–26
perioperative risk factors for, 525b
pharmacological management of supraventricular tachyarrhythmias (SVTs), 526
reentrant SVTs, 525–26
telehealth, tipping point of, 10
telehealth virtual visits, 11
telemedicine, 11
telemedicine visit, 8, 9t
telephone triage, 6
testosterone
conversion to estradiol, 478f, 478
injectable, 478–79
See also anabolic steroid use

therapeutic radiation, electromagnetic interference risks, 468t
thoracic surgery, surgical blood order schedule, 29f
thrombocytopenia, 315
X-linked, 315
thromboelastography (TEG), 156
thrombosis risk, perioperative management of antiplatelet medications, 58t
thyroidectomies
preoperative clinic for, 78
thyroid diseases and, 437
Timed Up and Go (TUG) test, 125, 128, 129t
tizanidine, autistic patient, 440–41
tongue swelling, 433, 434
total hip replacement (THR)
case and key questions, 84–85
components of multidisciplinary prehabilitation pathway, 89f
elective procedure, 85
enhanced recovery after surgery (ERAS) prehabilitation model of care, 85–86
ERAS protocol, 85, 86, 89
exercise and nutrition, 89
multidisciplinary team, 86, 89f
osteoarthritis as indication for, 85
patient satisfaction, 85
physiotherapy and patient education program, 86
prehabilitation pathway, 89
preoperative care pathway, 86–89
review questions, 90
smoking cessation, 85–86
studies of prehabilitation programs and their outcomes, 87t
total iron deficit (TID), 34
Toxoplasma, infection, 198
train natriuretic peptide (BNP), stress testing, 30
transarterial chemoembolization (TACE) therapies, hepatocellular liver cancer (HCC), 17
transcatheter aortic valve replacement (TAVR), 140
transcutaneous electrical nerve stimulator (TENS), electromagnetic interference risks, 468t
transcutaneous pacing, indications for, 524
transesophageal echocardiography (TEE), 60, 63, 336
Transfusion Requirements in Critical Care (TRICC) trial, 385
transient ischemic attacks (TIAs), 291
See also stroke
transplant surgery, surgical blood order schedule, 29f
transurethral resection of the prostate (TURP), electromagnetic interference risks, 468t
transverse rectus abdominus myocutaneous (TRAM) flap reconstruction, elective surgery, 249, 250
triage
algorithm, 11
overall process, 7f
Pre-Anesthesia Consultation Clinic (PACC) questionnaire at Cleveland Clinic, 7
telephone, 6
trial of labor after cesarean delivery (TOLAC), 360
triple aim, patient outcome, 24
Tulsky, James, 426
twin-to-twin transfusion syndrome, 360

U

University of California, Los Angeles (UCLA), 8–9
urinary problem, 46
US Department of Veteran Affairs
　chronic pain management, 71
　opioid therapy for chronic pain, 70
US Food and Drug Administration (FDA), 150–51
clozapine, 443
implanted cardiac devices, 473
US Supreme Court, 396
uterine scar dehiscence, 360

V

vaginal birth after cesarean delivery (VBAC), 360, 367
variable extrathoracic obstruction, pulmonary function test, 18f
Vascular Study Group of New England (VSGNE), 416, 419
venous thromboembolism (VTE)
　Caprini Score, 373
　obesity and pregnancy, 363
voluntariness, informed consent, 403, 408, 409, 412, 418

W

Wish-Worry-Wonder framework, difficult conversations, 428f, 428
women. *See* pregnant patient for non-obstetric surgery
World Allergy Organization, 436
World Health Organization, 362, 381
World War II, 396